Handbook of Experimental Pharmacology

Volume 93

Pharmacology of Antihypertensive Therapeutics

Contributors

W. Bartsch, H. Becker, A. Bilski, R. Casto, D.P. Clough, J. Conway, D.A. Eichler, D. Ganten, P. Gohlke, Lan-Shen Gong, M.-G. Gruber, R. Gryglewski, R. Henning, R.G. Hooper, L.G. Howes, A. Jödicke, N.M. Kaplan, W. Kaufmann, Y. Kawano, S. Kazda, A. Knorr, W. Kobinger, H.J. Kramer, E.M. Krieger, R. Lang, R.E. Lang, W.J. Louis, F.C. Luft, V.F. Mauro, J. Mehta, P.J. Mulrow, L.O.T. Nascimento, T. Omae, L. Pichler, K.H. Rahn, O.L. Ramos, J.I.S. Robertson, P.R. Saxena, B.A. Schölkens, G. Schröder, B.-G. Schulz, I.K. Shkhvatsabaya, G. Sponer, H.M. Steffen, G. Stock, T. Strasser, T. Unger, P.A. van Zwieten, A. Wagner, Hong Wang, A.H. Weston, L. Wilhelmsen, W. Wouters, A. Zanchetti, Wei-Zhong Zhang

Editors

Detlev Ganten and Patrick J. Mulrow

Springer-Verlag Berlin Heidelberg New York
London Paris Tokyo Hong Kong

Professor DETLEV GANTEN, M.D, Ph.D.

German Institute for High Blood Pressure Research
and Department of Pharmacology
University of Heidelberg
Im Neuenheimer Feld 366
D-6900 Heidelberg, FRG

Professor PATRICK J. MULROW, M.D.

Medical College of Ohio
C.S. # 10008
Toledo, OH 43699, USA

With 147 Figures

ISBN 3-540-50427-3 Springer-Verlag Berlin Heidelberg New York
ISBN 0-387-50427-3 Springer-Verlag New York Berlin Heidelberg

Library of Congress Cataloging-in-Publication Data. Pharmacology of antihypertensive therapeutics/editors, Detlev Ganten and Patrick J. Mulrow; contributors, W. Bartsch ... [et al.]. p. cm. — (Handbook of experimental pharmacology; v. 93) ISBN 0-387-50427-3 (U.S.): 1. Hypotensive agents. 2. Hypertension—Chemotherapy. I. Ganten, D. (Detlev), 1941– . II. Mulrow, Patrick J. (Patrick Joseph), 1926– . III. Series. QP905.H3 vol. 93 [RC685.H8] 615'.1 s—dc20 [615'.71] 89-26138 CIP

Typesetting: Best-set Typesetter Ltd., Hong Kong
Printing and bookbinding: Brühlsche Universitätsdruckerei, Giessen
2122/3130-543210 — Printed on acid-free paper

Professor DETLEV GANTEN, M.D, Ph.D.

German Institute for High Blood Pressure Research
and Department of Pharmacology
University of Heidelberg
Im Neuenheimer Feld 366
D-6900 Heidelberg, FRG

Professor PATRICK J. MULROW, M.D.

Medical College of Ohio
C.S. # 10008
Toledo, OH 43699, USA

With 147 Figures

ISBN-13:978-3-642-74211-8 e-ISBN-13:978-3-642-74209-5
DOI: 10.1007/978-3-642-74209-5

Library of Congress Cataloging-in-Publication Data. Pharmacology of antihypertensive therapeutics/editors, Detlev Ganten and Patrick J. Mulrow; contributors, W. Bartsch ... [et al.]. p. cm. — (Handbook of experimental pharmacology; v. 93) ISBN-13:978-3-642-74211-8 (U.S.): 1. Hypotensive agents. 2. Hypertension—Chemotherapy. I. Ganten, D. (Detlev), 1941- . II. Mulrow, Patrick J. (Patrick Joseph), 1926- . III. Series. QP905.H3 vol. 93 [RC685.H8] 615'.1 s—dc20 [615'.71] 89-26138 CIP

Softcover reprint of the hardcover 1st edition 1990

Typesetting: Best-set Typesetter Ltd., Hong Kong

2122/3130-543210 — Printed on acid-free paper

Preface

The previous volume on *Antihypertensive Agents* in the *Handbook of Experimental Pharmacology*, published in 1977, was edited by the late Franz Gross from the Department of Pharmacology in Heidelberg, who was one of the grand old men in hypertension research.

Now, more than 10 years later, it is necessary to update this volume. From the early days of antihypertensive drug treatment, starting about 30 years ago with drugs such as reserpine and guanethidine, the pharmacology of cardiovascular therapy has evolved into a highly sophisticated and effective therapeutic regimen.

The major breakthroughs in the 1960s were the introduction of diuretics and beta-blockers. Then, in the 1980s, came the calcium antagonists and converting enzyme inhibitors. It can be anticipated that the next decade will see a further expansion and sophistication of blood pressure lowering drugs.

This book provides a state-of-the-art discussion of chemical, experimental, and clinical pharmacological data as well as of practical experience with drugs which are presently being used or which are going to be introduced on the market in the near future. The purpose of this volume is to provide a complete discussion of antihypertensive agents. Each major class of antihypertensive drugs is treated exhaustively in a separate chapter, fully referenced with chemical formulae, and richly illustrated with figures and tables. International authorities were asked to contribute in their respective fields of expertise.

New areas of drug development are discussed: drugs acting on multiple receptors (Chap. 5), calcium antagonists (Chap. 9), converting enzyme inhibitors (Chap. 10), renin inhibitors (Chap. 11), prostaglandin agonists and antagonists (Chap. 12), serotonin antagonists (Chap. 13), interferences with dopamine receptors (Chap. 14), interferences with peptidergic mechanisms (Chap. 15) and ionic membrane channels (Chap. 16), and natural agents and extracts (Chap. 19). Special chapters are devoted to toxicity testing of antihypertensive drugs (Chap. 22) and traditions of antihypertensive therapy on different continents (Chap. 23). For practical use, a catalogue of antihypertensive drugs with useful cross-referencing of generic and trade names is also included.

The experimental pharmacologist will find detailed chemical and experimental information; the practicing physician will be able to obtain background information as well as practical advice for therapy with respect to differential therapy, side effects, combination of drugs, and contraindications. It is particularly important that the practicing physician have up-to-date and unbiased in-

List of Contributors

W. BARTSCH, Pharmacological Research, Boehringer Mannheim GmbH, Sandhofer Str. 116, P.O. Box 310120, D-6800 Mannheim 31

H. BECKER, Pharmakognosie and Analytische Phytochemie, Universität des Saarlandes, Fachrichtung 14.3, D-6600 Saarbrücken

A. BILSKI, ICI Pharmaceuticals Division, Mereside, Alderley Park, Macclesfield, Cheshire SK10 4TG, Great Britain

R. CASTO, Division of Pharmacology, Department of Medicine M 036, University of California at San Diego, La Jolla, CA 92092, USA

D. CLOUGH, Research Division, Roche Products Ltd., P.O. Box 8, Welwyn Garden City, Hertfordshire AL7 3AY, Great Britain

J. CONWAY, Cardiac Department, John Radcliffe Hospital, Headington, Oxford OX3 9DU, Great Britain

D.A. EICHLER, Research Division, Roche Products Ltd., P.O. Box 8, Welwyn Garden City, Hertfordshire AL7 3AY, Great Britain

D. GANTEN, German Institute for High Blood Pressure Research and Department of Pharmacology, University of Heidelberg, Im Neuenheimer Feld 366, D-6900 Heidelberg

P. GOHLKE, Department of Pharmacology, University of Heidelberg, Im Neuenheimer Feld 366, D-6900 Heidelberg

LAN-SHEN GONG, Shanghai Institute of Hypertension, 197 Ruijin Road II, Shanghai, L, 200025, People's Republic of China

M.-G. GRUBER, Department of Pharmacology, University of Heidelberg, Im Neuenheimer Feld 366, D-6900 Heidelberg

R. GRYGLEWSKI, Department of Pharmacology, Copernicus Academy of Medicine, 16 Grzegórzecka, 31531 Cracow, Poland

R. HENNING, PGU Heart-Circulation G838, Hoechst AG, Postfach 800320, D-6230 Frankfurt/M.80

R.G. HOOPER, Pharmacological Research, Boehringer Mannheim GmbH, Sandhoferstr. 116, Postfach 310120, D-6800 Mannheim 31

L.G. Howes, Department of Medicine, The University of Melbourne, Clinical Pharmacology and Therapeutics Unit, Austin Hospital, Heidelberg, Victoria 3084, Australia

A. Jödicke, Research Laboratories of Schering AG, Berlin (West) and Bergkamen, Müllerstr. 170–178, P.O. Box 650311, D-1000 Berlin 65

N.M. Kaplan, Department of Internal Medicine, University of Texas, Southwestern Medical School at Dallas, 5323 Harry Hines Boulevard, Dallas, TX 75235-9030, USA

W. Kaufmann, Krankenhaus Köln-Merheim, Medizinische Klinik, Lehrstuhl für Innere Medizin II der Universität Köln, Ostmerheimer Str. 200, D-5000 Köln 91

Y. Kawano, National Cardiovascular Center, Fujishirodai, Suita, Osaka 565, Japan

S. Kazda, Institute of Pharmacology, Bayer AG, Aprather Weg 18a, P.O. Box 101709, D-5600 Wuppertal 1

A. Knorr, Institute of Pharmacology, Bayer AG, Aprather Weg 18a, P.O. Box 101709, D-5600 Wuppertal 1

W. Kobinger, Abteilung Pharmakologie, Ernst Boehringer Institut für Arzneimittelforschung, Bender+Co GesmbH, Dr. Boehringer-Gasse 5–11, A-1121 Wien

H.J. Kramer, Medizinische Universitäts-Poliklinik, Wilhelmstr. 35–37, D-5300 Bonn

E.M. Krieger, Heart Institute, University Hospital — Faculty of Medicine, University of Sao Paulo, P.O. Box 11.450, 05499 Sao Paulo, SP-Brazil

R. Lang, Frankenklinik der Landesversicherungsanstalt Unterfranken, Menzelstr, 5–7, D-8730 Bad Kissingen

R.E. Lang, Department of Pharmacology, University of Heidelberg, Im Neuenheimer Feld 366, D-6900 Heidelberg

W.J. Louis, Department of Medicine, University of Melbourne, Clinical Pharmacology and Therapeutics Unit, Austin Hospital, Heidelberg, Victoria 3084, Australia

F.C. Luft, Department of Nephrology, IV Medical Clinic, Krankenhausstr. 12, D-8520 Erlangen

V.F. Mauro, College of Pharmacy, University of Toledo, 2801 W. Bancroft Street, Toledo, OH 43606, USA

J. Mehta, Division of Cardiovascular Medicine, University of Florida, Box Y 277, Gainesville FL, USA

P.J. Mulrow, Department of Medicine, Medical College of Ohio, CS10008, 300 Arlington Avenue, Toledo, OH 43699, USA

L.O.T. Nascimento, Heart Institute, University Hospital — Faculty of Medicine, University of Sao Paulo, P.O. Box 11.450, 05499 Sao Paulo, SP-Brazil

T. Omae, National Cardiovascular Center, 5-7-1 Fujishiro-dai, Suita, Osaka 565, Japan

L. Pichler, Department of Pharmacology and Toxicology, IMMUNO AG, Industriestr. 67, A-1220 Wien

K.H. Rahn, Department of Medicine D, University of Münster, Albert-Schweitzer-Str. 33, D-4400 Münster

O.L. Ramos, Division of Nephrology, Paulista School of Medicine, Rue Botucatu, 740-04023-Sao Paulo, SP-Brazil

J.I.S. Robertson, Department of Medicine, Prince of Wales Hospital, Chinese University of Hong Kong and Janssen Research Foundation, Turnhoutseweg 30, B-2340 Beerse

P.R. Saxena, Department of Pharmacology, Faculty of Medicine and Health Sciences, Erasmus University Rotterdam, Post Box 1738, NL-3000 DR Rotterdam

B.A. Schölkens, PGU Heart-Circulation H821, Hoechst AG, Postfach 800320, D-6230 Frankfurt 80

G. Schröder, Research Laboratories of Schering AG, Berlin (West) and Bergkamen, Müllerstr. 170–178, P.O. Box 650311, D-1000 Berlin 65

B.-G. Schulz, Research Laboratories of Schering AG, Berlin (West) and Bergkamen, Müllerstr. 170–178, P.O. Box 650311, D-1000 Berlin 65

I.K. Shkhvatsabaya, The All-Union Cardiology Research Centre, 3rd Cherepkovskaya st., 15-a, Moscow, 121552 USSR

G. Sponer, Pharmacological Research, Boehringer Mannheim GmbH, Sandhoferstr. 116, Postfach 310120, D-6800 Mannheim 31

H.M. Steffen, Krankenhaus Köln-Merheim, Medizinische Klinik, Lehrstuhl für Innere Medizin II der Universität Köln, Ostmerheimer Str. 200, D-5000 Köln 41

G. Stock, Research Laboratories of Schering AG, Berlin (West) and Bergkamen, Müllerstr. 170–178, Postfach 650311, D-1000 Berlin 65

T. Strasser, World Hypertension League, 20, avenue du Bouchet, CH-1209 Geneva

T. Unger, Department of Pharmacology, University of Heidelberg, Im Neuenheimer Feld 366, D-6900 Heidelberg

P.A. van Zwieten, Division of Pharmacotherapy, Academic Medical Centre, University of Amsterdam, Meibergdreef 15, NL-1105 AZ Amsterdam

A. Wagner, PGU Heart-Circulation G838, Hoechst AG, Postfach 800320, D-6230 Frankfurt 80

Hong Wang, Shanghai Institute of Hypertension, 280 South Chongquing Road, Shanghai, People's Republic of China

A.H. Weston, Department of Physiological Sciences, Medical School, University of Manchester, Stopford Building, Oxford Road, Manchester M13 9PT, Great Britain

L. Wilhelmsen, Department of Medicine, University of Gothenburg, Östra Sjukhuset, CK Plan 2, S-416 85 Göteborg

W. Wouters, Department of Pharmacology, Duphar B.V., Post Box 2, NL-1380 AA Weesp

A. Zanchetti, Istituto di Clinica Medica Generale e Terapia Medica, Università di Milano, Centro di Fisiologia Clinica e Ipertensione, Ospedale Maggiore, Via F. Sforza 35, I-20122 Milano

Wei-Zhong Zhang, Shanghai Institute of Hypertension, 280 South Chongquing Road, Shanghai, People's Republic of China

formation on the many new drugs which are being developed and will soon be introduced on the market such as renin inhibitors, angiotensin and other peptide receptor antagonists, and drugs developed from natural agents and extracts so that he can understand the developments in the hypertensive drug market in the coming years. Different attitudes towards treatment of hypertension on various continents and in different culture may also lead to different perspectives for the treating physician.

The medical care a physician provides his patient includes much more than just the prescription of an effective drug. We have therefore felt it particularly important to include a discussion of non-pharmacological treatment of high blood pressure in this volume. This is especially important in mild hypertension. The latest results of a consensus conference of the International Society of Hypertension (ISH) and World Health Organization (WHO) have been incorporated in these recommendations. Since pathophysiological and clinical knowledge is the basis for all antihypertensive therapeutic measures, this is also briefly discussed in an introductory chapter.

If this book helps to improve care and treatment of patients with high blood pressure, the efforts of the editors and our editorial assistants Dr. LYNN LINDPAINTNER and DORIS M. WALKER were not in vain.

Heidelberg and Toledo

D. GANTEN
P.J. MULROW

Contents

CHAPTER 1

Basis for the Treatment of Hypertension: Some Considerations Concerning the Epidemiology, Pathophysiology, Treatment, and Prevention of Hypertension

D. GANTEN and P.G. MULROW

CONTENTS

1 Introduction

Hypertension is a worldwide health problem. Its prevalence is between 10% and 20% of the population. These figures vary depending on the level of blood pressure at which a person is classified as hypertensive and on the technical procedures of blood pressure measurement. Hypertension occurs more frequently in European countries, Japan, and North America than in less industrialized countries and rural societies. It is generally anticipated that the prevalence of hypertension will increase if no specific measures with respect of prevention or improved treatment are taken.

Before starting to treat hypertension, one has to define the boundary of normality. According to PICKERING (1968), hypertension represents the right end of the Gaussian curve for mean arterial blood pressure which is controlled by a multifactorial biological system. Furthermore, mean arterial pressure is not a fixed entity even in a given individual. Sleep, exercise, emotions, and food can all have profound effects on blood pressure and shift the levels from normal to abnormal or vice versa (BEVAN et al. 1969; MILLAR-CRAIG et al. 1978; PICKERING 1977). It is not the level of blood pressure per se that is important but rather its consequences such as damage to the blood vessels or heart. Possibly due to differences in genetic background, some patients can withstand elevated blood pressure better than others. In the animal world, the giraffe is an excellent example. In order to supply its brain, which is high above the heart when the giraffe is feeding on tree tops, it must maintain a mean arterial pressure of 250 mmHg. No obvious harm results from this pressure to its massively thick-walled cardiovascular system.

The variability in blood pressure makes separation of normotension from hypertension difficult. Presumably, the average mean arterial pressure over many years is what determines the damage to the cardiovascular system, and this damage is influenced by genetic factors. If the clinician had a way of predicting accurately who will develop complications for a certain mean arterial pressure, then treatment could be tailored for a given individual, and many patients with mild hypertension would not need to be treated. To a certain extent we do employ some predictors in our assessment plan. Age, sex, race, smoking, cholesterol level, and presence of diabetes are used, but these are not sufficiently precise to have a major impact on the selection of patients to treat. In this chapter we will discuss some introductory personal views on this topic. For further information the reader is also referred to some excellent publications (GENEST et al. 1983; PAGE 1987; GROSS 1977; SCRIABINE 1980; ANTONACCIO 1984).

2 Classification

The term primary hypertension is being touted as a better term than essential or idiopathic hypertension, and it distinguishes primary from secondary hypertension, the latter being due to known causes such as adrenal tumors or renal disease. Primary hypertension is by far the most common form; it is the diagnosis in over 95% of all hypertensive patients. Hypertension can be classified in different ways, e.g., by etiology (primary or secondary) or by classifications according to severity such as mild, moderate, labile, stable or malignant hypertension.

The World Health Organization (WHO) has developed definitions of blood pressure categories:

(a) Normotension-systolic less than 140 mmHg and diastolic less than 90 mmHg.
(b) Borderline hypertension-systolic from 140 to 160 mmHg and diastolic between 90 and 95 mmHg.
(c) Hypertension-systolic greater than 160 mmHg and/or diastolic greater than 95 mmHG.

These are consensus numbers and do not take into account all the other factors which influence morbidity due to an elevated blood pressure. For some experts the numbers may be too high. In large population studies, morbidity from blood pressure appears to be linear from low blood pressure to high blood pressure with the slope increasing in the high blood pressure range.

The U.S. Joint National Committee on Detection, Evaluation, and Treatment of High Blood Pressure defined normotension as diastolic less than 85 mmHg. Diastolic pressure between 85 and 89 mmHg was considered "high normal".

3 Mild Hypertension is the Problem

When looking at hypertension as a chronic disease in the population, mild hypertension is more frequent than severe hypertension. This is the reason why a joint committee of the International Society of Hypertension (ISH) and the WHO was convened under the theme "Mild hypertension is the problem" (Strasser and Ganten 1987). This is certainly true, because most people who have raised blood pressure fall into this category, the percentage varying between 75% and 85%. Hence, with respect to community health care, mild hypertension is of major significance and also presents a substantial financial burden to the community ("community risk"). For the individual, severe hypertension poses the greater problem ("individual risk"), which, however, may be solved more easily by conventional therapeutic medical approaches.

Mild hypertension in adults is officially defined as a persistent resting level of diastolic blood pressure (phase V) between 90 and 104 mmHg (12–14 kPa). "Borderline" hypertension is included in this definition and accounts for about half of the total. With repeated measurements over periods of 3–6 months, the diastolic pressure of almost half of those within the mild range falls to levels below this range. This finding indicates the importance of long-term blood pressure measurements before a patient is classified and "labelled" as hypertensive and before chronic treatment is started. The diagnostic value of repeated measurements over 24-h periods is presently being investigated.

People whose resting values of diastolic blood pressure remain persistently above 90 mmHg after repeated measurement are at increased relative risk of cardiovascular mortality and morbidity, and the risk clearly increases with the level of the diastolic blood pressure. Between 12% and 15% of such patients will develop moderate or severe hypertension (diastolic blood pressure at or above 105 mmHg) within 3–5 years, with a worse prognosis, while the remaining patients remain within the mild range.

It has to be kept in mind that there is a continuum of cardiovascular risk associated with blood pressure level: The higher the pressure, the higher the risk. The dividing line between "normotension" and "hypertension" is not fixed. The definition of mild hypertension as a diastolic pressure of 90/104 mmHg is completely artificial and historically results from statistical deliberations when planning therapeutic trials. Calculations of the number of patients to be included in such studies partly determined the limits of blood pressure. For practical and didactical purposes mild hypertension should be redefined to even numbers (above 90 mmHg and below 100 mmHg diastolic) which also take into account the precision (or lack of it) of blood pressure measurements in the physicians' practice or at the patients' home.

To achieve this we have therefore intentionally changed and simplified the guidelines of the WHO/ISH committee for the classification and management of patients with mild hypertension, keeping, however, the essentials of these recommendations unchanged and partly verbatim.

The goals in the management of patients with mild hypertension is to provide a safe classification (without false "labelling" of the patients) and to decrease the diastolic blood pressure to below 90 mmHg and systolic blood pressure to below 140 mmHg.

The classification and decision on treatment without or with drugs should be done with great patience over a period of 6 months or even longer in young people. High blood pressure usually develops over several years, and in general there is no hurry to classify and make drug therapeutic decisions unless there is a hypertensive emergency. However, it should be kept in mind that complications may occur during the observation period, so it is important that careful evaluation of the blood pressure and risk factors be maintained.

The time course of the different steps of classification and treatment is conveniently divided into the 1st month after initial screening and subsequently into 3-month periods of blood pressure monitoring (Fig. 1):

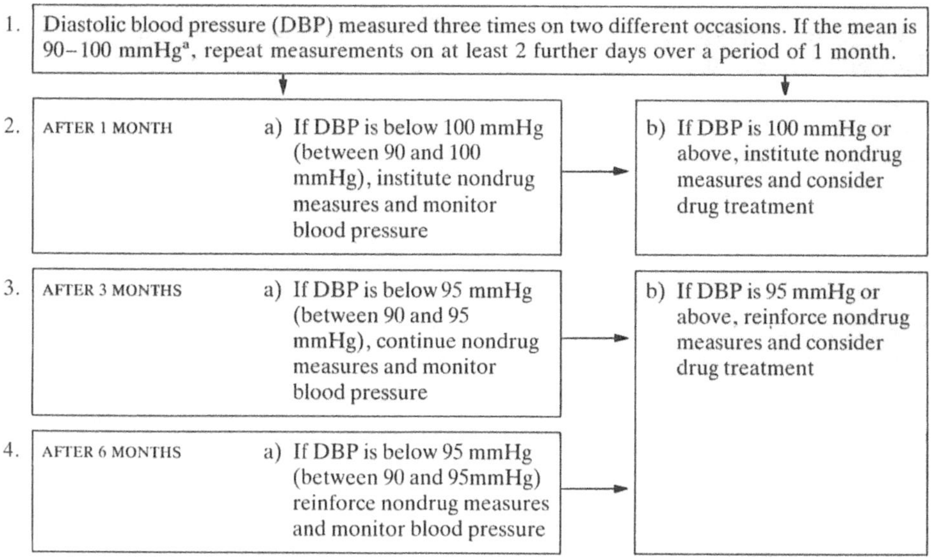

Fig. 1. Schematic outline of the definition, monitoring, and management of mild hypertension. The therapeutic goal is to decrease the diastolic blood pressure to below 90 mmHg and the systolic blood pressure to below 140 mmHG.

[a] Note that different approaches are necessary if DBP is above 100 mmHg at the first screening. Systolic blood pressure at 160 mmHg or above favors earlier start of drug treatment.

1. If the diastolic blood pressure, measured three times on two different occasions during the first screening, is 90 mmHg or above, repeated measurements on at least 2 further days over a period of 1 month are necessary.
2. (a) If 1 month after initial screening the diastolic blood pressure is below 100 mmHg (i.e., between 90 and 100 mmHg), nondrug measures should be instituted, and blood pressure monitored further.
   (b) If 1 month after initial screening the diastolic blood pressure is 100 mmHg or above, nondrug measures should be continued, and drug treatment has to be seriously considered.
3. (a) If after 3 months of blood pressure monitoring and possibly nondrug measures the diastolic blood pressure is still between 90 and 95 mmHg (below 95 mmHg), nondrug measures should be instituted and blood pressure monitored regularly.
   (b) If after 3 months of blood pressure monitoring and nondrug measures the diastolic blood pressure is still 95 mmHg or above, the nondrug measures should be reinforced, and drug treatment has to be seriously considered.
4. (a) If after 6 months of blood pressure monitoring and nondrug measures the diastolic blood pressure is still elevated between 90 and 95 mmHg (below 95 mmHg), the nondrug measures should be reinforced, and blood pressure has to be monitored regularly.
   (b) If after 6 months of blood pressure monitoring plus nondrug measures the diastolic blood pressure is still elevated at 95 mmHg or above, the nondrug measures have to be reinforced, and drug treatment should be started.

Patients whose diastolic pressure remains between 90 and 95 mmHg after prolonged observation also have an increased risk of cardiovascular disease. This is more marked when the systolic blood pressure is also elevated, as well as in smokers, diabetics, those with increased plasma cholesterol, and those with a family history of cardiovascular disease. Drug treatment should be considered for such patients at higher risk. Lower risk subjects, if not treated with drugs, should be further assessed at about 3-month intervals, and appropriate nondrug measures should be maintained or reinforced.

4 Nondrug Measures

Several nonpharmacological interventions have been shown to lower blood pressure in patients with mild hypertension. Weight reduction in overweight subjects, cessation of heavy alcohol consumption, regular exercise in sedentary patients, and, in some patients, sodium restriction are effective in lowering blood pressure. Efforts to reduce blood pressure using nonpharmacological methods should normally precede any decision about the necessity for drug treatment of mild hypertension—it should be noted that some of these measures may take several months to become fully effective. Furthermore, it must be recognized that these measures may be difficult to achieve in many patients. If a decision is made to begin drug treatment, a structured program of nonpharmacological intervention remains an essential component of the overall therapeutic regimen.

All the large-scale trials of treatment of mild hypertension have confirmed that treated hypertensive patients who smoke tobacco have a greater incidence of both stroke and coronary heart disease than equivalently treated hypertensive patients who do not smoke. Repeated advice as to how to discontinue smoking is therefore of major importance and will need to be coupled with particular efforts to prevent any consequent weight gain. Intensive advice programs are more effective than haphazard admonitions.

Serum cholesterol levels and clinical diabetes also unfavourably influence the long-term prognosis of hypertensive sufferers; nutritional counselling and, when appropriate, drug treatment are indicated to control these risk factors. If dietary measures are to be successful, a careful program of motivation, dietary instruction, and follow-up should be instituted. Since increased physical activity is also likely to reduce the risk of cardiovascular disease, it is appropriate for mildly hypertensive patients.

5 The Aim Is Prevention

One could rephrase the theme of the above-mentioned ISH/WHO meeting into: "Mild hypertension represents a unique opportunity". The cardiovascular disease prevention programs are all aimed at reducing the risk factors in the population. On the other hand, we know that not all but only a portion of those obese, inactive, salt-eating smokers develop hypertension, stroke, and heart attack. This makes it difficult to impose strict cardiovascular prevention methods upon the population in general. The individual person will not understand why he should give up his old habits if he cannot be assured that he himself will benefit from the risk factor reduction. This is the point at which mild hypertension plays an important role and may indeed represent an opportunity for the prevention programs from a medical and psychological point of view.

It can be assumed that subjects with one or several of the above-mentioned risk factors who present with mild hypertension are, in the majority of cases, the ones who are sensitive to these civilization-specific risks for genetic or other reasons and in whom, therefore, preventive measures are particularly meaningful and probably effective. Detection of and care for mildly hypertensive subjects thus provides us with a unique opportunity to reach about 20% of the adult population at a time when preventive measures are readily understood. Prevention at this point will be particularly meaningful because there is already the beginning of a disease, but organ damage has probably not yet occurred or is still reversible. In such a situation the doctor will be more persuasive and the patient more easily convinced that certain curative or preventive measures are meaningful. The detection of these persons at risk is easy: blood pressure measurement can be done not only in the physician's office but also at the work site, at home, in schools, etc.

In addition, since one blood pressure measurement does not classify the person in question as a hypertensive subject, repeated measurements have to be performed. This is an excellent opportunity for the physician to test whether the patient is willing and able to do something about his risk factors and reduce weight, salt and fat intake, smoking, and physical inactivity.

The reduction of blood pressure together with the reduction of those risk factors which can be monitored and controlled by the patient will then be a convincing argument for the effectiveness of such health measures for the patient himself, for his family, and his social milieu.

Thus, as a "side effect", a mild hypertension program will, without additional efforts, be effective also with respect to the reduction of other diseases, such as cancer and diabetes, if we are successful in reducing obesity, physical inactivity (diabetes), and smoking (cancer).

It is clear that much more research is necessary to support some of the above statements, and this view may be too optimistic. Mild hypertension does represent, however, a risk factor which gives us a unique opportunity to demonstrate the value and the success of more comprehensive cardiovascular prevention programs to the physician and to the general population. Comprehensive preventive general health programs are needed and are to be preferred to programs attacking just one risk factor. Since the hypertensive patient frequently presents with several risk factors, the psychological approach to the patient (and the physician) may be facilitated by singling out hypertension as a starter.

However, the physician should never forget that mild hypertension is a risk factor and that changing one's life-long habits is very difficult and often impossible for many patients. Furthermore, the years of public education about the dangers of high blood pressure have made patients aware of the risk. In many cultures, patients expect a drug from the physician to cure their illness. Physicians therefore must educate their patients about the importance of the evaluation period so that the patients do not "drop out" only to return later with the complications of untreated hypertension.

6 Pathophysiological Considerations

To treat primary hypertension intelligently, one needs to know the pathogenesis of the elevated blood pressure. In the adult, when hypertension has been stable for several years, the cardiovascular hemodynamics are well-defined (Freis 1960; Frohlich 1977). The peripheral resistance is elevated (Conway 1963), the cardiac output is normal, plasma volume is normal or slightly decreased, and the baroreceptor function (McCubbin et al. 1956; Sleight 1980) is reset at a higher level. Renal vascular resistance is increased with a decrease in renal blood flow and an increase in the filtration fraction due to efferent arteriole vasoconstriction. At this stage, the problem is in the resistance vessels, the precapillary arterioles (Follow 1982; Halpern et al. 1978). These vessels exhibit hypertrophied smooth muscle with decreased luminal radius and increased sensitivity to a variety of vasomotor stimuli (Mulvary et al. 1978; Suwa and Takahaski 1971). Despite the resetting of the cardiovascular system, the system can still regulate itself. Factors which contrive to raise the blood pressure are promptly counteracted by compensatory mechanisms: the kidney rapidly excretes sodium and water, and the baroreceptors dampen the rise by reflex mechanisms.

In view of the cardiovascular hemodynamics, it seems logical at this phase to treat the factor maintaining the elevated blood pressure, the increased peripheral resistance. Direct vasodilators such as hydralazine, calcium channel blockers, converting enzyme (CE) inhibitors, and inhibitors of the adrenergic system (from α_1-adrenoreceptor inhibitors to CNS inhibitors) are effective. It does not make physiological sense to lower cardiac output with β-adrenoreceptor blockers or lower plasma volume with diuretics. Yet clearly both are quite effective in lowering blood pressure alone or in combination with the direct vasodilators. In fact, the β-adrenoreceptor blockers lower blood pressure but raise at least transiently the abnormal peripheral resistance. Chronic diuretic treatment on the other hand is associated with reduced peripheral resistance by an unknown mechanism.

While the characteristics of the hemodynamics in established primary hypertension are agreed upon by most experts, there is considerable disagreement regarding the beginning phase. In chronic diseases like hypertension, it is always difficult to observe the beginning since it has so insidious an onset. Indeed, the cardiovascular system of those predisposed to develop hypertension may be abnormal at birth. Children with higher blood pressure are more prone to have higher blood pressure as adults. The heart and blood vessels of SHR are hypertrophied at birth compared with appropriate controls. A Dahl salt-sensitive rat has a slightly higher blood pressure than a Dahl salt-resistant rat at a young age, before hypertension is present. The main question at the beginning phase is what causes the peripheral resistance to increase. This obviously is an extremely important question since the early treatment and prevention of hypertension could be carried out more rationally if we understood the pathogenesis. There are several attractive, although controversial hypotheses.

6.1 The Autoregulatory Hypothesis

First proposed by BORST and expanded by GUYTON and his group (see GUYTON et al. 1972, 1974; GUYTON 1977), the essence of this hypothesis is that cardiac output is first increased, and the enhanced flow to the tissue leads to reflex vasoconstriction throughout the vascular system. The cardiac output then returns to normal, but the peripheral vasoconstriction persists. With time, there is hypertrophy of the small resistance vessels, which maintains the blood pressure level despite a normal cardiac output. The latter may be inappropriately high considering the elevated peripheral resistance. What leads to the increased cardiac output? Guyton and his group claim it is the result of a defect in the kidney which leads to sodium and water retention, increased plasma volume, and increased cardiac output.

The ensuing elevated pressure induces a pressure natriuresis and a decrease in volume towards normal. According to this hypothesis, the hypertensive kidney has an intrinsic defect so that it needs a higher pressure in order to excrete sodium and water to maintain volume homeostasis. The pressure natriuresis curve is shifted to the right (LEDINGHAM and COHEN 1964). Initial support for this hypothesis came from rat studies. Hypertension was produced by clipping one renal artery, and then the subsequent hemodynamics were followed. There was a transient increase in salt retention, volume expansion, and cardiac output, followed by a second phase of a persistent increase in peripheral resistance. A similar pattern was found in partially nephrectomized dogs which were volume-expanded with normal saline (COLEMAN et al. 1971).

6.2 The Neurogenic Hypothesis

Championed by FOLKOW and others (FOLKOW 1982, 1983), this hypothesis is somewhat similar, but the initiating event is not an intrinsic defect in the kidney; rather it is an increase in neurogenic activity leading to increased venous tone, vascular resistance, and heart rate. The increased venous tone shifts blood from the capacitance vessels, which contain about 70% of the blood volume, to the central system. This increase in central blood volume and the resulting tachycardia increases cardiac output which in turn results in whole body autoregulation. In this model increased sympathetic activity to the kidney can lead to increased sodium retention and volume expansion.

There is support for the neurogenic theory in human hypertension. Studies in young and labile hypertensive patients have noted increased cardiac output, normal peripheral resistance, and tachycardia. These hyperkinetic hypertensive patients respond well to β-adrenoreceptor blockade. The studies by LUND-JOHANSEN (1967, 1977, 1980, 1984) are particularly important in this regard. He followed early hyperkinetic hypertensive patients for 10 years and found that untreated borderline hypertension changed from a high cardiac output and normal peripheral resistance phase to a raised peripheral resistance and normal cardiac output phase. Resting heart rate also fell. Normotensive subjects in the same group showed no significant hemodynamic change over the 10 years. Further evidence for a primary neurogenic component is the response of adolescents of hypertensive parents to mental stress (FALKNER et al. 1979). These adolescents had higher basal heart rates and increased pressure and heart rate responses to stress. A hyperactive sympathetic system is evident in young SHR as well (FOLKOW et al. 1981; HALLBACK and FOLKOW 1974; JUDY et al. 1976).

It is clear from both the experimental hypertensive animal strains and humans that there is a strong genetic component in hypertension. Those who support the autoregulatory hypothesis believe there is a genetic defect in the kidney for sodium excretion, and in fact renal transplantation experiments in SHR and Dahl salt-sensitive rats support this concept (DAHL et al. 1974). Those supporting the neurogenic hypothesis believe there is a major genetic abnormality in the autonomic nevous system and perhaps the CNS (FOLKOW 1982).

It is important, of course, to know which is the primary event since our understanding of the pathogenesis of hypertension will lead to more specific treatment. If the failure of the kidney to excrete sodium adequately is the primary event, then a low sodium diet or diuretic therapy would be the proper treatment. If on the other hand, the CNS or autonomic system is abnormal, then drugs aimed at controlling the CNS or the peripheral response would be reasonable. It is also possible, even probable, that in different individuals the primary event may be a failure of sodium excretion while in others it is hyperactivity of the sympathetic nervous system.

A third hypothesis attempting to explain initial events in primary hypertension is a defect in sodium transport. This theory is a derivative of the autoregulatory hypothesis. The defect in sodium transport in vascular smooth muscle leads to increased intracellular sodium which in turn results in increased intracellular calcium (BLANSTEIN 1980). The latter increases vascular tone and elevates peripheral resistance. However, the presence of an abnormal sodium pump in cells from hypertensive patients is still controversial. Furthermore, the initial event still appears to be a defect in sodium excretion by the kidney which is followed by volume expansion and secretion of a natriuretic hormone (DE WARDENER 1977; DE WARDENER and MACGREGOR 1980). This hormone enhances sodium excretion by the kidney and inhibits sodium potassium ATPase in vascular smooth muscle, resulting in abnormal intracellular ion levels and vasoconstriction.

7 Hereditary Aspects

There is a general consensus that the predisposition to high blood pressure is hereditary. The evidence for this emerged from records of single families, studies of family histories, and investigations in identical and nonidentical twins. Strong support for the genetic origin of hypertension also comes from the various hypertensive rat strains (RASCHER et al. 1982). The polygenic or multifactorial hypothesis of inheritance assumes that multiple factors, both inherited and acquired, will lead to an elevation of blood pressure. The distribution of the hypertension phenotype will then be continuous in the population at large and is the expression of "major" and "minor" genes and their interactions with the environment.

Epidemiological studies confirm that the distribution of levels of blood pressure in relatives of hypertensive patients is significantly higher than in relatives of normotensive control populations. The higher the pressure of the proband, the higher the pressure of the relative; this relationship is linear with a correlation coefficient of 0.23 against an expected coefficient of 0.50 for the total genetic determination of hypertension. It is assumed that three to six major genes and several polygenes (plus environment) determine hypertension (see GROSS and ROBERTSON 1979). The genes involved have not yet been identified, but molecular biological techniques are available to study these problems at the DNA level. Differences in gene structure and DNA sequences between normotensive nd hypertensive subjects can be investigated by different techniques, one of which is restriction fragment length polymorphism (RFLP). This technique enables us to define areas of the genome that are associated with blood pressure differences. Genes (and gene differences) that are causally related to hypertension will remain associated with high blood pressure in genetically segregating populations of normotensive and hypertensive subjects.

One of the obvious systems to be investigated in this respect is the renin-angiotensin system. Indeed, RFLPs have been described for the renin gene and the angiotensinogen gene in two different strains of hypertensive rats. The localization of the renin RFLP on a regulatory 5-portion of the gene in one study (LINDPAINTNER et al. 1988) and the cosegregation with blood pressure in another study (RAPP et al. 1989) indicate the potential pathogenetic relevance of these findings.

These and other molecular biological findings exemplify new approaches to the study of the pathophysiology of hypertension (CAMUSSI and BIANCHI 1988). "Hypertension genes" can now be isolated, sequenced, and characterized in vitro, in cell culture, and in vivo, e.g., using transgenic animals. This will in the future not only increase our pathophysiological knowledge but will also make new therapeutic approaches possible, and we will be able to define subjects who are genetically at risk or not; this will lead eventually to true predictive and preventive medicine.

8 Consequences of Elevated Blood Pressure

The blood pressure per se is not the problem but rather the effect of the elevated blood pressure on the vascular system. Most likely, it is the sustained elevation of blood pressure rather than intermittent peak elevations that is important. In population studies the rate of morbid events is related to the height and the duration of hypertension. However, there is considerable variation in risk among hypertensive patients. Genetic background, blood cholesterol levels, diabetes, smoking history, age of the patient, sex, and race all influence the response of the vascular system to elevated blood pressure (Hypertension Detection and Follow Up Cooperative Group I 1979; Multiple Risk Factor Intervention Trial Research Group 1982).

The major sites of the cardiovascular system affected by hypertension are the heart, cerebral vessels, kidney, eyes, abdominal aorta, and lower extremity vessels. Several changes occur in the heart. Left ventricular hypertrophy is secondary to the increased peripheral resistance and initially is an important compensatory response, but later the heart becomes overloaded and decompensates, and congestive heart failure ensues. The coronary vessels become atherosclerotic; hypertensive patients have a higher incidence of death from myocardial infarction. In fact, with control of the hypertension, mortality from other causes such as stroke and renal failure decreases significantly, while that from heart disease decreases to a much lesser extent, and it becomes thus the leading cause of death.

Hypertension is a major cause of cerebral vascular disease. The cerebral vessels develop atherosclerosis which can result in brain infarcts. The cerebral vessels also develop microaneurysms that may rupture and cause intracranial hemorrhages. In severe hypertension, encephalopathy due to brain edema may occur. In addition to strokes from abnormalities in the cerebral vessels, strokes may occur as a result of atherosclerosis of the extracranial vessels. The internal carotid arteries often develop atheromatous lesions and fragments of the atheromata may dislodge and embolize to the cerebral vessels with subsequent brain infarction.

Hypertension is also a major risk factor in developing vascular disease in the larger blood vessels. The vast majority of patients with abdominal aortic dissection have hypertension. Atheromata of the large vessels in the lower extremities cause claudication, a common occurrence in patients with long-standing hypertension.

The kidney not only plays an important etiological role in the pathogenesis of hypertension but is also damaged by the elevated pressure. Initially, the renal blood vessels participate in the generalized increase in peripheral resistance, which results in functional changes such as increased filtration rate and decreased renal blood flow. Early renal involvement is not easily demonstrated. Nocturia and albuminuria, usually mild, reflect vascular sclerosis with hyalinization of the glomerulus and damage of the tubules. Renal damage is slowly progressive. With severe hypertension about 10% of patients progress to uremia, and in malignant hypertension there is a rapid deterioration of function. Nevertheless, most patients with mild hypertension do not develop severe renal failure.

The evidence is quite clear that treatment of hypertension reduces the incidence of strokes, heart failure, renal failure, and large vessel disease, but it does not lessen coronary artery disease to the same extent. The reasons for this are not evident, but one popular idea is that some of the antihypertensive agents raise plasma lipid levels or have other secondary effects which offset the benefit of lowering blood pressure.

9 When to Treat and How to Treat

We have discussed above the definition of hypertension and the lower limit of high blood pressure which necessitates a decision whether or not to treat with drugs. The most important point is that medical care for the hypertensive patient does not automatically mean drug treatment.

In patients with moderate to severe hypertension the decision to begin drug treatment rarely poses a problem. The situation is less clear in patients with mild hypertension. Factors additional to diastolic hypertension will influence the therapeutic strategy. Isolated systolic hypertension is not uncommon, especially in the elderly patient, and at any level of diastolic blood pressure increasing systolic pressure carries an additional risk. Controlled therapeutic trials are presently under way to study the value of therapy more precisely.

Old age is no bar to drug treatment, but caution is needed since side effects may be severe. In elderly patients, however, blood pressure elevation can often be controlled by low-dose medication. The benefits of hypertensive therapy are more conspicuous in older subjects, but those who are in good general health should probably be treated in the same way as younger patients. The lowering of blood pressure should be attempted even more slowly than is recommended in younger patients; to reach goal pressure may take several months. Elderly hypertensive patients with cardiac failure benefit significantly from antihypertensive drug treatment, even if given over a short period of time. There is, however, as yet no evidence that long-term antihypertensive treatment is of benefit in people aged 80 years and over.

Men have a greater risk of cardiovascular disease, and the evidence of benefit from treatment is less strong in white women. Clinical, electrocardiographic, echocardiographic, or radiological evidence of left ventricular hypertrophy or clinical, electrocardiographic, or angiographic evidence of ischemic heart disease is a clear indication to begin drug treatment. A history of cerebrovascular disease (e.g., transient cerebral ischemia or stroke) is also a clear indicator to begin treatment.

If there are signs of renal disease, e.g., raised plasma creatinine, hematuria, or proteinuria, drug treatment should be started. A strong family history of stroke, heart disease, or sudden death should influence the decision towards early drug treatment. Continued smoking, elevated fasting glucose, elevated serum cholesterol, or creatinine all markedly increase the cardiovascular risk associated with high blood pressure and should influence the decision toward the intensive use of appropriate nondrug measures and early drug treatment.

10 Profiles of Antihypertensive Drugs

Fortunately, there is a wide variety of drugs with different actions available to treat hypertension. Treatment should be adatped to the needs of the individual patient. Different patients may respond to one drug better than to others. One of the main factors influencing effective treatment is patient compliance. Frequency of dose, side effects, and cost all play important roles in determining patient compliance.

In addition to blood pressure lowering agents, control of those risk factors which aggravate the effect of hypertension is important. Hyperlipidemia, diabetes, cigarette smoking, obesity, excessive alcohol and salt intake should be controlled. In mild forms of hypertension, relaxation techniques may be beneficial and can lead to control of blood pressure without drug therapy, but with persistent hypertension, pharmacotherapy is the treatment of choice. At what level of blood pressure treatment should begin is discussed above.

10.1 Diuretics

The mainstay of therapy is the diuretic, the most commonly used drug in the world to treat hypertension. If sodium retention by kidney is the initial event leading to the development of hypertension then it makes sense to use a drug to interfere with sodium reabsorption. Diuretics, especially the thiazides, have many advantages. Cost is low, once a day treatment is usually sufficient, and low doses may be used in the typical hypertensive patient, thus lessening the side effects, especially the renal loss of potassium. Although the efficiency of diuretics in lowering blood pressure is well-known, the precise mechanism is still unclear. Acutely, diuretics lower plasma volume and decrease cardiac output, but with chronic therapy these parameters return to normal while peripheral resistance is reduced by mechanisms that are unknown. One hypothesis is that by decreasing plasma volume, diuretics reduce the concentration of the natriuretic hormone. Subsequently, the vascular smooth muscle vasoconstriction is reduced.

In addition to their use as a primary agent, diuretics are frequently used in combination with other drugs, and both drugs together are more antihypertensive than either drug alone. A diuretic is especially useful in preventing the edema that often accompanies vasodilator therapy. The potent diuretics such as furosemide ae particularly effective in treating hypertension in patients with chronic renal failure. Volume-dependent hypertension is clearly important in this group of patients. Since renal function decreases with age, volume expansion may also be an important mechanism contributing to hypertension of the elderly, and diuretics are effective in this group.

Diuretics are fairly safe drugs when used in low doses. Electrolyte disturbances are a major problem, especially hypokalemia, ventricular ectopics, and impotence, but these complications can usually be managed and are frequently avoided with low doses. Mild abnormalities in carbohydrate tolerance may also occur. The lipid disturbances are of concern today. Diuretics cause a modest increase in serum triglycerides and cholesterol, including LDL cholesterol, but this appears to be transient. There is concern, nevertheless, that these lipid abnormalities may be the reason for the failure of hypertensive treatment to lower coronary artery disease efficiently.

10.2 Adrenergic System Inhibitors

These drugs constitute a large class of antihypertensive agents and can be divided into several subclasses: (a) peripheral neuronal inhibitors, (b) central α_2-adrenoreceptor stimulators, (c) α-adrenoreceptor inhibitors, (d) β-adrenoreceptor inhibitors, and (e) combined α- and β-adrenoreceptor inhibitors.

Of the peripheral neuronal inhibitors reserpine is the only one that is still in common use in many countries. They lost favor because of an inaccurate cancer scare and because of their side effects, especially mental depression. It is now clear that the side effects are mild when low doses, which are sufficient in treating hypertension, are used. Reserpine is an effective, cheap, administered once daily drug. It was one of the drugs used in the original Veterans Administration cooperative trial showing the efficacy of drug therapy. Reserpine is usually combined with a diuretic. This combination can control blood pressure in a large percentage of patients. Once daily treatment plus the low cost encourage compliance.

The two most common central α-adrenergic stimulators are α-methyldopa and clonidine. This class of drug lowers blood pressure by decreasing the activity of the sympathetic nervous system. The most annoying side effect is drowsiness.

Since these drugs often lead to sodium retention, they are best given with a diuretic. At low doses they are well-tolerated, safe, and useful drugs.

α-Adrenoreceptor blockers form an important class of drugs for controlling blood pressure. Since the chronic phase of hypertension is characterized by increased peripheral resistance, drugs which lower peripheral resistance seem indicated. The classical α-adrenoreceptor antagonist phentolamine has not proven successful in the long-term control of high blood pressure. However, the selective α_1-adrenoreceptor prazosin and related compounds have proven to be useful as antihypertensive agents. One of the major advantages of these drugs is a lack of reflex tachycardia. α_1-Receptor antagonism causes arterial and venous dilatation. This latter function may help in the treatment of heart failure. The venous vasodilatation probably explains the orthostatic hypertension, which is known as the "first dose" effect. It can be prevented by using a small starting dose. The advantage of the α_1-receptor class of drugs is their lack of effect on carbohydrate tolerance and their improvement of blood lipid levels with an increase in HDL and a decrease in LDL cholesterol. Like all vasodilators, these drugs may cause fluid retention and therefore are usually given with a diuretic.

The widespread use of β-blockers in the treatment of asymptomatic hypertension attests to their freedom from serious toxic effects. Selective antagonists such as atenolol and nonselective ones such as propranolol appear to have the same effect on lowering blood pressure and relatively similar side effects. The explanation for their mechanism of action is still controversial, but decreased cardiac output appears to be the major mechanism. Peripheral resistance initially rises and then returns towards pretreatment levels, which in the hypertensive patient is higher than normal. In some patients a lowering of plasma renin activity may also be important. These drugs have many advantages, a relative lack of side effects, and a decrease in heart rate with a decrease in contractility which makes them useful in preventing aortic dissection. Their use is associated with a reduction in incidence of heart attacks, reversal of left ventricular hypertrophy, and a mild increase in serum potassium. They are contraindicated in patients with asthma or diabetes on insulin with frequent episodes of hypoglycemia and in patients with serious cardiac conduction defects.

In young hypertensive patients with high cardiac outputs and overactive sympathetic activity, β-blockers are the initial drug of choice. They are frequently given with diuretics and by reducing secondary stimulation of renin and aldosterone levels may lessen the hypokalemic action of diuretics.

Labetalol is the prototype of a class of drugs which have the advantage of acting as an α_1-inhibitor, leading to vasodilatation, and as β-blocker, decreasing cardiac output. This drug has a rapid onset of action and can be used in hypertensive emergencies. Clinical experience with it in the treatment of chronic hypertension is still limited.

10.3 Calcium Channel Antagonists

The numerous calcium channel antagonists are chemically heterogeneous compounds having a similar mechanism of action and therapeutic effect in hypertension. By inhibiting transmembrane calcium influx in vascular smooth muscle they reduce peripheral vascular resistance. In addition, these drugs have a mild natriuretic action through a direct tubular effect. In monotherapy, the calcium channel blockers are as effective as diuretics or β-blcokers. Side effects are frequent but mild and reversible, and each of the drugs has its own peculiar side effects. They are frequently used in combination with other drugs and can be prescribed for asthmatic as well as diabetic patients. Since they are effective in treating angina pectoris, they are indicated in patients with angina and hypertension.

10.4 Converting Enzyme Inhibitors

The use of converting enzyme (CE) inhibitors has increased significantly over the past few years. These substances lower blood pressure by decreasing peripheral resistance through inhibition of the enzyme that converts angiotensin I to angiotensin II. In addition, the concentrations of the potent vasodilator bradykinin may also increase. The CE inhibitors are especially effective in lowering blood pressure in patients with high plasma renin concentrations. By lowering renal glomerular pressure the CE inhibitors may reduce urinary protein excretion and slow the progression of the glomerular lesion in patients with nephritis. However, in some patients with renal disease, especially those with bilateral renal artery stenosis, the CE inhibitors can produce renal failure, which is usually, however, reversible. It is therefore advisable to measure renal function at appropriate time intervals.

Because of their ability to reduce afterload, these drugs have been successful in treating congestive heart failure and may even prolong the life-span of patients with this disease.

Except for the occasional deleterious effect on the kidney, the CE inhibitors are well-tolerated and do not alter blood lipid levels.

10.5 Direct Vasodilators

The prototype type in this group is hydralazine, which has a long history of effective use in the treatment of hypertension. This class of drugs is not regularly used as monotherapy but in combination with other drugs. The main side effect is a reflex tachycardia which can be prevented by a combination with reserpine or a β-blocker. A reversible lupus syndrome occurs in about 5% of patients on high doses of hydralazine.

For a discussion of the other drugs, the reader is referred to the respective chapters in this volume.

11 Cost of Antihypertensive Treatment and the Market

A major factor determining compliance with pharmacotherapy is the cost of the drug to the patient. In those countries in which the patient must pay for medication, cost often determines which drug is prescribed. Prices are a particularly serious problem for the elderly hypertensive patient living on a pension and with multiple medical problems. These patients may be taking four or more drugs and are likely to stop costly antihypertensive drugs since hypertension usually does not cause acute symptoms. Some method must be developed to provide appropriate medication for all hypertensive patients. From a purely economic viewpoint, the prevention of the complications of hypertension would save enormous sums of money from hospitalization, rehabilitation, disability payments, and lost productivity.

For the pharmaceutical industry the cardiovascular market is one of the most important, with a worldwide volume of approximately US $20 billion in 1988, of which antihypertensive drugs have the biggest share at about 55%. Of the 10 leading drugs worldwide a calcium antagonist (US $900 million), a CE inhibitor (US $ 700 million), and a β-blocker (US $ 700 million) occupy places 3, 4, and 5, respectively, preceded only by two histamine H_2-blockers (US $1.8 billion and US $1.3 billion).

More important may be the percentage market share of the many classes of antihypertensive substances in 1988: Calcium antagonists make up 27%, closely followed by the β-blocking agents (26%); diuretics make up 18%, CE inhibitors 17%, and other antihypertensive drugs 12%.

It is obvious from Chap. 23 that the use of drugs has specific regional peculiarities. Taking the relatively new CE inhibitors as an example, the total share in 1988 was about US $ 2 billion, of which 30% were sold in the USA, 17% in Japan, 16% in France, 14% in Italy, 6% in Germany (FRG), 3% in the UK, and 14% in the rest of the world.

There are major fluctuations to be noted. Comparing the 1986 and the 1988 worldwide data, β-blockers have decreased from 31% in 1986 to 26% in the 1988 market share, and diuretics decreased from 22% to 18% over the same period. In contrast, calcium antagonists increased from 21% in 1986 to 27% in 1988, and CE inhibitors more than doubled from 8% in 1986 to 17% in 1988.

12 Do We Already Have Too Much? Do We Need More?

The achievements of antihypertensive therapy in the year 1990 compared with 1960 when many patients were doomed to die of malignant hypertension are undisputed. Overtreatment may, however, today be as much a problem as insufficient treatment.

The cardiovascular risk of a patient with treated and controlled hypertension is, however, still higher than that of a normotensive person. Therefore, antihypertensive therapy cannot as yet be considered ideal. The quest for new antihypertensive drugs is on, and some of the new approaches are discussed in this volume. The major challenges are to improve the effectiveness of antihypertensive therapy on coronary heart disease prevention and the prevention and regression of atherosclerosis and blood vessel lesions, to develop drugs with greater effectiveness, to improve their profile with respect to metabolic actions in a larger percentage of the patients, and to improve their acceptability with respect to subjective and objective side effects and quality of life.

Hypertension is a multifactorial disease expressed in individual patients. It can be predicted that there will be no one ideal drug for all patients; rather, there will be a series of antihypertensive agents with different properties and mechanisms of action which need to be used with intelligence and responsibility for individualized therapy. The schematic "stepped care" approach will be advanced to "alternative substitution"; the first choice, low-dose drug remains under trial and depending on the patient's response is modified or substituted. New drugs will improve individualized therapy.

The real problem is the fact that hypertension is a chronic disease and its sequelae (and their regression) develop very slowly. It is increasingly difficult with the newer drugs to test them against the decades of experience with well-known, first-line antihypertensive agents and their proven efficacy with respect to morbidity, mortality, and relative subjective acceptability. The purpose of this handbook is meant to provide the basis for an educated choice and also to indicate future development in the therapy of hypertension.

References

Antonaccio MJ (ed) (1984) Cardiovascular Pharmacology. Raven, New York

Bevan AT, Honour AJ, Stott FH (1969) Direct arterial pressure recording in unrestricted man. Clin Sci 36:329–344

Blaustein MP (1980) How does sodium cause hypertension? A hypothesis. In: Zumkley H, Losse H (eds) Intracellular electrolytes and arterial hypertension. Thieme, Stuttgart; pp 151–157

Borst JGG, Borst De Geus A (1963) Hypertension explained by Starling's theory of circulatory homeostasis. Lancet i: 677–682

Camussi A, Bianchi G (1988) Genetics of essential hypertension. From the unimodal-bimodal controversy to molecular technology. Hypertension 12:620–628

Coleman TG, Granger HJ, Guyton AC (1971) Whole body circulatory autoregulation and hypertension. Circ Res 28–29 [Suppl II]: 76–86

Conway J (1963) A vascular abnormality in hypertension. A study of blood flow in the forearm. Circulation 27:520–529

Dahl LK, Heine M, Thompson K (1974) Genetic influence of the kidneys on blood pressure. Evidence from chronic renal homografts in rats with opposite predispositions to hypertension. Circ Res 34:94–101

De Wardener HE (1977) Natriuretic hormone. Clin Sci Mol Med 53:1–8

De Wardener HD, Macgregor GA (1980) Dahl's hypothesis that a saluretic substance may be responsible for a sustained rise in arterial pressure: its possible role in essential hypertension. Kidney Int 18:1–9

Falkner B, Onesti G, Angelakos ET, Fernandes M, Langman C (1979) Cardiovascular response to mental stress in normal adolescents with hypertensive parents. Hypertension 1:23–30

Folkow B (1982) Physiological aspects of primary hypertension. Physiol Rev 62(2): 347–503

Folkow B (1983) Personal views on the mechanisms of primary hypertension. In: Genest J, Kuchel O, Hamet P, Cantin M (eds) Hypertension: pathophysiology and treatment. McGraw-Hill, New York, pp 646–658

Folkow B, Hallback-Nordlander M, Lundin S, Ricksten SE, Thoren P (1981) Neurogenic elements in rat primary hypertension-differences between SHR and MHS. In: Laragh JH (ed) Frontiers in hypertension research. Springer-Verlag, New York, pp 367–369

Freis ED (1960) Hemodynamics of hypertension. Physiol Rev 40:27–54
Frohlich ED (1977) Hemodynamics of hypertension. In Genest J, Koiw E, Kuchel O (eds) Hypertension. McGraw-Hill, New York, pp 15–48
Genest J, Kuchel O, Hamet P, Cantin M (eds) (1983) Hypertension, 2nd edn. McGraw-Hill, New York
Gross F (ed) (1977) Antihypertensive agents. Springer, Berlin Heidelberg New York
Gross FH, Robertson JIS (eds) (1979) Arterial hypertension. Pitman, London
Gross F, Strasser T (eds) (1983) Mild hypertension. Recent advances. Raven, New York
Guyton AC (1977) Personal views on mechanisms of hypertension. In: Genest J, Koiw E, Kuchel O (eds) Hypertension. McGraw-Hill, New York, pp 566–575
Guyton AC, Coleman TG, Cowley AW, Scheel KW, Manning RD, Normal RA (1972) Arterial pressure regulation. Am J Med 52: 584–594
Guyton AC, Coleman TG, Cowley AD JR, Manning RD JR, Norman RA JR, Ferguson JD (1974) A systems analysis approach to understanding long-range arterial blood pressure control and hypertension. Circ Res 35: 159–176.
Hallback M, Folkow B (1974) Cardiovascular response to acute mental stress in spontaneously hypertensive rats. Acta Physiol Scand 90:648–698
Halpern W, Mulvany NJ, Warshaw DW (1978) Mechanical properties of smooth muscle cells in the walls of arterial resistance vessels. J Physiol [Lond] 275:85–101
Hypertension Detection and Follow Up Cooperative Group I (1979) Reduction in mortality of persons with high blood pressure including mild hypertension. JAMA 242:2562–2771
Judy WV, Watanabe AM, Henry DP, Besch HR, Murphy WR, Hockel KM (1976) Sympathetic nerve activity. Role in regulation of blood pressure in the spontaneously hypertensive rats. Circ Res 38 [Suppl II]:21–29
Lardinois CL, Neuman SL (1988) The effects of antihypertensive agents on serum lipids and lipoproteins. Arch Intern Med 148:1280–1286
Ledingham JM, Cohen RC (1964) Changes in the extracellular fluid volume and cardiac output during the development of experimental renal hypertension. Can Med Assoc J 90:292–294
Lindpaintner K, Takanashi S, Metzger R, Murakami K, Ganten D (1988) Restriction fragment length polymorphism (RFLP) of the renin gene distinguishes hypertensive and normotensive rat strains. Hypertension 12(3):359
Lund-Johansen P (1967) Hemodynamics in early essential hypertension. Acta Med Scand 183[Suppl 482]:1–105
Lund-Johansen P (1977) Hemodynamic alterations in hypertension-spontaneous changes and effects of drug therapy. A review. Acta Med Scand [Suppl]603:1–14
Lund-Johansen P (1980) Haemodynamics in essential hypertension. State of the art review. Clin Sci 59:343s–354s
Lund-Johansen P (1984) Hemodynamic effects of antihypertensive agents. In: Doyle AE (ed) Handbook of hypertension, vol 5. Clinical pharmacology of antihypertensive drugs. Elsevier, Amsterdam, pp 39–66
McCubbin JW, Green JH, Page IH (1956) Baroreceptor function in chronic renal hypertension. Circ Res 4:205–210
Millar-Craig MW, Bishop CN, Raftery EB (1978) Circadian variation of blood pressure. Lancet 1:795–797
Multiple Risk Factor Intervention Trial Research Group (1982) Multiple risk factor intervention trial: risk factor changes and mortality results. JAMA 248:1465–1477
Mulvany MJ, Hansen PK, Aalkjaer C (1978) Direct evidence that the greater contractility of resistance vessels in spontaneously hypertensive rats is associated with a narrower lumen, a thicker media and a larger number of smooth muscle cell layers. Circ Res 43:854–864
Page IH (ed) (1987) Hypertension mechanisms. Grune and Stratton, New York
Pickering GW (1968) High blood pressure 2nd edn. Churchill, London
Pickering GW (1977) Personal views on mechanisms of hypertension. In: Genest J, Koiw E, Kuchel O (eds) Hypertension. McGraw-Hill, New York, pp 598–606
Rapp JP, Wand S-M, Dene H (1989) A genetic polymosphism in the renine gene of Dahl rats cosegregates with blood pressure. Science 243:542–544

Rascher W, Clough D, Ganten D (eds) (1982) Hypertensive mechanisms. Schattauer, Stuttgart
Reid JL (1988) Hypertension 1988: present challenges and future strategies. J Hypertens 6:3–8
Rettig R, Ganten D, Luft F (eds) (1989) Salt and hypertension. Springer, Berlin Heidelberg New York
Scriabine A (ed) (1980) Pharmacology of antihypertensive drugs. Raven, New York
Sleight P (ed) (1980) Arterial baroreceptors and hypertension. Oxford Univ Press, London
Strasser T, Ganten D (eds) (1987) Mild hypertension. From drug trials to practice. Raven, New York
Suwa N, Takahashi T (1971) Morphological and morphometrical analysis of circulation in hypertension and ischemic kidney. Urban & schwarzenberg, Berlin
Thomas CB (1973) Genetic pattern of hypertension in man. In: Onesti G, Kim KE, Moyer JH (eds) Hypertension: mechanisms and management. Grune & Stratton, New York, pp 67–73

CHAPTER 2

Diuretics

H.J. KRAMER

CONTENTS

1 Introduction

Diuretics have been used successfully as antihypertensive drugs for over 30 years. In 1957, chlorothiazide was introduced into clinical trials to treat hypertensive patients (HOLLANDER and WILKINS 1957). Although their antihypertensive mechanisms are not yet fully understood, diuretics are recommended for first-step treatment of hypertension. In fact, they may be more effective than β-adrenergic blocking agents in controlling blood pressure in hypertensive patients. They are not only powerful antihypertensive agents but also enhance the antihypertensive activity of other drugs. In recent years, however, their efficacy, long-term safety, and position in therapeutic schemes have been challenged since new antihypertensive drugs have been developed. This debate relates to a number of unwanted side-effects, which mainly result from the relatively high doses frequently used in the past. With increasing understanding of the pathogenesis of hypertension and with improved knowledge of their mode of action, potency, and the reasons for side effects, their usefulness and efficacy as antihypertensive drugs can now be reconsidered in a more sophisticated way.

The following chapter will summarize the chemical nature, pharmacokinetics, metabolism, pharmacodynamics, as well as the renal and antihypertensive mechanisms of action of the most representative diuretic agents presently available for the oral treatment of hypertension. Although acetazolamide is no longer used as diuretic or antihypertensive agent, it is included for historical and pharmacological reasons. Not included in this chapter are other diuretic agents which are no longer used in antihypertensive treatment such as organomercurials, the potent loop diuretic muzolimine, and the uricosuric agents indacrinone and ticrynafen (tienilic acid). In the second part of this chapter the therapeutic aspects of the use of diuretics as antihypertensive agents will be discussed including dosages, combination drug therapy with other antihypertensive agents, and special indications for differential usage of individual diuretics. Their side effects and contraindications as well as their interactions with other drugs which may interfere with their diuretic and antihypertensive actions will be discussed.

2 Chemistry

2.1 Chemical Structure of Diuretics

According to their chemical structures diuretic agents presently used in clinical medicine can be divided into five chemical classes (Fig. 1): (a) sulfonamide derivatives, (b) thiazolidone derivatives, e.g., etozolin, (c) aryloxyacetic acids, e.g., phenoxyacetic acid derivatives, (d) pyrazine and pyrimidine derivatives, i.e., pteridine derivatives, and (e) aldosterone antagonists.

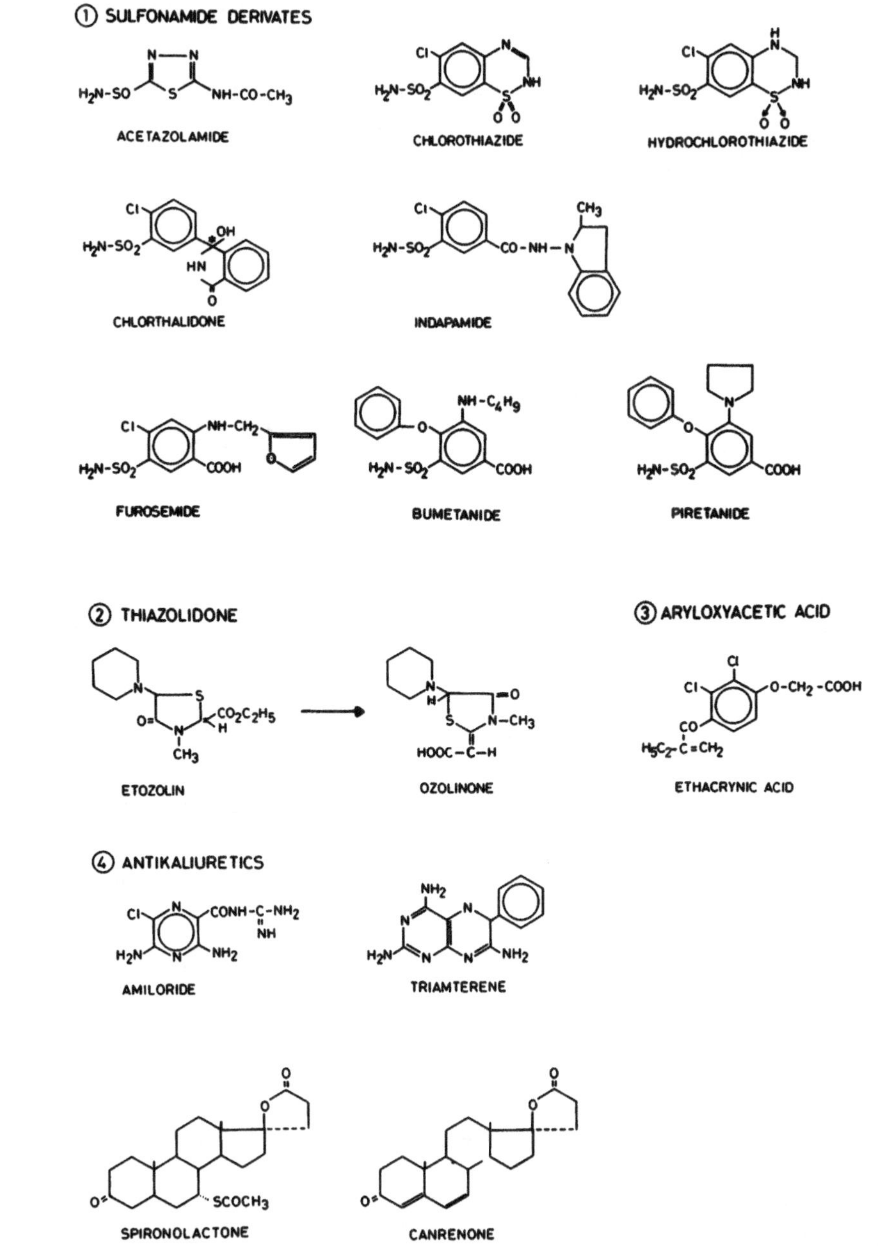

Fig. 1. Chemical structures of representative compounds of different groups of diuretics

Sulfonamide derivatives can be subdivided into three subclasses: (a) carbonic anhydrase inhibitors, (b) benzothiadiazine derivatives, e.g., thiazides and hydrothiazides, and (c) thiazide analogues with two subgroups, namely the thiazide-like sulfonamides and the potent chloruretic sulfonamides, i.e., loop diuretics. The chemistry of diuretics (Table 1) has been extensively reviewed by

Table 1. Type, generic name and chemical structure of representative diuretics for oral use

Diuretic type		Generic name	Chemical structure
Sulfonamide diuretics	Carboanhydrase inhibitor	Acetazolamide	2-acetylamino-1,3,4-thiadiazole-5-sulfonamide
	Benzothiadiazines (thiazides)	Chlorothiazide	6-chloro-2*H*-1,2,4-benzothiadiazine-1,1-dioxide-7-sulfonamide
		Hydrochlorothiazide	6-chloro-3,4-dihydro-2*H*-1,2,4-benzothiadiazine-1,1-dioxide-7-sulfonamide
	Thiazide-like sulfonamides	Chlorthalidone	2-chloro-5-(1-hydroxy-3-oxo-1-isoindolinyl-benzo-sulfonamide
		Indapamide	4-chloro-*N*-(2-methylindoline-1-yl)-3-sulfamoyl-benzamide
		Furosemide	4-chloro-5-sulfamoyl-*N*-furfuryl-anthranilic acid
		Bumetanide	3-*n*-butylamino-4-phenoxy-5-sulfamoyl-benzoic acid
		Piretanide	4-phenoxy-3-(1-pyrrolidinyl)-5-sulfamoyl-benzoic acid
Thiazolidone		Etozolin (ozolinone)	(3-methyl-4-oxo-5-(1-piperidyl)-2-thiazolidinylidin) acetic acid ester
Aryloxyacetic acid		Ethacrynic acid	2,3-dichloro-4-(2-methylenebutyryl)-phenoxyacetic acid
Pteridine derivatives		Amiloride	3,5-diamino-6-chloropyrazine-2-(*N*-amidinocarbonamide)-HCI
		Triamterene	2,4,7-triamino-6-phenylpteridine
Aldosterone antagonist		Spironolactone	3-(7a-acetylthio-17ß-hydroxy-3-oxo-4-androstene-17a-yl)-propionic acid-γ-lactone

CRAGOE (1978) and therefore only more recently introduced compounds will be referenced in this section.

The first sulfonamide derivative which could be administered orally was acetazolamide, a carbonic anhydrase inhibitor (ROBLIN and CLAPP 1950). Benzothiadiazines and thiazide analogues are derived from the carbonic anhydrase inhibitors but lack this enzyme-inhibiting property and therefore do not produce significant metabolic acidosis.

The first thiazide introduced about 30 years ago for clinical trials was chlorothiazide (HOLLANDER and WILKINS 1957; NOVELLO and SPRAGUE 1957) which was soon followed by hydrochlorothiazide having a more than ten times greater diuretic potency (DE STEVENS et al. 1958). Numerous benzothiadiazine derivatives have since been introduced in which modification of the thiadiazine ring (Fig. 1) has led to greater lipid solubility or slower degradation and elimination, resulting in a far more potent and longer acting diuretic activity on a milligram-for-milligram basis. They include bendroflumethiazide, cyclothiazide, cyclopenthiazide, methyclothiazide, benzthiazide, hydroflumethiazide, trichlormethiazide, and polythiazide. Thiazide analogues with thiazide-like action are benzothiadiazine-related heterocyclics which include phthalimidines such as chlorthalidone, quinazolinones such as quinethazone and metolazone, benzene sulfonamides such as mefruside, and chlorobenzamides such as clopamide, indapamide, and xipamide. Indapamide has the unique characteristic of possessing vasodilator properties similar to calcium channel blockers at low nonnatriuretic doses (MORLEDGE 1983).

Thiazide analogues also include the highly potent (high-ceiling) chloruretic sulfonamide derivatives, known as loop diuretics, e.g., the sulfamoylbenzoates furosemide (STURM et al. 1966), bumetanide (FEIT 1971; OSTERGAARD et al. 1972), piretanide, (MERKEL et al. 1976), azosemide (KRÜCK et al. 1978), and torasemide (LAMEIRE and DIDION 1988). Azosemide, which has a phenylsulfanilamide structure, and torasemide are closely related to furosemide. With bumetanide and piretanide the chlorine atom on the benzoic acid ring of furosemide was replaced by a phenoxy group (Fig. 1) which strongly increased their diuretic potency on a milligram-for-milligram basis (FEIT 1981). Both agents demonstrate a similar dose-response curve to that of furosemide, however.

The thiazolidone etozolin is a heterocyclic compound which contains no benzene ring or sulfonamide group in its molecule (Fig. 1). Because of its site and potency of action etozolin belongs to the loop diuretics (GREVEN et al. 1980).

From the group of aryloxyacetic acids ethacrynic acid (SCHULTZ et al. 1962) (Fig. 1) is the only phenoxyacetic acid derivative presently released for diuretic treatment. Because of its main site of action at the ascending limb of Henle's loop and its strong diuretic potency, it belongs to the loop diuretics.

The group of pyrazine and pyrimidine derivatives, i.e., pteridine derivatives, includes the potassium-sparing diuretics amiloride (CRAGOE et al. 1967) and triameterene (WIEBELHAUS et al. 1965) (Fig. 1).

Aldosterone antagonists act by competition with the binding site of aldosterone for its receptor protein. Spironolactone is at present the only very effective aldosterone antagonist when taken orally. (DODSON and TWEIT 1959) (Fig. 1).

2.2 Pro-drugs

Examples of diuretic pro-drugs, which have to undergo biotransformation to develop their diuretic action fully, are the loop diuretic etozolin, the potassium-sparing triamterene, and the aldosterone antagonist spironolactone.

Etozolin undergoes extensive first-pass metabolism essentially to its 2-methylene-carboxylic acid ozolinone, which displays greater diuretic potency (HEIDENREICH et al. 1964). From the two optical isomers of ozolinone only the

(-)enantiomer has diuretic activity and acts on the thick ascending limb of Henle's loop (GREVEN et al. 1980).

Triamterene is converted rapidly and almost completely into *p*-hydroxytriamterene after its ingestion. This phase I-metabolite and the phase II-metabolite *p*-hydroxytriamterene sulfuric acid ester (LEHMANN 1965) are at least as potent diuretics as the parent compound.

The aldosterone antagonist spironolactone undergoes extensive metabolism, resulting in canrenone as the active circulating metabolite (SADÉE et al. 1972).

3 Pharmacology

3.1 Renal Sites and Mechanisms of Action of Diuretics

According to their site of action diuretics can be subdivided into four groups acting at:

(a) the proximal tubule which represents the target site for carbonic anhydrase inhibitors, e.g., acetazolamide
(b) the ascending limb of Henle's loop which is the target site of the so-called loop diuretics, e.g., furosemide, bumetanide, piretanide, etozolin, and ethacrynic acid
(c) the early distal convoluted tubule which represents the site of action of benzothiadiazine derivatives and of thiazide-like acting sulfonamide derivatives
(d) the late distal convoluted tubule and cortical collecting duct which are the tubular target sites for the potassium-sparing diuretics amiloride and triamterene and the aldosterone antagonist spironolactone

3.1.1 Tubular Sites and Mechanisms of Fluid and Electrolyte Reabsorption and the Action of Diuretics

Since the site of action of diuretics is one major determinant of their diuretic, natriuretic, and chloruretic potencies as well as of their effects on tubular calcium and magnesium reabsorption and on potassium secretion, tubular handling of fluid and electrolytes within the nephron (Fig. 2) will be shortly reviewed (KOKKO 1984).

Two-thirds of the glomerular filtrate is reabsorbed isosmotically in the proximal tubule (site I). Approximately one-third of this amount is reabsorbed via active sodium reabsorption driven by the sodium pump located in the basolateral cell membrane of proximal tubular cells. Another one-third of proximal tubular fluid reabsorption depends on the sodium-hydrogen exchange at the luminal cell membrane which is coupled to bicarbonate reabsorption and depends on the carbonic anhydrase activity (PITTS 1968); it is located in the luminal brush border, intracellularly, and in peritubular cell membranes (PITTS and ALEXANDER 1945; WISTRAND and KINNE 1977). These are the target sites for carbonic anhydrase inhibitors. The last third of isosmotic reabsorption is ascribed to solvent drag. The high sodium concentration resulting from active

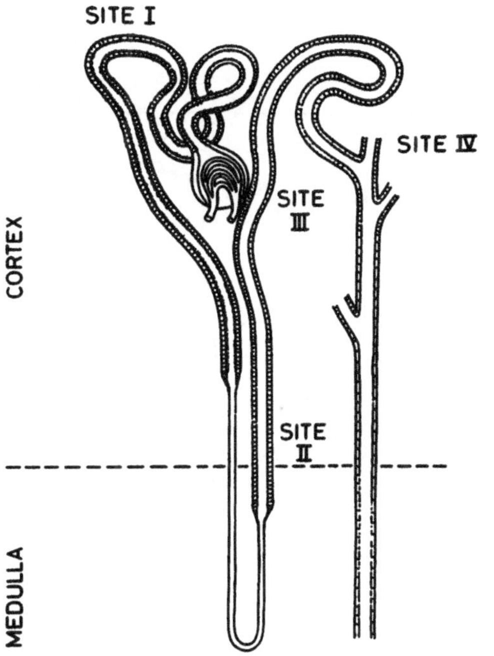

Fig. 2. Tubular sites of action of diuretics: *site I*, proximal tubule; *site II*, thick ascending limb of Henle's loop, *site III*, early convoluted tubule; *site IV*, late distal and early cortical collecting duct

sodium transport out of the proximal tubular cell into the lateral and basal infoldings sets up an osmotic gradient which causes passive transfer of water from the tubular lumen via the tight junctions into the lateral spaces between the proximal tubular cells. Fluid reabsorption out of this compartment is then determined by oncotic and hydrostatic pressure in the peritubular vasculature (Fig. 3). The extent of reabsorption in this segment is thus dependent on physical factors as well as possibly on other humoral or hormonal factors related to the state of extracellular fluid volume. Approximately 25% of the filtered sodium chloride reaching the ascending limb of Henle's loop (site II) is reabsorbed in the thick segment. At this site sodium follows the active chloride absorption via a 2 Cl-1 Na-1 K-carrier (Burg 1982; Greger and Schlatter 1983) located in the luminal cell membrane which represents the receptor for loop diuretics such as furosemide, ethacrynic acid, and ozolinone (Fig. 4). Extrusion of sodium out of the cell is subsequently driven by the sodium pump present in high density within the basolateral cell membrane. Approximately 60% of filtered magnesium (Quamme and Dirks 1980) and a large part of filtered calcium (Agus et al. 1981) are also reabsorbed in this segment.

Sodium reabsorption continues in the early distal convoluted tubule, i.e., site III. In the late distal convoluted tubule and in the cortical collecting duct, i.e., site IV, sodium is reabsorbed from the tubular fluid in exchange for potassium and hydrogen ions in amounts of up to 5% of the filtered load of sodium

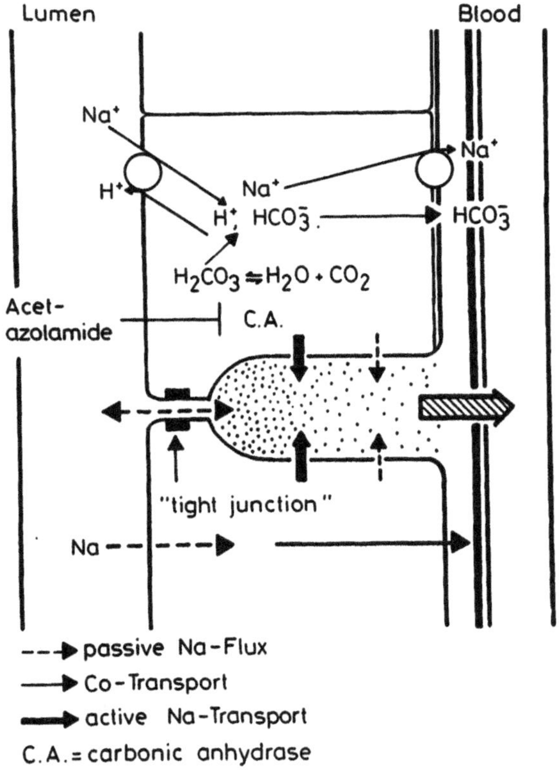

Fig. 3. Proximal tubular sodium reabsorption and target site for carbonic anhydrase inhibitors

(JAMISON et al. 1982; WRIGHT and GIEBISCH 1985). Reabsorption in these segments is enhanced by aldosterone, which controls the sodium pump at the basolateral cell surface as well as the carrier for sodium entrance at the luminal cell surface. This action of aldosterone is competitively inhibited by spironolactone. The sodium channel in the luminal cell membrane represents the target site for the potassium-sparing diuretics amiloride and triamterene. Blockade of this channel inhibits sodium reabsorption as well as potassium and hydrogen ion secretion (HROPOT et al. 1985) (Fig. 4).

3.1.2 Natriuretic Potency of Diuretics According to Their Tubular Site of Action

A major determinant of the potency of diuretic drugs is the site of their action within the renal tubule (SELDIN et al. 1966) (Fig. 5). With a few exceptions, e.g. chlorothiazide, most diuretics are extensively bound to plasma proteins (see Table 5), and most of them are weak acids. Therefore, they reach the tubular lumen by active secretion via the organic anion pump located in the proximal tubule rather than through glomerular filtration. This secretory process also guarantees high concentrations of diuretics reaching their site of action at the

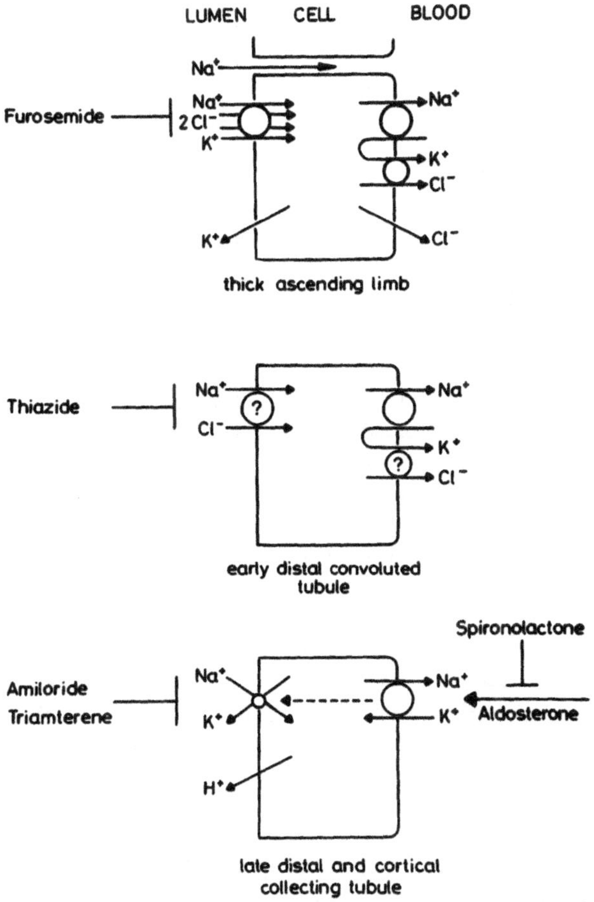

Fig. 4. Transport mechanisms for sodium, chloride, and potassium in the thick ascending limb of Henle's loop (*above*), the early distal convoluted tubule (*middle*), and the late distal and cortical collecting tubule (*below*) of the nephron as well as the respective target sites for loop diuretics, thiazides, and potassium-sparing diuretics, respectively

luminal cell surface. According to the above classification carbonic anhydrase inhibitors such as acetazolamide act at the proximal tubule since carbonic anhydrase is almost exclusively concentrated in this region of the nephron with very little activity in the distal convoluted tubule. Although relatively large amounts of sodium are reabsorbed in the proximal tubule via sodium-hydrogen exchange, inhibition of carbonic anhydrase will only lead to a fractional sodium excretion of approximately 5% because of a compensatory rise in reabsorption of sodium at more distal tubular sites. According to the amount of sodium reabsorbed in the cortical diluting segment of Henle's loop and the early distal tubule, thiazides and thiazide-like sulfonamides will result in a similar fractional sodium excretion of approximately 5% of the filtered load. Potassium-sparing diuretics including spirolactone, which act at the late distal convoluted tubule

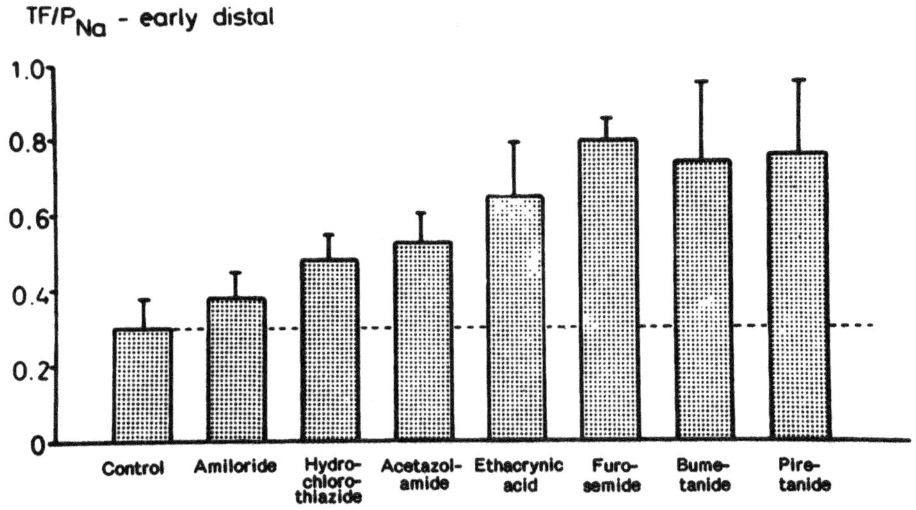

Fig. 5. Ratios of tubular fluid/plasma-sodium concentrations (TF/P_{Na}) in the early distal tubule after administration of various diuretics in the rat (DEETJEN 1980)

and the cortical collecting duct, will result in an even smaller fractional sodium excretion of approximately 3% of the filtered load. In contrast, loop diuretics, which inhibit chloride and sodium reabsorption in the ascending limb of Henle's loop are the most potent (high-ceiling) diuretics, resulting in a fractional sodium excretion of approximately 25% or more depending on the amount of tubular fluid reaching this segment (Table 2).

The relative potency of individual diuretics (Fig. 6) not only depends on their site of action but also on their chemical structure and especially on their lipid solubility and distribution coefficient (Table 3). Thus, diuretics with high lipid

Table 2. Sites of action and relative potency of representative diuretics

Potency	Diuretic	Major site of action	Fractional sodium excretion (%)
Medium potency	Acetazolamide	Proximal tubule	5
	Thiazides	Early distal tubule	5–8
	Chlorthalidone		
	Indapamide		
High potency	Furosemide	Ascending limb of Henle's loop	20–25
	Bumetanide		
	Piretanide		
	Etozolin		
Potassium sparing	Spironolactone	Late distal and cortical collecting tubule	3
	Triamterene		3
	Amiloride		3

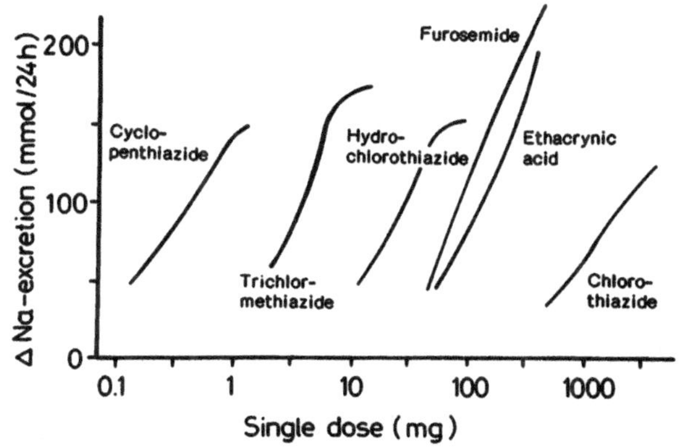

Fig. 6. Dose-effect curves of representative diuretics administered to nonedematous subjects (MENG and LOEW 1974)

solubility may recirculate within the kidney and thereby maintain high local concentrations to inhibit transport processes.

3.1.3 Effects of Diuretics on Renal Hemodynamics

Diuretic treatment will generally result in extracellular fluid volume contraction, which is often associated with a decrease in renal blood flow and glomerular filtration rate. Thus, administration of thiazides or thiazide-like sulfonamides is accompanied usually by a temporary moderate fall in renal perfusion and glomerular filtration (VAN BRUMMELEN et al. 1979). In contrast, loop diuretics such as furosemide (DATA et al. 1978), bumetanide (OLSEN and AHNFELT-RONNE 1976), and ethacrynic acid (WILLIAMSON et al. 1976) were found to reduce renal vascular resistance and to increase renal blood flow as well as to increase or to maintain glomerular filtration rate. These hemodynamic effects are presumed to be mediated at least in part by activation of the renal prostaglandin system. Since the renal vascular endothelium produces predominantly the potent

Table 3. Relative natriuretic potency of two groups (a and b) of diuretics as related to their ether/water distribution coefficient (Meng and Loew 1974)

Diuretic	Distribution coefficient ether/water at pH 7.4	Relative natriuretic potency
a) Chlorothiazide	0.08	1
Hydrochlorothiazide	0.37	10
Trichlormethiazide	1.6	100
Cyclopenthiazide	10.2	1000
b) Furosemide	0.025	1
Bumetanide	0.43	40–60

vasodilator prostacyclin (BOGLER et al. 1978) and only small amounts of PGE_2, it is interesting to note that higher doses of furosemide in the dog resulted in a significant diuresis, natriuresis, and increase in plasma renin activity as well as a significant rise in effective renal plasma flow which was accompanied by a strong rise in the excretion of 6-keto-$PGF_{1\alpha}$, the stable metabolite of prostacyclin. In contrast, small doses of furosemide, while resulting in a diuresis and natriuresis, had no effect on plasma renin activity or renal plasma flow and did not alter urinary excretion of 6-keto-$PGF_{1\alpha}$ (WILSON et al. 1982). Thus, the hemodynamic effects of loop diuretics may be dose-related and depend on stimulation of the vascular prostacyclin synthesis. Another explanation for maintenance of the glomerular filtration rate and renal perfusion in the presence of loop diuretics, in contrast to thiazides, may relate to the fact that loop diuretics such as furosemide were shown to inhibit the tubulo-glomerular feedback mechanism (WRIGHT and SCHNERMANN 1974). This mechanism normally results in a reduction of glomerular filtration when increased amounts of fluid and sodium chloride are delivered to the macula densa site.

The rise in renal blood flow, which is associated with the administration of loop diuretics and probably mediated by increased prostaglandin synthesis, will also result in a redistribution of intrarenal blood flow with an increase in medullary perfusion (DATA et al. 1978; LUCAS et al. 1975; DUCHIN and HUTCHEON 1978). The subsequent rise in interstitial pressure with decreased sodium reabsorption may therefore contribute to the potent natriuretic activity of these diuretics.

It is of interest to note that the diuretic ozolinone, which is the active main metabolite of etozolin, exhibits unique properties with regard to its renal tubular and hemodynamic effects. The two optical isomeres of ozolinone are both secreted by the proximal tubule into the tubular lumen, but only the (-) enantiomer is diuretic and natriuretic, while both enantiomers increase renal blood flow (GREVEN et al. 1980).

3.1.4 Antihypertensive Action of Diuretics

Cardiac output, which depends on blood volume and arterial baroreceptor function, and peripheral vascular resistance are the determinants of arterial pressure. It is obvious, therefore, that no single abnormality can be responsible for the development of arterial hypertension. It appears, however, that hypertension will not develop even in the presence of excessive vasoconstrictor hormone activities unless there is sufficient body sodium and extracellular fluid volume.

In various forms of hypertension extracellular fluid volume expansion may result from a genetic intrinsic or an acquired inability of the kidney to eliminate excessive sodium and water from the body adequately (Fig. 7). Thus, high activities of the adrenergic system in pheochromocytoma, of angiotensin II in renal artery stenosis, of aldosterone in primary aldosteronism, or the reduced nephron population in renal parenchymal disease as well as the lack of local hormones such as prostaglandins (KRAMER 1987) or kinins (KRAMER et al. 1980)

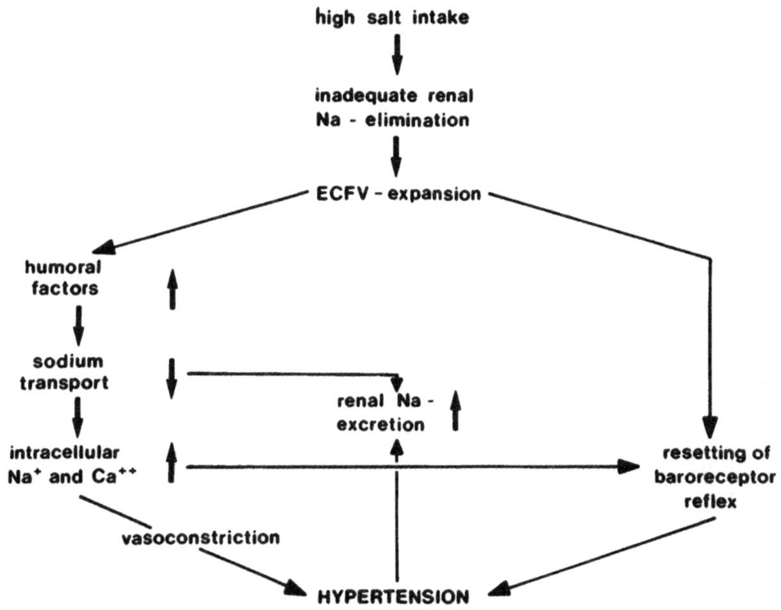

Fig. 7. Synopsis of the pathogenetic mechanisms of volume-dependent hypertension (KRAMER et al. 1984) (*ECFV*, extracellular fluid volume)

which promote renal sodium excretion all may cause renal fluid and sodium retention.

The early stage of essential hypertension in young subjects is most frequently associated with sympathetic overdrive. Simple negative stimuli, such as stress or pain, will lead within the kidney to excessive vasoconstriction which may outlast these stimuli by a relatively long period of time (BROD 1973; HOLLENBERG et al. 1981; LIGHT et al. 1983). Eventually, this will result in a positive salt and water balance and will change the sympathetically mediated rise in blood pressure to volume-dependent hypertension. Pressure diuresis subsequently reestablishes normal sodium and fluid balance. Nevertheless, central blood volume may remain increased because of a progressive decrease in the compliance of the venous capacitance vessels (LONDON and SAFAR 1985).

Central blood volume expansion suppresses arterial baroreceptor function and is assumed to stimulate the secretion of an endogenous sodium pump inhibitor (KRAMER 1981a). Thus, a number of recent studies have shown directly or indirectly the presence of a circulating endogenous inhibitor of the sodium pump or of a vascular sensitizing factor in hypertensive men and hypertensive animals (KRAMER 1986). These findings were recently incorporated into the pathogenetic scheme of essential hypertension which is based on the original experiments of DAHL et al. (1974) who showed that hypertension can be transferred by renal transplantation from a hypertensive into a normotensive rat. These authors were also the first to postulate a circulating hypertensinogenic factor on the basis of experiments with parasymbiotic rats (DAHL et al. 1967). If this hypertensinogenic factor is indeed an inhibitor of the sodium pump then, according to Blaustein's hypothesis (BLAUSTEIN 1977), and a much earlier postulate by WILBRANDT (1955), inhibition of the sodium pump at the level of the vascular smooth muscle cell will lead not only to a loss of intracellular potassium and accumulation of sodium but also to an increase in intracellular calcium. This, in turn, then mediates the rise in the basal tone of the vascular wall and also enhances the response of the vascular smooth muscle cell to vasoconstrictor hormones. Decreased baroreceptor reflex sensitivity in the presence of increased central blood volume (VATNER et al. 1975) and vasoconstriction resulting from enhanced vascular sensitivity to vasoconstrictor hormones will then result in a rise in systemic arterial pressure (KRAMER 1988a).

If disturbed renal volume homeostasis with increased extracellular fluid and central blood volume is a major determinant of hypertension, especially in so-called salt-sensitive hypertensive subjects (FUJITA et al. 1980), then diuretics may have a compensatory action on the kidney by directly promoting diuresis and natriuresis. Thereby, they create a state of slightly negative sodium balance.

Antihypertensive treatment with diuretics is know to exert a relatively acute as well as a more slowly developing blood pressure lowering effect. In the *early phase* (Table 4) systolic and diastolic blood pressure decrease in response to the reduction in plasma volume and cardiac output despite a temporary activation of catecholamines, the renin-angiotensin system, and other vasoconstrictor and sodium-retaining hormones, and is associated with a rise in total peripheral vascular resistance. With continuous administration of the diuretic, plasma volume and cardiac output return to normal whereas blood pressure remains low or even continues to decrease further. This *second phase* of the blood pressure lowering effect of diuretics reflects their indirect or direct vascular action (KRAMER 1985) (Table 4). In this regard, animal experiments have shown that diuretics reduce the vascular responsiveness to noradrenaline (ZSOTER et al. 1970) and angiotensin II (WEINBERGER et al. 1972). In addition, in hypertensive patients it was shown that long-term administration of diuretics desensitizes the vasculature in its response to endogenous vasoconstrictor hormones. In the presence of diuretics significantly higher doses of noradrenaline were necessary to increase blood pressure to the same degree than were needed before diuretic treatment (WEIDMANN et al. 1981). This reduction in the vascular response to vasoconstrictor hormones such as noradrenaline, angiotensin II, and vasopressin may be related to a decrease in intracellular sodium concentration. In fact, diuretics were found to reduce red blood cell sodium to normal levels in parallel with their antihypertensive effect in patients with essential hypertension (GESSLER 1962). Finally, diuretic-induced vascular secretion of endogenous vasodilators, especially of prostacyclin, PGE_2, and also of kinins (see below), may contribute to the blood pressure lowering effect of diuretics (Table 4). Along these lines, we have previously shown that furosemide, hydrochlorothiazide, and spironolactone stimulate the renal excretion of PGE_2 (KRAMER et al. 1980), a natriuretic and vasodilating eicosanoid. The stimulation of prostacyclin, the most potent vasodilating eicosanoid of vascular origin, by furosemide has been discussed in the previous section. The mechanism by which loop diuretics stimulate prosta-

Table 4. Antihypertensive mechanisms of diuretics

Early phase:	Sodium and volume depletion Decrease in extracellular fluid volume (ECFV) Decrease in blood volume Decrease in cardiac output (CO) Decreased secretion of membrane transport inhibitors
Late phase:	Decrease in vascular resistance Decrease in intracellular sodium concentration Reduced vascular response to vasoconstrictors (AII, NA, AVP) Increased secretion of vasodilators (PG, kinins) Normalisation of ECFV, CO, and baroreceptor sensitivity

AII, angiotensin II; NA, noradrenaline; AVP, arginine-vasopressin; PG, prostaglandin.

glandin metabolism has not yet been completely elucidated. Decreased degradation of prostaglandins in the presence of loop diuretics was suggested by in vitro studies which showed that furosemide inhibits 15-OH-PG-dehydrogenase (PAULSRUD and MILLER 1974) and 9-keto-reductase (STONE and HART 1976). On the other hand, in vivo (WEBER et al. 1977) and in vitro-ex vivo-studies (KATAYAMA et al. 1984) have shown that furosemide might stimulate the release of arachidonic acid by activation of phospholipase. Interestingly, FUJITA et al. (1980) have shown that salt-sensitive hypertensive patients respond to diuretic treatment with a rise in urinary PGE_2 excretion, whereas the prostaglandin system of salt-insensitive patients is unresponsive to diuretic treatment.

Increasing evidence suggests an intimate link between the renal kinin and prostaglandin systems, both agents causing renal vasodilation, diuresis and natriuresis when infused into the renal artery. Some effects ascribed to the renal kinin system may be mediated by intrarenal prostaglandins (MCGIFF et al. 1975), since kinins activate phospholipase A_2 (ANTONELLO et al. 1978) and prostaglandin synthesis (BLUMBERG et al. 1977). Similar to prostaglandins, infusions of kinins increase total renal blood flow with a predominant increase in deep cortical and medullary flow (STEIN et al. 1971).

With the exception of spironolactone, diuretics such as furosemide were reported to increase kallikrein release from the kidney associated with a reduction in renal kallikrein activity (JOHNSTON et al. 1976). HALUSHKA et al. (1979), however, were unable to demonstrate a rise in urinary kallikrein excretion after an oral dose of 40 mg furosemide in healthy female volunteers or patients with mild essential hypertension. Thus, results concerning baseline kallikrein excretion in hypertensive patients as well as the effect of diuretics on urinary kallikrein excretion are controversial and inconclusive. Diuretic-induced urinary kallikrein excretion may represent a non-specific effect such as tubular wash-out with increased urinary flow or, more likely, may be related to altered renin and/or circulating aldosterone activity (KRAMER 1979/80). Thus, furosemide increases the urinary kallikrein excretion parallel to the rise in plasma renin activity (ABE et al. 1978; JOHNSTON et al. 1976). In contrast, spironolactone was shown to suppress kallikrein release from renal cortical cells in vitro (KAIZU and

MARGOLIUS 1975), to prevent the rise in urinary kallikrein excretion during a low salt diet, and to abolish increased enzyme excretion in patients with primary aldosteronism (MARGOLIUS et al. 1974).

Despite the equivocal results concerning the role of the kinin system in the pathogenesis of hypertension, it remains possible that the vascular effects of diuretics may partly be due to stimulation of the potent vasodilating kinin and prostaglandin systems.

3.2 Pharmacokinetics and Metabolism of Diuretics

3.2.1 Intestinal Absorption

Bioavailability of orally administered diuretics is essentially dependent on the degree of intestinal absorption, but in some instances also on subsequent biotransformation of a pro-drug into its active metabolite. Most diuretics are extensively absorbed in the gastrointestinal tract, but in some instances the rate of absorption is slow, e.g. that of chlorthalidone. Absorption by the intestinal wall greatly depends on the lipid solubility of the individual diuretics. Thus, chlorothiazide reveals a relatively smaller intestinal absorption than hydrochlorothiazide and chlorthalidone. These latter drugs, like furosemide and amiloride, show a degree of absorption in the range between 50% and 70%. Spironolactone is 70% absorbed from the intestinal tract, whereas most other diuretics are more than 80% or even 90% absorbed (Table 5). A decrease in absorption may occur by interference with other drugs, e.g., furosemide in the presence of phenylhydantoin (FINE et al. 1977), or in the presence of food intake, as with amiloride (SCHMID and FRICKE 1969).

3.2.2 Protein-Binding

Protein binding of diuretics also depends on their lipid solubility since lipophilic drugs are bound to plasma proteins to a greater extent than hydrophilic drugs. Thus, chlorothiazide, etozolin, amiloride, and triamterene are bound to plasma proteins to a degree between 35% and 50%. Hydrochlorothiazide, chlorthalidone, indapamide, and furosemide show protein binding between 65% and 80%, whereas the remaining diuretics are bound to proteins by more than 90% (Table 5). In some instances diuretics may be bound to a large degree to blood cell membranes, e.g., chlorthalidone to human red blood cells (DIETERLE et al. 1976).

3.2.3 Lipid Solubility and Distribution

Lipid solubility and the distribution coefficient depend on the pK_a values of the individual diuretics (Table 5). Diuretics with a pK_a greater than 7.4 are quite lipid soluble and therefore are distributed to a large degree in tissue compartments. Thus, the individual diuretic potency and duration of action clearly depend on lipid solubility and the distribution coefficient (see Table 3). They determine extracellular distribution and accumulation also in renal tissue, specifically in the renal cortex, outer medulla, and papilla.

Table 5. Bioavailability, protein binding, pk_a, and plasma elimination half-life of diuretics

	Bioavailability (%)	Protein binding (%)	pk_a	Plasma elimination half-life (h)
Acetazolamide		92	7.4	4
Chlorothiazide	25–40	45	6.7	1
Hydrochlorothiazide	50–70	65	8.8	5
Chlorthalidone	64	76		24–50
Indapamide	94	79	8.3	18–24
Furosemide	50–65	98	3.80	1
Bumetanide	95	95	3.60	1–1.5
Piretanide	90	90	4.10	1–1.5
Etozolin (Ozolinone)	>90	35		7–10
Ethacrynic acid		95	3.50	
Amiloride	50	>50		6–9
Triamterene	>80	50		4
Spironolactone (canrenone)	70 (25)	98		10–35

3.2.4 Metabolism and Biotransformation

Acetazolamide (MAREN 1969), chlorothiazide (BRETTELL et al. 1960), and hydrochlorothiazide (BEERMANN et al. 1976) undergo little endogenous metabolism, and chlorthalidone is more than 85% excreted as the unchanged molecule (BEERMANN et al. 1975). On the other hand, indapamide is extensively metabolized so that only 4% of the unchanged substance appears in the urine (CAMPBELL and PHILLIPS 1974).

Furosemide is metabolized mainly to its glucuronide ester and less than 1% to 4-chloro-5-sulfamoyl-anthranylic acid (SÖRGEL et al. 1979). Bumetanide is excreted 60% as unaltered substance (PENTIKAINEN et al. 1977). As a pro-drug etozolin undergoes extensive metabolism to the two optical isomers of ozolinone (VON HODENBERG et al. 1977), of which only the (-) enantiomer possesses diuretic activity (GREVEN et al. 1980). Ethacrynic acid is approximately 50% excreted as cysteine metabolites (BEYER et al. 1965; KLAASSEN and FITZGERALD 1974).

Amiloride is not subjected to endogenous metabolism (WEISS et al. 1969), whereas triamterene, after its intestinal absorption, is rapidly and extensively metabolised to *p*-hydroxytriamterene and *p*-hydroxytriamterene sulfate ester (LEHMANN 1965), which are at least as potent as the parent compound (GREBIAN et al. 1978; KRAMER et al. 1981). Triamterene is excreted as *p*-hydroxytriamterene sulfate (LEHMANN 1965). As mentioned earlier, the aldosterone antagonist spironolactone undergoes extensive metabolism to result in canrenone as its active metabolite which is excreted more than 99% as the glucuronide (SADÉE et al. 1972).

3.2.5 Elimination

Many diuretics are eliminated via the biliary tract and thereby may undergo enterohepatic recirculation. Biliary excretion of these compounds will increase with decreasing renal excretory function (BAER et al. 1959). Chlorothiazide (BAER et al. 1959), hydrochlorothiazide (BEERMANN et al. 1976), and ethacrynic acid were shown to be excreted via the biliary tract at rates of 20% (HART and SCHANKER 1966), up to 9% (PRATT and AIKAWA 1962), and up to more than 40% (KLAASSEN and FITZGERALD 1974), respectively, whereas the biliary excretion of furosemide is negligible (HÄUSSLER and HAJDU 1964).

Renal excretion of diuretics results essentially from proximal tubular secretion as glomerular filtration is negligible because of the extensive protein binding of most diuretics. All thiazides and thiazide-like sulfonamides and other diuretics (BEYER and BAER 1961; BEYER et al. 1965; GAYER 1965) except for canrenone, are actively secreted by the organic anion pump in the proximal tubule. Acidic diuretics will be secreted into the tubular luminal fluid to a much greater degree than basic diuretics. Lipid solubility will also determine the rate of diffusion into the tubular lumen. In addition, high lipid solubility will result in reabsorption and intrarenal accumulation, thereby delaying renal excretion of individual diuretics.

The elimination half-life in most instances determines the duration of action of a diuretic. Thus, furosemide and other loop diuretics, which have the shortest elimination half-life since they are rapidly excreted, also have the shortest duration of action. In contrast, it is well-known that for the same reasons chlorthalidone and canrenone exhibit the longest duration of action of all diuretics, due to their extremely long elimination half-life (Table 5).

3.2.6 Onset, Peak, and Duration of Action of Diuretics

After oral administration the onset of action of diuretics depends on (a) the rate of intestinal absorption, (b) the time to reach the target site at a sufficient concentration, and in some instances, (c) the rate of biotransformation into the active metabolite. The most rapid onset of action is exhibited by the loop diuretics furosemide, bumetanide, piretanide, and ethacrynic acid. Their diuretic and natriuretic effects appear within 0.5–1 h after oral administration. The onset of action of the thiazides, thiazide-like sulfonamides, etozolin, and the potassium-sparing diuretics amiloride and triamterene extends from approximately 1 to 3 h after oral administration. Only spironolactone, a specific aldosterone antagonist, exhibits a delayed onset of action of 24–48 h after oral administration, which may be related to the hormonal action of aldosterone and the associated receptor protein metabolism (FANESTIL and KIPNOWSKI 1982) as well as to the biotransformation of spironolactone to canrenone (SADEE et al. 1972) (Table 6).

The peak of diuretic and natriuretic activities of the various diuretics parallels their onset of action, i.e., 1–2 h for most of the loop diuretics, 2–8 h for most of the remaining diuretics except for a possibly later peak of action for chlorthalidone and for spironolactone (Table 6).

The shortest duration of action is exhibited by the classic loop diuretics,

Table 6. Comparative time course of action of diuretic drugs after oral administration (h)

Drug	Onset	Peak	Duration
Acetazolamide	1–2	2–4	8–12
Chlorothiazide	1–2	4–6	6–12
Hydrochlorothiazide	1–2	4–6	6–18
Chlorthalidone	2–3	4–24	48–72
Indapamide	3	4–6	36
Furosemide	0.5–1	1–2	4–8
Bumetanide	0.5–1	1–2	4–6
Piretanide	0.5–1	1–2	4–8
Etozolin	0.5–1	1–2	4–8
Ethacrynic acid	2	4–8	12–18
Amiloride	1–2	4–8	12–24
Triamterene	1–2	2–8	12–24
Spironolactone	24–48	48–72	72–96

whereas most of the other diuretics exhibit a duration of action between 6 and 12–24 h, again with the exception of chlorthalidone and spironolactone which exhibit the longest duration of action of 48–96 h (Table 6). This duration of action of the individual diuretics depends on their pharmocokinetic properties, especially on their elimination half-life (see Sect. 3.2.5), which is shortest for loop diuretics. This, in turn, also depends on their lipid solubility and pK_a values, which mainly determine their distribution volume (Table 5). All diuretics with a pK_a greater than 7.0 have a longer duration of action than those with pK_a less than 7.0 (MENG and O'DEA 1973). Diuretics with a higher pK_a reveal a higher nonionic diffusion, e.g., tubular reabsorption and an intrarenal recirculation. Loop diuretics such as furosemide and ethacrynic acid thus show small back-diffusion at physiological pH and are therefore rapidly excreted (see below) (DEETJEN 1966).

4 Therapeutic Use of Diuretics in Hypertension

4.1 Dosage

The average daily dose ranges of the most representative diuretics, when administered orally, are summarized in Table 7. As a general rule, the lowest effective dose of diuretics should be employed to avoid unwanted side effects. Thereby clinically relevant hypokalemia with its consequences of metabolic alkalosis and decreased glucose tolerance, hypomagnesemia, hyponatremia, hyperuricemia, and hyperlipidemia as well as orthostatic hypotension can be

Table 7. Oral dosages of representative diuretics

Diuretic	Dose/day (mg)
Thiazides	
Chlorothiazide	250–2000
Hydrochlorothiazide	12.5–100
Thiazide-like sulfonamides	
Chlorthalidone	25–100
Indapamide	50–150
Loop diuretics	
Furosemide	20–500
Bumetanide	0.5–2
Piretanide	3–18
Etozolin	400–800
Ethacrynic acid	50–400
Potassium-sparing diuretics	
Amiloride	2.5–20
Triamterene	25–100
Spironolactone	25–200

avoided in most cases. Elderly patients, who often have pre-existing extracellular fluid volume contraction leading to a decrease in cardiac output, decreased vascular responsiveness, increased peripheral vascular resistance, decreased baroreceptor function, and altered autoregulation of cerebral blood flow are especially susceptible to hypotensive episodes potentially leading to reduced organ perfusion and organ damage, e.g., myocardial infarction, stroke, and renal failure. It is therefore recommended to titrate the dose of diuretics starting with a low dose, e.g., 12.5 mg hydrochlorothiazide per day. Doses at the upper limit of the dose range should be avoided for the above reasons. If blood pressure is not well controlled, combination therapy with other antihypertensive drugs of different mechanisms of action should be initiated (see Sect. 4.3). However, decreased renal function may at times requires the administration of high doses of, for example, loop diuretics (see Sect. 4.2.2).

4.2 Differential Therapy with Diuretics for Hypertension

4.2.1 Diuretics in Patients with Normal Renal Function

In principal, all diuretics may be used for antihypertensive treatment, i.e., thiazides, thiazide-like sulfonamides, loop diuretics, and also potassium-sparing diuretics.

Thiazides, because of their longer duration of action, may have a greater blood pressure lowering effect in patients with mild to moderate hypertension than do loop diuretics. But because of their larger total sodium excretion per 24 h at least within the first period of treatment, they may cause a larger fall in serum potassium concentration. In elderly patients with normal renal function, thiazides or thiazide-like sulfonaides may be preferred because of their somewhat slower onset of action as compared with loop diuretics, since these elderly patients are often sensitive to changes in body fluid volume, i.e fluid volume contraction which may already be present.

Thiazides and thiazide-like sulfonamides may be used preferentially in hypertensive patients who have hypercalciuria or are renal stone formers. This group of diuretics decreases urinary calcium concentration (see below) because of enhanced distal as well as proximal tubular calcium reabsorption associated with thiazide-induced natriuresis. There will also be a tendency to acid urine in the presence of thiazides because of enhanced distal hydrogen ion secretion at least as long as no major blood alkalosis occurs. Finally, their protective effect against renal stone formation may be related to the rise in urinary magnesium excretion, since magnesium has an antilithogenic action (see Sects. 4.4.1.3 and 4.4.1.4).

Loop diuretics are more effective than thiazides in patients with advanced stages of hypertension and kidney involvement, especially when the serum creatinine concentration ranges above 2 mg per 100 ml, i.e., endogenous creatinine clearance is below 30 ml/min. Loop diuretics in these patients may also maintain renal blood flow and glomerular filtration rate in contrast to thiazides, which reveal a tendency to decrease the glomerular filtration rate in the presence of volume contraction. Loop diuretics are also helpful in severe hypertension when treatment with angiotensin converting enzyme (ACE) inhibitors is indicated. ACE inhibitors in these situations will eliminate the consequence of secondary hyperaldosteronism, usually associated with the administration of short-acting loop diuretics. Furosemide or other loop diuretics may also be used as adjuvant therapy in patients with hypertensive crisis.

Spironolactone has been used as single-drug therapy in essential hypertension but has its special indication in patients with primary aldosteronism. Amiloride and triamterene may be used as well in this latter condition, but their greatest usefulness is in combination with conventional diuretics to avoid urinary potassium loss (DÜSING and KRAMER 1977; KRAMER 1987).

4.2.2 Diuretics in Patients with Impaired Renal Function

Diuretics which are predominantly eliminated via renal excretion may accumulate with decreasing renal function. Therefore, on the one hand, their dose or dose interval should be adapted to renal excretory function. On the other hand, with a decreasing number of functional nephrons, proximal tubular secretion of diuretics will be lower than normal. Higher doses of, for example, furosemide are then necessary to reach sufficiently high intratubular concentrations for adequate inhibition of tubular sodium reabsorption. A significant increase in the half-life of furosemide has been observed with advanced renal failure (HUANG et al. 1974).

Many diuretics are also excreted by the biliary tract. Increased biliary excretion will therefore compensate for decreased renal function and thereby avoid drug accumulation (BAER et al. 1959).

As already mentioned, thiazides and thiazide-like sulfonamides are not potent enough diuretics to induce a diuresis and natriuresis when the glomerular filtration rate has decreased to values below 20–30 ml/min. In patients with advanced renal failure, therefore, loop diuretics must be used to achieve an adequate diuresis and natriuresis resulting in a negative sodium balance.

Potassium-sparing diuretics must not be administered to patients with serum creatinine concentrations above 1.5–2 mg/100 ml, sine in these patients distal tubular potassium secretion is the major pathway to eliminate excess potassium from the body (GONICK et al. 1971). Inhibition of this secretory process may cause life-threatening hyperkalemia. Triamterene represents a special problem in advanced renal failure. Triamterene is rapidly and largely converted into its phase-I-metabolite *p*-hydroxytriamterene, which is as active as the parent drug. Triamterene is mainly excreted as *p*-hydroxytriamterene sulphuric acid ester (LEHMANN 1965), a unique phase-II-metabolite. This metabolite still possesses a strong antikaliuretic activity. It is excreted via the kidney and therefore will accumulate with decreasing renal function.

4.2.3 Resistance to Diuretics

It is well-known that the continuous administration of acetazolamide results in a progressive metabolic acidosis. With the development of acidosis the diuretic and natriuretic effect of acetazolamide ceases, thus inducing a resistance to the diuretic.

With increasing contraction of extracellular and plasma fluid volume and the resulting effects on renal hemodynamics, diuretics acting at the ascending limb of Henle's loop or at more distal segments may become ineffective. This is because enhanced proximal tubular reabsorption may result in the delivery of insufficient fluid, sodium, and chloride to the distal tubule under these circumstances.

In this situation, even high doses of the very powerful loop diuretic furosemide may be ineffective. Under such circumstances administration of ethacrynic acid may still be effective in inducing sufficient diuresis and natriuresis. Metolazone may also be effective in these situations as it might have an additional effect on proximal tubular reabsorption (PUSCHETT and RASTEGAR 1974). In addition, a combination of a loop diuretic with acetazolamide might be helpful in the diuretic resistant state.

4.3 Use of Diuretics in Combination with Other Antihypertensive Drugs

Because of the well-known multifactorial pathogenesis of primary hypertension, normalization of blood pressure in hypertensive patients by a single antihypertensive drug can be achieved in only approximately 50% of unselected patients. Therefore, the step-wise and combined use of antihypertensive agents is generally recommended.

Approximately 40% of hypertensive patients can be identified as being salt-sensitive (FUJITA et al. 1980), whereas the remainder appears to be salt-insensitive. The former group therefore can be expected to respond to diuretic treatment much better than the latter. If blood pressure cannot be normalized at low or medium doses of diuretics, combined therapy with other antihypertensive agents of a different mechanism of action should be initiated at an early stage. Thus, the combination of a diuretic with a β-receptor blocking agent will increase the responder rate to more than 80% as compared with 40%–50% when treated with a diuretic alone. (Noncardio-selective β-blockers will also blunt the rise in PRA induced by diuretics.) This responder rate will further increase to approximately 95% when the diuretic is combined with a β-receptor blocking agent and a vasodilator agent. The most common combination with vasodilators is that of a diuretic, a β-blocking agent, and hydralazine or dihydralazine. The use of direct vasodilators such as hydralazine, dihydralazine, or minoxidil requires the simultaneous administration of a diuretic to avoid tachyphylaxia due to fluid retention, which is associated with the administration of all direct vasodilators.

Diuretics may be combined with all other types of antihypertensive agents, such as pre- and postsynaptic α-blockers, centrally acting sympatholytics, calcium channel blockers, and ACE inhibitors. The advantages of such a combination therapy consists not only in the avoidance of drug-induced side effects because of the low-dose efficacy of each component drug but also in the potentiation of the action of nondiuretic antihypertensive agents by the simultaneous use of diuretics. This is especially true for ACE inhibitors in the presence of loop diuretics.

Fixed combinations of individual drugs from the above-mentioned groups of antihypertensive agents have the advantage of greater compliance by the patient because of the reduced number of tablets to be administered daily but may be associated with some hazard since the treating physician may not always be aware of the action of single compounds of such a combination therapy, e.g., administration of a combination containing a β-receptor blocking agent to a patient with obstructive lung disease.

4.4 Side Effects of Diuretics

Diuretic-induced side effects include electrolyte disturbances, metabolic alterations, and unwanted hemodynamic effects. Rarely they may cause allergic, toxic, or other adverse reactions.

Electrolyte disturbances
- Hypokalemia (+ hypochloremic alkalosis)
- Hypomagnesemia
- Hypercalciuria (loop diuretics)
- Hypocalciuria (thiazides)
- Hyponatremia

Metabolic disturbances
- Hyperuricemia
- Glucose intolerance
- Plasma lipid changes

Hemodynamic disturbances
Orthostatic hypotension
Decreased renal perfusion (prerenal azotemia)
Others
Ototoxicity (loop diuretics)
Urolithiasis (triamterene)

4.4.1 Electrolyte Disturbances

4.4.1.1 Diuretic-Induced Hypokalemia

Hypokalemia represents the most often encountered electrolyte disturbance associated with diuretic treatment. The kidney is the most important organ in maintaining normal potassium balance (JAMISON et al. 1982). Urinary potassium excretion is mainly determined by potassium balance, aldosterone secretion rate, acid base status, and sodium balance. Thus, secretion of potassium in the distal convoluted tubule is determined by intracellular potassium concentration, the amount of sodium within the tubular lumen reaching the distal convoluted tubule, and the urinary flow rate. Since aldosterone increases the intracellular potassium concentration via the active Na/K pump at the basolateral membrane and also modifies the Na channel at the luminal membrane of the distal convoluted tubular cell (FANESTIL and KIPNOWSKI 1982), this hormone modifies distal tubular potassium secretion. Therefore, any diuretic which increases the delivery of sodium out of the ascending limb of Henle's loop and increases urinary flow rate within this tubular segment will cause significant potassium secretion. In other words, the more effective a diuretic drug is in increasing sodium excretion, the greater the degree of potassium excretion in the urine (PUSCHETT and RASTEGAR 1974) (Fig. 8). Loop diuretics, such as furosemide, which act throughout the ascending limb of Henle's loop are more powerful diuretics than thiazides, which only act in the cortical diluting segment. However, the total loss of sodium over a 24-h period after injection of furosemide is significantly smaller than that observed after a single dose of thiazide. This relates to the short duration of action of loop diuretics in contrast to the longer duration of action of the thiazides. In addition to this direct effect of diuretics on potassium secretion via the increase in sodium and fluid delivery to the distal convoluted tubule, the loss of volume will stimulate renin secretion, thereby causing secondary hyperaldosteronism which then provokes an additional kaliuresis by facilitating distal tubular potassium and hydrogen ion secretion in exchange for sodium reabsorption. Extracellular fluid volume depletion also causes enhanced proximal bicarbonate reabsorption. This, in addition to the distal loss of hydrogen ions as titratable acid and ammonium, will result in metabolic alkalosis. Subsequently, the increased delivery of poorly reabsorbable bicarbonate to the distal tubule will further accelerate potassium and hydrogen secretion in this nephron segment. (GIEBISCH 1981). Hypokalemia, hypochloremia, and metabolic alkalosis, therefore, are the well-known consequences of long-term diuretic treatment (Fig. 9). Depending on the type of diuretic and on the dose administered the incidence of serum potassium concentrations below

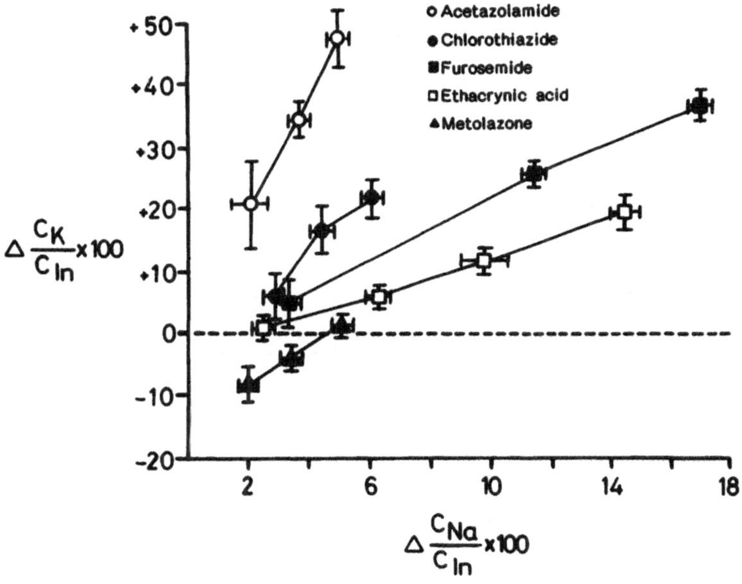

Fig. 8. Relationship of fractional potassium excretion to fractional sodium excretion in the presence of some representative diuretics (PUSCHETT and RASTEGAR 1974)

3.5 mmol/l has been found to range between 2% and 11% (Table 8) but may go up to more than 25%, as reported by others. The lowest incidence is observed with lowest doses of the diuretic (LIGHT et al. 1983). Hypokalemia in risk patients with normal renal function can be prevented most effectively by combination with a potassium-sparing diuretic (KRAMER 1987).

During long-term diuretic therapy an initial decrease in total body potassium of 5%–10% may be observed, whereas at later stages no significant changes in total body potassium can be detected (WILKINSON et al. 1975) (Table 9).

With regard to the intracellular potassium concentration, controversal results were reported. In red and white blood cells normal or reduced potassium concentrations were observed (Table 9). In our patients a decrease in intracellular potassium of leucocytes was found only with severe hypokalemia of less than 3.2 mmol/l (SCHLEBUSCH et al. 1983). In skeletal muscle cells normal, reduced, or even increased potassium concentrations were observed with diuretic treatment (Table 9).

4.4.1.2 Effects of Potassium Balance on Blood Pressure

In hypertensive patients potassium depletion may have pressor as well as depressor effects. Pressor effects may relate to direct vasoconstriction due to potassium depletion, causing sodium retention with an increased intracellular sodium content, stimulation of plasma renin activity, and rise in the number of angiotensin II receptors. The vasodepressor effect of potassium depletion may be related to a decrease in aldosterone and vasopressin secretion and a decreased affinity of angiotensin II receptors (KAPLAN 1985) possibly due to an increased receptor occupancy. The blunted response to angiotensin II may also

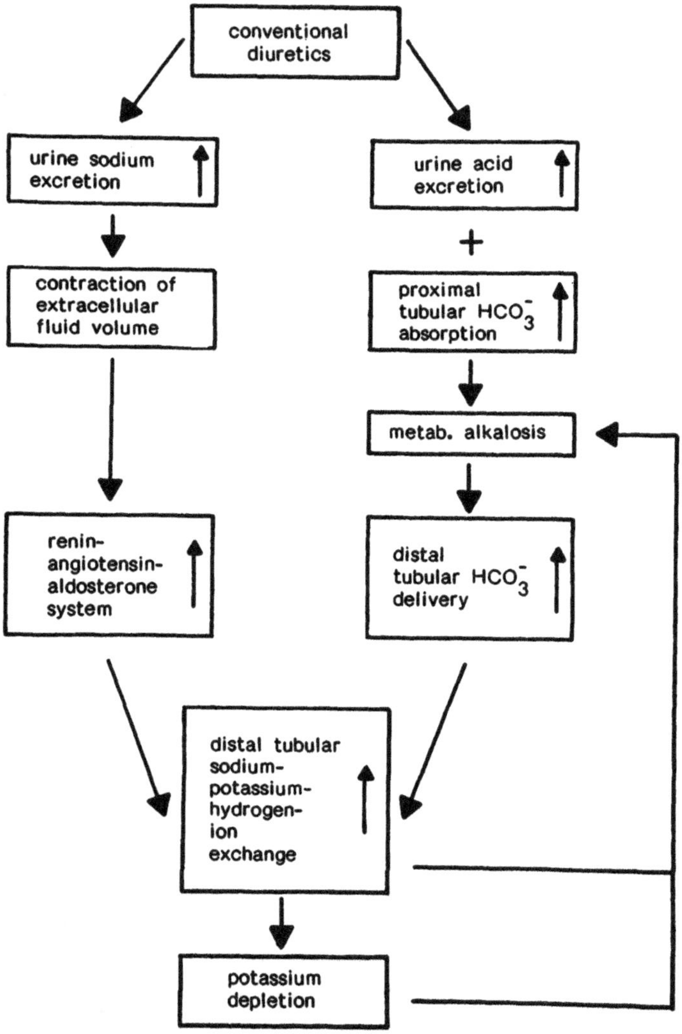

Fig. 9. Schematic presentation of mechanisms leading to diuretic-induced potassium depletion (modified according to GIEBISCH 1981)

be due to the enhanced prostaglandin synthesis in response to potassium depletion (DÜSING et al. 1980). Finally, potassium itself may have a blood pressure lowering effect by acutely increasing sodium excretion, suppressing renin secretion, decreasing sympathetic activity, and enhancing baroreceptor sensitivity. Thus, potassium supplementation has been shown to blunt the rise in blood pressure during a sodium chloride load, to decrease blood pressure in patients with diuretic-induced hypokalemia, to suppress sympathetic activity induced by sodium restriction or administration of diuretics (KAPLAN 1985), and to enhance baroreceptor sensitivity (GLÄNZER et al. 1983; for review see also TOBIAN 1989).

Table 8. Incidence of hypokalemia (serum potassium < 3.5 mmol/l) as related to the dose of diuretics during antihypertensive treatment. LIGHT et al. (1983)

Diuretic	Dose (mg/day)	Incidence (%)	No. of patients
Hydrochlorothiazide	50	11.0	500
Chlorthalidone	25	8.1	37
Furosemide	40	3.5	284
Hydrochlorothiazide	25	2.2	183

LIGHT et al. (1983)

4.4.1.3 Hypokalemia as a Risk Factor in Hypertension

The extra-/intracellular potassium concentration gradient, which determines the cardiac membrane action potential, is altered to a much greater degree by changes in extracellular potassium concentration than by intracellular changes. Electrocardiographic changes in hypokalemic patients include prolongation of the PR and QT intervals, ST-T wave abnormalities and the occurrence of U-waves. Most concern relates to the fact that hypokalemia in hypertensive patients treated with diuretics may be associated with an increased incidence of cardiac arrhythmias and sudden death. Patients with baseline electrocardiographic abnormalities, a preexisting abnormal rhythm, left ventricular hypertrophy, cardiac failure, preexisting coronary artery disease, acute myocardial infarction, or those on digitalis therapy are more susceptible to life-threatening arrhythmias or sudden death due to hypokalemia than are healthy subjects (LIEF et al. 1984).

There is a significantly higher percentage of these events in patients with serum potassium levels below 3.5 mmol/l or an even higher risk when potassium levels are below 3.1 mmol/1 than in patients with potassium levels above 3.5

Table 9. Effects of diuretics on potassium balance in healthy subjects and in patients with hypertension

Total body potassium		
normal	GRAYBIEL and SODE	1971
	DARGIE et al.	1974
	WILKINSON et al.	1975
	LEEMHUIS et al.	1976
Skeletal muscle		
increased	VILLAMIL et al.	1963
reduced	BERGSTRÖM and HULTMAN	1966
normal	BEVEGARD et al.	1977
	DYCKNER and WESTER	1978
Leucocyte		
reduced		
normal	DONALDSON et al.	1976
	EDMONDSON et al.	1974

mmol/l (see Weinberger 1988). Severe hypokalemia is often accompanied by loss of magnesium which may not only strongly contribute to the risk of cardiac arrhythmias and sudden death, but magnesium repletion in addition to potassium replacement may be required to reverse hypokalemia and/or its associated cardiac risks (see Sect. 4.4.1.3). Some forms of hypertension, cardiac failure, and myocardial infarction are associated with high plasma catecholamine levels, and diuretics may additionally increase catecholamine release; this may produce a shift of potassium out of the extracellular space and thereby alter the cardiac action potential. In patients with normal renal function, the risk of ventricular ectopic activity can be prevented by the combination of thiazides or thiazide-like diuretics with potassium-sparing diuretics (Holland et al. 1988).

4.4.1.4 Diuretic-Induced Magnesium Loss

Since 60% of filtered magnesium is reabsorbed in the ascending limb of Henle's loop (Quamme and Dirks 1980), loop diuretics and thiazides increase urinary magnesium excretion (Abdelhamid et al. 1969) and may reduce body magnesium content in patients receiving long-term treatment (Sheehan and White 1982). The incidence of hypomagnesemia during treatment with these diuretics may be less than 10% (Laake et al. 1978). Normal or decreased magnesium content was observed in muscle cells. Magnesium depletion, which often accompanies diuretic-induced hypokalemia, may induce cardiac arrhythmias such as "torsades de pointes" in patients with coronary artery and/or myocardial disease, especially in those on digitalis therapy (fish 1973). Prevention or correction of hypomagnesemia is therefore needed in these patients. This can be achieved with potassium-sparing diuretics which do not enhance magnesium excretion (Abdelhamid et al. 1969) (Fig. 10).

4.4.1.5 Effects of Diuretics on Serum Calcium Concentration

Loop diuretics such as furosemide increase urinary calcium excretion (Suki et al. 1970) but in general do not lead to hypocalcemia. In contrast, thiazide diuretics reduce urinary calcium excretion (Yendt and Cohanim 1978), possibly due to enhanced calcium reabsorption in the distal tubule (Costanzo and Windhager 1978) and also to enhanced calcium absorption in the proximal tubule as a consequence of volume contraction (Brickman et al. 1972). Hypercalcemia will occur only exceptionally and may then suggest the presence of primary hyperparathyroidism (Balizit 1973).

4.4.1.6 Diuretic-Induced Hyponatremia

Hyponatremia is seldom encountered in hypertensive patients treated with diuretics in the absence of cardiac or hepatic failure or a nephrotic syndrome. In elderly patients, however, diuretic-induced hyponatremia has been observed repeatedly (Ashouri 1986). In some of these patients hyponatremia may persist despite cessation of the diuretic treatment because of a resetting of central osmoreceptors (Ghose 1977). Volume contraction as a nonosmotic stimulus for

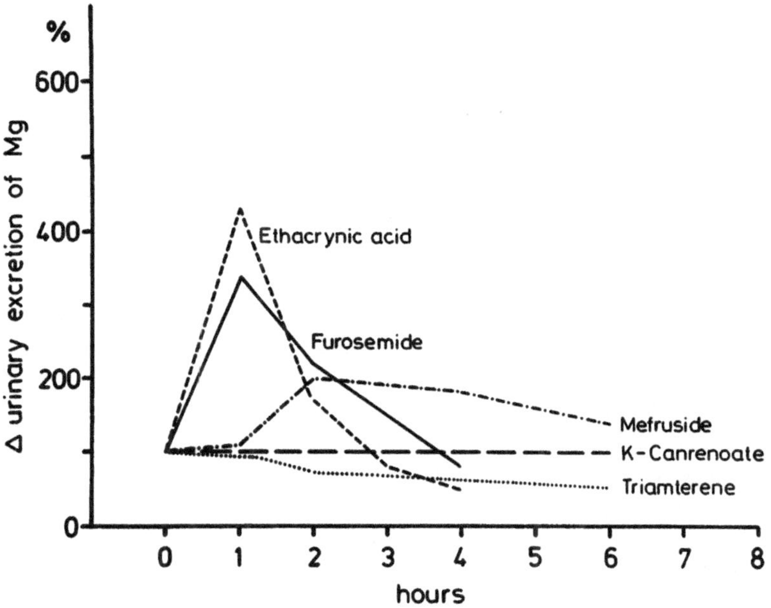

Fig. 10. Renal magnesium excretion after a single oral dose of mefruside, furosemide, ethacrynic acid, and triamterene as well as after a single intravenous dose of K-canrenoate (ABDELHAMID et al. 1969)

excessive vasopressin secretion may contribute to this hyponatremia, which can also be observed in other clinical states associated with decreased effective plasma volume.

4.4.2 Metabolic Side-Effects

4.4.2.1 Hyperuricemia

An increase in plasma uric acid concentration may be observed in up to 30% of hypertensive patients treated with diuretics, but in a significantly smaller percentage of patients plasma concentration of uric acid rises above 7.0 mg/100 ml. Rarely, the level of uric acid will reach values high enough to represent a risk for gouty attacks, which are actually uncommon in diuretic-treated hypertensive patients without a previous history of gout. Two mechanisms may be responsible for the diuretic-induced rise in plasma uric acid concentration. First, uric acid is secreted in the proximal tubule by the organic anion pump. Therefore, diuretics as weak acids, which are also secreted via the organic anion pump, may compete with uric acid for this secretory process. This interaction between diuretics and uric acid for secretion into the tubular lumen may be of relatively minor importance since volume repletion in the presence of diuretics prevents the rise in plasma uric acid concentration. The second mechanism, therefore, i.e., diuretic-induced volume contraction with enhanced proximal tubular reabsorption including uric acid reabsorption, is probably the major factor responsible for diuretic-induced hyperuricemia (LANG et al. 1977).

4.4.2.2. Altered Glucose Metabolism

Impaired carbohydrate metabolism with a decrease in glucose tolerance and hyperglycemia is often observed in patients undergoing thiazide treatment for hypertension. Hypokalemia and the decrease in total body potassium have been incriminated as the major mechanism for this metabolic disturbance, since hypokalemia can be shown to result in a delayed insulin secretion. However, a direct effect of thiazides or thiazide-like sulfonamides upon insulin secretion or glucagon secretion by alpha-cells cannot be excluded (HOSKINS and JACKSON 1978). Whereas impaired carbohydrate metabolism is often observed during short-term diuretic treatment, equivocal observations have been made during long-term antihypertensive therapy with thiazide diuretics. Similar to total body potassium, which returns into the normal range with long-term diuretic treatment, glucose metabolism was found to be normal in hypertensive patients treated with thiazides or thiazide-like sulfonamides for more than 1 year. There may be differences between different types of diuretics in their effects on glucose metabolism since no evidence of glucose intolerance was found in patients treated with loop diuretics. This again may be related to the potassium balance, which may be less affected by short-acting diuretics.

4.4.2.3 Effects on Lipid Metabolism

Small and moderate but statistically significant increases in plasma concentrations of cholesterol, triglycerides, or low density lipoprotein cholesterol were reported in patients during long-term treatment with thiazides or thiazide-like sulfonamides (WEIDMANN et al. 1985). Most clinical trials have demonstrated that treatment of hypertension reduces total cardiovascular morbidity and/or mortality by prevention of stroke and congestive heart failure. In contrast, coronary events could not be reduced, although coronary disease is more common than stroke in mild hypertension. This points to additional causes of coronary artery disease which may not be adequately controlled by antihypertensive treatment with diuretics. In fact, treatment with thiazide diuretics but not with the indoline diuretic indapamide was generally found to be associated with a small rise in total cholesterol and significant rises in low (LDL-C) and very low (VLDL-C) density lipoprotein cholesterol without changes in high density lipoprotein cholesterol (HDL-C). Most of the studies concerned with lipid-related side effects of diuretics lasted less than 1 year and used relatively high doses of thiazides or thiazide-like diuretics. Although it appears that lipid alterations persist throughout diuretic treatment, it cannot be definitely decided therefore on the basis of these studies if this is correct and whether lower doses of diuretics may induce smaller alterations in lipid metabolism (see AMES 1988). Thus, taken together, neither the mechanisms underlying this metabolic impairment nor its clinical significance as a risk factor for ischemic heart disease can be exactly delineated at the present time. Combined treatment with a diuretic and a β-receptor blocking agent with intrinsic sympathetic activity was found to avoid changes in plasma lipid concentrations.

4.4.3 Hemodynamic Side-Effects

4.4.3.1 Orthostatic Hypotension

As a consequence of the decrease in extracellular fluid and plasma volume, orthostatic hypotension may be encountered in patients in whom initial high doses of diuretics have caused acute urinary fluid and sodium losses. Orthostatic hypotension due to acute volume contraction may be especially hazardous in elderly hypertensive patients who often have a reduced extracellular fluid and plasma volume and decreased vascular distensibility. Elderly hypertensive patients also may show resetting as well as decreased sensitivity of baroreceptor function. Since they are less able to counterregulate a sudden fall in blood pressure due to acute volume contraction, acute fluid losses may impair organ perfusion. Diuretic therapy in the elderly should therefore start with very small doses of a diuretic without abrupt onset of action, e.g., 12.5 mg hydrochlorothiazide.

4.4.3.2 Prerenal Azotemia

Prerenal azotemia also represents a hemodynamic consequence of extracellular fluid and plasma volume contraction which occurs especially during administration of thiazides. This happens less frequently in the presence of loop diuretics. Patients with advanced stages of hypertension and renal involvement or elderly patients with nephrosclerosis who still have normal serum creatinine concentrations may be more susceptible to volume contraction than younger patients without renal involvement. Serum creatinine concentration will rise above the normal upper range when the glomerular filtration rate decreases below 50% of normal. In hypertensive patients with renal involvement loop diuretics such as furosemide, bumetanide, or piretanide, which maintain renal blood flow and glomerular filtration rate even in the presence of moderate volume contraction by there action on the tubulo-glomerular feedback (see 3.1.3), may be more suitable than the administration of thiazide diuretics.

4.4.4 Other Side-Effects

4.4.4.1 Ototoxicity

The occurrence of ototoxicity, in the form of reversible loss of hearing, has repeatedly been reported in the past in patients with advanced chronic renal failure who received high doses of loop diuretics, e.g., furosemide (Heidland and Wigand 1970). Accumulation of furosemide and of some of its metabolites may inhibit extrarenal transport processes such as the one responsible for production of endolymph, thereby causing the reversible hearing loss. A more serious ototoxic effect may result from the simultaneous administration of furosemide or ethacrynic acid with aminoglycoside antibiotics (Mathog and Klein 1969). As shown by animal studies, loop diuretics may produce a reversible decrease in the cochlear microphonic potential and an irreversible hair cell damage at high doses (Brown et al. 1979).

4.4.4.2 Nephrolithiasis

In recent years, several reports (Ettinger et al. 1980) have shown that triamterene administration may be associated with formation of renal or urinary calculi, and tubular deposition of crystals has been observed. As stated earlier, *p*-hydroxytriamterene sulfate is the major urinary metabolite of triamterene. This phase-II metabolite was shown to have a very low solubility coefficient at urinary pH values between 5 and 7 (Werness et al. 1982).

Additional rare side effects of diuretics are:

Thiazides and thiazide-like sulfonamides
- Leukopenia, thrombocytopenia, pancytopenia, hemolytic anemia of newborns
- Exanthema, photosensitization
- Necrotizing vasculitis
- Gastrointestinal symptoms, acute hemorrhagic pancreatitis, hepatic coma in cirrhosis
- Acute pulmonary alterations
- Interstitial nephritis
- Antinuclear antibodies

Furosemide
- Loin pain
- Epidermolysis bullosa

Ethacrynic acid
- Gastrointestinal symptoms, bleeding, icterus
- Agranulocytosis
- Necrotizing hemorrhagic changes (legs), purpura

Spironolactone
- Hyperkalemia, hyperchloremia, acidosis
- Gastrointestinal symptoms
- Gynecomastia, galactorrhea, libido loss, impotence, amenorrhea
- Vertigo, headache, dizziness
- Maculopapular exanthema, skin pigmentation, alopecia
- Raynaud's symptoms

Amiloride, triamterene
- Hyperkalemia, hyperchloremic acidosis
- Gastrointestinal symptoms
- Headache
- Exanthema

4.5 Contraindications

Aside from a contraindication to the use of sulfonamide derivatives as antihypertensive diuretics in patients with known sulfonamide hypersensitivity, there are very few absolute contraindications for the administration of diuretics.

One such contraindication may pertain to the patient who is already volume-contracted. Potassium-sparing diuretics are definitely not indicated and may be hazardous in patients with reduced renal function and serum creatinine concentrations above 1.5 mg/100 ml. The reason for the development of potentially life-threatening hyperkalemia in these patients has been outlined above. Potential hazards for the development of hyperkalemia may result from combined therapy with ACE inhibitors and potassium-sparing diuretics. Such therapy may be necessary in an exceptional patient with persistent hypokalemia but should be performed under close supervision. (KRAMER 1988b).

4.6 Drug Interactions

With regard to diuretics, drug interactions may be divided into interactions by which diuretics alter the action of other drugs and those in which the efficacy of diuretics is altered in the presence of other drugs. In both situations the interactions can be of a pharmacokinetic or pharmacodynamic type, but the former is most often the case.

Diuertic-induced volume contraction results in an increased proximal tubular reabsorption of uric acid. Thus, diuretic treatment may partially blunt the efficacy of uricosuric agents. A similar mechanism underlies the reduced renal excretion of lithium in the presence of volume contraction (PETERSEN et al. 1974). Furthermore, diuretic-induced hypokalemia with its effect on glucose tolerance may decrease the efficacy of oral hypoglycemics. Furosemide and ethacrynic acid potentially enhance the ototoxic action of aminoglycosides (MATHOG and KLEIN 1969) mentioned earlier. Finally, diuretics may compete with other drugs, e.g., warfarin, for protein-binding and thereby enhance the anticoagulant action of this cumarol. The simultaneous administration of ACE inhibitors with potassium-sparing diuretics may result in hyperkalemia.

Intestinal reabsorption of diuretics may be reduced in the presence of cholestyramine (GALLO et al. 1965) or phenhydantoin (FINE et al. 1977) as in the case of reduced furosemide reabsorption. Clofibrate may competitively reduce protein binding of diuretics (KOCH-WESER, 1976); thus their potency of action may be enhanced, but the duration of action can be shortened. A major pharmacokinetic problem results from interference at the level of the organic anion pump within the proximal tubule. Thus, probenecid (BENET 1979) and nonsteroidal antiinflammatory drugs (CHENNAVASIN et al. 1980) which are also transported by this secretory process may inhibit the secretion of diuretics and thereby reduce the concentration in the luminal fluid reaching their target site.

Nonsteroidal antiinflammatory drugs are widely used, and therefore their interference with the action of diuretics is of practical importance. PATAK et al. (1975) first demonstrated in hypertensive patients that indomethacin blunts the antihypertensive and renin secretion-stimulating actions of furosemide. These observations have been confirmed in human and animal studies (BERG and LOEW 1977) (CHENNAVASIN et al. 1980; KRAMER et al. 1980; OLIW et al. 1978). Although the results of some studies were controversial, inhibition of prostaglandin synthesis by nonsteroidal antiinflammatory drugs such as acetylsalicylic

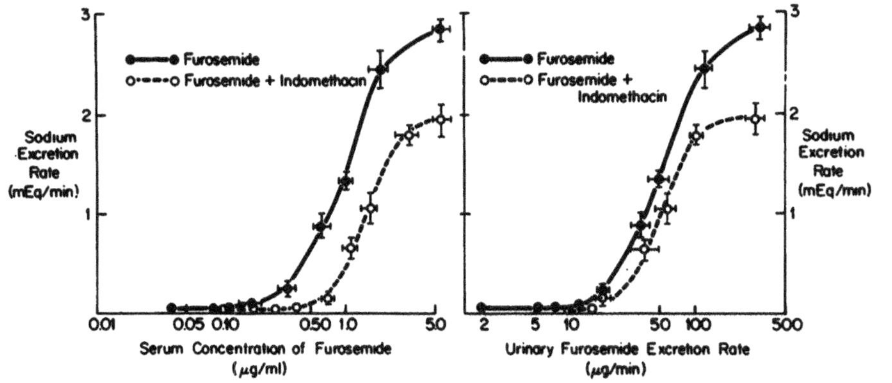

Fig. 11. Shift of the dose-response curve of furosemide in the presence of indomethacin (CHENNAVASIN et al. 1980)

acid, meclofenamate or indomethacin may at least partially blunt the action of loop diuretics (KRAMER et al. 1985a). Several factors may be responsible for this drug interference, namely, (a) a decrease in the concentration of the diuretic reaching its target site within the tubule, (b) drug interference resulting in a decrease in the duration of action, i.e., the time the diuretic acts at its target site, and (c) the dose/efficacy relation may be altered. The first two factors relate to pharmacokinetic drug interactions. The alteration in the dose/efficacy relationship presents a pharmacodynamic problem. As already mentioned, diuretics, as well as indomethacin, are weak acids which compete for secretion by the organic anion pump. This pharmacokinetic interaction results in a decreased renal clearance of furosemide (CHENNAVASIN et al. 1980; DATA et al. 1978). Since indomethacin not only decreases the renal but also the extrarenal clearance of furosemide, increased plasma concentrations of furosemide will result, which in turn lead to an unaltered total excretion of furosemide in the urine (CHENNAVASIN et al. 1980). Therefore, increased plasma concentrations of furosemide are necessary to result in the same efficacy of the drug in the tubular lumen at the ascending limb of Henle's loop, i.e., a shift of the dose-efficacy curve to the right is observed (Fig. 11). In some instances, however, even high concentrations of furosemide within Henle's loop resulted in a decreased natriuresis in the presence of indomethacin, indicating a pharmacodynamic interaction (DÜSING et al. 1982). This could occur on the tubular or vascular level (KRAMER et al. 1987). A direct interaction at the tubular level would be consistent with a direct effect of PGE_2 on tubular sodium reabsorption (STOKES 1979; STOKES and KOKKO 1977). On the vascular level, it is known that prostaglandins enhance (LUCAS et al. 1975) and indomethacin decreases (KIRSCHENBAUM et al. 1974) medullary blood flow which, probably by changes in interstitial pressure, may result in a decrease or increase of sodium reabsorption, respectively. Thus, indomethacin may blunt the diuretic-induced natriuresis by suppressing the furosemide-dependent rise in total renal and medullary blood flow (BAILIE et al. 1975; SPITALEWITZ et al. 1982).

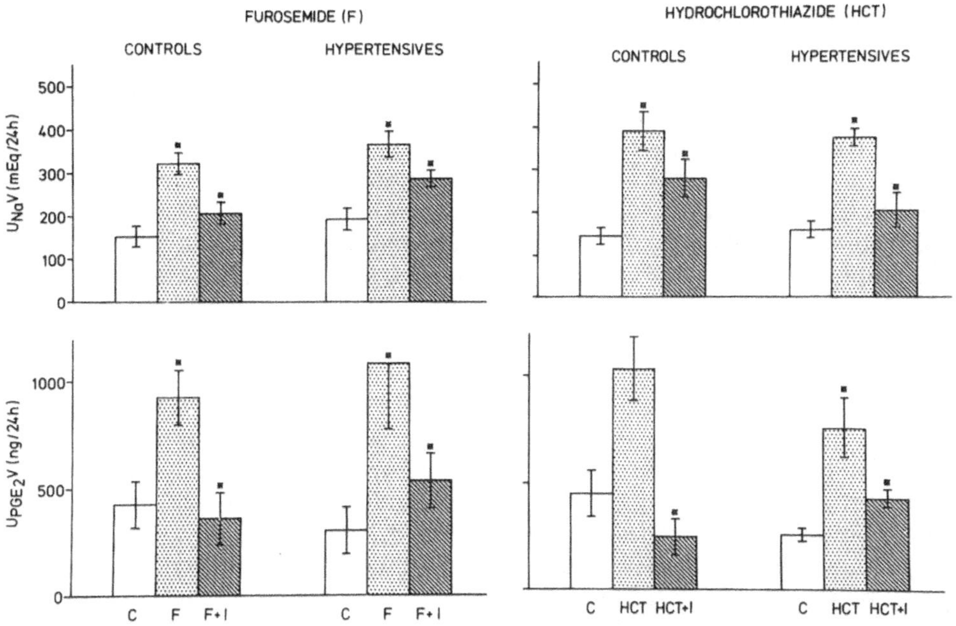

Fig. 12. Effects of indomethacin (I) on furosemide- and hydrochlorothiazide-induced natriuresis and increased prostaglandin E_2 excretion in healthy subjects and in patients with essential hypertension (KRAMER et al. 1981b)

We have observed that indomethacin not only interferes with the action of furosemide but also with that of hydrochlorothiazide and of spironolactone (KRAMER et al. 1980; TWEEDDALE and OGILVIE 1973). Furosemide, hydrochlorothiazide, and spironolactone increased urinary excretion of PGE_2. Indomethacin reduced not only urinary PGE_2 excretion significantly but also the furosemide- and hydrochlorothiazide-induced natriuresis. It abolished the potassium-sparing effect of spironolactone as well and partially suppressed the diuretic-induced rise in plasma renin activity. Furosemide- and hydrochlorothiazide-induced natriuresis and the rise in urinary PGE_2 excretion were also partially blunted in hypertensive subjects receiving indomethacin (Fig. 12). From our studies it appears that, under conditions of a stimulated renin-angiotensin system, inhibition of prostaglandin synthesis by nonsteroidal antiinflammatory agents will blunt the renal actions of diuretics, especially those of loop diuretics. Inhibition of prostaglandin synthesis interferes less with the renal natriuretic response in the presence of a suppressed renin-angiotensin system (KRAMER et al. 1985b).

Summary

Since 1957, when hydrochlorothiazide was first released for treatment of hypertensive patients, diuretics have been used most widely as effective antihypertensive drugs. Despite the development of numerous potent antihypertensive drugs with different and often very specific mechanisms of action, diuretics still belong to the first step category of antihypertensive agents.

In the first and second parts of this chapter the chemical nature, pharmacokinetics, metabolism, and pharmacodynamics as well as the renal and antihypertensive mechanisms of action of diuretic agents are summarized. These include their intrarenal hemodynamic effects and tubular sites and mechanisms of action which determine their diuretic and natriuretic potencies. Pharmacokinetic aspects and metabolism of diuretics include intestinal absorption, protein binding, lipid solubility, biotransformation, and elimination which determine onset, peak, and duration of action of diuretics. Their antihypertensive action is characterized by an early phase of reduction of plasma and extracellular fluid volume and of cardiac output. During a second phase, when plasma volume and cardiac output again tend to return towards control levels, indirect vascular effects prevail, namely a decrease in total peripheral vascular resistance and a blunted vascular response to vasoconstrictor hormones which may be related to changes in intracellular electrolyte activity and the activation of systemic and local vasodilator hormones such as prostanoids and kinins.

Diuretic treatment is probably most effective in volume-dependent forms of hypertension, e.g., in salt-sensitive hypertensive patients who often have low renin hypertension. As discussed in the third part, in other forms of hypertension diuretics are effective when combined with other antihypertensive drugs whose blood pressure lowering effect may be greatly enhanced in the presence of a diuretic. The chapter concludes with the differential use of individual diuretics, their unwanted side-effects and contraindications, and finally with the potential interaction of diuretics with other drugs, e.g., nonsteroidal antiinflammatory agents, which are widely used in general clinical practice.

Acknowledgements: Part of the author's studies cited in this chapter was supported by research grants No FA-7604, FA-8676 and FA-9214 from the Ministerium für Wissenschaft und Forschung NRW, FRG. The author gratefully acknowledges the technical assistance of Mrs A Bäcker and the secretarial assistance of Mrs L Mehrem.

References

Abdelhamid S, Seyberth H, Hänze S (1969) Untersuchungen zur Wirkung verschiedener Diuretika und Aldosteronantagonisten auf die renale Magnesiumausscheidung. Verh Dtsch Ges Inn Med 75:935–938

Abe K, Irokawa N, Yasujima M, Seino M, Chiba S, Sakurai Y, Yoshinaga K, Saito T (1978) The kallikrein-kinin system and prostaglandins in the kidney. Their relation to furosemide-induced diuresis and to the renin-angiotensin-aldosterone system in man. Circ Res 43:254–260

Ames RP (1988) Antihypertensive drugs and lipid profiles. Am J Hypertens 1:421–427

Antonello A, Tremolada C, Baggio B, Buin F, Favaro S, Piccoli A, Borsatti A (1978) In vivo activation of renal phospholipase activity by bradykinin in the rat. Prostaglandins 16:23–29

Agus ZS, Goldfarb S, Wasserstein A (1981) Calcium transport in the kidney. Rev Physiol Biochem Pharmacol 90:155–169

Ashouri OS (1986) Severe diuretic-induced hyponatremia in the elderly. Arch Intern Med 146:1355–1357
Baer JE, Leidy HL, Brooks AV, Beyer KH (1959) The physiological disposition of chlorothiazide (Diuril) in the dog. J Pharmacol Exp Ther 125:295–302
Bailie MD, Barbour JA, Hook JB (1975) Effects of indomethacin on furosemide-induced changes in renal blood flow. Proc Soc Exp Biol Med 148:1173–1176
Balizit L (1973) Recurrent parathyroid adenoma associated with prolonged thiazide administration. JAMA 225:1238
Beermann B, Hellström K, Lindström B, Rosen A (1975) Binding-site interaction of chlorthalidone and acetazolamide, two drugs transported by red blood cells. Clin Pharmacol Ther 17:424–432
Beermann B, Groschinsky-Grind M, Rosen A (1976) Absorption, metabolism, and excretion of ^{14}C-hydrochlorothiazide. Clin Pharmacol Ther 19:531–537
Benet LZ (1979) Pharmacokinetics/pharmacodynamics of furosemide in man: a review. J Pharmacokinet Biopharm 7:1–27
Berg KJ, Loew D (1977) Inhibition of furosemide-induced natriuresis by acetylsalicylic acid in dogs. Scand J Clin Lab Invest 37:125–131
Bergström J, Hultman E (1966) The effect of thiazides, chlorthalidone and furosemide on electrolytes and muscle glycogen in normal subjects. Acta Med Scand 180:363–376
Bevegard S, Castenfors J, Danielson M, Bergström J (1977) Effect of saluretic therapy on muscle content of water and electrolytes in relation to hemodynamic variables. Acta Med Scand 202:379–384
Beyer KH, Baer JE (1961) Physiological basis for the action of newer diuretic agents. Pharmacol Rev 13:517–562
Beyer KH, Baer JE, Michaelson JK, Russo HF (1965) Renotropic characteristics of ethacrynic acid; a phenoxyacetic saluretic-diuretic agent. J Pharmacol Exp Ther 147:1–22
Blaustein MV (1977) Sodium ions, calcium ions, blood pressure regulation, and hypertension: a reassessment and a hypothesis. Am J Physiol 232:C165-C173
Blumberg AL, Denny SE, Marshall GR, Needleman P (1977) Blood vessel-hormone interactions. Angiotensin, bradykinin, and prostaglandins. Am J Physiol 232: H305-H310
Bogler PM, Eisner GM, Ramwell PW, Slotkoff EJ (1978) Renal actions of prostacyclin. Nature 271:467–469
Brettell HR, Aikawa JK, Gordon GS, Harms DR (1960) Studies with chlorothiazide tagged with radioactive carbon (C^{14}) in human beings. Arch Intern Med 106:57
Brickman AS, Massry SG, Coburn JW (1972) Changes in serum and urinary calcium during treatment with hydrochlorothiazide. Studies on mechanism. J Clin Invest 51:945–954
Brod J (1973) The kidney. Butterworths, London
Brod J, Bahlmann J, Cachovan M, Pretschner P (1983) Development of hypertension in renal disease. Clin Sci 64:141–152
Brown RD, Manno JE, Duigneault EA, Manno BR (1979) Comparative acute toxicity of intravenous bumetanide and furosemide in the pure-bred beagle. Toxicol Appl Pharmacol 48:157–169
Burg MB (1982) Thick ascending limb of Henle's loop. Kidney Int 22:454–464
Campbell DB, Phillips EM (1974) Eur J Clin Pharmacol 7:407–414 Short-term effects and urinary excretion of the new diuretic, indapamide, in normal subjects.
Chennavasin P, Seiwell R, Brater DC (1980) Pharmacokinetic-dynamic analysis of the indomethacin-furosemide interaction in man. J Pharmacol Exp Ther 215:77–81
Costanzo LS, Windhager EE (1978) Calcium and sodium transport by the distal convoluted tubule of the rat. Am J Physiol 235:F492-F506
Cragoe EJ (1978) Diuretic agents. Am Chem Soc, Washington DC
Cragoe EJ, Woltersdorf OW, Bicking JB, Kwong SF, Jones JH (1967) Pyrazine diuretics. II. N-amidino-3-amino-5-substituted 6-halopyrazinecarboxamides. J Med Pharm Chem 10:66–75
Dahl LK, Knudsen KD, Heine M, Leitl G (1967) Effects of chronic excess salt ingestion: genetic influence on the development of salt hypertension in parabiotic rats: evidence

for a humoral factor. J Exp Med 126:687–699
Dahl LK, Heine M, Thompson K (1974) Genetic influence of the kidneys on blood pressure: evidence from chronic renal homografts in rats with opposite predispositions to hypertension. Circ Res 34:94–101
Dargie HJ, Boddy K, Kennedy AC, King PC, Read PR, Ward DM (1974) Body potassium in long-term frusemide therapy: is potassium supplementation necessary? Br Med J 4:316–319
Data JL, Rane A, Gerkens J, Wilkinson GR, Nies AS, Branch RA (1978) The influence of indomethacin on the pharmacokinetics, diuretic respone and hemodynamics of furosemide in the dog. J Pharmacol Exp Ther 206:431–438
Deetjen P (1966) Micropuncture studies on site and mode of diuretic action of furosemide. Ann N Y Acad Sci 139:408–415
Deetjen P (1980) Die Wirkungsweise diuretischer Substanzen in Abhängigkeit von ihrer renalen Behandlung. In: Krück F, Schrey A (eds) Diuretika III. Springer, Berlin Heidelberg New York, pp 35–41
De Stevens G, Werner LH, Halamandairs A, Ricca S (1958) Dihydrobenzothiadizine dioxides with polent diuretic effect. Experientia 14:463
Dieterle W, Wagner J, Faigle JW (1976) Binding of chlorthalidone (Hygroton) to blood components in man. Eur J Clin Pharmacol 10:37–42
Dodson RM, Tweit RC (1959) Addition of alkanethiolic acids to $\Delta^{1,4}$-3-oxo- and $\Delta^{4,6}$-3-oxosteroids. J Am Chem Soc 81:1224
Donaldson EK, Patrick J, Sivapragasm S, Woo Ming MO, Alleyne GAO (1976) Effect of triamterene on leukocyte sodium and potassium levels in heart disease. Br Med J 1:1254–1255
Duchin KL, Hutcheon DE (1978) Distribution of intracortical renal blood flow induced by bumetanide in the dog. J Pharmacol Exp Ther 204:135–140
Düsing R, Kramer HJ (1977) Triamteren in der Hochdruckbehandlung mit Hydrochlorothiazid und Propranolol. Dtsch Med Wochenschr 102:1541–1546
Düsing R, Bartter FC, Gill JR, Harrison L, Bhathena SJ, Recant L, Kramer HJ (1980) Experimentelle Hypokaliämie beim Menschen. Klin Wochenschr 58:881–887
Düsing R, Nicolas V, Glänzer K, Kipnowski J, Kramer HJ (1982) Prostaglandins participate in the regulation of NaCI absorption in the diluting segments of the nephron in vivo: effects of furosemide. Renal Physiol 5:115–123
Dyckner T, Wester PO (1978) The relation between extra- and intracellular electrolytes in patients with hypokalemia and/or diuretic treatment. Acta Med Scand 204:269–282
Edmondson RPS, Hilton PJ, Thomas RD, Patrick J (1974) Leucocyte electrolytes in cardiac and non-cardiac patients receiving diuretics. Lancet 1:12–14
Ettinger B, Oldroyd NO, Sörgel F (1980) Triamterene nephrolithiasis. JAMA 244: 2243–2245
Fanestil DD, Kipnowski J (1982) Molecular action of aldosterone. Klin Wochenschr 60:1180–1185
Feit PW (1971) Aminobenzoic acid diuretics. II. 4-substituted 3-amino-5-sulfamylbenzoic acid derivatives. J Med Chem 14:432–439
Feit PW (1981) Bumetanide—the way to its chemical structure. J Clin Pharmacol 21:531–536
Fine A, Henderson IS, Morgan DR, Tilstone WJ (1977) Malabsorption of furosemide caused by phenytoin. Br Med J 2:1061–1062
Fish C (1973) Relation of electrolyte disturbances to cardiac arrhythmias. Circulation 47:408–419
Fujita T, Henry WL, Bartter FC, Lake CR, Delea CS (1980) Factors influencing blood pressure in salt-sensitive patients with hypertension. Am J Med 69:334–344
Gallo DG, Bailey KR, Sheffner AL (1965) The interaction between cholestyramine and drugs. Proc Soc Exp Biol Med 120:60–65
Gayer J (1965) Die renale Exkretion des neuen Diureticum Furosemid. Klin Wochenschr 43:898–902
Gessler U (1962) Intra- und extrazelluläre Elektrolytveränderungen bei essentieller Hypertonie vor und nach Behandlung. Z Kreislaufforsch 51:177
Ghose RR (1977) Reset of osmostat after diuretic treatment. Br Med J 2:1063

Giebisch G (1981) Kaliummangelsyndrom durch Diuretika. In: Krück F, Schrey A (eds) Diuretika II. Wolf, Munich, pp 120–133

Glänzer K, Kramer HJ, Adams O, Düsing R, Sorger M, Krück F (1983) High dietary potassium attenuates the vasoconstrictor effect of ouabain and enhances baroreceptor sensitivity. J Hypertens 1 [Suppl 2]:214–216

Gonick HC, Kleeman CR, Rubini ME, Maxwell MH (1971) Functional impairment in chronic renal disease. III. Studies of potassium excretion. Am J Med Sci 261:281

Graybiel AL, Sode J (1971) Diuretics, potassium depletion, and carbohydrate intolerance. Lancet II:265

Grebian B, Geissler HE, Knauf H, Mutschler E, Schnippenkoetter I, Völger KD, Wais U (1978) On the pharmakokinetics of triamterene and its active metabolites in renal insufficiency. Drug Res 28:1420–1425

Greger R, Schlatter E (1983) Cellular mechanism of the action of loop diuretics on the thick ascending limb of Henle's loop. Klin Wochenschr 61;1019–1027

Greven J, Defrain W, Glaser K, Meywald K, Heidenreich O (1980) Studies with the optically active isomers of the new diuretic drug ozolinone. I. Differences in stereoselectivity of the renal target structures of ozolinone. Pflügers Arch 348:57–60

Halushka PV, Margolius HS, Allen H, Conradi EC (1979) Urinary excretion of prostaglandin E like material and kallikrein. Effects of furosemide. Prostaglandins 18:359–368

Hart LG, Schanker LS (1966) Active transport of chlorothiazide into bile. Am J Physiol 211:643–646

Häussler A, Hajdu P (1964) Untersuchungen mit dem Salidiuretikum 4-Chlor-N-furylmethyl)-5-sulfamyl-anthranilsäure. Arzneimittelforschung (Drug Res) 15:81

Heidenreich O, Gharemani G, Keller P, Kook Y, Schmiz K (1964) Die Wirkungen von 2-Carbäthoxymethylen-3-methyl-5-N-piperidinothiazolidon-4 auf die Nierenfunktion von Ratten und Hunden. Arzneimittelforschung 14:1242–1248

Heidland A, Wigand ME (1970) Einfluß hoher Furosemiddosen auf die Gehörfunktion bei Urämie. Klin Wochenschr 48:1052–1056

Holland OB, Kuhnert L, Pollard J, Padia M, Anderson RJ, Blomqvist G (1988) Ventricular ectopic activity with diuretic therapy. Am J Hypertens 1:380–385

Hollander W, Wilkins R (1957) Chlorothiazide: a new type of drug for the treatment of arterial hypertension. Boston Med Q 8:69–73

Hollenberg NK, Williams GH, Adams DF (1981) Essential hypertension: abnormal renal vascular and endocrine responses to a mild psychological stimulus. Hypertension 3:11–17

Hoskins B, Jackson CM III (1978) The mechanism of chlorothiazide-induced carbohydrate intolerance. J Pharmacol Exp Ther 206:423–430

Hropot M, Fowler N, Karlmark B, Giebisch G (1985) Tubular action of diuretics: distal effects on electrolyte transport. Kidney Int 28:477–489

Huang CM, Atkinson AJ, Levin M, Levin NW, Quintanilla A (1974) Pharmacokinetics of furosemide in advanced renal failure. Clin Pharmacol Ther 16:659–666

Jamison RL, Work J, Schafer JA (1982) New pathways for potassium transport in the kidney. Am J Physiol 242:F297

Johnston CI, Matthews PG, Dax E (1976) Renin-angiotensin and kallikrein-kinin systems in sodium homeostasis and hypertension in rats. Clin Sci Mol Med 51:283s-286s

Kaizu T, Margolius HS (1975) Studies on rat renal cortical cell kallikrein. I. Separation and measurement. Biochim Biophys Acta 411:305–315

Kaplan NM (1985) Potassium supplementation ameliorates hypertension in patients with diuretic-induced hypokalaemia. Klin Wochenschr 63[Suppl 3]:122–124

Katayama S, Attallah AA, Stahl RA, Bloch DL, Lee JB (1984) Mechanism of furosemide-induced natriuresis by direct stimulation of renal prostaglandin E_2. Am J Physiol 247:F555-F561

Kirschenbaum MA, White N, Stein JH, Ferris TF (1974) Redistribution of renal cortical blood flow during inhibition of prostaglandin synthesis. Am J Physiol 227:801–805

Klaassen CD, Fitzgerald TJ (1974) Metabolism and biliary excretion of ethacrynic acid. J Pharmacol Exp Ther 191:548–556

Koch-Weser J (1976) Medikamentöse Wechselwirkungen in der kardiovaskulären Ther-

apie. Schweiz Med Wochenschr 106:1531–1538
Kokko JP (1984) Site and mechanism of action of diuretics. Am J Med [Suppl] Nov 5:11–17
Kramer HJ (1979/80) The renal kallikrein-kinin system. Renal Physiol 2:107–121
Kramer HJ (1981a) Natriuretic hormone—a circulating inhibitor of sodium- and potassium-activated adenosine triphosphatase. Its potential role in body fluid and blood pressure regulation. Klin Wochenschr 59:1225–1230
Kramer HJ (1981b) Wechselwirkung zwischen Diuretika und renalem Prostaglandin- und Kininsystem: Untersuchungen bei gesunden Probanden und bei Patienten mit essentieller Hypertonie. In: Krueck F, Schrey A (eds) Diuretika II. Wolf, Munich, pp 184–201
Kramer HJ (1985) Neue Aspekte der Hochdruckpathogenese—Rationale Basis für den Einsatz von Diuretika. In Krück F, Schrey A (eds) Diuretika III. Springer, Berlin, Heidelberg New York, pp 148–156
Kramer HJ (1986) Endogenous inhibitors of sodium- and potassium-activated adenosine triphosphatase: a potential role for body fluid and blood pressure regulation. In: Krück F, Thurau K (eds) Endocrine regulation of electrolyte balance. Springer, Berlin, Heidelberg New York, pp 136–147
Kramer HJ (1987) Diuretic-induced hypokalaemia. Royal Soc Med Serv Int Congr Symp Ser 102:37–42
Kramer HJ (1988a) Zur Rolle der Niere in der Pathogenese des Bluthochdrucks. Z Kardiol 77:139–144
Kramer HJ (1988b) Inhibition of angiotensin-converting enzyme—effects on renal function and electrolyte balance. Z Kardiol 77 (Suppl 3): 39–45
Kramer HJ, Düsing R, Stinnesbeck B, Prior W, Bäcker A, Eden J, Kipnowski J, Glänzer K, Krück F (1980) Interaction of conventional and antikaliuretic diuretics with the renal prostaglandin system. Clin Sci 59:67–70
Kramer HJ, Rörig M, Völger KD (1981) Effects of triamterene and its phase I and phase II metabolites on sodium transport of the isolated frog skin. Pharmacology 23: 149–155
Kramer HJ, Glänzer K, Freitag T, Schönfeld J, Sorger M, Düsing R, Krück F (1984) Studies on the role of Na-K-ATPase inhibition in the pathogenesis of human hypertension. Changes in vascular and cardiac function following inhibition of the sodium pump in normotensive subjects and effects of calcium entry blockade. Klin Wochenschr 63:32–36
Kramer HJ, Kipnowski J, Düsing R (1985a) Interaktion von Furosemid und renalem Prostaglandin-System. Nieren Hochdruckkr 14:229–234
Kramer HJ, Stinnesbeck B, Klautke G et al. (1985b) Interaction of renal prostaglandins with the renin-angiotensin and renal adrenergic nervous systems in healthy subjects during dietary changes in sodium intake. Clin Sci 68:387–393
Kramer HJ, Kipnowski J, Düsing R (1987) The role of renal prostaglandins in the regulation of renal sodium excretion. Agents Actions 22 [Suppl]:61–72
Krück F, Bablok W, Besenfelder E et al. (1978) Clinical and pharmacological investigations of the new saluretic azosemide. Eur J Clin Pharmacol 14:153–161
Laake K, Horvei C, Aspöy B, Foss OP (1978) Hypomagnesaemia during treatment with diuretics. Curr Ther Res Clin Exp 23:730
Lameire N, Didion L (1988) Acute and chronic effects of torasemide in healthy volunteers. Drug Res 38:167–171
Lang F, Greger R, Deetjen P (1977) Effect of diuretics on uric acid metabolism and excretion. In: Siegenthaler W, Beckerhoff R, Vetter W (eds) Diuretics in research and clinics. Thieme, Stuttgart, pp 213–224
Leemhuis MP, van Damme KJ, Struyvenberg A (1976) Effects of chlorthalidone on serum and total body potassium in hypertensive patients. Acta Med Scand 200: 37–45
Lehmann K (1965) Trennung, Isolierung und Identifizierung von Stoffwechsel-Produkten des Triamteren. Drug Res 15:812–816
Licht JH, Haley RJ, Pugh B, Lewis SB (1983) Diuretic regimens in essential hypertension. A comparison of hypokalemic effects, BP control, and cost. Arch Intern

Med 143:1694–1699
Lief PD, Belizon I, Matos J, Bank N (1984) Diuretic-induced hypokalemia does not cause ventricular ectoppy in uncomplicated hypertension. Kidney Int 25:203 (abstr)
Light KC, Koepke JP, Obrist PA, Willis PW IV (1983) Psychological stress induces sodium and fluid retention in men at high risk for hypertension. Science 220:429–431
London GM, Safar ME (1988) Renal haemodynamics, sodium balance and the capacitance system in essential hypertension. Clin Sci 74:449–453
Lucas C, Chang T, Splawinski JA, Oates JA, Nies AS (1975) Enhanced renal prostaglandin production in the dog. II. Effects on intrarenal hemodynamics. Circ Res 36:204–207
Maren TH (1969) Renal carbonic anhydrase and the pharmacology of solfonamide inhibitors. In: Herken H (ed) Diuretica. Springer, Berlin Heidelberg New York, pp 195–256 (Handbook of experimental pharmacology, vol 24)
Margolius HS, Horwitz D, Pisano JJ, Keiser HR (1974) Urinary kallikrein excretion in hypertensive man. Relationship to sodium intake and sodium-retaining steroids. Circ Res 35:820–825
Mathog RH, Klein WJ (1969) Ototoxicity of ethacrynic acid and aminoglycoside antibiotics in uremia. N Engl J Med 280:1223–1224
McGiff JC, Itskovitz HD, Terragno NA (1975) The actions of bradykinin and eledoisin in the canine isolated kidney: relation to prostaglandins. Clin Sci 49:125–132
Meng K, Loew D (1974) Diuretika. Chemie, Pharmakologie, Therapie. Thieme, Stuttgart
Meng K, O' Dea K (1973) Peritubular and intraluminal concentrations of diuretics affecting isotonic fluid absorption in the kidney tubule. Pharmacology 9:193–200
Merkel W, Bormann D, Mania D et al. (1976) Piretanide (Hoe 118) a new high ceiling salidiuretic. Eur J Med Chem Chim Ther 5:399–406
Morledge JH (1983) Clinical efficacy and safety of indapamide in essential hypertension. Am Heart J 106:229–237
Novello FC, Sprague JM (1957) Benzothiadiazine dioxides as novel diuretics. J Am Chem Soc 79:2028–2029
Oliw E, Kover G, Larsson C, Anggard E (1978) Reduction by indomethacin of furosemide effects in the rabbit. Eur J Pharmacol 38:95–100
Olsen UB, Ahnfelt-Ronne I (1976) Bumetanide induced increase in renal blood flow in conscious dogs and its relation to local hormones (PGE, kallikrein and renin). Acta Pharmacol Toxicol 38:219–228
Ostergaard EH, Magnussen MP, Nielsen CK, Eilertsen E, Frey HH (1972) Pharmacological properties of 3-n-butyl-amino-4-phenoxy-5-sulfamylbenzol acid (Bumetanide), a new potent diuretic. Arzneimittel forschung 22:66–72
Patak RV, Mookerjee BK, Bentzel CJ, Hysert PE, Babej M, Lee JB (1975) Antagonism of the effects of furosemide by indomethacin in normal and hypertensive man. Prostaglandins 10:649–659
Paulsrud JR, Miller ON (1974) Inhibition of 15-OH prostaglandin dehydrogenase by several diuretic drugs. Fed Proc 33:590 (abstr)
Pentikäinen PJ, Penttilä A, Neuvonen PJ, Gothoni G (1977) Fate of [^{14}C]-bumetanide in man. Br J Clin Pharmacol 4:39–44
Petersen V, Hvidt S, Thomsen K, Schou M (1974) Effect of prolonged thiazide treatment on renal lithium clearance. Br Med J 3:143–145
Pitts RF, Alexander RS (1945) The nature of the renal tubular mechanism for acidifying the urine. Am J Physiol 144:239
Pitts RF (1968) *The physiology of the kidney and body fluids*. Year Book, Chicago
Pratt EB, Aikawa IK (1962) Secretion and effect of hydrochlorothiazide in bile and pancreatic juice. Am J Physiol 202:1083
Puschett JB, Rastegar A (1974) Comparative study of the effects of metolazone and other diuretics on potassium excretion. Clin Pharmacol Ther 15:397–405
Quamme GA, Dirks JH (1980) Magnesium transport in the nephron. Am J Physiol 239:F393–401
Roblin RO, Clapp JW (1950) The preparation of heterocyclic sulfonamides. J Am Chem Soc 72:4890

Sadée W, Dagcioglu M, Schröder R (1972) Pharmacokinetics of Aldectone in humans. In: Brendel W et al. (eds) Extrarenal activity of aldosterone and its antagonists. Exerpta Medica Amsterdam, p 40–42
Schlebusch H, Sorger M, Höck A, Krück F (1983) An improved method for the determination of potassium in leucocytes. Clin Sci 64:505–510
Schmid E, Fricke G (1969) Studies on urinary excretion of the potassium-retaining diuretic amiloride (desmethyl-pipazuroyl-guanidine, MK 870) in man. Pharmacol Clin 1:110
Schultz EM, Cragoe EJ, Bicking JB, Bolhofer WA, Sprague JM (1962) a,ß-unsaturated ketone derivatives of aryloxyacetic acids, a new class of diuretics. J Med Pharm Chem 5:660
Seldin DW, Eknoyan G, Suki WN, Rector FC Jr (1966) Localization of diuretic action from the pattern of water and electrolyte excretion. Ann N Y Acad Sci 139: 328–343
Sheehan J, White A (1982) Diuretic-associated hypomagnesiaemia. Br Med J 285:1157
Sörgel F (1978) Experimentelle Untersuchungen Fur biochemischen und pharmakologischen Cherekterisierung von Solidiuretika bei Mensch und Tier. Inaugural-Dissertation, Johann-Wolfgang Goethe Universität, Frankfurt/Main
Spitalewitz S, Chou SY, Faubert PF, Porush JG (1982) Effects of diuretics on inner medullary hemodynamics in the dog. Circ Res 51:703–710
Stein JA, Ferris TF, Huprich JE, Smith TC, Osgood RW (1971) Effects of renal vasodilatation on distribution of cortical blood flow in the kidney of the dog. J Clin Invest 50:1429–1438
Stokes JB (1979) Effect of prostaglandin E on chloride transport across the thick ascending limb of Henle. Selective inhibition of the medullary portion. J Clin Invest 64:495–502
Stokes JB, Kokko JP (1977) Inhibition of sodium transport by prostaglandin E across the isolated perfused rabbit collecting tubule. J Clin Invest 49:1099–1104
Stone KJ, Hart M (1976) Inhibition of renal PGE_2-9-ketoreductase by diuretics. Prostaglandins 12:197–207
Suki WN, Yium JJ, von Minden M, Saller-Hebert C, Eknoyan G, Martinez-Maldonado M (1970) Acute treatment of hypercalcemia with furosemide. N Engl J Med 283:836–840
Tobian L (1988) High potassium diets during hypertension reduce arterial endothelial injury, stroke mortality rate, arterial hypertrophy and renal lesions without lowering blood pressure in: Rettig R, Ganten D, Luft F (eds) Salt and hypertension. Springer, Heidelberg, 218–234
Tweeddale MG, Ogilvie RI (1973) Antagonism of spironolactone-induced natriuresis by aspirin in man. N Engl J Med 289:198–200
Van Brummelen P, Woerlee M, Schalekamp MA (1979) Long-term versus short-term effects of hydrochlorothiazide on renal haemodynamics in essential hypertension. Clin Sci Mol Med 56:463–469
Vatner SF, Boettcher DH, Heyndrick GR, McRitchie RJ (1975) Reduced baroreflex sensitivity with volume loading in conscious dogs. Circ Res 37:236–242
Villamil MF, Yeyati N, Enero MA, Rubians C, Tacquinin AC (1963) Effect of long-term treatment with hydrochlorothiazide on water and electrolytes of muscle in hypertensive subjects. Am Heart J 65:294
Von Hodenberg A, Vollmer KO, Klemisch W, Liedtke B (1977) Metabolismus von Etozolin bei Ratte, Hund und Mensch. Drug Res 27:1776–1785
Weber PC, Scherer B, Larsson C (1977) Increase of free arachidonic acid by furosemide in man as the cause of prostaglandin and renin release. Eur J Pharmacol 41:329–332
Weidmann P, Beretta-Piccoli C, Meier A, Keusch G, Glueck Z (1981) Untersuchungen zum antihypertensiven Mechanismus von Diuretika. In: Krück F, Schrey A (eds) Diuretika II. Wolf, Munich, pp 58–76
Weidmann P, Uehlinger DE, Gerber A (1985) Antihypertensive treatment and serum lipoproteins. J Hypertens 3:297–306
Weinberger MH (1988) Diuretics and their side effects. Dilemma in the treatment of hypertension. Hypertension 11 [Suppl II]:II-16–II-20

Weinberger MH, Ramsdell JW, Bosner DR (1972) Effect of chlorothiazide and sodium on vascular responsiveness to angiotensin II. Am J Physiol 223:1049–1052
Weiss P, Hersey RM, Dujovne CA, Bianchine JR (1969) The metabolism of amiloride hydrochloriole in man. Clin Pharmacol Ther 10:401–406
Werness PG, Bergert JH, Smith LH (1982) Triamterene urolithiasis: solubility, pK, effect on crystal formation, and matrix binding of triamterene and its metabolites. J Lab Clin Med 99:254–262
Wiebelhaus VD, Weinstock J, Maas AR, Brennan FT, Sosnowski G, Larsen T (1965) The diuretic and natriuretic activity of triamterene and several related pteridines in the rat. J Pharmacol Exp Ther 149:397–403
Wilbrandt W (1955) Zum Wirkungsmechanismus der Herzglykoside. Schweiz Med Wochenschr 85:315–320
Wilkinson PR, Hesp R, Issler H, Raftery EB (1975) Total body and serum potassium during prolonged thiazide therapy for essential hypertension. Lancet I:759–762
Williamson HE, Marchand GR, Bourland WA, Farley DB, van Orden DE (1976) Ethacrynic acid-induced release of prostaglandin E to increase renal blood flow. Prostaglandins 11:519–522
Wilson TW, Loadholt CB, Privitera PJ, Halushka PV (1982) Furosemide increases urine 6-keto-prostaglandin $F_{1a}\alpha$. Relation to natriuresis, vasodilation, and renin release. Hypertension 4:634–641
Wistrand PJ, Kinne R (1977) Carbonic anhydrase activity of isolated brush border and basal-lateral membranes of renal tubular cells. Pflügers Arch 370:121–126
Wright FS, Giebisch G (1985) Regulation of potassium excretion. In: Seldin DW, Giebisch G (eds) The kidney: physiology and pathophysiology. Raven, New York, pp 1223–1249
Wright FS, Schnermann J (1974) Interference with feedback control of glomerular filtration rate by furosemide, triflocin and cyanide. J Clin Invest 53:1695–1708
Yendt ER, Cohanim M (1978) Prevention of calcium stones with thiazides. Kidney Int 13:397–409
Zsoter TT, Hart F, Radde IC (1970) Mechanism of antihypertensive action of prolonged administration of hydrochlorothiazide in rabbit and dog. Circ Res 27:717–725

CHAPTER 3

β-Blockers

J. CONWAY and A. BILSKI

CONTENTS

1 History

Over the past 20 years β-blockers have proved to be singularly effective in the treatment of ischaemic heart disease, hypertension and several other conditions. So enormous is the literature surrounding these agents that it is impossible to review it comprehensively or to do justice to the many β-blockers recently introduced. This article therefore highlights the major developments and attempts to illustrate principles. The choice of references has per force had to be selective. For a fuller account of β-blockers, readers are referred to the comprehensive book by Cruickshank and Prichard (1987), and we acknowledge the help that this work has been to us.

The emergence of β-blockers as therapeutic agents is a final practical step at the end of a long and fascinating trail of outstanding basic research. The journey began with the pioneering work of Langley (1905) and Dale (1906) who between them described the anatomy and function of the autonomic nervous system. Elliot (1905) noted a similarity between the effects of injected adrenaline and sympathetic nervous responses and suggested that adrenaline might be a transmitter substance.

Today the notion of chemical transmission is so much a part of biological thinking that it is easy to forget how inherently difficult it was to accept that a chemical process, which was thought to be a slow one, might be a vital link in an electrical process. However, Otto Loewi (1921), in simple and elegant experiments, proved conclusively that the chemical link existed. He suspended two perfused frog hearts in tandem. The second one received the perfusate from the first. The nerve to the first heart was intact. Upon stimulation of this the rate and force of the first heart beat was changed, and this was followed, after an appropriate delay, by an identical response in the second heart. Thus, the existence of chemical transmission was established, and later Cannon and Rosenblueth (1933) promoted the idea that sympathetic nerve endings released either a stimulating substance (sympathin E) or an inhibitory substance (sympathin I), which then had the appropriate actions on the tissues. The functions of the sympathetic part of the autonomic nervous system were encapsulated by Cannon's concept that it prepared the organism for "fight or flight".

The next major contribution was made by Ahlquist (1948), who, from an analysis of the potency and actions of six sympathetic agonists, postulated the existence of two types of sympathetic receptor which he called "alpha" and "beta". The α-receptor, by and large, produced predominantly excitatory actions, except for the intestine where they were inhibitory. The β-receptors generally produced inhibitory effects, except for the heart where the action was excitatory. Because of these exceptions, full acceptance of the α and β classification was delayed until antagonists specific for each class of receptor had been found. The first β-adrenoceptor antagonist to be discovered was dichloroisoprenaline (DCI; SLATER and POWELL 1957). This compound antagonised both catecholamine stimulation of the heart and relaxation of the guinea pig tracheal smooth muscle (MORAN and PERKINS 1958).

The crucial stage in the understanding of the β-receptor trail was the appreciation by James Black that an agent which would effectively inhibit adrenaline could be of value in ischaemic heart disease by reducing myocardial oxygen

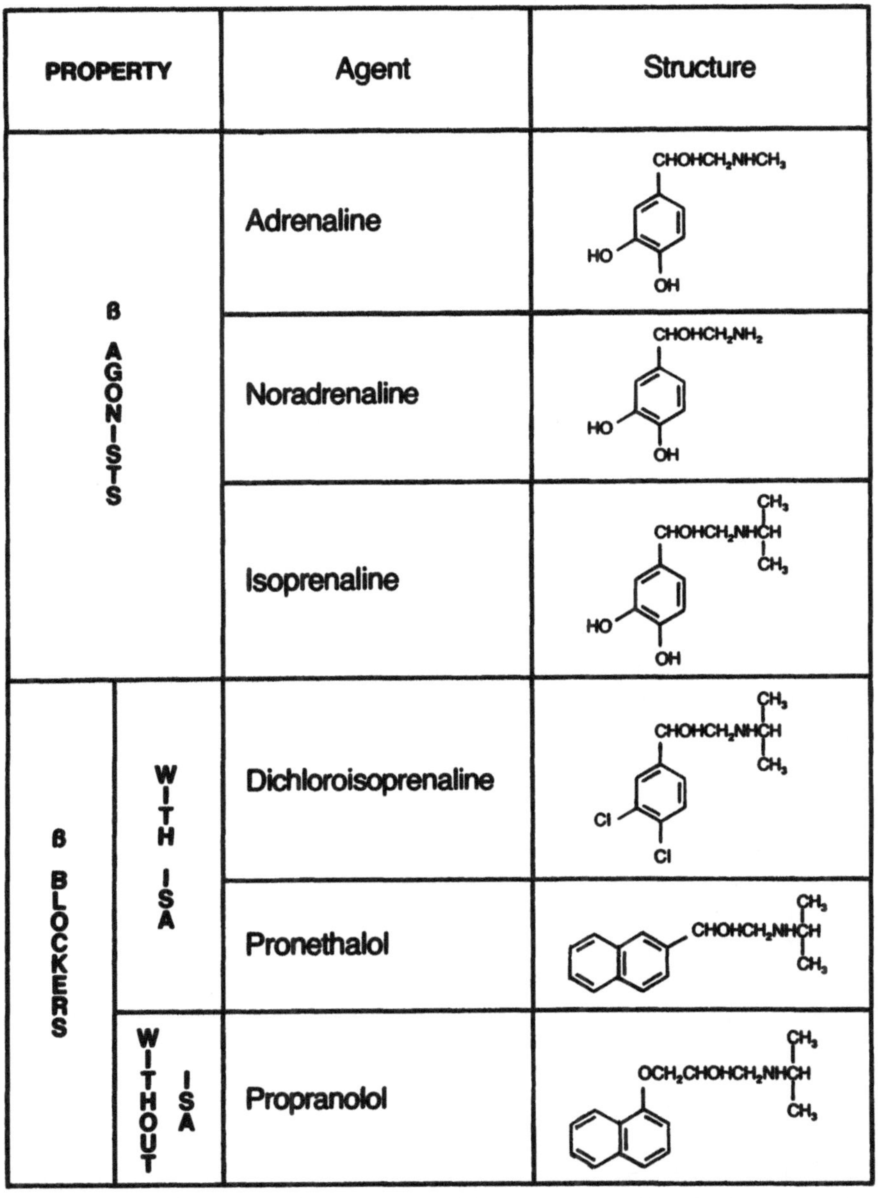

Fig. 1. Chemical structure of β-agonists and the first three β-blockers, dichloroisoprenaline, pronetholol and propranolol

consumption (Black 1976). DCI was not effective enough as a blocker, and it possessed stimulant actions of its own (partial agonist activity). The first effective β-blocker, pronethalol, was discovered by Black and his colleagues at ICI (Black and Stephenson 1962) (Fig. 1). From the initial development of the first β-blocker, there followed the discovery of a great many other agents whose prime effect was to prevent the natural agonists adrenaline and noradrenaline from stimulating the β-receptor.

Finally, Lands, from studies of the different effects of bronchodilators, postulated that there were two subtypes of β-receptors which he called β_1 and β_2 (Lands et al. 1967).

2 Chemistry

β-Blocker substances compete at the receptor site for the naturally occurring transmitters, adrenaline and noradrenaline. Three general structural requirements have been described as necessary for β-adrenoceptor antagonism (Main and Tucker 1985).

(a) An ethanolamine or oxypropanolamine side-chain. With few exceptions, most β-blockers possess the latter side-chain (Fig. 2). DCI possesses an ethanolamine side-chain. In general, the oxypropanolamine side-chain confers greater antagonist potency on the molecule than the ethanolamine side-chain, e.g. propranolol is ten times more potent as an antagonist than pronethalol.
(b) An aromatic ring which may be benzenoid (e.g. atenolol), bicyclic aromatic (e.g. propranolol), heterocyclic (e.g. timolol) or benzoheterocyclic (e.g. pindolol).
(c) An amine substituent which is a branched chain alkyl group. The isopropyl and tertiary-butyl groups have been found to confer optimum potency.

2.1 Intrinsic Sympathomimetic Activity

Full agonism is generally observed if the catechol moiety in the aromatic ring is retained. Loss of one or both hydroxyl groups results in partial agonism. The level of intrinsic sympathomimetic activity (ISA) is reduced with large *ortho* substituents; thus oxprenolol (o-OCH_2CHCH_2) has only modest ISA. Partial agonism is also observed with hydroxy amidic and ether substituents in the *para* position (e.g. practolol $p$$NHCOCH_3$). However, ISA is lost when a methylene group is inserted between the aromatic ring and these functions, as with atenolol and metoprolol.

The degree of agonism can also be governed by the side-chain — ethanolamines tend to have more ISA than oxypropanolamines. In addition, the level of ISA can be finely tuned by changing the substituents in the acyl portion of an acylaminoalkyl side-chain. This method was used to find the partial agonist epanolol. Partial agonism will be discussed more fully below.

oxypropanolamines

$R_1 = OCH_2CHOHCH_2NHCH(CH_3)_2$

$R_3 = OCH_2CHOHCH_2NHC(CH_3)_3$

$R_2 = OCH_2CHOHCH_2NHCH_2CH_2NHCOCH_2$ 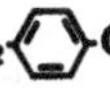 OH

$R_4 = OCH_2CHOHCHCH_3NHCH(CH_3)_2$

Property		Agent	Structure
B_1 SELECTIVE	WITHOUT ISA	Atenolol	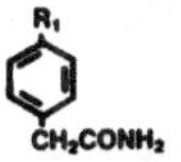
		Metoprolol	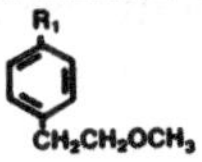
	WITH ISA	Practolol	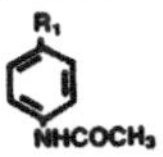
		Acebutolol	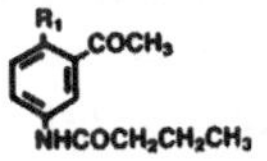
		Epanolol	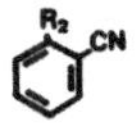
NON SELECTIVE	WITHOUT ISA	Propranolol	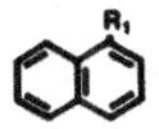
		Timolol	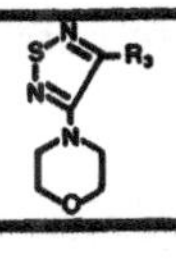
	WITH ISA	Oxprenolol	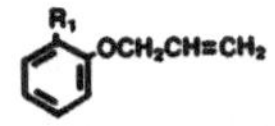
		Pindolol	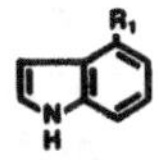
B_2 SELECTIVE	WITHOUT ISA	ICI 118551	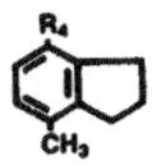

Fig. 2. Chemical structures of 10 β-blockers classified according to their selectivity and intrinsic activity

2.2 Cardioselectivity

The suggestion by Lands that the β-receptors can be subdivided into two chemically distinct classes raised the possibility that agents might be developed which would selectively affect one type of receptor rather than the other. The word cardioselectivity is used because the most prominent effect of the β-receptor is manifested by the heart. Selectivity for this receptor seems to depend upon substitution in the *para* position of an oxypropanolamine type of compound with either an amidic group (e.g. practolol, atenolol and acebutolol) or other moieties capable of participating in hydrogen bond formation (metoprolol) (L.H. SMITH 1978). Selectivity can also be governed by amidic substitution into the amine component of the oxypropranolamine side-chain; thus, epanolol is highly cardioselective probably by virtue of the amidic substituent, -NHCO-, in its side-chain.

2.3 Isomerism

A steric relationship is required for the interaction between the receptor and the agonist or antagonist. β-blockers contain an asymmetric carbon atom, so they exist as pairs of optical isomers. In the oxypropanolamine series, activity generally resides with the *S*-enantiomer. This is usually some 50–150 times more potent as an antagonist at the cardiac β-receptor than the corresponding *R*-enantiomer (KAUMANN and BLINUS 1980; BARRETT and CULLUM 1968). Interestingly, the enantiomeric antagonist ratio for the β_2-receptor is less than it is for the β_1, suggesting different steric requirements for the two subtypes (WALTER et al. 1984). Recent work has shown that the isomers of pindolol express the same degree of ISA, although potency values (expressed as EC_{50}) are different (WALTER et al. 1984). Whether this finding extends to other β-adrenoceptor partial agonists remains to be seen.

3 Pharmacokinetics and Metabolism

The effect of a β-blocker on its receptor depends upon the logarithm of the concentration in the tissue. In the intact animal this is adequately represented by the plasma level of a compound (AMERY et al. 1977; MCAINSH 1977). β-Blocker compounds vary considerably in their lipid solubility, with penbutolol and propranolol being extremely lipophilic and atenolol and sotalol being primarily hydrophilic. The distribution of compounds between the lipid and aqueous phases is conveniently measured by the ratio of their distribution between octanol and water. The log partition coefficient of propranolol is 3.65, and at the other extreme atenolol is 0.23 (CRUICKSHANK 1980). The partition coefficient dominates the absorption, distribution and rate of metabolism of each compound and the mode of excretion. Most β-blockers, which are weak bases, are minimally absorbed from the stomach. The major site of absorption is in the small intestine where by virtue of the environmental pH and the great surface area, approximately 90% of the more lipophilic compounds are absorbed. For hydrophilic agents such as atenolol and nadolol intestinal absorption is limited to about 30%–50%. With these compounds the time to achieve a maximum blood level is about 4 h whereas with lipophilic compounds the peak is usually achieved in about 0.5–2 h. There are several different types of sustained release formulations for the more rapidly absorbed compounds, which delay absorption and extend their duration of action. Food decreases the absorption of some compounds like atenolol and sotalol, and it enhances that of propranolol and metoprolol (MELANDER et al. 1977, 1979). Other substances may also affect absorption. For example, aluminium hydroxide decreases the absorption of atenolol (KIRCH et al. 1981), and for reasons that are not entirely clear ampicillin substantially reduces the absorption of atenolol (SCHAFER-KORTING et al. 1983), and frusemide increases plasma propranolol levels (CHIARIELLO et al. 1979).

3.1 Hepatic Metabolism

Material absorbed from the gut is delivered at its highest concentration via the splanchnic circulation to the liver and is metabolised to varying extents. Alprenolol and propranolol are extensively metabolised (NIES and SHAND 1975). This first pass effect depends critically upon the dose since the relevant enzymes can be come saturated (SHAND et al. 1973). At the usual clinical doses liver metabolism reduces the bioavailability of propranolol to about 30%. However, this is not the end of the story, since the primary metabolites are biologically active. 4-hydroxy propranolol, for example, is as potent as the parent compound. The process of absorption and metabolism of propranolol leads to considerable variability in the peak and trough blood levels between individuals (SHAND 1974). The efficiency in metabolism of drugs by the liver is genetically determined, and the ratio of high to normal metabolisers in the population varies between different races. Poor metabolisers tend to have higher levels in the blood, and this applies particularly to alprenolol, propranolol, metoprolol and timolol (SHAH et al. 1982; DAYER et al. 1982). Substances which may affect hepatic enzymes (cytochrome oxidase P450) will also affect the rate of metabolism and hence blood level of different drugs. Thus, interactions are seen between propranolol and metropolol and cimetidine (HEAGERTY et al. 1981) and diazepam (HAWKSWORTH et al. 1984).

3.2 Distribution

Lipophilic agents are distributed more widely in the tissues than the hydrophilic ones. The volume of distribution of hydrophilic agents is similar to that of the extracellular fluid. Lipophilicity confers an ability to enter the CNS, and hence neurogenic side effects tend to be greater with these agents (BETTS and ALFORD 1985). The distribution of lipophilic compounds may, however, be limited in some degree by their greater binding affinity to plasma proteins.

3.3 Excretion

The hydrophilic compounds like atenolol, sotalol and nadalol are excreted by glomerular filtration, practically unchanged (WARREN et al. 1983), and the elimination half-lives are of the order of 6–12 h. The dose of these compounds therefore has to be adjusted in the presence of renal failure or in older subjects as the filtration rate declines (ZECH et al. 1977). Lipid soluble compounds are handled primarily by the liver, either by biliary excretion or by metabolism.

4 Mechanism of Action

4.1 Cellular Processes

β-Receptors exist in the membrane of many cells, and as a general rule those which have a close innervation are of the β_1-type, and those which are stimulated by circulating agonists are the β_2 type (Table 1). The receptors have a con-

Table 1. Predominant β-receptor types in various tissues and their actions

System		Response
Heart	β_1	Increase in heart rate
	β_1	Increase in conduction velocity
	β_1	Increase in excitability
	β_1	Increase in force of contraction
	β_2	Hypertrophy (trophic effect)
Blood vessels	β_1	Dilatation of coronary arteries
	β_2	Dilatation of most artieries
Lung	β_2	Bronchodilatation
Skeletal muscle	β_2	Tremor
	β_2	Stimulation of Na/K ATPase
Uterus	β_2	Relaxation
Gut	β_1	Relaxation
Platelets	β	Aggregation promoted
Eye: Intraocular pressure	β_1	Increase in intraocular pressure
Tear secretion	β_2	Increased basic secretion
Nervous system:		
Locus coerulus	β_2	Blood pressure regulation, alerting response
Hypothalamic	β_1	Blood pressure regulation
Noradrenaline release	β_2	Facilitated
Metabolism:		
Glycogenolysis	β_2	Promoted
Lipolysis (white adipocytes)	$\beta_1 > \beta_2$	Promoted
Calorigenesis (brown adipocytes)	β?	Promoted
Hormone secretion:		
Insulin	β_2	Secreted
Parathyroid hormone	β_1	Secreted
Renin	β_1	Secreted
Mast cells	β	Inhibition of release of mediators of anaphylaxis

figuration which binds stereo-specifically to the agonists noradrenaline and adrenaline. When the agonist attaches itself to this receptor structure, it initiates a cascade of events starting with the activation of a membrane-bound enzyme, adenylate cyclase. This leads to the conversion of adenosine triphosphate to adenosine-3,5-cyclic monophosphate (cAMP). In turn, this leads to the activation of a further enzyme, protein kinase, which is responsible for the final cellular effect through the phosphorylation of specific substrates and hence to the action of the compound. It is possible to purify the receptor substances and determine their structure (LEFKOWITZ and HOFFMAN 1980 a,b).

β-Blockers bind to the appropriate receptor and prevent agonists from initiating the cascade of events which leads to cellular activity. This results in a characteristic shift to the right of the concentration response curve by the β-blocker (Fig. 3). A parallel shift indicates that there is competitive binding at the receptor, but a sufficient concentration of an agonist can displace the blocker. The specificity of their action is the property above all else which makes the β-blockers so successful as therapeutic agents. Thus, none of the known β-blockers affect other surface receptors, having negligible affinity for cholinergic, histaminergic and dopaminergic receptors. Propranolol, however, does interact

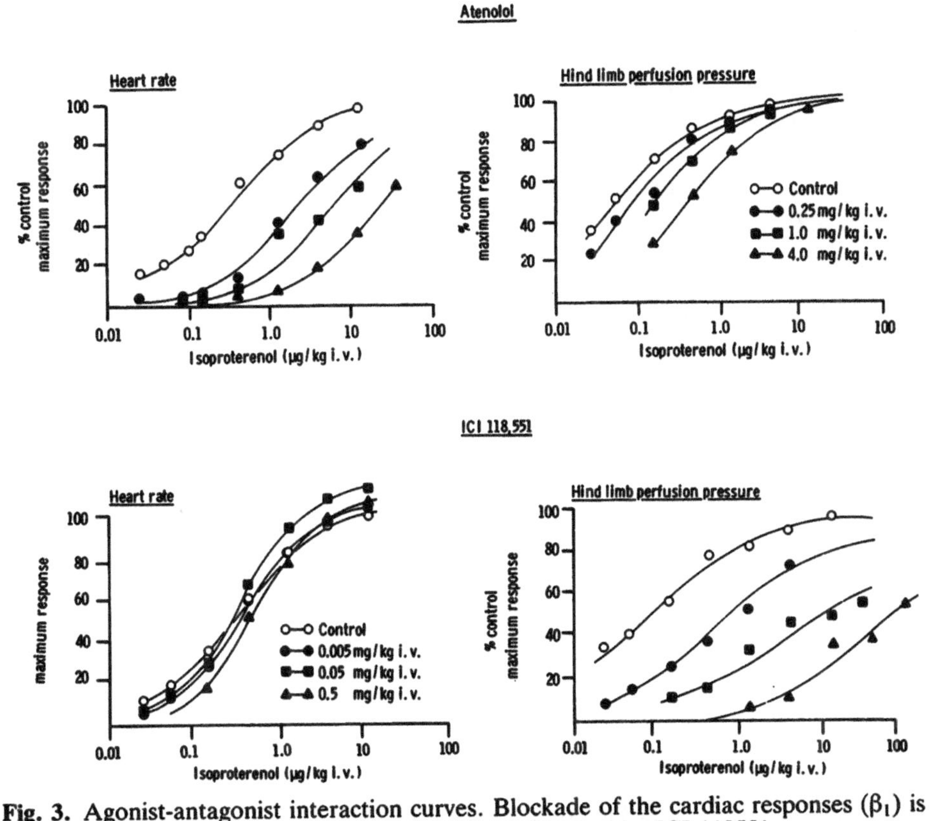

Fig. 3. Agonist-antagonist interaction curves. Blockade of the cardiac responses (β_1) is seen with atenolol while the limb vessels (β_2) are blocked by ICI 118551

with some classes of serotonin receptor (WEINSTOCK et al. 1977). An estimate of the antagonist potency of an agent can be determined from its activity against the responses to an agonist. Potencies are expressed either as the ED_{50} (which is the concentration of antagonist required to reduce the maximum effect by 50%), the pA2 (which is the negative logorithm of the molar antagonist concentration which necessitates a doubling of the agonist concentration to regain the control response) or the equilibrium dissociation constant, K_B (which is derived from a Schild plot relating the concentration of β-blocker with the dose ratio shift). The pA_2 values of number of β-blockers are shown in Table 2; the higher the pA2 value, the more potent the drug is as an antagonist. Potencies of drugs can also be derived from radioligand binding studies (expressed as equilibrium dissociation constants), which also give receptor number and proportion of receptor subtypes within a tissue.

Receptor numbers can change; in general, they vary inversely with the concentration of the agonist. Thus, it is possible to account for the well-known phenomenon of denervation hypersensitivity (CANNON and ROSENBLUETH 1949) by an increase in the number of receptors (up-regulation) and for the phenomenon of tachyphylaxis which develops in the presence of high concentrations of the agonist (down-regulation). The administration of most β-blockers leads to an increase in the number of receptors (AARONS and MOLINOFF 1982; WHYTE et al. 1987), and this may be clinical importance in producing a state of hypersensitivity to sympathetic agonists after the withdrawal of β-blockers.

β_1-Receptors exist in the heart and in the coronary arteries. β_2-receptors are prominent in arteries in the lungs and in skeletal muscle. (Table 1). The distributions are not absolute; there are β_2-receptors in the heart and β_1-receptors in the lungs, although the proportions are low. The relative ratios of the two subtypes in a given tissue depend upon the species, the levels of circulating hormones and the disease. It has also been shown that although the small proportion of β_2-receptors in the human ventricle are capable of producing a major proportion of the increase in cAMP, they are not capable of producing a full agonist response. In contrast, β_1-receptors do exert a full response (KAUMANN and LEMOINE 1987). The physiological and pathological significance of these findings has yet to be determined. There are β_2-receptors in the central nervous system and on peripheral nerves (see Sect. 4.10).

Table 2. β-Blocking actions of atenolol, practolol, epanolol, propranolol and pindolol expressed as pA_2 (mean + SEM) in isolated guinea pig cardiac and tracheal preparations

	pA_2		
	Right atrium	Trachea	Cardioselectivity ratio
Atenolol	7.27 + 0.11	5.21 + 0.06	115
Practolol	6.49 + 0.01	4.61 + 0.08	76
Epanolol	8.42 + 0.11	6.33 + 0.139	123
Propranolol	8.30 + 0.09	7.66 + 0.13	4
Pindolol	8.9 + 0.09	8.8 + 0.04	1

4.2 Heart

In isolated atria, adrenaline and noradrenaline cause an increase in the frequency and force of contractions. These are prevented by β-blockers. Bradycardia is produced by decreasing the rate of spontaneous repolarisation of the pacemaker potentials which determine the spontaneous beating of the sinus node. Sinus node recovery time and atrial refractory period are prolonged and atrioventricular conduction delayed (SEIDES et al. 1974; HOMBACH et al. 1982). These actions form the basis of the effect of β-blockers in controlling supraventricular arrhythmias. In isolated papillary muscle there is a decrease in the force of cardiac contraction with prolongation of the contraction and relaxation times. Depending upon the level of sympathetic stimulation, β-blockers either increase, decrease or produce no change in stroke volume, although they always produce a decrease in cardiac output. A functional consequence of the decrease in force of contraction is an increase in heart size. The rate of development of peak tension and the rates of ejection and filling are slower (SONNENBLICK et al. 1965; WOLFSON and GORLIN 1969). β-Blockade reverses all the effects of agonists in a dose-dependent manner, irrespective of whether the stimulation is produced by sympathetic nerves to the heart or by circulating agonist (DUNLOP and SHANKS 1968). As β-blockers are competitive antagonists, it follows that in the absence of stimulation they have little effect. Thus in humans there may be only a small fall in heart rate and cardiac output at rest, but during exercise the effect progressively increases (REYBROUCK et al. 1977). There is very little difference between cardioselective and non-selective blockers in their cardiac effects. β_2-blockers have also been reported to produce a small fall in heart rate (VINCENT et al. 1985; B. DAHLOF et al. 1983). Compounds with intrinsic stimulant activity, like pindolol, can prevent the fall in cardiac output and heart rate (MAN IN'T VELD and SCHALEKAMP 1982; see Sect. 4.18).

After the injection of a β-blocker the heart rate falls quite quickly and reaches a minimum in 30–90 min. Cardiac output falls over the same period of time (LUND-JOHANSEN 1974; SVENDSEN et al. 1979). It is important to note this timing since cardiac β-blockade is achieved without an appreciable change in blood pressure. The dissociation in time between the development of full cardiac β-blockade and fall in blood pressure will be considered in more detail in discussion of the antihypertensive action of β-blockers (Sect. 4.20).

Finally, in addition to its dual effects on the heart, noradrenaline has an indirect effect through its trophic action on cells (BLAES and BOISSEL 1983). β-Blockers prevent the cardiac hypertrophy induced by exercise (OSTMAN-SMITH 1981) and reverse ventricular hypertrophy in hypertension (ROWLANDS et al. 1982; DUNN et al. 1987).

4.3 Peripheral Blood Vessels

The blood vessels supplying muscle beds have a rich supply of β_2-receptors. The difference between a cardioselective agent and a β_2-selective one can be shown by comparing the responses to isoprenaline in the heart and hind limb (Fig. 3). The increase in heart rate is blocked by the cardioselective antagonist (atenolol) whilst the vasodilation is preferentially blocked by the β_2-antagonist (ICI 118551).

Infusing propranolol into the brachial artery leads to a small reduction in resting flow (BRICK et al. 1966; HARTLING et al. 1980). It also inhibits the dilator effect of isoprenaline infusions and converts the vasodilator response of adrenaline to a constrictor one. When propranolol is given orally, forearm and muscle blood flow falls. A reduction in skin blood flow has been seen with all the β-blockers that have been examined, whether they are of β_1- or β_2-type (GILLAM and PRICHARD 1966; MCSORLEY and WARREN 1978). The fall in skin blood flow is almost certainly due to a reflex response initiated by the fall in cardiac output and not due to the direct effect of β-blockade per se.

The fall in cardiac output leads to a uniform reduction in blood flow to all tissues, and the distribution of blood flow is not greatly altered (NIES et al. 1973). The reduction in coronary blood flow by β-blockers (WOLFSON and GORLIN 1969) is due partly to a direct effect and partly to the decreased oxygen requirement of the heart. The splanchnic area suffers the same reduction in flow as other parts of the body (PRICE et al. 1966), but here it appears that non-selective agents may have a greater effect than those affecting only β_1-receptors.

4.4 Renal Effect

β-Blockers affect the kidney in several ways. Some effects are secondary to the circulatory changes and others, to a local action. In humans renal plasma flow and glomerular filtration rate are reduced (DELEEUW and BIRKENHÄGER 1983). This also applies to dogs and rats (NIES et al. 1971; LEES 1968; SMITS et al. 1982). Nadolol and timolol may be exceptions, since renal blood flow appears to be preserved (BERNSTEIN and O'CONNOR 1984; DUPONT et al. 1985). The reasons for these exceptions are not clear.

Subjects who experience a fall in blood pressure with propranolol show little decline in renal plasma flow and glomerular filtration rate, whereas those who fail to respond suffer a decrease in both (DELEEUW and BIRKENHÄGER 1982). Reductions in renal plasma flow and filtration rate tend to be greater after acute β-blockade than after chronic therapy (VAN BAAK et al. 1985).

The effect of β-blockers on renal tubular function and electrolyte excretion is unclear. Although the renal tubules are innervated by the sympathetic nervous system, a direct tubular action of β-blockers has not been demonstrated. However, whether by a direct or indirect action, β-blockers can affect sodium excretion. Sodium excretion falls acutely after propranolol in anaesthetised dogs (NIES et al. 1971), but a short-lived diuresis occurs in rats (LEES 1968; SMITS et al. 1982). In humans sodium balance is usually unaffected by β-blockade (WEBER and DRAYER 1980; WILKINSON 1982). This is interesting since it would be expected that the reduction in cardiac output induces sodium retention. It is possible, therefore, that a direct action producing diuresis is matched by an increase in sympathetic tone acting in the opposite direction. Changes in electrolyte excretion are not great enough to influence body fluid volumes (SEDERBERG OLSEN and IBSEN 1972; BAUER 1983; TSUKIYAMA et al. 1983; MATUNAGA et al. 1977).

4.5 Plasma Renin Activity

β-Blockers lower resting and stimulated plasma renin activity, and this is achieved at modest doses (WINER et al. 1969; BUHLER et al. 1972; MICHELAKIS and MCALLISTER 1972; ESLER et al. 1977; LEONETTI et al. 1975). The importance of this in the antihypertensive effect of β-blockers will be discussed in Sect. 4.20.2. The effect on renin is a β_1-action. However, renin release is affected by two mechanisms independent of the sympathetic nerves; the sodium content of proximal tubular fluid and renal perfusion pressure. It is not surprising, therefore, that β-blockers only halve the prevailing level of plasma renin activity. First, plasma aldosterone will fall, and second, the glomerular and tubular effects of angiotensin will be reduced. The fall in aldosterone might be off-set by the reduced hepatic blood flow.

4.6 Catecholamines

A small increase in plasma catecholamines occurs with blockade (RAHN et al. 1978; ESLER et al. 1981). This effect is not found consistently, probably because it depends upon the level of autonomic tone prevailing at the time of the study (GROBECKER et al. 1977; DE CHAMPLAIN et al. 1977). The rise in catecholamines induced by exercise and mental stress may be exaggerated (N.J. CHRISTENSEN et al. 1975; GROBECKER et al. 1977; TRAP-JENSEN et al. 1982). Likewise, the raised adrenaline levels resulting from hypoglycaemia are exaggerated by β-blockade (SCHLUTER et al. 1982). This is a β_2-effect.

4.7 Peripheral Autonomic Nerves

The nerve terminals of the autonomic nervous system possess receptors which modify the quantity of transmitter released with each nerve impulse (STARKE 1977). Presynaptic β_2-receptors enhance the released of noradrenaline (MAJEWSKI et al. 1980). Thus, isoprenaline leads to an increase in plasma noradrenaline, an effect which is blocked by propranolol (VINCENT et al. 1982). Adrenaline has a greater affinity than noradrenaline for the β_2-receptor. Having been secreted by the adrenal gland, this catecholamine can either have a direct effect on transmitter release or, being taken up by the nerve terminals, have an indirect effect when it is release again by nerve stimulation (MAJEWSKI et al. 1980). Increased adrenaline levels occur in some hypertensive patients (FRANCO-MORSELLI et al. 1977; AMANN et al. 1981; DOMINIAK and GROBECKER 1982). A non-selective β-blocker would prevent the presynaptic action of this adrenaline. The possible role of presynaptic blockade in lowering blood pressure will be considered in Sect. 4.20.1.

4.8 Nerve Activity

The effects of β-blockers on sympathetic nerve activity are conflicting. P.J. LEWIS and HAEUSLER (1975) reported that propranolol decreases splanchnic nerve activity in conscious rabbits. MAJCHERCZYK et al. (1987) on the other hand have shown that propranolol and metoprolol increase renal nerve activity in conscious rats. β-blockers reduce the level of tyrosine hydroxylase in sympathetic ganglia after chronic propranolol administration (RAINE and CHUBB 1977), which would be consistent with a decrease in nerve activity. Neural sympathetic activity, which can be measured in humans from the peroneal nerve, is increased acutely after intravenous metoprolol (SUNDLOF et al. 1983) at a time when it is known that peripheral resistance increases. After chronic therapy, however, sympathetic activity falls back to pretreatment levels or little below it (WALLIN et al. 1984).

4.9 Baroreflex

DUNLOP and SHANKS (1969) observed that the pressor response to carotid occlusion was reduced after chronic treatment with propranolol in animals, although there was no change after a single dose. Baroreceptor discharge appears to fall with β-blockade (DORWARD and KORNER 1978; SCOTT and WILLIAMS 1982). In humans the position regarding the sensitivity of the baroreflex to β-blockade is confused. Some observers have indicated that with acute administration of these agents there is a reduction in the sensitivity of the reflex (PICKERING et al. 1972; TAKESHITA et al. 1975), although this has not been confirmed (SIMON et al. 1977; WATSON et al. 1979). Using the neck chamber method, an increase in the sensitivity of the reflex has been reported (ECKBERG et al. 1960). After chronic treatment there seems to be agreement that the sensitivity of the reflex is unchanged (SIMON et al. 1977; KREDIET and DUNNING 1979; WATSON et al. 1979; PARATI et al. 1983).

4.10 Chemoreflexes

Aortic chemoreceptors are stimulated primarily by hypoxia. β-Receptor agonists such as isoprenaline stimulate these receptors, and it has been proposed that oxygen chemoreception is dependent on β-adrenergic mechanisms (BARCROFT et al. 1957; BUTLAND et al. 1982; FOLGERING et al. 1982). This proposal has been challenged by MULLIGAN et al. (1986). They showed that although propranolol could block the effects of isoprenaline on chemoreceptor responses, it failed to affect the response of aortic chemoreceptors to hypoxia and hypotension, which suggests that β-receptors are not an integral part of oxygen chemoreception. However, the situation is complicated by the fact that β-agonists also decrease plasma potassium levels, an effect which will decrease chemoreceptor responsiveness; hyperkalaemia stimulates aortic chemoreceptors and hence respiration (BAND and LINTON 1986). Thus, the contribution of the direct and indirect effects of β-agonists on chemoreceptor responses has still to be fully evaluated. The stimulant effect of carbond dioxide on breathing is reduced by β-blockers (MUSTCHIN et al. 1976; PATRICK et al. 1978). However, the stimulant action of potassium on the chemoreceptors is reduced by β-blockers (PATERSON and NYE 1988).

4.11 Central Nervous Effects

β-Receptors are to be found in the brain, particularly in the ascending reticular formation (IVERSEN 1977). Both β_1- and β_2-receptors are present in the posterior hypothalamus, but only β_1-receptors appear to be concerned with cardiovascular control (PHILIPPU and STROEHL 1978). In the locus coeruleus, an area of the brain concerned with alertness and cardiovascula regulation, the receptors are mainly of the β_2-subtype, and chronic treatment with propranolol reduces the firing rate of the neurons found in this region (C. DAHLOF 1981). β-Blockers produce EEG changes (ROUBICEK 1976), and the CNS side effects of insomnia and vivid dreams suggest a central action (TYRER and LADER 1974). β-blockers also have an anxiolytic effect (SUZMAN 1981). All these actions are more prominent with the lypophilic, non-selective agents.

4.12 Tremor

Benign essential tremor, although present in everyone, is prominent in a certain proportion of subjects. It is made worse by emotional stress or movement. It is known that i.v. infusion of either adrenaline or isoprenaline exaggerates the tremor. This is almost certainly due to an effect on β_2-receptors since tremor can be produced by β_2-selective agonists, such as salbutamolol, and is blocked by propranolol and the selective β_2-blocker, ICI 118551 (ARNOLD et al. 1983; ABILA et al. 1985). The coarse tremor produced by Parkinson's disease almost certainly uses some mechanisms in common with physiological tremor, and there is evidence that it is improved somewhat by non-selective β-blockers. Cerebellar tremor on the other hand is not influenced by β-blockers.

4.13 Respiratory Effects

Bronchial smooth muscles are innervated by the sympathetic nervous system to induce bronchial dilatation. The receptors involved are predominantly of the β_2-type (LANDS et al. 1967), especially in humans, in whom there is little evidence for β_1-receptors (CARSWELL and NAHORSKI 1983; CARSTAIRS et al. 1985). In other species the proportion of β_2- to β_1-receptors in the lung can vary. In normal subjects β-blockers produce very little effect on the resistance to air flow (TATTERSFIELD et al. 1973). However, in asthmatics, with sensitised bronchial smooth muscle, in whome the calibre is critically dependent upon inhibitory sympathetic tone, β-blockers increase airways resistance (JOHNSSON et al. 1975; ASTROM 1975; MCNEILL 1964). Non-selective β-blockers also tend to prevent the dilator response to bronchodilators, especially β_2-stimulants (JOHNSSON et al. 1975). Asthmatic subjects, in a quiescent phase, will usually tolerate β_1-blockers (ASTROM 1975; BENSON et al. 1978), and if bronchospasm occurs they will respond to β-stimulants (DECALMER et al. 1978). Patients with chronic bronchitis and emphysema may not tolerate non-selective β-blockers. The cilia lining the airways down to the terminal bronchi are also affected by β-stimulants and blocked by non-selective agents (DOROW et al. 1984; PAVIA et al. 1986).

Partial stimulant activity (ISA) can, in some degree, prevent bronchoconstriction induced by non-selective blockers (C.C. Christensen et al. 1978). These agents, however, still appear to impair the relaxation produced by β-stimulants (Benson and Graf 1977; C.C. Christensen et al. 1978; Lammers et al. 1985).

4.14 Glucose Metabolism

The sympathetic nervous system can influence carbohydrate metabolism by many different mechanisms, and it is very difficult to define the exact role and subtype of α- and β-receptor involved in this process. However, catecholamines stimulate glycogenolysis in muscle and liver, and adrenaline-induced hyperglycaemia can be blocked by a combination of non-selective α- and β-blockers (Lant 1980). It is known that glucose formation in the liver from blood lactate is also affected by β_2-receptors (Garber et al. 1976). Overall, β-blockers produce little effect on blood glucose (Shand 1975), but hypoglycaemia can occur when the glycogen reserve of the liver is reduced during fasting or in subjects under stress. The hgypoglycaemic response to insulin is prolonged by non-selective agents (U. Smith and Lager 1978). These effects have implications for the treatment of diabetic patients with non-selective β-blockers.

Lactate production by working muscle is impaired by β-blockers (Hartling et al. 1980), and this applies to heart muscle as well as to skeletal muscle (Mueller et al. 1974).

Finally, insulin secretion is in some degree under the control of β_2-receptors (Harms et al. 1978). β_2-selective antagonists, such as ICI 118551, inhibit the release of insulin induced by isoprenaline, whereas β_1-selective blockers such as atenolol and epanolol have negligible effects at β_1-selective doses. None of these antagonists affected resting plasma insulin levels (H.J. Smith et al. 1983). The overall control, therefore, of diabetes is not directly affected by β-blockers, but a response to hypoglycaemia may be blunted. It is interesting to note that the high insulin levels associated with insulinoma can be reduced by β-blockers (Blum et al. 1983).

4.15 Lipid Metabolism

Triglycerides stored in fat cells are hydrolysed to fatty acids and glycerol and then transported to the liver or to muscle for metabolism. The hormone activating the lipolytic process is stimulated by catecholamines. Although the receptors mediating lipolysis were classified as the β_1-subtype (Lands et al. 1967), work by Ablad et al. (1975) suggests that in humans there may be a mixture of β_1 and β_2. Catecholamines, given by injection or released by stress, increase free-fatty acid levels, an effect which is blocked by both types of β-antagonists (Harms et al. 1978; J.L. Day et al. 1982).

Plasma triglyceride levels increase with both selective and non-selective β-blockers (England et al. 1978; J.L. Day et al. 1982), and the ratio of HDL is reduced in relation to LDL (J.L. Day et al. 1982; Weidman et al. 1983).

Non-shivering thermogenesis, which results in a high rate of metabolism in brown fat, is stimulated by adrenaline and by insulin. The type of receptor involved in this process has not been properly characterised, but it appears to be neither of the β_1- nor β_2-type (ARCH et al. 1984). Propranolol inhibits thermogenesis in rats but not in humans (SEATON et al. 1985).

4.16 Thyroid

Some of the manifestations of thyrotoxicosis respond to β-blockade. For example, tremor and tachycardia are reduced, and the sense of well-being is restored. However, β-blockers do not restore elevated oxygen consumption to normal and fail to affect exophalmos. β-Blockers also affect the tissue conversion of thyroxine (T4) to triiodothyronine (T3) (FEELY et al. 1979).

In thyrotoxicosis there appears to be a preference for non-selective blockers, although compounds with intrinsic activity are not as effective as others (McDEVITT and NELSON 1978).

4.17 Serum Potassium

The administration of adrenaline causes an initial rise in serum potassium followed by a prolonged fall (D'SILVA 1934; BROWN et al. 1983). The initial increase is mediated by activation of hepatic α- and β-receptors, whilst the hypokalaemic effect is mediated by stimulation of β_2-receptors in skeletal muscle and liver. During exercise, serum potassium rises (LINTON et al. 1984). In the presence of β-blockade, the resting serum potassium level tends to rise (BATEMAN et al. 1979), and the rise with exercise is accentuated (LINTON et al. 1984). The rise in serum potassium is greater with the non-selective agents. The fall in serum potassium may be of considerable practical importance since the adrenaline-induced hypokalaemia is reversed by non-selective and β_2-selective blockers but only partially modified by cardioselective blockers (STRUTHERS et al. 1983). Since there is evidence that hypokalaemia increases the incidence of ventricular arrhythmias, it may well be that the benefit from β-blockade treatment in myocardial infarct is in part due to the reduction in adrenaline-induced hypokalaemia. Of therapeutic interest is the fact that the rise in serum potassium resulting from β-blockade nicely balances the loss induced by diuretics (BATEMAN et al. 1979).

4.18 Intrinsic Sympathomimetic Activity

After occupying the β-receptor, some compounds are able to stimulate the receptor and produce a response that is less than that produced by a full agonist. At the same time these compounds, known as partial agonists, prevent full agonists such as noradrenaline and adrenaline from occupying the receptor and exerting their effects. Thus, dichlorisoprenaline is capable of producing nearly the full effect of isoprenaline, and yet it blocks the response of this agent. Compounds can therefore be classified according to the maximal effect they will

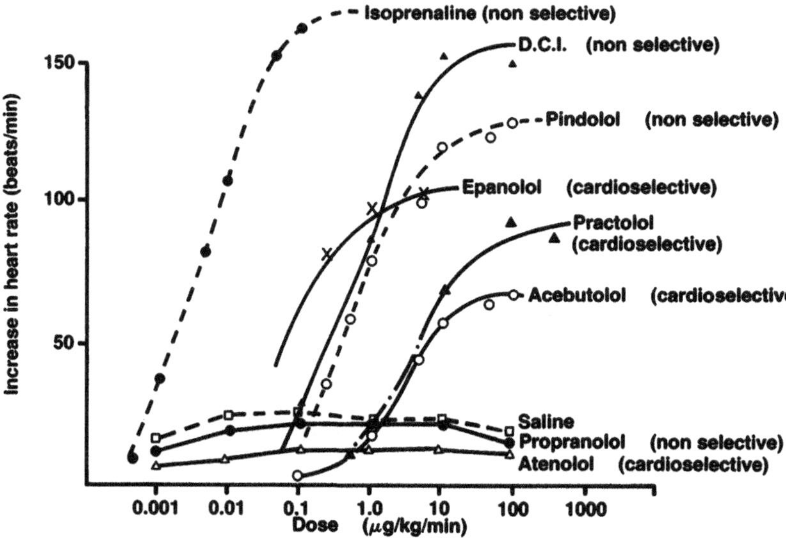

Fig. 4. Quantitative assessment of intrinsic sympathomimetic activity in rat atria

produce on a tissue as compared with isoprenaline (Fig. 4). To measure the amount of intrinsic stimulant activity (ISA) it is advisable first to abolish resting sympathetic activity. This can be done in the laboratory by pretreatment of an animal with syrosingopine, which depletes the tissues of catecholamines.

Using heart rate as the response in anaesthetised rats, it can be shown that the scale of ISA is dichloroisoprenaline > pindolol > epanolol > practolol > acebutolol (Bilski et al. 1979). The measurement of ISA depends to some extent upon the species, the preparation and the conditions under which the measurement is made. It can be shown, however, that measurement of heart rate in rats reasonably predicts the rank order of intrinsic activity in humans. This was beautifully demonstrated by Svendsen et al. (1981, 1987), who showed that in humans the reduction in resting cardiac ouput inversely correlated with the ISA level of the compound (Fig. 5). The partial agonist pindolol has also been compared with propranolol over a 24-h period on resting heart rate in humans. In awake subjects pindolol has a smaller effect than propranolol. However, during sleep, when sympathetic activity is minimal, heart rate actually rises above control with pindolol. This is in contrast to propranolol which produces a fall at that time (Floras et al. 1982).

Although pindolol is the most potent β-blocker and has the highest ISA amongst the compounds listed in Table 3, the order of ISA strength does not correspond to the antagonist potency of these compounds as β-blockers. A further complication to understanding ISA is provided by the demonstration that for some compounds the dose required for ISA may differ from that required for β-blockade. For example, pindolol, oxprenolol and acebutolol all produce blockade alone at the lowest doses, and ISA emerges with increasing doses (non-classical ISA) (Fig. 6). By contrast practolol and epanolol produce

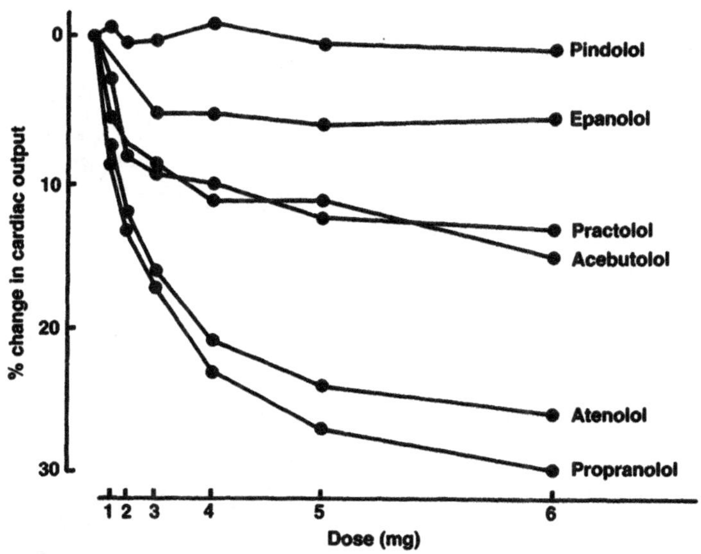

Fig. 5. Effect of intrinsic activity on cardiac output. *Note*: With pindolol, cardiac output is maintained by two mechanisms, cardiac stimulation and β_2-dilatation. For epanolol, practolol and acebutolol, it is sustained by cardiac stimulation. Epanolol does not lower blood pressure. Practolol and acebutolol are less effective, and the greatest fall is achieved by the two non-stimulant agents, propranolol and atenolol. (Data from the work of SYENDSEN et al. 1979, 1981)

Table 3. β-Blocker pharmacological profile

Approved name	Approx. potency (propranolol)	Daily dose range (mg)	Cardio-selectivity	Intrinsic sympathomimetic activity
Acebutolol	0.3	400–1200	+	+
Alprenolol	0.3	40–400	–	+
Atenolol	1.0	50–100	++	–
Epanolol	1.0	50–200	++	++
Labetalol	0.3	200–800	–	–
Metoprolol	0.8–1.0	100–400	++	–
Nadolol	0.5–1.0	40–240	–	–
Oxprenolol	0.5–1.0	120–480	–	++
Penbutolol	4.0	40–80	–	+
Pindolol	6.0	15–45	–	+++
Propranolol	1.0	30–320	–	–
Sotalol	0.3	120–600	–	–
Timolol	6.0	10–60	–	–

blockade and stimulation at the same doses (BILSKI et al. 1988). This is typical for classical partial agonists. The anomalous behaviour of non-classic compounds can best be explained by postulating that there are at least two types of cardiac receptor with differing efficacy and/or affinity for the agonist activity. It is misleading therefore to classify β-blockers only according to the presence or

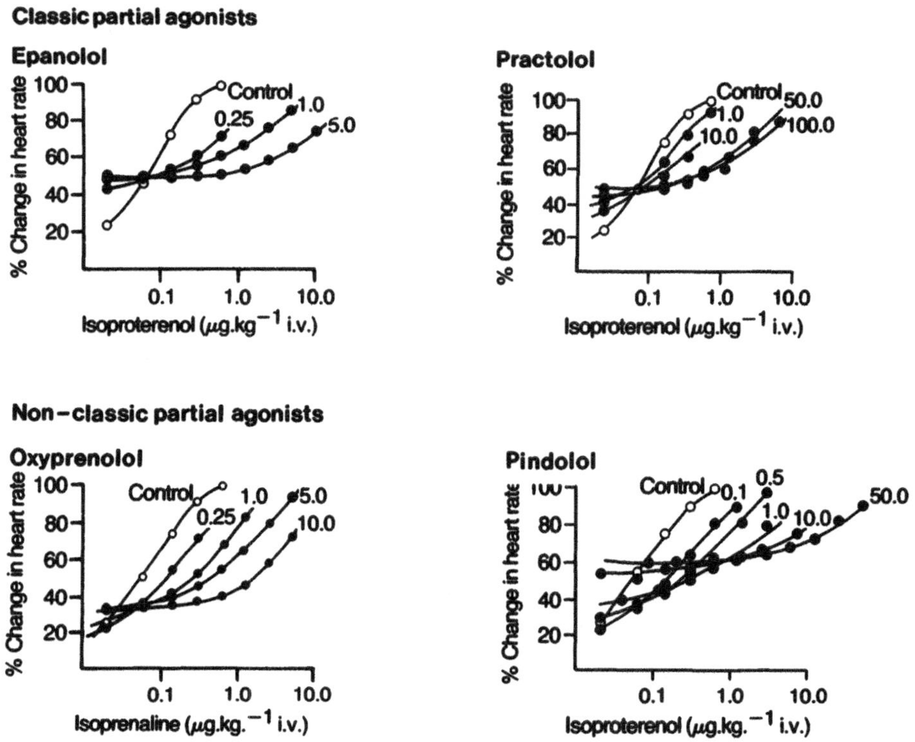

Fig. 6. Classic and non-classic intrinsic activity tested in rat atria

degree of ISA (FITZGERALD 1969). The ratio of blockade to stimulant activity at different doses is important. To avoid confusion, compounds should be analysed at the doses at which they are to be used clinically. The findings in this rat preparation have been broadly confirmed in humans. Pindolol in small doses has been shown to reduce heart rate, whereas higher doses produce blockade without affecting heart rate (ANDREN and HANNSON 1982). A similar picture is seen with oxprenolol, with which a reduction in heart rate during exercise is similar to that produced by propranolol when low doses are used, but higher doses have significantly less effect (HARRY et al. 1979).

ISA can vary according to tissue subtype; for example, xamoterol has partial agonist activity at the cardiac β_1-receptor (43% of the maximum increase produced by isoprenaline) but no agonist activity at the vascular β_2-receptor (NUTTALL and SNOW 1982). By contrast, pindolol has agonist activity on both the receptors, although the level of this activity at the two receptors is different. This plays a part in the unusual haemodynamic profile of pindolol, which is unique in reducing resistance in the forearm (ATTERHOG et al. 1977).

In conclusion, ISA is an important property of some β-blockers, and it determines in a large degree the effect that each compound will have on heart rate, cardiac output and vascular and bronchial resistances, particularly at rest when ISA is low. In order to identify the pharmacological profile of a β-blocker with ISA it is necessary to determine both its agonist and antagonist selectivities as well as the subtype of its intrinsic agonist activities. These properties may have important clinical relevance to the treatment of ischaemic heart disease, and, as will be shown later (Sect. 4.20.3), it has a bearing on our understanding of the antihypertensive activity of these molecules.

4.19 Other Actions

β-Receptors are to be found in various tissue membranes throughout the body. The function of many of these, for example those on red cells, is obscure. However, the uterus, which contains β_2-receptors, is relaxed by β_2-agonists. These agents have been used to inhibit premature labour. Paradoxically, however, β-blockers do not appear to induce premature labour (RUBIN 1981). Likewise, although the gut contains many β_2-receptors, which raise the possibility of motility problems with these agents, only occasional digestive symptoms occur during treatment.

Tear production and intra-orbital pressure are reduced (POTTER 1981), and platelet aggregation is inhibited (MEHTA et al. 1978) by non-selective blockers. Thromboxane production is also reduced (MEHTA et al. 1983; JACKSON and CAMPBELL 1981). It is not certain whether this action is in fact due to β-blockade, and the clinical relevance of this finding has yet to be assessed.

4.20 Mechanism of Action in Lowering Blood Pressure

When β-blockers were first introduced, it was not generally accepted that they lowered blood pressure. However, PRICHARD and GILLAM (1964, 1969) and later ZACHARIAS and COWEN (1970) proved conclusively that this group of agents does in fact possess antihypertensive properties. Their mode of action in lowering blood pressure has been the subject of controversy, although with the accumulation of more information, a clearer picture is now emerging. Details of the antihypertensive effects of individual β-blockers is given in an excellent review article by VAN BAAK et al. (1975).

The characteristics of the blood pressure response to β-blockers is important for any discussion of their mode of action. Blood pressure falls both in the recumbent and standing positions in equal degree, although unexpectedly the blood pressure variability is not reduced (WATSON et al. 1979). The effect on blood pressure is present both by day and by night (FLORAS et al. 1982), but it is more prominent when sympathetic tone is high, for example during exercise (SHINEBOURNE et al. 1967; LUND-JOHANSEN 1974; REYBROUCK et al. 1977). During sleep, when sympathetic tone is low, the effect is minimal (FLORAS et al. 1982). Cardiac output falls as heart rate declines (TARAZI and DUSTAN 1972; LUND-JOHANSEN 1974; SVENDSEN et al. 1979; TSUKIYAMA et al. 1982). There is no difference in the effectiveness of selective as compared with non-selective β-blockers in lowering blood pressure (ÅMERY et al. 1976b; CRUICKSHANK 1980), although under circumstances in which circulating adrenaline levels are raised, for example after smoking, during stress or hypoglycaemia, the selective agents are superior to the non-selective (VAN HERWAARDEN et al. 1977; TRAP JENSEN et al. 1979). It should be mentioned here that the fall in cardiac output and heart rate, which occurs about 30 min after oral administration, is not accompanied by a fall in blood pressure. This follows some hours later. This delay has to be considered in any theory regarding the mechanism for this action, as does the fact that β_1-blockade alone is sufficient to lower blood pressure.

4.20.1 Nervous Action

It has been suggested that β-blockers exert their effects through a central action since administration into the cerebral ventricular system lowers blood pressure (H.D. DAY and ROACH 1974). However, this effect is probably due to a spill-over of the β-blocker into the systemic circulation (SMITS 1979, 1980). β-Blockers probably do not reduce sympathetic tone since circulating levels of catecholamines tend to rise rather than fall after β-blockade (see Sect. 4.6 and a review by MAN IN'T VELD and SCHALEKAMP 1983). Sympathetic nerve discharge in the peroneal nerve rises immediately after the administration of β-blocker and subsequently falls to about the control level. Also, although the β-receptors in the CNS are not of uniform subtype, in the locus coeruleus, an important adrenergic area concerned with the control of blood pressure, they are of the β_2-subtype (C. DAHLOF 1981). It could thus be expected that non-selective β-blockers are more effective than selective agents, which is not the case.

It has also been suggested that β-blockers exert their effects by a peripheral presynaptic action, which lowers blood pressure by reducing the release of noradrenaline (MAN IN'T VELD and SCHALEKAMP 1982). There are several problems with this theory. First, there is no delay in the onset of the presynaptic blockade. Second, the presynaptic receptors are of the β_2-type (C. DAHLOF 1981), and a β-blocker which selectively antagonises the β_2-receptor (ICI 118551) has little effect on blood pressure (B. DAHLOF et al. 1983; ROBB et al. 1985). VINCENT et al. (1985) have shown a small fall in blood pressure, but this was accompanied by a small fall in heart rate.

So how do β-blockers lower blood pressure? Central nervous and peripheral presynaptic actions seem unlikely mechanisms. It is known that selective β_1-blockers are effective in lowering blood pressure whilst β_2-blockers are not. It is therefore possible that the organs most likely to be involved in the fall in blood pressure are those which contain mainly β_1-receptors, namely the kidney and the heart. The activities of the β-receptors in these two organs will now be reviewed.

4.20.2 Plasma Renin Activity

β-Blocking agents lower renin levels (Sect. 4.5), and it has been suggested that the fall in blood pressure with β-blockers results from this fall in renin. Although there is a delay in the fall in blood pressure after the fall in plasma renin, renin involvement is still possible, since blood vessels contain renin with a slower turnover than that of plasma. Subjects with low renin levels show little reduction in blood pressure whilst those with high renin levels show a greater reduction

(BUHLER et al. 1972, 1973; AMERY et al. 1976b). A renin mechanism for the antihypertensive effect of β-blockers is nevertheless disputed (e.g. PEDERSEN and KORNERUP 1977; BRAVO et al. 1975; MORGAN et al. 1975). The reason for this is that the demonstrated relationship between the fall in blood pressure and plasma renin activity is determined by the extremes. These extremes form a small proportion of the population of hypertensive patients. For the majority, a relationship between the fall in renin and the change in blood pressure cannot be found. The plasma concentrations of β-blocker required to reduce renin is much smaller than that required to lower blood pressure (LEONETTI et al. 1975). Although low plasma concentrations of β-blocker reduce both renin and blood pressure, higher concentrations produce a further fall in blood pressure with little change in plasma renin activity (ESLER et al. 1977; HOLLIFIELD et al. 1976). This is the clearest evidence that at least two effects of β-blockers are involved in the fall in blood pressure.

4.20.3 Cardiovascular Effects

With intravenous or oral administration of β-blockers, heart rate and cardiac output fall within about 30 min. However, blood pressure does not change (FITZGERALD 1978) but falls 3–8 h later (FITZGERALD et al. 1978; LEONETTI et al. 1980; COLFER et al. 1984). Total peripheral resistance rises initially to compensate for the fall in cardiac output. However, it then declines over a period of time.

In SHR following oral β-blockade, cardiac output falls and total peripheral resistance rises, as it does in humans. The rise in total peripheral resistance is due to reflex vasoconstriction initiated by the baroreceptor since, if the buffer nerves are cut, the delay in the fall in blood pressure is greatly reduced (STRUYKER BOUDIER et al. 1982; SMITS and STRUYKER BOUDIER 1982). Thus, the fall in cardiac output triggers the baroreceptor reflex to sustain blood pressure by increasing sympathetic vasoconstriction (Sect. 4.9). However, with time this reflex activity wanes, and though cardiac output remains depressed total peripheral resistance falls to pretreatment levels (TARAZI and DUSTAN 1972; AMERY et al. 1976a). The major problem in understanding the mechanisms responsible for the fall in blood pressure is to understand why in some subjects the baroreceptor control wanes while in others it sustains blood pressure at its pretreatment levels.

In rats it has been shown that a natriuresis helps to lower blood pressure (SMITS et al. 1982), and in this species catecholamine release from the adrenal medulla maintains blood pressure immediately after β-blockade (BUCKINGHAM and HAMILTON 1980). The importance of this α-receptor-mediated sympathetic tone occurring immediately after β-blockade can be demonstrated by studies with labetolol, which is a β-blocker with α-sympathetic antagonist properties. With this agent, blood pressure falls immediately (ROSEI et al. 1975).

The pattern observed after 24 h of β-blockade is then sustained over a period of years of treatment with β-blockers (LUND JOHANSEN 1974, 1979). Stroke volume tends, however, to return towards normal, and cardiac output rises a little (WIKSTRAND et al. 1983), and this may be a result of regression of the cardiac and vascular hypertrophy (ROWLANDS et al. 1982; DUNN et al. 1987).

The blood pressure reduction induced by β-blockers results from the fall in heart rate and cardiac output. This mechanism of action has been disputed because β-blockers with ISA tend to lower blood pressure with minimal effects on cardiac output (MAN IN'T VELD and SCHALEKAMP 1983). However, this finding rests very much on the effects of pindolol, which tends to lower blood pressure to the same degree as other β-blockers while cardiac output does not fall. Pindolol has other properties besides ISA for the heart. It has β_2-stimulant activity, which dilates peripheral blood vessels, and this action will sustain cardiac output and lower blood pressure (ATTERHOG et al. 1977; MAAREK et al. 1986; see Sect. 4.3). The mechanism of action of agents with non-selective β-stimulant properties differs from other compounds.

To test whether a fall in cardiac output is essential for a reduction in blood pressure, it is necessary to administer classic partial agonists, differing only in the level of β_1-agonist activity on the heart. There are fortunately three compounds, practolol, epanolol and acebutolol, which with atenolol provide a range of ISA from none with atenolol to a high level with epanolol. There is a profound fall in cardiac output with atenolol and a lesser effect with the compounds according to the level of ISa (Fig. 5). It can be shown that atenolol is the most effective agent in lowering blood pressure, whereas epanolol has little effect (SYENDSEN et al. 1987; B. DAHLOF et al. 1983; LEONETTI et al. 1985).

In conclusion, therefore, the antihypertensive action of β-blockers depends upon at least two actions. The first, observed at low doses, is due to a reduction in renin. The second is almost certainly due to a fall in cardiac output and heart rate. Subjects with high levels of sympathetic tone, as evidence by high plasma renin activity and elevated plasma noradrenaline levels, tend to have the greatest fall in blood pressure. (ESLER et al. 1976; MYERS and DE CHAMPLAIN 1983).

5 Therapeutic Use

5.1 Characteristics of the Antihypertensive Effect of β-Blockers

The demonstration by PRICHARD and GILLAM (1964) of the antihypertensive effect of β-blockers has been confirmed in numerous studies, and these agents are now the most commonly used first line therapy for hypertension. The reported falls in blood pressure vary considerably, ranging from 17–24 mmHg systolic to 7–15 mmHg diastolic. The effects are smaller during sleep than they are in the awake state and are greater during exercise (SHINEBOURNE et al. 1967; REYBROUCK et al. 1977). All forms of hypertension respond reasonably well, except with very low renin hypertnsion (BUHLER et al. 1973). There is a limit to the fall in blood pressure, and troublesome hypotension does not commonly occur. This is an advantage of this particular group of antihypertensive drugs.

Argument has surrounded several points in their usage: the dosage required, the proportion of subjects in a population responding, the type of subject likely to respond and possible benefits of therapy other than lowering blood pressure. Blood pressure estimations in the clinic are so variable that accurate dose-response relationships to any antihypertensive agent is difficult to establish. While early studies recommended rather high doses of propranolol (PRICHARD and GILLAM 1969; ZACHARIAS et al. 1972), the effective dose for the majority of patients has been shown to be lower than that originally employed (PETRIE et al. 1983).

Although most subjects show some fall in blood pressure with β-blockers, estimations vary regarding the proportion of patients who wil respond adequately to them. The effect depends critically upon the population studied, and estimations of the proportion of responders can only be gained from large-scale trials. Very roughly, these show that an adequate response occurs in approximately 50% of the population (Veterans Administration 1977; Medical Research Council 1985). Thus, the proportion of patients responding to β-blockers does not differ from other commonly used antihypertensive agents.

As the plasma renin level falls with age, it follows that older subjects should respond less well to β-blockade (BUHLER et al. 1972). This generalisation is not strong enough, however, to be a guide to the treatment of individual subjects, and the largest trial done has shown that the blood pressure response in older subjects was in fact greater than in the young (Medical Research Council 1985). Patients with high levels of sympathetic tone tend to respond well to β-blockers. Black patients, who tend to have low plasma renin levels, respond poorly to β-blockers (RICHARDSON et al. 1968), although Asian subjects respond as well as Caucasians (SEEDAT et al. 1973). β-Blockers are effective and safe in the treatment of hypertension in pregnancy (REDMAN 1980; RUBIN 1981). There is no evidence for tolerance to the antihypertensive effect of β-blockers with time (RICHARD and GILLAM 1969; ZACHARIAS 1976). Sodium retention, however, can occur, and when this happens blood, pressure control is lost (AMERY et al. 1976a).

5.2 Therapeutic Benefit

Lowering blood pressure controls hypertensive heart failure, arrests renal damage and reduces the incidence of stroke. In addition, after myocardial infarction β-blockers will reduce the incidence of renal infarction. (HJALMARSON et al. 1981, Norwegian Multi-Centre Study Group 1981; Beta-Blocker Heart Attack Trial Research Group 1982). There is also the suggestion that β-blockers may have a role in the primary prevention of myocardial infarction (STEWART 1976; LAMBERT 1977; CRUICKSHANK et al. 1987). Although some trials have failed to demonstrate this, the trend is certainly discernible when evidence from all the trials is examined.

A further beneficial effect of β-blockers is their ability to reverse left ventricular hypertrophy. This has been demonstrated in animal preparations (VAUGHAN WILLIAMS and RAINE 1974) and in humans (ROWLANDS et al. 1982; TARAZI 1985; DUNN et al. 1987). Vascular hypertrophy is also reversed (WEISS et al. 1974).

6 Combinations

The use of β-blockers with diuretics is a logical combination since it is known that the failure to respond to diuretics results from the rise in plasma renin activity caused by a loss of sodium. In general, β-blockers produce greater falls in blood pressure than diuretics, but in combination their effects are additive (PETRIE et al. 1975; ANDERSEN 1982). In the more severe form of hypertension combined treatment is likely to control about 60% of patients (ZACHARIAS et al. 1977, CRUICKSHANK et al. 1987).

The reflex tachycardia observed with vasodilators, particularly hydralazine and minoxidol, is well suppressed with β-blockers (GILMORE et al. 1970; ZACHEST et al. 1972), and in combination they produce an additional fall in blood pressure. Although tachycardia is less commonly seen with calcium antagonists, the blood lowering effects are additive with β-blockade. One note of caution with this combination is that β-blockers prolong the P-R interval, a property which they share with the dihydropyridine calcium antagonist verapamil, and their combined use can precipitate heart block. The combination, however, of β-blockers and calcium antagonists is advantageous is that the troublesome side-effects of headache and flushing produced by calcium antagonists are reduced by β-blockers (DANIELS and OPIE 1986; DE DIVITIIS et al. 1985). β-Blockers and methyldopa in combination also produce a greater effect than either drug alone (WEBSTER et al. 1977).

7 Interactions

7.1 Pharmacokinetic Interactions

Lipophilic agents like propranolol which require hepatic metabolism will inevitably be affected by other substances which are also metabolised in the liver. Enzyme-inducing agents like phenobarbitone and rifampicin increase the rates of metabolism and hence reduce the bioavailability of propranolol. Occasionally, it works the other way, in that one agent will reduce the metabolism of another. Hence, chlorpromazine reduces the clearance of propranolol (PEET et al. 1981) as does hydralazine, which appears to reduce the first pass effect (BYRNE et al. 1984; SCHNECK and VRAY 1984). Cimetidine (HEAGERTY et al. 1981) and frusemide (CHIARIELLO et al. 1979) also increase the plasma level of propranolol. β-Blockers may also alter the metabolism and concentration of other compounds. Thus, they increase the blood levels of lignocaine (SCHNECK et al. 1984) and diazepam (HAWKSWORTH et al. 1984).

7.2 Pharmacodynamic Interactions

One of the most clinically important interactions of β-blockers is with the non-steroidal anti-inflammatory drugs. These inhibit the synthesis of renal vasodilator prostaglandins, which may be the reason why they raise diastolic blood pressure by about 15 mmHg and antagonise the antihypertensive action of β-blockers (Watkins et al. 1980). Sulindac, which does not inhibit renal prostaglandin synthesis, shows no such interaction (R.V. Lewis et al. 1986).

Vasoconstrictor substances which may be used for the symptoms of a common cold can achieve blood levels which have a pharmacological action, and the presence of a β-blocker will allow the uninhibited α-vasoconstrictor actions of these agents. This effect is greater with a non-selective than a selective β-blocker. Hypertension upon withdrawal from clonidine is exaggerated for the same reason as the effect of ergot compounds for the treatment of migraine. Smoking raises the plasma adrenaline level, and this leads to a rise in blood pressure in the presence of propranolol (Trap-Jensen et al. 1979).

7.3 Contraindications

Most contraindications to β-blockers arise as a consequence of their pharmacodynamic action. The molecules themselves appear to be relatively free from other toxic effects. The most important absolute contraindication to β-blockers is asthma and bronchitis, in which there are elements of increased bronchial tone. This applies whether asthma is clinically evident or whether there is just a history of it (Benson et al. 1978). Cardioselective blockers carry an advantage as far as pulmonary disease is concerned, since subjects retain a response to β_2-stimulants (Johnsson et al. 1975; Decalmer et al. 1978).

Bradycardia of sufficient degree to produce symptoms can occur with β-blockers, especially if atrioventricular conduction is already compromised by disease or by drugs. A specific example is the sick-sinus syndrome which is an absolute contraindication of β-blockers. When β-blockers were introduced, it was felt that there would be a renal danger of the development of heart failure in subjects with hypertension, but this has in fact not substantially materialised. However, the danger is still a possibility, and the adequacy of the cardiac reserve should be considered in choosing an antihypertensive agent. With the sodium and water retention which accompanies heart failure, blood pressure control is lost (Amery et al. 1976a).

An enhanced level of sympathetic tone or high levels of circulating adrenaline are absolute contraindications to the use of β-blockers unless treatment has been preceded by an α-blocker. Such conditions may be found in the rebound after clonidine medication or with phaeochromocytoma (Conolly et al. 1972; Rosei et al. 1976).

Diabetic patients suffering hypoglycaemic episodes with high levels of circulatory adrenaline may experience a pressor response to non-selective β-blockers. Insulin-dependent diabetes is therefore a relative contraindication to the use of non-selective β-blockers (Armitstead et al. 1983).

8 Side Effects and Toxicity

8.1 Side Effects

The widespread acceptance of β-blockers in the treatment of hypertension attests to their relative freedom from side effects. The occasional unwanted effects resulting directly from the cardiovascular actions of β-blockers have already been considered. In a large therapeutic trial in hypertension, the reasons for withdrawal from treatment with propranolol were lethargy, dyspnoea, nausea, dizziness or headache, impotence and cold hands and feet (Medical Research Council 1985). Vivid dreams have also been reported, and their incidence is probably higher with the lipid soluble agents (BETTS and ALFORD 1985; LEWIS et al. 1984). In an extensive review of the adverse effects on atenolol, a similar range of side effects was reported (CRUICKSHANK 1981; CRUICKSHANK and PRICHARD 1987).

8.2 Toxicity

The widespread acceptance of β-blockers in the treatment of an asymptomatic condition like hypertension attests to their relative freedom from unwanted actions. Some β-blockers, being lipid soluble, have a measure of membrane-stabilising activity. Although there was once a suggestion that some of the actions of propranolol might be due to this effect, this property is clinically irrelevant. However, in suicidal or accidental overdosage, the quinidine-like effect will be evident and depress the heart. It will also contribute to central nervous manifestations of overdosage such as respiratory failure, coma and seizure (WERMUT and WOJCICKI 1973). Sotalol possesses class III antiarrhythmic activity (SINGH and VAUGHAN WILLIAMS 1970), which can lead to a prolonged Q-T interval and a tendency to ventricular extrasystoles and fibrillation (LAAKSO et al. 1981). A high level of ISA can modify the effects of overdosage. For example, with pindolol bradycardia may not occur. This does not appear to be the case with other agents possessing ISA (ELKHARRAT and BISMUTH 1982) and may be dependent upon the level of agonist activity. With practolol, a β-blocking agent which is no longer available, a unique syndrome of keratoconjunctivitis sicca, hyperkeratosis and sclerosing peritonitis occurred (WRIGHT 1974, 1975; FELIX and IVE 1974). This was an immunological phenomenon (AMOS et al. 1975) which has not been fully elucidated. Fortunately, it has not been seen with other β-blockers. Acebutolol, however, is capable of inducing raised antinuclear factor levels (CODY et al. 1979; BURGESS RECORD 1981).

Myalgia and cramps have been reported with β-blockers (YAMAOKI et al. 1983). These can be due to a proximal myopathy, and in some instances muscle enzymes (CPK) levels are elevated. The reported cases have mainly been observed with non-selective β-blockers (FORFAR et al. 1979; IMATAKA et al. 1981).

Acknowledgement. We would like to thank Dr. B. Main of ICI Pharmaceuticals for help with the chemical aspects of this paper.

Summary

The introduction of β-blockers was the practical outcome of basic research into chemical transmission of impulses from nerve endings to the effector cells. The blocking molecules have structural similarities with natural transmitters;

adrenaline and noradrenaline compete with these substances for the β-receptor sites in the membranes of many tissues. There are two types of β-receptors. β_1-receptors are found predominantly in the heart and kidney and are closely innervated. The β_2-receptors are more widely distributed but are concentrated mainly in the lungs and peripheral vasculature. They are stimulated by circulating agonists. β_2-subtypes are also be found in the peripheral nerve terminals where they modulate the release of noradrenaline.

Many β-blockers affect both types of receptor, but selective agents have been developed for each of the subtypes. The β_1-receptor blockers, called cardioselective agents, lower blood pressure, whereas the β_2-blockers have little effect on it.

Some β-blockers have various degrees of stimulant activity in addition to their blocking properties. This stimulant activity can be selective or non-selective. There are also complex relationships between the dose-response relationships for stimulation and blockade, and these have to be considered when describing the pharmacological properties of these agents. Both the non-selective and the cardioselective β-blockers lower blood pressure to approximately the same degree. The fall in blood pressure is not the immediate consequence of β-blockade since this effect appears to follow cardiac and renal blockade by 2–6 h. At low doses the fall in blood pressure may partially be due to a decrease in plasma renin activity. In the majority of subjects, with normal plasma renin levels, the fall in blood pressure is not related to the fall in renin. There is no convincing evidence that a neurogenic effect, peripheral or central, contributes to the fall in blood pressure. The fall can almost certainly be attributed to a reduction in heart rate and cardiac output, since there is a direct relationship between the changes in these parameters and the fall in blood pressure. This association has been derived from clinical data using β-blockers with differing degrees of intrinsic activity.

Some β-blockers with β_2-stimulant activity lower blood pressure and at the same time increase blood flow to the tissues. The relative contributions of cardiac blockade and peripheral dilatation with these agents is difficult to assess.

References

Aarons RD, Molinoff PB (1982) Changes in the density of beta-adrenergic receptors in rat lymphocytes, heart and lung after chronic treatment with propranolol. J Pharmacol Exp Ther 22:439–443

Abila B, Wilson JF, Marshall RW, Richens A (1985) Tremorolytic action of beta-adrenoceptor blockers in essential, physiological and isoprenaline-induced tremor is mediated by beta-adrenoceptors located in a deep periphereal compartment. Br J Clin Pharmacol 20:369–376

Ablad B, Borg KO, Carlsson E, Ed L, Johnsson J, Malmfors T, Regardh C-G (1975) A survey of the pharmacological properties of metoprolol in animals and man. Acta Pharmacol Toxicol 36[Suppl 5]:7–23

Ahlquist RP (1948) A study of the adrenotropic receptors. Am J Physiol 153:586–600

Amann FW, Bolli P, Kiowski W, Buhler FR (1981) Enhanced alpha-adrenoceptor mediated vasoconstriction in essential hypertension. Hypertension 3:1–119

Amery A, Billiet L, Boel A, Fagard R, Reybrouck T, Williems J (1976a) Mechanism of

hypotensive effect during beta-adrenergic blockade in hypertensive patients. Am Heart J 91:634–642
Amery A, De Plaen JF, Fagard R, Lijnen P, Reybrouck T (1976b) The relationship between beta-blockade, hyporeninaemic and hypotensive effect of two beta-blocking agents. Postgrad Med J 52[Suppl 4]:102–108
Amery A, De Plaen JF, Lijnen P, McAinsh J, Reybrouck T (1977) Relationship between blood level of atenolol and pharmacologic effect. Clin Pharmacol Ther 21:691–699
Amos HE, Brigden WD, McKerron RA (1975) Untoward effects associated with practolol: demonstration of antibody binding to epithelial tissue. Br Med J 1 598–600
Andersen GS (1982) Antihypertensive treatment of elderly patients in general practice (preliminary results). Acta Med Scand [Suppl] 676:151–160
Andren L, Hannson L (1982) Positive relationship between the dosage of pindalol and its antihypertensive effect. J Cardiovasc Pharmacol 4:32–33
Arch JRS, Ainsworth AT, Cawthorne MA et al. (1984) Atypical beta-adrenoceptor on brown adipocytes as target for anti-obesity drugs. Nature 309:163–165
Armitstead JG, Lightman SL, Brown MJ, Causon RC, Vaughan NJA (1983) The effect of selective and non-selective beta-adrenoceptor blockade, and of naloxone infusion, on the hormonal mechanisms of recovery from insulin-induced hypoglycaemia in man. Br J Clin Pharmacol 16:718–721
Arnold JMO, Johnston GB, Harron DWG, Shanks RG, McDevitt DG (1983) The effect of ICI118551 on isoprenaline-induced beta-adrenoceptor responses in man. Br J Clin Pharmacol 15:133–134
Astrom H (1975) Comparison of the effects on airway conductance of a new selective beta-adrenergic blocking drug, atenolol, and propranolol in asthmatic subjects. Scand J Respir Dis 56:292–296
Atterhog J-H, Duner H, Pernow B (1977) Hemodynamic effect of long-term treatment with pindolol in essential hypertension with special reference to the resistance and capacitance vessels of th forearm. Acta Med Scand 202:517–521
Band DM, Linton RA (1986) The effect of potassium on carotid body chemoreceptor discharge in the anaesthetised cat. J Physiol (Lond) 381:39–47
Barcroft H, Basnayake V, Celander O, Cobbold AF, Cunningham DJC, Jukes MG, Young IM (1957) The effect of carbon dioxide on the respiratory response to noradrenaline in man. J Physiol (Lond) 137:365–373
Barrett AM, Cullum VA (1968) The biological properties of the optical isomers of propranolol and their effects on cardiac arrhythmias. Br J Pharmacol 35:43–51
Bateman DN, Dean CR, Mucklow JC, Bulpitt CJ, Dollery CT (1979) Atenolol and chlorthalidone in combination for hypertension. Br J Clin Pharmacol 7:357–363
Bauer JH (1983) Effects of propranolol therapy on renal function and body fluid composition. Arch Intern Med 143:927–931
Benson MK, Graf PD (1977) Bronchial reactivity: interaction between vagal stimulation and inhaled histamine. J Appl Physiol Respir Environ Exercise Physiol 43:643–647
Benson MK, Berrill WG, Cruickshank JM, Sterling GS (1978) A comparison of four beta-adrenoceptor antagonists in patients with asthma. Br J Clin Pharmacol 5:415–419
Bernstein KN, O'Connor DT (1984) Antiadrenergic antihypertensive drugs: their effect on renal function. Annv Rev Pharmacol Toxicol 24:105–120
Beta-Blocker Heart Attack Trial Research Group (1982) A randomised trial of propranolol in patients with acute myocardial infarction. JAMA 247:1707–1713
Betts TA, Alford C (1985) Beta-blockers and sleep: a controlled trial. Eur J Clin Pharmacol 28 [Suppl]:65–68
Bilski A, Robertson HH, Wale JL (1979) A study of the relationship between cardiac beta-adrenoceptor blockade and intrinsic sympathomimetic activity in rats depleted of catecholamines. Clin Exp Pharmacol Physiol 6:1–9
Bilski AJ, Hadfield SE, Wale JL (1988) The pharmacology of epanolol (ICI 141292)—a new β1-selective adreneceptor partial agonist. J Cardiovasc Pharmacol 12:227–232
Black JW (1976) Ahlquist and the development of beta-adrenoceptor antagonists. Postgrad Med J 52 [Suppl 4]:11–13

Black JW, Stephenson JS (1962) Pharmacology of a new adrenergic beta-receptor blocking compound (Nethalide). Lancet ii:311–314
Blaes N, Boissel JP (1983) Growth-stimulating effect of catecholamines on rat aortic smooth muscle cells in culture. J Cell Physiol 116:167–172
Blum I, Rusecki Y, Doron M, Lahav M, Laron Z, Atsmon A (1983) Evidence for a therapeutic effect of dl-propranolol in benign and malignant insulinoma: report of three cases. J Endocrinol Invest 6:41–45
Bravo EL, Tarazi RC, Dustan HP (1975) Beta-adrenergic blockade in diuretic treated patients with essential hypertension. N Engl J Med 292:66–70
Brick I, Glover E, Hutchison KJ, Roddie IC (1966) Effects of propranolol on peripheral vessels in man. Am J Cardiol 18:329
Brown MJ, Brown DC, Murphy MB (1983) $Beta_2$-receptor stimulation by circulating epinephine causes prolonged hypokalemia. N Engl J Med 309:1414–1419
Buckingham RE, Hamilton TC (1980) Comparison of the antihypertensive response to beta-adrenoceptor blocking drugs in intact and adrenal demedullated spontaneously hypertensive rats. Br J Pharmacol 68:667–676
Buhler FR, Laragh JH, Baer L, Vaughan ED, Brunner HR (1972) Propranolol inhibition of renin secretion. A specific approach to diagnosis and treatment of renin dependent hypertensive diseases. N Engl J Med 287:1209–1214
Buhler FR, Laragh JH, Vaughan ED, Brunner HR, Gavras H, Baer L (1973) Anti-hypertensive action of propranolol. Am J Cardiol 32:511–522
Burgess Record N (1981) Acebutolol-induced pleuropulmonary lupus syndrom. Ann Intern Med 95:326–327
Butland RJA, Pang JA, Geddes DM (1982) The selectivity of the beta-adrenoceptor for ventilation in man. Br J Clin Pharmacol 14:707–711
Byrne AJ, McNeil JJ, Harrison PM, Louis W, Tonkin AM, McLean AJ (1984) Stable oral availability of sustained release propranolol when coadministered with hydralazine or food: evidence implicating substrate delivery rate as a determinant of presystemic drug interactions. Br J Clin Pharmacol 17[Suppl 1]:45S-50S
Cannon WB, Rosenblueth A (1933) Studies on conditions of activity in endocrine organs; Sympathin E and Sympathin I. Am J Physiol 104:557–574
Cannon WB, Rosenblueth A (1949) The supersensitivity of denervated structures: a law of denervation. Macmillan, New York
Carstairs JR, Nimmo AJ, Barnes PJ (1985) Autoradiographic visualization of beta-adrenoceptor subtypes in human lung. Am Rev Respir Dis 132:541–547
Carswell H, Nahorski SR (1983) Beta-adrenoceptor heterogeneity in guinea-pig airways: comparison of functional and receptor labelling studies. Br J Pharmacol 79:965–971
Chiariello M, Volpe M, Rengo F, Trimarco B, Violini R, Ricciardello B, Condorelli M (1979) Effect of furosemid on plasma concentration and beta-blockade by propranolol. Clin Pharmacol Ther 26:433–436
Christensen CC, Boye NP, Erikson H, Hansen G (1978) Influence of pindolol (Visken) on respiratory function in 20 asthmatic patients. Eur J Clin Pharmacol 13:9–12
Christensen NJ, Trap-Jensen J, Clausen MP, Noer I, Krogsgaard AR, Larsen OA (1975) Effect of beta-receptor blockade on heart rate, hepatic blood flow and circulating noradrenaline during exercise in man. Acta Physiol Scand 95(2):62A-63A
Cody RJ, Calabrese LH, Clough JD, Tarazi RC, Bravo EL (1979) Development of antinuclear antibodies during acebutolol therapy. Clin Pharmacol Ther 25:800–805
Colfer HT, Cottier C, Sanchez R, Julius S (1984) Role of cardiac factors in the initial hypotensive action by beta-adrenoreceptor blocking agents. Hypertension 6:145–151
Conolly ME, Briant RH, George CF, Dollery CT (1972) A crossover comparison of clonidine and methyldopa in hypertension. Eur J Clin Pharmacol 4:222–227
Cruickshank JM (1980) The clinical importance of cardioselectivity and lipophilicity in beta-blockers. Am Heart J 100:160–178
Cruickshank JM (1981) Beta-blockers, bradycardia and adverse effects. Acta Therapeutica 7:309–321
Cruickshank JM, Prichard BNC (1987) Beta-blockers in clinical practice. Churchill Livingstone, Endinburg

Cruickshank JM, Pennert K, Sorman AE, Thorp JM, Zacharias FM, Zacharias FJ (1987) Low mortality from all causes, including myocardial infarction, in well-controlled hypertensives treated with a beta-blocker plus other antihypertensives. J Hypertens 5:489–498

Dahlof B, Andren L, Svensson A, Hansson L (1983) Antihypertensive mechanism of beta-adrenoceptor antagonism—the role of beta$_2$-blockade. J Hypertens [Suppl 2]: 112–115

Dahlof C (1981) Studies on B-adreneoceptor mediated facilitation of sympathetic neurotransmission. Acta Physiol Scand [Suppl] 500:1–147

Dale HH (1906) On some physiological actions of ergot. J Physiol (Lond) 34:160–206

Daniels AR, Opie LH (1986) Atenolol plus nifedipine for mild to moderate systemic hypertension after fixed doses of either agent along. Am J Cardiol 57:965–970

Day JL, Metcalfe J, Simpson CN (1982) Adrenergic mechanisms in control of plasma lipid concentrations. Br Med J 284:1145–1148

Day MD, Roach AG (1974) Cardiovascular effects of beta-adrenoceptor blocking agents after intracerebroventricular administration in conscious normotensive cats. Clin Exp Pharmacol Physiol 1:333–339

Dayer P, Kubli A, Kupfer A, Courvoisier F, Balant L, Fabre J (1982) Defective hydroxylation of bufuralol associated with side effects of the drug in poor metabolisers. Br J Clin Pharmacol 13:750–752

Decalmer PBS, Chatterjee SS, Cruickshank JM, Benson MK, Sterling GM (1978) Beta-blockers and asthma. Br Heart J 40:184–189

De Champlain J, van Ameringen MR, Cousineau D, Marc-Aurele J, Yamaguchi N (1977) The role of the sympathetic system in experimental and human hypertension. Postgrad Med J 53 [Suppl 3]:15–30

De Divitiis O, Petitto M, Di Somma S, Galderisi M, Villari B, Santomauro M, Fazio S (1985) Nitrendipine and atenolol: comparison and combination in the treatment of arterial hypertension. Arzneimittel forschung 35:727–729

De Leeuw PW, Birkenhäger WH (1982) Renal response to propranolol treatment in hypertensive humans. Hypertension 4:125–131

De Leeuw PW, Birkenhäger WH (1983) Renal effects of beta-blockade in essential hypertension. Eur Heart J 4[Suppl D]:13–17

Derkx FHM, Schalekamp MADH (1985) Compound ICI 118551, a beta$_2$-adrenoceptor antagonist lowers blood pressure. J Hypertens 3:S247-S249

Dominiak P, Grobecker H (1982) Elevated plasma catecholamines in young hypertensive and hyperkinetic patients: effect of pindolol. Br J Clin Pharmacol 13:381S-390S

Dorow P, Weiss T, Felix R, Schmutzler H (1984) The influence of propranolol, metoprolol, and mepindolol on mucociliary clearance in coronary heart disease patients without pulmonary disease. Int J Clin Pharmacol Ther Toxicol 22:108–111

Dorward PK, Korner PI (1978) Effect of d,l-propranolol on renal sympathetic baroreflex properties and aortic baroreceptor activity. Eur. J. Pharmacol 52:51–71

D'Silva, JH (1934) The actions of adrenaline on serum potassium. J Physiol (Lond) 82:393–398

Dunlop D, Shanks RG (1968) Selective blockade of adrenoceptive beta-receptors in the heart. Br J Pharmacol Chemother 32:201–218

Dunlop D, Shanks RG (1969) Inhibition of the carotid sinus reflex by the chronic administration of propranolol. Br J Pharmacol 36:132–143

Dunn FG, Ventura HO, Messerli FH, Kobrin I, Frohlich ED (1987) Time course of regression of left ventricular hypertrophy in hypertensive patients treated with atenolol. Circulation 76:254–258

Dupont AG, Vanderniepen P, Bossuty AM, Jonckheer MH, Six RO (1985) Nadolol in essential hypertension: effect on ambulatory blood pressure, renal haemodynamics and cardiac function. Br J Clin Pharmacol 20:93–99

Eckberg DL, Abboud FM, Mark AL (1960) Modulation of carotid baroreflex responsiveness in man: effects of posture and propranolol. J Appl Physiol 41:383–387

Elkharrat D, Bismuth C (1982) Acute intoxication by beta-blocking agents: mortality in 40 cases. Int J Clin Pharmacol Res II:207–210

Elliot TR (1905) The action of adrenalin. J Physiol (Lond) 32:401–467

England JDF, Hua ASP, Shaw J (1978) Beta-adrenoreceptor blocking agents and lipid metabolism. Clin Sci Mol Med 55[Suppl 4]:323s-324s
Esler M, Julius S, Randall O, DeQuattro V, Zweifler A (1976) High-renin essential hypertension: adrenergic cardiovascular correlates. Clin Sci Mol Med 51:181s-184s
Esler MD, Zweifler A, Randall O, DeQuattro V (1977) Pathophysiologic and pharmacokinetic determinants of the antihypertensive response to propranolol. Clin Pharmacol Ther 22:299–308
Esler M, Jackman G, Leonard P, Skews H, Bobik A, Jennings G (1981) Effect of propranolol on noradrenaline kinetics in patients with essential hypertension. Br J Clin Pharmacol 12:375–380
Feely J Isles TE, Ratcliffe WA, Crooks J (1979) Propranolol, triiodothyronine, reverse triiodothyronine and thyroid disease. Clin Endocrinol (Oxf) 10:431
Felix RH, Ive FA (1974) Skin reactions to practolol. Br Med J 2:333
Fitzgerald JD (1969) Perspectives in adrenergic beta-receptor blockade. Clin Pharmacol Ther 10:292–306
Fitzgerald JD, Ruffin R, Smedstad, KG:, Roberts, R., McAinsh, J. (1978) Studies on the pharmacokinetics and pharmacodynamics of atenolol in man. Eur J Clin Pharmacol 13:81–89
Floras JS, Jones JV, Hassan MO, Sleight P (1982) Ambulatory blood pressure during once-daily randomised double-blind administration of atenolol, metoprolol, pindolol, and slow-release propranolol. Br Med J 285:1387–1392
Folgering H, Pointe J, Sadig T (1982) Adrenergic mechanisms and chemoreception in the carotid body of the cat and rabbit. J Physiol (Lond) 325:1–21
Forfar JC, Brown GJ, Cull RE (1979) Proximal myopathy during beta-blockade. Br Med J 2:1331–1332
Franco-Morselli R, Elghozi JL, Joly E, Di Giulio S, Meyer P (1977) Increased plasma adrenaline concentrations in benign essential hypertension. Br Med J 2:1251–1254
Garber AJ, Cryer PE, Santiago JV, Haymond MW, Pagliara AS, Kipnis DM (1976) The role of adrenergic mechanisms in the substrate and hormonal response to insulin-induced hypoglycaemia in man. J Clin Invest 58:7–15
Gillam PMS, Prichard BNC (1966) Propranolol in the therapy of angina pectoris. Am J Cardiol 18:366–369
Gilmore E, Weil J, Chidsey C (1970) Treatment of essential hypertension with a new vaso-dilator in combination with beta-adrenergic blockade. N Engl J Med 282:521–527
Grobecker H, McCarty R, Saavedra JM, Chiueh CC, Kopin IJ (1977) Dopamine-beta-hydroxylase activity and catecholamine concentrations in plasma: experimental and essential hypertension. Postgrad Med J 53 [Suppl 3]:43–48
Harms HH, Gooren L, Spoelstra AJG, Hesse C, Verschoor L (1978) Blockade of isoprenaline-induced changes in plasma free fatty acids, immunoreactive insulin levels and plasma renin activity in healthy human subjects, by propranolol, pindolol, practolol, atenolol, metoprolol and acebutolol. Br J Clin Pharmacol 5:19–26
Harry JD, Knapp MF, Linden RJ, Stoker JB, Newcombe C (1979) Effects of four beta-adrenoceptor blocking drugs on blood pressure and exercise heart rate in hypertension. Eur J Cardiol 10:131–141
Hartling OJ, Nower I, Svendsen TL, Clausen JP, Trap-Jensen J (1980) Selective and non-selective beta-adrenoceptor blockade in the human forearm. Clin Sci 58:279–286
Hawksworth G, Betts T, Crowe A et al. (1984) Diazepam/beta-adrenoceptor antagonist interactions. Br J Clin Pharmacol 17[Suppl 1]:69S-76S
Heagerty AM, Donovan MA, Castleden CM, Pohl JF, Patel L, Hedges A (1981) Influence of cimetidine on pharmacokinetics of propranolol. Br Med J 282:1917–1919
Hjalmarson A, Herlitz J, Malek I et al. (1981) Effect of mortality of metroprolol in acute myocardial infarction. Lancet ii:823–826
Hollifield JW, Sherman K, Vander Zwaag R, Shand DG (1976) Proposed mechanisms of propranolol's antihypertensive effect in essential hypertension. N Engl J Med 295:68–73
Hombach V, Braun V, Hopp H-W, Gil-Sanchez D, Behrenbeck DW, Tauchert, M, Hilger, HH: (1982) Electrophysiological effects of cardioselective and non-cardio-

selective beta-adrenoceptor blockers with and without ISA at rest and during exercise. Br J Clin Pharmacol 13:285S-293S
Imataka K, Seki A, Takahashi N et al. (1981) Elevation of serum creatine phosphokinase during pindolol treatment. J Jpn Soc Int Med 70:580–585
Iversen LL (1977) Catecholamine-sensitive adenylate cyclase in nervous tissues. J Neurochem 29:5–12
Jackson KE, Campbell WB (1981) A possible antihypertensive mechanism of propranolol: antagonism of angiotensin II enhancement of sympathetic nerve transmission through prostaglandins. Hypertension 3:23–33
Johnsson G, Svedmyr N, Thiringer G (1975) Effects of intravenous propranolol and metoprolol and their interaction with isoprenaline on pulmonary function, heart rate and blood pressure in asthmatics. Eur J Clin Pharmacol 8:175–180
Kaumann AJ, Blinks JR (1980) B-adrenoceptor blocking agents as partial agonists in isolated heart muscle: dissocation of stimulation and blockade. Naunyn Schmiedeberg's Arch Pharmacol 311:237–248
Kaumann AJ, Lemoine H (1987) B_2-adrenoceptor-mediated positive inotropic effect of adrenaline in human ventricular myocardium. Naunyn Schmiedeberg's Arch Pharmacol 335:403–411
Kirch W, Schafer-Korting M, Axthelm T, Kohler H, Mutschler E (1981) Interaction of atenolol with furosemide and calcium and aluminium salts. Clin Pharmacol Ther 30:429–435
Krediet RT, Dunning AJ (1979) Baroreflex sensitivity in hypertension during beta-adrenergic blockade. Br Heart J 41:106–110
Laakso M, Pentikainen PJ, Pyorala K, Neuvonen PJ (1981) Prolongation of the Q-T interval caused by sotalol—possible association with ventricular tachyarrhythmias. Eur Heart J 2:353–358
Lambert DMD (1977) Long-term effects of propranolol on morbidity and mortality in patients with angina pectoris. Cardiovasc Med 2:253–260
Lammers JWJ, Folgering HTM, van Herwaarden CLA (1985) Ventilatory effects of long-term treatment with pindolol and metoprolol in hypertensive patients with chronic obstructive lung disease. Br J Clin Pharmacol 20:205–210
Lands AM, Arnold A, McAuliff JP, Luduena FP, Brown TG (1967) Differentiation of receptor systems activated by sympathomimetic amines. Nature 214:597–598
Langley JN (1905) On the reaction of cells and of nerve-endings to certain poisons, chiefly as regards the reaction of striated muscles to nicotine and to curare. J Physiol (Lond) 33:374–413
Lant A (1980) The influence of beta-blockade on intermediary metabolism. Topics Therapeutics 6:53–66
Lees P (1968) The influence of beta-adrenoceptive blocking agents on urinary function in the rat. Br J Pharmacol 34:429–444
Lefkowitz RJ, Hoffman BB (1980a) New directions in adrenergic receptor research pt I. Trends Pharmacol Sci 1:314–318
Lefkowitz RJ, Hoffman BB (1980b) New directions in adrenergic receptor research pt II. Trends Pharmacol Sci 1:369–372
Leonetti G, Mayer G, Morganti A et al. (1975) Hypotensive and renin suppressing activities of propranolol in hypertensive patients. Clin Sci Mol Med 48:491–499
Leonetti G, Terzoli L, Bianchini C, Sala C, Zanchett A (1980) Time course of the antihypertensive action of atenolol: comparison of response to first dose and to maintained oral administration. Eur J Clin Pharmacol 18:365–374
Leonetti G, Sampieri L, Cuspidi C et al. (1985) Does $beta_1$-selective agonistic activity interfere with the antihypertensive efficacy of $beta_1$-selective blocking agents? J Hypertens 3[Suppl 3]:S243-S245
Lewis PJ, Haeusler G (1975) Reduction in sympathetic nervous activity as a mechanism for hypotensive effect of propranolol. Nature 256:440
Lewis RV, Jackson PR, Ramsay LE (1984) Quantification of side-effects of beta-adrenoceptor blockers using visual analogue scales. Br J Clin Pharmacol 18:325–330
Lewis RV, Toner JM, Jackson PR, Ramsay LE (1986) Effects of indomethacin and sulindac on blood pressure of hypertensive patients. Br Med J 292:934–935

Linton RAF, Lim N, Wolff CB, Wilmshurst P, Band DM (1984) Arterial plasma potassium measured continuously during exercise in man. Clin Sci 66:427–431
Loewi O (1921) Über humorale Übertragbarkeit der Herznervenwirkung. Pflügers Arch Gesamte Physiol Menschen Tiere 189:239–242
Lund-Johansen P (1974) Haemodynamic changes at rest and during exercise in long-term beta-blocker therapy of essential hypertension. Acta Med Scand 195:117–121
Lund-Johansen P (1979) Hemodynamic consequences of long-term beta-blocker therapy: a 5-year follow-up study of atenolol. J Cardiovasc Pharmacol 1:487–495
Maarek B, Simon AC, Levenson J, Merli I, Bouthier J (1986) Chronic effects of pindolol on the arterioles, large arteries, and veins of the forearm in mild to moderate essential hypertension. Clin Pharmacol Ther 39:403–408
Main BG, Tucker H (1985) Recent advances in beta-adrenergic blocking agents. In: Ellis GP, West GB (eds) Progress in medicinal chemistry, vol 22. Elsevier, Amsterdam, pp 122–164
Majcherczyk S, Mikulski A, Sjolander M, Thoren P (1987) Increase of renal sympathetic nerve activity of spontaneously hypertensive rats. Br J Pharmacol 91:711–714
Majewski H, McCulloch MW, Rand MJ, Story DF (1980) Adrenaline activation of prejunctional beta-adrenoceptors in guinea pig atria. Br J Pharmacol 71:435–444
Man in't Veld AJ, Schalekamp MADH (1982) How intrinsic sympathomimetic activity modulates the haemodynamic responses to beta-adrenoceptor antagonists. A clue to the nature of their antihypertensive mechanism. Br J Clin Pharmacol 13:245S-257S
Man in't Veld AJ, Schalekamp MADH (1983) Hemodynamic consequences of intrinsic sympathomimetic activity and cardioselectivity in beta blocker therapy for hypertension. Eur Heart J 4 [Suppl D]:31–41
Matunaga M, Hara A, Ogino K, Motokara S, Saito M, Yamamoto J, Pak CH (1977) Effects of beta-adrenergic blocking agents on the blood pressure, plasma renin activity and hemodynamics of hypertensive patients. Jpn Heart J 18:24–30
McAinsh J (1977) Clinical pharmacokinetics of atenolol. Postgrad Med J 53[Suppl 3]: 74–78
McDevitt DG, Nelson JK (1978) Comparative trial of atenolol and propranolol in hyperthyroidism. Br J Clin Pharmacol 6:233–237
McNeill RS (1964) Effect of a beta-adrenergic blocking agent, propranolol, on asthmatics. Lancet ii:1101–1102
McSorley PD, Warren DJ (1978) Effects of propranolol and metoprolol on the peripheral circulation. Br Med J 2:1598–1600
Medical Research Council Working Party (1985) MRC trial of treatment of mild hypertension: principal results. Br Med J 291:97–104
Meekers J, Missotten A, Fagard R et al. (1975) Predictive value of various parameters for the antihypertensive effect of the beta-blocker ICI 66,082. Arch Int Pharmacodyn (1978) 213:294–306
Mehta J, Mehta P, Pepine CJ (1978) Platelet aggregation in aortic and coronary venous blood in patients with and without coronary disease. 3. Role of tachycardia stress and propranolol. Circulation 58:881–886
Mehta J Mehta P, Ostrowski N (1983) Influence of propranolol and 4-hydroxypropranolol on platelet aggregation and thromboxane A_2 generation Clin. Pharmacol. Therap. 34:559–564
Melander A, Danielson K, Schersten B, Wahlin E (1977) Enhancement of the bioavailability of propranolol and metoprolol by food. Clin Pharmacol Therap 22:108–112.
Melander A, Stenbury P, Liedholm H, Schirsten B, Watkin-Boll E 1979 Food-induced reduction in bioavailability of atenolol. Eur J Clin Pharmacol 16:327–330
Michelakis AM, McAllister RG (1972) The effect of chronic adrenergic receptor blockade on plasma renin activity in man. J Clin Endocrinol Metab 34:386–394
Moran NC, Perkin ME (1958) Adrenergic blockade of the mammalian heart by a dichloro analogue of isoproterenol. J Pharmacol Exp Ther 124:223–237
Morgan TO, Roberts R, Carney SL, Louis WJ, Doyle AE (1975) Beta-adrenergic receptor blocking drugs, hypertension and plasma renin. Br J Clin Pharmacol. 2:169–164
Mueller HS, Ayres SM, Religa A, Evans RG (1974) Propranolol in the treatment of

acute myocardial infarction. Circulation 49:1078–1087
Mulligan E, Lahiri S, Mokashi A, Matsumoto S, McGregor KN (1986) Adrenergic mechanisms in oxygen chemoreception in the cat aortic body. Resp Physiol 63: 375–382
Mustchin CP, Gribbin HR, Tattersfield AE, George CG (1976) Reduced respiratory responses to carbon dioxide after propranolol: A central action. Br Med J Nov 20th:1229–1231
Myers MG, De Champlain J: Effects of atenolol and hydrochlorothiazide on blood pressure and plasma catecholamines in essential hypertension. Hypertension. 5(4): 591–596.
Nies AS, McNeil JS, Schrier RW (1971) Mechanism of increased sodium reabsorption during propranolol administration. Circulation. 44(4):596–604
Nuttall A, Snow HM (1982) The cardiovascular effects of ICI 118,587: A beta 1-adrenoceptor partial agonist. Br J Pharmacol 77(2):381–8
Ostman Smith I (1981) Cardiac sympathetic nerves as the final common pathway in the induction of adaptive cardiac hypertrophy. Clin Sci 61(3):265–72
Parati G, Pomidossi G, Grassi G, Gavazzi C, Ramirez A, Gregorini, L, Mancia G (1983) Mechanisms of antihypertensive action of beta-adrenergic blocking drugs: evidence against potentiation of baroreflexes. Eur Heart J 4(D):19–25
Paterson DJ, Nye PC (1988) The effect of beta adrenergic blockade on the carotid body response to hyperkalaemia in the cat. Respir Physiol 74(2):229–37
Patrick JM, Tutty J, Pearson SB (1978) Propranolol and the ventilatory response to hypoxia and hypercapnia in normal man. Clin Sci Mol Med 55:491–497
Pavia D Bateman JRM, Lennard-Jones AM, Agnew JE, Clarke SW (1986) Effect of selective and non-selective beta-blockade on pulmonary function and tracheobronchial mucociliary clearance in healthy subjects. Thorax. 41:301–305
Pedersen EB, Kornerup HJ (1977) Plasma renin concentration in essential hypertension during beta-adrenergic blockade and vasodilator therapy. Eur J Clin Pharmacol. 12:93–96
Peet M, Middlemiss DN, Yates RA (1981) Propranolol in schizophrenia. II. Clinical and biochemical aspects of combining propranolol with chlorpromazine. Br J Psychiatry 139:112–117
Petri JC, Galloway DB, Webster J, Simpson WT, Lewis JA (1975) Atenolol and bendrofluazide in hypertension. Br Med J 4:133–135
Petrie JC, Jeffers TA, Scott AK, Webster J (1983) Dose and duration of response to beta-blockers in the treatment of hypertension. Drugs (Symposium on beta-blockers in the 1980's) 25[Suppl 2]:26–29
Philippu A, Stroehl U (1978) Beta-adrenoreceptors of the posterior hypothalamus. Clin Exp Hypertens [A] 1:25–38
Pickering TG, Gribbin B, Petersen ES, Cunningham DJC, Sleight P (1972) Effects of autonomic blockade on the baroreflex in man at rest and during exercise. Circ Res 30:177–185
Potter DE (1981) Adrenergic pharmacology of aqueous humor dynamics. Pharmacol Rev 33(3):133–153
Price HL, Deutsch S, Davidson IA, Clement AJ, Behar MC, Epstein RM (1966) Can general anaesthesia produce splanchnic visceral hypoxia by reducing regional blood flow? Anesthesiology 27:24
Prichard BNC, Gillam PMS (1964) Use of propranolol in the treatment of hypertension. Br Med J 2:725–727
Prichard BNC, Gillam PMS (1969) Treatment of hypertension with propranolol. Br Med J 1:7–16
Rahn KH, Gierlichs HW, Planz G, Planz R, Schols M, Stephany W (1978) Studies on the effects of propranolol on plasma catecholamine levels in patients with essential hypertension. Eur J Clin Invest 8:143–148
Raine AEG, Chubb IW (1977) Long-term beta-adrenergic blockade reduces tyrosine hydroxylase and DBH activities in sympathetic ganglia. Nature 267:265–267
Redman CWG (1980) Treatment of hypertension in pregnancy. Kidney Int 18:267–278
Reybrouck T, Amery A, Billiet L (1977) Haemodynamic response to graded exercise

after chronic beta-adrenergic blockade. J Appl Physiol Respir Environ Exercise Physiol 42:133–138
Richardson DW, Freund J, Gear AS, Mauck HP, Preston LW (1968) Effect of propranolol on elevated arterial blood pressure. Circulation 37:534–542
Robb OJ, Petrie JC, Webster J, Harry J (1985) ICI 118551 does not reduce BP in hypertensive patients responsive to atenolol and propranolol. Br J Clin Pharmacol 19:541P-542P
Rosei EA, Trust PM, Brown JJ, Lever AF, Robertson JIS (1975) Intravenous labetalol in severer hypertension. Lancet ii:1093–1094
Rosei EA, Brown JJ, Lever AF, Robertson AS, Robertson JIS, Trust RM (1976) Treatment of phaeochromocytoma and of clonidine withdrawal hypertension with labetalol. Br J Clin Pharmacol 3[Suppl]:809–815
Roubicek J (1976) The effect of beta-adrenoceptor blocking drugs on EEG. Br J Clin Pharmacol 3:661–665
Rowlands DB, Glover DR, Stallard TJ, Littler WA (1982) Control of blood pressure and reduction of echocardiographically assessed left ventricular mass with once-daily timolol. Br J Clin Pharmacol 14:89–95
Rubin PC (1981) Beta-blockers in pregnancy. N Engl J Med 305:1323–1326
Schafer-Korting M, Kirch W, Axthelm T, Kohler H, Mutschler E (1983) Atenolol interaction with aspirin, allopurinol, and ampicillin. Clin Pharmacol Ther 33:283–288
Schluter KJ, Aellig WH, Petersen K-G, Rieband H-Ch, Wehrli A, Kerp L (1982) The influence of beta-adrenoceptor blocking drugs with and without intrinsic sympathomimetic activity on the hormonal responses to hypo- and hyperglycaemia. Br J Clin Pharmacol 13:407S-417S
Schneck DW, Vary JE (1984) Mechanism by which hydralazine increases propranolol bioavailability. Clin Pharmacol Ther 35:447–453
Schneck DW, Luderer JR, Davis D, Vary J (1984) Effects of nadolol and propranolol on plasma lidocaine clearance. Clin Pharmacol Ther 36(5):584–587
Scott EM, Williams EK (1982) The effect of atenolol on aortic nerve discharge in the anesthetized cat. Br J Pharmacol 77:325
Seaton TB, Welle S, Campbell RG (1985) Thermogenesis in brown adipose tissue. N Engl J Med 312:1062–1063
Sederberg-Olsen P, Ibsen H (1972) Plasma volume and extracellular fluid volume during long-term treatment with propranolol in essential hypertension. Clin Sci 43:165–170
Seedat YK, Stewart-Wynne EG, Reddy J, Randeree M (1973) Experiences with beta-adrenergic blockade drugs in hypertension. S Afr Med J 47:259–262
Seides SF, Josephson ME, Batsford WP, Wesifogel GM, Lau SH, Damato AN (1974) The electrophysiology of propranolol in man. Am Heart J 88:733–741
Shah RR, Oates NS, Idle JR, Smith RL (1982) Beta-blockers and drug oxidation status. Lancet i:508–509
Shand DG (1974) Pharmacokinetic properties of the beta-adrenergic receptor blocking drugs. Drugs 7:39–47
Shand DG (1975) Propranolol. N Engl J Med 293:280
Shand DG, Branch RA, Evans GH, Nies AS, Wilkinson GR (1973) The disposition of propranolol. VII. The effects of saturable hepatic tissue uptake on drug clearance by the perfused rat liver. Drug Metab Dispos 1:679–686
Shinebourne E, Fleming J, Hamer J (1967) Effects of beta-adrenergic blockade during exercise in hypertensive and ischaemic heart disease. Lancet ii:1217–1220
Simon G, Kiowski W, Julius S (1977) Effect of beta-adrenoceptor antagonists on baroreceptor reflex sensitivity in hypertension. Clin Pharmacol Ther 22:293–298
Singh BN, Vaughan Williams EM (1970) A third class of antiarrhythmic action. Effects on atrial and ventricular action potentials and other pharmacological actions on cardiac muscle, of MJ 1999 and AH 3474. Br J Pharmacol 39:675–687
Slater IH, Powell CE (1957) Blockade of adrenergic inhibitory receptor sites by 1-(3′-4′-dichloro-phenol)-2-isopropyl-aminoethanol hydrochloride. Fed Proc 16:336
Smith HJ, Halliday SE, Earl DCN, Stribling P (1983) Effects of selective (beta-1 and beta-2) and nonselective beta adrenoceptor antagonists on the cardiovascular and metabolic responses to isoproterenol: comparison with ICI 141292. J Pharmacol Exp

Ther 226:211–216
Smith LH (1978) Cardio-selective B-adrenergic blocking agents. J Appl Chem Biotechnol 28:201–212
Smith U, Lager I (1978) Beta-blockade in diabetes. N Engl J Med 299:1467–1469
Smits JFM, Struyker Boudier HAJ (1982) The mechanisms of antihypertensive action of the adrenergic receptor blocking druts. Clin Exp Hypertens [A] 4:71–86
Smits JFM, van Essen H, Struyker-Boudier HAJ (1980) Is the antihypertensive effect of propranolol caused by an action with the central nervous system? J Pharmacol Exp Ther 215(1):221–225
Smits JFM, Coleman TG, Smith TL, Kasbergen CM, van Essen H, Struyker-Boudier HAJ (1982) Antihypertensive effect of propranolol in conscious spontaneously hypertensive rats: central hemodynamics, plasma volume and renal function during beta-blockade with propranolol. J Cardiovasc Pharmacol 4:903–914
Sonnenblick EB, Braunwald E, Williams JF, Glick G (1965) Effects of exercise on myocardial force-velocity relations in intact unanesthetized man: Relative roles of changes in heart rate, sympathetic activity, and ventricular dimensions. J Clin Invest 44:2051–2062
Starke K (1977) Regulation of NA release by presynatpic receptor systems. Rev Physiol Biochem Pharmacol 77:1–125
Stewart I McD G (1976) Compared incidence of first myocardial infarction in hypertensive patients under treatment containing propranolol or excluding beta-receptor blockade. Clin Sci Mol Med 51:509s-511s
Struthers AD, Reid JL, Whitesmith R, Rodger JC (1983) The effects of cardioselective and non-selective beta-adrenoceptor blockade on the hypokalaemic and cardiovascular responses to adrenomedullary hormones in man. Clin Sci 65:143–147
Struyker-Boudier HAJ, Evenwel RT, Smits JFM, van Essen H (1982) Baroreflex sensitivity during the development of spontaneous hypertension in rats. Clin Sci 62: 589–594
Sundlof G, Wallin BG, Stromgren E, Nerhed C (1983) Acute effects of metroprolol on muscle sympathetic activity in hypertensive humans. Hypertension 5:749–756
Suzman MM (1981) Use of beta-adrenergic receptor blocking agents in psychiatry. In: Neuropharmacology of central nervous system and behavioural disorders, chap 14. Academic, New York, pp 339–391
Svendsen TL, Hartling O, Trap-Jensen J (1979) Immediate haemodynamic effects of propranolol, practolol, pindolol, atenolol and ICI 89,406 in healthy volunteers. Eur J Clin Pharmacol 15:223–228
Svendsen TL, Hartling OJ, Trap-Jensen J, McNair A, Bliddal J (1981) Adrenergic beta-receptor blockade: haemodynamic importance of intrinsic sympathomimetic activity at rest. Clin Pharmacol Ther 29:711–718
Svendsen TL, Lyngbourg K, Mehlsen J, Trap-Jensen J (1987) Immediate haemodynamic effects of a novel partial partial agonist, B1-adrenoceptor blocking drug ICI 141292. After intravenous administration to healthy young volunteers and patients with ischaemic heart disease. Br J Clin Pharmacol 23:35–40
Takeshita A, Tanaka S, Kuroiwa A et al. (1975) Reduced baroreceptor sensitivity in borderline hypertension. Circulation 51:738–742
Tarazi RC (1985) The heart in hypertension. N Engl J Med 312:308–309
Tarazi RC, Dustan HP (1972) Beta-adrenergic blockade in hypertension. Am J Cardiol 29:633–640
Tattersfield AE, Leaver DG Pride N (1973) Effects of beta-adrenergic blockade and stimulation on normal human airways. J Appl Physiol 35:613–619
Trap-Jensen J, Carlsen JE, Lysbo Svendsen T, Christensen NJ (1979) Cardiovascular and adrenergic effects of cigarette smoking during immediate non-selective and selective beta-adrenoceptor blockade in humans. Eur J Clin Invest 9:181–183
Trap-Jensen J, Carlsen JE, Hartling OJ, Svendsen TL, Tango M, Christensen NJ (1982) Beta-adrenoceptor blockade and psychic stress in man. A comparison of the acute effects of labetalol, metoprolol, pindolol and propranolol on plasma levels of adrenaline and noradrenaline. Br J Clin Pharmacol 13:391S-395S

Tsukiyama H, Otsuka K, Higuma K (1982) Effects of beta-adrenoceptor antagonists on central haemodynamics in essential hypertension. Br J Clin Pharmacol 13:269S-278S
Tsukiyama H, Otsuka K, Morii M, Yoshii Y, Hatori Y, Nakamura Y, Nemoto E, Yamato T, Sakai T, Yamamoto Y (1983) Possible significance of the pharmacological differentiation of beta-blocking agents in hemodynamic effects in essential hypertension. Jpn Circ J 47:313–322
Tyrer PJ, Lader MH (1974) Response to propranolol and diazepam insommatic and psychic anxiety. Br Med J 2:14–16
Van Baak MA, Struyker Boudier HAJ, Smits JFM (1985) Antihypertensive mechanisms of beta-adrenoceptor blockade: a review. Clin Exp Hypertens [A]7(1):1–72
Van Herwaarden CLA, Fennis JFM, Binkhorst RA, van't Laar A (1977) Haemodynamic effects of adrenaline during treatment of hypertensive patients with propranolol and metoprolol. Eur J Clin Pharmacol 12:397–402
Vaughan Williams EM, Raine AEG (1974) Effect of prolonged beta-receptor blockade on dry weight and electrophysiological responses of rabbit hearts. Lancet ii:1048–1049
Veterans Administration Cooperative Study Group on Antihypertensive Agents (1977) Propranolol in the treatment of essential hypertension. JAMA 237(21):2303–2310
Vincent HH, Man in't Veld AJ, Boomsma F, Wenting GH, Schalekamp MADH (1982) Elevated plasma noradrenaline in response to beta-adrenoceptor stimulation in man (propranolol, atenolol). Br J Pharmacol 13(5):717–721
Vincent HH, Man in't Veld AJ, Boomsma F, Derkx F, Schalekamp ADH (1985) Compound ICI 118551, a beta-2-adrenoceptor antagonist lowers blood pressure. J Hypertens 3[Suppl 3]:S247-S249
Waal-Manning HJ (1979) Atenolol and three nonselective beta-blockers in hypertension. Clin Pharmacol Ther 25:8–18
Wallin G, Sundlof G, Stromgren E, Aberg H (1984) Sympathetic outflow to muscles during treatment of hypertension with metoprolol. Hypertension 6:557–562
Walter M, Lemoine H, Kaumann AJ (1984) Stimulant and blocking effects of optical isomers of pindolol on the sinoatrial node and trachea of guinea pig. Role of B-adrenoceptor subtypes in the dissociation between blockade and stimulation. Naunyn Schmiedeberg's Arch Pharmacol 327:159–175
Warren DJ, Waller DG, McAinsh J (1983) Beta-blockers and renal function. Drugs 25[Suppl 2]:108–112
Watkins J, Abbot EC, Hensby CN, Webster J, Dollery CT (1980) Attenuation of hypotensive effect of propranolol and thiazide diuretics by indomethacin. Br Med J 281:702–705
Watson RDS, Stallard TJ, Littler WA (1979a) Effects of beta-adrenoceptor antagonists on sino-aortic baroreflex sensitivity and blood pressure in hypertensive man. Clin Sci 57:241–247
Watson RDS, Stallard TJ, Littler WA (1979b) Influence of once-daily administration of beta-adrenoceptor (antagonists on arterial pressure and its variability. Lancet 1:1210–1213
Weber MA, Drayer JIM (1980) Renal effects of beta-adrenoceptor blockade. Kidney Int. 18:686–699
Webster J, Jeffers TA, Galloway DB, Petrie JC, Barker NP (1977) Atenolol, methyldopa, and chlorthalidone in moderate hypertension. Br Med J 1:76–78
Weidmann P, Gerber A, Mordasini R (1983) Effects of antihypertensive therapy on serum lipoproteins. Hypertension 5[Suppl III]:III-120-III-131
Weinstock M, Weiss C, Gitter S (1977) Blockade of 5 hydroxytryptamine receptors in the central nervous system by beta-adrenoceptor antagonists. Neuropharmacology 16:273–276
Weiss L, Lundgren Y, Folkow B (1974) Effects of prolonged treatment with adrenergic beta-receptor antagonists on blood pressure, cardiovascular design and ractivity in spontaneously hypertensive rats (SHR). Acta. Physiol. Scand. 91:447–457
Wermut W, Wojcicki M (1973) Suicidal attempt with propranolol. Br Med J 3:591.
Whyte K, Jones CR, Howie CA, Deighton N, Sumner DJ, Reid JL (1973) Haemodynamic, metabolic, and lymphocyte beta$_2$-adrenoceptor changes following chronic

beta-adrenoceptor antagonism. Eur J Clin Pharmacol
Wikstrand J, Trimarco B, Buzzett G, Ricciardelli B, de Luca N, Volpe M, Condorelli M (1983) Increased cardiac output and lowered peripheral resistance during metoprolol treatment. Acta Med Scand 672:105–110
Wilkinson R (1982) Beta-blockers and renal function. Drugs 23:195–206
Winer N, Chokshi DS, Yoon MS, Freedman AD (1969) Adrenergic receptor mediation of renin secretion. J Clin Endocrinol Metab 29:1168–1175
Wolfson S, Gorlin R (1969) Cardiovascular pharmacology of propranolol in man. Circulation 40:501–511
Wolfson S, Heuler RA, Herman MV, Kemp HG, Sullivan JM, Gorlin R (1966) Propranolol in angina pectoris. Am J Cardiol 18:345–352
Wright P (1974) Skin reactions to practolol. Br Med J 2:560
Wright P (1975) Untoward effects associated with practolol administration: oculomucocutaneous syndrome. Br Med J 1:595–598
Yamaoki K, Imataka K, Seki A, Takayama Y, Fujii J (1983) Muscle symptoms in patients treated with pindolol. Igaku no Ayumi 126:233–234
Zacest R, Gilmorek E, Koch-Weser J (1972) Treatment of essential hypertension with combined vasodilation and beta-adrenergic blockade. N Engl J Med 286:617–622
Zacharias FJ (1976) Patient acceptability of propranolol and the occurrence of side effects. Postgard Med J 52[Suppl 4]:87–89
Zacharias FJ, Cowen KJ (1970) Controlled trial of propranolol in hypertension. Br Med J 1:471–474
Zacharias FJ, Cowen KJ, Vickers J, Wall BG (1972) Propranolol in hypertension. A Study of long-term therapy 1964–1970. Am Heart J 83:755–761
Zacharias FJ, Cuthbertson PJR, Prestt J et al. (1977) Atenolol in hypertension: a study of long-term therapy. Postgrad Med J 53[Suppl 3]:102–110
Zech PY, Labeeuw M, Pozet N, Hadj-Aissa A, Sassar J, McAinsh J (1977) Response to atenolol in arterial hypertension in relation to renal function, pharmacokinetics and renin activity. Postgard Med J 53[Suppl 3]:134–141

CHAPTER 4

α-Adrenoceptor Antagonists

P.A. VAN ZWIETEN

CONTENTS

1 Introduction

Ever since the development of α-adrenoceptor antagonistic drugs (α-blockers), attempts have been made to treat arterial hypertensive disease with such compounds. This approach would seem logical since α-adrenoceptor antagonists are vasodilators with a very strong action in the arteriolar vascular bed; in addition it should be realized that elevated total peripheral resistance is the most consistent hemodynamic change in established essential hypertension. Treatment with vasodilator drugs thus seems a rational route to lower blood pressure in hypertensive patients.

However, classic α-adrenoceptor antagonists, such as phentolamine, phenoxybenzamine, tolazoline, and hydrogenated ergot alkaloids have not proved useful in the long-term control of blood pressure in hypertensive patients. Reflex tachycardia, fluid and sodium retention, and difficulties in dosage adjustment have limited the use of these agents, particularly phentolamine, to the preoperative preparation of patients with pheochromocytoma.

More recently, phentolamine has been studied as an experimental "unloading drug" in patients with congestive heart failure (GEORGOPOULOS et al. 1978; GOULD et al. 1980).

Indoramin has been studied as a potential antihypertensive drug and shown to be effective, although its adverse reactions proved considerable (STOKES et al. 1979; MARSHALL et al. 1980). At present it cannot be judged whether or not indoramin is likely to become a useful antihypertensive drug.

A renaissance of interest in α-adrenoceptor antagonists as antihypertensive drugs was triggered by the development of the selective α_1-adrenoceptor blocking agent prazosin, which proved to be a much better antihypertensive than the aforementioned classic α-blockers. One of the major advantages over the classic α-blockers is the virtual absence of reflex tachycardia during treatment with prazosin and related selective α_1-blockers. Prazosin and subsequently a series of similar successor drugs have not only proven to be useful antihypertensives but have also gained considerable fundamental importance as pharmacologic tools, owing to their selectivity for α_1-adrenoceptors. For those reasons our emphasis in the present chapter will be on prazosin and closely related drugs. Some attention will be paid to drugs which display additional pharmacologic activities besides their α_1-blocking potency, such as urapidil, labetalol, and ketanserin.

2 Chemistry

The chemical structures of those α-adrenoceptor antagonists which are of interest for clinical, fundamental, or historical reasons are depicted in Figs. 1 and 2. Phenoxybenzamine is a phenylethylamine derivative and as such is chemically related to the endogenous catecholamines, noradrenaline and adrenaline. Phentolamine, however, is an imidazoline derivative, and attempts have been made to relate its activity to that of clonidine, a centrally acting hypotensive with an imidazolidine structure. Indoramin, a compound with miscellaneous activities, contains an indole moiety. The prazosin molecule shows some resemblance to both papaverine and the aminopyrimidine moiety of cAMP and cGMP. This structural resemblance was introduced deliberately, since prazosin was originally designed to be a vasodilator with a direct action on vascular smooth muscle. Direct vasodilatation is indeed induced by prazosin, but only in doses well beyond the therapeutic level (CONSTANTINE et al. 1973). Furthermore, the inhibition of phospodiesterase by prazosin, an activity suggested by its chemical structure, also occurs only at much higher doses than those used therapeutically (HESS 1974; SANDS and JORGENSEN 1979). Doxazosin, trimazosin, and terazosin are the successor drugs to prazosin and as such are also selective antagonists of postsynaptic α_1-adrenoceptors. They show a close chemical resemblance to prazosin. Piperazino substitution at position 2 and 6,7-dimethoxy substitution in the aromatic ring proved to be requirements for optimal antihypertensive activity. As is obvious from the structures of the successor drugs, further substitution at the piperazino moiety can be largely varied without losing antihypertensive activity. In prazosin this substituent is a furan moiety, whereas in the closely related terazosin it is a tetrahydrofuran nucleus, in doxazosin, a benzdioxan moiety, and in trimazosin an ester with a hydroxy-substituted tertiary $-CH_2-C(CH_3)_2-$ moiety.

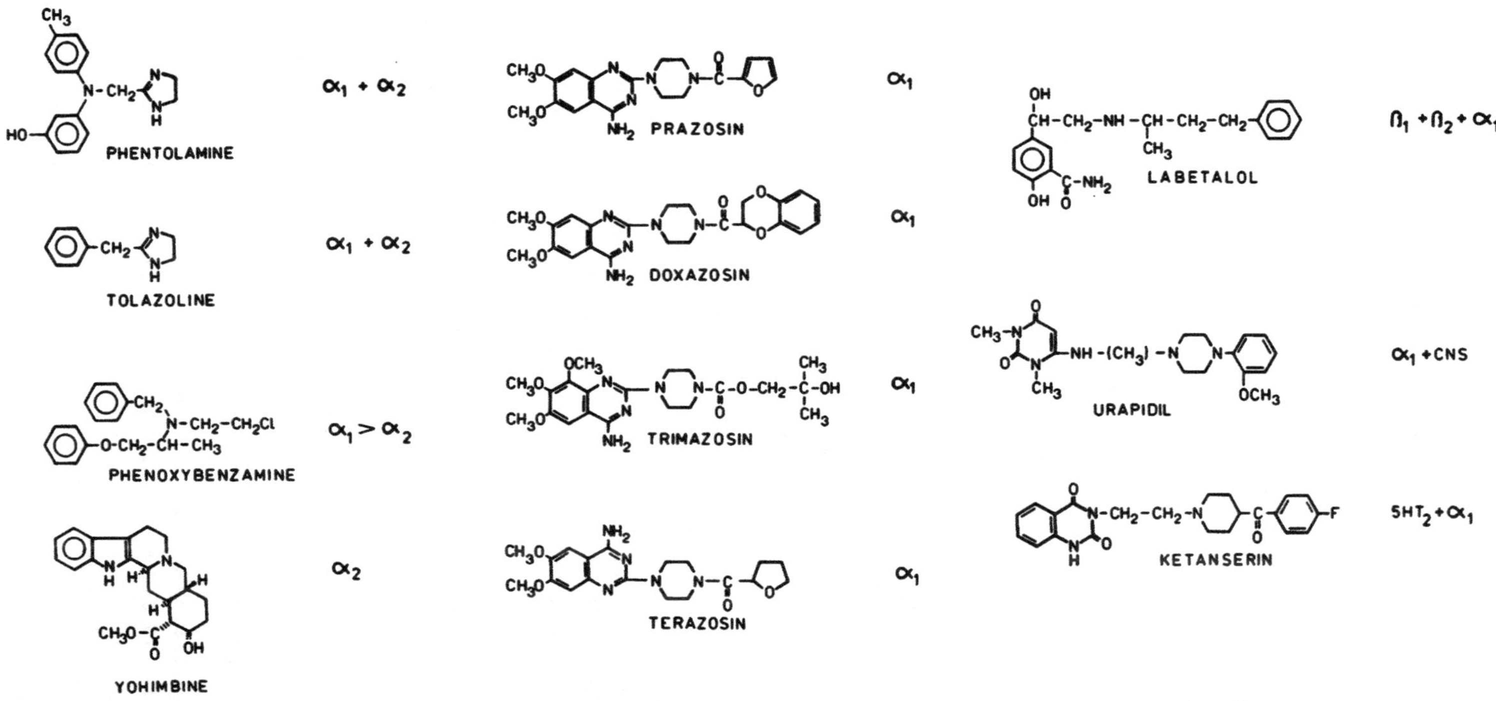

Fig. 1. Chemical structures of nonselective ($\alpha_1 + \alpha_2$)-adrenoceptor antagonists (*left*) and selective α_1-blockers (*right*). *Urapidil, ketanserin,* and *labetalol* are selective blockers of α_1-adrenoceptors, but they possess additional pharmacological activities not related to α-adrenoceptors

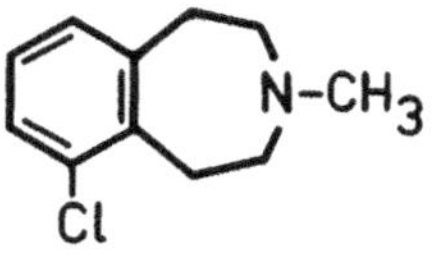

SK & F 86466

Fig. 2. Chemical structure of 6-chloro-*N*-methyl-2,3,4,5-tetrahydro-1-*H*-3-benzazepine (*SK&F 86466*), a selective α_2-adrenoceptor antagonist with hypotensive potency in animal experiments (Roesler et al. 1986)

Concerning the α_1-adrenoceptor drugs with ancillary activities, to be discussed in more detail in Sect. 4, urapidil appears to be chemically derived from uracil. It should be emphasized here that this molecule does not contain any stereoisomers, no asymmetric carbon atoms being available. Labetalol, a combined α- and β-adrenoceptor blocker, is a derivative of salicylamide. The molecule contains a phenylalkyl moiety and also resembles the classic β-blocker structures found in propranolol and related drugs. As a result of two asymmetric carbon atoms, the labetalol molecule has four stereoisomers, with differing pharmacologic properties.

Ketanserin is a selective antagonist of $5HT_2$-receptors with additional, modest affinity for α_1-adrenoceptors. Its chemical structure is largely different from that of the various α-adrenoceptor blockers discussed in this chapter.

α_2-Adrenoceptor blocking agents have been of use as tools in pharmacological studies only. Yohimbine, rauwolscine, and idazoxan are the prototypes of more or less selective α_2-adrenoceptor antagonists. Yohimbine and rauwolscine are diasteromeric rauwolfia alkaloids. The experimental compound SK&F 86466 (Roesler et al. 1986), which is also a selective α_2-adrenoceptor blocking agent, has been shown to lower blood pressure in some animal models of hypertension and will be studied in humans. The structure of this compound is shown in Fig. 2.

In general it is striking how little relationship between chemical structure and pharmacological activity the α-adrenoceptor blocking agents demonstrate, although within certain subgroups, for instance the prazosin-related drugs, such relationships appear to exist. This lack of structure-activity relationship (SAR) clearly contrasts with that of the β-adrenoceptor blocking drugs, where a SAR is easily detectable and adheres to quantitative criteria.

3 Pharmacokinetics and Metabolism

We shall emphasize prazosin and its successor drugs here, since these are the most relevant α-adrenoceptor blocking agents. The kinetic behavior of phenoxybenzamine and phentolamine may be briefly summarized as follows.

After oral administration approximately 30% of the administered *phenoxybenzamine* is absorbed. Inactivation occurs both through biotransformation in the liver and by renal excretion. Phenoxybenzamine has a long duration of action, thus requiring a once daily dosage schedule. It is known from clinical experience that a patient should be maintained on one particular dose for at least 3 days before this dose is increased.

Phentolamine is characterized by a fast oral absorption and rapid development of its hypotensive action. The drug is predominantly and quickly inactivated by biotransformation in the kidney, hence its duration of action is short, requiring a new dose every 4 h when given orally (IMHOF et al. 1976).

Prazosin is approximately 60% absorbed following oral administration (GRAHAM and PETTINGER 1979). The drug is subject to a substantial first pass effect in the liver. Maximal plasma concentrations are achieved 1–2 h after oral ingestion. In both animals and humans, prazosin is subject to extensive biotransformation in the liver: Mainly *O*-dealkylation and conjugation with glucuronic acid occur in humans, while 6-*O*-demethylprazosin is the main metabolite in dogs (TAYLOR et al. 1977). Less than 1% of the unchanged drug is excreted via the kidney. As shown with ^{14}C-labeled prazosin, the drug and its metabolites are rapidly taken up by various tissues. The highest concentrations were found in the lungs, various blood vessels, and the heart, whereas the brain level remained rather low in spite of its lipophilic character (HESS 1974; TAYLOR et al. 1977). In dogs, the plasma half-life amounts to 1–2 h (HESS 1974), whereas in humans a half-life of almost 3 h is found (BATEMAN et al. 1979). Following intravenous injection there is a correlation between plasma levels and hypotensive effect but only in the early phase of treatment (BATEMAN et al. 1979). However, after oral ingestion the plasma half-life (3–4 h) (WOOD et al. 1976) is shorter than that of the therapeutic, hypotensive effect. In the steady state approximately 97% of the drug is bound to plasma albumin.

For orally administered *trimazosin* the bioavailability has been reported to be approximately 60%. The drug is extensively metabolized in the liver (REID et al. 1983), and its major metabolite (CP 23445) in humans is an alkyl-hydroxylated derivative. According to REID et al. (1983) the pharmacokinetic profile of trimazosin is best described by a two-compartment model. The terminal half-life of trimazosin proved to be 2.73 ± 0.90 h, that of the metabolite (CP 23445), 1.47 ± 0.65 h. A similar elimination half-life after oral and intravenous administration was found.

Relatively few detailed pharmacokinetic data on *doxazosin* are available at present. In healthy, normotensive subjects the major pharmacokinetic difference between prazosin and doxazosin has been found in the elimination half-life, which for doxazosin was significantly longer (11 h; ELLIOTT et al. 1982) than for prazosin (2.5 h; ELLIOTT et al. 1981).

Upon oral administration terazosin is reported to be 90% absorbed (SONDERS 1986; TITMARSCH and MONK 1987), which is higher than observed for prazosin (60%). Food appeared to have no significant influence on oral absorption. The maximal plasma concentration was achieved 1–2 h after oral administration. A good correlation appeared to exist between administered dose and plasma concentration. Protein binding in plasma amounted to 90%–94%. Terazosin is extensively metabolized in the liver, according to the following pathways (SONDERS 1986): (a) hydrolysis at the amide bond, to yield the free piperazine derivative; (b) smaller portions of the drug are subject to *O*-demethylation and *N*-dealkylation, respectively, as well as cleavage of the piperazine ring. The biliary tract is a major route of excretion, as concluded from the observation that approximately 60% of the radioactive material is recovered from the feces of healthy volunteers who had received ^{14}C-terazosin by mouth. Approximately a third of the drug was recovered in the unchanged form from both faces and urine after oral administration.

After either oral or intravenous administration the half-life of plasma elimination has been reported in the range of 10–18 h, with an average of 12 h (KONDO et al. 1982; SONDERS 1986). Accordingly, the drug is eliminated more slowly than prazosin, thus allowing a once daily dosage in the treatment of hypertension. SONDERS (1986) demonstrated that the half-life of elimination of terazosin was significantly prolonged in subjects over 70 years of age compared with those 39 years old.

Hypertensive disease and congestive heart failure do not appear to cause relevant changes in the kinetic behavior of the drug.

After oral administration to healthy volunteers *urapidil* was reported to have an average bioavailability of 78%. A first pass effect is assumed to occur. Peak concentrations in plasma are achieved 4–6 h after ingestion of the currently used slow-release preparation (standard capsule).

The time course of the plasma concentration after an i.v. bolus injection could be described by means of a two-compartment model, with half-lives of 35 min and 2.7 h, reflecting distribution and elimination, respectively. Approximately 80% of the drug appears to be protein bound.

The half-life of elimination after oral administration amounts to 3.1 h. Approximately 50%-70% of the drug is eliminated via the renal route, consisting of 15% parent compound and the rest as metabolites (for review, see ZECH et al. 1986).

In humans *p*-hydroxylated urapidil appears to be the major metabolite (M_1). *O*-methylated (M_2) and *N*-demethylated (M_3) urapidil are also demonstrable but quantitatively of less importance. M_1 appears to be biologically inactive, whereas M_2 may contribute to the drug's blood pressure-lowering effect. M_2 has a longer half-life than urapidil and may therefore become more important upon prolonged treatment.

In the elderly enteral absorption was not different from that in younger adults. However, the half-life of elimination was clearly prolonged in elder hypertensive patients, and it would seem prudent to use lower doses of urapidil in the treatment of the elderly.

For *labetalol* and *ketanserin* see the respective chapters. 5 and 13.

4 Mechanism of Action, Pharmacodynamics, and Hemodynamic Effects

α-Adrenoceptors are generally recognized to be a vital component of the transmission process in the synapses of the sympathetic nervous system. They have been studied extensively over the past decade with respect to their molecular, pharmacological, and pathophysiological characteristic. The role of α-adrenoceptors in hypertensive disease has been studied in the past few years, although as yet no clear answers have been obtained. Nevertheless, the blockade of α-adrenoceptors by appropriate antagonistic drugs is known to be effective in lowering blood pressure, in particular with selective α_1-antagonists like prazosin and related drugs.

Before discussing the mode of action of the α-adrenoceptor antagonists as antihypertensives, it would seem useful to summarize current views on the subdivision and classification of α-adrenoceptors, as well as current opinions on their possible role in hypertensive disease.

4.1 Classification and Function of α-Adrenoceptors

α-Adrenoceptors can be divided into α_1- and α_2-subtypes (BERTHELSEN and PETTINGER 1977; STARKE 1981; TIMMERMANS and VAN ZWIETEN 1981). This subclassification is based on the affinity of selective agonists and antagonists for these two subtypes, whereas the subdivision into presynaptic and postsynaptic (prejunctional and postjunctional) α-adrenoceptors defines the localization with respect to the synapse (Fig. 3). Presynaptic receptors are located on the sympathetic nerve ending and postsynaptic receptors on the target organ, such as blood vessel (LANGER 1981; VAN ZWIETEN and TIMMERMANS 1983; VAN ZWIETEN

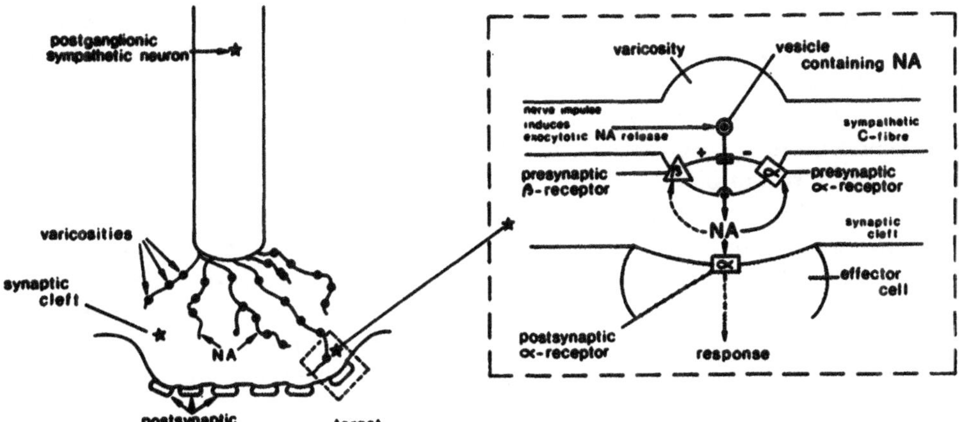

Fig. 3. Adrenergic synapse. Nerve activity releases the endogenous neurotransmitters noradrenaline (*NA*) and adrenaline from the varicosities. Noradrenaline and adrenaline reach the postsynaptic α- (or β-) adrenoceptors on the cell membrane of the target organ by diffusion. Upon receptor stimulation, a physiologic or pharmacologic effect is initiated. At postsynaptic sites both α_1- and α_2-adrenoceptors are present. Their stimulation in blood vessels causes vasoconstriction. At presynaptic sites predominantly α_2-adrenoceptors occur. Their stimulation causes a reduction of the noradrenaline release from the nerve ending. Noradrenaline release from presynaptic sites is enhanced when prejunctional α_2-adrenoceptors are blocked by selective α_2-adrenoceptor blocking agents or by nonselective (α_1 + α_2)-adrenoceptor antagonists

1984). Noradrenaline and adrenaline are nonselective agonists, that is, they stimulate α_1- and α_2-adrenoceptors equally well. Similarly, classic α-adrenoceptor blockers, like phentolamine, are nonselective compounds that antagonize both α_1- and α_2-adrenoceptors. At present we have a variety of agonists and antagonists at our disposal that are selective for either of the two receptor subtypes (Table 1). These selective compounds are useful tools in experimental pharmacology, but some of them—the selective blocker of α_1-adrenoceptor prazosin, for instance—have become valuable drugs in the treatment of hypertension and more recently in congestive heart failure as well.

Presynaptic α-adrenoceptors are almost exclusively of the α_2-subtype, judging by their affinity for selective α_2-receptor agonists and antagonists. However, both α_1- and α_2-adrenoceptors occur in comparable numbers at postsynaptic sites. Stimulation of presynaptic α_2-adrenoceptors reduces the release of endogenous noradrenaline from the nerve ending. Stimulation of vascular postsynaptic α_1- and α_2-adrenoceptors by their respective agonists causes vasoconstriction (VAN ZWIETEN and TIMMERMANS 1983; VAN ZWIETEN 1984; LANGER et al. 1980).

α-Adrenoceptors of both subtypes are found in a variety of organs and tissues. We shall limit the discussion to those tissues in which the α-adrenoceptors are targets for antihypertensive drugs. Peripheral α_1- and α_2-adrenoceptors at postsynaptic sites are involved functionally in the constriction of precapillary arterioles (resistance vessels), which is brought about by the endogenous neurotransmitters noradrenaline and adrenaline. It seems likely that the postsynaptic α_2-adrenoceptors are not innervated; in other words, their location is extrasynaptic rather than inside the synapse. Accordingly, they may be considered as hormone receptors, reacting to circulating catecholamines rather than to the neurotransmitter (noradrenaline) that is released from presynaptic structures (LANGER et al. 1980; WILFFERT et al. 1982). The stimulation of both α_1- and α_2-adrenoceptors at postsynaptic sites by appropriate agonists causes vasoconstriction and a rise in blood pressure. Accordingly, the vasoconstriction caused by noradrenaline and adrenaline is an effect based upon both α_1- and α_2-adrenoceptor stimulation. The concept of the postsynaptic α_2-adrenoceptor is rather new, and it has considerably changed our views on the distribution and functional role of α-adrenoceptors. Recent experiments have demonstrated that postsynaptic α_2-adrenoceptors probably play an important role in maintaining vascular tone in human resistance vessels (JIE et al. 1984; VAN BRUMMELEN et al. 1985).

The modulation of noradrenaline release from presynaptic sites by presynaptic α_2-adrenoceptors may be involved in physiologic regulation, particularly of blood pressure and heart rate. α_2-Adrenoceptors have been found in the heart, both at presynaptic and postsynaptic sites. Their functional role in regulating the circulation is unclear; however, presynaptic α_2-receptors may play a part in bradycardia induced by clonidine and related drugs (DE JONGE et al. 1981; TIMMERMANS and VAN ZWIETEN 1982). However, the role of these receptors in sympathetic regulation of heart rate is speculative.

In the CNS, α-adrenoceptors are located in the brain stem, specifically the

Table 1. α-Adrenoceptor agonists and antagonists: characterization with respect to their selectivity for α_1- and α_2-adrenoceptors and possible therapeutic applications

Agents	Receptor stimulated or blocked	Application
Agonists		
Noradrenaline (neurotransmitter)	$\alpha_1 + \alpha_2 + \beta_1$	Vasoconstrictor ($\alpha_1 + \alpha_2$)
Adrenaline	$\alpha_1 + \alpha_2 + \beta_1 + \beta_2$	Vasoconstrictor ($\alpha_1 + \alpha_2$)
Phenylephrine	$\alpha_1 > \alpha_2$	Vasoconstrictor (α_1), decongestant (α_1)
Cirazoline	α_1	Vasoconstrictor
Methoxamine	α_1	Vasoconstrictor
Clonidine	$\alpha_2 + \alpha_1$	Antihypertensive (central α_2)
Guanfacine	$\alpha_2 > \alpha_1$	Antihypertensive (central α_2)
Azepexole (B-HT 933)	α_2	Experimental antihypertensive (central α_2)
B-HT 920	α_2 + DA	Experimental
UK-14,304	α_2	Experimental
Antagonists		
Phentolamine (Regitine)	$\alpha_1 + \alpha_2$	Pheochromocytoma preoperative phase ($\alpha_1 + \alpha_2$)
Tolazoline	$\alpha_2 > \alpha_1$	Vasodilator ($\alpha_1 + \alpha_2$)
Prazosin (Minipress)	α_1	Antihypertensive (peripheral α_1)
Doxazosin	α_1	Antihypertensive (peripheral α_1)
Terazosin	α_1	Antihypertensive (peripheral α_1)
Trimazosin	α_1	Antihypertensive (peripheral α_1)
Corynanthine } Diastereoisomers	α_1	Experimental
Rauwolscine } Diastereoisomers	α_1	Experimental
Yohimbine } Diastereoisomers	α_2	Experimental
Idazoxan	α_2	Experimental
SK&F 86466	α_2	Experimental

nucleus tractus solitarii, the vasomotor center, and the nucleus of the vagal nerve. The region of the nucleus tractus solitarii shows a particularly high density of (nor)adrenergic synapses, suggesting a functional role of α-adrenoceptors. These receptors are mainly of the α_2-subtype, although the presence of α_1-adrenoceptors has been demonstrated by receptor-binding techniques.

The stimulation of central α_2-adrenoceptors by appropriate agonists induces a reduction of peripheral sympathetic tone. Arterial blood pressure and heart rate fall via the stimulation of an inhibitory neuron—probably the bulbospinal neuron. The stimulation of central α_2-adrenoceptors also induces an enhanced vagal tone, thus contributing to bradycardia. It seems likely that the central α_2-adrenoceptors are functionally involved in regulating blood pressure and heart rate. (For reviews on central α-adrenoceptors, their involvement in blood pressure regulation, and as targets of centrally acting antihypertensive drugs, see SCHMITT 1971; KOBINGER 1978; VAN ZWIETEN 1975; VAN ZWIETEN and TIMMERMANS 1984; REID et al. 1983; and Chapter 6 of this book.)

4.2 Role of α-Adrenoceptors in Hypertensive Disease

To date, a clear and consistent picture regarding the characteristics and density of α-adrenoceptors in human hypertensive disease has not emerged. This limitation is explained so far by methodological shortcomings, which do not allow investigation of α-adrenoceptors in vascular smooth muscle, virtually all studies being limited to α_2-adrenoceptors on ex vivo thrombocytes. Conflicting results have been reported with respect to the α_2-receptor density in thrombocytes of hypertensive patients. BRODDE et al. (1984, 1985) have repeatedly found significantly increased densities of α_2-adrenoceptors in the thrombocytes of hypertensive patients, as compared with those obtained from age- and sex-matched normotensive subjects. JONES et al. (1985), however, found a lower α_2-adrenoceptor density in platelets from hypertensives, whereas MOTULSKY et al. (1983) found no difference et al.

A hyperreactivity to pressor stimuli has been reported repeatedly in hypertensive patients (PHILIPP et al. 1978; AMANN et al. 1981; BUEHLER et al. 1985); the hyperreactivity already described for the systemic circulation was also found in the vascular bed of the human forearm (JIE et al. 1984, 1986; KIOWSKI et al. 1983). Again, the hyperreactivity was a general phenomenon for both α_1- and α_2-adrenoceptor-mediated vasoconstriction, as well as for both adrenaline and noradrenaline. These findings cast doubt upon the specificity of the hyperreactivity phenomenon encountered in hypertensive subjects. Whether highly specific or not, the hyperreactivity to vasoconstrictor stimuli in hypertensives appears a logical basis for drug treatment with α-adrenoceptor antagonistic drugs.

4.3 Antihypertensive Activity of α-Adrenoceptor Blocking Agents

α-Adrenoceptor antagonists cause vasodilatation and a fall in blood pressure because the endogenous agonists noradrenaline and adrenaline can no longer reach and stimulate the vascular α-receptor, which is occupied by the antagonist. Non-selective α_1- and α_2-adrenoceptor antagonists like phentolamine cause vasodilatation which is based upon the blockade of both α_1- and α_2-adrenoceptors. The administration of such drugs is accompanied by marked reflex tachycardia, triggered by the baroreceptor reflex system and the autonomic nervous system. Owing to presynaptic α_2-receptor blockade, treatment with phentolamine results in enhanced release of catecholamines from the nerve endings. Probably as a result of reflex sympathetic activation, phentolamine treatment induces the stimulation of the renin-angiotensin-aldosterone system, and plasma renin activity is increased, causing the retention of sodium and water.

The reflex tachycardia is a serious drawback in the use of non-selective (α_1 + α_2)-adrenoceptor blocking agents as antihypertensive agents. The introduction of the selective α_1-adrenoceptor blocking agent prazosin offers much better possibilities for antihypertensive treatment, reflex tachycardia being virtually absent. According to CONSTANTINE et al. (1978) prazosin does not cause reflex tachycardia in conscious dogs, although weak reflex tachycardia in rats has been described (GRAHAM and PETTINGER 1979; LEFÈVRE-BORG et al. 1979). Several authors have reported that in hypertensive patients continuously treated with prazosin no substantial reflex tachycardia is observed in the steady state (for reviews, see BROGDEN et al. 1977; GRAHAM and PETTINGER 1979; CAVERO and ROACH 1980; STANASZEK et al. 1983).

The absence of a marked reflex stimulation of the heart cannot be explained in detail. A partial explanation is offered by the absence of noradrenaline release via a presynaptic (α_2) mechanism. α_1-Adrenoceptors are found almost exclusively at postjunctional sites; prejunctional α-receptors are predominantly of the α_2 subtype. For this reason, it would be expected that prazosin should not significantly interfere with the release of endogenous noradrenaline mediated by presynaptic α_2-adrenoceptors. It has indeed been observed by various investigators that prazosin does not enhance the release of noradrenaline from sympathetic nerve endings, whereas classic, non-selective blockers of α_1- and α_2-adrenoceptors do stimulate the liberation of noradrenaline via a presynaptic mechanism.

The lack of a pronounced reflex tachycardia following prazosin treatment may be due to reduced baroreceptor modulation since it has been found that prazosin depresses the baroreflex function in cats (CAMBRIDGE et al. 1977), dogs (HARDEY and LOKHANDWALA 1979), and humans (SASSO and O'CONNOR, 1982). However, such an effect could not be established for prazosin in rabbits (CAVERO 1982). Prazosin (and indoramin) reduces sympathetic nerve discharges in cats (RAMAGE 1982) and rats (PERSSON et al. 1981). Furthermore, no increase in plasma dopamine-β-hydroxylase activity accompanied the fall in blood pressure caused by prazosin in humans, nor is an increase in plasma noradrenaline levels found following administration of prazosin in conscious dogs (SAEED et al. 1982). Finally, prazosin has very little influence on plasma renin, the levels of which are usually unchanged or occasionally somewhat reduced. Nevertheless, some retention of sodium and water may occur, although less than that observed after treatment with directly acting vasodilators or phentolamine.

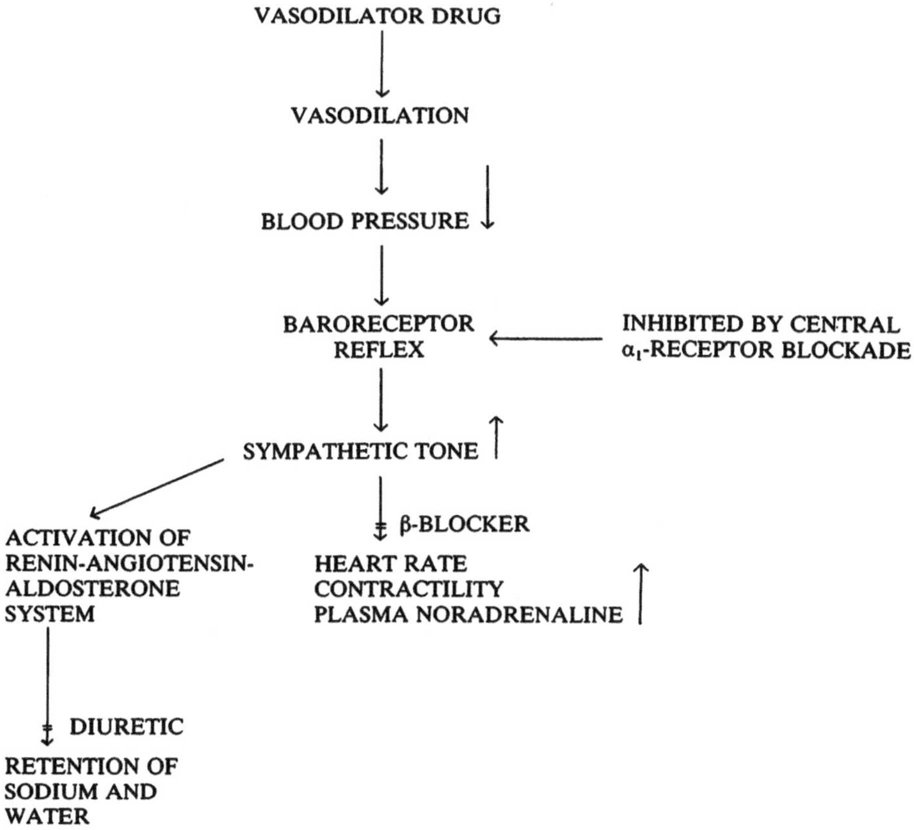

Fig. 4. Reflex activity, elicited by vasodilator drugs and mediated by the baroreceptor mechanism and the symathetic nervous system. Enhanced sympathetic activity causes elevated plasma noradrenaline levels, a rise in heart rate and contractility, and also the activation of the renin-angiotensin-aldosterone system, thus giving rise to the retention of sodium and water. The rise in heart rate can be counteracted with a β-blocker, the retention of sodium and water by a diuretic. Blockade of central α_1-adrenoceptors by selective α_1-adrenoceptor antagonists modulates the baroreceptor reflex mechanism and hence suppresses reflex tachycardia

A second mechanism which may help to explain the lack of reflex tachycardia during prazosin treatment is the blockade of central α_1-adrenoceptors. It has been demonstrated by Huchet et al. (1981) that this blockade, e.g., by prazosin, modulates baroreceptor reflex mechanisms and thus counteracts the reflex tachycardia evoked by prazosin-induced vasodilatation. For a schematic presentation of this mechanism, see Fig. 4. At present, there is general agreement that the reversible blockade of vascular postsynaptic α_1-adrenoceptors is the underlying cause of the vasodilating and hypotensive effect of prazosin.

Various other mechanisms involved in the hypotensive effect can be excluded. Prazosin does not interfere with transmission in peripheral sympathetic ganglia or neurons (Constantine et al. 1973). It does not clearly display acute central hypotensive activity (Constantine et al. 1973; Roach et al. 1978;

Timmermans et al. 1979), although blockade of central α_1-adrenoceptors in rat brain has been demonstrated. It has been reported by only one group that α_1-adrenoceptor antagonists such as prazosin can reduce blood pressure (and heart rate) in animals, not only via blockade of vascular α_1-adrenoceptors, but also as a result of a centrally mediated decrease in sympathetic tone (Persson et al. 1981).

Central α_2-adrenoceptor stimulation decreases sympathetic nervous activity and increases vagal tone. Conversely, it has recently been suggested that activation of central α_1-adrenoceptors increases sympathetic tone and reduces vagal activity (Huchet et al. 1981).

Inhibition of phosphodiesterase by prazosin as well as a direct vasodilator action apparently do not play a role at therapeutic doses of the drug (Brogden et al. 1977). Prazosin does not decrease cardiac output (Constantine et al. 1973). Its hypotensive effect is due solely to a decrease in total peripheral resistance, reflecting dilatation of the precapillary arterioles as a result of the blockade of vascular α_1-adrenoceptors. The selectivity of prazosin for α_1-adrenoceptors has been demonstrated on isolated, perfused, rabbit pulmonary artery (Cambridge et al. 1977), perfused cat spleen, rat brain slices, and other in vivo and in vitro preparations (Doxey et al. 1977; Timmermans et al. 1980). Receptor-binding studies using prazosin as the displacing drug (U'Prichard et al. 1978) or as a tritiated ligand (Greengrass and Bremner 1979; Cambridge et al. 1980; Hornung et al. 1979; Miach et al. 1980) have confirmed its marked affinity and selectivity for α_1-adrenoceptors.

Prazosin causes a relaxation of both resistance and capacitance vessels. The pronounced venous dilatation is understandable in view of the particular dependence of the veins on sympathetic stimulation (Lund-Johansen 1974; Robinson 1981). The venous dilatation is probably the cause of the "first dose" effect, i.e., the orthostatic hypotension observed after the first dose of prazosin. A dilator effect of prazosin on renal resistance vessels which is not associated with impairment of renal function has been described in hypertensive patients (Preston et al. 1979).

The successor drugs to prazosin, i.e., trimazosin, doxazosin, and terazosin, appear to have the same mode of action as prazosin, as far as can be judged at present.

Trimazosin is somewhat less selective for α_1-adrenoceptors than prazosin (Singleton et al. 1982), and in contrast to prazosin it shows weak direct vasodilator activity (Constantine and Hess 1981). It seems very likely that trimazosin, like prazosin, induces a hypotensive/antihypertensive effect and causes a reduction in total peripheral resistance, predominantly as a result of vascular postsynaptic α_1-adrenoceptor blockade. Since α_1-blockade by trimazosin is somewhat weaker than that caused by prazosin, it has been suggested that other mechanisms, possibly direct vasodilator activity, may contribute to the drugs' hypotensive effect (Reid et al. 1983). The possibility should also be considered that trimazosin's active metabolite (CP 23445) displays hypotensive activity as a result of direct vasodilator activity. Trimazosin does not significantly influence heart rate, probably for the same reasons as discussed for prazosin (see above).

Like prazosin, trimazosin causes dilatation of both resistance and capacitance vessels (Awan et al. 1982).

Doxazosin is also a selective α_1-adrenoceptor blocking agent in animal preparations (Timmermans et al. 1980; Vincent et al. 1983a) and in humans (Singleton et al. 1980; Elliot et al. 1982; Vincent et al. 1983b). It has a somewhat lower potency as an α_1-antagonist than prazosin (Hamilton et al. 1985). Probably for similar reasons as discussed for prazosin, it does not cause relevant reflex tachycardia. Concomitantly, its mode of action appears to be the same as that of prazosin, but doxazosin has a longer duration of action.

Terazosin displays the same degree of selectivity for α_1-adrenoceptors as prazosin, but on a molar basis its potency is threefold lower (Kyncl 1986; Titmarsch and Monk 1987; and quoted literature). It should be assumed, therefore, that terazosin's mode of hypotensive action is the same as that of prazosin. Terazosin has a longer duration of action than prazosin, and it is more hydrophilic. As with prazosin, doxazosin, and trimazosin, virtually no reflex tachycardia is observed during treatment with terazosin (Moser 1986).

Urapidil is a selective α_1-adrenoceptor antagonist with an additional central hypotensive action which is not fully understood. On a molar basis urapidil is less potent as an α_1-blocker than prazosin and also somewhat less selective. A

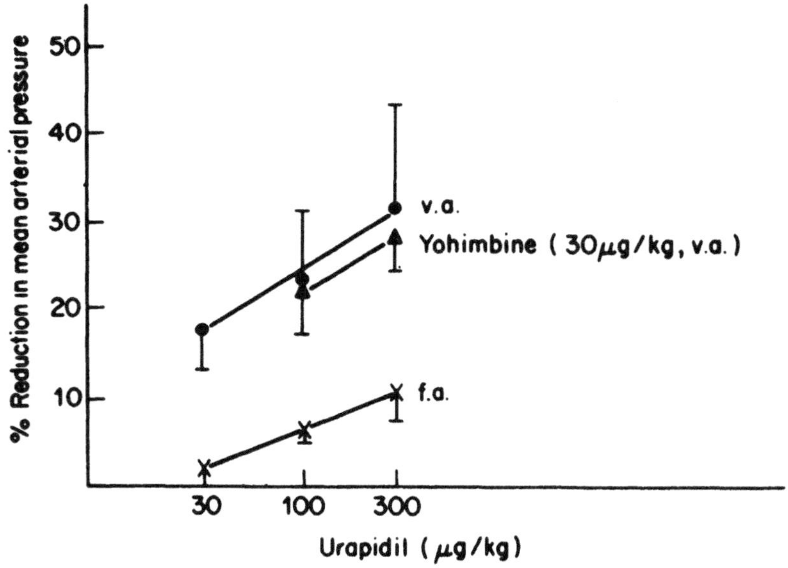

Fig. 5. Demonstration of the central hypotensive activity of urapidil. After infusion into the left vertebral artery, inducing perfusion of th brain stem with the drug, the hypotensive effect is much stronger than after systemic administration via a femoral artery. The central hypotensive effect of urapidil is not reduced by prior treatment with the α_2-adrenoceptor antagonist yohimbine. Dose-response curves for the reduction in mean arterial pressure of chloralose-anesthetized cats by urapidil after infusion via the vertebral artery (*v.a.*) or via the femoral artery (*f.a.*) and after infusion via the vertebral artery 15 min after v.a. infusion of *yohimbine* (30 μg/kg). Symbols represent mean values ±S.E.; $n = 4-5$; $\beta < 0.05$. Data from van Zwieten et al. (1985)

modest affinity of urapidil for β_1-adrenoceptors was found in both radioligand binding and functional studies with isolated organs. However, this β_1-adrenoceptor blocking activity does not play a role in the antihypertensive activity of urapidil in humans. In older studies urapidil had been said to possess a presynaptic α_2-adrenoceptor agonistic effect, but this could not be confirmed by several researchers. Since urapidil has very little affinity for α_2-adrenoceptors, as concluded from radioligand binding studies, a relevant presynaptic α_2-effect can hardly be expected.

Apart from its manifest α_1-adrenoceptor blocking activity, urapidil shows central hypotensive activity in several animal models, for instance, after injection into cerebral ventricles or into the vertebral artery (Fig. 5). Although difficult to demonstrate in human patients, the central mechanism can be expected to contribute to the drug's blood pressure-lowering effect. In contrast to classic centrally acting drugs like clonidine, guanfacine, and α-methyl-DOPA, the central effect of urapidil is not mediated by central α_2-adrenoceptors. It has been submitted recently that the central hypotensive activity of urapidil might be mediated by $5HT_{1A}$-receptors in the CNS. This view, which is mainly based upon a certain affinity of urapidil for $5HT_{1A}$-receptors in radioligand binding studies, has not been substantiated by conclusive pharmacological experiments so far (for reviews, see SCHOETENSACK et al. 1983; AMERY 1986).

In conclusion, urapidil should be considered a moderately selective α_1-adrenoceptor antagonist with an additional central hypotensive mechanism, which unlike clonidine does not involve central α_2-adrenoceptors. Urapidil's various pharmacological activities are shown schematically in Fig. 6.

For the modes of action of *labetalol* and *ketanserin* see Chap. 5 and 13, respectively.

4.4 Hemodynamic Profile of α-Adrenoceptor Antagonistic Drugs

Phentolamine and phenoxybenzamine both induce dilatation in the arterial as well as in the venous vascular bed, since in both types of blood vessels α-adrenoceptors are present and hence subject to blockade by an α-adrenoceptor antagonistic drug. Orthostatic hypotension is probably caused predominantly by venodilatation. I have already discussed the reflex tachycardia induced by these classic α-adrenoceptor blockers (see Sect. 4.3) as well as the retention of sodium and water due to sympathetic activation of the renin-angiotensin-aldosterone system. The hemodynamic profile of the selective α_1-adrenoceptor blockers, may be summarized as follows.

Prazosin and related drugs cause a reduction in total peripheral resistance and a fall in blood pressure as a result of dilatation of the precapillary arterioles (resistance vessels). Simultaneously, venodilatation occurs, owing to the blockade of α_1-adrenoceptors in the venous vascular bed. This effect is probably the reason for the well-known side effect of orthostatic hypotension. As discussed previously (see Sect. 4.3) prazosin and related drugs cause little or no reflex tachycardia. Fluid retention is observed upon prolonged treatment and usually requires the combined application of a natriuretic drug.

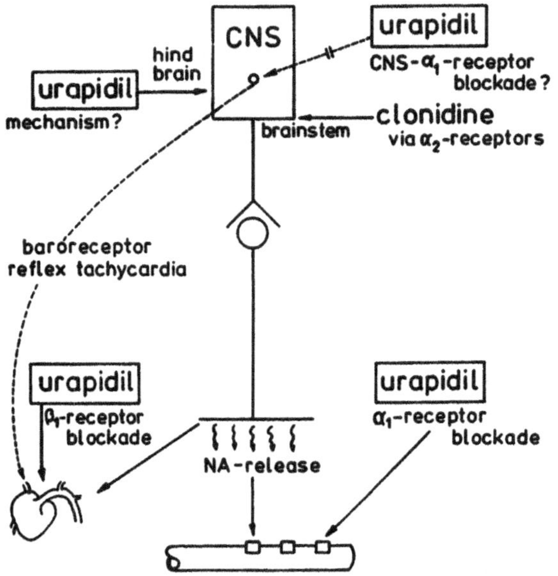

Fig. 6. Schematic representation of the mechanisms underlying the hemodynamic changes induced by urapidil. (1) *Blockade* of vascular postsynaptic α_1-adrenoceptors causes dilatation of the precapillary arterioles, a reduction in total peripheral resistance, and hence a fall in blood pressure. (2) A central hypotensive effect with a so far unknown mechanism is initiated probably at the level of the *hindbrain*. Accordingly, peripheral sympathetic tone is reduced, causing vasodilatation. (3) *Baroreceptor reflex tachycardia* is blunted, probably at a central level, possibly involving blockade of central α_1-adrenoceptors. (4) Urapidil shows modest antagonistic activity on cardiac *β_1-adrenoceptors*. This mechanism may offer a moderate contribution to the impairment of reflex tachycardia

The newer α_1-adrenoceptor blocking drugs, like doxazosin, trimazosin, and terazosin, display a hemodynamic profile which is very similar to that of prazosin.

It should be realized that the hemodynamic profile of α_1-blockers in hypertensive patients closely resembles that in normotensive volunteers. However, when used in patients with congestive heart failure the hemodynamic changes induced by α_1-adrenoceptor blocking agents are clearly different. For instance, it was shown for terazosin (LUI et al. 1985) that in patients with congestive heart failure this α_1-adrenoceptor antagonist significantly reduces left ventricular filling pressure and systemic vascular resistance, while increasing both heart rate and cardiac index.

Urapidil when administered i.v. to hypertensive patients displays a hemodynamic profile very similar to that of prazosin and related drugs (MESSERLI et al. 1986). Accordingly, the acute fall in arterial blood pressure is accompanied by an increase in systemic, renal, and splanchnic blood flow as well as transient reflex tachycardia as a result of sympathetic activation. In several patients treated with urapidil, orthostatic hypotension was observed, reflecting venous dilatation. This hemodynamic profile is virtually the same as that observed for i.v. administered prazosin (Kobrin et al. 1984; Stanaszek et al. 1983).

As with prazosin, reflex tachycardia does not occur during prolonged treatment with urapidil. A detailed hemodynamic analysis of the long-term effects of urapidil has not yet been performed.

For a discussion of the hemodynamic profiles of *labetalol* and *ketanserin* see Chaps. 5 and 13, respectively.

5 Therapeutic Use and Dosage

As stated previously the older α-blockers like *phentolamine* and *phenoxybenzamin* are only used in the preoperative phase of pheochromocytoma and during surgery. Phentolamine is given orally every 4 h in 20 mg doses, until the desired effect is achieved. Intravenously, doses of 5–10 mg are given preoperatively, to be repeated if necessary during surgery.

Phenoxybenzamine treatment is started with 10 mg oral doses which can be raised up to 20–60 mg daily, in three doses. As an i.v. infusion a dose of 0.5–1 mg/kg body weight is given over 2 h, 36h, and 12 h prior to surgical intervention. However intravenous phentolamine is the preferred drug during surgical intervention.

Prazosin's efficacy in mild to severe hypertension has been demonstrated in numerous therapeutic trials, against placebo and in comparison with other drugs. Follow-up studies have shown continued efficacy after 2–5 years of treatment. Its efficacy as monotherapy has been shown, but prazosin is frequently combined with a diuretic, a β-blocker, or both. Comparative studies have shown prazosin to be as effective as α-methyl-DOPA, clonidine, hydralazine, atenolol, indoramin, minoxidil, propranolol, and labetalol. Prazosin does not significantly change renal function and does not cause adverse effects on renal function in hypertensive patients with renal impairment. The virtual absence of reflex tachycardia was already discussed (see Sect. 4.3). Orthostatic hypotension, probably caused by dilatation of the venous vascular bed, is the basis of the so-called first dose effect. It can be largely avoided by starting the therapy with a very low dose of 0.5 mg, to be ingested at bed time, followed by a gradual build-up of the dosage schedule. The following dosage schedule is therefore recommended:

An initial dose of 0.5 mg in the evening, followed by 2–3 doses per day of 0.5 mg each during the following 3 days. If necessary the doses can be gradually increased to a maximum of 20 mg per day in divided doses.

A certain efficacy of prazosin as an unloading drug in the treatment of congestive heart failure has been described, usually in trials with a rather small number of patients. Most of the trials are rather short, and one would like to see more prolonged periods of observation to be convinced of the drugs's long-term efficacy in cardiac failure. For an extensive survey of the results with prazosin in clinical trials both in hypertension and in congestive heart failure, see Brogden et al. (1977) and Stanaszek et al. (1983).

A few reports in the literature suggest that prazosin can be useful in the preoperative treatment of pheochromocytoma, but it seems advisable to combine it with a β-blocker in those particular cases (Cubeddu et al. 1982).

The dose-related antihypertensive effect of *trimazosin* has been demonstrated both in double-blind, placebo-controlled and in open studies. Initially a thrice daily regimen was used, but later it was shown that a twice daily schedule gave an 80% response rate. Similarly, though initial dosing was typically 900 mg daily, it is now recognized that in most cases a satisfactory response is obtained at a daily dose of 300 mg. The duration of action of trimazosin is thus obviously longer than that of prazosin, although pharmacokinetic data would suggest that trimazosin should be administered thrice daily.

Both trimazosin and its most important metabolite are pharmacologically active. Its onset of action is slower than that of prazosin, and the first dose effect may also be expected to be milder than that of prazosin. Nevertheless, it would seem wise to titrate the dosage schedule of trimazosin as carefully as that of prazosin, until more clinical experience has been obtained with this newer drug.

No consensus has yet been reached concerning the dosage regimen of trimazosin. In mild to moderate essential hypertension the following schedule is proposed: begin with 50 mg two times daily, increase up to a maximal dosage of 300 mg daily, divided into two doses. Further clinical studies are required to establish such a schedule more firmly. For reviews on the clinical application of trimazosin, see Perry (1985) and Taylor et al. (1983).

Doxazosin: in the first two weeks 1 mg per day, to be gradually increased to 4 mg or maximally 8 mg once daily.

Terazosin has been studied in double-blind trials against placebo or against prazosin in periods of 4–13 weeks, in doses from 1 up to 40 mg daily given orally to patients with mild to moderate essential hypertension. Terazosin is significantly more effective than placebo in lowering blood pressure. In most cases no increase in heart rate is observed. As monotherapy, administered at a dosage up to 20 mg once daily terazosin displays an antihypertensive efficacy similar to prazosin up to 10 mg twice daily. Both drugs reduced supine mean systolic and diastolic blood pressures by 5–10 mmHg. In doses up to 10 mg once daily, however, terazosin proved less effective than hydrochlorothiazide 25–50 mg twice daily. Drayer et al. (1983) observed that terazosin produces a downward shift in the circadian pattern of blood pressure, confirming persistent antihypertensive effects for 24 h.

The available data suggest that terazosin can be applied as monotherapy in doses of 10–20 mg once daily, although a twice daily dose of terazosin appears to be well-tolerated. More clinical experience is required to establish its optimal dosage schedule and its final position in the management of essential hypertension. Terazosin might be anticipated to be of potential use in congestive heart failure. So far, beneficial effects were seen in small numbers of patients only.

For extensive reviews of the therapeutic efficacy of terazosin in hypertension see Moser (1986) and Titmarsh and Monk (1987).

Urapidil's efficacy has been demonstrated in several smaller and larger clinical trials, against placebo or against other drugs. Clinical trials including multicenter studies have been performed for periods of up to 2 years and lead to the conclusion that efficacy is maintained with prolonged treatment. In most cases sustained-release capsules of 30 mg have been used, which were usually given twice daily. Once daily administration is under investigation at present.

In smaller studies it has been shown that urapidil given intravenously as a bolus injection may be used to manage a hypertensive emergency. In a few small studies the impression has been obtained that urapidil may be beneficial as an unloading drug in the treatment of congestive heart failure.

For reviews on the clinical efficacy of urapidil, see SCHOETENSACK et al. (1983) and AMERY (1986).

For a discussion of the therapeutic efficacy of *labetalol* and *ketanserin* see Chaps. 5 and 13, respectively.

6 Combination with Other Drugs and Drug Interactions

The antihypertensive activity of α-adrenoceptor blocking agents is enhanced by a variety of current antihypertensive drugs. As a whole this should be considered as a mere additive effect which does not involve specific, receptor-triggered mechanisms, and potentiation does not occur.

With respect to *prazosin* a variety of different antihypertensive drugs can be combined with this α_1-adrenoceptor blocker (STANASZEK et al. 1983), but it is most frequently combined with a β-blocker and/or a diuretic. As such, prazosin is usually added to a combined therapy with a β-blocker and a diuretic. The diuretic in this triple therapy counteracts potential fluid retention induced by prazosin. In all studies reported prazosin appears to cause an additive decrease in blood pressure (for review, see STANASZEK et al. 1983).

Trimazosin, doxazosin, and terazosin can also potentially be combined with various other antihypertensive agents such as diuretics, β-blockers, or both to yield an additive antihypertensive action. However, such combinations have not been studied systematically.

There are only a few incidental reports on combined use of *urapidil* with other antihypertensives. At least on theoretical grounds a similar outcome as described for prazosin and its successor drugs may be anticipated, but further studies are required.

6.1 Drug Interactions

Specific interactions between α-adrenoceptor blocking agents and other drugs do not play a relevant role in the management of hypertension or congestive heart failure. However, volume depletion by diuretic therapy may accentuate their hypotensive action.

7 Contraindications

Absolute contraindications for α-adrenoceptor blocking agents are few, but caution appears to be advisable in certain clinical conditions. An abrupt hypotensive effect, as caused by intravenously administered α-adrenoceptor blockers (in particular phentolamine or phenoxybenzamine) may be deleterious in patients with cerebral or coronary ischemia and in general in the elderly. Orthostatic hypotension leading to falls is a potential risk of all α-adrenoceptor blocking drugs. Hypersensitivity, although a rare phenomenon, is a contraindication for prazosin.

In contrast to β-blockers prazosin can be safely used in patients with obstructive airways disease, diabetes mellitus, or peripheral vascular disorders. The same probably holds for its various successor drugs.

8 Side Effects and Toxicity

Most adverse reactions to α-adrenoceptor antagonists can be extrapolated from their vasodilator and α-blocking potency. Hypotension, dizziness, headache, reflex tachycardia, congestion of the nasal mucosa, and impaired ejaculation are logical side effects of the α-blockers, in particular of the non-selective ($\alpha_1 + \alpha_2$)-blockers.

The virtual absence of reflex tachycardia during treatment with prazosin and related α_1-selective drugs has already been discussed in Sect. 4.3. Postural hypotension, known as the first dose effect of prazosin, probably reflects venous dilatation. This phenomenon can be largely prevented by careful titration of the dosage.

Prazosin has been reported to influence favourably the profile of plasma lipids during long-term treatment of hypertension, with a tendency to improve the ratio HDL/LDL + VLDL-cholesterol, in the sense of increasing HDL and reducing LDL + VLDL-cholesterol. In some studies but not all, prazosin was found to decrease plasma triglyceride levels. Most studies on the influence of prazosin on lipid levels have included small numbers of patients, without adequate control of other factors influencing plasma lipids, such as diet and smoking habits. Studies with larger numbers of patients under carefully controlled conditions will be required to establish the influence of prazosin on the lipid profile. Prazosin appears not to influence glucose metabolism and can therefore be safely used for diabetic patients. Sexual dysfunction owing to prazosin is very rare and not firmly established. Renal and respiratory functions remain uninfluenced by prazosin. For extensive reviews on the side effects of prazosin, see Brogden et al. (1977) and Stanaszek et al. (1983).

It seems very likely that *trimazosin, doxazosin, and terazosin* display a pattern of side effects similar to that of prazosin. For review, see Titmarsh and Monk (1987).

Urapidil shows the usual side effects of a selective α_1-blocking agent as discussed above for prazosin, but a first dose effect has not clearly been recognized and described. Mild sedation is sometimes observed in the beginning of the treatment period but is usually transient. There are virtually no reports on sexual dysfunction caused by urapidil treatment. As a whole, urapidil appears to be well-tolerated. For reviews on its side effects, see Schoetensack et al. (1983).

Summary

Elevated peripheral resistance being the most consistent hemodynamic change in established essential hypertension, it would seem logical to treat hypertensive disease with vasodilator drugs, including α-adrenoceptor blockers.

Classic α-adrenoceptor antagonists like phenoxybenzamine and phentolamine are hardly useful as antihypertensives, apart from the preoperative treatment of pheochromocytoma. However, the selective α_1-adrenoceptor antagonists have proved useful, with an interesting and logical mode of action. In the present chapter a survey is given of the selective α_1-adrenoceptor antagonists, of which prazosin and its successor drugs trimazosin, doxazosin, and terazosin are the prototypes. Before discussing these drugs and their properties, we review the modern classification of α-adrenoceptors as well as their possible role in hypertensive disease.

The chemistry, pharmacokinetic and metabolic profiles, as well as their modes of action and hemodynamic effects of individual agents are discussed, with an emphasis on the mechanism of action. The clinical part of this chapter deals with the therapeutic activity and dosage, contraindications, combination with other drugs, and adverse reactions. Urapidil, a compound which is a selective α_1-adrenoceptor blocking agent with an additional central hypotensive mechanism (which is not understood in detail) is included in the discussions.

References

Amery A (ed) (1986) Treatment of hypertension with urapidil. Preclinical and clinical update. R Soc Med Serv 101:1–186

Amann FW, Bolli P, Kiowski W et al. (1981) Enhanced α-adrenoceptor-mediated vasoconstriction in essential hypertension. Hypertension 3(Suppl I):119–123

Awan N, Hermanovich J, Vera Z et al. (1982) Cardiocirculatory actions of trimazosin and sodium nitroprusside in ischemic heart disease. Clin Pharmacol Ther 31:290

Bateman DN, Hobbs DC, Twomey TM et al. (1979) Prazosin, pharmacokinetics and concentration effect. Eur J Clin Pharmacol 16:177–181

Berthelsen S, Pettinger WA (1977) A functional basis for classification of α-adrenergic receptors. Life Sci 21:595–606

Brodde OE, Daul AE, O'Hara N, Bock KD (1984) Increased density and responsiveness of α- and β-adrenoceptors in circulating blood cells of essential hypertensive patients. J Hypertens 2(Suppl 3):111–113

Brodde OE, Daul AE, O'Hara H, Khalifa AM (1985) Properties of α- and β-adrenoceptors in circulating blood cells of patients with essential hypertension. J Cardiovasc Pharmacol 7:S162-S167

Brogden RN, Heel RC, Speight TM, Avery GS (1977) Prazosin: a review of its pharmacological properties and therapeutic efficacy in hypertension. Drugs 14:163–197

Buehler FR, Bolli P, Erne P, Kiowski W, Mueller FB, Hulthén UL, Ji BH (1985) Adrenoceptors, calcium and vasoconstriction in normal and hypertensive humans. J Cardiovasc Pharmacol 7:S130-S136

Cambridge D, Davey MJ, Massingham R (1977) The pharmacology of antihypertensive drugs with special reference to vasodilators, α-adrenergic blocking agents and prazosin. Med J Aust (Suppl 2):2

Cambridge D, Davey MJ, Greengrass PM (1980) The pharmacology of antihypertensive drugs with special reference to vasodilators, α-adrenergic blocking agents and

prazosin. Prog Pharmacol 3:107
Cavero I (1982) Effects of prazosin on reflex changes in heart rate evoked by vasopressor and vasodepressor stimuli in conscious rabbits. J Cardiovasc Pharmacol 4(Suppl): S108
Cavero I, Roach AG (1980) The pharmacology of prazosin, a novel antihypertensive agent. Life Sci 27:1525–1533
Constantine JW, Hess HJ (1981) The cardiovascula effects of trimazosin. Eur J Pharmacol 74:227
Constantine JW, McShane WK, Scriabine A, Hess HJ (1973) Analysis of the hypotensive action of prazosin. In: Onesti G, Kim KE, Moyer JH (eds) Hypertension: mechanisms and management. Grune and Stratton, New York, p 429
Constantine JW, Weeks RA, McShane WK (1978) Prazosin and presynaptic α-receptors in the cardio-accelerator nerve of the dog. Eur J Pharmacol 50:51
Cubeddu LX, Zarate NA, Rosales CB, Zschaek W (1982) Prazosin and propranolol in preoperative management of phaeochromocytoma. Clin Pharmacol Ther 32:156–160
De Jonge A, Timmermans PBMWM, Van Zwieten PA (1981) Participation of cardiac presynaptic α_2-adrenoceptors in the bradycardiac effects of clonidine and analogues. Nauyn Schmiedebergs Arch Pharmacol 317:8–12
Doxey JC, Smith CFC, Walker JM (1977) Selectivity of blocking agents for pre- and postsynaptic α-adrenoceptors. Br J Pharmacol 60:91
Drayer JIM, Weber MA, De Young JL, Brewer DD (1983) Long term blood pressure monitoring in the evaluation of antihypertensive therapy. Arch Intern Med 143: 898–901
Elliott HL, McLean K, Sumner DJ et al. (1981) Immediate cardiovascular responses to oral prazosin—effects on current β-blockers. Clin Pharmacol Ther 29:303
Elliott HL, Meredith PA, Sumner DJ et al. (1982) A pharmacodynamic and pharmacokinetic assessment of a new α-adrenoceptor antagonist, doxazosin (UK 33274) in normotensive subjects. Br J Clin Pharmacol 13:699
Georgopoulos AJ, Valasidis A, Siourthas D (1978) Treatment of chronic heart failure with slow release phentolamine. Eur J Clin Pharmacol 13:325
Gould L, Becker WH, Macklin EE (1980) Effects of intravenous phentolamine on hemodynamics and restind pulmonary gas exchange in man. Angiology 31:120
Graham RM, Pettinger WA (1979) Prazosin. N Engl J Med 300:232–236
Greengrass PM, Bremner R (1979) Binding characteristics of ^{3}H-prazosin to rat brain α-adrenergic receptors. Eur J Pharmacol 55:323
Hamilton CA, Reid JL, Vincent J (1985) Pharmacokinetic and pharmacodynamic studies with two α-adrenoceptor antagonists, doxazosin and prazosin in the rabbit. Br J Pharmacol 86:79–87
Hardey DW, Lokhandwala MF (1979) Influence of prazosin on cardiac reflex function. Eur J Pharmacol 57:251
Hess HJ (1974) Biochemistry and structure-activity studies with prazosin. In: Cotton DKW (ed) Prazosin—evaluation of a new antihypertensive agent. Excerpta Medica, Amsterdam, p 5
Hornung R, Presek P, Glossman H (1979) Alpha-adrenoceptors in rat brain: direct identification with prazosin. Naunyn Schmiedebergs Arch. Pharmacol 308:223
Huchet AM, Velly J, Schmitt H (1981) Role of α_1- and α_2-adrenoceptors in the modulation of the baroreflex vagal bradycardia. Eur J Pharmacol 71:455–461
Imhof PR, Carnier B, Brunner L, Keller G, Rohrer T (1976) Human Pharmacology of orally administered phentolamine. In: Taylor SH (ed) Phentolamine in heart failure and other cardiac disorders. Huber, Bern, pp 11–22
Jie K, Van Brummelen P, Vermey P, Timmermans PBMWM, Van Zwieten PA (1984) Identification of vascular postsynaptic α_1- and α_2-adrenoceptors in man. Circ Res 54:447–452
Jie K, Van Brummelen P, Vermey P, Timmermans PBMWM, Van Zwieten PA (1986) α_1- and α_2-Adrenoceptor mediated vasoconstriction in the forearm of normotensive and hypertensive subjects. J Cardiovasc Pharmacol 8:190–196
Jones CR, Hamilton CA, Whyte KF, Elliott HL, Reid JL (1985) Acute and chronic

regulation of alpha(2)-adrenoceptor number and function in man. Clin Sci 68 (Suppl 10):129S-132S

Kiowski W, Hulthén UL, Ritz R, Buehler FR (1983) Alpha-2-adrenoceptor mediated vasoconstriction in human arterial vessels. J Clin Pharmacol Ther 34:565–569

Kobinger W (1978) Central α-adrenergic systems as targets for hypotensive drugs. Rev Physiol Biochem Pharmacol 81:40–100

Kobrin I, Gallo A, Kumar A, Pegram BL, Frohlich ED (1984) Immediate hemodynamic changes produced by urapidil in normotensive and spontaneously hypertensive rats. Clin Exp Hypertens A6:685–697

Kondo K, Ohashi K, Ebiwara A (1982) Pharmacokinetics and pharmacological effects of terazosin, a new alpha-blocker. Jpn J Clin Pharmacol Ther 13:137–138

Kyncl JJ (1986) The pharmacology of terazosin. Am J Med 80(Suppl 5B):12–19

Langer SZ (1981) Presynaptic regulation of the release of catecholamines. Pharmacol Rev 32:337–362

Langer SZ, Massingham R, Shepperson NB (1980) Presence of postsynaptic α_2-adrenoceptors of predominantly extrasynaptic location in the vascular smooth muslce of the dog hind limb. Clin Sci 59(Suppl 6):225S-228S

Lefèvre-Borg F, Roach AG, Gomeni R, Cavero I (1979) Mechanism of antihypertensive activity of orally administered prazosin in spontaneously hypertensive rats. J Cardiovasc Pharmacol 1:31

Lund-Johansen P (1974) Hemodynamic changes at rest and during exercise in long-term prazosin therapy of essential hypertension. In: Cotton DKW (ed) Prazosin—evaluation of a new antihypertensive agent. Excerpta Medica, Amsterdam, p 43

Lui HK, Awan NA, Needham K, Mason DT (1985) Comparative evaluation of the new oral systemic vasodilator terazosin and nitroprusside in severe chronic heart failure. Clin Res 33:207A

Marshall AJ, Kettle MA, Barritt DW (1980) Evaluation of indoramin added to oxprenolol and bendrofluazide as a third agent in severe hypertension. Br J Clin Pharmacol 10:217

Messerli FH, Kobrin I, Amodeo C, Ventura HO, Frohlich ED (1986) Immediate cardiovascular effects of urapidil in essential hypertension. In: Amery A (ed) Treatment of hypertension with urapidil. Roy Soc Med Serv 101:87–91

Miach PJ, Dausse JP, Cardot A, Meyer P (1980) ^{3}H-Prazosin binds specifically to α_1-adrenoceptors in rat brain. Naunyn Schmiedebergs Arch Pharmacol 312:23

Moser M (ed) (1986) Advances in the management of hypertension: focus on terazosin, a new alpha-1-adrenergic antagonist. Am J Med 80(5B):1–105

Motulsky HJ, O'Connor DT, Insel PA (1983) Platelet α_2-adrenergic receptors in treated and untreated essential hypertension. Clin Sci 64:265–272

Perry RS (1985) Trimazosin. Drugs Today 21:243–252

Persson B, Yao T, Thoren P (1981) Correlation between decreased heart rate and central inhibition of sympathetic discharges after prazosin administration in the spontaneously hypertensive rat. Clin Exp Hypertens 3:245–250

Philipp T, Distler A, Cordes U (1978) Sympathetic nervous system and blood pressure control in essential hypertension. Lancet 2:959–963

Preston RA, O'Connor DT, Stone RA (1979) Prazosin and renal hemodynamics: arteriolar vasodilatation during therapy of essential hypertension in man. J Cardiovasc Pharmacol 1:277

Ramage AG (1982) Why do α_1-adrenoceptor antagonists fail to cause reflex tachycardia? Br J Pharmacol 77(Suppl):323P

Reid JL, Meredith PA, Elliott H (1983) Pharmacokinetics and pharmacodynamic of trimazosin in man. Am Heart J 106:1222–1228

Roach AG, Gomeni R, Mitchard M et al. (1978) The blood pressure lowering effects of intravenous versus intracerebroventricular prazosin in anesthetized cats. Eur J Pharmacol 49:271–274

Robinson BF (1981) Drugs acting directly on vascular smooth muscle: circulatory and secondary effects. Br J Pharmacol 12:5S

Roesler JM, McCafferty JP, De Marinis RM, Matthews WD, Hieble JP (1986) Characterization of the antihypertensive activity of SK&F 86466, a selective α_2-antagonist in the rat. J Pharmacol Exp Ther 236:1–7

Saeed M, Sommer O, Holtz J, Bassenge E (1982) α-Adrenoceptor blockade by phentolamine causes β-adrenergic vasodilatation by increased catecholamine release due to presynaptic α-blockade. J Cardiovasc Pharmacol 4:44–48

Sands H, Jorgensen R (1979) Effects of prazosin on cyclic nucleotide content and blood pressure of the spontaneously hypertensive rat. Biochem Pharmacol 28:685–687

Sasso EH, O'Conner DT (1982) Prazosin depression of baroreflex function in hypertensive man. Eur J Clin Pharmacol 22:7–9

Schmitt H (1971) Action des α-sympathomimétiques sur les structures nerveuses. Actual Pharmacol 24:93–113

Schoetensack W, Bruckschen EG, Zech K (1983) Urapidil. In: Scriabine W (ed) New drugs annual: Cardiovascular drugs. Raven, New York, pp 19–48

Singleton W, Saxton CAPD, Hernandez R, Ferrer RS, Pritchard BNC (1980) Alpha blocking effect of prazosin, trimazosin and UK-33,274 in man. In: Turner P (ed) World conference on clin pharmac ther Abs. MacMillan, London

Singleton W, Sexton CAPD, Hernandez J, Prichard BN (1982). Postjunctional selectivity of α-blockade with prazosin, trimazosin and UK-33,274 in man. J Cardiovasc Pharmacol 4:S145–S155

Sonders RC (1986) The pharmacokinetics of terazosin. Am J Med 80: (Suppl 5B): 77–81

Stanaszek WF, Kellerman D, Brogden RN (1983) Romankiewicz. Prazosin update. A review of its pharmacological properties and therapeutic use in hypertension and congestive heart failure. Drugs 25:339–384

Starke K (1981) α-Adrenoceptor subclassification. Rev Physiol Biochem Pharmacol 88:199–236

Stokes GS, Frost GW, Graham RM, MacCarthy EP (1979) Indoramin and prazosin as adjuncts to beta-adrenoceptor blockade in hypertension. Clin Pharmacol Ther 25: 783–785

Taylor CR, Leader JP, Singleton MB, Munster EW, Falkner FC (1983) Profile of trimazosin: an effective and safe antihypertensive agent. Am Heart J 106:1269–1285

Taylor LA, Twomey TM, Schuch von Wintenau M (1977) The metabolic fate of prazosin. Xenobiotica 7:357–364

Timmermans PBMWM, Van Zwieten PA (1981) The postsynaptic α_2-adrenoceptor. J Auton Pharmacol 1:171–183

Timmermans PBMWM, Van Zwieten PA (1982) α_2-Adrenoceptors: classification, localisation, mechanisms and targets for drugs. J Med Chem 25:1389–1401

Timmermans PBMWM, Lam E, Van Zwieten PA (1979) The interaction between prazosin and clonidine at α-adrenoceptors in rats and cats. Eur J Pharmacol 49: 271–276

Timmermans PBMWM, Kwa HY, Karamat Ali F, Van Zwieten PA (1980) Prazosin and its analogues UK-18,596 and UK-33,274: a comparative study on cardiovascular effects and α-adrenoceptor blocking activities. Arch Int Pharmacodyn 245:218

Titmarsch S, Monk JP (1987) Terazosin. A review of its pharmacodynamic and pharmacokinetic properties, and therapeutic efficacy in essential hypertension. Drugs 33:461–477

U'Prichard DC, Charness ME, Robertson D, Snyder S (1978) Prazosin: differential affinities for two populations of α-adrenergic receptor binding sites. Eur J Pharmacol 50:87

Van Brummelen P, Jie K, Timmermanns PBMWM, Van Zwieten PA (1985) Postjunctional α-adrenoceptors and the regulation of arteriolar tone in humans. J Cardiovase Pharmacol 7:S149-S152

Van Zwieten PA (1975) Antihypertensive drugs with a central action. Prog Pharmacol 1:1–63

Van Zwieten PA (1984) Role of α-adrenoceptors in hypertension and antihypertensive drug treatment. Am J Med 77:17–25

Van Zwieten PA, Timmermans PBMWM (1983) Cardiovascular α_2-adrenoceptors. J Mol Cell Cardiol 15:717–733

Van Zwieten PA, Timmermans PBMWM (1984) Pharmacological basis for the hypoten-

sive activity and side-effects of α-methyl-DOPA, clonidine and guanfacine. Hypertension (Suppl 6):28–33
Van Zwieten PA, De Jonge A, Wilffert B, Timmermans PBMWM, Beckeringh JJ, Thoolen MJMC (1985) Cardiovascular effects and interaction with adrenoceptors of urapidil. Arch Int Pharmacodyn 276:180–201
Vincent J, Hamilton CA, Sumner DJ, Reid JL (1983a) A comparison of the hypotensive activity and in vitro and in vivo α_1-adrenoceptor antagonist properties of prazosin, trimazosin and doxazosin in the rabbit. Br J Pharmacol 79 (Suppl):388P
Vincent J, Elliott HL, Meredith PA, Reid JL (1983b) Doxazosin, an α_1-adrenoceptor antagonist. Pharmacokinetics and concentration effect relationships in man. Br J Clin Pharmacol 15:719–725
Wilffert B, Timmermans PBMWM, Van Zwieten PA (1982) Extrasynaptic location of α_2- and non-innervated β_2-adrenoceptors in the vascular system of the pithed normotensive rat. J Pharmacol Exp. Ther 221:762–768
Wood AJ, Bolli P, Simpson FO (1976) Prazosin in normal subjects: plasma levels, blood pressure and heart rate. Br J Pharmacol 3:199–202
Zech K, Steinijans VW, Radtke HW (1986) Pharmacokinetics of urapidil in normal subjects. In: Amery A (ed) Treatment of hypertension with urapidil. Roy Soc Med Serv 101:29–38

CHAPTER 5

Drugs Acting on Multiple Receptors: β-Blockers with Additional Properties

G. SPONER, W. BARTSCH, and R.G. HOOPER

CONTENTS

1 Introduction

The main haemodynamic disorder in the majority of patients with established arterial hypertension is abnormally high peripheral vascular resistance. The most rational goal of any drug therapy should therefore be to restore normal haemodynamic conditions at rest and under physical or emotional stress, while reducing blood pressure to normotensive levels. Consequently, any strategy for the treatment of established hypertension should include vasodilator drugs. However, therapy solely with a variety of vasodilators is not reasonable, because they also induce activation of counter-regulatory mechanisms such as reflex tachycardia and stimulation of the renin-angiotensin-aldosterone system. These compensatory responses may limit the antihypertensive activity of the drugs. On the other hand, chronic monotherapy with most β-adrenergic receptor blockers does not reduce total peripheral resistance in hypertensive patients and does not correct abnormal haemodynamics, particularly during exercise (Frohlich et al. 1968; Tarazi and Dustan 1972; Hansson 1977; Lund-Johansen 1983a). Moreover, the blood pressure of some hypertensive patients treated with β-blockers cannot be controlled because of adrenergic vasoconstriction (Birkenhäger and De Leeuw 1983).

The combined use of vasodilating agents and β-blockers comes closer to the goal of restoration of normal haemodynamics in hypertension, because the undesired effects of the individual components compensate for each other, and, additionally, the responder rate is increased (Sannerstedt et al. 1972; Zacest et al. 1972; Pape 1974; Eggertsen and Hansson 1985). This concept sparked the development of drugs that possess both of the desired pharmacological activities in one molecule. Labetalol was the first member of this new class of antihypertensive agents. Its efficacy in the treatment of hypertension has been confirmed by a considerable number of a clinical investigations. In the past few years a variety of other compounds that also combine β-receptor blocking and vasodilating properties has been developed and are available—up to now in a few countries—or are under advanced investigations. These drugs exhibit a broad spectrum of pharmacological activity as their vasodilating activities are mediated by various mechanisms.

2 General Chemistry of β-Blocking Compounds with Additional Properties

The different mechanisms of vasodilation have been reflected by the broad variety of chemical structures of the individual compounds. The common structure of all of them is an ethanolamine or isopropanolamine moiety which is essential for the β-adrenoceptor blocking activity. Thus, the β-blockers with additional properties can be divided into arylethanolamines:

$$\mathrm{Ar{-}\underset{\displaystyle OH}{\underset{|}{CH}}{-}CH_2{-}NH{-}R} \qquad (1)$$

and aryloxyisopropanolamines:

$$\mathrm{Ar{-}O{-}CH_2{-}\underset{\displaystyle OH}{\underset{|}{CH}}{-}CH_2{-}NH{-}R} \qquad (2)$$

Many of compounds have been synthesised with special substituents on the aryl (Ar)-site and/or the amine (R)-site in order to introduce additional vasodilating properties into the molecules.

2.1 Arylethanolamines

Bufuralol is a compound with a benzofuryl-(2)-group at the aromatic Ar-site, whereas the amine moiety $—NH—C(CH_3)_3$ does not differ from that of some other classical β-blocking agents.

On the other hand, the substitution of the isopropyl or tert. butyl moiety of classic β-blockers by arylalkyls or aryloxyalkyls also provides the possibility of modifying the pharmacological profile of these compounds. The augmentation

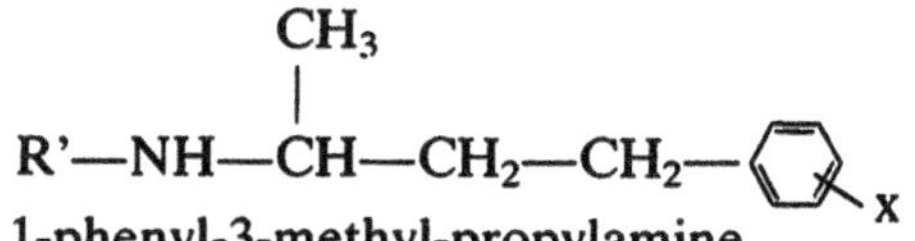

1-phenyl-3-methyl-propylamine (3)

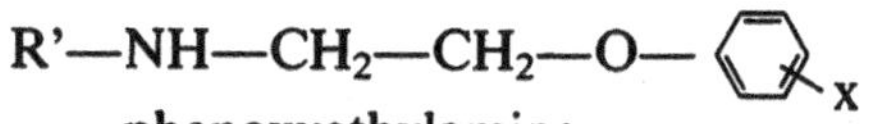

phenoxyethylamine (4)

of the carbon chain to 1-phenyl-3-methyl-propylamines (3) or phenoxyethylamines (4), configurations with well-known affinities to adrenoceptors, or their ring substitution (x) induce a vasodilatory component into the entity, which can be mediated by α-adrenoceptor blocking activity (Table 1). A typical example of the former is labetalol, the best known β-blocking compound with additional properties, and its *R*,*R*-stereoisomer, dilevalol. Chemically related to labetalol is medroxalol. An example of the latter is amosulalol.

2.2 Aryloxyisopropanolamines

Compounds have been synthesised with substituents on the Ar-site having some structural similarities to well-known vasodilating agents (Table 2). Examples include: nipradilol containing a nitrate configuration, prizidilol containing a moiety resembling hydralazine, BW A575C with a moiety related to enalapril, and MK 761 with an aryl-substituent related to nicotinic acid.

Arotinolol is a thioisopropanolamine; its aryl-substituent has no relation to well-known vasodilating properties.

The aryl-substitution of celiprolol produces a compound which is related to the conventional β-adrenoceptor blocker acebutolol but does not have similarities to structures with well-known vasodilating properties.

The possibility of introducing additional vasorelaxing potential by modifying the R-moiety, as discussed for the arylethanolamines, can also be transferred to the aryloxyisopropranolamines. Examples of these approaches are bucindolol, adimolol, carvedilol and bevantolol.

2.3 Stereospecificity

The compounds mentioned above have, like pure β-blockers, at least one chiral centre. Some of them (nipradilol, labetalol, medroxalol) have a further chiral centre, with the consequence that the compounds are mixtures of equal portions of two or four stereoisomers. The only exception to be a pure stereoisomer is dilevalol, the *R*,*R*-isomer of labetalol (Sybertz et al. 1981).

The optical isomers of some compounds have been shown to differ in their pharmacological profiles, in particular with respect to their β-blocking or α-blocking activity (Nakagawa et al. 1980; Brittain et al. 1982). It also seems conceivable that the enantiomers have different pharmacokinetic properties.

Table 1. β-Adrenoceptor blockers with additional vasodilating properties (arylethanolamines) ranked according to the variations on the amine moiety. The asterisk shows the position of the optical centre of the compounds

$$R_1-\overset{*}{C}H(OH)-CH_2-NH-R_2$$

Compound	R_1	R_2	Manufacturer	Stage
Bufuralol (Ro 3–4787)	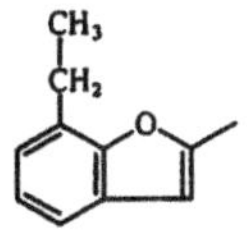	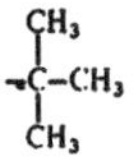	Roche (CH)	dis-continued
Arotinolol (S 596)	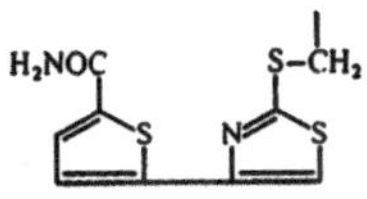	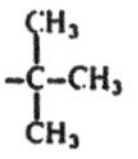	Sumitomo (J)	available in Asia
Labetalol (AH 5158)	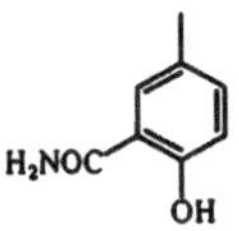	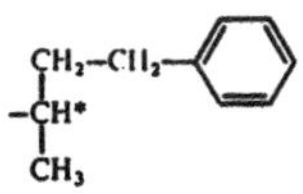	Allen–Hanbury (UK) Schering–Plough (USA)	available world-wide
Dilevalol (SCH 19 927)	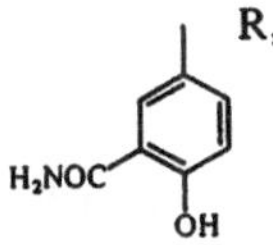 R, R–Isomer of Labetalol	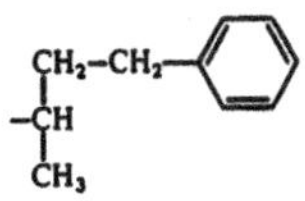	Schering–Plough (USA)	Phase III
Medroxalol (RMI 81968)	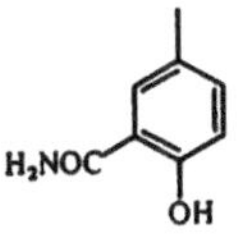	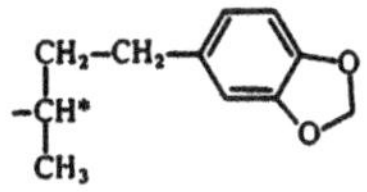	Richardson–Merell (USA)	dis-continued
Amosulalol (YM 09538)	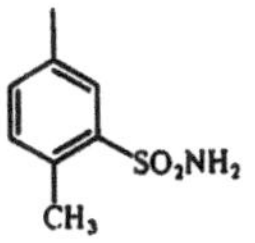	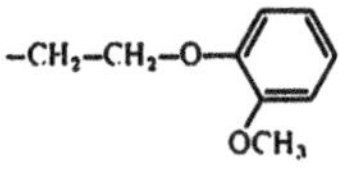	Yamanouchi (J)	available in Japan
Sulfinalol (WIN 40808)	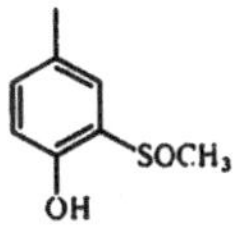	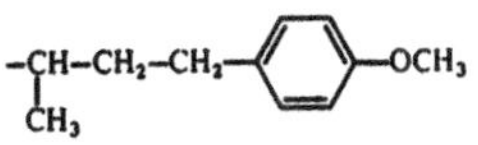	Sterling–Wintrop (USA)	dis-continued

Table 2. β-Adrenoceptor blockers with additional vasodilating properties (aryloxyisopropranolamines) ranked according to the variations on the amine moiety. The asterisk shows the position of the optical centre of the compounds

$$R_1-O-CH_2-\underset{OH}{\overset{*}{C}}H-CH_2-NH-R_2$$

Compound	R_1	R_2	Manufacturer	Stage
MK 761	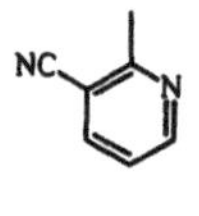	$-\underset{CH_3}{\overset{CH_3}{C}}-CH_3$	Merck, Sharp & Dohme (USA)	dis-continued
Celiprolol (ST 1396)	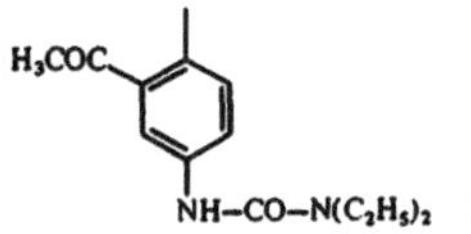	$-\underset{CH_3}{\overset{CH_3}{C}}-CH_3$	Chemie Linz (A) Revlon (USA)	broadly available in Europe
Prizidilol (SK+F 92657)	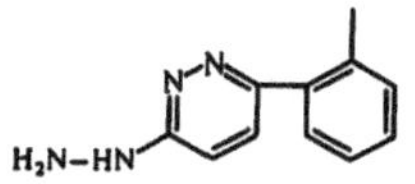	$-\underset{CH_3}{\overset{CH_3}{C}}-CH_3$	SK + F (UK)	dis-continued
Nipradilol (K 351)	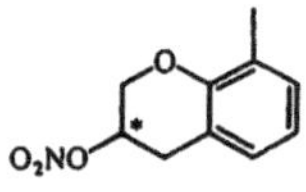	$-\underset{CH_3}{\overset{CH_3}{C}}H$	KOWA (J)	available in Japan
BW A 575 C	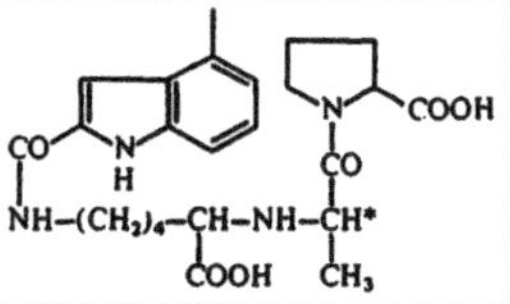	$-\underset{CH_3}{\overset{CH_3}{C}}H$	Wellcome (UK)	Phase I
Bucindolol (MJ 13 105)	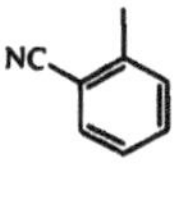	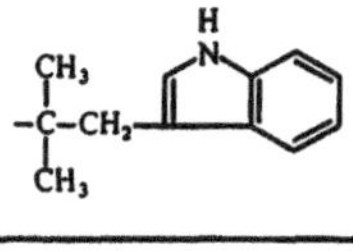	Mead–Johnson (USA)	discon-tinued for hyper-tension
Adimolol (MEN 935)	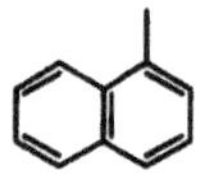	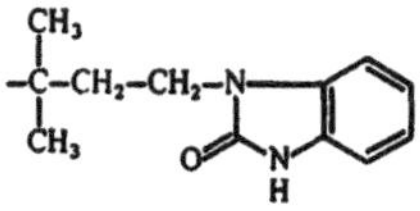	Boehringer Ingelheim (FRG)	dis-continued
Bevantolol (Cl 775)	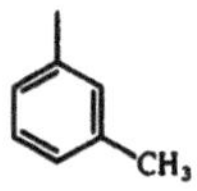	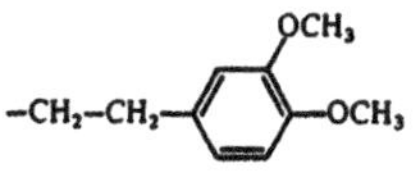	Parke–Davis (USA)	available in Denmark
Carvedilol (BM 14.190)	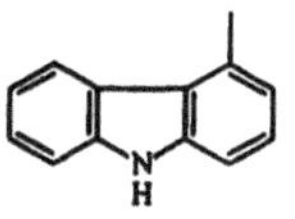	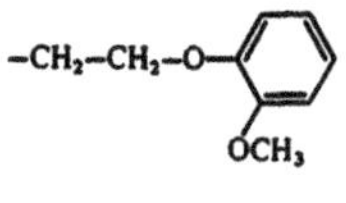	Boehringer Mannheim (FRG)	Phase III

This could result in broad individual variations of the pharmacodynamic profile. However, the knowledge of the differences between enantiomers with respect to their pharmacodynamic and pharmacokinetic properties are based solely upon data generated from animal experiments.

The enantiomers of β-adrenoceptor blockers differ in their pharmacodynamic profiles. Only one of the enantiomers possesses β-blocking properties. With respect to α-adrenoceptor properties, there does not seem to be a simple rule. For example, the four diastereoisomers of labetalol exert different α-adrenoceptor blocking activities, but both enantiomers of carvedilol induce almost identical effects (Brittain et al. 1982; Erb et al. 1989).

From the purely scientific point of view, racemic hybrids may be classified as "fixed ratio combinations" of two compounds with different pharmacological profiles (Ariens 1984). On the other hand, it should be mentioned that hybrid molecules have also been screened in their racemic forms and selected according to their balanced profile for the desired activities. Nevertheless, it seems to be reasonable to obtain information on the pharmacodynamic and pharmacokinetic profile of the enantiomers at an early phase in the development of a new drug. Proceeding in this manner may enable conclusions to be drawn for the further development of such drugs.

The pharmacological and pharmacokinetic profiles, as well as clinical data on the individual compounds, will be discussed in the following sections. In accordance with the long clinical experience and worldwide use, labetalol will be reviewed extensively, whereas data on compounds currently undergoing advanced stages of development will be discussed briefly. Compounds discontinued from further development will not be discussed.

3 Individual Compounds

3.1 Labetalol

3.1.1 Chemistry

Labetalol is a salicylamide derivative. In contrast to conventional β-blockers, the isopropyl group has been replaced by an aralkyl substituent. Woods and Robinson (1981) found a distribution coefficient at pH 7.4 and 37°C between *n*-octanol/buffer of 11.5 for labetalol and 20.2 for propranolol. The chloroform/water partition coefficent is 1.2, compared with 9 for propranolol (Martin et al. 1976). Labetalol is thus more polar and has a lower lipid solubility than propranolol. The protein binding of labetalol in human plasma is about 50% (Martin et al. 1976). The original fluorimetric method for determination of labetalol in plasma was described by Martin et al. (1976). The more sensitive and specific HPLC assay has a detection limit of 4–10 ng/ml (Dusci and Hackett 1979; Meredith et al. 1982; Alton et al. 1984).

Labetalol has two optical centres and thus consists of equal proportions of the four resulting enantiomers. Each of these has been synthesised, and they have been shown to differ in their α- and β-blocking activity (Brittian et al. 1982).

3.1.2 Experimental and Clinical Pharmacology

3.1.2.1 Pharmacodynamics and Mode of Action

3.1.2.1.1 Receptor Binding

The interaction of labetalol with α- and β-adrenoceptors has been demonstrated in binding studies. The drug displaces the binding of [^{3}H]prazosin, [^{3}H]WB 4101, [^{3}H]dihydroergocryptine and [^{3}H]dihydroalprenolol in membrane preparations from rat brain, liver or heart (AGGERBECK et al. 1978; DEVOTO et al. 1980). The K_i values for the heart are 77 n*M* for the β-sites and 510 n*M* for the α-sites. Thus, the affinity of labetalol is about 10 times higher for the β- than for the α-receptor. Furthermore, its affinity for the different adrenergic receptors is about 10 times less than that of the specific antagonists propranolol and phentolamine (AGGERBECK et al. 1978). The binding of the α_2-agonists [^{3}H]clonidine in guinea pig splenic membranes and [^{3}H]guanfacine in rat cortex homogenates is only very weakly affected by labetalol (BAUM and SYBERTZ 1983a).

3.1.2.1.2 In Vitro Experiments Demonstrating α- and β-Blockade

Using a variety of experimental in vitro models, labetalol has been shown to be a specific and competitive antagonist of both α- and β-adrenoceptors. The β_1-blockade has been confirmed by the rightward shift of the curve of increases in force of contraction or rate of isolated guinea pig atria versus the concentration of isoprenaline (FARMER et al. 1972; BRITTAIN and LEVY 1976; LEVY and RICHARDS 1980; LOUIS et al. 1984). The β_2-adrenoceptor blockade has been shown by the inhibition of the relaxant effect of isoprenaline in guinea pig tracheal preparations contracted with carbachol. The pA_2 values generated from these experiments in different laboratories are summarised in Table 3. It can be concluded that labetalol blocks β_1- and β_2-adrenoceptors to a similar extent and that it is approximately 1.5 to 18 times less potent than propranolol (FARMER et al. 1972; BRITTAIN and LEVY 1976).

Labetalol inhibits the contractile responses to α-receptor agonists such as phenylephrine in various isolated tissues, e.g. aortic strips. The inhibition is specific and does not extend to serotonin, acetylcholine or barium. Labetalol is approximately four to eight times less potent in blocking α-receptors than β-receptors in isolated tissues (BRITTAIN and LEVY 1976).

Table 3. Adrenoceptor blocking activity of β-adrenoceptor blockers with additional properties and of propranolol. Data represent pA_2 values, the negative logarithms of the antagonist concentrations that require twice as much agonist to be added to elicit the same response achieved without the antagonist

Compound	β_1	β_2	α_1	Reference
Labetalol	7.35	7.54	6.99	FARMER et al. (1972)
Propranolol	8.40	–	–	
Labetalol	8.31	8.10	7.44	BRITTAIN and LEVY (1976)
Propranolol	8.81	8.33	4.00	

Table 3. (continued)

Compound	β_1	β_2	α_1	Reference
Arotinolol	8.48	8.56	–	Hara et al. (1979)
Propranolol	8.33	7.56	–	
Labetalol	7.62	7.84	6.77	Nakagawa et al. (1980)
Labetalol	7.68	7.40	6.99	Brittain et al. (1982)
Dilevalol	8.26	8.52	5.87	
Labetalol	8.13	–	6.45	Takenaka et al. (1982a)
Amosulalol	7.56	–	7.67	
Propranolol	8.76	–	–	
Nipradilol	8.92	8.33	6.85	Uchida et al. (1983)
Celiprolol	8.0	6.77	–	Pittner (1983a)
Celiprolol	7.55	5.95	6.5	R.D. Smith and Wolf (1984)
Labetalol	7.68	–	7.21	Monopoli et al. (1984)
Propranolol	8.38	–	–	
Dilevalol	8.28	–	6.40	
Carvedilol	–	–	7.5	Moulds et al. (1984)
Labetalol	7.46	7.30	7.42	Miyagishi et al. (1984)
Arotinolol	8.69	8.40	6.91	
Propranolol	7.76	7.87	–	
Arotinolol	9.31	9.09	–	Nagatomo et al. (1984)
Nipradilol	8.59	8.53	–	
Labetalol	7.72	6.88	6.48	Matsunaga et al (1986a)
Dilevalol	8.40	7.14	5.90	
Propranolol	8.56	8.01	–	
Labetalol	8.13	7.47	7.00	Honda et al. (1986)
Amosulalol	7.56	7.04	7.97	
Propranolol	8.76	8.82	–	
Labetalol	7.48	7.16	6.22	Takayanagi et al. (1987)
Bevantolol	7.75	6.69	4.77	
Labetalol	7.5	7.7	7.5	Louis et al. (1988)
Propranolol	8.3	8.0	5.5	
Dilevalol	8.3	8.5	5.9	
Carvedilol	8.8	8.8	6.8	
Arotinolol	8.0	8.0	7.2	
Labetalol	8.2	–	6.5	Hofferber et al. (1988)
Dilevalol	8.3	–	5.6	
Carvedilol	9.0	–	7.3	

3.1.2.1.3 In Vivo Experiments Demonstrating α- and β-Blockade

The adrenoceptor blocking activity of labetalol has also been demonstrated in intact individuals. Investigations have been performed in a variety of experiments in animals (Farmer et al. 1972; Brittain and Levy 1976; Sybertz et al. 1981; Baum and Sybertz 1983a) as well as in healthy volunteers (Collier et al. 1972; Richards et al. 1977a; Richards and Prichard 1978) and in hypertensive patients (Mehta and Cohn 1977). Shifts of the dose-response curves of isoprenaline with respect to increase in heart rate are similar in magnitude to those of vasorelaxation or reductions in diastolic blood pressure. This confirms that labetalol exerts a non-selective β-adrenoceptor blocking effect (Richards et al. 1978; Baum and Sybertz 1983a). Interestingly, isoprenaline-induced tachycardia is more effectively inhibited than isoprenaline-induced inotropism (Cohn et al. 1982). From investigations with intact individuals, labetalol has been assessed to be 3 to 7 times less active than propranolol (Farmer et al. 1972; Richards et al. 1978). Tachycardia induced by tilting, Valsalva's manoeuvre or physical exercise is also reduced by labetalol (Collier et al. 1972; Richards et al. 1977a; Fagard et al. 1979).

Labetalol inhibits the vasopressor response induced by sympathetic nerve stimulation or by i.v. injection of α-sympathomimetics in a variety of experimental models (Brittain and Levy 1976). In intact individuals it displaces the dose-response curve of phenylephrine but not that of angiotensin II (Brittain and Levy 1976; Sybertz et al. 1981; see Fig. 1). Drew et al. (1981) found a correlation between the decrease in basal blood pressure produced by 10–100 mg/kg labetalol and the inhibition of pressor responses to phenylephrine in DOCA-hypertensive rats, indicating that α_1-blockade plays an important role in the acute hypotensive activity of labetalol. The α_1-blocking activity of labetalol has been confirmed by the observation that in hypertensive patients the phenylephrine response is reduced by 30%-50% after a few weeks' treatment (average dose 1.6 g/day) (Fagard et al. 1979). However, labetalol is a relatively ineffective antagonist to vasopressor responses to norepinephrine in animals and in humans (Kennedy and Levy 1975; Richards et al. 1979a; Reid et al. 1981). In dogs, cats, pithed rats and spinal dogs, the pressor response to norepinephrine is inhibited only slightly by labetalol in doses up to 1 mg/kg; larger doses do not exert any further effect. This "self-limiting" effect cannot be observed in dogs pretreated with cocaine (Farmer et al. 1972; Kennedy and Levy 1975; Baum and Sybertz 1983a). There is, therefore, some evidence that labetalol blocks the re-uptake processes for norepinephrine (Richards et al. 1979a; Levy and Richards 1980). On the other hand, labetalol releases norepinephrine from some tissues (for review, see Levy and Richards 1980).

The results of in vivo experiments provide the possibility of calculating the ratio of α- to β-blocking potency of labetalol. This has been reported to be between 1 : 16 (Brittain and Levy 1976) and 1 : 39 (Sybertz et al. 1981) after i.v. injection into anaesthetised dogs. The ratio in humans obviously depends on the dose level. After an oral dose of 400–1600 mg labetalol, the ratio ranges from 1 : 2.9 (Richards et al. 1976) to 1 : 4.6 (Mehta and Cohn 1977). If

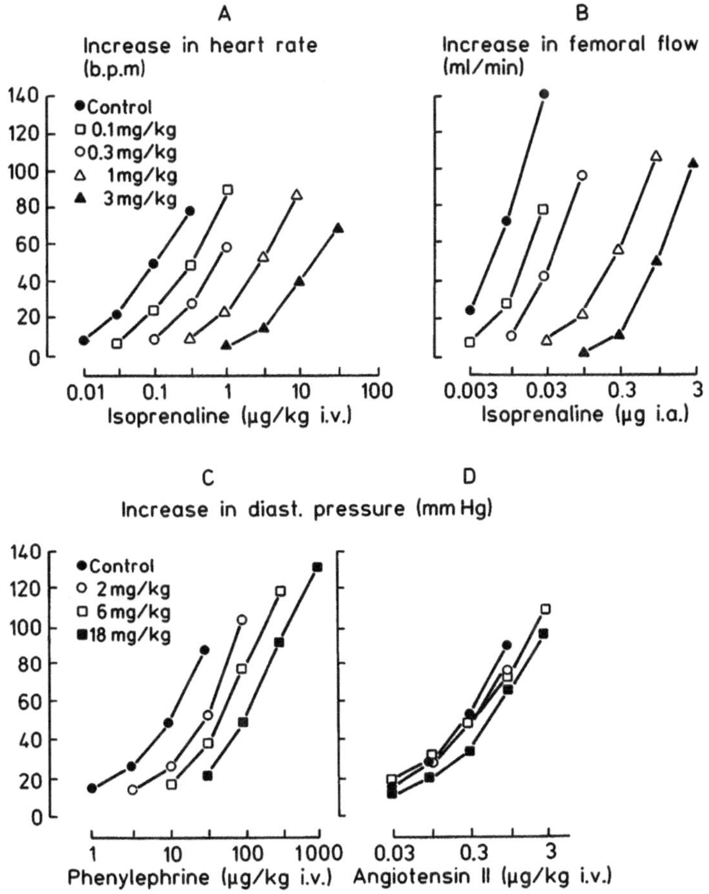

Fig. 1A–D. β- and α-adrenoceptor blocking activity of labetalol in pentobarbital-anaesthetised dogs. **A** (β_1): Increases in heart rate in response to i.v. injection of isoprenaline before (0) and after increasing doses (0.1–3 mg/kg i.v.) of labetalol; $n = 6$ ganglionically blocked dogs. **B** (β_2): Increase in femoral flow in response to intra-arterial injection of isoprenaline before (0) and after increasing doses (0.1–3 mg/kg i.v.) of labetalol; $n = 4$ ganglionically blocked dogs. **C** (α_1): Increase in blood pressure in response to i.v. injection of phenylephrine before (0) and after increasing doses (2–18 mg/kg i.v.) of labetalol; $n = 6$ vagotomized dogs. **D** (direct): Increase in blood pressure in response to i.v. injection of angiotensin II before (0) and after increasing doses of labetalol; $n = 6$ vagotomized dogs. (According to SYBERTZ et al. 1981)

administered i.v., it is 1 : 2.5 after 40 mg, 1 : 6.9 after 113 mg (= 1.5 mg/kg) and 1 : 9.8 after 160 mg (RICHARDS et al. 1977a). Interestingly, the shift in the dose-response curve of phenylephrine has been reported to be almost identical after 113 mg and 160 mg labetalol. This indicates that the dose-response curves for α- and β-blockade do not have the same pattern (Fig. 2).

SEMPLICINI et al. (1983) investigated the influence of short-term and long-term treatment with 600 mg labetalol daily on the dose-response curves to

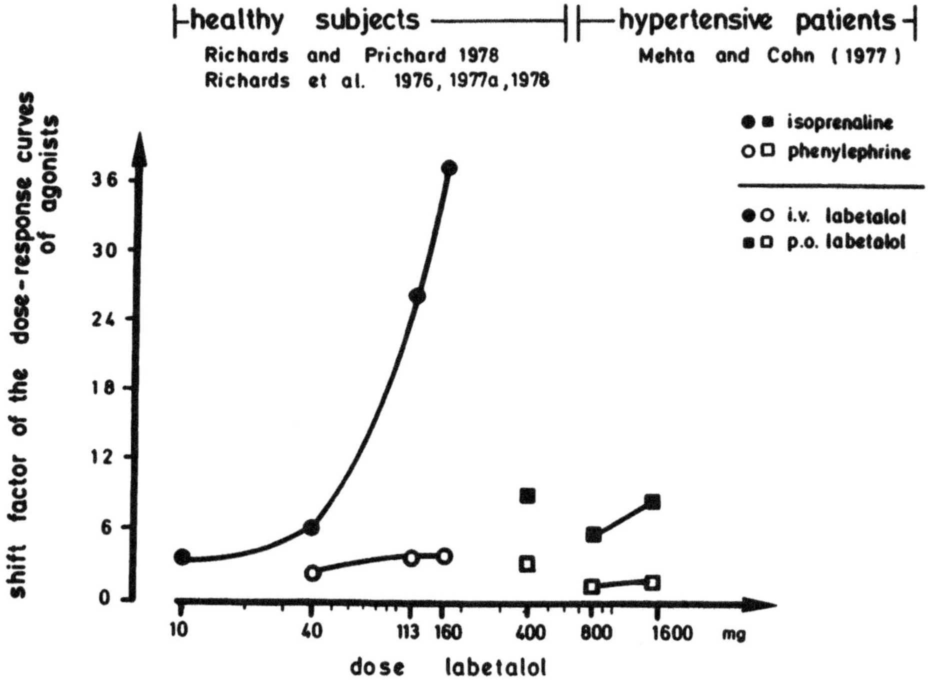

Fig. 2. Shift factors of the dose-response curves of isoprenaline (*filled symbols*) and phenylephrine (*open symbols*) after intravenous (*circles*) or oral (*squares*) administration of labetalol. The shift factor represents the multiple of the agonist dose required to produce a given effect under the influence of the dose of the antagonist. (According to data reported by RICHARDS et al. 1976, 1977a, 1978; RICHARDS and PRICHARD 1978; METHA and COHN 1977). Note: The β-blocking activity of labetalol has a steep dose-response curve after i.v. administration when compared with that of the α_1-blocking activity

isoprenaline and phenylephrine. The almost identical response to isoprenaline on the 3rd day and 6th month of treatment indicates a constant β-blocking activity. In contrast, there was a progressive decline in the α-blocking activity: after 1 month's treatment with labetalol, the dose-response curve of phenylephrine was almost the same as that before treatment. The authors suggest, therefore, that the decline of the α-blocking activity might account for the disappearance of postural hypotension in the course of chronic treatment with labetalol. On the other hand, the sustained haemodynamic profile observed in a considerable number of long-term clinical trials argues against the loss of α-blocking activity of labetalol during long-term therapy.

3.1.2.1.4 Further Investigations on the Mode of Vasodilatory Action

In contrast to its lack of selectivity on β-adrenoceptors, labetalol is a selective antagonist of α_1- as opposed to α_2-adrenoceptors. Labetalol does not antagonise the clonidine-induced attenuation of responses to sympathetic nerve stimulation in the rat vas deferens (LEVY and RICHARDS 1980) or the clonidine-induced inhibition of the twitch response in the guinea pig ileum (DREW 1978). Labetalol is also ineffective in preventing clonidine-induced sedation in rats, an effect mediated via α_2-adrenoceptors in the central nervous system (DREW et al. 1977).

Labetalol has been reported to be devoid of intrinsic α-adrenoceptor agonist activity, as judged by its inability to cause contractions of guinea pig mesenteric vein (FARMER et al. 1972), rabbit and rat aortic strips (BRITTAIN and LEVY 1976) and cat splenic strips (BLAKELY and SUMMERS 1977). However, after cardiac autonomic blockade with propranolol and scopolamine, labetalol produced a positive inotropic response in conscious rabbits which has been interpreted as a possible partial α-adrenoceptor agonist action (MCRITCHIE and CHALMERS 1981). Furthermore, under certain circumstances, labetalol may stimulate α-adrenoceptors indirectly by releasing norepinephrine from sympathetic nerves (DOGGRELL and PATON 1978) or by its inhibition of neuronal re-uptake (BLAKELEY and SUMMERS 1977).

Even though the concentrations required to produce α-adrenoceptor blockade and acute blood pressure response are in the same range (LEVY and RICHARDS 1980), there is some evidence that further mechanisms contribute to the vasorelaxing and antihypertensive activity of labetalol.

Labetalol does not exert β_1-sympathomimetic activities in dogs pretreated with syrosingopine (FARMER et al. 1972; BRITTAIN and LEVY 1976), but partial β_1-agonistic activities have been found in spinal cats and in adrenolectomised, reserprinised cats (TADEPALLI and NOVAK 1986). Strong evidence, however, exists that labetalol possesses intrinsic activity on β_2-adrenoceptors. Labetalol relaxes guinea pig tracheal preparations (CARPENTER 1981) and inhibits the spontaneous contraction of uteri removed from rats during spontaneous oestrus; this effect can be blocked by propranolol (CAREY and WHALLEY 1979). In anaesthetised cats labetalol decreases bronchoconstriction induced by serotonin or $PGF_{2\alpha}$ at doses of 0.01–3 mg/kg i.v.; these effects have been reported to be reversed by propranolol but not by practolol (LEVY and RICHARDS 1980). However, it is not clear to what extent the intrinsic activity on β_2-adrenoceptors contributes to the blood pressure lowering activity of labetalol.

Moreover, there is some evidence that direct vasodilatation contributes to the hypotensive activity of labetalol in addition to the adrenoceptor-mediated effect. JOHNSON et al. (1977) reported that labetalol causes both relaxation in Ba^{2+}-contracted rabbit portal veins and a hypotensive effect in dogs after pretreatment with high doses of propranolol and phentolamine.

Additional evidence for a direct vasodilator effect may be derived from experiments in which labetalol was administered i.v. following elimination of the neurogenic sympathetic tone with hexamethonium bromide. Under these circumstances propranolol does not reduce blood pressure, whereas labetalol in low doses (0.01–0.1 mg/kg) causes significant decreases. The response is probably the result of vasodilatation since these doses cannot be expected to reduce cardiac output. Hydralazine also reduces blood pressure in these experiments (BAUM and SYBERTZ 1983a).

DAGE and HSIEH (1980) reported a labetalol-induced (0.3–10 mg intraarterially), dose-dependent decrease in perfusion pressure of isolated perfused gracilis muscles of dogs pretreated with 1 mg/kg propranolol and 10–15 mg/kg phentolamine. In separate experiments, labetalol (0.1–10 mg/kg i.v.) elicited decreases in blood pressure in adrenalectomised, vagotomised spinal dogs. Finally, it has been demonstrated that the femoral blood flow of anaesthetised dogs is increased after intra-arterial injection of labetalol or dilevalol, both in innervated and in acutely sympathetically denervated limbs, whereas prazosin or phentolamine is active only in innervated limbs. The vasodilator response to labetalol or dilevalol is attenuated but not abolished by i.v. pretreatment with propranolol (BAUM et al. 1981).

Thus, a β-adrenoceptor-mediated or direct vasodilatory mechanism may be involved in the vasodilating or antihypertensive activity of labetalol.

3.1.2.2 Acute Blood Pressure Response and Haemodynamics

3.1.2.2.1 Investigations in Animals

In contrast to propranolol, labetalol decreases dose-dependently the arterial blood pressure in conscious renal hypertensive dogs, DOCA-hypertensive rats, renal hypertensive rats or SHR (BRITTAIN and LEVY 1976; GULATI and GULATI 1980; BAUM et al. 1981; DREW et al. 1981).

The haemodynamic effects of labetalol and propranolol were compared at doses between 0.01 and 3 mg/kg in anaesthetised, bivagotomised dogs. Labetalol, like propranolol, reduces heart rate, cardiac contractility and cardiac output. These effects can be attributed to the β-adrenoceptor blockade of the compounds. Labetalol had no effect on the total peripheral resistance (TPR) at low doses and reduced it at higher doses. In contrast, propranolol increased TPR over the whole dose range tested. Consequently, labetalol caused larger decreases in blood pressure than propranolol at equipotent cardiac β-adrenoceptor blocking doses. The differences between the two drugs were attributed to a peripheral vasodilating action of labetalol, probably resulting from its vascular α_1-adrenoceptor blocking activity (FARMER et al. 1972; BRITTAIN and LEVY 1976). The results of this study were confirmed by further experimental investigations. Small differences between the results can be attributed to the individual experimental situation, depending on the balance of autonomic influences (MAXWELL 1973; BAUM et al. 1981).

3.1.2.2.2 Investigations in Humans

Haemodynamic studies in healthy subjects and in hypertensive patients have confirmed that the additional α-blocking properties of labetalol result in a haemodynamic profile unlike that of propranolol and other pure β-adrenoceptor blocking agents (for review, see LUND-JOHANSEN 1984). A *single dose* of labetalol induces, like a combination of propranolol plus hydralazine (PRICHARD et al. 1975), a rapid decrease in blood pressure via a reduction of TPR. The heart rate is almost unchanged or slightly reduced (PRICHARD et al. 1975; JOEKES and THOMPSON 1976; KOCH 1977; OMVIK and LUND-JOHANSEN 1982; MEHTA et al. 1983), occurring as a result of dilatation of arterioles combined with a blockade of reflex tachycardia. Labetalol does not decrease the peripheral blood flow

(BERTONI et al. 1985), whereas the acute effect of pure β-blockers is a decrease in cardiac output and peripheral blood flow and an increase in TPR with only a small effect on the arterial blood pressure (TARAZI and DUSTAN 1972; PRICHARD et al. 1975; RICHARDS et al. 1978; HOLTZMAN et al. 1986). In labetalol-treated patients, pulmonary, coronary and renal resistance, as well as pulmonary capillary wedge pressure and right atrial pressure, have been shown to be unchanged or slightly reduced at rest in a supine or sitting position (KOCH 1977, 1979a; FAGARD et al. 1979; SVENDSON et al. 1980; MEHTA et al. 1983). Left ventricular pressure and stroke volume/filling pressure ratio are unchanged, but systolic blood pressure × heart rate is lowered, particular during exercise (KOCH 1979b; FEIT et al. 1985). Myocardial oxygen consumption and coronary sinus flow decrease after i.v. administration of labetalol 0.6 mg/kg to hypertensive patients (MEHTA et al. 1983). In patients with coronary artery disease labetalol 1.5 mg/kg i.v. induces an increase in coronary blood flow and a decrease in coronary resistance (GAGNON et al. 1982).

Forearm blood flow (BAHLMANN et al. 1979) and cerebral blood flow (PEARSON et al. 1979) are not reduced by labetalol.

In hypertensive patients without impairment of renal function, a single dose of 50 mg labetalol i.v. induces a reduction of glomerular filtration rate and renal blood flow by about 10%, whereas the excretion of water and sodium is reduced by 25%-40%. This effect is probably due to a reduced perfusion pressure (KOCH 1979c).

Remarkably, MALINI et al. (1982) found, in contrast to KEUSCH et al. (1980), an increase in effective renal plasma flow and glomerular filtration rate after chronic treatment, whereas the renal vascular resistance was decreased. The opposite was observed after treatment with propranolol.

Long-term oral treatment of hypertensive patients with labetalol is associated with maintained blood pressure control, even over a 6-year period of treatment (LUND-JOHANSEN 1983b). In principle, the haemodynamic profile is similar to that observed after a single dose; some effects are, however, more pronounced. In particular, the stroke index has been reported to be increased by about 10%-15%, whereas the TPR decreases by about 15%-20% (EDWARDS and RAFTERY 1976; JOEKES and THOMPSON 1976; KOCH 1976, 1979a, 1981; SVENDSON et al. 1980; COHN et al. 1982; MEHTA et al. 1983). Thus, central haemodynamics have been normalised by labetalol. This may reflect the regression of structural changes in the heart and in the resistance vessels. The alterations seen with labetalol are opposite to what has been observed in untreated hypertensive patients or in those treated with pure β-blockers (LUND-JOHANSEN 1979, 1983a).

Haemodynamic investigations during exercise have shown that labetalol decreases the basal heart rate and inhibits the exercise-induced increase in heart rate, cardiac index and blood pressure after acute and sustained administration (KOCH 1977; BALASUBRAMANIAN et al. 1979b; FAGARD et al. 1979; LUND-JOHANSEN 1983b; MEHTA et al. 1983). The decrease in TPR observed at rest is also maintained during exercise. Similar observations have been made in investigations in which the haemodynamic changes were produced by emotional stress (TRAP-JENSEN et al. 1980; BAHLMANN et al. 1980).

Labetalol, but not propranolol, reduced the hypertensive response to isometric exercise or to orgasm in female subjects (NYBERG et al. 1979; NYBERG AND BERGLUND 1982; RILEY and RILEY 1981; MEHTA et al. 1983). This is not unexpected, since the blood pressure response under these conditions is mediated by an increase sympathetic tone, mainly via α-receptors.

Investigations in patients with hypertension and heart failure show that labetalol does not produce deterioration of left ventricular function (JOHNSON et al. 1984). In contrast to atenolol, an improvement of diastolic filling has even been demonstrated in mildly hypertensive patients (DIANZUMBA et al. 1987).

3.1.2.3.3 Influence of Labetalol on Catecholamines and Renin-Angiotensin-Aldosterone System

The presence of labetalol or its metabolities interferes with the fluorimetric and spectrophotometric methods of assaying for catecholamines and their 0-methylated metabolites. Using these methods in labetalol-treated patients when screening for phaeochromocytoma may therefore lead to a false-positive diagnosis (MIANO et al. 1979; LEVY and RICHARDS 1980). To avoid such errors it is advisable in these cases to measure the urinary excretion of 4-hydroxy-3-methoxy-mandelic acid. If it is raised, urinary or plasma catecholamines should be measured by radioenzymatic methods or by HPLC. When such sensitive and specific methods are used, labetalol does not substantially increase the plasma or urine concentrations of catecholamines (HAMILTON et al. 1978; CHRISTENSEN et al. 1978; LOUIS et al. 1978a; KOLLOCH et al. 1979; RICHARDS et al. 1979a, b; LIJNEN et al. 1979; KORNERUP et al. 1980; KEUSCH et al. 1980; EISALO and VIRTA 1982). LOUIS et al. (1978a) did not find any changes in plasma renin activity within 12 h after i.v. injection of 100 mg labetalol. During chronic treatment, some investigators observed a decrease in plasma renin activity and plasma aldosterone concentration (WEIDMANN et al. 1978; LIJNEN et al. 1979; SALVETTI et al. 1979; FAGARD et al. 1982), but HAUGER-KLEVENE (1981) did not find any influence of labetalol on the plasma renin concentration. This effect is obviously mediated by the expansion of plasma volume and can be prevented by diuretics. Indeed, during combined treatment with labetalol and diuretics, no increase in renin activity or plasma aldosterone has been found (WEIDMANN et al. 1978; KORNERUP et al. 1980).

3.1.2.3 Toxicology

The results of toxicological investigation have been reviewed by LEVY and RICHARDS (1980) and MACCARTHY and BLOOMFIELD (1983).

3.1.2.4 Pharmacokinetics and Metabolism

3.1.2.4.1 Absorption and Bioavailability

Labetalol is rapidly absorbed from the gastrointestinal tract of rabbits, rats and humans. The peak plasma concentration is reached about 1 h after administration (MARTIN et al. 1976; MARONDE et al. 1983). From measurements of the total plasma radioactivity it has been shown that labetalol is well absorbed, but only a small fraction of the parent compound reaches the systemic circulation (LEITZ et al. 1982). Most of the drug undergoes metabolism during its first passage through the liver and possibly in the gut wall as well. Plasma concentrations are therefore considerably lower after oral than after intravenous administration of the same dose (MARTIN et al. 1976).

The degree of bioavailability of labetalol varies greatly among different subjects (LOUIS et al. 1978a; MCNEIL et al. 1979; KANTO et al. 1981); a range from 11% to 86% with a mean of 33% has been reported by MCNEIL et al. (1979).

There is evidence that the bioavailability of labetalol increases with increasing age. KELLY et al. (1982) reported an average bioavailability of about 30% in the 30- to 40-year age group and 60%–70% in their subset of patients of approximately 80 years. There was also a slight trend towards longer half-lives in the elderly patients.

When labetalol is administrered with food, the bioavailability increases slightly (MÄNTYLÄ et al. 1980; DANESHMEND and ROBERTS 1982), but the rate of absorption is slowed with the consequence of increased time to reach maximum plasma drug concentrations. The administration of labetalol with food may, thus, circumvent the incidence of postural hypotension.

The bioavailability of labetalol has been reported to be increased from 30% to 54% by concomitant treatment with cimetidine (DANESHMEND and ROBERTS 1981).

3.1.2.4.2 Distribution

The total apparent volume of distribution of labetalol has been reported to be 567–805 litres in healthy volunteers (HOMEIDA et al. 1978; DANESHMEND and ROBERTS 1982) and 392 litres in hypertensive patients (MCNEIL et al. 1979) with a wide range between 188 and 747 litres. The discrepancy between the mean results of these two studies may be related to the fact that MCNEIL et al. (1979) used a higher i.v. dose for their study and at this dose level some of the tissue binding sites might have become saturated. Labetalol may concentrate within tissues; the extent to which it does varies considerably among different subjects. The high plasma clearance (1500 ml/min) also suggests an extensive biotransformation and/or tissue uptake (MCNEIL et al. 1979).

Autioradiographic and radiochemical studies in rats and dogs using [^{3}H]labetalol have shown that negligible amounts of the drug enter the brain or the fetuses of pregnant rats. Thus, labetalol does not readily penetrate the blood-brain barrier or the placental barrier. The highest concentrations of radioactivity have been found in the lungs, liver and kidneys (MARTIN et al. 1976).

Labetalol, but not its metabolities, has been reported to be bound reversibly to the melanin pigment of the eyes. In special long-term studies with detailed ophthalmological and histological examinations, no changes were found that indicate oculotoxicity (POYNTER et al. 1976).

3.1.2.4.3 *Elimination*

Labetalol and its metabolites are rapidly and completely excreted in the urine and bile of animals and humans. The proportion of radioactivity found in the urine of different species ranges between 48% and 66%. The percentage of the dose excreted in the urine as unchanged drug is 2% in rabbits, 5% in humans and 19% in dogs (MARTIN et al. 1976). The rest are mostly glucuronyl conjugates (LEVY and RICHARDS 1980).

The elimination half-life of unchanged labetalol has been reported to range in animals and humans between 3 and 5 h after i.v. administration (MARTIN et al. 1976; MCNEIL et al. 1979). REID et al. (1981), MARONDE et al. (1983) and CHUNG et al. (1986) concluded from their data that the pharmacokinetics of labetalol fit an open two-compartment model. The half-life after oral administration was between 5 and 8 h during acute and chronic treatment. The mean total plasma clearance has been calculated to be 24.8 ml $\times$ min^{-1} $\times$ kg^{-1} (KANTO et al. 1981). WOOD et al. (1982) observed no significant differences between paients with severe renal failure and controls for any pharmacokinetic parameter. They concluded therefore that no modification of labetalol dosage is required in patients with impaired renal function.

3.1.2.4.4 *Steady State Kinetics*

Steady state concentrations of labetalol during chronic treatment have been found to be 1.7 times higher than those predicted from single-dose pharmacokinetics. The reason for this is unknown, but a small decline in the rate of clearance of labetalol with long-term administration has been suggested (MCNEIL et al. 1982). In contrast, when MARONDE et al. (1983) and CHUNG et al. (1986) investigated pharmacokinetics after acute and chronic treatment, the predictd and observed values during the steady state were in good agreement.

A close correlation between daily doses and mean steady state plasma concentrations indicates dose-linear kinetics (SANDERS et al. 1979; BLOOMFIELD et al. 1983; CHUNG et al. 1986). However, MCNEIL et al. (1982) and SANDERS et al. (1979) have also found a large variation in the plasma concentration during sustained therapy, probably due to differences between individuals in bioavailability and clearance.

3.1.2.4.5 *In Pregnancy*

In a pharmacokinetic study, a single i.v. dose of 50 mg labetalol was given to pregnant women in the third trimester and again 3–4 months post-partum. There were no significant differences in plasma concentrations, volume of distribution, clearance or half-life, which suggests that the dose regimen for pregnant patients need not differ from that of other patients (RUBIN et al. 1983). However, no information is available for pregnant patients regarding plasma concentration following oral administration, either after a single dose or during sustained treatment.

The concentration of labetalol has also been determined in infant cord blood at the time of delivery (MICHAEL 1979) and in breast milk of lactating women

(MICHAEL 1979; LEITZ et al. 1983). The concentrations have been found to be 20%–60% of that of the plasma concentration.

3.1.2.4.6 Chronic Liver Disease and Renal Disease

As metabolic clearance plays an important role in the elimination of labetalol, it might be expected that impaired hepatic function would affect its disposition. HOMEIDA et al. (1978) showed that the average bioavailability of labetalol in 10 patients with chronic liver diseases was nearly double (63%) that of 7 normal controls of similar age (33%). Higher plasma concentrations of labetalol and greater blood pressure responses indicate that the dosage of labetalol should be reduced in such patients. In contrast, pharmacokinetic patterns have been reported to be unchanged in patients with impaired renal function (WOOD et al. 1982; WALSTADT et al. 1981).

3.1.2.4.7 Relation Between Plasma Concentration and Blood Pressure Effects

DREW et al. (1981) found a close correlation ($r = 0.73$) between the decrease in diastolic blood pressure and plasma concentration in DOCA-hypertensive rats treated with oral doses of between 10 and 100 mg/kg labetalol.

The plasma concentrations of free labetalol required for a hypotensive effect in hypertensive rats, dogs or humans has been calculated to be about $5 \times 10^{-8}\,M - 10^{-7}\,M$ (LEVY and RICHARDS 1980).

RICHARDS et al. (1977b) reported a linear correlation ($r = 0.84$) between the maximum inhibition of exercise-induced tachycardia and the logarithm of the plasma concentration 2 h after an oral dose of 100, 200, and 400 mg labetalol.

SANDERS et al. (1979) found a close correlation ($r = 0.72$) under steady state conditions between the plasma concentration of labetalol and its β-blocking activity, whereas no relationship existed between concentration and blood pressure response.

KANTO et al. (1980a, 1981), MCNEIL et al. (1981) and MARONDE et al. (1983) demonstrated that the mean plasma concentrations and the mean hypotensive effect on blood pressure in the upright position declined in parallel with time in hypertensive patients treated with doses ranging from 200 to 1200 mg. A clear relationship between hypotensive activity of a single dose and plasma concentration has also been reported in pregnant women (RUBIN et al. 1983). MCNEIL et al. (1979) reported an inverse correlation between the fall in plasma labetalol concentration and maximal fall in supine diastolic blood pressure in the 1st h after intravenous administration. This suggests that the more rapid the distribution, the greater the effect on blood pressure. These observations therefore raised the possibility of labetalol acting on a deep tissue compartment or, alternatively, that an active metabolite contributes to its effect.

The correlation coefficient between mean log plasma concentration and decrease in mean standing blood pressure was $r = 0.96$ in Maronde's study. However, they pointed out the wide inter-patient variation which limits the predictive value of labetalol plasma levels with respect to expected blood pressure lowering effects. Taking into account the fact that individual sensitivity to labetalol's antihypertensive action may obscure any plasma concentration-response relationship, it is not surprising that other investigators (LUND-JOHANSEN and BAKKE 1979; SANDERS et al. 1979) have claimed that no such relationship exists. Also, MCNEIL and LOUIS (1984) did not find any correlation in a series of 12 individuals treated with a single dose of 100 mg labetalol when the individual values of area under the plasma concentration-time curves were plotted against area under the mean blood pressure-time curve (MCNEIL et al. 1979; MCNEIL and LOUIS 1984). They also found no correlation between bioavailability and blood pressure response.

3.1.2.4.8 Metabolism

Labetalol is extensively metabolised in animals and in humans. Studies in different species suggest that the metabolites are formed by first-pass metabolism during passage through the intestinal wall and liver. This can be concluded from the fact that only 5% of the total radioactivity in the plasma can be attributed to the parent compound. However, the metabolites have been identified only in the urine (MARTIN et al. 1976). The major metabolites in the urine are glucuronide conjugates, in humans mainly the alcoholic glucuronide (MARTIN et al. 1976; LEVY and RICHARDS 1980). It is therefore not surprising that the metabolites do not exhibit pharmacological activity in animals after oral administration (MARTIN et al. 1976).

3.1.3 Therapeutic Use

3.1.3.1 Acute Use

In contrast to pure β-blocking agents, labetalol has been shown to decrease high blood pressure promptly (AGABITI-ROSEI et al. 1977).

This property of labetalol has been utilised in the management of hypertensive emergencies. The mode of action of labetalol should make it especially suitable for the treatment of severe hypertension due to excessive secretion of catecholamines, as with phaeochromocytoma or following clonidine withdrawal.

It even seems possible to reduce the blood pressure of patients with severe hypertension markedly with single oral doses of 300–400 mg labetalol (GHOSE 1979). Intravenous administration should be preferred, since this procedure provides more reliable control of the pressure in the individual situation.

After i.v. injection or rapid infusions, the blood pressure falls sharply within a few minutes and usually remains at the lower level for several hours (RONNE-RASMUSSEN et al. 1976; TRUST et al. 1976). In contrast to diazoxide, this effect is not accompanied by activation of the renin-angiotensin system or by an increase in heart rate or cardiac output.

The degree of blood pressure reduction after i.v. administration of labetalol appears to be related to the pretreatment basal plasma norepinephrine concentration and also to the age of the patients (PAPADEMETRIOU et al. 1982; AGABITI-ROSEI et al. 1983).

The maximum dose for i.v. administration of labetalol is 300 mg. Intravenous dosage regimens used have included single rapid injections of 1–2 mg/kg (PEARSON and HAVARD 1976, 1978; TRUST et al. 1976; CUMMING et al. 1979b), infusions of 1–2 mg/min until reaching the therapeutic goal (MAZZOLA et al. 1981; LEBEL et al. 1985), repeated bolus injections of 20–80 mg at 10–15 min intervals (J.J. BROWN et al. 1977; PAPADEMETRIOU et al. 1982) and incremental infusions in steps between 20 and 160 mg/h (CUMMING et al. 1979a). Some investigators recommend giving a loading dose of 20–100 mg before starting the graded dosages (DAL PALU et al. 1982; WILSON et al. 1983). The advantage of a graded dosing schedule is that the blood pressure is reduced more smoothly. Some side effects can therefore be prevented, and the pressure can be better titrated to the required level.

Although incremental infusion of labetalol is usually safe and effective, some patients remain resistant. There is a dispute as to whether the response to labetalol in hypertensive emergencies may be less satisfactory if the patients are already receiving other antihypertensive drugs, in particular other adrenergic blocking agents (PEARSON and HAVARD 1976; MCGRATH et al. 1978; ANDERSON and GABRIEL 1978; MACCARTHY et al. 1978; YEUNG et al. 1979; WILSON et al. 1983). One case report describes a pressor response after i.v. administration of labetalol in a man pretreated with other drugs, including high doses of propranolol (CROFTON and GABRIEL 1977). However, the overall response rate of 70%-90% compares favourably with that observed for diazoxide (KEUSCH et al. 1983; RUMBOLDT et al. 1983).

A precipitous decrease in blood pressure may sometimes occur unpredictably. Close and continuous supervision of all patients receiving labetalol as i.v. injection or infusion is therefore essential. CUMMING et al. (1982) pointed out additionally that labetalol, as a compound with α- and β-blocking activity, may be hazardous in patients with congestive heart failure who are not digitalised. When purely left heart failure is present and evidently the result of severe hypertension, the use of a loop diuretic such as furosemide concurrently with labetalol is advisable. However, in WILSON's study (1983) labetalol was effective and safe in the treatment of severe hypertension associated with acute left ventricular failure, acute myocardial infarction, angina pectoris, stable congestive heart failure, atrial fibrillation and left ventricular hypertrophy. The patients tolerated labetalol i.v. without clinical deterioration of their underlying condition.

The adverse reactions reported after i.v. administration of labetalol are mostly mild and transient and do not require discontinuation (WILSON et al. 1983). They include nausea, vomiting, sweating, flushing, headaches, faintness despite recumbency and excessive hypotension. These symptoms can be reduced at least partly by stopping the infusion, by elevating the foot of the bed and by i.v. administration of fluids. In order to avoid postural hypotension, patients should always be in a supine position during and for some hours after i.v. administration (CUMMING et al. 1982; WILSON et al. 1983). Severe adverse reactions such as syncope with symptoms of myocardial ischaemia or focal neurological deficits as the result of too precipitous hypotension occur very seldom with labetalol if it is administered in graded dosages (J.J. BROWN et al. 1977; DAL PALU et al. 1982; WILSON et al. 1983; LEBEL et al. 1985).

The absence of neurological symptoms during blood pressure lowering with labetalol may be due to the lack of reduction of cerebral blood flow with this compound. The α-blocking activity of labetaolol may prevent the sympathetic vasoconstriction of larger cerebral arteries that can compromise cerebral blood flow during a fall in systemic blood pressure (D.N.W. GRIFFITH et al. 1979; PEARSON et al. 1979).

3.1.3.2 Chronic Use in Treatment of Hypertension

Labetalol has been extensively investigated in clinical trials. The results of many open or double-blind studies versus placebo or other antihypertensive medications confirm the hypotensive activity of labetalol (for review, see BROGDEN et al. 1978; MACCARTHY and BLOOMFIELD 1983; PRICHARD 1984; LOUIS and MCNEIL 1984; KANTO 1985). Some studies have been continued for many years, and they have shown that labetalol maintains reduction of peripheral resistance with consequent control of blood pressure without the development of tolerance (PRICHARD et al. 1979; WAAL-MANNING and SIMPSON 1982; KANE 1982; TAKEDA et al. 1982; LUND-JOHANSEN 1983b; ÖHMAN and ASPLUND 1984).

Furthermore, it has been observed in a considerable number of studies that patients with severe and previously uncontrolled hypertension responded satisfactorily to labetalol (DARGIE et al. 1976; MORGAN et al. 1978; PRICHARD et al. 1979; L.C. WILLIAMS et al. 1979; MYERS et al. 1980; KRISTENSEN and LA COUR PETERSEN 1980; MACDONALD et al. 1980; HAUGER-KLEVENE 1981; KANE 1982; WAAL-MANNING and SIMPSON 1982; WALLIN et al. 1983). However, OMVIK and LUND-JOHANSEN (1982) observed a fading of the antihypertensive efficacy of labetalol in severely hypertensive patients.

The dosages stated to be appropriate for achieving the desired blood pressure level vary greatly, probably due to the wide interindividual variation in the pharmacokinetic patterns and the inhomogeneous groups of patients. In some individuals 100–300 mg per day are sufficient to control the blood pressure (HANSSON and HÄNEL 1976; PRICHARDS and BOAKES 1976; LOUIS et al. 1978b; PRICHARD et al. 1979; TAKEDA et al. 1982; MCNEIL et al. 1982; WAAL-MANNING and SIMPSON 1982), whereas in some patients daily doses of 2400 mg, or even up to 8000 mg, have been used (PRICHARD and BOAKES 1976; DARGIE et al. 1976; KRISTENSEN and LA COUR PETERSEN 1980). The individual daily doses within the trials have been reported to range between 100 and 2400 mg (WAAL-MANNING and SIMPSON 1982; WILSON et al. 1983), and the average doses of various clinical trials are mostly in the range from 600 to 900 mg daily. However, also lower (GOMEZ and PHILLIPS 1980; OLIVIER et al. 1980; TAKEDA et al. 1982; ARINSOY and ORAM 1986) and higher (DARGIE et al. 1976; PRICHARD et al. 1979; ERICHS et al. 1980; KORNERUP et al. 1980) doses have been reported. This wide variation in the dosages indicates that a careful, but inconvenient, upward titration is necessary to find the adequate dose for an individual patient.

Since the bioavailability of labetalol is increased in elderly patients, and in addition they may react more sensitively to α-blockers or other vasodilators, careful titration is appropriate in this special subset of patients in particular. EISALO and VITRA (1982) found in a well-conducted, long-term study a good blood pressure response in patients aged from 59 to 72 years at a daily dose from 100 to 600 mg. Of 24 patients 14 were controlled for 1 year with 200 mg labetalol daily, remarkably without orthostatic side effects. Similar results have been reported from a double-blind, placebo-controlled study performed in 50 elderly patients (NUGENT et al. 1985). A comparative study was performed by ABERNETHY et al. (1987) in younger and older patients, including cases of isolated systolic hypertension. Labetalol was well-tolerated in both groups; in particular postural hypotension was not observed, and labetalol was at least as effective in the elderly as in the younger subset. The dose required to achieve blood pressure control was relatively lower in the elderly patients (mean 245 mg daily).

Most clinical studies have been performed with a thrice daily dosing schedule. There are clinical studies with intra-arterial blood pressure monitoring that indicate that thrice daily and even twice daily is satisfactory for controlling the blood pressure over the whole day without a rise in the early morning (BALASUBRAMANIAN et al. 1979a; MANCIA et al. 1982; BELLAMY et al. 1983). From the few preliminary reports it is not possible to draw clear conclusions as to whether a single-dose regimen can control blood pressure for 24 h (VAN SCHOOR 1979; ROSSI et al. 1982). BRECKENRIDGE et al. (1982) stated according to their own experience that from the pharmacodynamic and pharmacokinetic points of view, labetalol can be administered once daily, but postural hypotension after a large dose may limit the usefulness of this dose regimen. They therefore recommend a twice daily dosing schedule.

The chronic antihypertensive effect of labetalol has been compared with that of other compounds in a variety of well-conducted studies using fixed and titrated doses.

Labetalol was compared in double-blind studies with diuretics. In these studies in mildly hypertensive patients treated with low doses (maximum: 600 mg daily), labetalol was only more effective on the standing blood pressure. The combination produced a larger fall in pressure than either drug alone (DAWSON et al. 1979; HORVATH et al. 1979; LECHI et al. 1982; BLOOMFIELD et al. 1983; Labetalol/hydrochlorothiazide multicenter study group 1985).

It has been observed in some studies that patients whose blood pressure had been inadequately controlled by previous β-blocker therapy achieved better control of blood pressure with labetalol.

In a considerable number of double-blind trials, partly as within-patient studies, labetalol was compared with different pure β-blockers such as propranolol, pindolol, metoprolol, atenolol, alprenolol and acebutolol. Generally, the mean reduction in resting supine blood pressure of mildly or moderately hypertensive patients did not differ between the labetalol-treated patients and those treated with the other compounds, but the decrease in sitting or standing blood pressure was more pronounced with labetalol, whereas the heart rate was more reduced by the pure β-blockers, both at rest and during exercise (PUGSLEY et al. 1976, 1979; MCNEIL and LOUIS 1979; NICHOLLS et al. 1980; KOFOD et al. 1980; BJERLE et al. 1980; WEST et al. 1980; BACKHOUSE 1981; THULIN et al. 1981; WALSTADT et al. 1982; FRISHMAN et al. 1983; KUBIK and COOTE 1984; WEBER et al. 1984; ROMO et al. 1984). However, in Kofod's double-blind, crossover study, 22 of 32 of the labetalol-treated patients reached the target blood pressure, whereas satisfactory control of the blood pressure was achieved by only 11 alprenolol-treated patients. Also HUNYOR et al. (1980) found labetalol to be superior to propranolol in lowering supine and standing blood pressure. In some of the trials mentioned, individual dose titration was not possible, which may lead to inconclusive results with respect to efficacy. In a further study in which doses were individually titrated, labetalol at doses up to 800 mg/day induced a significantly greater decrease in supine arterial blood pressure than the same doses of acebutolol (THIBONNIER et al. 1980). In this study, higher doses of labetalol (1200–1600 mg daily) had the same potency as the combination of acebutolol (400–800 mg daily) plus dihydralazine (50–100 mg daily).

Further studies show that labetalol is equal to or even superior to the combination of β-adrenoceptor blockers plus vasodilators (J.G. WILLIAMS et al. 1978; BARNETT et al. 1978; MIDTBO and HALS 1981; COLOMBO et al. 1982; VAN DER VEUR et al. 1982) in terms of the control of supine and standing blood pressure, but other trials have not demonstrated the advantages of labetalol in comparison with such combinations (LEHTONEN et al. 1979; WEST et al. 1980).

When compared with methyldopa in double-blind trials, labetalol was equipotent in mild or moderate hypertension (SANDERS et al. 1978) but definitely more potent in patients with severe hypertension regardless of additional therapy with furosemide (WALLIN et al. 1983). ÖHMAN et al. (1985) compared the efficacy of labetalol, nifedipine and their combination in a doube-blind, crossover study. Both supine and standing blood pressure were decreased more by labetalol than by nifedipine, whereas the combination was more effective than either agent given alone. The effects of labetalol (mean dose 500 mg twice daily) and prazosin (mean dose 5.6 mg twice daily) on blood pressure and heart rate were compared in a double-blind study of essential hypertension using automated ambulatory monitoring. Labetalol had significantly greater effects on blood pressure during daily activity than prazosin. The heart rate and pressure-rate product was reduced only by labetalol (GRAY et al. 1988). Finally, LILJA et al. (1982) compared labetalol with clonidine in a within-patient study in patients inadequately treated with bendrofluazide. Blood pressure control was similar when using either drug, but side effects, in particular tiredness and dry mouth, were much more common with clonidine.

The efficacy of labetalol in black hypertensive patients deserves special interest since this population generally responds poorly to β-adrenoceptor blockers. EL-ACKAD et al. (1984b) observed in a comparative study of labetalol and propranolol that both drugs had similar modest antihypertensive effects but that the labetalol effect was better maintained. JENNINGS and PARSONS (1976) found a satisfactory response to labetalol in Caucasian patients but not in those from African or West Indian origin. However, the compliance of the latter group was suspect, and there was some indication that these patients did not adhere reliably to their prescribed therapy. FRISHMAN et al. (1983) also saw in his small subset of black patients only a slight decrease in blood pressure when labetalol was administered as monotherapy. On the other hand, W.B. SMITH et al. (1983) reported a fall in blood pressure from 209/143 to 140/93 mmHg in 19 black patients after i.v. injection of labetalol in doses between 20 and 300 mg. Wallin (1983), Cubberly (1985) and Due et al. (1986b) pointed out that their black patients responded well to labetalol. In two studies from South Africa, major racial disparity has not been observed (Seedat 1979; Olivier et al. 1980). In a controlled comparative study with propranolol in black and white hypertensive patients, equal efficacy was shown in whites, but in the black patients labetalol was more effective than propranolol, and supplementary diuretics had to be added less often (Flamenbaum et al. 1985). In a further double-blind study on patients unsatisfactorily controlled with hydrochlorothiazide, whites and blacks responded equally to the additional therapy with labetalol (Labetalol/hydrochlorothiazide multicentre study group 1985). Finally, labetalol and methyldopa were equally effective in Nigerian hypertensive patients (Mabadeje et al. 1982).

3.1.3.3 Special Indications

3.1.3.3.1 Renal Hypertension and Hypertension Associated with Impaired Renal Function

A considerable number of well-conducted studies in hypertensive patients with impaired renal function show that labetalol can be used effectively alone or in combination with a diuretic for lowering arterial blood pressure.

Moreover, on the basis of studies in patients with or without impairment of renal function, it can be concluded that labetalol does not have any deleterious effect on renal function (Craswell et al. 1977; Thompson et al. 1977, 1978; J.G. Williams et al. 1978; Bailey 1979b; Rasmussen and Nielsen 1981; Valvo et al. 1981; Watson et al. 1981; Malini et al. 1982; Wood et al. 1982; Wallin 1983; Weber et al. 1984). In renal hypertensive patients, labetalol is more effective than a combination of conventional β-blocker plus hydralazine, but less effective than minoxidil (J.G. Williams et al. 1978).

In contrast to propranolol, which decreases renal plasma flow and glomerular filtration rate during exercise, labetalol has no effect on these parameters (Valvo et al. 1981; Larsen and Pedersen 1980).

3.1.3.3.2 Hypertension in Pregnancy

A number of studies have shown that labetalol is effective and safe in the treatment of hypertension in pregnancy (Michael 1979, 1982). In this study, blood pressure was controlled in 79 of 85 patients with doses up to 1200 mg daily. There were no significant maternal or fetal side effects. Two infants were stillborn, 24 of 89 live births had intrauterine growth retardation. Labetalol, however, seems to exert a beneficial effect on fetal lung maturation. There was a low perinatal mortality of 4.4%, which compares very favourably with other series in comparably affected patients. This may be traced back to the fact that the uteroplacental flow does not fall after labetalol administration (Lunell et al. 1982), as demonstrated in a group of eight pre-eclamptic women. In comparative studies with methyldopa (Lamming et al. 1980; Plouin et al. 1987) or atenolol (Lardoux et al. 1983), labetalol was at least as effective as the standard drugs in lowering blood pressure, but more pregnant patients had spontaneous labour in the labetalol group than in the methyldopa group (LAMMING et al. 1980), and the birth weights in the labetalol group were significantly higher than those in the atenolol group. Renal function improved during labetalol treatment, whereas in the methyldopa-treated patients proteinuria developed in five women. Despite the improvement in renal function, labetalol, in contrast to methyldopa, increased the serum uric acid concentration (LAMMING et al. 1980). In situations in which rapid reduction of blood pressure is required, such as in severe pre-eclampsia, labetalol can be administered by the intravenous route with satisfactory results (LAMMING et al. 1980; LILFORD 1980; LUNELL et al. 1981; GARDEN et al. 1982).

3.1.3.3.3 Phaeochromocytoma and Clonidine Withdrawal

Because of early negative results (BRIGGS et al. 1978; FITZGERALD 1978; HURLEY et al. 1979; FEEK and EARNSHOW 1980) labetalol was previously considered not to be the optimal drug for treatment in these conditions. The limited efficacy may be the consequence of its relatively weak α-blocking activity (LOUIS and MCNEIL 1984). Nevertheless, there are reports showing that labetalol has been successfully used in patients with hypertensive attacks due to phaeochromocytoma or in the chronic treatment of this disease (AGABITI-ROSEI et al. 1976a, b; BAILEY 1979a; REACH et al. 1980; TAKEDA et al. 1982). In these patients labetalol has been titrated up to 6400 mg daily. In particular, labetalol provides satisfactory cover of surgery for removal of such tumours at doses of 50 mg i.v. (AGABITI-ROSEI et al. 1976a, b; KAUFMAN 1979). Acute hypertension induced by abrupt clonidine withdrawal can also be prevented with labetalol. ROSENTHAL et al. (1981) successfully prevented any rise in blood pressure under these conditions when labetalol was given orally at the first symptoms of blood pressure rise. The total dosages were up to 1200 mg over 3 days. On the basis of their results they recommended the use of labetalol prophylactically whenever clonidine is being withdrawn. However, it is necessary to monitor the blood pressure closely and ensure that adequate labetalol doses are given, since too small doses will not block post-clonidine hypertension (HURLEY et al. 1979).

3.1.3.3.4 Tetanus

Hypertension induced by tetanus has been successfully treated with labetalol. In one case report, the drug was administered in doses at 1–2 mg/min for 17 days (DUNDEE and MORROW 1979). In a series including 15 patients labetalol was given by intermittent i.v. injection of 5–75 mg or by infusion of 1–10 mg/h or by daily oral administration of doses of 200–800 mg. Even though the results were variable, 12 of 15 patients responded with a decrease in blood pressure (WESLEY et al. 1983).

3.1.3.3.5 Controlled Hypotensive Anaesthesia

It has been reported that labetalol attenuates the hypertensive response due to endotracheal intubation (MAHARAJ et al. 1983). Results obtained with labetalol in association with halothane-anaesthesia suggest that it is a useful adjunct to controlled hypotensive anaesthesia (COPE and CRAWFORD 1979; KAUFMAN 1979; SCOTT et al. 1976; SCOTT 1982; HUNTER 1979; JONES 1979; KANTO et al. 1980b). An initial dose of intravenous labetalol of 20 mg was followed by further increments of 5–10 mg until the desired level of systolic blood pressure of 60–80 mmHg and a heart rate of 60 bpm was achieved. In order to keep the haemodynamic conditions constant, the halothane concentration was reduced and adjusted individually by about 1%. Of particular value is the fact that on completion of surgery the patient's blood pressure and heart rate can be easily returned to normal by reducing the halothane concentration and/or i.v. injection of atropine 0.6 mg. Because of the α- and β-blocking properties of labetalol, the usual indicators of acute blood loss may be masked during such a combined procedure for anaesthesia.

3.1.3.3.6 Myocardial Infarction with Systemic Hypertension

MARX and REID (1979) investigated the effect of labetalol in 13 hypertensive patients with acute myocardial infarction and 2 patients with unstable angina. The drug was infused in incremental doses; the total doses varied between 30 and 440 mg. The systemic blood pressure was safely and effectively lowered from 184/122 mmHg to 118/84 mmHg. Heart rate, left ventricular filling pressure, cardiac index and TPR decreased, whereas the stroke index was almost unchanged. No side effects occurred, and all 15 patients survived and were discharged from the hospital (MARX and REID 1979). Similar results have been reported by TIMMIS et al. (1980), CANTELLI and BRACCHETTI 1981 and RENARD et al. (1983). NELSON et al. (1982), however, observed a slight decrease in blood pressure, cardiac output and stroke index without any change in heart rate and left ventricular filling pressure in patients in the early stages of uncomplicated myocardial infarction during infusion of labetalol (0.5 mg/kg·h). The authors felt that these haemodynamic changes may be advantageous in such a situation because of the reduced oxygen consumption.

It has been shown in an experimental study that labetalol effectively reduces infarct size in rats (CHIARIELLO et al. 1980). This could, however, not be confirmed in a well-conducted clinical study in 160 normotensive patients suffering from myocardial infarction. In these patients, labetalol was able to reduce the heart rate and to keep the blood pressure at normotensive levels, but on the basis of indices of myocardial necrosis, such as CKMB-enzyme release and R-wave score, the labetalol-treated patients did not benefit from this therapy. The authors, therefore, did not recommend the use of labetalol as a routine treatment for normotensive patients admitted to hospital with suspected myocardial infarction (HEBER et al. 1987b).

3.1.3.4 Adverse Reactions

There are some reviews from various countries dealing with the types and incidence of adverse reactions induced by labetalol (GOMEZ and PHILLIPS 1980; WAAL-MANNING and SIMPSON 1982; TAKEDA et al. 1982; TCHERDAKOFF 1983; MICHELSON et al. 1983) (see Table 4). Apart from the Japanese report, most

Table 4. Labetalol-induced side effects reported in reviews from various countries

Reference	WAAL-MANNING and SIMPSON 1982[a]	TCHERDAKOFF 1983[a]	MICHELSON et al. 1983[a]	GOMEZ and PHILLIPS 1980	TAKEDA et al. 1982
Country	New Zealand	France	USA	UK	Japan
Method of evaluation	inquiry	questionaire	patient's report	patient's report	patient's report
Number of patients	163	251	337	1286	239
Averaged daily dose	700	654	600	477	336
Range (mg)	100–2400	100–2400	200–2400	50–1600	150–1200
Duration of treatment	up to 6.5 years	6–18 months	1–20 months	up to 2 years	3–12 months
Bronchospasm, dyspnoea	5	5	6	9	1
Heart failure, fluid retention	3	–	10	–	1
Disturbed peripheral circulation	7	–	–	–	2
Dreams (nightmares, depression)	7	3	–	–	4
Postural hypotension	28	3	28	20	2
Dizziness, tiredness	17	17	42	9	–
Fatigue, light-headedness	–	2	46	–	22
Headaches	6	1	14	6	5
Nasal stuffiness; dry mouth	6	16	40	–	1
Urogenital side effects	4	26	29	7	1
Gastrointestinal side effects	24	11	79	9	6
Scalp tingling	13	53	23	4	1
Skin rash	9	2	–	6	–
Nuclear-specific antibodies	4	–	–	–	–
Transaminase increase	–	–	14	–	–
Others	20	9	29	23	5
Withdrawn due to side effects	45	25	32	93	7
Patients without side effects	77	125	83	651	211

[a] Most of the patients were previously treated with other antihypertensives. They changed over to labetalol because of unsatisfactory blood pressure control, side-effects or both.
Most of the side-effects were reported to be mild and transient.

patients included in these reviews had been previously treated with other agents and were changed over to labetalol because the previous therapy was not effective enough or because of side effects. The figures for labetalol-induced side effects in these reviews may not therefore reflect the true incidence of adverse events in general practice. Interestingly, the incidence and distribution of side effects vary considerably between the reports (see Table 3).

Adverse reactions induced by labetalol can be assigned to two categories:

(a) those related to adrenoceptor blockade,
(b) those that are non-specific, i.e. not related to adrenoceptor blockade.

In general, adverse reactions to labetalol are more frequent during the first few days or weeks of treatment than later (KANE 1982). Obviously, the relatively rapid lowering of blood pressure induced by labetalol provokes unwanted reactions which decline with time. Moreover, the increase in blood volume occurring during prolonged treatment (HUNYOR et al. 1982; WEIDMANN et al. 1978) tends to reduce any side effect associated with vascular α-receptor blockade.

3.1.3.4.1 Adverse Reactions Due to Adrenoceptor Blockade

Generally, adverse reactions caused by the β-blocking property of labetalol are less than those induced by "pure" β-blocking agents (WAAL-MANNING and SIMPSON 1982; DUE et al. 1986a). This might be expected, as the additional α-blockade contributes to the antihypertensive activity of labetalol, and therefore relatively less β-blockade is needed for a given effect. Moreover, some of the adverse reactions due to β-blockade would be reduced by concomitant blockade of the α-adrenoceptors.

On the other hand, NICHOLLS et al. (1980) reported, on the basis of a well-conducted and controlled comparison of labetalol with propranolol, the same profile of adverse reactions, but a slight tendency for a higher incidence during labetalol treatment, whereas the blood pressure was reduced to the same extent.

Obviously, airway obstruction is a rare adverse reaction to labetalol. Patients, however, with a history of bronchospasm can encounter trouble with labetalol (TCHERDAKOFF 1983). GOMEZ and PHILLIPS (1980) had to withdraw labetalol in 9 of 54 patients due to exacerbated airway obstruction. LARSSON (1982) and ANAVEKAR et al. (1982) also observed some instances of deterioration of airway obstruction in predisposed patients. Other investigators have not observed any deterioration in patients with chronic obstructive airway disease (SKINNER et al. 1975; MACONOCHIE et al. 1977; ADAM et al. 1982; GEORGE et al. 1983; LIGHT et al. 1983). JACKSON and BEEVERS (1983) compared in a double-blind, placebo-controlled study the effect of 100 mg atenolol and 300 mg labetalol. They did not find any significant differences between the drugs with respect to the reduction of FEV_1. However, labetalol reduced significantly the effect of inhaled salbutamol on FEV_1. EL ACKAD et al. (1984a) compared labetalol with metoprolol in seven patients with bronchial asthma sensitive to propranolol in a double-blind, crossover study. After 100 mg of labetalol only one patient had a fall in FEV_1 of more than 10%; after 200 mg of metoprolol, FEV_1 was reduced in all patients by more than 10%. Thus, labetalol seems to have at least less overall effect on airways than non-cardioselective β-blockers. This may be caused by the additional α-blockade (Patel 1976), which may at least partly reduce the effect of β-blockade on the bronchi.

Only a few cases of symptoms of peripheral vascular disturbances have been reported. On the other hand, it has been reported that circulatory disturbances induced by other β-blockers were improved or disappeared after a change over to labetalol (Waal-Manning and Simpson 1982; Tcherdakoff 1983). De Cesaris et al. (1985) observed, on the basis of thermographic measurements, that labetalol markedly improved the peripheral vascularisation of the hands, while atenolol did not exert such an effect.

Tiredness, dizziness and fatigue are common adverse reactions of antihypertensive agents, including adrenoceptor blocking agents. The effects may be attributable to a central effect or they may be the consequence of blood pressure reduction, in particular in the first few weeks of treatment. These symptoms have been reported to be relatively frequent (Waal-Manning and Simpson 1982; Kane 1982; Michelson et al. 1983; Tcherdakoff 1983).

Postural hypotension is a very common adverse reaction induced by α-receptor blocking agents, especially at the beginning of therapy. It might therefore be expected also in patients treated with labetalol. Postural related dizziness and hypotension have indeed been reported from a considerable number of clinical trials. It seems to be the most troublesome adverse reaction that occasionally necessitates the withdrawal of labetalol. The overall incidence of postural hypotension after labetalol, however, seems to be less than that during therapy with α-blockers alone. This may be due to the fact that labetalol lowers blood pressure both by its α- and β-blocking activity. Postural hypotension tends to occur more frequently with higher doses of labetalol (Dargie et al. 1976; Maronde et al. 1983) and in patients treated additionally with diuretics (Bolli et al. 1976; Pugsley et al. 1976; McNeil et al. 1981), particularly during the early stages of treatment. It is therefore important to initiate therapy with low doses—e.g. 100 mg twice daily—of labetalol, to titrate upwards slowly and to decrease the dosage when adding a diuretic.

Remarkably, some investigators reported an extremely low incidence of postural hypotension during chronic treatment with labetalol (Prichard et al. 1979; Balasubramanian et al. 1979b; Hauger-Klevene 1981; Wallin et al. 1983; Davidov et al. 1983; Gomez and Phillips 1980; Tcherdakoff 1983; Koch 1979a). Louis et al. (1978b) also pointed out the generally low incidence of postural symptoms, but they had two patients who were previously unsatisfactorily treated with other agents. They experienced weakness and faintness within 2 h after the first dose of 200 mg labetalol. The measurement of the plasma concentration suggested that this hypersensitivity probably resulted from unexpectedly high plasma concentrations. They could be well controlled chronically with 100 mg labetalol twice daily. The authors stated that there is a need for caution when starting new patients on labetalol. Individual dose titration is recommended in order to circumvent problems that may arise as the result of unpredictably high bioavailability.

Urogenital symptoms have been reported, in particular in the American survey (MICHELSON et al. 1983). Some 14% of the male patients suffered from ejaculation failure, impotence, decreased libido and strangury. Similar symptoms have been reported also by WAAL-MANNING and SIMPSON (1982), BAILEY (1977) and TCHERDAKOFF (1983). However, some patients in the last study had pre-existing sexual difficulties. DUE et al. (1986a) reported a lower incidence of erectile problems in labetalol-treated patients than in propranolol-treated subjects. In a single dose study of 100 and 300 mg in volunteers labetalol gave a dose-dependent delay in ejaculation and detumescence whereas erection was not affected (RILEY et al. 1982). In women, labetalol reduced vaginal lubrication but did not appear to affect other aspects of the sexual response (RILEY and RILEY 1981).

3.1.3.4.2 Non-specific Adverse Reactions

Headache is one of the most frequently reported complaints (KANE 1982; MICHELSON et al. 1983). However, it is not clear in all cases whether labetalol is responsible for this adverse reaction.

A broad spectrum of gastrointestinal disorders such as nausea, vomiting, abdominal pain and diarrhoea has been reported in the most studies.

A very distinctive adverse reaction induced by labetalol is that of formication (BAILEY 1977; COULTER 1979). The most common description is that of a tingling sensation of the scalp skin, especially when exposed to sunlight or to the heat of a hairdryer (WAAL-MANNING and SIMPSON 1982; TCHERDAKOFF 1983). HUA et al. (1977) described this sensation as resembling that of insects crawling under the scalp. It is not completely clear whether the skin itch described in some reports should be attributed to the above-mentioned tingling sensation of the scalp.

WAAL-MANNING and SIMPSON (1982) reported seven patients who were nuclear-specific antibody-negative prior to labetalol and who became positive (titre higher than 1:80) during therapy on labetalol and a diuretic. However, the patients did not exhibit symptoms of immunological diseases. Patients positive for nuclear-specific antibodies have been reported in two further studies (BOLLI et al. 1976; PUGSLEY et al. 1976), but the significance of these findings is not clear as the investigators did not suggest a positive association with labetalol.

There are isolated reports of cases of systemic lupus erythematosus (SLE; I.D. GRIFFITH and RICHARDSON 1979; R.C. BROWN et al. 1981; New Zealand Hypertension Study Group 1981) and bullous lichen planus (GANGE and WILSON-JONES 1978; MICHELSON et al. 1983) and other cutaneous reactions (BRANFORD et al. 1978).

There have been no reports of ophthalmological effects related to labetalol. In some studies (BOLLI et al. 1976; JENNINGS and PARSONS 1976) eye toxicity has been specifically stated to be absent after appropriate investigation.

MICHELSON et al. (1983) reported asymptomatic transaminase elevations in 14 of 337 patients. The increases were greater than twice normal, and they were accompanied by an increase in gamma glutamyl transpeptidase, whereas bilirubin was not affected. Labetalol therapy was discontinued in a total of five patients because of transaminase elevations. Levels were increased 10 to 15 times normal in three of these patients. Of the patients in whom therapy was discontinued, three were rechallenged; in each case, mild to moderate transaminase elevations recurred weeks thereafter, which again resolved when labetalol therapy was discontinued. Another patient from the New Zealand survey showed SLE symptoms and indications of abnormal liver function.

Other changes in laboratory parameters have not been found. In particular, labetalol does not appear to alter triglycerides, total cholesterol or high-density lipoproteins (HDL) (McGonigle et al. 1981; de Sommers et al. 1981; Frishman et al. 1983; Novo et al. 1984). Only Weber et al. (1984) observed a slight increase in the serum concentration of HDL.

During treatment with labetalol, a small increase in fasting blood glucose levels has been found, but no alterations in insulin activity or response to an oral glucose tolerance test (Andersson et al. 1976; Pagnan et al. 1979; Barbieri et al. 1981).

In patients with essential hypertension, prolonged therapy with labetalol caused a slight reduction in the previously elevated plasma concentration of the prostacyclin metabolite 6-keto-$PGF_{1\alpha}$, but no effect on plasma thromboxane concentration (Roy et al. 1983).

3.2 Celiprolol

3.2.1 Chemistry

Celiprolol (for structure, see Table 2) is a diethylurea-substituted β-adrenergic receptor blocking agent with the conventional tert. butyl side chain. The distribution coefficient of 0.152 (*n*-octanol/buffer at pH 7.4) characterises the substances as highly hydrophilic (Hippmann and Takacz 1983) and fits with the low protein binding rate of about 20% (Pruss et al. 1986). The assay for the determination of celiprolol in plasma or urine is based on HPLC. The limit of detection is 10 ng/ml (Buskin et al. 1982; Hippmann and Takacs 1983).

3.2.2 Pharmacology

3.2.2.1 Pharmacodynamics and Mode of Action

Using a variety of receptor preparations of mammalian tissues and different radiolabelled ligands, it has been demonstrated that celiprolol binds with a higher affinity to the β_1- than to the β_2-adrenoceptors. The K_i values for binding to the mebranes of rat hearts (β_1) and guinea pig lungs (β_2) are 0.33 μM and 1.9 μM, respectively. The binding potency of celiprolol to the β_1-receptors is about two orders of magnitude less than that of propranolol but similar to that of metoprolol (van Inwegen et al. 1984). In contrast to other β-blockers, celiprolol binds more to the α_2-receptors (K_i = 48 μM) than to the α_1-receptor (K_i = 500 μM). However, to what extent the binding to the α_2-receptor contributes to pharmacological effects such as bronchodilatation or vasorelaxation still needs to be investigated.

The β-blocking potency of celiprolol has been demonstrated in vitro and in vivo by its antagonism of isoprenaline actions. The pA_2 values are given in

Table 3; they indicate preferential β_1-adrenoceptor blockade (PITTNER 1983a; R.D. SMITH and WOLF 1984). The cardioselective properties of celiprolol have been confirmed in investigations in dogs, rats and humans. The doses required to prevent isoprenaline-induced decreases in diastolic blood pressure were much higher than those required to prevent the tachycardiac or inotropic effects of isoprenaline. This pattern resembles that of metoprolol and acebutolol, whereas propranolol had no preferential effect (PITTNER 1983a, b; BERGMANN et al. 1983). The β-blocking activity of celiprolol has been demonstrated in healthy subjects by its inhibitory effect on the tachycardia induced by exercise or isoprenaline (BERGMANN et al. 1983; PITTNER and BONELLI 1983).

The intrinsic sympathomimetic activity (ISA) of celiprolol has been demonstrated in a considerable number of investigations (for review, see PITTNER 1985). Celiprolol increases the heart rate and contractile force of cat atria. This effect can be shifted by preincubation with propranolol. The heart rate of reserpinised rats and reserpinised, vagotomised and adrenolectomised cats increases dose-dependently to the same extent as that induced by pindolol (PITTNER 1985). The observation that celiprolol reduces myocardial contractility to a lesser extent than propranolol, atenolol, metoprolol or acebutolol at equipotent β-blocking doses may also be attributed to its sympathomimetic activity (PITTNER 1983b). Finally, a study in hypertensive patients with 24-h monitoring of blood pressure and heart rate revealed that the heart rate decreases during the daytime but increases at night (PARATI et al. 1988).

The vasorelaxing and bronchodilating activities of celiprolol can also be explained (at least partly) by its ISA. Human arteries and veins precontracted with serotonin or potassium have been shown to relax after incubation with pindolol or celiprolol. This effect could be attenuated by preincubation with propranolol (THULESIUS et al. 1982). Celiprolol relaxes dose-dependently tracheal chains derived from guinea pigs or cattle; the concentration-response curves were shifted to the right by pretreatment with propranolol (PITTNER 1985). Finally, the decreased density of β-adrenoceptors of lymphocytes from patients treated with celiprolol indicates a considerable ISA at the β_2-receptor site (BRODDE et al. 1985, 1986; DAUL et al. 1986).

There is some evidence that celiprolol induces cardiostimulant and bronchodilating effects independently of its ISA. The mechanism responsible for these effects has not yet been identified (PRUSS et al. 1986). The increase in heart rate and myocardial contractility observed in ganglionic-blocked dogs can be attenuated but not abolished by propranolol (SHLEVIN et al. 1983; R.D. SMITH and WOLF 1984). In conscious dogs pretreated with propranolol and with a constant heart rate (triggered by electrical pacing) celiprolol 3 mg/kg i.v. increased preload independently of the left ventricular contractility by 16% (NGANELE et al. 1988).

In cats, celiprolol induced dose-dependently a decrease of the airway resistance elevated by pretreatment with serotonin. This bronchodilatory effect of celiprolol is obviously not related to its ISA since both enantiomers are equieffective and, moreover, pretreatment of the animals with propranolol did not inhibit the response (GORDON et al. 1983; PRUSS et al. 1986).

3.2.2.2 Haemodynamics

Haemodynamic investigations in anaesthetised dogs show a dose-related reduction of the heart rate and a slight decrease in blood pressure, cardiac output and myocardial contractility. TPR is increased less than that after propranolol or atenolol (PITTNER 1983b). This lack of decrease in TPR may distinguish celiprolol from other vasodilating β-blockers.

In healthy subjects, a single intravenous dose of 15 mg celiprolol increased the heart rate and systolic blood pressure slightly (BONELLI et al. 1978). In other clinicopharmacological studies, however, no changes in these parameters have been observed (PITTNER 1985). MANCIA et al. (1986) noted in hypertensive patients an increased forearm blood flow after celiprolol despite a decrease in systemic blood pressure. Likewise, renal plasma flow and glomerular filtration rate did not change, whereas the renal vascular resistance was significantly reduced (LUCARINI and SALVETTI 1988). In a double-blind, crossover trial with hypertensive patients, celiprolol decreased blood pressure via a decrease in TPR after 6 weeks' treatment, whereas metoprolol decreased blood pressure by a reduction of cardiac output as the result of a decreased heart rate (TRIMARCO et al. 1988).

3.2.2.3 Toxicology

The results of toxicological investigations have been reviewed by WENDTLANDT and PITTNER (1983).

3.2.2.4 Pharmacokinetics and Metabolism

Peak plasma concentrations are reached about 2–3 h after oral administration of celiprolol. The AUCs increase non-linearly with dosage as shown by investigations with doses between 100 and 600 mg (CARUSO et al. 1985; NORRIS et al. 1986). The bioavailability after 100 mg is about 30%, after 400 mg, about 74% (HITZENBERGER et al. 1983; CARUSO et al. 1985). Celiprolol, thus, manifests non-linear absorption characteristics. Studies up to now have not elucidated the reasons for this non-linearity. Moreover, wide inter-individual variations in maximum plasma concentrations and in the AUCs have been observed (GLUTH et al. 1983).

The bioavailability of celiprolol can be reduced by concomitant intake of food (CARUSO et al. 1985). The administration of the drug 1 h before or 2 h after food is therefore recommended. There is some evidence that the bioavailability of celiprolol is reduced by concomitant administration of chlorthalidone (RIDDELL et al. 1987).

Celiprolol is eliminated via bile and urine, mainly as unchanged compound. It is metabolised only to a limited extent. A small amount of mono- and didealkylated products have been found in rats and dogs but not in humans (HITZENBERGER et al. 1983).

The elimination half-life after oral administration of celiprolol is about 4–5 h irrespective of the dose (CARUSO et al. 1985), but GLUTH et al. (1983) reported an elimination half-life of 8.5–13.5 h.

In patients with varying degrees of renal impairment, renal excretion of a 200 mg dose of celiprolol is reduced to 2.6% compared with 18% in healthy subjects (SCHMIDT et al. 1985). The dose of celiprolol should therefore be decreased if renal function is markedly impaired.

No marked differences between young and elderly subjects have been found with respect to the pharmacokinetics (NORRIS et al. 1986).

3.2.3 Therapeutic Use

The antihypertensive effect of celiprolol has been demonstrated in a considerable number of well-designed clinical investigations. The efficacy of celiprolol has been compared with that of placebo or other β-adrenoceptor blockers, in particular with that of propranolol or atenolol (for reviews, see R.D. SMITH and WOLF 1984; RIDDELL et al. 1987). Obviously, there were no differences in the antihypertensive potency of the different drugs, but celiprolol reduced the heart rate to a lesser extent than the other β-adrenoceptor blockers. Celiprolol has been used in daily doses of between 100 and 600 mg, mostly on a once a day dosing schedule. The antihypertensive action of 400 mg celiprolol once daily has been investigated in a study with 24-h blood pressure monitoring. The reduction in blood pressure has been claimed to be evident even throughout the night and to be maintained 24 h after administration (PARATI et al. 1988). However, analysis of the data presented shows that statistically significant differences between the blood pressures following placebo and active treatment do not exist between 11 p.m. and 8 a.m.

Significant decreases in blood pressure without any adverse effects on carbohydrate metabolism have been reported in 40 diabetic patients with essential hypertension (JANKA et al. 1983). In another study with celiprolol in diabetic patients, there was no difference found in insulin requirements between patients treated with placebo or 300 mg celiprolol. In patients treated with sulphonylureas, both 120 mg propranolol and 300 mg celiprolol daily reduced blood glucose concentrations slightly but significantly in the middle of the afternoon (KRITZ et al. 1983).

Herrmann et al. (1988a; HERRMANN and MAYER 1988) investigated the influence of 12 months' treatment with celiprolol on the lipid profile of hypertensive patients. They found a reduction of the pathologically elevated pretreatment lipid values to levels within the normal range. Additionally, an increase in the HDL fraction and a decrease in the LDL fraction resulted in an improved lipid profile. A 2-year study with celiprolol, mepindolol, propranolol and bisoprolol showed that only celiprolol reduced the triglycerides in the blood and improved the LDL/HDL ratio significantly (FOGARI 1988). Decreases in the concentration of total cholesterol (from 282 to 262 mg/100 ml) and triglycerides (from 238 to 216 mg/100 ml) in the blood of patients with elevated lipids were also observed in a multicentre survey (HERRMANN et al. 1988b). An increase in the HDL-fraction in patients with Fredrickson type II or IV hyperlipidaemia has also been observed by PRISTAUTZ and STRADNER (1986).

The most striking property of celiprolol seems to be its bronchosparing

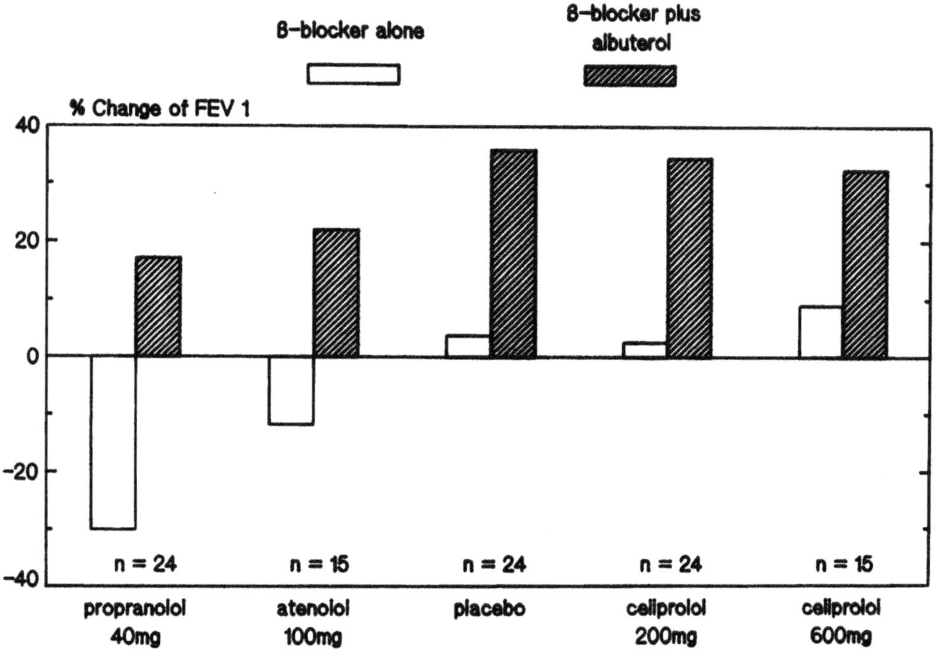

Fig. 3. Effect of propranolol, atenolol and celiprolol with and without additional albuterol on forced expiratory volume (FEV_1) of asthmatic patients. (Adapted from DOSHAN et al. 1986a,b)

activity, which has been demonstrated in a considerable number of comparative studies on asthmatics with or without hypertension (for review, see RIDDELL et al. 1987; DOROW 1988). At dosages usually used to treat hypertension, celiprolol did not inhibit the bronchodilatation induced by different bronchodilating compounds, including β_2-sympathomimetics (Fig. 3). In normotensive asthmatics suffering from bronchoconstriction after a single dose of 80 mg propranolol, 200 or 400 mg celiprolol did not cause any deterioration of pulmonary function (MATTHYS et al. 1985). In hypertensive patients with reversible bronchoconstriction, there was no difference in the incidence of respiratory symptoms or requirement for bronchodilator therapy during 12 weeks of treatment with celiprolol or chlorthalidone. Neither drug had any clinically significant effect on spirometric values (DOROW et al. 1986). Controlled comparative studies with celiprolol (200–600 mg), propranolol (40 mg), atenolol (100 mg) and metoprolol (200 mg) showed that celiprolol does not reduce FEV_1 and vital capacity and does not enhance airway resistance, whereas the other β-blockers do. Interestingly, only celiprolol did not affect the bronchodilatory effect of albuterol or isoprenaline (SCHINDL et al. 1986; DOSHAN et al. 1986a, b; BRUSCHI et al. 1988). However, it should be mentioned that celiprolol significantly increased airway resistance in some asthmatic patients (KAIK 1980). Celiprolol, too, should therefore be given with care to asthmatic patients, even if it appears to cause minimal interference with pulmonary function in most predisposed patients.

In an open study of 17 hypertensive patients with peripheral obliterative disease, no worsening of the symptoms was reported after 6 weeks' treatment with 200 mg celiprolol daily, but there was a slight increase in the pain-free walking distance (DIEHM 1988). It might be speculated whether these unexpected results can be explained by a small but significant reduction of the serum fibrinogen concentration (from 288 to 253 mg/dl) observed in another study (HERRMANN and MEYER 1988). This effect can result in an improved blood viscosity.

The side effects reported for celiprolol resemble those of other β-adrenoceptor blockers. Specific adverse reactions for celiprolol have not been reported.

A post-marketing surveillance study including 2311 patients treated for longer than 3 weeks with celiprolol showed that no unknown side effects for β-blockers were reported. Even the typical unwanted effects of β-blockade such as bradycardia, heart failure, fatigue, cold extremities and central nervous system disturbances have been reported to be relatively infrequent. Only 58 patients (2.15%) discontinued the treatment because of adverse effects, including gastrointestinal disturbances (13), insomina (8), rash (8), vertigo (6), fatigue (6), headache (4), Raynaud's syndrome (4) and impotence (3). Of the 122 patients with chronic obstructive airways disease included in the survey, treatment had to be discontinued in only 3, and only 1 of 148 patients with peripheral arterial disease who entered the study experienced worsening of their symptoms. In addition to these patients a further 282 subjects (12%) reported mild and transient side effects that did not lead to discontinuation. Again, the most common adverse reactions, also known for conventional β-blockers, were gastrointestinal symptoms, insomnia and fatigue. They occurred mostly in the first 2 weeks of treatment (HOFFMANN and HOFFMANN 1985, 1986). In a further survey of 15 256 patients treated for 6 weeks with celiprolol a similar profile of adverse reactions has been found (HERRMANN et al. 1988b). Remarkably, the incidence of some of the complaints existing before treatment were reduced during therapy with celiprolol.

Some 1169 hypertensive patients treated with celiprolol were included in comparative studies with a double-blind protocol. The incidence for discontinuation due to side effects was 2% in patients treated with placebo or celiprolol, and 4% in those treated with propranolol. However, 21% of the patients treated with celiprolol and 19% treated with placebo reported side effects, but only 13% of the propranolol-treated patients (CAPONE and GARUTTI 1986). The complaints resembled those of Hoffmann's survey. No clinically meaningful or consistent trends in any of the haematological, biochemical or urinalysis parameters were noted for the celiprolol-treated patients (CAPONE and GARUTTI 1986).

3.3 Bevantolol

3.3.1 Chemistry

Bevantolol (for chemical structure, see Table 2) is a compound with a dimethyloxy-phenethylamino moiety. It is a weak base with a pKa of 8.1 and octanol/

buffer distribution coefficient of 13 at pH 7.0 (KAPLAN 1986). The protein binding is 95% (FRISHMAN et al. 1988). Bevantolol can be determined in body fluids by a gas-chromatographic method using electron capture detection. The detection limit is about 10–20 ng/ml (McNEIL et al. 1986). NATTEL et al. (1987) used HPLC with a fluorescence detection for assaying bevantolol in plasma or urine. The limit of detection was 50 ng/ml.

3.3.2 Pharmacololgy

Radioligand studies reveal that bevantolol interacts with the different types of adrenergic receptors. Using [^{3}H]-dihydroalprenolol and [^{3}H]-WB 4101 as ligands, IC_{50} values can be estimated as 0.06 μM for the β_1-receptors and 2 μM for the α_1-receptors. The importance of the binding to the α_1-receptors remains unclear since the affinity of bevantolol resembles that of norepinephrine or phenylephrine, but it is 100 or 1000 times lower than that of prazosin or labetalol (KAPLAN 1986).

3.3.2.1 Pharmacodynamics and Mode of Action

The β-adrenoceptor blocking activity of bevantolol has been demonstrated by parallel shifts of the dose-response curves of isoprenaline to the right in in vitro and in vivo experiments and by inhibition of isoprenaline-induced responses in various species. The potency of β-blockade was calculated as the apparent dissociation constant of the antagonist receptor complex (K_b) derived from experiments in isolated guinea pig atria and trachea. The K_b values of bevantolol were for the atria 0.9×10^{-8} M and for the trachea 3.0×10^{-7} M. This corresponds to pA_2 values of 8.04 and 6.52 (HASTINGS et al. 1977). Thus, bevantolol was about 32 times more potent in blocking β_1- than β_2-receptors. In the same experiments, propranolol was almost as active as bevantolol on the atrial preparation but did not show cardioselectivity (ratio 0.65). TAKAYANAGI et al. (1987) investigated the adrenoceptor antagonistic activity of bevantolol in vitro. The pA_2 values calculated from these experiments are 7.75 for the β_1-, 6.69 for β_2- and 4.77 for the α_1-receptors. The data indicate a lower cardioselectivity than for atenolol in the same study, as well as a very low α_1-adrenoceptor antagonistic activity.

In vivo tests to determine β-adrenoceptor blocking potency were performed in several species and by various routes of administration. With the exception of rat experiments with oral administration, bevantolol was ⅓ to ⅛ as potent as propranolol in mice, rats, dogs or pigs.

β-Blocking activity has also been confirmed in humans. Single doses of 0.2–0.9 mg/kg i.v. or 50–100 mg orally have been shown in healthy volunteers to inhibit the exercise-induced increases in heart rate or systolic blood pressure (LAMMERS et al. 1985; TRIEB and SIGWART 1978; FRISHMAN et al. 1988).

Whereas in anaesthetised dogs isoprenaline-induced tachycardia was only slightly more antagonised than hypotension (HASTINGS et al. 1977), in conscious dogs bevantolol was consistently more effective in blocking the cardiostimulatory effects of isoprenaline than the vasodepressor responses (KAPLAN et al.

1985). Bevantolol's cardioselectivity was confirmed in an animal bronchospasm model. The compound interfered only slightly with the protective action of isoprenaline against histamine-induced lethal bronchospasm in intact guinea pigs, whereas propranolol completely blocked the protective action of isoprenaline (KAPLAN et al. 1985).

Bevantolol does not exert intrinsic sympathomimetic activity. This can be deduced from the bradycardiac action observed in isolated rabbit atria or pithed rats and by the lack of tachycardia in catecholamine-depleted animals (HASTINGS et al. 1977; DUKES and VAUGHAN-WILLIAMS 1985).

On the basis of the results obtained in the mouse-tail pinch test, bevantolol can be assessed as having only a weak local anaesthetic activity (HASTINGS et al. 1977).

Bevantolol exerts a weak α_1-blocking activity. In antagonising the constrictor response to phenylephrine, the compounds has been reported to be four times less potent than labetalol (VAUGHAN-WILLIAMS 1987). On the other hand, the results from other investigations suggest that bevantolol may have partial α-adrenoceptor agonist activity, since in pithed rats it caused a dose-dependent increase in blood pressure which was inhibited by phentolamine (DUKES and VAUGHAN-WILLIAMS 1985). However, these results could not be reproduced by other laboratories (KAPLAN 1986). Further investigations were performed in four healthy volunteers in order to study the interactions of bevantolol with the α-adrenoceptors. The compound did not exert any effect on the pressor response to phenylephrine infusion, but increases in plasma growth hormone concentrations may indicate central α_2-adrenoceptor stimulation (FRISHMAN et al. 1988). Thus, the significance of the interaction of bevantolol with α-adrenoceptors remains unclear up to now and requires additional investigations, in particular with respect to its haemodynamic profile and clinical usefulness.

3.3.2.2 Haemodynamics

Doses of bevantolol up to 10 mg/kg i.v. induce, like propranolol, a slight decrease in the arterial blood pressure of anaesthetised dogs (HASTINGS et al. 1977). Extensive haemodynamic investigations have been performed in anaesthetised pigs at doses between 0.5 and 1.5 mg/kg i.v. Bevantolol decreased dose-dependently the heart rate, mean arterial pressure, cardiac output, stroke volume and left ventricular myocardial contractility, whereas the TPR rose (VERDOUW et al. 1986). Thus, this haemodynamic profile resembles more that of a pure β-blocking agent than that of a compound with additional vasodilating properties (Fig. 4).

Single oral or intraperitoneal doses of 50–100 mg/kg bevantolol have been shown to reduce the heart rate less and to decrease the arterial blood pressure of hypertensive rats more than the same doses of propranolol (KAPLAN et al. 1985; KAPLAN 1986). Since the β-blocking properties were not characterised in the same experimental model, it remains to be established whether the observed differences can be attributed to cardioselectivity or some other activity for bevantolol.

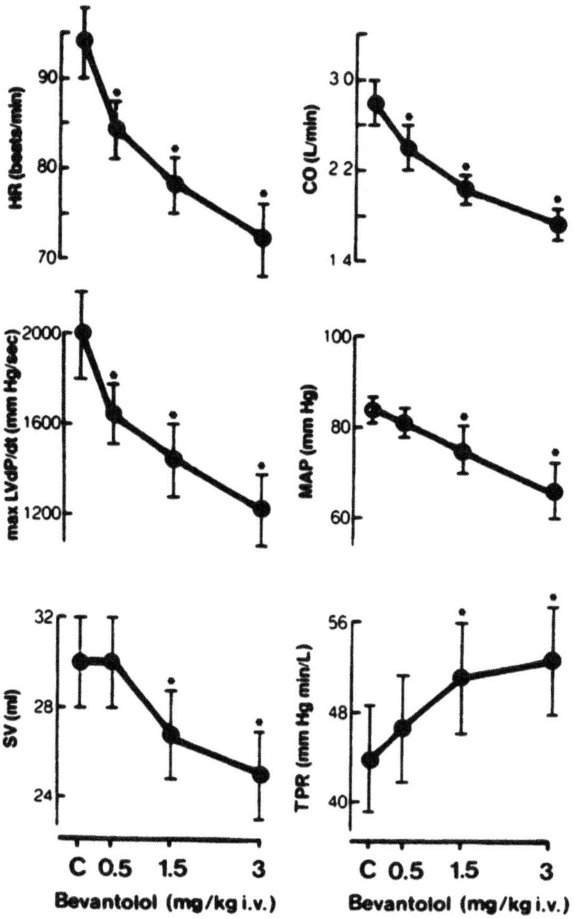

Fig. 4. Effects of increasing doses of bevantolol (total dose: 3 mg/kg i.v.) on the haemodynamics in anaesthetised pigs. *HR*, heart rate; *CO*, cardiac output; *max LVdP/dt*, maximum rate of left ventricular pressure; *MAP*, mean arterial blood pressure; *SV*, stroke volume; *TPR*, total peripheral resistance. (Adapted from VERDOUW et al. 1986)

An investigation of patients with hypertension showed that bevantolol increases the resting TPR, but this was affected to the same extent after bevantolol or placebo during exercise (TRIEB and SIGWART 1978).

Results of a controlled crossover study in healthy subjects reveal that 7 days' treatment with bevantolol 200 mg/day slightly increases the muscle blood flow and skin blood flow, whereas 100 mg atenolol reduces them (COOKE et al. 1987). However, in hypertensive patients treated for 8 weeks with the same dose, no differences between bevantolol and atenolol were observed with respect to resting supine blood pressure, heart rate, forearm blood flow and resistance or plasma concentrations of renin, aldosterone or catecholamines (SNEDDEN and FERNANDEZ 1988).

It has been demonstrated in studies in animal models of experimental myocardial ischaemia that bevantolol reduces the extent of experimentally induced myocardial infarction, improves the regional contractile function of the ischaemic zones and redistributes the flow to the ischaemic subendocardium (GROSS et al. 1979; WARLTIER et al. 1980). While the clinical implications of these observations remain to be established, it appears that bevantolol, in addition to reducing oxygen demands, may also reduce myocardial ischaemia by improving transmural blood flow redistribution.

3.3.2.3 Toxicology

The results of toxicological investigations have been reviewed by KAPLAN et al. (1985).

3.3.2.4 Pharmacokinetics and Metabolism

Following oral administration to laboratory animals or human subjects, bevantolol is rapidly and almost completely absorbed from the gastrointestinal tract. Peak plasma concentrations are reached within 2 h after dosing (KAPLAN et al. 1985). There is some evidence that the rate of absorption of bevantolol is slowed by food, but the total amount of the drug absorbed seems to be unaffected (TOOTHAKER et al. 1987; MCNEIL et al. 1986). Since bevantolol undergoes presystemic metabolic elimination after oral administration, the averaged absolute bioavailability has been calculated to be between 57% (MCNEIL et al. 1986) and 80% (VERMEJ and VAN BRUMMELEN 1986). MCNEIL et al. (1986) found a wide variation of the bioavailability (range 26%–98%) coupled with a threefold range of the peak plasma concentrations.

Tissue distribution after administration to laboratory animals was highest in the liver and kidney, with decreasing concentrations in lung, plasma, heart, spleen, body fat, red blood cells, muscle and brain. The concentrations declined in parallel with those in plasma, indicating the absence of significant retention in any tissue (VAUGHAN-WILLIAMS 1987). This fits with the relatively low volume of distribution of 1 to 1.5 l/kg (LATTS 1986; MCNEIL et al. 1986; VERMEJ and VAN BRUMMELEN 1986).

Bevantolol is rapidly eliminated by hepatic metabolism prior to its excretion in the urine in the form of conjungated metabolities. Results from a study with radiolabelled material show that in human volunteers approximately 75% of the administered radioactivity is excreted in the urine and 15% is recovered in the faeces in a 5-day period (LATTS 1986). Only 1% of unchanged bevantolol is excreted in the urine (MCNEIL et al. 1986). The elimination half-life of bevantolol in the plasma has been calculated to be about 1.5 h (LATTS 1986; MCNEIL et al. 1986; VERMEJ and VAN BRUMMELEN 1986).

Further pharmacokinetic studies show that after doses of 100–400 mg bevantolol peak plasma concentrations and AUC are proportional to the dose administered (LATTS 1986) and that accumulation does not occur after repeated administration (KAPLAN et al. 1985; VERMEJ and VAN BRUMMELEN 1986). However, in some subjects accumulation to a small extent has been found with repeated doses of bevantolol 200 mg daily. This is probably due to the contribution of a late and more persistent terminal elimination phase that was discernible in only certain individuals (Selen et al. 1986).

Pharmacokinetic investigations have been performed in patients with impaired renal function. Half of the subjects with a creatinine clearance of less than 50 ml/min had a longer elimination half-life, higher peak plasma levels and trough concentrations than those observed in healthy volunteers. Therefore, the monitoring of bevantolol concentrations is recommended in patients with moderate or severe renal impairment (Solimon et al. 1986; Randinitis et al. 1987).

A single oral dose of 200 mg bevantolol has been shown to induce the same peak plasma concentrations in patients with hepatic cirrhosis as in controls, but the absorption is slowed, and the elimination half-life is prolonged to 6.3 h. This is reflected by the longer bradycardiac effect in the patients with cirrhosis. Therefore, bevantolol should be used with care in patients with severe liver diseases, and a reduction of the dose is recommended (Nattel et al. 1987).

A comparative pharmacokinetic study showed that only small differences in the pharmacokinetics of bevantolol occur in young and elderly subjects during single or repeated dosing of 200 mg bevantolol daily (Selen et al. 1986). Slightly higher maximum concentrations and AUCs in elderly subjects do not have any clinical relevance.

Bevantolol is extensively metabolised after oral administration. Several products have been identified in human urine. The main metabolite is formed by oxidation of the methyl group on the phenoxy moiety of the molecule. Other metabolites are formed by hydroxylation or hydroxymethylation of the phenolic components. The metabolites are excreted as conjugates in the urine (Latts 1986). No attempt has been made to identify metabolites in the plasma or in the bile. One of the metabolites has β-adrenergic receptor blocking activity in dogs, but because of the small quantity formed in humans, it is not thought to contribute to the pharmacological effect in patients (Latts 1986).

McNeil et al. (1986) found a good correlation ($r = 0.79$, $n = 133$) between the logarithm of the bevantolol plasma concentration and the percentage inhibition of exercise-induced tachycardia. Similarly, the time course of the effect on exercise heart rate was similar to the profile of the plasms concentrations.

3.3.3 Therapeutic Use

The blood pressure lowering activity of bevantolol has been demonstrated in clinical investigations. Some of them have not been published but cited in reviews (see Vaughan-Williams 1987; Frishman et al. 1988).

Okawa (1986) concluded from the results of a multicentre, placebo-controlled, double-blind, dose-titration study that doses of 200–400 mg/day in equally divided doses control the blood pressure of patients with mild to moderate hypertension. However, marked differences have not been found between the different doses. Jain (1986) compared the results of two further, placebo-controlled, double-blind, multicentre trials on patients with mild to moderate hypertension. The two studies were identical in design and differed only in once daily or twice daily dose administration. The averaged decreases in home diastolic blood pressure at trough and the values determined in the clinic were more favourable in the bevantolol-treated patients (7–10 mmHg) than in the placebo-treated subjects (2–4 mmHg). There were no differences between the two dosing schedules. Similarly, AL-KHAWAJA et al. (1986) investigated the antihypertensive effect of bevantolol once or twice daily by means of 24-h blood pressure recording in ambulant patients. The total daily dose (200–600 mg) was administered at 8 p.m. and/or 8. a.m. for 6 weeks. Both systolic and diastolic blood pressures were significantly reduced over 24 h to the same extent by both dosing schedules. Remarkably, the early morning rise in blood pressure was blunted.

Bevantolol has been compared with both propranolol and atenolol in multicentre, double-blind studies. Whereas no significant differences have been found between bevantolol and propranolol with respect to a decrease in blood pressure and heart rate, bevantolol caused fewer adverse effects than propranolol (MACLEAN 1988). In another study, atenolol tended to be more effective than bevantolol in controlling blood pressure at the beginning of therapy (FAIRHURST 1986; FRISHMAN et al. 1988).

Hypertensive patients previously unsatisfactorily controlled with thiazides have been reported to respond with a decrease in blood pressure and heart rate after additional administration of bevantolol or propranolol. The effects were almost identical in Caucasian and in black patients (LUCAS et al. 1985; SNEDDEN et al. 1987).

Special populations of hypertensive patients have been treated with bevantolol. In a double-blind study on hypertensive, non-insulin-dependent diabetics, bevantolol 200–400 mg/day and propranolol 80–160 mg/day induced similar decreases in blood pressure and heart rate, but the compounds did not influence the fasting blood glucose or glucose tolerance (CHIODINI et al. 1985). In patients with impaired renal function, bevantolol did not significantly affect the clearances of inulin or PAH (SOLIMON et al. 1986).

LÖFDAHL et al. (1984) observed in a double-blind, crossover study the effects of low doses of bevantolol (75 or 100 mg) and propranolol (40 mg) on asthmatic patients. Both compounds reduced basal FEV_1. Whereas bevantolol shifted the dose-response curve of terbutaline to the right, propranolol almost completely blocked the effect of terbutaline. The effects of 400 mg bevantolol and 100 mg atenolol on ventilatory effects in asthmatic patients have been investigated in a further, double-blind, placebo-controlled study. At rest, neither placebo nor atenolol affected FEV_1 or peak expiraratory flow rate (PEFR), but bevantolol caused a significant decrease of both variables. During therapy with 400 mg bevantolol, the dose-response curves with terbutaline for FEV_1 and PEFR shifted downwards in comparison with placebo or atenolol, indicating less β_1-adrenoceptor selectivity for bevantolol than for atenolol at the dosages used (LAMMERS et al. 1985). The same tendency has been found in another study with a similar design using fenoterol as bronchodilating agent (PHILIP-JOET et al. 1986). The effects of cumulative doses of bevantolol (from 18.75 to 150 mg) or metoprolol (from 12.5 to 100 mg) were compared in a double-blind, randomised, crossover study with 15 asthmatic patients. Dosing was stopped if the symptoms warranted it or if there was a fall of more than 20% in FEV_1. Seven patients were withdrawn prematurely. In these patients, the averaged maximum tolerated cumulative doses were 45.5 mg bevantolol and 26.8 mg metoprolol; these doses are lower than those usually required for therapeutic activity. Therefore, the authors state that the respiratory response to both drugs could not be predicted, and asthmatic patients should be treated with care even with cardioselective β-adrenoceptor blockers (WILCOX et al. 1986).

The influence of bevantolol on the lipid profile does not show any uniform pattern. The plasma concentrations of total cholesterol and triglycerides have been reported to be unchanged in hypertensive patients, whereas a significant reduction (8%) of the HDL-cholesterol has been found (KOSKINEN and PELLINEN 1987). On the other hand, in a study of patients with coronary heart disease treated with bevantolol, SALONEN et al. (1986) observed a tendency for an increase in triglyceride concentration but an increase in HDL and decrease in LDLs, resulting in an improved HDL/LDL ratio. This beneficial effect was not found with atenolol in the same study.

The side effects reported for bevantolol resemble those of other β-adrenoceptor blockers. Specific adverse reactions for bevantolol have not been reported. BRAY (1986) reviewed the side effects experienced during eight, multicentre, double-blind, placebo-controlled trials with bevantolol. Some 579 patients being treated for hypertension or coronary heart disease were included in these studies. During short-term treatment, headache, fatigue, nausea, dizziness and gastrointestinal symptoms were the most reported adverse reactions. However, there were no marked differences between the placebo-treated or bevantolol-treated patients. Of the 378 patients continued on long-term bevantolol treatment, 18 patients (4.8%) were withdrawn due to side effects, mainly because of gastrointestinal disturbances, bronchospasm, depression, fatigue and dizziness. Bevantolol did not cause any clinically significant effects on laboratory variables or ophthalmological function (BRAY 1986). In a comparative study of bevantolol versus propranolol, the incidence of side effects and withdrawals with propranolol was less than with bevantolol, but the profiles were very similar in both groups (KOSKINEN and PELLINEN 1987; MACLEAN 1988).

3.4 Arotinolol

3.4.1 Chemistry

Arotinolol (for chemical structure, see Table 1) is a thiopropanolamine with a tert. butyl moiety. The physicochemical characteristics of the compound have not been published in English up to now. Arotinolol can be assayed by fluorodensitometry using TLC. The limit of detection is 5 ng/ml (NISHIDA et al. 1985). A method for the separate determination of the enantiomers of arotinolol and its metabolite by HPLC is described by DOI et al. (1985).

3.4.2 Pharmacology

3.4.2.1 Pharmacodynamics and Mode of Action

The binding of arotinolol to β_1-, β_2- and α_1-receptor sites has been investigated in radioligand studies. The compound has been shown to have about a three times higher affinity to the β_1-receptor sites than propranolol. K_i values are 1.52 ± 0.88 n*M* (NAGATOMO et al. 1984) or 2.7 ± 0.2 n*M* (HASHIMOTO et al. 1984) for the β_1-receptor sites and 4.3 ± 0.6 n*M* for the β_2-receptor sites. The K_i value calculated for the α_1-receptor sites (1050 ± 50 n*M*) indicates that the compound has a definitely lower affinity for the α_1- than for the β-receptor sites. This figure fits with the pharmacological data obtained from isolated organs in which the antagonistic potencies were investigated. The pA_2 values for the β-blockade derived from isolated right atrial and tracheal preparations of guinea pigs are between 9.31 and 8.48 for the β_1-blockade and between 9.09 and 8.40 for the β_2-blockade, indicating lack of cardioselectivity (HARA et al. 1979; NAGATOMO et al. 1984; MIYAGISHI et al. 1984). This pattern has been confirmed in anaesthetised, vagotomised cats and anaesthetised dogs, in which the doses have been determined that are required to inhibit isoprenaline-induced tachycardia and hypotension. Both doses were about ten times less than those of propranolol (MIYAGISHI et al. 1984; HARA et al. 1978). Further investigations showed that arotinolol does not possess intrinsic sympathomimetic activities or membrane-stabilising properties (HARA et al. 1978, 1979).

The vasorelaxing activity of arotinolol has been demonstrated in a variety of investigations on isolated organs such as rat aortic strips (MIYAGISHI et al. 1983, 1984) or dog coronary arteries (SAKANASHI et al. 1983, 1984b).

The pA_2 value for the α_1-blockade derived from experiments on rat aortic strips using phenylephrine as agonist is 6.91 (MIYAGISHI et al. 1984). The concentrations required for relaxing coronary arteries depolarised with potassium chloride or precontracted with norepinephrine, $PGF_{2\alpha}$ or PGE_2 are greater than 10^{-5} *M* (SAKANASHI et al. 1983, 1984b). Thus, arotinolol possesses only a weak vasorelaxing potency, and therefore the concentrations required for inducing this effect are much higher than those for causing β-adrenoceptor blockade. This has been confirmed by in vivo investigations in conscious rats and anaesthetised rabbits, cats and dogs. The doses required for decreasing the basal blood pressure and for inhibiting the phenylephrine-induced pressor response are about 100 times higher than those for antagonising the isoprenaline-induced effects (HARA et al. 1983; MIYAGISHI et al. 1983, 1984; HASHIMOTO et al. 1984; NAKAHARA et al. 1985b).

TAKEKOSHI et al. (1983) tried to determine the ratio of β- to α-blockade in healthy volunteers. Two hours after administration, a single oral dose of 15 mg arotinolol shifted the dose-response curve of isoprenaline for the increase in heart rate to the right by a factor of 15.6. The dose-response curve of noradrenaline for the increase in heart rate was shifted to the right by a factor of 1.96. Four hours after administration, no effect on the noradrenaline response was detectable.

There is some evidence that the acute antihypertensive activity of high doses of arotinolol are mainly mediated by its α_1-blocking property. In anaesthetised dogs arotinolol attenuates the pressor response to phenylephrine without any effect on the response to angiotensin II (HASHIMOTO et al. 1984). In anaesthetised rats, low doses of arotinolol reduce the renal sympathetic nerve impulses like propranolol, whereas high doses enhance the discharges like phentolamine (NAKAHARA et al. 1985b).

The α-blocking activity of arotinolol can also be deduced from the results of investigations in anaesthetised cats, in which contractions of the nictating membrane induced by electrical stimulation of the preganglionic and postganglionic superior cervical nerve are reduced and the responses to tyramine and noradrenaline are depressed (MIYAGISHI et al. 1984).

In order to clarify the mode of action, NAKAHARA et al. (1985a) compared the pressor responses to phenylephrine at equipotent antihypertensive doses of arotinolol and prazosin. The results of these investigations are, however, not conclusive, as the hypotensive effect of arotinolol may be the result of reduction of the cardiac output via β-blockade and additionally the inhibition of the counter-regulatory increase in total peripheral resistance mediated by α-blockade, whereas the hypotensive effect of prazosin is exclusively mediated by α-blockade.

It has been demonstrated that the arotinolol-induced vasorelaxation could be restored by adding Ca^{2+} to the bath solution. This observation indicates that a non-specific effect may contribute additionally to the α-adrenoceptor blockade to the vasorelaxing and antihypertensive activity of arotinolol (SAKANASHI et al. 1983).

3.4.2.2 Haemodynamics

Acute bradycardiac and antihypertensive activities of arotinolol have been demonstrated after oral administration in conscious hypertensive rats of different types. The reduction in heart rate is obviously more pronounced than that of the blood pressure. The doses required to cause the latter effect range between 20 and 100 mg/kg, whereas 5 mg/kg is sufficient to abolish the isoprenaline-induced effects (HARA et al. 1983; MIYANO et al. 1984; NAKAHARA et al. 1985b). This pattern is in contrast to other vasodilating β-blockers and may be explained by the fact that the two properties are evoked at different dose ranges.

The development of hypertension in SHRSP has been reported to be retarded slightly by daily oral intake of arotinolol 80 mg/kg, whereas the increase in heart rate was inhibited completely, histopathological lesions were prevented, the elevation of blood urea nitrogen was diminished, and the levels of catecholamines in heart and adrenal gland were reduced (MATSUO et al. 1984; SEKINE et al. 1984; IZUMI et al. 1985).

In other investigations, arotinolol was not able to retard the development of DOCA-salt hypertension in rats when administered at daily oral doses of 100 mg/kg, whereas propranolol and hydrochlorothiazide were effective (HARA et al. 1983).

KISHI et al. (1985) treated SHR for 12 weeks with arotinolol (20 or 100 mg/kg daily) or propranolol (100 mg/kg daily). The blood pressure determined by the tail cuff method did not show any decrease. However, at the end of treatment, the intra-arterially measured blood pressure was lowered in the arotinolol group to a greater degree than in the propranolol group. Both compounds reduced the heart rate and diminished significantly the incidence of vascular lesions in the kidneys and in the splanchnic region.

The antihypertensive activity of arotinolol could therefore be demonstrated only in some rat experiments, and substantial differences from classic β-blockers are scarcely evident.

Extensive haemodynamic investigations have been performed in anaesthetised dogs. Cardiac output and heart rate decreased at doses above 0.003 mg/kg, whereas the blood pressure decreased at doses higher than 0.3 mg/kg. Additionally, a dose-dependent decrease in cardiac contractility and coronary blood flow and increase in total peripheral resistance (TPR) have been observed (HASHIMOTO et al. 1984). In another investigation, arotinolol markedly decreased the heart rate and the arterial blood pressure of anaesthetised dogs in a dose-dependent manner. The TPR and the resistance in various vascular beds were not decreased but rather partly increased by arotinolol. The blood pressure response to arotinolol correlated with the plasma renin activity. The renal vasoconstrictor response to renal nerve stimulation was attenuated by arotinolol at low frequences like propranolol, the responses at high frequences or to local norepinephrine injection was diminished by arotinolol like prazosin (SUZUKI-KUSABA et al. 1988).

Haemodynamic investigations were also performed in healthy volunteers and in hypertensive patients after a single dose of 15 mg arotinolol. TAKEKOSHI et al. (1983) did not see changes in blood pressure, heart rate, right atrial pressure and pulmonary arterial end-diastolic pressure. However, the cardiac index tended to decrease, and the TPR tended to increase.

In other haemodynamic studies using echocadiography, arotinolol slightly reduced the resting systolic blood pressure, ejection fraction and cardiac output and increased the shortening fraction and TPR. The pre-ejection period showed a slight increase, and resting heart rate and left ventricular dimension were unchanged. During exercise, heart rate, blood pressure, double-product, shortening fraction and cardiac output were reduced, the left ventricular end-systolic dimension was enlarged, but the end-diastolic dimension was unaltered. The effect on the heart rate response lasted for more than 12 h. Thus, arotinolol has little effect on resting left ventricular performance and behaved, at least under exercise, like a long-acting, pure β-blocking agent (NAKASHIMA and OGUCHI 1982; NISHIDA et al. 1985).

TSUKIYAMA and OTSUKA (1984) showed in hypertensive patients that treatment with arotinolol decreased blood pressure by reduction of the cardiac index. It behaved like propranolol and differed from labetalol, which reduced the total peripheral resistance. Even after 6 months' treatment, the blood pressure decreasing effect is accompanied by a decrease in cardiac output, whereas TPR is increased. The inhibition of the pressure and heart rate responses to bicycle-ergometer exercise, but the lack of the inhibition of pressor responses to cold and isometric exercise, indicate that arotinolol acts as a pure β-blocking agent (KANDA 1985).

3.4.2.3 Pharmacokinetics and Metabolism

Detailed data regarding absorption, distribution, metabolism and elimination of arotinolol in animals or humans have not yet been published in English. NAKASHIMA and OGUCHI (1982) showed that arotinolol has an elimination half-life of 7.2 h.

3.4.3 Therapeutic Use

The only clinical study with arotinolol reported in English shows a blood pressure decreasing effect at daily doses of 10–30 mg. In patients with glucose intolerance, no changes of the lipid profile or of the plasma lipoprotein or apolipoprotein concentrations have been found (KAZUMI et al. 1988).

3.5 Amosulalol

3.5.1 Chemistry

Amosulalol is an ethanolamine (for structure, see Table 1). The octanol/water partition coefficient at pH 7.0 is 2.70 (TAKENAKA 1987). Amosulalol can be determined in body fluids by HPLC or gas chromatography. The latter method is more sensitive and has a limit of detection of 0.2 ng/ml (KAMIMURA et al. 1981, 1983).

3.5.2 Pharmacology

3.5.2.1 Pharmacodynamics and Mode of Action

The binding of amosulalol to the α_1-, α_2-, β_1- and β_2-receptor sites has been investigated in radioligand studies. The pK_i values are as follows: $\alpha_1 = 8.23$, $\alpha_2 = 5.14$, $\beta_1 = 7.64$, $\beta_2 = 7.26$ (TAKENAKA 1987). Similar values have been found by ASANO et al. (1983). Thus, the affinity of amosulalol for the α_1-adrenoceptors is about 1200 times higher than that for the α_2-adrenoceptors, but it has almost the same affinities for both β_1- and β_2-adrenoceptors. These values fit very well with the pharmacological data obtained from isolated organs in which the antagonistic potencies were investigated. The pA_2 values (see also Table 3) are as follows: $\alpha_1 = 7.97$, $\alpha_2 = 5.25$, $\beta_1 = 7.56$, $\beta_2 = 7.04$ (TAKENAKA et al. 1982a; HONDA et al. 1986).

In contrast to other drugs acting on multiple receptors, amosulalol has a higher selectivity for α_1-adrenoceptors than for β-adrenoceptors. Amosulalol is more potent as an α_1-adrenoceptor antagonist and less potent as a β-adrenoceptor antagonist than labetalol. Detailed investigations on rabbit pulmonary arteries and other tissues have shown that amosulalol exerts no relevant presynaptic α_2-adrenoceptor blockade (TAKENAKA et al. 1984; FUJOKA and SUZUKI 1985).

The adrenoceptor blocking activity of amosulalol has been confirmed in vivo by antagonism of the vasopressor response to phenylephrine and the positive chronotropic response to isoprenaline. In anaesthetised rats or dogs, amosulalol was about 10–20 times more potent as an α-adrenoceptor than labetalol, but only half as effective as labetalol as a β-adrenoceptor blocking agent (Takenaka et al. 1982a, b). The doses of amosulalol required to produce a tenfold shift of the dose-response curves of the agonists are almost identical after i.v. or oral administration (Takenaka et al. 1982a; Honda et al. 1985). Amosulalol has no effect on the pressor response to angiotensin II, indicating that the compound does not possess direct vasodilating activities (Takenaka et al. 1982b). Since neither the heart rate of reserpinised rats is increased nor the blood pressure response to amosulalol is prevented by propranolol, amosulalol can be considered to have no ISA at β-receptor sites. As amosulalol does not cause contraction of rabbit aortic strips or inhibit twitch responses to field stimulation of rat vas deferens, amosulalol also has no ISA at α-adrenoceptor sites (Takenaka et al. 1982b; Cohen and Hynes 1983; Honda et al. 1985; Takenaka 1987).

Pharmacological investigations in hypertensive patients show that the phenylephrine-induced and isoprenaline-induced responses were inhibited in humans. The blockade of the α-adrenoceptors in patients was also slightly more pronounced than that of the β-adrenoceptors (McNay et al. 1985).

Studies with the enantiomers of amosulalol indicate that the α_1-adrenoceptor blocking activity resides predominantly in the *S*(+)isomer, whereas the β-blocking activity is found predominantly in the*R*(−)isomer (Honda et al. 1986; Doggrell 1987).

3.5.2.2 Haemodynamics

A dose-dependent antihypertensive activity of amosulalol has been demonstrated in SHR after i.v. injection and single or repeated oral administration. The compound is about twice as potent as labetalol (Takenaka et al. 1982a; Honda et al. 1985). When the drug was administered to SHRSP, amosulalol was able to inhibit the development of hypertension and to reduce the incidence and severity of vascular lesions (Izumi et al. 1985).

Amosulalol decreased dose-dependently the arterial blood pressure of conscious normotensive and renal hypertensive dogs after single or repeated oral administration. Reflex tachycardia has not been observed. The antihypertensive effect correlated with the inhibition of the phenylephrine-induced response, indicating that the α_1-blockade is responsible for its blood pressure lowering activity (Takenaka 1987).

Haemodynamic investigations in anaesthetised dogs revealed that the decrease in blood pressure was accompanied by a reduction of heart rate, cardiac output, total peripheral resistance, myocardial contractility and pulmonary arterial pressure, whereas femoral and coronary blood flow were increased (Takenaka et al. 1982b).

Haemodynamic investigations in healthy volunteers showed that amosulalol at a dose of 0.16 mg/kg i.v. induced a decrease in the arterial blood pressure and heart rate, whereas the blood flow in fingers and limbs was increased. Data from echocardiographic investigations showed that the pre-ejection period, left ventricular ejection time, ejection fraction and cardiac output were not influenced (TAKENAKA 1987). Haemodynamic investigations with amosulalol during chronic oral treatment in hypertensive patients (10–40 mg twice daily) showed almost the same results. Thus, the blood pressure of the patients was reduced by a decrease in total peripheral resistance (NODA and FUJITA 1983; SAITO et al. 1985; OHTA et al. 1986; cited in TAKENAKA 1987).

3.5.2.3 Toxicology

The results of toxicological investigations have been reviewed by TAKENAKA (1987).

3.5.2.4 Pharmacokinetics and Metabolism

Peak plasma concentrations are reached about 2–4 h after oral administration of amosulalol to humans. There is a linear relation between the AUC and dose administered, indicating dose-linear kinetics. The systemic bioavailability calculated by the ratio of AUCs after i.v. and oral dosing is more than 93% in humans. This figure characterises amosulalol as a compound not subject to first-pass metabolism. The elimination half-life in humans is about 2.8 h after i.v. and about 5 h after oral administration. About 16%–26% of the parent compound is excreted in urine, and 13% is excreted as the sulphate conjugate of the para-hydroxylated compound (NAKASHIMA et al. 1984; KAMIMURA et al. 1985). Under steady-state conditions no indication of drug accumulation has been found (NAKASHIMA et al. 1985, cited in TAKENAKA 1987). A close correlation between the log plasma concentrations of unchanged amosulalol and adrenoceptor blocking activities has been described by TAKENAKA (1987).

3.5.3 Therapeutic Use

There are some reports in the literature of the use of amosulalol in the preoperative management of the hypertensive state in patients with phaeochromocytoma (MATSUURA et al. 1982; MANABE et al. 1984; OHASHI et al. 1986; OISHI et al. 1988). From these results it is deduced that amosulalol has a greater antihypertensive effect than labetalol in patients with phaeochromocytoma. This could be expected from its greater α_1-adrenoceptor antagonistic property.

Results from clinical studies of patients with primary hypertension have been published so far only by Japanese investigators, some of the trials having an open, multicentre design (TAKENAKA 1987). Generally, therapy was started at a dose of 5 or 10 mg twice daily; the dose was then increased at 3- to 5-day intervals to the final dose of 5–40 mg twice daily. Amosulalol caused significant decreases in systolic and diastolic blood pressure over a 24-h period without tachycardia or severe bradycardia. The normal shape of the circadian blood pressure profile was preserved (TAKENAKA 1987).

Amosulalol was compared with labetalol in a randomised, double-blind study in 374 outpatients. Both compounds significantly lowered blood pressure to the same extent, irrespective of whether the compounds were used as monotherapy or in combination with diuretics. There were no statistically significant differences in the incidence of adverse reactions; common side effects of both drugs were headache and dizziness. Skalp tingling, however, was not noted in the amosulalol-treated patients (IKEDA et al. 1986).

A survey of side effects in 750 hypertensive patients is given by TAKENAKA (1987). Dizziness (3.6%), headache (1.6%), fatigue or weakness (0.8%), anorexia (0.8%), nausea or vomiting (0.7%) and nasal congestion (0.7%) were those most often reported. Interestingly, despite the fact that amosulalol blocks vascular α_1-receptors, the incidence of dizziness was very low, and postural hypotension accompanied by fainting was not reported. No consistent changes in biochemical or haematological parameters have been observed (TAKENAKA 1987). The rate of discontinuation of treatment due to side effects has not been reported.

3.6 Dilevalol

3.6.1 Chemistry

Dilevalol is the *R,R*-isomer of labetalol. The chemical structure is given in Table 1. ALTON et al. (1988) described an assay for dilevalol in body fluids using HPLC. The limit of detection is about 4 ng/ml.

3.6.2 Pharmacology

3.6.2.1 Pharmacodynamics and Mode of Action

Receptor binding studies on human cardiovascular tissues indicate that dilevalol binds about 1000 times more to the β_1- than to the α_1-receptors. The binding constant (K_i) for the β-receptor is 6.5 n*M* and for the α_1-receptors, 6.5–15 μ*M* (BEVILACQUA et al. 1988).

In vitro investigations have shown that dilevalol is about four times more potent as a β_1-blocker and at least six times less potent as an α_1-blocker than labetalol (BRITTAIN et al. 1982; MONOPOLI et al. 1984; MATSUNAGA et al. 1986a); pA_2 values are given in Table 3. Investigations in anaesthetised dogs and rats as well as in healthy volunteers showed that the dose-response curves of isoprenaline and salbutamol are displaced by dilevalol. The data reveal that the compound is a potent blocker of β_1- and β_2-adrenoceptor but a weak α-blocking agent (SYBERTZ et al. 1981; GOLD et al. 1982; WHITEHEAD et al. 1988).

MATSUNAGA et al. (1986b) observed in their experiments on SHR that a single dose of dilevalol attenuated the responses to phenylephrine and isoprenaline, whereas in chronic experiments only the response to isoprenaline was inhibited. Therefore, it has been suggested that α-adrenoceptor antagonism contributes only to the acute but not to the chronic antihypertensive effect of dilevalol. The fact that labetalol and dilevalol differ markedly in their α- and β-blocking potency but induce nearly identical blood pressure lowering activities in SHR and conscious dogs even after acute administration (BAUM et al. 1981; GOLD et al. 1982; MONOPOLI et al. 1984; MATSUNAGA et al. 1986b) has raised the possibility that a mechanism other than α_1-blockade is responsible for the vasorelaxing and acute blood pressure lowering activity of dilevalol. This suggestion has been supported by the results obtained from investigations in anaesthetised dogs. Intra-arterial injection of dilevalol induced a dose-dependent increase in blood flow both in innervated and denervated femoral vascular beds, whereas the α-blockers prazosin and phentolamine are completely inactive in denervated beds (BAUM et al. 1981). Since the vasodilating and acute hypotensive effects as well as the effect of dilevalol on aortic compliance were inhibited by propranolol or by the specific β_2-adrenoceptor blocking agent ICI 118.551, it can be concluded that the β_2-receptor agonistic activity is mainly responsible for the vasodilation induced by dilevalol (BAUM et al. 1981; WATKINS et al. 1988a, b; MATSUNAGA et al. 1986b, 1988). The intrinsic β-sympathomimetic activity has been confirmed in investigations in guinea pig tracheal preparations, in which dilevalol inhibited histamine-induced bronchoconstriction. This effect was attenuated by preincubation with propranolol (MATSUNAGA et al. 1985).

Even though the intrinsic sympathomimetic activity of dilevalol is directed more to the β_2-receptors (BAUM and SYBERTZ 1983b; WATKINS et al. 1988a), a slight increase in the heart rate of pithed rats (LOUIS et al. 1988) and in the sleeping heart rate of normal volunteers indicates a weak agonistic activity also at the β_1-receptor site (RIDDELL et al. 1988).

Electrophysiological investigations in urethane-anaesthetised dogs show that dilevalol in β-adrenergic receptor blocking and antihypertensive doses does not suppress sinoatrial or atrioventricular nodal function. The electrophysiological spectrum of dilevalol thus differs from that of other pure β-adrenergic receptor antagonists (LYNCH et al. 1986).

3.6.2.2 Haemodynamics

Haemodynamic investigations in anaesthetised dogs show a dose-dependent decrease in blood pressure due to a decrease in total peripheral resistance (TPR) (BAUM et al. 1981).

Single or repeated oral doses of 400–800 mg dilevalol decrease the resting blood pressure in healthy subjects or hypertensive patients due to a decrease in TPR without reduction of heart rate, cardiac output (CO) or pulmonary capillary wedge pressure (PCWP). In contrast, during exercise the increases in blood pressure, heart rate and CO were reduced, while the increase in PCWP was pronounced, and TPR was slightly increased or unchanged (ATKINS 1986; BUGNI 1988; CLIFTON et al. 1988). Thus, the haemodynamics of dilevalol at rest are primarily related to its vasodilating effects, whereas during exercise the β-adrenoceptor blocking properties predominate. Similarly, in patients with mild hypertension and left ventricular dysfunction (ejection fraction below 0.45), dilevalol administered at a mean daily dose of 444 mg for 2 weeks decreased resting blood pressure and heart rate, whereas the ejection fraction increased from 0.32 to 0.37. Changes in systolic time intervals indicated an improved left ventricular performance. Under symptom-limited peak exercise, only systolic blood pressure and heart rate were reduced, but the ejection fraction was not changed (KINHAL et al. 1987). In a study in elderly hypertensive patients with normal left ventricular function, dilevalol had no substantial effect on a variety of parameters of left ventricular function (SCHOENBERGER et al. 1988b).

3.6.3 Therapeutic Use

In patients with severe hypertension, dilevalol decreased systolic and diastolic pressure from 184/124 to 143/95 mmHg after i.v. bolus injection (averaged total dose 417 mg), whereas the heart rate was not affected (WALLIN et al. 1988).

A dose-dependent decrease in diastolic blood pressure has been found in a study with single and 5-day administration of dilevalol at oral doses of between 200 and 800 mg. No differences between supine and standing blood pressure have been found, indicating a low risk for orthostatic hypotension (AFFRIME et al. 1987). The acute and chronic blood pressure lowering effect of dilevalol under resting and exercise conditions has been confirmed in some clinical trials. The individual daily oral doses have been established mostly by titration; the range used in Caucasians is between 100 and 1600 mg (MATERSON et al. 1988; SCHOENBERGER et al. 1988a, b), and in Japanese populations between 50 and 400 mg (TAKEDA et al. 1988). The mean daily doses in the different trials ranged between 153 mg (TAKEDA et al. 1988) and 617 mg (SCHOENBERGER et al. 1988a, b). A once a day dosing schedule was mostly used.

The efficacy of dilevalol has been compared in controlled clinical studies with that of propranolol (SCHOENBERGER et al. 1988b), metoprolol (MATERSON et al. 1988), atenolol (COOK et al. 1986), carteolol (BABA et al. 1988a) and captopril (FOGARI et al. 1988). Marked differences between the pure β-blockers and dilevalol have not been observed. In a comparative double-blind, between-patient study with dilevalol (mean dose 280 mg once daily) and captopril (50 mg twice daily), dilevalol lowered blood pressure at 4 h and trough more than captopril. In particular, the exercise-induced increase in blood pressure and heart rate was better controlled by dilevalol than by captopril (FOGARI et al. 1988).

Comparative, controlled studies of dilevalol with placebo or with metopolol, atenolol or carteolol in hypertensive patients with normal or mildly impaired renal function show that dilevalol does not affect or reduces renal vascular resistance, renal plasma flow, glomerular filtration rate or filtration fraction (FF), whereas the conventional β-blockers induce, at least at peak plasma concentrations, a slight decrease in glomerular filtration rate and FF. Thus, dilevalol produces, in contrast to other β-blockers, no effect on renal function following acute or chronic oral administration (COOK et al. 1986, 1988; BABA et al. 1988a, b; CLIFTON et al. 1988).

A survey of the side effects on the basis of 117 patients treated with dilevalol and 60 patients treated with propranolol show that the adverse reactions reflect the known pharmacological profile of the drugs (SCHOENBERGER et al. 1988a).

There is some evidence from this study as well as from two further comparative trials with metoprolol (Materson et al. 1988) and labetalol (Ishii et al. 1988) that the incidence of side effects and discontinuations are lower in dilevalol-treated patients than in those treated with the standard drugs. In particular, fatigue, bradycardia, depression, impotence and cold extremities were less frequent but gastrointestinal disturbances more frequent in dilevalol-treated patients. Remarkably, no postural hypotension has been reported. In tilting experiments, the blood pressure response to postural change was maintained in patients treated for 2 weeks with 800 mg dilevalol twice daily (Atkins 1986). Analysis of biochemical parameters reveals that labetalol increases triglycerides and HDL slightly, but total cholesterol and LDL are unchaged; in 2% of the patients, elevations of transaminases have been recorded (Materson et al. 1988). Plasma renin activity slightly decreased or remained unchanged and catecholamines increased after i.v. administration of dilevalol (Wallin et al. 1988).

A double-blind, comparative investigation with dilevalol, metoprolol and placebo in asthmatic patients showed that a single oral dose of 400 mg dilevalol reduces FEV_1 less than 200 mg metoprolol. Thus, dilevalol seems not to exert more bronchial side effects than cardioselective β-blockers. Nevertheless, it has to be considered that all β-blockers must be used with extraordinary care in asthmatic patients (Chodosh et al. 1988).

3.7 Carvedilol

3.7.1 Chemistry

Carvedilol (for structure, see Table 2) is a compound with a high lipid solubility. The octanol/buffer distribution coefficient at pH 7.3 is 226; protein binding is 95% (von Möllendorff et al. 1987a). Carvedilol can be determined in body fluids by HPLC with fluorimetric detection (Varin et al. 1986; Reiff 1987). A modification of this enables the separate assaying of the stereo-isomers (Eisenberg et al. 1989; Fujimaki et al. 1988). The detection limit of these methods is about 1 ng/ml.

3.7.2 Pharmacology

3.7.2.1 Pharmacodynamics and Mode of Action

The β-blocking activity of carvedilol has been documented by radioligand studies, by a parallel shift of the dose-response curves of isoprenaline to the right in in vitro and in vivo experiments and by inhibition of isoprenaline-induced tachycardia in various species (Sponer et al. 1987a). With regard to β-adrenoceptor blockade, carvedilol behaves like propranolol with respect to non-cardioselectivity, membrane-stabilising properties and lack of intrinsic sympathomimetic activity. The β-blocking potency of carvedilol has been demonstrated in some in vitro and in vivo experiments to be higher, equal or lower than that of propranolol (species-dependent). The pA_2 values for the β_1-blocking activity have been calculated to range between 8.24 and 9.0 (SPONER et al. 1987a; HOFFERBER et al. 1988; LOUIS et al. 1988). On the basis of equipotent β-blocking concentrations or doses, carvedilol is over ten times more active than labetalol (SPONER et al. 1987a).

The vasorelaxing activity of carvedilol has been confirmed in a variety of experiments using isolated human digital arteries and metatarsal veins (MOULDS et al. 1984), rat aortic strips (SPONER et al. 1987a, b; STREIN et al. 1987) and canine coronary arteries (HATTORI et al. 1989). Carvedilol relaxed blood vessels precontracted by different stimuli such as norepinephrine, serotonin, potassium chloride or Bay k 8644. In vitro experiments using a selective α_1-agonist, e.g. phenylephrine, have not been published. Norepinephrine-precontracted strips reacted most sensitively. Carvedilol and its enantiomers shifted equally the concentration-response curves of norepinephrine to the right. Even though the criteria for calculation of pA_2 values of α-blockade (parallel shift, unchanged maximum effect of the agonist) were not strictly fulfilled in some cases (MOULDS et al. 1984; SPONER et al. 1987b), pA_2 values were calculated from experiments in human, rat or rabbit arteries and range between 6.8 and 7.5 (MOULDS et al. 1984; HOFFERBER et al. 1988; LOUIS et al. 1988). It can be concluded from electrophysiological investigations on canine mesenteric arteries and veins that carvedilol exerts α_1- but not α_2-blocking activities (SEKI et al. 1988). As carvedilol binds competitively to the α_1-receptor and no other mode of action could be found at concentrations lower than 10^{-6} *M*, it can be assumed that its vasodilatory action is mediated predominantly by α_1-blockade. This has been confirmed in clinical pharmacological studies in which the phenylephrine-induced pressure response was attenuated, whereas that of angiotensin II was not influenced (CUBEDDU et al. 1987a, b).

However, other mechanisms obviously contribute to the vasodilatory activity of carvedilol. This can be concluded from in vitro and in vivo experiments in which carvedilol has been shown to inhibit the vasoconstrictor response to potassium chloride or Bay k 8644, indicating calcium entry blockade at least at high concentrations (SPONER et al. 1987a; HATTORI et al. 1989; A. NICHOLS and R. RUFFOLO, personal communication). Furthermore, it has been demonstrated that the local vasodilating effect of carvedilol in isolated perfused hind limbs of rabbits was reduced but not abolished by systemic pretreatment by α- and β-blockade, whereas the effect of prazosin was completely blocked (SPONER et al. 1988).

An additional vasodilatory mechanism besides α_1-blockade can be deduced from clinical pharmacological studies in which the vasoconstrictor response of locally infused norepinephrine or $PGF_{2\alpha}$ in human dorsal hand veins was attenuated equally by pretreatment with an oral dose of 50 mg carvedilol (BELZ et al. 1988).

TOMLINSON et al. (1988) investigated the influence of single oral doses of carvedilol (50, 100 mg), labetalol (400 mg) or propranolol plus hydralazine (80 mg + 50 mg) on the blood pressure response to phenylephrine, angiotensin II, handgrip, tilting and cold-pressor tests. Resting supine or tilting blood pressure was lowest after 100 mg carvedilol, but changes in tilting pressure and reduction of pressor responses to hand grip, cold and phenylephrine were greatest after labetalol. The angiotensin II pressor response was not influenced by labetalol but attenuated by carvedilol and the combination of propranolol plus hydralazine. These results also indicate that an additional non-specific vasodilator effect may be involved.

Indirect evidence that α_1-adrenoceptor blockade is not the only mechanism responsible for the vasodilation is derived also from investigations in tilting experiments. Even at high doses, the blood pressure response to orthostasis was influened in conscious rabbits to a lesser extent by carvedilol than by prazosin or labetalol (BARTSCH et al. 1987). This is in agreement with results from a clinical study in which no postural hypotension during tilting was observed (HEBER et al. 1987a).

3.7.2.2 Haemodynamics

The acute blood pressure lowering effect of carvedilol was evaluated in various experimental models, such as anaesthetised and conscious animals, in hypertensive animal models, e.g. SHR, and also in normotensive animals (SPONER et al. 1987a; TANAKA et al. 1987). This distinguishes carvedilol from classic β-adrenoceptor antagonists such as propranolol, which do not acutely lower arterial blood pressure in animals even at high doses. Furthermore, it is striking that carvedilol exhibits β-adrenoceptor blocking and acute blood pressure lowering activities in the same dose range, as demonstrated in conscious SHR or dogs. Haemodynamic investigations show that the changes in blood pressure mainly reflect the effect of the drug on the TPR, which is reduced by carvedilol but slightly increased by propranolol (see Fig. 5) (SPONER et al. 1987a; VON MÖLLENDORFF et al. 1987a; TANAKA et al. 1987).

The results obtained from animal pharmacology studies have been confirmed in humans. In healthy subjects, single oral doses of carvedilol between 25 and 100 mg lower supine and standing systolic and diastolic blood pressures. The exercise-induced increases in heart rate and stystolic blood pressure were significantly lowered (TOMLINSON et al. 1985). Compared with propranolol, carvedilol induced a greater reduction in supine resting blood pressure despite considerably less β-adrenoceptor antagonism. It differs also from labetalol, which produces mainly a fall in standing blood pressure (TOMLINSON et al. 1986, 1987). WENDT et al. (1987) found decreases in arterial or pulmonary pressure due to decreases in resistances during rest or exercise after a single oral dose of 50 mg carvedilol. The vasodilatory activity of carvedilol has been confirmed in healthy subjects as well as in patients using plethysmographic methods (EGGERTSEN et al. 1984a, b; VON MÖLLENDORFF et al. 1986; SUNDBERG et al. 1987; WENDT et al. 1987; MORGAN et al. 1987). The differences from pure β-blockers are obvious. In contrast to propranolol or metoprolol, carvedilol decreases blood pressure and forearm vascular resistance 90 min or 2 h after dosing on the 1st and 29th day, indicating that even during chronic therapy carvedilol's vasore-

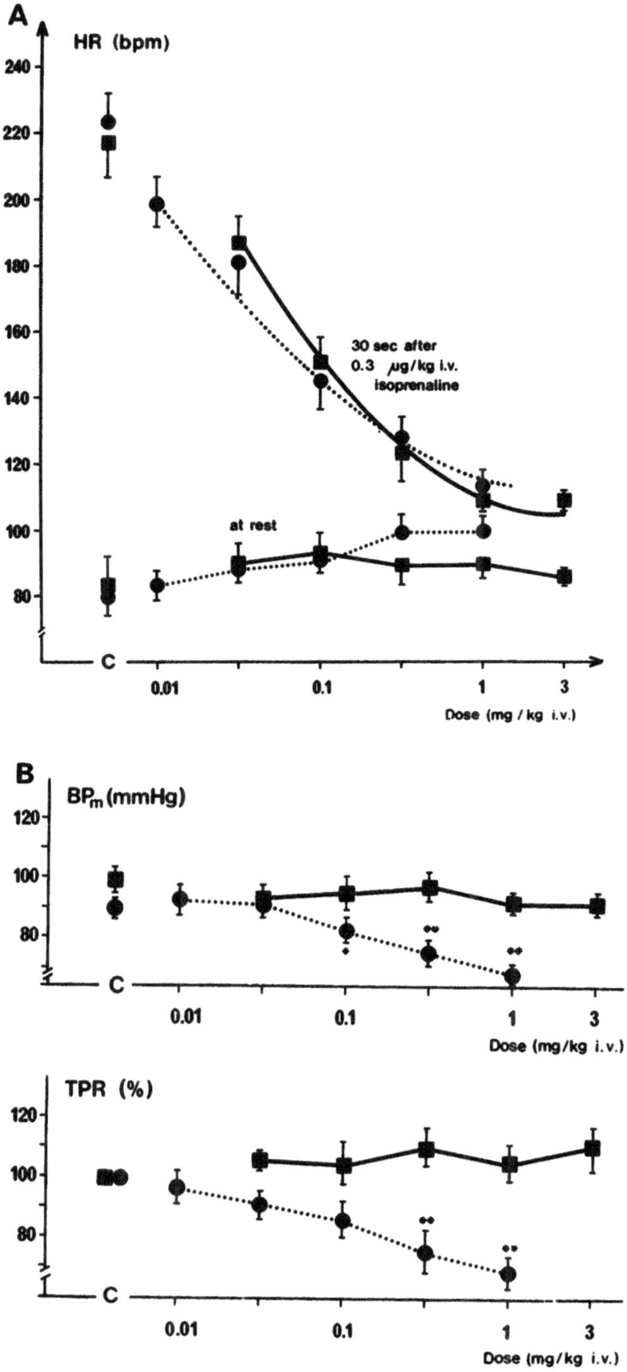

Fig. 5A,B. Effects of increasing doses of carvedilol (*circles*) and propranolol (*squares*) in conscious dogs (means ± SEM, $n = 10$). **A** Effects on heart rate (*HR*) at rest and on isoprenaline-induced tachycardia. **B** Effects on mean arterial blood pressure (BP_m) and total peripheral resistance (*TPR*)

laxing component contributes to the antihypertensive activity (Eggertsen et al. 1984b; Morgan et al. 1987).

Chronic experimental studies in SHR (Kohno et al. 1988b) and the results of a double-blind, placebo-controlled trial in patients with essential hypertension show that carvedilol decreases renal vascular resistance and does not influence renal blood flow (RBF) and glomerular filtration rate (GFR) (Dupont et al. 1987). An increase in RBF despite systemic hypotension and a stable GFR have also been observed in anaesthetised dogs after intrarenal infusion of carvedilol, whereas propranolol decreases GFR and RBF (Tamaki et al. 1988). In an experimental model, carvedilol exerted protective effects against the development of renal failure (Nakamoto et al. 1988).

Heber et al. (1987a) found that chronic treatment of hypertensive patients with carvedilol caused a considerable decrease in end-systolic and end-diastolic left ventricular volume, while the ejection fraction was not depressed. Using radionuclide ventriculography, it has been shown that in patients with coronary heart disease the ejection fraction, filling rate index and ⅓ filling fraction were increased after chronic treatment with 50 mg carvedilol daily, indicating that carvedilol improves the systolic and diastolic left ventricular function in contrast to pure β-blockers (Lahiri et al. 1987, 1988).

3.7.2.3 Toxicology

The results of toxicological investigations have been reviewed by von Mölllendorff et al. (1987a).

3.7.2.4 Pharmacokinetics and Metabolism

The pharmacokinetics of carvedilol have been investigated in healthy young (Neugebauer et al. 1987; von Möllendorff et al. 1987b) and elderly subjects (Louis et al. 1987; Morrison et al. 1987) as well as in patients with liver cirrhosis (Neugebauer et al. 1988) and hypertensive patients with renal failure (Hakusui and Fujimaki 1988). Peak plasma concentrations were reached about 1–1.5 h after oral administration (Neugebauer et al. 1987; Louis et al. 1987). Food does not affect absorption (Louis et al. 1987), and no deviation from linear kinetics has been observed. The absolute bioavailability is about 25% in healthy volunteers, but in patients with liver cirrhosis it is about 80% (Neugebauer et al. 1988). In dogs as well as in humans, concentrations of total radioactivity considerably exceed those of the parent drug, indicating a hepatic first-pass effect (von Möllendorff et al. 1987b). Its volume of distribution has been calculated to be 132 litres in non-cirrhotic and 321 litres in cirrhotic patients, indicating considerable tissue distribution (Neugebauer et al. 1987, 1988). Its serum concentration-time profiles can be fitted best to a three-compartment model (Varin et al. 1986).

The drug is almost completely eliminated by hepatic metabolism and excreted mainly via the bile (von Möllendorff et al. 1987b). The total clearance of the parent drug reaches about 600 ml/min, but in patients with liver cirrhosis this is only 390 ml/min. A mean elimination half-life of 2–2.5 h after i.v. administration and 6.4 h after oral administration of non-sustained release formulation has been reported (CUBEDDU et al. 1987b; NEUGEBAUER et al. 1987), while in patients with liver cirrhosis it was 7.1 h. The terminal elimination half-life of radioactivity ranged between 23 and 52 h in humans (VON MÖLLENDORFF et al. 1987b). Whereas the pharmacokinetic profile of carvedilol is not modified in patients with renal failure (HAKUSUI and FUJIMAKI 1988), the increased volume of distribution and bioavailability and the decreased clearance in patients with severe liver disease made it necessary to reduce the dose of carvedilol to 1/5 of normal in these persons (NEUGEBAUER et al. 1988).

Concomitant treatment with carvedilol and hydrochlorothiazide did not change the pharmacokinetics of carvedilol (RUDORF et al. 1988).

The main metabolic pathway of carvedilol consists of aromatic ring oxidation, aliphatic side chain oxidation and conjugation, in particular glucuronide and sulphate formation. The majority is eliminated via the faeces, and about 16% of the metabolites is cleared renally. The metabolites do not contribute to the haemodynamic efficacy of the drug (VON MÖLLENDORFF et al. 1987a; NEUGEBAUER et al. 1987).

3.7.3 Therapeutic Use

The acute and chronic blood pressure lowering effects of carvedilol under resting and exercise conditions have been confirmed in a considerable number of clinical trials. Dose-finding studies reveal that daily doses of 25–50 mg for European and American populations and 10–20 mg for Japanese people are appropriate for chronic antihypertensive therapy (RITTINGHAUSEN 1988; MCPHILLIPS et al. 1988; OGIHARA et al. 1988). The inter-individual range for the dose of carvedilol is obviously smaller than that reported for labetalol. In most clinical trials carvedilol was administered twice daily, but studies with 20–24 h monitoring show that a once a day dosing schedule is able to control blood pressure throughout the day with an additional reduction of the circadian variabiliy (OGIHARA et al. 1987; MEYER-SABELLEK et al. 1985, 1987a, b, 1988; RITTINGHAUSEN 1988; DE CESARIS et al. 1988). Carvedilol is able to reduce the early morning rise in pressure which is thought to provoke myocardial infarction (MEYER-SABELLEK et al. 1987a, b; HEBER et al. 1987a).

The effectiveness of carvedilol on blood pressure and heart rate has been compared with conventional β-blockers in a variety of controlled, chronic studies. In some studies, carvedilol was reported to be equally effective to propranolol or pindolol in decreasing blood pressure, but in contrast to conventional β-blockers it hardly reduced the heart rate (EGGERTSEN et al. 1984a, b; MORGAN et al. 1987; RITTINGHAUSEN 1988). In others, 50 mg carvedilol lowered the resting diastolic blood pressure or attenuated the pressure response to exercise during chronic treatment more than 100 mg atenolol or 200 mg metoprolol (FRANZ et al. 1984; DE CESARIS et al. 1988; MEYER-SABELLEK et al. 1985, 1987b). In particular, patients who did not respond satisfactorily to metoprolol could be controlled with carvedilol (FRANZ et al. 1984).

The combined use of carvedilol and thiazides induces a more pronounced blood pressure lowering effect than either individual component alone without causing significant side effects (Rudorf et al. 1988; Yasujima et al. 1988).

Carvedilol has been investigated in certain special hypertensive populations. In a study on hypertensive patients with serum creatinine above 2 mg/dl, carvedilol reduced the arterial blood pressure from 172/101 mmHg to 150/87 mmHg without changing the laboratory parameters, suggesting no deterioration of renal function (Kohno et al. 1988a). In hypertensive patients with non-insulin dependent diabetes, carvedilol reduced blood pressure but did not change the concentrations of fasting or postprandial blood glucose and haemoglobin A_1; hypoglycaemia did not occur (Ehmer et al. 1988). A double-blind study revealed that carvedilol and pindolol were very effective in elderly patients; both drugs were well tolerated and did not produce any safety problems (Staiger et al. 1988).

A survey of the first studies with respect to side effects have been given by Abshagen (1987). In 111 of 908 treated patients a total number of 265 adverse reactions has been observed. Headache and dizziness were the most frequently reported complaints. Postural hypotension was a rare adverse reaction in this survey (15 patients). However, in some clinical studies a few cases of excessive fall in blood pressure or orthostatic hypotension have been reported (Morgan et al. 1987; Louis et al. 1987; Schnurr et al. 1987; McPhillips et al. 1988). The results of a dose-finding study reveal that the side effects, in particular postural hypotension, are dose-related. In patients treated with 25 mg carvedilol daily, 4 of 52 patients experienced various kinds of side effects but not orthostatic hypotension, whereas 15 of 52 patients treated with 100 mg carvedilol daily reported adverse reactions (Rittinghausen 1988). Neither water and salt retention with subsequent weight gain nor changes in carbohydrate, lipid metabolism or other clinicochemical parameters have been reported (Schnurr et al. 1987; Higaki et al. 1988). In particular, the lipid profile was not adversely influenced by carvedilol (Staiger et al. 1988).

Acute or chronic oral dosing does not affect the resting plasma adrenaline concentration (Meyer-Sabellek et al. 1985; Leonetti et al. 1987; Higaki et al. 1988), but the standing or exercise levels of norepinephrine were slightly increased (Meyer-Sabellek et al. 1985). Plasma renin activity and plasma aldosterone decreased slightly (Meyer-Sabellek et al. 1985; Dupont et al. 1987; Morgan et al. 1987; Leonetti et al. 1987).

3.8 Nipradilol

3.8.1 Chemistry

Nipradilol (for chemical structure, see Table 2) is an entity with a nitrate moiety. It has low lipophilicity. The octanol/buffer partition coefficient at pH 7.4 is 0.85. The protein binding is about 30% (Uchida et al. 1987).

3.8.2 Pharmacology

3.8.2.1 Pharmacodynamics and Mode of Action

The β-blocking potency of nipradilol has been investigated in isolated right atrial and tracheal preparations of guinea pigs. The pA_2 values calculated from the competitive antagonism against isoprenaline were 8.92 for the β_1-blockade and 8.33 for the β_2-blockade, indicating lack of cardioselectivity. Nipradilol was about 2–3 times as potent as propranolol and about 10 times as potent as denitro-nipradilol (SHIRASAWA et al. 1982; UCHIDA et al. 1983). Investigations on tissues derived from reserpinised animals revealed that nipradilol exerts no sympathomimetic activity (UCHIDA et al. 1983). Like propranolol, the compound has membrane-stabilising activity. Furthermore, at concentrations greater than 30 μM it prolongs the action potential duration of canine Purkinje fibres, indicating slight class III antiarrhythmic properties (NAKAYA et al. 1984). However, these properties have not been found in preparations from rabbits or guinea pigs (KODAMA et al. 1985).

The vasorelaxing activity of nipradilol has been confirmed in various vascular beds, such as mesenteric arteries or veins or coronary arteries of dogs (UCHIDA et al. 1983; SAKANASHI et al. 1984a). Remarkably, larger coronary arteries reacted more sensitively than smaller ones. The pA_2 values in K^+-depolarised mesenteric arteries and veins were 6.35 and 6.23 (UCHIDA et al. 1983). Thus, nipradilol was about 100 times less active as a vasodilating agent than as β-blocker. This high ratio has been confirmed in in vivo investigations. In anaesthetised dogs, the doses required for inhibition of isoprenaline-induced responses can be estimated to be about 0.005 mg/kg and for that of phenylephrine, about 0.5 mg/kg (UCHIDA et al. 1983; FUJII et al. 1986). Denitro-nipradilol did not exert any vasorelaxing activity up to 10^{-4} M (UCHIDA et al. 1983; KOU and SUZUKI 1983; NANJO and KITAMURA 1984).

Vasodilatation induced by nipradilol was not accompanied by changes in electrical properties of the smooth muscle membranes. It inhibits contractions produced by high potassium solution or depolarising current pulses. This indicates that the vasodilating reaction of nipradilol is similar to that of glyceryl trinitrate (SHIRASAWA et al. 1982; KOU and SUZUKI 1983).

The venodilating effect of nipradilol has been demonstrated in a variety of experiments. The compound increases the diameter of brachiocephalic veins (UCHIDA et al. 1987), dilates venous capacitance vessels and decreases the central venous pressure of pithed rats pretreated with dihydroergotamine (SHIRASAWA et al. 1985). After chronic administration, the venous distensibility of SHR is increased by nipradilol (M. NAKAMURA et al. 1984). The effects on the myocardial preload can be assumed to be mediated by the nitrate configuration.

In additional to the glyceryl trinitrate-like vasodilatation, nipradilol obviously also has presynaptic α-adrenoceptor blocking activities, as demonstrated in a variety of in vitro investigations (ASADA et al. 1982; KOU et al. 1982; SHIRASAWA et al. 1982; UCHIDA et al. 1983; NANJO and KITAMURA 1984; OHIRA et al. 1985). The compound inhibits both the extra-junctional and the intra-junctional adrenoceptors, whereas prazosin inhibits only the extra-junctional α_1-receptors (KOU et al. 1982). The pA_2 values calculated from results obtained in isolated canine mesenteric arteries or veins using norepinephrine as α-adrenoceptor agonist are 6.85 or 6.68 (Uchida et al. 1983). Similar results have been found in guinea pig aortic strips using norepinephrine or phenylephrine as agonists (Ohira et al. 1985). The postsynaptic α_1-adrenoceptor blocking activity of nipradilol has been confirmed in investigations on pithed rats and in anaesthetised dogs in which it induced a parallel rightward shift of the pressure response curve of phenylephrine (Nakagawa et al. 1985; Fujii et al. 1986). Nipradilol has little or no presynaptic α_2-adrenoceptor blocking activity (Ohira et al. 1985).

Nevertheless, it seems doubtful whether the α_1-adrenoceptor blocking activity characterised in in vitro experiments contributes to the acute blood pressure lowering activity of nipradilol in vivo. The slight antihypertensive effect of nipradilol in pithed rats persisted even in the presence of propranolol plus prazosin or propranolol plus yohimbine (Nakagawa et al. 1985). The clear-cut antihypertensive effect induced by oral administration of 30 mg/kg nipradilol to conscious SHR was not accompanied by any modification of the pressor response to phenylephrine (Nakahara et al. 1985a).

In anaesthetised dogs, the haemodynamic effect of nipradilol has been attenuated by pretreatment with indomethacin (Hisa et al. 1984). However, the real role of the prostaglandin system for the vasodilatory and antihypertensive activity of nipradilol remains to be elucidated.

3.8.2.2 Haemodynamics

The blood pressure decreasing effect of nipradilol has been confirmed in a variety of experimental models. Doses higher than 1 mg/kg orally produce a long-lasting decrease in arterial blood pressure of SHR after acute and chronic administration (Shimizu et al. 1982; M. Nakamura et al. 1984; Uchida et al. 1983; Watanabe et al. 1985). Obviously, this effect can at least partly be attributed to the improvement of venous compliance since both effects occur in the same dose range (M. Nakamura et al. 1984).

However, the available literature does not provide information on whether the doses required for β-blockade and acute blood pressure response are in the same range.

In anaesthetised dogs, i.v. injection of nipradilol at doses between 0.01 and 1 mg/kg induced a sustained decrease in systolic and diastolic blood pressure, left ventricular pressure and its derivative d*p*/d*t*, cardiac output, venous return, mesenteric blood flow, heart rate and renin secretion rate. TPR was increased slightly, while left ventricular end-diastolic pressure (LVEDP) and renal blood flow were not affected significantly. Coronary sinus outflow and myocardial oxygen consumption were reduced on the basis of metabolic autoregulation due to diminished requirements; TPR and total coronary resistance were calculated to be increased (Hisa et al. 1984; Sakanashi et al. 1985; Fujii et al. 1986; Kawada et al. 1986). The close correlation found between the plasma renin activity and the decrease in systemic blood pressure may indicate that the suppression of the renin-angiotensin system is involved in its antihypertensive mechanism (HISA et al. 1984). KAWASHIMA et al. (1984) found in rabbits that 1 mg/kg i.v. abolished isoprenaline-induced tachycardia, reduced markedly the basal heart rate but exerted only weak antihypertensive activity. Thus, nipradilol behaved to a certain degree like a pure β-blocking agent. This may be based on the fact that the dose required for the β-blocking activity is obviously much lower than that required for acute vasodilatation. However, a transient reduction of TPR and LVEDP has been found directly after i.v. injection of doses between 0.1 and 1 mg/kg in similar investigations in anaesthetised as well as in conscious dogs (UCHIDA 1982; FUJII et al. 1986). Furthermore, the vasodilating effect of nipradolol has been demonstrated in anaesthetised dogs pretreated with propranolol, in which nipradilol caused a decrease in arterial blood pressure and central venous pressure, while TPR was reduced (FUJII et al. 1986; KAWADA et al. 1986).

In healthy volunteers and hypertensive patients treated with nipradilol, arterial blood pressure, heart rate and cardiac output decreased (KONDO et al. 1984). Whereas SAITO et al. (1985) reported a tendency for reduced TPR, TSUKIYAMA et al. (1985) did not observe any significant change.

3.8.2.3 Toxicology

The results of toxicological investigations have been reviewed by UCHIDA et al. (1987).

3.8.2.4 Pharmacokinetics and Metabolism

After oral administration, nipradilol is rapidly and well absorbed from the gastrointestinal tract. Peak plasma concentrations are reached within 2 h after oral administration to different species, including humans (YOSHIMURA et al. 1985a, b, c; KIMATA et al. 1985). Studies on bioavailability of nipradilol in dogs show that the relatively low systemic availability of the drug is mostly attributable to the metabolism of nipradilol in the liver, intestinal tract, or both. The systemic availability in humans is about 35% (YOSHIMURA et al. 1985a, b, c). In humans, the peak plasma concentrations and the AUCs increased in proportion to the orally administered dose. Remarkably, there was only a small interindividual variation of these two variables. Nipradilol has a large apparent volume of distribution in humans (5.6 l/kg) and is subject to considerable first pass metabolism. The peak plasma concentrations are therefore only 1 ng/ml per 1 mg oral dose (YOSHIMURA et al. 1985c). The mean elimination half-life of nipradilol has been reported to be 0.7–1.6 h in different species and 3.7 hours in humans (YOSHIMURA et al. 1985a, c; KIMATA et al. 1985). The renal and total plasma clearances were estimated to be 0.18 and 1.04 l/min in humans (YOSHIMURA et al. 1985c).

In rats, about 40% of orally administered radioactivity was excreted in the urine and 6% in the bile; enterohepatic circulation was minimal (KABUTO et al. 1985). The amount of parent drug excreted in the urine was less than 2% in animals, and about 6% in human. The major metabolites were denitronipradilol, 4-hydroxy-nipradilol generated by hydroxylation of the benzopyran skeleton, oxidative degradation of the β-blocking side chain and their glucuronidation (Kabuto et al. 1985; Yoshimura et al. 1985d). Denitration takes place mainly in the liver. The rate of degradation of nipradilol is markedly lower than that of glyceryl trinitrate or isosorbide dinitrate (Kabuto et al. 1986). There is some evidence from investigations with rats that the metabolic degradation is subject to a saturable process (Kimata et al. 1985; Kabuto et al. 1985).

After multiple oral administration of nipradilol in dogs and humans, the experimental plasma concentrations of nipradilol were in accordance with a computer fit for repeated administration, indicating no accumulation and no increase in the elimination half-life (Yoshimura et al. 1985a, c).

3.8.3 Therapeutic Use

Up to now, only few data are available concerning the usefulness of nipradilol as an antihypertensive agent. In particular, it does not seem to be clear to what extent the vasodilating component contributes to the antihypertensive activity. The observation that blood pressure starts to decrease 2 weeks after the beginning of treatment is similar to that obtained with pure β-blockers (Kondo et al. 1984; Saito et al. 1985; Tsukiyama et al. 1985; Ueda et al. 1987; Yamada et al. 1986). The doses for chronic antihypertensive therapy are 6–18 mg/day twice daily. Comparative, controlled studies with propranolol (60–120 mg/day thrice daily) or pindolol (15–30 mg/day thrice daily) show that nipradilol was nearly as effective as conventional β-blockers (Ueda et al. 1987; Yamada et al. 1986).

During a long-term study on five patients for 30–46 weeks, nipradilol was administered at doses between 6 and 12 mg twice daily (N. Nakamura et al. 1985). During the first few days of treatment, the circadian variation in blood pressure was not influenced by the compound. The blood pressure responses in the cold pressure test and during mental arithmetic did not change significantly, and the plasma renin activity and plasma aldosterone concentration tended to decrease gradually after the administration of nipradilol. The antihypertensive effect of nipradilol was maintained during chronic treatment; development of tolerance did not, therefore, occur (N. Nakamura et al. 1985).

In addition to the studies in hypertensive patients nipradilol has been investigated extensively in patients with coronary heart disease (for review, see Uchida et al. 1987).

3.9 BW A575C

3.9.1 Chemistry

BW A575C is an entity chemically related to pindolol and enalapril (for chemical structure, see Table 2). The two active moieties are linked by a proteolytically stable secondary amide bond, which is stable both in vitro and in vivo. The molecule contains two chiral centres, one in the side chain associated with the β-adrenoceptor antagonist activity and the other in the peptide structure associated with the ACE inhibition. Therefore, the compound consists of a mixture of four diastereoisomers.

3.9.2 Pharmacology

BW A575C produced competitive inhibition of responses to isoprenaline in guinea pig right atrial preparation with a pK_b of 7.18 ± 0.05 (cf. pindolol 8.9 ± 0.07). BW A575C inhibited the partially purified preparation of ACE from rabbit lung with an IC_{50} of 10.7 ± 2.1 n*M* (cf. enalaprilat 4.4 ± 0.8 n*M*) (Allan et al. 1987a).

The β-blocking activity and ACE-inhibiting activity have been investigated in vivo in pithed rats and in conscious individuals. Both angiotensin I-induced pressor responses and isoprenaline-induced tachycardia were displaced dose-dependently to the right (0.015–1.5 mg/kg i.v.) by BW A575C. In pithed rats, the compound was approximately 100 times more active as an ACE-inhibitor than as a β-adrenoceptor blocking agent. In conscious dogs and rats, however, BM A575C was only 2 to 10 times more active as an ACE inhibitor than as a β-blocker (Allan et al. 1987a; Cambridge et al. 1987).

The recovery time course of the inhibition of the responses to isoprenaline and angiotensin I is almost identical. About 4 h after administration, 80% of the pretreatment responses to the challenges have been restored. With respect to angiotensin I, no basic difference between enalapril and BW A575C exist (Allan et al. 1987a; Cambridge et al. 1987).

BW A575C does not decrease the arterial blood pressure at doses of 1 mg/kg i.v. in conscious normotensive rats or dogs. However, in conscious, instrumented, acute renovascular hypertensive dogs, BW A575C induces a decrease in arterial blood pressure within a few minutes after i.v. injection of 1 mg/kg, and the effect is sustained for up to 4 h (Allan et al. 1986a, 1987a; Cambridge et al. 1987).

Comparative haemodynamic investigations have been performed in anaesthetised dogs. In contrast to propranolol or pindolol, BW A575C in equipotent β-blocking doses decreased blood pressure, induced renal vasodilatation, improved renal function but had less cardiodepressive activity. In contrast to enalapril, BW A575C decreased heart rate and left ventricular contractility at equipotent ACE-inhibiting doses (Allan et al. 1986b).

Preliminary data with the *S,S,S,S*-stereoisomer (BW B385C) on rats and dogs show that this compound is approximately ten times more active as an ACE-inhibitor than as β-adrenoceptor blocker agent (Allan et al. 1987b). The arterial blood pressure of renal hypertensive rats and SHR decreases after a single i.v. dose of 1 mg/kg of BW B385C (Cambridge and Butterfield 1988).

Data with respect to pharmacokinetics and to clinical use have not been published up to now.

3.10 Various Other Compounds

Besides the compounds described in detail in the previous sections, there are a considerable number of further compounds for which action on multiple receptors may be suggested. Some of these compounds have been withdrawn from further development as antihypertensive agents for various reasons. For other entities only limited information from preclinical investigations are available up to now. Therefore, these compounds will be mentioned only with their name and chemical structure (see Tables 1, 2 and 5): adimolol, bometolol, bucindolol, bufuralol, chinoin-103, dramedilol, epanolol, medroxalol, pacrinolol, primidolol, prizidilol, ridazolol, sulfinalol, teoprolol, tolamolol, B24/76, ICI 89.406, ICI 89.963, ICI 141292, KF-577, KF-4317, MK 761, N 1518, P-0160 A.

4 Summary and Conclusions

The final conclusions on compounds acting on multiple receptors can be made mainly upon the data available for labetalol. For most of the other compounds (e.g. arotinolol, amosulalol, nipradilol, dilevalol) mentioned in this chapter, only pharmacological results and some clinical data have been published. They do not allow a final assessment with respect to their position as antihypertensive agents.

There is some evidence that not all compounds mentioned in this chapter fulfill exactly the requirements of a compound with a dual mechanism of action. For example, the doses required for inducing both components of action differ for arotinolol and nipradilol with the consequence that their haemodynamic profile resembles that of a pure β-adrenoceptor blocker. Also, the significance of the interaction of bevantolol or celiprolol with the α-adrenoceptors remains to be established.

It seems to be clear that compounds acting in the same dose range on multiple receptors, i.e. β-adrenoceptor blocking agents with additional vasorelaxing properties, are very effective antihypertensive agents with a favourable haemodynamic profile. They have been reported to be able to control the blood pressure of patients who were previously unsatisfactorily treated with other antihypertensive drugs.

Labetalol has been reported to be useful in particular in severe or resistant hypertensive patients and in special indications such as pregnancy, phaeochromocytoma and hypertensive emergencies. There is some evidence that it is more effective in black patients than plain β-adrenoceptor blockers.

Many well-conducted comparative clinical trials have been performed with these compounds in mild to moderate hypertensive patients, some of which were designed as crossover, double-blind studies. However, the blood pressure response and the incidence of side effects generally did not differ markedly from standard drugs.

The most convincing evidence for the beneficial action of the compounds is their favourable haemodynamic profile. They are able to compensate for the main haemodynamic disturbances in arterial hypertension. They normalise the increased TPR without activation of counter-regulatory mechanisms. Furthermore, in contrast to conventional β-blockers, they preserve coronary and renal blood flow and maintain effective cardiac output. Although studies with respect to the influence of the compounds on the morbidity and mortality of patients during long-term treatment do not exist, it may be anticipated that they are at least as good as pure β-blockers. This assumption can be made on the basis of their pharmacological profile and their lack of adverse effects on blood lipids.

Table 5. Further compounds with proposed dual mode of action. They have either been withdrawn from further development or only limited information from preclinical investigations is available

$$R_1\text{–O–}CH_2\text{–}\underset{\displaystyle OH}{CH}\text{–}CH_2\text{–NH–}R_2$$

Compound	R_1	R_2	Manufacturer
Pacrinolol Hoe–224	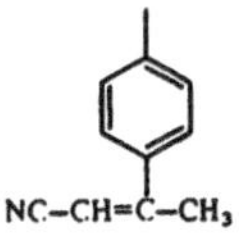	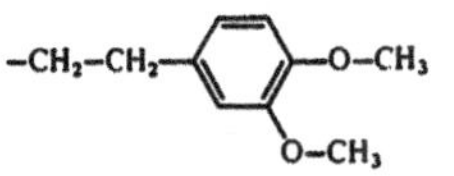	Hoechst (FRG)
Epanolol ICI–141292	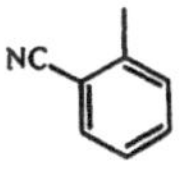	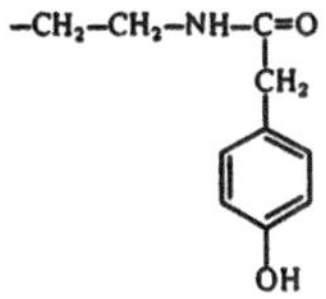	ICI (UK)
Tolamolol UK–6558	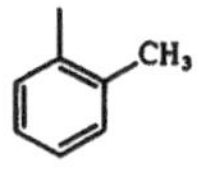	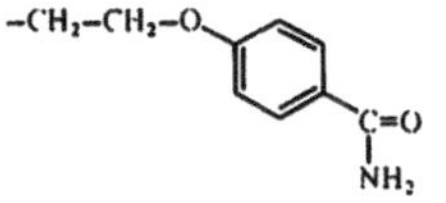	Pfizer (UK)
Primidolol UK–11443	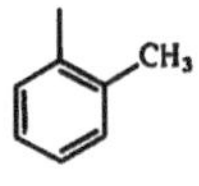	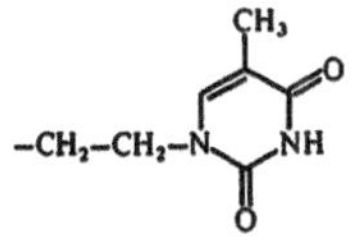	Pfizer (UK)
Ridazolol CAS–413	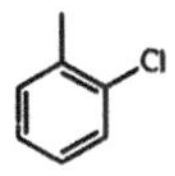	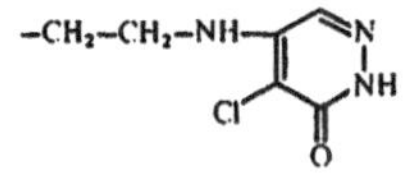	Cassella (FRG)

Table 5. (continued)

$$R_1{-}O{-}CH_2{-}\underset{\displaystyle OH}{\underset{|}{C}H}{-}CH_2{-}NH{-}R_2$$

Compound	R_1	R_2	Manufacturer
ICI–89406	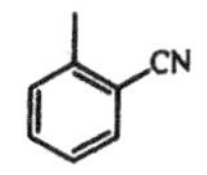	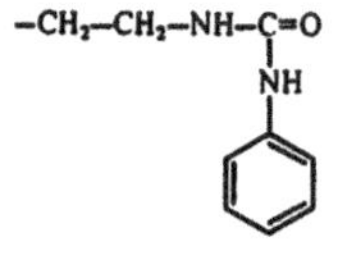	ICI (UK)
B 24/76	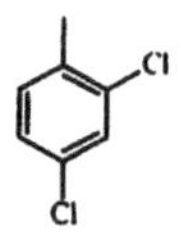	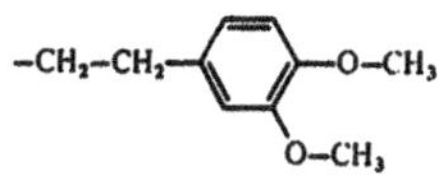	Arzneimittelwerk Dresden (GDR)
ICI–89963	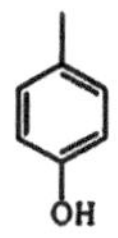	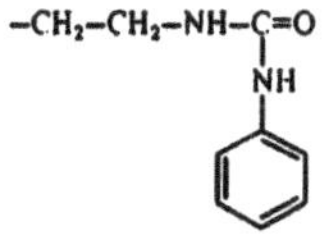	ICI (UK)
Dramedilol ISF–3382	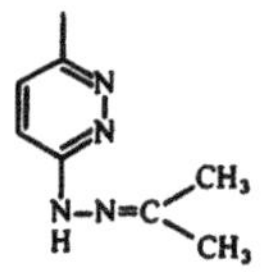	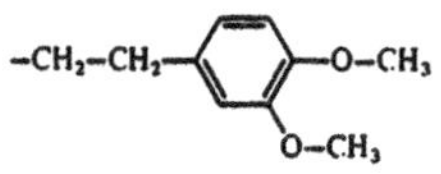	ISF (I)
Bometolol OPC–1427	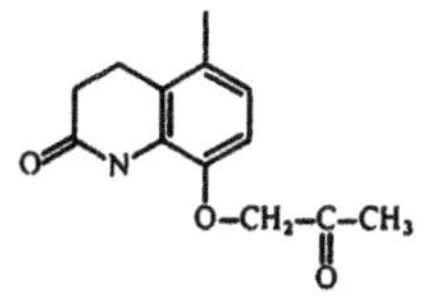	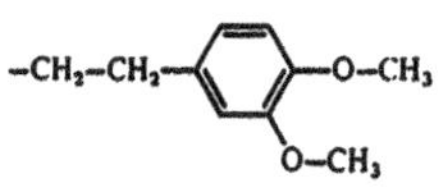	Otsuka (J)

Table 5. (continued)

$$R_1-O-CH_2-CH(OH)-CH_2-NH-R_2$$

Compound	R_1	R_2	Manufacturer
Teoprolol D 13.312	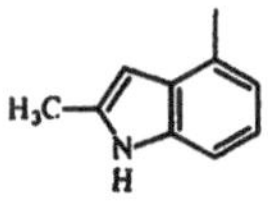	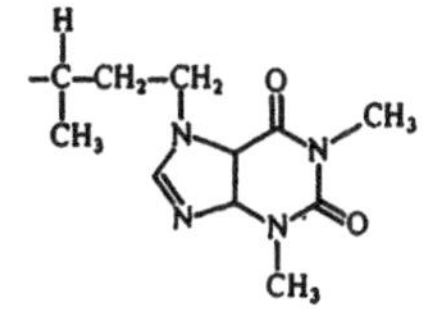	Asta Pharma (FRG)
P–0160 A	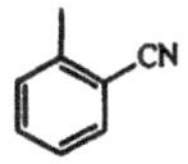	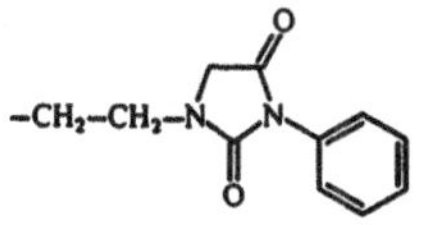	Pierrel (I)
N–1518	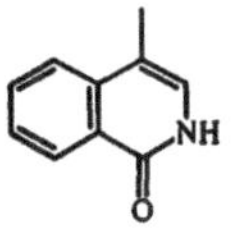	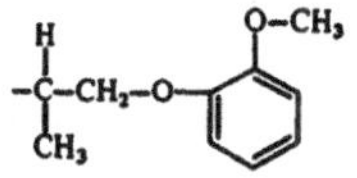	Nisshin (J)
KF–4317	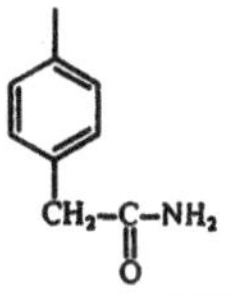	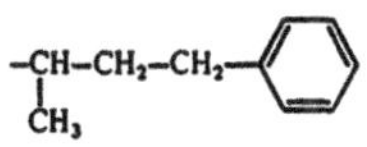	Kyowa (J)

$$R_1-O-CH_2-CH(OH)-CH_2-CH_2-NH-R_2$$

Compound	R_2	R_1	Manufacturer
Chinoin–103 TE–176	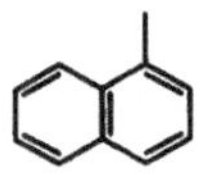	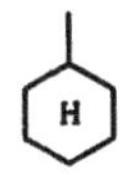	Chinoin (H)

Compounds acting on multiple receptors have in principle the possibility of a broad spectrum of side effects, namely those related to the different pharmacological components, and additional side effects not related to their pharmacological profile. On the other hand, the incidence of side effects related to the specific pharmacological mechanisms, e.g. α- or β-adrenoceptor blockade, seems to be lower than that during treatment with compounds acting only on one receptor site, because some of the adverse reactions may be compensated for by the dual mode of action.

Drugs acting on β- and α-adrenoceptors should be used with caution or avoided in patients crucially dependent on their sympathetic tone to maintain cardiovascular homeostasis. In instances in which the β-adrenoceptor blocking action could prove to be harmful, such as in patients with asthma, β-blockers with additional properties should also be used with caution or avoided. In order to diminish the potential for a pressure response to the drug in patients with phaeochromocytoma, it seems preferable to use labetalol or some other α-blocking agents i.v. before using the drugs orally.

Postural hypotension, in particular during the early phase of treatment after administration of high doses, seems to be the most troublesome side-effect of some of these compounds. However, this may be prevented by a slow upward titration in order to find the optimal dose. The wide range of the individual dosages—between 100 and 2400 mg daily for labetalol—makes such a titration procedure inconvenient for the patient and for the physician. This may be the reason why labetalol has not found wider acceptance in general practice despite its favourable pharmacological and haemodynamic profile. It remains to be established whether the newer compounds will find a higher acceptance due to their modified pharmacological and pharmacokinetic properties.

Acknowledgement. We would like to thank Ms. A. Ragaller for the patience, care and accuracy with which she typed this manuscript.

References

Abernethy DR, Bartos P, Plachetka JR (1987) Labetalol in the treatment of hypertension in elderly and younger patients. J Clin Pharmacol 27:902–906

Abshagen U (1987) A new molecule with vasodilating and β-adrenoceptor blocking properties. J Cardiovasc Pharmacol 10 [Suppl 11]:S23–S32

Adam WR, Meagher EJ, Barter CE (1982) Labetalol, beta-blockers and acute deterioration of chronic airways obstruction. Clin Exp Hypertens 4:1419–1428

Affrime MB, Perentesis GP, Patrick JE, Kramer WG (1987) Multiple-dose steady-state evaluation of dilevalol in hypertensive patients. In: 3rd European Meeting on Hypertension, Milan, 14–16 June 1987 (abstr no 5)

Agabiti-Rosei E, Brown JJ, Lever AF, Robertson AS, Robertson JIS, Trust PM (1976a) Treatment of phaeochromocytoma and of clonidine withdrawal hypertension with labetalol. Br J Clin Pharmacol 3 [Suppl]: 809–815

Agabiti-Rosei E, Brown JJ, Fraser R, Lever AF, Morton JJ, Robertson JIS, Trust PM (1976b) Labetalol (AH 5158), a competitive alpha- and beta-receptor blocking drug in the management of hypertension. Aust N Z J Med 6 [Suppl 3]:83–88

Agabiti-Rosei E, Fraser R, Morton JJ, Brown JJ, Lever AF, Robertson JIS, Trust PM (1977) Labetalol an alpha- and β-adrenergic blocking drug in the treatment of hypertension. Am Heart J 93:125–126

Agabiti-Rosei E, Alicandri CL, Beschi M, Castellano M, Fariello R, Montini E, Muisan ML, Romanelli G, Muisan G (1983) The acute and chronic hypotensive effect of labetalol and the relationship with pretreatment plasma noradrenaline levels. Br J Clin Pharmacol 13 [Suppl]:87S–92S

Aggerbeck M, Guellaen G, Hanoune J (1978) Biochemical evidence for the dual action of labetalol on alpha- and β-adrenoceptors. Br J Pharmacol 62:543–548

Al-Khawaja IM, Carnana MP, Prince H, Whittington J, Raftery EB (1986) Once- and twice-daily bevantolol for systemic hypertension using 24-hour ambulatory intraarterial blood pressure recording. Am J Cardiol 58 [Suppl]:17E–20E

Allan G, Cambridge D, Hardy GW, Follenfant MJ, Ford A, Oliver PL (1986a) BW A575C, a novel antihypertensive agent with converting enzyme inhibition and beta-blocking properties. J Hypertens 4 [Suppl 6]:S131–S133

Allan G, Cambridge D, Whiting MV (1986b) The cardiac and renovascular effects of BW A575C, a novel angiotensin converting enzyme inhibitor and beta-adrenoceptor antagonist. Br J Pharmacol 89 [Suppl]:488p (abstr)

Allan G, Cambridge D, Hardy GW, Follenfant MJ (1987a) BW A575C, a chemically novel agent with angiotensin converting enzyme inhibitor and β-adrenoceptor-blocking properties. Br J Pharmacol 90:609–615

Allan G, Ashton D, Cambridge D, Follenfant MJ, Hardy GM, Mills G (1987b) The preclinical pharmacology of a novel dual-acting antihypertensive agent, BW B385C. Br J Pharmacol 92 [Suppl]:571 P (abstr)

Alton KB, Leitz F, Bariletto S, Jaworsky L, Desrivieres D, Patrick J (1984) High-performance liquid chromatographic assay for labetalol in human plasma using a PRP-1 column and fluorometric detection. J Chromatogr Biomed Appl 311:319–328

Alton KB, Petruzzi RF, Patrick JE (1988) High-performance liquid chromatographic assay for dievalol in human plasma and urine using a PRP-1 column and fluorometric detection. J Chromatogr Biomed Appl 425:363–372

Anavekar SN, Barter C, Adam WR, Doyle AE (1982) A double-blind comparison of verapamil and labetalol in hypertensive patients with coexisting chronic obstructive airways disease. J Cardiovasc Pharmacol 4 [Suppl 3]:S374–S377

Anderson CC, Gabriel R (1978) Poor hypotensive response and tachyphylaxis following intravenous labetalol. Curr Med Res Opin 5:424–426

Andersson O, Berglund G, Hanssen L (1976) Antihypertensive action, time of onset and effects of carbohydrate metabolism of labetalol. Br J Clin Pharmacol 3 [Suppl]: 756–761

Ariens EJ (1984) Stereochemistry, a basis for sophisticated nonsense in pharmacokinetics and clinical pharmacology. Eur J Clin Pharmacol 26:663–668

Arinsoy T, Oram E (1986) Results of labetalol administration in the treatment of hypertension. Curr Ther Res 40:1123–1128

Asada H, Nanjo T, Itoh T, Suzuki H, Kuriyama H (1982) Effects of 3,4-dihydro-8-(2-hydroxy-3-isopropylaminopropoxy)-3-nitroxy-2H-1-b enzopyran (K-351) on smooth muscle cells and neuromuscular transmission in guinea pig vascular tissues. J Pharmacol Exp Ther 223:560–572

Asano H, Hashimoto H, Nakashima M (1983) Affinities for alpha- and beta-adrenoceptor subtypes of YM-09538, a new combined alpha- and beta-adrenoceptor antagonist, by radioligand binding assay. Arch Int Pharmacodyn Ther 262:34–46

Atkins JM (1986) The hemodynamic effects of dilevalol, the R-R'-isomer of labetalol. In: 11th Scientific Meeting of the International Society of Hypertension, Heidelberg, 31 Aug–6 Sept 1986 (abstr no 140)

Baba T, Murabayashi S, Tomiyama T, Takebe K (1988a) Comparison between short-term renal effects of dilevalol and carteolol in essential hypertenson: a cross-over study. In: Satellite symposium of the 12th Scientific Meeting of the International Society of Hypertension: dilevalol: combined beta-blockade and $beta_2$-stimulation in the treatment of hypertension, Kyoto, 21 May 1988

Baba T, Murabayashi S, Aoyagi K, Ishizaki T (1988b) Effects of dilevalol, an R,R-isomer of labetalol, on blood pressure and renal function in patients with mild to moderate essential hypertension. Eur J Clin Pharmacol 35:9–15

Backhouse CI (1981) A double-blind comparison of labetalol (Trandate) and propranolol

in general practice. Clin Trials J 18:241–253
Bahlmann J, Brod J, Hubrich W, Cachovan M, Pretschner P (1979) Effect of an alpha- and beta-adrenoceptor-blocking agent (labetalol) on haemodynamics in hypertension. Br J Clin Pharmacol 8 [Suppl]:113S–117S
Bahlmann J, Brod J, Hubrich W, Prestschner P (1980) Beeinflussung der hämodynamischen Streßreaktion bei Hypertonikern durch eine kombinierte alpha- und betablockade mit Labetalol. Dtsch Med Wochenschr 105:1414–1418
Bailey RR (1977) Scalp tingling and difficulty in micturition in patients on labetalol. Lancet ii:720–721
Bailey RR (1979a) Labetalol in the treatment of a patient with phaeochromocytoma: a case report. Br J Clin Pharmacol 8 [Suppl]:141S–142S
Bailey RR (1979b) Labetalol in the treatment of patients with hypertension and renal functional impairment. Br J Clin Pharmacol 8 [Suppl]:135S–140S
Balasubramanian V, Mann S, Raftery EB, Miller-Craig NW, Altman D (1979a) Effect of labetalol on continuous ambulatory blood pressure. Br J Clin Pharmacol 8 [Suppl]: 119S–123S
Balasubramanian V, Mann S, Miller-Craig NW, Raftery EB (1979b) Effect of labetalol in hypertension during exercise and postural changes. Br J Clin Pharmacol 8 [Suppl]: 95S–100S
Barbieri C, Ferrari C, Caldara R, Crossignani RM, Bertazzoni A (1981) Endocrine and metabolic effects of labetalol in man. J Cardiovasc Pharmacol 3:986–991
Barnett AJ, Kalowski S, Guest C (1978) Labetalol compared with pindolol plus hydralazine in the treatment of hypertension. Med J Austr 1:105–109
Bartsch W, Sponer G, Strein K, Böhm E, Hooper RG (1987) Evaluation of the risk for drug-induced postural hypotension in an experimental model: investigations with carvedilol, prazosin, labetalol and guanethidine. J Cardiovasc Pharmacol 10 [Suppl 11]:S49–S51
Baum T, Sybertz EJ (1983a) Pharmacology of labetalol in experimental animals. Am J Med 75 [Suppl 4A]:15–23
Baum T, Sybertz EJ (1983b) Antihypertensive actions of an isomer of labetalol and other vasodilator-β-adrenoceptor blockers. Fed Proc 42:176–181
Baum T, Watkins RW, Sybertz EJ, Vemulapalli S, Pula KK, Eynon E, Nelson S, Vliet GV, Glennon J, Moran RM (1981) Antihypertensive and hemodynamic actions of SCH 19927, the R,R-isomer of labetalol. J Pharmacol Exp Ther 218:444–452
Bellamy GR, Hunyor SN, Roffe D, Massang J (1983) Magnitude and mechanism of the antihypertensive action of labetalol, including ambulatory assessment. Br J Clin Pharmacol 16:9–16
Belz GG, Beermann C, Neugebauer G (1988) Influence of oral carvedilol in the responsiveness of human hand veins to noradrenaline and dinoprost (short communication). Drugs 36 [Suppl 6]:69–74
Bergmann H, Tabassi D, Rasser W, Necek S, Pittner H (1983) Beeinflussung der Kreislaufwirkungen von Isoprenalin durch den neuen β-Rezeptoren-Blocker Celiprolol an gesunden freiwilligen Versuchspersonen. Arzneimittelforschung 33:53–55
Bertoni T, de Ambroggi L, Niutta E, Peloso A, Ghezzi M (1985) Comparison of the effects of propranolol and labetalol on peripheral blood-flow in hypertensive patients. Clin Trials J 22:71–78
Bevilacqua M, Monopoli A, Vago T, Baldi G, Ongini E, Norbiato G (1988) Characterization of dilevalol affinity for beta- and alpha$_1$-adrenergic receptors of human cardiovascular tissues. J Cardiovasc Pharmacol 11 [Suppl 2]:S25–S27
Birkenhäger WH, De Leeuw PW (1983) Adrenergic vasoconstriction as a cause of inadequate hypotensive response to beta-adrenergic blockade. Hypertension 5 [Suppl III]:31–35
Bjerle P, Fransson L, Koch G, Lindström B (1980) Pindolol and labetalol in hypertension; comparison of their antihypertensive effects with particular respect to conditions in the upright posture and during exercise. Curr Ther Res 27:516–525
Blakeley AGH, Summers RJ (1977) The effects of labetalol (AH 5158) on adrenergic transmission in the cat spleen. Br J Pharmacol 59:643–650
Bloomfield SS, Lucas CP, Gantt Cl, Poland MC, Medakovicz M (1983) Step II treatment

with labetalol for essential hypertension. Am J Med 75 [Suppl 4A]:81–86
Bolli P, Waal-Manning HJ, Wood AJ, Simpson FO (1976) Experience with labetalol in hypertension. Br J Clin Pharmacol 3 [Suppl]:765–771
Bonelli VJ, Magometschnigg D, Hitzenberger G, Kaik G (1978) Hämodynamische Charakterisierung eines neuen Beta-Rezeptorenblockers: Celiprolol (ST 1396) in Ruhe und unter Ergometerbelastung, verglichen mit Propranolol (Inderal). Wien Klin Wochenschr 90:350–354
Branford WA, Hunter JAA, Muir Al (1978) Cutaneous reaction to labetalol. Practitioner 221:765–767
Bray JS (1986) Safety profile of bevantolol. Angiology 37:248–253
Breckenridge A, Omre M, Serlin MJ, Maciver M (1982) Labetalol in essential hypertension. Br J Clin Pharmacol 13 [Suppl]:37S–39S
Briggs RSJ, Birtwell AJ, Pohl JEF (1978) Hypertensive response to labetalol in phaeochromocytoma. Lancet i:1045–1046
Brittain RT, Levy GP (1976) A review of the animal pharmacology of labetalol, a combined alpha- and beta-adrenoceptor blocking drug. Br J Clin Pharmacol 3 [Suppl]:
Brittain RT, Drew GM, Levy GP (1982) The alpha- and beta-adrenoceptor blocking potencies of labetalol and its individual stereoisomers in anaesthetized dogs and in isolated tissues. Br J Pharmacol 77:105–114
Brodde OE, Daul A, Stuka N, O'Hara N, Borchard U (1985) Effects of β-adrenoceptor administration on β_2-adrenoceptor density in human lymphocytes. The role of the "intrinsic sympathomimetic activity". Naunyn-Schmiedeberg's Arch Pharmacol 328: 417–422
Brodde OE, Schemuth R, Brinkmann M, Wang XL, Daul A, Borchard U (1986) Beta-adrenoceptor antagonists (non-selective as well as β_1-selective) with partial agonist activity decrease β_2-adrenoceptor density in human lymphocytes. Evidence for a β_2-agonist component of the partial agonistic activity. Naunyn-Schmiedeberg's Arch Pharmacol 333:130–138
Brown JJ, Lever AF, Cumming AM, Robertson JIS (1977) Labetalol in hypertension. Lancet i:1147
Brown RC, Cooke J, Losowski MS (1981) SLE syndrome, probably induced by labetalol. Postgrad Med J 57:189–190
Bruschi C, Casali L, Cerveri I, Peona V, Zoia MC (1988) Effects of celiprolol on the bronchial reactivity in asthma. Am J Cardiol 61[Suppl]:53C–54C
Buck JD, Gross GJ, Warltier DC, Jolly SR, Hardman HF (1979) Comparative effects of cardioselective versus noncardioselective beta-blockade on subendocardial blood flow and contractile function in ischemic myocardium. Am J Cardiol 44:657–663
Bugni WJ (1988) The hemodynamic effects of dilevalol in patients with mild hypertension. J Cardiovasc Pharmacol 11 [Suppl 2]:S36 (abstr)
Buskin JN, Upton RA, Sörgel F, Williams RU, Lang E, Benet LZ (1982) Specific and sensitive assay of celiprolol in blood, plasma and urine using high-performance liquid chromatography. J Chromatogr Biomed Appl 230:454–460
Cambridge D, Butterfield LJ (1988) Acute antihypertensive effects of BW B385C in the conscious hypertensive rat. Br J Pharmacol 95 [Suppl]:709P (abstr)
Cambridge D, Allan G, Hardy GW, Follenfant MJ, Ford A, Oliver PL (1987) BW A575C Pharmacological profile in vivo of a novel angiotensin-converting enzyme inhibitor and β-blocker. J Cardiovasc Pharmacol 10[Suppl 11]:S64–S68
Cantelli I, Bracchetti D (1981) Haemodynamic effects of intravenous labetalol in patients with acute myocardial infarction and systemic arterial hypertension. Curr Ther Res 30:1043–1054
Capone P, Garutti R (1986) Side effect profile of celiprolol in hypertensive patients. In: Satellite symposium of the 11th Scientific Meeting of the International Society of Hypertension: hypertension into the nineties, Heidelberg, 6 Sept 1986
Carey B, Whalley ET (1979) Labetalol possesses β-adrenoceptor agonist action on the isolated rat uterus. J Pharm Pharmacol 31:791–792
Carpenter JR (1981) Intrinsic activity of labetalol on guinea-pig isolated trachea. J Pharm Pharmacol 33:806–807

Caruso FS, Doshan HD, Hernandez PH, Costello R, Applin W, Neiss ES (1985) Celiprolol: pharmacokinetics and duration of pharmacodynamic activity. Br J Clin Pract 39 [Suppl 40]:12–16

Chiariello M, Brevetti, G, De Rosa G, Acunzo R, Petillo F, Rengo F, Condorelli M (1980) Protective effects of simultaneous alpha- and beta-adrenergic receptor blockade on myocardial cell necrosis after coronary arterial occlusion in rats. Am J Cardiol 46:249–254

Chiodini G, Bertolini S, Elicio N, Reggiani E, Valice S (1985) Bevantolol versus propranolol in hypertensive non-insulin-dependent diabetics. Curr Ther Res 38: 586–591

Chodosh S, Tuck J, Blasucci DJ (1988) The effects of dilevalol, metoprolol, and placebo on ventilatory function in asthmatics. J Cardiovasc Pharmacol 11 [Suppl 2]:S18–S24

Christensen NJ, Trap-Jensen J, Svendsen TL, Rasmussen S, Nielson PE (1978) Effect of labetalol on plasma noradrenaline and adrenaline in hypertensive man. Eur J Clin Pharmacol 14:227–230

Chung M, Leitz FH, Maier G, Patrick JE, Gural RP, Symchowitz S (1986) Rising multiple-dose pharmacokinetics of labetalol in hypertensive patients. J Clin Pharmacol 26:248–252

Clifton GG, Poland M, Cook ME, Wallin JD (1988) The effect of single dose dilevalol treatment on blood pressure and renal function of normotensive male volunteers. Curr Ther Res 44:86–93

Cohen ML, Hynes LM (1983) Effect of labetalol and YM-09538 on neuronal uptake of ^{3}H-norepinephrine in the rat vas deferens. Clin Exp Hypertens [A]5:563–575

Cohn JN, Mehta J, Francis GS (1982) A review of the haemodynamic effects of labetalol in man. Br J Clin Pharmacol 13 [Suppl]:19S–26S

Collier JG, Dawney NAH, Nachev C, Robinson BF (1972) Clinical investigation of an antagonist of alpha- and β-adrenoceptor-AH 5158. Br J Pharmacol 44:286–293

Colombo G, Fea F, Planca E, Savioli G, Pellicciolí I (1982) Antihypertensive activity of labetalol and propranolol plus hydralazine association in severe essential hypertension. Curr Ther Res 32:834–843

Cook ME, Clifton GG, Poland MP, Flamenbaum W, Wallin JD (1986) Effects of dilevalol and atenolol on renal function and haemodynamics of patients with mild to moderate hypertension. J Hypertens 4 [Suppl 5]:S504–S506

Cook ME, Wallin JD, Clifton GG, Poland M (1988) Renal function effect of dilevalol, a nonselective beta-adrenergic blocking drug with beta$_2$-agonist activity. Clin Pharmacol Ther 43:393–399

Cooke ED, Maltz MB, Smith RE, Bowcok SA, Watkins CJ, Camm AJ (1987) Peripheral vascular effects of β-adrenoceptor blockade: comparison of two agents. Br J Clin Pharmacol 24:359–366

Cope DHP, Crawford MC (1979) Labetalol in controlled hypotension. Administration of labetalol when adequate hypotension is difficult to achieve. Br J Anaesth 51:359–365

Coulter DM (1979) A comparison of scalp tingling, thirst and polyuria in patients on labetalol and metoprolol. N Z Med J 90:397

Craswell P, Williams J, de Voss K (1977) Labetalol in chronic renal failure with hypertension. Aust N Z J Med 7:441–442

Crofton M, Gabriel R (1977) Pressor response after intravenous labetalol. Br Med J 2:737

Cubberly RB (1985) Labetalol as monotherapy in hypertensive black patients. J Clin Hypertens 4:304–314

Cubeddu LX, Fuenmayor N, Varin V, Villagra VG, Colindres RE, Powell JR (1987a) Clinical pharmacology of carvedilol in normal volunteers. Clin Pharmacol Ther 41:31–44

Cubeddu LX, Fuenmayor N, Varin F, Villagra VG, Colindres RE, Powell JR (1987b) Mechanism of vasodilatory effect of carvedilol in normal volunteers: a comparison with labetalol. J Cardiovasc Pharmacol 10 [Suppl 11]:S81–S84

Cumming AMM, Brown JJ, Fraser R, Lever AF, Morton JJ, Richards DA, Robertson JIS (1979a) Blood pressure reduction by incremental infusion of labetalol in patients with severe hypertension. Br J Clin Pharmacol 8:359–364

Cumming AMM, Brown JJ, Lever AF, Mackay A, Robertson JIS (1979b) Treatment of severe hypertension by repeated bolus injection of labetalol. Br J Clin Pharmacol 8 [Suppl]:199S–204S

Cumming AMM, Brown JJ, Lever AF, Robertson JIS (1982) Intravenous labetalol in the treatment of severe hypertension. Br J Clin Pharmacol 13 [Suppl]:93S–96S

Dage RC, Hsieh CP (1980) Direct vasodilatation by labetalol in anaesthetized dogs. Br J Pharmacol 70:287–293

Dal Palu C, Pessina AC, Semplicini A, Hlede M, Morandin F, Palatini P, Sperti G, Rossi GP (1982) Intravenous labetalol in severe hypertension. Br J Clin Pharmacol 13 [Suppl]:97S–99S

Daneshmend TK, Roberts CJC (1981) Cimetidine and bioavailability of labetalol. Lancet i:565

Daneshmend TK, Roberts CJC (1982) The influence of food on the oral and intravenous pharmacokinetics of a high clearance drug: a study with labetalol. Br J Clin Pharmacol 14:73–78

Dargie HJ, Dollery CT, Daniel J (1976) Labetalol in resistant hypertension. Br J Clin Pharmacol 3 [Suppl]:751–755

Daul A, Wang XL, Borchard U, Bock KD, Brodde OE (1986) Differential changes in lymphocyte β_2-adrenoceptor density by β-blocker administration: role of intrinsic sympathomimetic activity. J Cardiovasc Pharmacol 8 [Suppl 4]:S93–S96

Davidov ME, Moir GD, Poland MP, Maloy J, Medakovic M (1983) Monotherapy with labetalol in the treatment of mild hypertension: a double-blind study. Am J Med 75 [Suppl 4A]:47–53

Dawson A, Johnson BF, Smith IK, Munro-Faure AD (1979) A comparison of the effects of labetalol, bendrofluazide and their combination in hypertension. Br J Clin Pharmacol 8:149–154

DeCesaris R, Grimaldi A, Balestrazzi M, Ranieri G, Chiarappa R, Avantaggiato F (1985) Changes in blood pressure and thermographic values resulting from use of a beta-blocker plus diuretic and of an alpha-beta-blocker plus diuretic. Drugs Exp Clin Res 11:725–729

De Cesaris R, Ranieri G, Chiarappa R, Assereto R, Garzelli P, Martignoni U, Nazzaron P, Pettricione A, Bedoschi D (1988) Comparison of antihypertensive efficacy of carvedilol, a new vasodilating β-blocker, versus atenolol. Drugs 36 [Suppl 6]:102–105

de Sommers, K, de Villiers LS, van Wyk M, Schoeman HS (1981) The effect of labetalol and oxprenolol on blood lipids. S Afr Med J 60:379–380

Devoto P, Stefanini E, Marchisio AM, Vernaleone F, Collu R (1980) Labetalol blockade of central alpha- and beta-noradrenergic receptors in rat brain homogenates. Pharmacol Res Commun 12:177–182

Dianzumba SB, Di Pette DJ, Weber E, Cornman C, Townsend R, Joyner CR (1987) The role of alpha-adrenergic blockade on left ventricular diastolic filling in mild hypertension. Clin Res 35:440 (abstr)

Diehm C (1988) Vasodilating effects of celiprolol in patients with peripheral obliterative arterial disease. J Int Med Res 16 [Suppl 1]:34A–38A

Doggrell SA (1987) Effects of (+)- and (−)-amosulalol on the rat isolated right ventricle. J Cardiovasc Pharmacol 9:213–218

Doggrell SA, Paton DM (1978) Release of noradrenaline by labetalol in the rat anococcygeus muscle. Naunyn-Schmiedeberg's Arch Pharmacol 305:103–108

Doi T, Kobayshi A, Maeda K (1985) Separation of enantiomers of arotinolol hydrochloride and its metabolite by high performance liquid chromatography. Yakugaku Zasshi 105:1145–1149

Dorow P (1988) Celiprolol—review of airway studies. Am J Cardiol 61 [Suppl]:23C–26C

Dorow P, Clauzel AM, Capone P, Mayol R, Mathieu M (1986) A comparison of celiprolol and chlorthalidone in hypertensive patients with reversible brochial obstruction. J Cardiovasc Pharmacol 8 [Suppl 4]:S102–S104

Doshan HD, Rosenthal RR, Brown R, Slutsky A, Applin WJ, Caruso FS (1986a) Celiprolol, atenolol and propranolol: a comparison of pulmonary effects in asthmatic patients. J Cardiovasc Pharmacol 8 [Suppl 4]:S105–S108

Doshan HD, Brown R, Applin WJ, Kapoor M, Caruso FS (1986b) Effects of high doses

of celiprolol in asthmatic patients. J Cardiovasc Pharmacol 8 [Suppl 4]:S109–S111
Drew GM (1978) Pharmacological characterisation of the presynaptic alpha-adrenoceptors regulating cholinergic activity in the guinea-pig ileum. Br J Pharmacol 64: 293–300
Drew GM, Gower AJ, Marriott AS (1977) Pharmacological characterisation of alpha-adrenoceptors which mediate clonidine-induced sedation. Br J Pharmacol 61:468 P (abstr)
Drew GM, Hildtich A, Levy GP (1981) The relationships between the cardiovascular effects, alpha- and beta-adrenoceptor blocking actions and plasma concentration of labetalol in DOCA-hypertensive rats. Clin Exp Hypertens 1:597–611
Due DL, Gigueric GC, Plachetka JR (1986a) Postmarketing comparison of labetalol and propranolol in hypertensive patients. Clin Ther 8:624–631
Due DL, Bradshaw MH, Sirgo MA, Plachetka JR (1986b) Equal antihypertensive efficacy of labetalol in blacks and non-blacks. Curr Ther Res 40:181–190
Dukes ID, Vaughan-Williams EM (1985) Cardiovascular effects of bevantolol, a selective β_1-adrenoceptor antagonist with a novel pharmacological profile. Br J Pharmacol 84:365–380
Dundee JW, Morrow WFK (1979) Labetalol in severe tetanus. Br Med J 1:1121–1122
Dupont AG, van der Niepen P, Taeymans Y, Ingels M, Piepsz A, Bossuyt A, Block P, Six RO, Jonckheer MH, Vanhaelst L (1987) Effect of carvedilol on ambulatory blood pressure, renal hemodynamics and cardiac function in essential hypertension. J Cardiovasc Pharmacol 10 [Suppl 11]:S130–S136
Dusci LJ, Hackett LP (1979) Determination of labetalol in human plasma by high-performance liquid chromatography. J Chromatogr 175:208–210
Edwards RC, Raftery EB (1976) Haemodynamic effects of long-term oral labetalol. Br J Clin Pharmacol 3 [Suppl 3]:733–736
Eggertsen R, Hansson L (1985) Vasodilators in hypertension—a review with special emphasis on the combined use of vasodilators and beta-adrenoceptor blockers. Int J Clin Pharmacol Ther Toxicol 23:411–423
Eggertsen R, Andren L, Sivertsson R, Hansson L (1984a) Acute haemodynamic effects of carvedilol (BM 14.190), a new combined beta-adrenoceptor blocker and precapillary vasodilating agent, in hypertensive patients. Eur J Clin Pharmacol 27:19–22
Eggertsen R, Sivertsson R, Andren LL, Hansson L (1984b) Haemodynamic effects of carvedilol, a new beta-adrenoceptor blocker and precapillary vasodilator in essential hypertension. Hypertension 2:529–534
Ehmer B, van der Does R, Rudorf J (1988) Influence of carvedilol on blood glucose and glycohaemoglobin A_1, in non-insulin dependent diabetics. Drugs 36 [Suppl 6]: 136–140
Eisalo A, Virta P (1982) Treatment of hypertension in the elderly with labetalol. Acta Med Scand [Suppl 665]:129–133
Eisenberg EJ, Patterson WR, Kahn GC (1989) High performance liquid chromatographic method for the simultaneous determination of the enantiomers of carvedilol and its O-desmethyl metabolite in human plasma after chiral derivatization. J Chromatogr Biomed Appl 493:105–115
El Ackad TM, Zeitz HJ, Medacovic M, Samter M (1984a) The effects of labetalol and metoprolol on ventilatory function in patients with bronchial asthma sensitive to propranolol. Clin Res 32:330A (abstr)
El Ackad TM, Curry CL, Hind JE, Roper KO, Saunders EB, Medakovic M (1984b) Comparison of the antihypertensive efficacy of labetalol with that of propranolol in black hypertensive patients. Clin Res 32:330A (abstr)
Erb JM, Sponer G, Bartsch W, Böhm E, Martin U, Strein K (1989) Ratio of alpha:beta-blocking activity of some vasodilating β-blockers in pithed rats and their relation to the hypotensive activity in SHR. Naunyn-Schmiedeberg's Arch Pharmacol 339 [Suppl]:R51 (abstr no 203)
Erichs M, Rothgardt NP, Andersson E (1980) Long-term treatment of hypertension with labetalol. Postgrad Med J 56[Suppl 2]:53–56
Fagard R, Amery A, Reybrouck T, Lijnen P, Billiet L (1979) Response of the systemic

and pulmonary circulation to alpha- and beta-receptor blockade (labetalol) at rest and during exercise in hypertensive patients. Circulation 60:1214–1219

Fagard R, Lijnen P, Amery A (1982) Response of the systemic pulmonary circulation to labetalol at rest and during exercise. Br J Clin Pharmacol 13 [Suppl]:13S–17S

Fairhurst GJ (1986) Comparison of bevantolol and atenolol for systemic hypertension. Am J Cardiol 58 [Suppl]:25E–27E

Farmer JB, Kennedy I, Levy GP, Marshall RJ (1972) Pharmacology of AH 5158:a drug which blocks both alpha- and β-adrenoceptors. Br J Pharmacol 45:660–675

Feek CM, Earnshow PM (1980) Hypertensive response to labetalol in phaochromocytoma. (letter) Br Med J 281:387

Feit A, Holtzman R, Cohen M, El-Sharif N (1985) Effect of labetalol on exercise tolerance and double product in mild to moderate essential hypertension. Am J Med 78:937–941

Fitzgerald GA (1978) Hypertensive response to labetalol in phaeochromocytoma. Lancet i:1259

Flamenbaum W, Weber MA, McMahon FG, Materson BJ, Carr AA, Poland M (1985) Monotherapy with labetalol compared with propranolol: differential effects by race. J Clin Hypertens 1:59–69

Fogari R (1988) The clinical performance and therapeutic potential of celiprolol: effects on lipid metabolism. In: Satellite symposium of the 10th Congress of the European Society of Cardiology: the therapeutic potential of third generation beta-adrenergic receptor blockers, Vienna, 31 Aug 1988

Fogari R, Poletti L, Tettamanti F, Civardi M, Savonitto S (1988) Rest and exercise evaluation of the antihypertensive efficacy of dilevalol and captopril. J Cardiovasc Pharmacol 11 [Suppl 2]:S28–S31

Franz IW, Wievel D, Ketelhut R (1984) Antihypertensiver Effekt einer β-blockierend und vasodilatorisch wirkenden Substanz auf Ruhe- und Belastungsblutdruck im Vergleich zur alleinigen β-Rezeptorenblockade. Verh Dtsch Ges Inn Med 90:750–752

Frishman WH, Michelson EL, Johnson BF, Poland MP (1983) Multiclinic comparison of labetalol to metoprolol in treatment of mild to moderate systemic hypertension. Am J Med 75 [Suppl 4A]:54–67

Frishman WH, Goldberg RJ, Benfield P (1988) Bevantolol. A preliminary review of its pharmacodynamic and pharmacokinetic properties, and therapeutic efficacy in hypertension and angina pectoris. Drugs 35:1–21

Frohlich ED, Tarazi RC, Dustan HP, Page IH (1968) The paradox of beta-adrenergic blockade in hypertension. Circulation 37:417–423

Fujii M, Shirasawa Y, Kondo S, Sawanobori K, Nakamura M (1986) Cardiovascular effects of nipradilol, a beta-adrenoceptor blocker with vasodilating properties. Jpn Heart J 27:233–250

Fujimaki M, Murakoski Y, Hakusui H (1989) Assay and disposition of carvedilol enantiomers in human and monkey: evidence of stereoselective pre-systemic metabolism. J Pharm Sci (in press)

Fujoka M, Suzuki H (1985) Effects of amosulalol on the electrical response of guinea pig vascular smooth muscle to adrenoceptor activation. Br J Pharmacol 84:489–497

Gagnon RM, Morisette M, Presant S, Savard D, Lemire J (1982) Hemodynamic and coronary effects of intravenous labetalol in coronary artery disease. Am J Cardiol 49:1267–1269

Gange RW, Wilson-Jones E (1978) Bullous lichen planus caused by labetalol. Br Med J 1:816–817

Garden A, Devey DA, Dommisse J (1982) Intravenous labetalol and dihydralazine in severe hypertension in pregnancy. Clin Exp Hypertens [B] 1:371–373

George RB, Manocha K, Buford JG, Conrad SA, Kinasewitz GT (1983) Effect of labetalol in hypertensive patients with chronic obstructive pulmonary disease. Chest 83:457–460

Ghose RR (1979) Acute management of severe hypertension with oral labetalol. Br Clin Pharmacol 8 [Suppl]:189S–193S

Gluth WP, Sörgel F, Geldmacher M, Mallinkrodt M (1983) Celiprolol kinetics in healthy volunteers after oral dosing. Naunyn-Schmiedeberg's Arch Pharmacol 324 [Suppl]:

R77 (abstr no 308)
Gold EH, Chang W, Cohen M, Baum T, Ehrreich S, Johnson G, Prioli N, Sybertz EJ (1982) Synthesis and comparison of some cardiovascular properties of the stereoisomers of labetalol. J Med Chem 25:1363–1370
Gomez G, Phillips LA (1980) Labetalol (Trandate) in hypertension: a multicentre study in general practice. Curr Med Res Opin 6:677–684
Gordon RJ, Wolf PS, Pruss TP, Travis J, Sweeney D, Leibowitz M (1983) Further studies on the bronchodilator properties of celiprolol hydrochloride (RHC 5320-A), a cardioselective beta-blocker. Pharmacologist 25:121 (abstr no 109)
Gray JM, Silberman MH, Gorwit JI (1988) Comparison of labetalol and prazosin in hypertensive patients using automated ambulatory monitoring. Am J Med 84: 904–910
Griffith DNW, James IM, Newbury PA, Woollard ML (1979) The effect of β-adrenergic receptor blocking drugs on cerebral blood flow. Br J Clin Pharmacol 7:491–494
Griffith ID, Richardson J (1979) Lupus-type illness associated with labetalol. Br Med J 2:496–497
Gross GJ, Buck JD, Warltier DC, Hardman HF (1979) Beneficial actions of bevantolol on subendocardial blood flow and contractile function in ischemic myocardium. J Cardiovasc Pharmacol 1:139–147
Gulati OP, Gulati N (1980) Effects of labetalol in chronic two-kidney Goldblatt hypertension (2-KGH) in rats. Arch Int Pharmacodyn 243:255–260
Hakusui H, Fujimaki M (1988) Pharmacokinetics of carvedilol in hypertensive patients with renal failure (short communication). Drugs 36 [Suppl 6]:144–147
Hamilton CA, Jones DH, Dargie HJ, Reid JL (1978) Does labetalol increase excretion of urinary catecholamines? Br Med J 2:800
Hansson L (1977) Effects of beta adrenoceptor blocking agents on haemodynamic parameters. Acta Med Scand [Suppl] 606:49–54
Hansson L, Hänel B (1976) Antihypertensive effect of labetalol, a new alpha- and beta-adrenergic blocking agent. Int J Clin Pharmacol 14:195–198
Hara Y, Sato E, Miyagishi A, Aisaka A, Hibino T (1978) Synthesis and β-adrenoceptor blocking action of a new thiazylthiopropanolamine derivative. J Pharm Sci 67: 1334–1335
Hara Y, Sato E, Miyagishi A, Aono S, Nakatani H (1979) Pharmacological properties of dl-2-(3′-t-butylamino-2′-hydroxypropylthio)-4-(5′-carbamoyl-2′-thienyl)thiazole hydrochloride (S-596), a new β-adrenergic blocking agent. Folia Pharmacol Jpn 75:707–720
Hara Y, Nakahara H, Miyagishi A, Nakatani H (1983) Antihypertensive effect of arotinolol (S-596), a new adrenergic β-blocking agent, in experimental hypertensive rats. Folia Pharmacol Jpn 82:103–116
Hashimoto H, Asano M, Hayashi T, Oguro Y, Takiguchi Y, Nakashima M (1984) Hemodynamic effects of arotinolol in anaesthetized dogs and its affinity for adrenoceptors in vitro. Arch Int Pharmacodyn 267:23–34
Hastings SG, Smith RD, Corey RM, Essenburg AD, Pettway CE, Tessman DK (1977) Pharmacological evaluation of CI-775, a cardioselective beta-adrenergic antagonist. Arch Int Pharmacodyn 226:81–99
Hattori Y, Nakaya Y, Endou M, Nakao Y, Kanno M (1989) Vascular effects of carvedilol, a new beta-adrenoceptor antagonist with vasodilating properties in isolated canine coronary artery. J Cardiovasc Pharmacol 13:572–579
Hauger-Klevene JH (1981) Treatment of severe essential hypertension with labetalol: effect on active and inactive renin. Pharmacotherapeutica 3:46–54
Heber ME, Brigden GS, Caruana MP, Lahiri A, Raftery EB (1987a) Carvedilol for systemic hypertension. Am J Cardiol 59:400–405
Heber ME, Rosenthal E, Thomas N, Haskett VL, Burwood RD, Lutkin J, Vincent R, Chamberlain DA (1987b) Effect of labetalol on indices of myocardial necrosis in patients with suspected acute infarction. Eur Heart J 8:11–18
Herrmann JM, Mayer EO (1988) A long-term study of the effects of celiprolol on blood pressure and lipid associated risk factors. Am Heart J 116:1416–1421
Herrmann JM, von Heyman F, Freischütz G (1988a) Lipid profile improvement following

celiprolol. J Int Med Res 16 [Suppl 1]:39A–46A
Herrmann JM, Zieseniss E, Freischütz G (1988b) Betablocker-Therapie der Hypertonie und koronaren Herzkrankheit. Ergebnisse einer 6wöchigen Multizenter-Studie mit Celiprolol an 15256 Patienten. Münch Med Wochenschr 130:735–740
Higaki J, Ogihara T, Nakamaru M, Morishita R, Kumakara Y (1988) Effects of carvedilol on plasma hormonal and biochemical factors and renal function in Japanese patients with essential hypertension (short communication). Drugs 36 [Suppl 6]: 64–68
Hippmann D, Takacs F (1983) Eine quantitative Methode zur Bestimmung von Celiprolol im biologischen Material mit Hilfe der Hochleistungsflüssigchromatographie unter Verwendung eines Fluoreszenz-Detektors. Arzneimittelforschung 33:8–12
Hisa H, Suzuki M, Kamijo T, Satoh S (1984) Effects of K-351 on hemodynamics and renin release in anaesthetized dogs. Arch Int Pharmacodyn 271:169–176
Hitzenberger G, Takacs F, Pittner H (1983) Pharmakokinetik des Beta-Rezeptoren-Blockers Celiprolol nach einmaliger intravenöser und oraler Gabe am Menschen. Arzneimittelforschung 33:50–52
Hofferber E, Jacobitz P, Armah BI (1988) Vasodilating β-receptor antagonists. comparison of labetalol, carvedilol, dilevalol and brefanolol. Naunyn Schmiedeberg's Arch Pharmacol 338 [Suppl]:R65 (abstr no 207)
Hoffmann W, Hoffmann H (1985) Ergebnisse der Selectol-Feldstudie in Österreich. Wien Med Wochenschr 135 [Suppl 93]:3–12
Hoffmann W, Hoffmann H (1986) Results of the Austrian celiprolol postmarketing suveillance study. J Cardiovasc Pharmacol 8 [Suppl 4]:S88–S90
Holtzman JL, Finley D, Johnson B, Berry DA, Sirgo MA (1986) The effects of single-dose atenolol, labetalol and propranolol on cardiac and vascular function. Clin Pharmacol Ther 40:268–273
Homeida M, Jackson L, Roberts CJC (1978) Decreased first-pass metabolism of labetalol in chronic liver disease. Br Med J 2:1048–1050
Honda K, Takenaka T, Shiono K, Miyata-Osawa A, Nakagawa C (1985) Autonomic and antihypertensive activity of oral amosulalol (YM-09538), a combined alpha- and beta-adrenoceptor blocking agent in conscious rats. Jpn J Pharmacol 38:31–41
Honda K, Takenaka T, Miyata-Osawa A, Terai M (1986) Adrenoceptor blocking properties of the stereoisomers of amosulalol (YM-09538) and the corresponding desoxy-derivative (YM-11133). J Pharmacol Exp Ther 236:776–783
Horvath JS, Caterson RJ, Collet P, Duggin GG, Kelly DH, Tiller DJ (1979) Labetalol and bendrofluazide: comparison of their antihypertensive effects. Med J Aust 1: 626–628
Hua ASP, Thomas GW, Kincaid-Smith P (1977) Scalp tingling in patients on labetalol. Lancet ii:295
Hunter JM (1979) Synergism between halothane and labetalol. Anaesthesia 34:257–259
Hunyor SN, Bauer GE, Ross M, Larkin H (1980) Labetalol and propranolol in mild hypertensives. Comparison of blood pressure and plasma volume effects. Aust N Z J Med 10:162–166
Hurley DM, Vandongen R, Beilin LJ (1979) Failure of labetalol to prevent hypertension due to clonidine withdrawal. Br Med J 1:1122
Ikeda M, Masuyama Y, Yoshinaga K, Inagaki Y, Ishii M, Kajiwara N, Kuramoto K, Saruta T, Ogiwara T, Kubo S, Nishio I, Kuramochi M (1986) Clinical response to amosulalol (YM-09538) in essential hypertension: double blind controlled study of amosulalol and labetalol with or without diuretic therapy. Igaku No Ayumi 139: 425–453
Ishii M, Kaneko Y, Omae T (1988) Clinical evaluation of the overall efficacy and safety of dilevalol. In: Satellite symposium of the 12th Scientific Meeting of the International Society of Hypertension; dilevalol: combined beta-blockade and beta$_2$-stimulation in the treatment of hypertension, Kyoto, 21 May 1988
Izumi R, Kunisada K, Niwa M, Ozaki M, Sekine I, Matsuo K, Nishimori I (1985) Effects of chronic administration of arotinolol (ARL, S-596) on stroke-prone spontaneously hypertensive rats (SHRSP). 1st: blood pressure, heart rate and biochemical values. Pharmacometrics 28:455–458

Izumi R, Ozaki M, Sekine I, Nishimori I (1985) Antihypertensive effect of chronic treatment with amosulalol in stroke-prone spontaneously hypertensive rats (SHRSP). Pharmacometrics 29:863–871

Jackson SHD, Beevers DG (1983) Comparison of the effects of single doses of atenolol and labetalol on airway obstruction in patients with hypertension and asthma. Br J Clin Pharmacol 15:533–536

Jain A (1986) Effectiveness of bevantolol in the treatment of hypertension: once-daily versus twice-daily evaluation of home blood pressure measurements. Angiology 37:239–245

Janka HU, Petschke H, Standl A, Mehnert H (1983) Kohlehydrat-und Lipid-Stoffwechsel unter der β-Blocker Therapie mit Celiprolol. Eine Doppelblind-Studie mit Sulfonylharnstoff-behandelten Diabetikern mit Hypertonie. Arzneimittelforschung 33:76–79

Jennings K, Parsons V (1976) A study of labetalol in patients of European, West Indian and West African origin. Br J Clin Pharmacol 3 [Suppl]:773–775

Joekes AM, Thompson FD (1976) Acute haemodynamic effects of labetalol and its subsequent use as an oral hypotensive agent. Br J Clin Pharmacol 3 [Suppl]:789–793

Johnson GL, Prioli NA, Ehrreich SJ (1977) Antihypertensive effects of labetalol (SCH 15719W, AH 5168A). Fed Proc 36:1049 (abstr no 4091)

Johnson LL, Escala EL, Feder J, Stone JE, Weiss MB (1984) Experience with labetalol in patients with hypertension and heart failure. Clin Res 32:A334 (abstr)

Jones SEF (1979) Coarctation in children. Controlled hypotension using labetalol and halothane. Anaesthesia 34:1052–1055

Kabuto S, Kimata H, Yonemitsu M, Koide T, Nakao H, Suzuki J (1985) Pharmacokinetics of the new antihypertensive agent nipradilol in rats. 1st communication: metabolism and disposition after single oral administration of ^{14}C-nipradilol. Arzneimittelforschung 35:1674–1679

Kabuto S, Kimata H, Yonemitsu M, Suzuki J (1986) Metabolism of nipradilol by liver homogenates from different spezies. I. Comparative studies on denitration of nipradilol and other organic nitrates. Xenobiotika 16:307–315

Kaik G (1980) Beta-Rezeptorenblocker und obstruktive Atemwegserkrankung. 6: Celiprolol. In: Kaik G (ed) Bronchospasmolytika und ihre klinische Pharmakologie. Urban and Schwarzenbeck, Munich, pp 428–435

Kamimura H, Sasaki H, Kawamura S (1981) Determination of the alpha, β-adrenoceptor blocker YM-09538 in plasma by high-performance liquid chromatography with fluorescence detection. J Chromatogr 225:115–121

Kamimura H, Sasaki H, Kawamura S, Shimizu M, Matsumoto H, Kobayashi Y (1983) Determination of the alpha, β-adrenoceptor blocker YM-09538 in urine by gas chromatography with a nitrogensensitive detector. J Chromatogr 275:81–87

Kamimura H, Sasaki H, Kawamura S (1985) Metabolism of amosulalol hydrochloride in man: quantitative comparison with laboratory animals. Xenobiotica 15:413–420

Kanda K (1985) Efficacy in lowering blood pressure and influence on various tests of the alpha, beta-blocker arotinolol. Kiso to Rinsyo 19:2733–2744

Kane JA (1982) Labetalol in general practice. A review. Br J Clin Pharmacol 13 [Suppl]:59S–63S

Kanto JH (1985) Current status of labetalol, the first alpha- and beta-blocking agent. Int J Clin Pharmacol Ther Toxicol 23:617–628

Kanto J, Allonen H, Lekonen A, Mäntylä R, Pekkanen A (1980a) Clinical and pharmacokinetic studies in alpha- and beta-blocking drug labetalol. Ther Drug Monit 2:145

Kanto J, Pekkanen A, Allonen H, Kleimola T, Mäntylä R (1980b) The use of labetalol as a moderate hypotensive agent in otological operations—plasma concentrations after intravenous administration. Int J Clin Pharmacol Ther Toxicol 18:191–194

Kanto J, Allonen H, Kleimola T, Mäntylä R (1981) Pharmacokinetics of labetalol in healthy volunteers. Int J Clin Pharmacol Ther Toxicol 19:41–44

Kaplan HR (1986) Bevantolol hydrochloride. Preclinical pharmacological profile. Angiology 37:254–262

Kaplan HR, Chang T, Eckerson HW, Tessman DK (1985) Bevantolol hydrochloride. In:

Scriabine A (ed) New drugs annual: cardiovascular drugs vol 3. Raven, New York, pp 85–97
Kaufman L (1979) Use of labetalol during hypotensive anaesthesia and in the management of phaeochromocytoma. Br J Clin Pharmacol 8 [Suppl]:229S–232S
Kawada M, Satoh K, Taira N (1986) Cardiohemodynamic effects of nipradilol (K-351) in the dog: comparison with propranolol, nadolol and prazosin. Jpn J Pharmacol 42: 9–18
Kawashima K, Watanabe TX, Sokabe H (1984) Pharmacodynamic and pharmacokinetic studies on prizidilol and nipradilol (K-351), antihypertensive drugs with combined vasodilator and beta-adrenoceptor blocking actions in rabbits. Jpn J Pharmacol 36:519–526
Kazumi T, Yoshino G, Okutani T, Kato J, Kasama T, Matsuba K, Iwai M, Yoshida M, Baba S (1988) Short-term effects of arotinolol, a new alpha- and beta-adrenoceptor blocking agent, on plasma lipoproteins and apolipoproteins in hypertensive patients with glucose intolerance. Curr Ther Res 44:40–45
Kelly JG, McGarry K, O'Malley K, O'Brien ET (1982) Bioavailability of labetalol increases with age. Br J Clin Pharmacol 14:304–305
Kennedy I, Levy GP (1975) Combined alpha- and beta-adrenoceptor blocking drug AH 5158: further studies on alpha-adrenoceptor blockade in anaesthetized animals. Br J Pharmacol 53:585–592
Keusch G, Weidmann P, Ziegler WH, de Chatel R, Reubi FC (1980) Effect of chronic alpha- and beta-adrenoceptor blockade with labetalol on plasma catecholamines and renal function in hypertension. Klin Wochenschr 58:25–29
Keusch G, Schiffl H, Binswanger K (1983) Diazoxide and labetalol in acute hypertension during haemodialysis. Eur J Clin Pharmacol 25:523–527
Kimata H, Kabuto S, Yonemitsu M, Koide T, Nakao H, Suzuki J (1985) Pharmacokinetics of the new antihypertensive agent nipradilol in rats. 2nd communication: a single oral administration of ^{14}C-nipradilol to spontaneously hypertensive rats. Arzneimittelforschung 35:1680–1684
Kinhal V, Kulkarni A, Pozerac R (1987) Hemodynamic effects of dilevalol in patients with hypertension and left ventricular dysfunction. In: 3rd European Meeting on Hypertension, Milan 14–17 June, 1987 (abstr no 276)
Kishi K, Kawashima K, Sokabe H, Saito K (1985) Chronic effects of arotinolol (S-596) in spontaneously hypertensive rats. J Pharmacobiodyn 8:50–55
Koch G (1976) Haemodynamic effects of combined alpha- and β-adrenoceptor blockade after intravenous labetalol in hypertensive patients at rest and during exercise. Br J Clin Pharmacol 3 [Suppl]:725–728
Koch G (1977) Acute hemodynamic of an alpha- and β-blocking agent (AH 5158) on the systemic and pulmonary circulation at rest and during exercise in hypertensive patients. Am Heart J 93:585–591
Koch G (1979a) Haemodynamic adaptation at rest and during exercise to long-term antihypertensive treatment with combined alpha- and beta-adrenoceptor blockade by labetalol. Br Heart J 41:192–198
Koch G (1979b) Cardiovascular dynamics after acute and long term alpha- and beta-adrenoceptor blockade at rest supine and standing and during exercise. Br J Clin Pharmacol 8 [Suppl]:101S–105S
Koch G (1979c) Effect of combined alpha- and β-receptor blockade on renal hemodynamics, excretory function, plasma renin and plasma catecholamines in man. Pflüger's Arch 373 [Suppl]:R33 (abstr no 101)
Koch G (1981) Hemodynamic changes after acute and long-term combined alpha-/beta-adrenoceptor blockade with labetalol as compared with beta-receptor blockade. J Cardiovasc Pharmacol 3 [Suppl 1]:S30–S41
Kodama I, Anno T, Toyama J, Yamada K (1985) Electrophysiological effects of nipradilol (K-351) on isolated rabbits hearts and guinea pig ventricular muscles. J Cardiovasc Pharmacol 7:1013–1019
Kofod P, Kjaer K, Veljo S, Hvidt S (1980) Labetalol and alprenolol: a comparative investigation of antihypertensive effect. Postgrad Med J 56 [Suppl 2]:69–74
Kohno M, Takeda T, Ishii M, Saruta T, Mizuno Y, Yoshimura M, Kubo S, Fukiyama K,

Fujishima M (1988a) Therapeutic benefits and safety of carvedilol in the treatment of a renal hypertension: An open short term study. Drugs 36 [Suppl 6]:129–135
Kohno M, Murakawa K, Okamura M, Yasunari K, Yokokawa K, Horio T, Inoue T, Takeda T (1988b) Effects of long term administration of carvedilol on renal hemodynamics and functions in DOCA-salt induced accelerated hypertension of spontaneously hypertensive rats (short communication). Drugs 36 [Suppl 6]:165–168
Kolloch R, Miano L, De Quattro V (1979) Labetalol and urinary catecholamines. Br Med J 1:268–269
Kondo K, Oka T, Okashi K (1984) Pharmacodynamics and pharmacology of nipradilol (K-351) in healthy volunteers in comparison with propranolol. Jpn J Clin Pharmacol Ther 15:9–10
Kornerup HJ, Pedersen EB, Pedersen A, Pedersen G, Christansen NJ (1980) Plasma catecholamines, renin and aldosterone during combined alpha- and beta-adrenoceptor blockade in patients with severe arterial hypertension. Postgrad Med J 56 [Suppl 2]: 49–52
Koskinen P, Pellinen TJ (1987) Effects of bevantolol and propranolol on blood pressure, serum lipids and lipoproteins in essential hypertension. Curr Ther Res 41:952–960
Kou K, Suzuki H (1983) The effects of 3,4-dihydro-8-(2-hydroxy-3-isopropylaminopropoxy)-3-nitroxy-2H-1-benzopyran (K-351) and its denitrated derivative on smooth muscle cells of the dog coronary artery. Br J Pharmacol 79:285–295
Kou K, Kuriyama H, Suzuki H (1982) Effects of 3,4-dihydro-8-(2-hydroxy-3-isopropylaminopropoxy)-3-nitroxy-2H-1-benzopyran (K-351) on smooth muscle cells and neuromuscular transmission in the canine mesenteric artery. Br J Pharmacol 77: 679–689
Kristensen BO, La Cour Petersen E (1980) Effects of long-term high-dose labetalol on blood pressure in patients with severe hypertension resistant to previous therapy. Postgrad Med J 56 [Suppl 2]:57–59
Kritz H, Najemnik C, Irsigler K (1983) Beta-Rezeptoren-Blockade und Diabetes mellitus: Effekt von Celiprolol auf Blutzucker und Insulin-Bedarf bei Typ I- und Typ II-Diabetikern. Arzneimittelforschung 33:72–76
Kubik MM, Coote JH (1984) Propranolol vs metoprolol vs labetalol: a comparative study in essential hypertension. Eur J Clin Pharmacol 26:1–6
Labetalol Hydrochlorothiazide Multicenter Study Group (1985) Labetalol and hydrochlorothiazide in hypertension. Clin Pharmacol Ther 38:24–27
Lahiri A, Rodrigues AE, Al-Khawaja I, Raftery EB (1987) Effects of a new vasodilating beta-blocking drug, carvedilol, on left ventricular function in stable angina pectoris. Am J Cardiol 59:769–774
Lahiri A, Rodrigues AE, Heber ME, van der Does R, Raftery EB (1988) Effects of carvedilol on left ventricular function in essential hypertension and ischemic heart disease (short communication). Drugs 36 [Suppl 6]:141–143
Lammers JWJ, Folgering HTM, van Herwaarden CLA (1985) Ventilatory effects of atenolol and bevantolol in asthma. Clin Pharmacol Ther 38:428–433
Lamming GD, Broughton Pipkin F, Symonds EM (1980) Comparison of the alpha- and beta-blocking drug, labetalol, and methyldopa in the treatment of moderate and severe pregnancy-induced hypertension. Clin Exp Hypertens [A] 2:865–895
Lardoux H, Gerard J, Blazquez G, Fluovat B (1983) Which beta-blocker in pregnancy-induced hypertension? Lancet ii:1194
Larsen JS, Pedersen EB (1980) Comparison of the effects of propranolol and labetalol on the renal haemodynamics at rest and during exercise in essential hypertension. Eur J Clin Pharmacol 18:135–139
Larsson K (1982) Influence of labetalol, propranolol and practolol in patients with asthma. Eur J Respir Dis 63:221–230
Latts JR (1986) Clinical pharmacokinetics and metabolism of bevantolol. Angiology 37:221–225
Lebel M, Langlois S, Belleau LJ, Grose JH (1985) Labetalol infusion in hypertensive emergencies. Clin Pharmacol Ther 37:615–618
Lechi A, Pomari S, Berto R, Buniotto P, Parinello A, Marini F, Cago L, Tomasi A, Baretta G (1982) Clinical evaluation of labetalol alone and combined with chlor-

thalidone in essential hypertension: a double-blind multicentre controlled study. Eur J Clin Pharmacol 22:289–293
Leitz F, Bariletto S, Chung M, Gural M, Jaworsky L, Maier G, Patrick J, Symchowitz S (1982) Bioavailability/pharmacokinetics of labetalol in normotensive male volunteers. Fed Proc 41:1557 (abstr)
Leitz F, Bariletto S, Gural R, Jaworsky L, Patrick J, Symchowicz S (1983) Secretion of labetalol in breast milk of lactating woman. Fed Proc 42:378 (abstr)
Lehtonen A, Allonen H, Kleimola T (1979) Antihypertensive effect and plasma levels of labetalol. A comparison with propranolol and dihydrallazine. Int J Clin Pharmacol Biopharm 17:71–75
Leonetti G, Sampieri L, Cuspidi C, Boselli L, Terzoli L, Rupoli L, Zanchetti A (1987) Resting and postexercise hemodynamic effects of carvedilol, a β-adrenergic blocker and precapillary vasodilator in hypertensive patients. J Cardiovasc Pharmacol 10 [Suppl 11]:S94–S96
Levy GP, Richards DA (1980) Labetalol. In: Scriabine A (ed) Pharmacology of antihypertensive drugs. Raven, New York, p 325–347
Light RW, Chetty KG, Stansbury DW (1983) Comparison of the effects of labetalol and hydrochlorothiazide on the ventialtory function of hypertensive patients with mild chronic obstructive pulmonary disease. Am J Med 75 [Suppl 4A]:109–114
Lijnen PJ, Amery AK, Fagard RH, Reybrouck TM, Moerman EJ, De Schaepdryver AF (1979) Effects of labetalol on plasma renin, aldosterone and catecholamines in hypertensive patients. J Cardiovasc Pharmacol 1:625–632
Lilford RJ (1980) Letter to the editor. Br Med J 281:1635–1636
Lilja M, Jounela AJ, Karppanen H (1982) Comparison of labetalol and clonidine in hypertension. Eur J Clin Pharmacol 21:363–367
Löfdahl CG, Svedmyr K, Svedmyr N (1984) Selectivity of bevantolol hydrochloride, a β_1-adrenoceptor antagonist, in asthmatic patients. Pharmacotherapy 4:205–210
Louis WJ, McNeil JJ (1984) 7. Labetalol. In: Doyle AE (ed) Clinical pharmacology of antihypertensive drugs. Elsevier, Amsterdam, pp 225–245 (Handbook of hypertension, vol 5)
Louis WJ, Christophidis M, Brignell M, Vijayasekaran V, McNeil JJ, Vajda FJE (1978a) Labetalol: bioavailability, drug plasma levels, plasma renin and catecholamines in acute and chronic treatment of resistant hypertension. Aust N Z J Med 8:602–609
Louis WJ, Brignell MJ, McNeil JJ, Christophidis N, Vajda FJE (1978b) Labetalol in hypertension. Lancet i:452–453
Louis WJ, McNeil JJ, Drummer OH (1984) Pharmacology of combined alpha-beta-blockade I. Drugs 28 [Suppl 2]:16–34
Louis WJ, McNeil JJ, Workman BS, Drummer OH, Conway EL (1987) A pharmacokinetic study of carvedilol (BM 14.190) in elderly subjects: Preliminary report. J Cardiovasc Pharmacol 10 [Suppl 11]:S89–S93
Louis WJ, Drummer OH, Tung LH (1988) Actions of dilevalol on adrenoceptors. J Cardiovasc Pharmacol 11 [Suppl 2]:S5–S11
Lucarini A, Salvetti A (1988) Systemic and renal hemodynamic effects of celiprolol in essential hypertensives. Am J Cardiol 61 [Suppl]:45C–48C
Lucas CP, Morledge JH, Tessman DK (1985) Comparison of hydrochlorothiazide and hydrochlorothiazide plus bevantolol in hypertension. Clin Ther 8:49–60
Lund-Johansen P (1979) Comparative haemodynamic effects of labetalol, timolol, prazosin and the combination of tolamolol and prazosin. Br J Clin Pharmacol 8 [Suppl]:107S–111S
Lund-Johansen P (1983a) Central haemodynamic effect of beta-blockers in hypertension. A comparison between atenolol, metoprolol, timolol, penbutolol, alprenolol, pindolol, and bunitrolol. Eur Heart J 4 [Suppl D]:1–12
Lund-Johansen P (1983b) Short- and long-term (six year) hemodynamic effects of labetalol in essential hypertension. Am J Med 75 [Suppl 4A]:24–31
Lund-Johansen P (1984) Pharmacology of combined alpha- beta-blockade. II Haemodynamic effects of labetalol. Drugs 28 [Suppl 2]:35–50
Lund-Johansen P, Bakke OM (1979) Haemodynamic effects and plasma concentrations of labetalol during long-term treatment of essential hypertension. Br J Clin

Pharmacol 7:169–174
Lunell NO, Hjemdahl P, Fredholm BB, Nisell B, Persson B, Wager J (1981) Circulatory and metabolic effects of a combined alpha- and beta-adrenoceptor blocker (labetalol) in hypertension of pregnancy. Br J Clin Pharmacol 12:345–348
Lunell NO, Nylund L, Lewander R, Sarby B (1982) Acute effect of an antihypertensive drug, labetalol, on uteroplacental blood flow. Br J Obstet Gynaecol 89:640–644
Lynch JJ, Montgomery DG, Lucchesi BR (1986) Cardiac electrophysiological actions of SCH 19927 (dilevalol), the R,R-isomer of labetalol. J Pharmacol Exp Ther 239: 719–723
Mabadeje AFB, Okuwobi BO, George BO, Jaiyeola BAO (1982) Crossover trial between labetalol and methyldopa among hypertensive Nigerians. Clin Exp Hypertens [A] 4:330–331
MacCarthy EP, Bloomfield SS (1983) Labetalol, a review of its pharmacology, pharmacokinetics, clinical use and adverse effects. Pharmacotherapy 4:193–219
MacCarthy EP, Frost GW, Stokes GS (1978) Labetalol in hypertensive emergencies. Med J Aust 1:399–400
MacDonald I, Hua ASP, Thomas GW, Woo KT, Withworth JA, Kincaid-Smith P (1980) Use of labetalol in moderate to severe hypertension. Med J Aust 1:325–327
Maclean D (1988) Bevantolol vs propranolol: a double-blind controlled trial in essential hypertension. Angiology 39:487–496
Maconochie JG, Woodings EP, Richards DA (1977) Effects of labetalol and propranolol on histamine-induced bronchoconstriction in normal subjects. Br J Clin Pharmacol 4:157–162
Maharaj RJ, Thompson M, Broch-Utne JG, Williamson R, Downing JW (1983) Treatment of hypertension following endotracheal intubation: a study comparing the efficacy of labetalol, practolol and placebo. S Afr Med J 63:691–694
Malini PL, Strocchi E, Negroni S, Abrosioni E, Magnani B (1982) Renal haemodynamics after chronic treatment with labetalol and propranolol. Br J Clin Pharmacol 13 [Suppl]:123S–126S
Manabe K, Amano K, Hiraaki K, Koga S, Kishikawa H, Takabe S, Kato N, Shigemoto K, Ookubo T (1984) A case of pheochromocytoma-clinical use of YM-09538. Annu Rep Kitakyushu Gen Hosp 1:69–75
Mancia G, Pomidossi G, Parati G, Bertinieri G, Grassi G, Navone F, Ferrari A, Gregorini L, Zanchetti A (1982) Blood pressure response to labetalol on twice and three times daily administration during 24-hour period. Br J Clin Pharmacol 13 [Suppl]:27S–35S
Mancia G, Grassi G, Parati G, Pomidossi G, Sabadini E, Giannattassio C, Bolla G, Zanchetti A (1986) Effects of celiprolol on reflex control of the cardiovascular system in essential hypertension. J Cardiovasc Pharmacol 8 [Suppl 4]:S67–S74
Mäntylä R, Allonen H, Kanto J, Kleimola T, Sellman R (1980) Effect of food on the bioavailability of labetalol. Br J Clin Pharmacol 9:435–437
Maronde RF, Robinson D, Vlachakis ND, Barr JW, Chung M, Zampaglione N, Medakovic M (1983) Study of single and multiple dose pharmacokinetic pharmacodynamic modeling of the antihypertensive effects of labetalol. Am J Med 75 [Suppl 4A]:40–46
Martin LE, Hopkins R, Bland R (1976) Metabolism of labetalol in animals and man. Br J Clin Pharmacol 3 [Suppl]:695–710
Marx PG, Reid DS (1979) Labetalol infusion in acute myocardial infarction with systemic hypertension. Br J Clin Pharmacol 8 [Suppl]:233S–238S
Materson BJ, Lucas CP, Vlachakis ND, Glasser S, Ramanathan KB, Ahmad S, Moreledge JH, Saunders E, Payton CE, Schnaper HW, Maxwell M (1988) Dilevalol compared to metoprolol for treatment of hypertension: a multicenter trial. J Cardiovasc Pharmacol 11 [Suppl 2]:S37 (abstr)
Matsunaga K, Nakamura K, Ueda M (1985) Intrinsic β-sympathomimetic activity of dilevalol, R,R-isomer of labetalol. J Pharmacobiodyn 8:785–787
Matsunaga K, Nakamura K, Ueda M (1986a) Alpha- and beta-blocking activities of dilevalol, R,R-isomer of labetalol, in isolated guinea pig tissues. Pharmacometrics 31:437–439
Matsunaga K, Nakamura K, Ueda M (1986b) Antihypertensive effect of dilevalol in the

experimental hypertensive rat. Pharmacometrics 32:789–799
Matsunaga K, Hara S, Ueda M (1988) The role of beta$_2$-vasodilation of dilevalol in the acute hypotensive effect in spontaneously hypertensive rats. In: Satellite symposium of the 12th Scientific Meeting of the International Society of Hypertension: dilevalol: combined beta-blockade and beta$_2$-vasodilation in the treatment of hypertension, Kyoto, 21 May 1988
Matsuo K, Sekine I, Nishimori I, Kunisada K, Izumi R, Niwa M, Ozaki M (1984) Effects of chronic administration of arotinolol (ARL, S-596) on stroke-prone spontaneously hypertensive rats (SHRSP). 3rd: studies on catecholamine contents in heart and adrenal gland. Pharmacometrics 28:467–471
Matsuura H, Koyama M, Tsuchioka N, Kurogane H, Yoshida M, Kajiyama G, Miyoshi A, Sugihara T, Inoue T (1982) The effects of alpha- and β-adrenoceptor blocking agent (YM-09538) upon the clinical features of a patient with pheochromocytoma. Hormon Rinsho 30:1439–1446
Matthys H, Doshan HD, Rühle KH, Braig H, Pohl M, Applin WJ, Caruso FS, Neiss ES (1985). The bronchosparing effect of celiprolol, a new beta$_1$-, alpha$_2$-receptor antagonist on pulmonary function of propranolol-sensitive asthmatics. J Clin Pharmacol 25: 354–359
Maxwell GM (1973) Effect of an alpha- and beta-adrenoceptor antagonist (AH 5158) upon general and coronary hemodynamics of intact dogs. Br J Pharmacol 49:370–372
Mazzola C, Ferrario N, Calzavara MP, Guffanti E, Vaccarella A (1981) Acute antihypertensive and antiarrhythmic effects of labetalol. Curr Ther Res 29:613–633
McGonigle RJS, Williams L, Murphy MJ, Parsons V (1981) Labetalol and lipids. Lancet i:163
McGrath BP, Matthews PG, Walter NM, Maydom BW, Johnston CI (1978) Emergency treatment of severe hypertension with intravenous labetalol. Med J Aust 2:440–441
McNay LJ, Smith D, Leenen FHH (1985) LY 137224 produces greater alpha$_1$-than beta-adrenoceptor blockade in hypertensive patients. Clin Pharmacol Ther 37:211 (abstr no B49)
McNeil JJ, Louis WJ (1979) A double-blind cross-over comparison of pindolol, metoprolol, atenolol and labetalol in mild to moderate hypertension. Br J Clin Pharmacol 8 [Suppl]:163S–166S
McNeil JJ, Louis WJ (1984) Clinical pharmacokinetics of labetalol. Clin Pharmacokinet 9:157–167
McNeil JJ, Anderson AE, Louis WJ, Morgan DJ (1979) Pharmacokinetics and pharmacodynamic studies of labetalol in hypertensive subjects. Br J Clin Pharmacol 8 [Suppl]:157S–161S
McNeil JJ, Anderson AE, Louis WJ (1981) An analysis of the blood pressure response to labetalol in hypertensive patients. Clin Sci 61[Suppl]:449S–452S
McNeil JJ, Anderson AE, Louis WJ, Raymund K (1982) Labetalol steady state pharmakocinetics in hypertensive patients. Br J Clin Pharmacol 13 [Suppl]:75S–80S
McNeil JJ, Drummer OH, Anderson AIE, Louis WJ (1986) Pharmacokinetics and concentration-effect relationships of bevantolol (CI-775) in normal volunteers. J Cardiovasc Pharmacol 8:1201–1207
McPhillips JJ, Schwemer GT, Scott DI, Zinny M, Patterson D (1988) Effect of carvedilol on blood pressure in patients with mild to moderaty hypertension: a dose response study. Drugs 36 [Suppl 6]:82–91
McRitchie RJ, Chalmers JP (1981) Paradoxical inotropic effects of clonidine and labetalol in the conscious rabbit. J Cardiovasc Pharmacol 3: 818–827
Mehta J, Cohn JN (1977) Hemodynamic effects of labetalol, an alpha- and beta-adrenergic blocking agent, in hypertensive subjects. Circulation 55:370–375
Mehta J, Feldman RL, Marx JD, Kelly GA (1983) Systemic, pulmonary and coronary hemodynamic effects of labetalol in hypertensive subjects. Am J Med 75 [Suppl 4A]:32–39
Meredith PA, McSharry LP, Elliot HL, Reid JL (1982) The determination of labetalol in plasma by high performance liquid chromatography using fluorescent detection. J Pharmacol Methods 6:309–314
Meyer-Sabellek W, Schulte KL, Kloppenburg-Steineke F, Peters P, Gotzen R (1985)

Effects of long-term treatment with carvedilol (BM 14.190) versus metoprolol on haemodynamic parameters. J Hypertens 3:422 (abstr)
Meyer-Sabellek W, Schulte KL, Distler A, Gotzen R (1987a) Follow up of a method of 24-hour indirect blood pressure monitoring: evaluation of carvedilol, a new antihypertensive agent. Nephron 47 [Suppl 1]:42–46
Meyer-Sabellek W, Schulte KL, Distler A, Gotzen R (1987b) Circadian antihypertensive profile of carvedilol (BM 14.190). J Cardiovasc Pharmacol 10 [Suppl 11]:S119–S123
Meyer-Sabellek W, Schulte KL, Streitberg B, Gotzen R (1988) Two years follow up of 24 hour indirect blood pressure monitoring: An open study: evaluation of once-daily and twice-daily regimens of carvedilol (short communication). Drugs 36 [Suppl 6] 106–112
Miano L, Kolloch R, de Quattro V (1979) Increased catecholamine excretion after labetalol therapy: a spurious effect of drug metabolites. Clin Chim Acta 95:211–217
Michael CA (1979) Use of labetalol in the treatment of severe hypertension during pregnancy. Br J Clin Pharmacol 8 [Suppl]:211S–215S
Michael CA (1982) The evaluation of labetalol in the treatment of hypertension complicating pregnancy. Br J Clin Pharmacol 13 [Suppl]:127S–131S
Michelson EL, Frishman WH, Lewis, JE, Edwards WT, Flanigan WJ, Bloomfield SS, Johnson BF, Lucas C, Freis ED, Finnerty FA, Sawin HS, Sabol SA, Long C, Poland MP (1983) Multicenter clinical evaluation of long-term efficacy and safety of labetalol in treatment of hypertension. Am J Med 75 [Suppl 4A]:68–80
Midtbo K, Hals O (1981) Labetalol compared with the combination of propranolol and hydralazine in the treatment of hypertension. Curr Ther Res 29:79–88
Miyagishi A, Nakahara H, Hara Y, Nakatomi H (1983) Effects of the new beta-adrenoceptor blocking agent, S-596 on the peripheral autonomic system and smooth muscles. Arch Int Pharmacodyn 261:222–237
Miyagishi A, Nakahara H, Hara Y (1984) Adrenoceptor blocking effects of arotinolol, a new combined alpha- and beta-adrenoceptor blocking agent. Arch Int Pharmacodyn 271:249–262
Miyano T, Miyagishi A, Hara Y (1984) Acute hypotensive action of a β-adrenoceptor blocking agent, arotinolol in normotensive DOCA-saline and renal hypertensive rats. Pharmacometrics 28:307–313
Monopoli A, Bamonte F, Forlani A, Ongini E, Parravicini L (1984) Effects of the R,R-isomer of labetalol, SCH 19927, in isolated tissues and in spontaneously hypertensive rats during a repeated treatment. Arch Int Pharmacodyn 272:256–263
Morgan T, Gillies A, Morgan G, Adam W (1978) The effect of labetalol in the treatment of severe drug-resistant hypertension. Med J Aust 1:393–396
Morgan T, Snowden R, Butcher L (1987) Effect of carvedilol and metoprolol on blood pressure, blood flow, and vascular resistance. J Cardiovasc Pharmacol 10 [Suppl 11]: S214–S219
Morrison PJ, Bradbrook JD, Mant TG, Robinson J, Altmann J (1987) The pharmacokinetic profile of carvedilol in young and elderly healthy volunteers. Document on file N 14, Boehringer, Mannheim
Moulds RFW, Stevens MJ, Lipe S, Medcalf RL, Iwanov V (1984) Effects of carvedilol on human isolated blood vessels. J Am Coll Cardiol 3, pt 2:566 (abstr)
Myers J, Morgan T, Waga S, Hodgson M, Adam W (1980) Long-term experiences with labetalol. Med J Aust 1:665–666
Nagatomo T, Tsuchihashi H, Sakaki M, Nakagawa Y, Nakahara M, Imai S (1984) Beta-receptor blocking potencies of the three newly synthetized β-antagonists (S-596, K-351, N-696) as assessed with the radioligand assay method in rat cardiac muscle membrane treated with neuraminidase. Jpn J Pharmacol 34:249–254
Nakagawa Y, Shimamoto N, Kakazawa M, Imai S (1980) Alpha- and beta-blocking activity of racemates of labetalol. Jpn J Pharmacol 30:743–745
Nakagawa Y, Nakahara H, Chin WP, Imai S (1985) Alpha-blockade and vasodilatation induced by nipradilol, arotinolol and labetalol in pithed rats. Jpn J Pharmacol 39: 481–485
Nakahara H, Nakazawa M, Takeda K, Imai S (1985a) Role of alpha-adrenergic blocking effect in the acute hypotensive effect of β-adrenergic blocking drugs with alpha-

blocking activities in conscious SHR. Jpn J Pharmacol 39:487–492
Nakahara H, Nakazawa M, Tsukada T, Imai S (1985b) Mechanism of the hypotensive effect of a new beta-adrenergic blocking drug arotinolol (S-596) in anaesthetized rabbits. Arch Int Pharmacodyn 277:253–263
Nakamoto H, Suzuki H, Katsumata H, Ohishi A, Saruta T, Sakaguchi H (1988) Effects of carvedilol on renal function and blood pressure in 3/5 nephrectomized spontaneously hypertensive rats loaded with high salt (short communication). Drugs 36 [Suppl 6]:160–164
Nakamura M, Fujii M, Matsumoto J, Shirasawa Y (1984) Effect of chronic administration of nipradilol (K-351) on altered venous function in spontaneously hypertensive rats. Jpn J Pharmacol 36:66p (abstr)
Nakamura N, Sakakida N, Kishikawa H, Uzawa H (1985) Clinical studies on hypotensive effect of nipradilol (K-351). Curr Ther Res 37:853–866
Nakashima M, Oguchi S (1982) Haemodynamics of a new alpha, beta-blocking agent. Rinsho-Yakuri 13:495–503
Nakashima M, Asano M, Ohguchi S, Hashimoto H, Seki T, Miyazaki M, Takenaka T (1984) Amosulalol, a combined alpha and beta adrenoceptor antagonist: kinetics after intravenous and oral doses. Clin Pharmacol Ther 36:436–443
Nakaya H, Kimura S, Nakao Y, Kanno M (1984) Effects of nipradilol (K-351) on the electrophysiological properties of canine cardiac tissues: comparison with propranolol and sotalol. Eur J Pharmacol 104:335–344
Nanjo T, Kitamura K (1984) Actions of nipradilol (K-351), a new alpha- and beta-adrenoceptor blocker, on the rabbit portal vein. Jpn J Pharmacol 35:359–369
Nattel S, Lawand S, Matthews C, McCans J (1987) Bevantolol disposition in patients with hepatic cirrhosis. J Clin Pharmacol 27:962–966
Nelson GIC, Ahnja RC, Hussain M, Silke B, Taylor SH (1982) Alpha- and beta-blockade with labetalol in acute myocardial infarction. J Cardiovasc Pharmacol 4:921–924
Neugebauer G, Akpan W, von Möllendorff E, Neubert P, Reiff K (1987) Pharmacokinetics and disposition of carvedilol in humans. J Cardiovasc Pharmacol 10 [Suppl 11]: S85–S88
Neugebauer G, Gabor M, Reiff K (1988) Pharmacokinetics and bioavailability of carvedilol in patients with liver cirrhosis (short communication). Drugs 36 [Suppl 6]: 148–154
New Zealand Hypertension Study Group (1981) A multicentre study of labetalol in hypertension. N Z Med J 93:215–218
Nganele DM, DeLeonardis VM, Hintze TH (1988) Celiprolol: a positive inotropic beta-adrenoceptor blocking agent in conscious dogs. Br J Pharmacol 93:501–508
Nicholls DP, Husaini MH, Bulpitt CJ, Stephans MDB, Butler AG (1980) Comparison of labetalol and propranolol in hypertension. Br J Clin Pharmacol 9:233–237
Nishida K, Niki S, Furukawa K, Yamada C, Sugihara H, Katsume H, Ijishi H (1985) Effects of S-596, a new beta-adrenoceptor blocking agent on left ventricular performance of normal subjects during exercise. Jpn Heart J 26:437–449
Norris RJ, Lee EH, Muirhead D, Sanders SW (1986) A pharmacokinetic evaluation of celiprolol in healthy elderly volunteers. J Cardiovasc Pharmacol 8 [Suppl 4]:S91–S92
Novo S, Giamporcaro A, Davi G, Adamo L, Strano A (1984) Chronic administration of labetalol in hypertensives with chronic heart disease (C.H.D.) does not influence plasma lipid concentrations. Curr Ther Res 36:532–536
Nugent CA, Bleicher JM, Plachetka JR, Thomas M (1985) Treatment of elderly hypertensives with labetalol. J Clin Pharmacol 25:634 (abstr)
Nyberg G, Berglund G (1982) Effect of labetalol on the peripheral circulation in hypertensive patients. Acta Med Scand [Suppl] 665:93–101
Nyberg G, Vedin A, Wilhelmsson C (1979) Effects of labetalol and propranolol on blood pressure at rest and during isometric exercise. Eur J Clin Pharmacol 16:299–303
Ogihara T, Ikeda M, Goto Y, Yoshinaga K, Kumahara Y, Iimura O, Ishii M, Murakami E, Takeda T, Kokubu T, Arakawa K (1987) The effect of low dose carvedilol on circadian variation of blood pressure in patients with essential hypertension. J

Cardiovasc Pharmacol 10 [Suppl 11]:S108–S112
Ogihara T, Goto Y, Yoshinaga K, Kumahara Y, Iimura O, Ishii M, Takeda T, Kokubu U, Arakawa K, Ikeda M (1988) Dose-effect relationship of carvedilol in essential hypertension. An open study. Drugs 36 [Suupl 6]:75–81
Ohashi T, Ohashi Y, Irie S et al. (1986) Clinical study on YM-09538 (amosulalol hydrochloride) for preoperative management of pheochromocytoma. Nishinihon J Urol 48:1461–1465
Ohira A, Wada Y, Nakamura M, Kasuya Y, Hamada Y, Shigenobu K (1985) Effects of nipradilol (K-351) on alpha-adrenoceptor mediated responses in various isolated tissues. Arch Int Pharmacodyn 278:61–71
Öhman KP, Asplund J (1984) Labetalol in primary hypertension: a long-term effect and tolerance study. Curr Ther Res 35:277–286
Öhman KP, Weiner L, von Schenck H, Karlsberg BE (1985) Antihypertensive and metabolic effects of nifedipine and labetalol alone and in combination in primary hypertension. Eur J Clin Pharmacol 29:149–154
Oishi S, Sasaki M, Ohno M, Umeda T, Sato T (1988) Periodic fluctuation of blood pressure and its management in a patient with pheochromocytoma. Case report and review of the literature. Jpn Heart J 29:389–399
Okawa KK (1986) Dose response studies of bevantolol in hypertensive patients. Angiology 37:233–238
Olivier LR, Retief JH, Buchel EH, van Niekerk FJ, Schoeman HS (1980) Evaluation of labetalol hydrochloride (Trandate) in hospital outpatients. Clin Trials J 17:75–79
Omvik P, Lund-Johansen P (1982) Acute hemodynamic effects of labetalol in severe hypertension. J Cardiovasc Pharmacol 4:915–920
Pagnan A, Pessina AC, Hlede M, Zanetti G, Dal Palu C (1979) Effects of labetalol on lipid and carbohydrate metabolism. Pharmacol Res Commun 11:227–236
Papademetriou V, Notargiacomo AV, Khatri IM, Freis EM (1982) Treatment of severe hypertension with intravenous labetalol. Clin Pharmacol Ther 32:431–435
Pape J (1974) The effect of alprenolol in combination with hydralazine in essential hypertension. Acta Med Scand [Suppl] 554:55–62
Parati G, Pomidossi G, Casadei R, Ravogli A, Trazzi S, Mutti E, Mancia G (1988) 24-h ambulatory non-invasive blood pressure monitoring in the assessment of the antihypertensive action of celiprolol. J Int Med Res 16 [Suppl 1]:52A–61A
Patel KR (1976) Alpha-adrenoceptor blocking drugs in asthma. Br J Clin Pharmacol 3:601–605
Pearson RM, Havard CWH (1976) Intravenous labetalol in hypertensive patients treated with beta-adrenoceptor blocking drugs. Br J Clin Pharmacol 3 [Suppl]:795–798
Pearson RM, Havard CWH (1978) Intravenous labetalol in hypertensive patients given by fast and slow injection. Br J Clin Pharmacol 5:401–405
Pearson RM, Griffith DNW, Woollard M, James IM, Havard CWH (1979) Comparison of effects on cerebral blood flow of rapid reduction in systemic arterial pressure by diazoxide and labetalol in hypertensive patients. Preliminary findings. Br J Clin Pharmacol 8 [Suppl]:195S–198S
Philip-Joet F, Saadjian A, Bruguerolle B, Arnaud A (1986) Comparative study of the respiratory effects of two β_1-selective blocking agents atenolol and bevantolol in asthmatic patients. Eur J Clin Pharmacol 30:13–16
Pittner H (1983a) Pharmakodynamische Wirkung von Celiprolol, einem cardioselektiven Beta-Rezeptorenblocker. Arzneimittelforschung 33:13–25
Pittner H (1983b) Hämodynamische Wirkungen von Celiprolol und anderen β-Rezeptorenblockern an narkotisierten Hunden. Arzneimittelforschung 33:26–29
Pittner H (1985) Die sympathomimetische Eigenwirkung und ihre Besonderheiten am Beispiel des β_1-Rezeptorenblockers Celiprolol. Wien Klin Wochenschr 97 [Suppl 162]:3–21
Pittner H, Bonelli J (1983) Dosis-Wirkungs-Beziehung von intravenös appliziertem Celiprolol in bezug auf Herzfrequenz und systolischen Blutdruck bei gesunden freiwilligen Versuchspersonen in Ruhe und unter Fahrradergometer-Belastung. Arzneimittelforschung 33:55–57
Plouin PF, Breart G, Milliard F, Papiernik E, Relier JP (1987) Comparison of labetalol

and methyldopa in the treatment of mild to moderate hypertension in pregnancy. J Hypertens 5 [Suppl 5]:S543–S545
Poynter D, Martin LE, Harrison C, Cook J (1976) Affinity of labetalol for ocular melanin. Br J Clin Pharmacol 3 [Suppl]:711–721
Prichard BNC (1984) Combined alpha- and β-receptor inhibition in the treatment of hypertension. Drugs 28 [Suppl 2]:51–68
Prichard BNC, Boakes AJ (1976) Labetalol in long-term treatment of hypertension. Br J Clin Pharmacol 3 [Suppl]:743–750
Prichard BNC, Thompson FO, Boakes AJ, Joekes AM (1975) Some haemodynamic effects of compound AH 5158 compared with propranolol, propranolol plus hydralazine and diazoxide: the use of AH 5158 in the treatment of hypertension. Clin Sci Mol Med 48 [Suppl]:97S–100S
Prichard BNC, Boakes AJ, Hernandes R (1979) Long-term treatment of hypertension with labetalol. Br J Clin Pharmacol 8 [Suppl]:171S–177S
Pristautz M, Stradner F (1986) Wirkung von Celiprolol und Metoprolol auf die Serumlipide bei Patienten mit verschiedenen Formen von Hyperlipoproteinämie. Wien Med Wochenschr 136:443–448
Pruss TP, Khandwala A, Wolf PS, Grebow P, Wong L (1986) Celiprolol: a new beta adrenoceptor antagonist with novel ancillary properties. J Cardiovasc Pharmacol 8 [Suppl 4]:S29–S32
Pugsley DJ, Armstrong BK, Nassim MA, Beilin LJ (1976) Controlled comparison of labetalol and propranolol in the management of severe hypertension. Br J Clin Pharmacol 3 [Suppl 3]:777–782
Pugsley DJ, Nassim MA, Armstrong BK, Beilin LJ (1979) A controlled trial of labetalol (Trandate), propranolol and placebo in the management of mild to moderate hypertension. Br J Clin Pharmacol 7:63–68
Randinitis EJ, Nelson C, Kinkel AW (1984) Gas chromatographic determination of bevantolol in plasma. J Chromatogr Biomed Appl 308:345–349
Randinitis EJ, Nelson C, Kinkel A, Campese V, Welling P (1987) Pharmacokinetics of bevantolol in patients with varying degrees of renal failure. Pharmaceutical Res 4 [Suppl]:S 89 (abstr no pp 641)
Rasmussen S, Nielsen PE (1981) Blood pressure, body fluid volumes and glomerular filtration rate during treatment with labetalol in essential hypertension. Br J Clin Pharmacol 12:349–353
Reach G, Thibonnier M, Chevillard C, Corvol P, Milliez P (1980) Effect of labetalol on blood pressure and plasma catecholamine concentrations in patients with phaeochromocytoma. Br Med J 280:1300–1301
Reid JL, Meredith PA, Elliot HL (1981) Labetalol and the management of hypertension. J Cardiovasc Pharmacol 3 [Suppl 1]:S60–S68
Reiff K (1987) High-performance liquid chromatographic method for the determination of carvedilol and its desmethyl metabolite in body fluids. J Chromatogr Biomed Appl 413:355–362
Renard M, Riviere A, Jacobs P, Bernard R (1983) Treatment of hypertension in acute stage of myocardial infarction. Haemodynamic effects of labetalol. Br Heart J 49: 522–527
Richards DA, Prichard BNC (1978) Concurrent antagonism of isoproterenol and norepinephrine after labetalol. J Clin Pharmacol Ther 23:253–258
Richards DA, Tuckman J, Prichard BNC (1976) Assessment of alpha- and beta-adrenoceptor blocking actions of labetalol. Br J Clin Pharmacol 3 [Suppl]:849–855
Richards DA, Prichard BNC, Boakes AJ, Tuckman J, Knight EJ (1977a) Pharmacological basis for antihypertensive effects of intravenous labetalol. Br Heart J 39:99–106
Richards DA, Maconochie JG, Bland RE, Hopkins R, Woodings EP, Martin LE (1977b) Relationship between plasma concentration and pharmacological effects of labetalol. Eur J Clin Pharmacol 11:85–90
Richards DA, Prichard BNC, Dobbs RJ (1978) Adrenoceptor blockade of the circulatory responses to intravenous isoproterenol. Clin Pharmacol Ther 24:264–273
Richards DA, Prichard BNC, Hernandez R (1979a) Circulatory effects of noradrenaline and adrenaline before and after labetalol. Br J Clin Pharmacol 7:371–378

Richards DA, Harris DM, Martin LE (1979b) Labetalol and urinary catecholamines. Br Med J 1:685
Riddell JG, Shanks RG, Brogden RN (1987) Celiprolol: a preliminary review of its pharmacodynamic and pharmacokinetic properties and its therapeutic use in hypertension and angina prectoris. Drugs 34:438–458
Riddell JG, McCaffrey PM, Shanks RG (1988) An assessment of the dose dependency of the partial agonist activity of dilevalol by its effect on sleeping heart rate in normal volunteers. In: 12th Scientific Meeting of International Society of Hypertension, Kyoto, 22–26 May 1988 (abstr no 1028)
Riley, AJ, Riley EJ (1981) The effect of labetalol and propranolol on the pressure response to sexual arousal in woman. Br J Clin Pharmacol 12:341–344
Riley AJ, Riley EJ, Davies HJ (1982) A method for monitoring drug effects on male sexual response: the effect of single dose labetalol. Br J Clin Pharmacol 14:695–700
Rittinghausen R (1988) Response rate with respect to blood pressure lowering effect of the vasodilating and β-blocking agent carvedilol. Drugs 36 [Suppl 6]:92–101
Romo M, Saarinen P, Sarna S (1984) Comparison of labetalol and pindolol in hypertension. Curr Ther Res 36:195–200
Ronne-Rasmussen JO, Anderson GS, Boewal-Jensen N, Andersson E (1976) Acute effect of intravenous labetalol in the treatment of systemic arterial hypertension. Br J Clin Pharmacol 3 [Suppl]:805–808
Rosenthal T, Rabinowitz B, Boichis E, Elazar E, Brauner A, Neufeld HN (1981) Use of labetalol in hypertensive patients during discontinuation of clonidine therapy. Eur J Clin Pharmacol 20:237–240
Rossi A, Ziacchi V, Lomanto B (1982) The hypotensive effect of a single daily dose of labetalol: a preliminary study. Int J Clin Pharmacol Ther Toxicol 20:438–445
Roy L, Metha J, Metha P (1983) Increased plasma concentration of prostacyclin metabolite 6-keto PGF_{1alpha} in essential hypertension. Influence on therapy with labetalol. Am J Cardiol 51:464–467
Rubin PC, Butters L, Kelman AW, Fitzsimons C, Reid JL (1983) Labetalol disposition and concentration-effect relationship during pregnancy. Br J Clin Pharmacol 15: 465–470
Rudorf JE, Ehmer B, van der Does R (1988) Pharmacokinetic and pharmacodynamic interactions of combined acute administration of carvedilol and hydrochlorothiazide in hypertensive volunteers (short communication). Drugs 36 [Suppl 6]:113–117
Rumboldt Z, Bagatin J, Vidovic A (1983) Diazoxide vs. labetalol: a crossover comparison of short term effects in hypertension. Int J Clin Pharmacol Res 3:47–54
Saito T, Yamamoto K, Sugiyama Y, Inagaki Y (1985) Haemodynamic effect of nipradilol (K-351) in essential hypertension. Jpn J Clin Pharmacol Ther 16:727–733
Sakanashi M, Miyamoto Y, Takeo S, Noguchi K (1983) Effects of a new beta-adrenoceptor blocking agent, S-596 (arotinolol), on isolated dog coronary arteries. Arch Int Pharmacodyn 263:208–216
Sakanashi M, Takeo S, Ito H, Naguchi K, Miyamato Y, Higa T (1984a) Effects of an antihypertensive agent, nipradilol, on isolated coronary artery of the dog. Pharmacology 29:241–246
Sakanashi M, Miyamoto Y, Ito H, Takeo S, Noguchi K, Higa T (1984b) Possible alpha-adrenoceptor activity of arotinolol (S-596), a new β-adrenoceptor blocking agent in isolated dog coronary artery. Pharmacology 29:204–209
Sakanashi M, Noguchi K, Takeo S, Ito H, Miyamoto Y, Kato T (1985) Effects of nipradilol (K-351) on cardiac function in anaesthetized open-chest dogs. Arch Int Pharmacodyn 274:47–55
Salonen JT, Taskinen E, Salonen R, Seppänen K, Venäläinen J, Rauramaa R (1986) Effects of bevantolol and atenolol on symptoms, exercise tolerance and metabolic risk factors in angina pectoris. Am J Cardiol 58 [Suppl]:35E–40E
Salvetti R, Pedrinelli R, Sassano P, Arzilli F (1979) Effects of increasing doses of labetalol on blood pressure, plasma renin activity and aldosterone in hypertensive patients. Clin Sci 57:401S–404S
Sanders GL, Routledge PA, Rao JG, Gales GM, Davies DM, Rawlins MD (1978)

Labetalol, a cross-over double-blind controlled trial. Eur J Clin Pharmacol 14: 301–304

Sanders GL, Routledge PA, Ward A, Davies DM, Rawlins MD (1979) Mean steady state plasma concentrations of labetalol in patients undergoing antihypertensive therapy. Br J Clin Pharmacol 8 [Suppl]:153S–155S

Sannerstedt R, Stenberg J, Vedin A, Wilhelmsson G, Werkö L (1972) Chronic beta-adrenergic blockade in arterial hypertension. Hemodynamic influences of dihydralazine on dynamic exercise and clinical effects of combined treatment. Am J Cardiol 29:718–723

Schindl R, Würtz J, Hoffmann M (1986) The effect of the cardioselective beta-blocker celiprolol on pulmonary function in asthmatic patients. J Cardiovasc Pharmacol 8 [Suppl 4]:S99–S101

Schmidt P, Takacs F, Pittner H, Minar E, Balke P, Zazgornik J, Deutsch E (1985) Vergleichende Pharmakokinetik des β_1-Rezeptoren-Blockers Celiprolol nach oraler Einzeldosis an Nierengesunde und Patienten mit eingeschränkter Nierenfunktion. Wien Klin Wochenschr 97:729–732

Schnurr E, Widmann L, Glocke M (1987) Efficacy and safety of carvedilol in the treatment of hypertension. J Cardiovasc Pharmacol 10 [Suppl 11]:S101–S107

Schoenberger J, Frishman W. Gorwit J, Wallin JD, Davidov M, Michelson E (1988a) Comparison of the side effect profile of dilevalol and propranolol. J Cardiovasc Pharmacol 11 [Suppl 2]:S39 (abstr)

Schoenberger J, Frishman W, Liebson P, Strom J (1988b) The effect of dilevalol on left ventricular performance in hypertensive elderly patients. J Cardiovasc Pharmacol 11 [Suppl 2]:S38 (abstr)

Scott DB (1982) The use of labetalol in anaesthesia. Br J Clin Pharmacol 13 [Suppl]: 133S–135S

Scott DB, Buckley FB, Drummond GB, Littlewood DG, Macrae WR (1976) Cardiovascular effects of labetalol during halothane anaesthesia. Br J Clin Pharmacol 3 [Suppl]: 817–821

Seedat YK (1979) Labetalol hydrochloride in the treatment of black and Indian hypertensive patients. Med Proc 25:53–57

Seki N, Nagao K, Komori K, Suzuki H (1988) Alpha- and beta-adrenoceptor blocking action of carvedilol in the canine mesenteric artery and vein. J Pharmacol Exp Ther 246:1116–1122

Sekine I, Matsuo K, Takagi Y, Shimizu K, Kishikawa M, Nishimori I, Kunisada K, Izumi R, Ozaki M (1984) Effect of chronic administration of arotinolol (ARL, S-596) on stroke-prone spontaneously hypertensive rats (SHRSP). 2nd: histopathological studies. Pharmacometrics 28:459–465

Selen A, Kinkel AW, Darke AC, Greene DS, Welling PG (1986) Comparative single dose and steady-state pharmacokinetics of bevantolol in young and elderly subjects. Eur J Clin Pharmacol 30:699–704

Semplicini A, Pessina AC, Rossi GP, Hlede M, Morandin F (1983) Alpha-adrenoceptor blockade by labetalol during long-term dosing. Clin Pharmacol Ther 33:278–282

Shimizu S, Yamauchi Y, Ikuta J, Nakamura M, Kuga H, Saito N (1982) Antihypertensive action of 3,4-dihydro-8-(2-hydroxy-3-isopropylamino)propoxy-3-nitroxy-2H-1-benzpyran (K-351) in hypertensive rats. Jpn J Pharmacol 32:135p (abstr)

Shirasawa Y, Fujii M, Nakazawa M, Kondo S, Ohira A, Nakamura M (1982) Vasodilating and β-adrenoceptor blocking actions of K-351, a new antihypertensive agent. Jpn J Pharmacol 32 [Suppl]:175P (abstr)

Shirasawa Y, Fujii M, Nakamura M (1985) Venodilating action of nipradilol (K-351) in pithed rats pretreated with dihydroergotamine. Jpn J Pharmacol 39:77–82

Shlevin HH, Barrett JA, Thompson GF, Wolf PS, Pruss TP, Smith RD (1983) Celiprolol HC1: propranolol-insensitive cardiostimulatory effects in anaesthetized dogs. Pharmacologist 25:836 (astr)

Skinner C, Gaddie J, Palmer KNV (1975) Comparison of intravenous AH 5158 (Ibidomide) and propranolol in asthma. Br Med J 2:59–61

Smith RD, Wolf PS (1984) Celiprolol. In: Scriabine A (ed) New drugs annual.

Cardiovascular drugs. Raven, New York, pp 19–35
Smith WB, Clifton GG, O'Neill WM, Wallin JD (1983) Antihypertensive effectiveness of intravenous labetalol in accelerated hypertension. Hypertension 5:579–583
Snedden W, Fernandez PG (1988) Cadiovascular and neurohumoral responses to chronic cardioselective beta antagonist therapy in hypertension. Clin Res 36 (3):433 A (abstr)
Snedden W, Fernandez PG, Nath C (1987) The blood pressure responses of thiazide-resistant hypertensives to a once-a-day bevantolol regimen. Can J Cardiol 3:322–325
Solimon M, Massry SG, Campese VM (1986) Renal hemodynamics and pharmacokinetics of bevantolol in patients with impaired renal function. Am J Cardiol 58 [Suppl]:21E–24E
Sponer G, Bartsch W, Strein K, Müller-Beckmann B, Böhm E (1987a) Pharmacological profile of carvedilol as a β-blocking agent with vasodilating and hypotensive properties. J Cardiovasc Pharmacol 9:317–327
Sponer G, Strein K, Müller-Beckmann B, Bartsch W (1987b) Studies on the mode of vasodilating action of carvedilol. J Cardiovasc Pharmacol 10 [Suppl 11]:S42–S48
Sponer G, Bartsch W, Strein K, Müller-Beckmann B, Kling L (1988) Mode of vasodilating action of carvedilol in isolated perfused hind limbs of rabbits (short communication). Drugs 36 [Suppl 6]:55–61
Staiger C, Steger W, Widmann L, Ehmer B, Holtbrügge W (1988) Double-blind, controlled clinical trial to evaluate the antihypertensive effect of carvedilol in elderly patients with mild to moderate hypertension (short communication). Drugs 36 [Suppl 6]:169–171
Strein K, Sponer G, Müller-Beckmann B, Barstsch W (1987) Pharmacological profile of carvedilol, a compound with beta-blocking and vasodilating properties. J Cardiovasc Pharmacol 10 [Suppl 11]:S33–S41
Sundberg S, Tiihonen K, Gordin A (1987) Vasodilatory effects of carvedilol and pindolol. J Cardiovasc Pharmacol 10 [Suppl 11]: S76–S80
Suzuki-Kusaba M, Hisa H, Kimura T, Satoh S (1988) Effects of arotinolol on hemodynamics and adrenergically induced renin release and renal vasoconstriction. Arzneimittelforschung 38:671–677
Svendson TL, Rasmussen S, Hartling OJ, Nielsen PE, Trap-Jensen J (1980) Acute and long-term effects of labetalol on systemic and pulmonary haemodynamics in hypertensive patients. Eur J Clin Pharmacol 17:5–11
Sybertz EJ, Sabin CS, Pula KK, Vliet GV, Glennon J, Gold EH, Baum T (1981) Alpha and beta adrenergic blocking properties of labetalol and its R,-R-isomer, SCH 19927. J Pharmacol Exp Ther 218:435–443
Tadepalli AS, Novak PJ (1986) Intrinsic sympathomimetic activity of labetalol. J Cardiovasc Pharmacol 8:44–50
Takayanagi I, Kizawa Y, Iwasaki S, Nakagoshi A (1987) (±)-1-[[2-(3,4-dimethoxphenyl) ethyl]amino]-3-(3-methylphenoxy)-2-propanol hydrochloride (bevantolol, NC-1400) as a β_1-selective adrenoceptor blocker with $alpha_1$-adrenoceptor blocking activity. Gen Pharmacol 18:87–89
Takeda T, Kaneko Y, Omae T, Yoshinaga K, Masuyama Y, Nukada T, Shigiya R (1982) The use of labetalol in Japan: results of multicentre clinical trials. Br J Clin Pharmacol 13 [Suppl]:49S–57S
Takeda T, Kaneko Y, Omae T (1988) Long term evaluation of the overall efficacy and safety of dilevalol. In: Satellite-symposium of the 12th Scientific Meeting of the International Society of Hypertension; dilevalol: combined beta-blockade and $beta_2$-vasodilatation in the treatment of hypertension, Kyoto, 21 May 1988
Takekoshi N, Murakami E, Matusi S, Murakami H, Emoto J, Hashimoto A (1983) Studies on concurrent alpha- and beta adrenoceptor blocking action of S-596 (arotinolol). Jpn Heart J 24:925–933
Takenaka T (1987) Amosulalol. In:Scriabine A (ed) New cardiovascular drugs 1987, vol 5. Raven, New York, pp 117–134
Takenaka T, Shiono K, Honda K, Asano M, Miyazaki I, Maeno H (1982a) Antihypertensive and adrenoceptor blocking properties of new sulfonamide-substituted phenylethylamines. Clin Exp Hypertens [A] 4:125–137
Takenaka T, Asano M, Berdeaux A, Guidicelli JF (1982b) Adrenoceptor blocking,

hemodynamic and coronary effects of YM 09538, a new combined alpha- and beta-adrenoceptor blocking drug, in anaesthetized dogs. Eur J Pharmacol 85:35–50

Takenaka T, Shiono K, Honda K, Maeno H (1984) Preferential blockade of postsynaptic alpha-adrenoceptors by amosulalol (YM-09538), a new combined alpha- and beta-blocking agent, in the pulmonary artery of the rabbit. Biogenic Amines 1:285–289

Tamaki T, Hasui K, Yamamoto A, Aki Y, Shoji T, Nakamura A, Kimura S, Fukui K, Iwao H, Abe Y (1988) Renal vasodilatory action of carvedilol in the dog (short communication). Drugs 36 [Suppl 6]:155–159

Tanaka M, Masumara H, Tanaka S, Akashi A (1987) Studies on the antihypertensive properties of carvedilol, a compound with beta-blocking and vasodilating effects. J Cardiovasc Pharmacol 10 [Suppl 11]:S52–S57

Tarazi RC, Dustan HP (1972) Beta adrenergic blockade in hypertension. Practical and theoretical implications of long-term hemodynamic variations. Am J Cardiol 29: 633–640

Tcherdakoff (1983) Side effects with long-term labetalol: an open study of 251 patients in a single centre. Pharmacotherapeutica 3:342–348

Thibonnier M, Lardoux MD, Corvol P (1980) Comparative trial of labetalol and acebutolol alone or associated with dihydralazine in treatment of essential hypertension. Br J Clin Pharmacol 9:561–567

Thompson FD, Joekes AM, Hussein MM (1977) Labetalol used as a hypotensive agent in the presence of renal disease. Kidney Int 11:287–288

Thompson FD, Joekes AM, Hussein MM (1978) Monotherapy with labetalol for hypertensive patients with normal and impaired renal function. Br J Clin Pharmacol 8 [Suppl]:129S–133S

Thulesius O, Gjöres JE, Berlin E (1982) Vasodilating properties of β-adrenoceptor blockers with intrinsic sympathomimetic activity. Br J Clin Pharmacol 13 [Suppl]: 229S–230S

Thulin T, Henningsen NC, Karlberg BE, Nilsson OR (1981) Clinical and metabolic effects of labetalol with atenolol in primary hypertension. Curr Ther Res 30:194–204

Timmis AD, Fowler MS, Jaggarao NSV, Chamberlain DA (1980) Labetalol infusion for the treatment of hypertension in acute myocardial infarction. Eur Heart J 1:413–416

Tomlinson B, Cronin CJ, Graham BR, Smith CCT, Prichard BNC (1985) Haemodynamics and pharmacokinetics of carvedilol (BM 14.190). Br J Clin Pharmacol 19: 566P (abstr)

Tomlinson B, Cronin CJ, Graham BR, Prichard BNC (1986) Acute haemodynamic effects of carvedilol compared to propranolol, labetalol and pindolol. Br J Clin Pharmacol 21:581P–582P (abstr)

Tomlinson B, Cronin CJ, Graham BR, Prichard BNC (1987) Haemodynamics of carvedilol in normal subjects compared with propranolol, pindolol, and labetalol. J Cardiovasc Pharmacol 10 [Suppl 11]:S69–S75

Tomlinson B, Bompart F, Graham BR, Liu J, Prichard BNC (1988) Vasodilating mechanism and response to physiological pressor stimuli at acute doses of carvedilol compared with labetalol, propranolol and hydralazine. Drugs 36 [Suppl 6]:37–47

Toothaker RD, Randinitis EJ, Nelson C, Kinkel AW, Goulet JR (1987) The influence of food on the oral absorption of bevantolol. J Clin Pharmacol 27:297–299

Trap-Jensen J, Clausen JP, Hartling OJ, Svendsen TL, Kroogsgard AR (1980) Immediate effect of labetalol on central, splanchnic-hepatic and forearm haemodynamics during pleasant emotional stress in hypertensive patients. Postgrad Med J 56 [Suppl 2]:34–42

Trieb G, Sigwart U (1978) Die Wirkung des neuen Beta-Rezeptorenblockers Bevantolol (CI 775) auf die linksventrikuläre Ruhe- und Belastungshämodynamik. Herz 3: 276–287

Trimarco B, Lembo G, DeLuca N, Ricciardelli B, Rosiello G, Volpe M, Orofino G, Condorelli M (1988) Long-term reduction of peripheral resistance with celiprolol and effects on left ventricular mass. J Int Med Res 16 [Suppl 1]:62A–72A

Trust PM, Rosei EA, Brown JJ, Fraser R, Lever AF, Morton JJ, Robertson JIS (1976) Effect of blood pressure, angiotensin II and aldosterone concentrations during treatment of severe hypertension with labetalol: comparison with propranolol. Br J Clin Pharmacol 3[Suppl]:799–803

Tsukiyama H, Otsuka K (1984) Hemodynamic effects of the alpha, beta blocker arotinolol and the alpha blockers bunazosin und prazosin in essential hypertension. Rinsho-Yakuri 15:341–354

Tsukiyama H, Otsuka K, Higuma K (1985) Haemodynamic effects of short term treatment with nipradilol in hypertension. Ther Res 3:1121–1129

Uchida Y (1982) Cardiovascular effect of [3,4-dihydro-8-(2-hydroxy-3-isopropylamino-propoxy)-3-nitrato-2H-benzopyran] (K-351). Jpn Heart J 23:981–988

Uchida Y, Nakamura M, Shimziu S, Shirasawa Y, Fujii M (1983) Vasoactive and β-adrenoceptor blocking properties of 3,4-dihydro-8-(2-hydroxy-3-isopropylamino) propoxy-3-nitroxy-2H-1-benzopyran (K-351), a new antihypertensive agent. Arch Int Pharmacodyn 262:132–149

Uchida Y, Nakamura M, Tsuruta T, Yoshimura M (1987) Nipradilol. In: Scriabine A (ed) New cardiovascular drugs 1987, vol 5. Raven, New York, pp 95–115

Ueda H, Kaneko Y, Kuramoto K, Yasuda H, Oyama Y, Kanazawa T, Yoshinaga K, Ishii M, Uchida Y, Inoue K (1987) Clinical effect of nipradilol (K-351) in combination with thiazide diuretic on essential hypertension. A multi-central double blind comparison with propranolol. Clin Eval 15:73–106

Valvo E, Previato G, Tessitore N, Oldrizzi L, Gammaro L, Corgnati A, Maschio G (1981) Effects of long-term administration of labetalol on blood pressure, hemodynamics and renal function in essential and renal hypertension. Curr Ther Res 29: 634–641

van der Veur E, ten Berge BS, Donker AJM, May JF, Wesseling H (1982) Comparison of labetalol, propranolol and hydralazine in hypertensive outpatients. Eur J Clin Pharmacol 21:457–460

van Inwegen RG, Khandwala A, Weinryb I, Pruss TP, Neiss E, Sutherland CA (1984) Effect of celiprolol (REV 5320), a new cardioselective beta-adrenoceptor antagonist, on in vitro adenylate cyclase, alpha- and beta-adrenergic receptor binding and lipolysis. Arch Int Pharmacodyn 272:40–55

van Schoor JJF (1979) A once a day dose of labetalol hydrochloride in the treatment of hypertension in general practice. Med Proc 25:59–61

Varin F, Cabeddu LX, Powell JR (1986) Liquid chromatographic assay and disposition of carvedilol in healthy volunteers. J Pharm Sci 75:1195–1197

Vaughan-Williams EM (1987) Bevantolol: a beta-adrenoceptor antagonist with unique additional actions. J Clin Pharmacol 27:450–460

Verdouw PD, Hartog JM, Saxena PR, Hugenholtz PG (1986) Systemic and regional hemodynamic, antiarrhythmic and antiischemic effects of bevantolol in anaesthetized pigs. Am J Cardiol 58 [Suppl]:8E–16E

Vermej P, van Brummelen P (1986) Pharmacokinetic parameters of bevantolol. Eur J Clin Pharmacol 30:375–377

von Möllendorff E, Abshagen U, Akpan W, Neugebauer G, Schröter E (1986) Clinical pharmacologic investigations with carvedilol a new beta-blocker with direct vasodilator activity. Clin Pharmacol Ther 39:677–682

von Möllendorff E, Sponer G, Strein K, Bartsch W, Müller-Beckmann B, Neugebauer G, Czerwek H, Bode G, Schnurr E (1987a) Carvedilol. In: Scriabine A (ed) New cardiovascular drugs 1987, vol 5. Raven, New York, pp 135–153

von Möllendorff E, Reiff K, Neugebauer G (1987b) Pharmacokinetics and bioavailability of carvedilol, a vasodilating beta-blocker. Eur J Clin Pharmacol 33:511–513

Waal-Manning HJ, Simpson FO (1982) Review of long term treatment with labetalol. Br J Clin Pharmacol 13 [Suppl]:66S–73S

Wallin JD (1983) Antihypertensives and their impact on renal function. Am J Med 75 [Suppl 4A]:103–108

Wallin JD, Wilson D, Winer N, Maronde RF, Michelson EL, Langford H, Maloy J, Poland M (1983) Treatment of severe hypertension with labetalol compared with methyldopa and furosemide. Result of a long-term, double-blind, multicenter trial. Am J Med 75 [Suppl 4A]:87–94

Wallin JD, Cook ME, Clifton GG, Blasucci DJ, Poland M (1988) Intravenous dilevalol. Effects of the R-R optical isomer of labetalol in patients with severe hypertension. Arch Intern Med 148:534–538

Walstadt RA, Nilsen OG, Berg KJ, Wessel-Aas T (1981) The pharmacokinetics and clinical effect of one single dose of labetalol in patients with normal and impaired renal function. Acta Pharmacol Toxicol 49 [Suppl 1]:54 (abstr F 27)

Walstadt RA, Berg KJ, Wessel-Aas T, Nilsen OG (1982) Labetalol in the treatment of hypertension in patients with normal and impaired renal function. Acta Med Scand [Suppl] 665:135–141

Warltier DC, Gross GJ, Jesmok GJ (1980) Protection of ischemic myocardium: comparison of effects of propranolol, bevantolol, and a dimethyl propranolol on infarct size following coronary occlusion in anaesthetized dogs. Cardiology 66:133–146

Watanabe T, Sokabe H, Kawashima K (1985) An analysis of blood pressure effects of nipradilol and prizidilol in normotensive and spontaneously hypertensive rats. Jpn J Pharmacol 38:273–279

Watkins R, Cadeno K, Cook J, McLeod R, Pula K, Tedesco R, Sybertz EJ (1988a) Role of beta$_2$-receptor stimulation in the peripheral vascular actions of the antihypertensive dilevalol. In: 12th Scientific Meeting of the International Society of Hypertension, Kyoto 22–26 May 1988 (abstr no 911)

Watkins RW, Sybertz EJ, Antonellis A, Pula K, Rivelli M (1988b) Effects of the antihypertensive dilevalol on artery compliance in anesthetized dogs. J Cardiovasc Pharmacol 12:42–50

Watson A, Maher K, Koegh JAB (1981) Labetalol and renal function. Ir J Med Sci 150:174–177

Weber MA, Drayer JIM, Kaufman CA (1984) The combined alpha- and beta-adrenergic blocker labetalol and propranolol in the treatment of high blood pressure: similarities and differences. J Clin Pharmacol 24:103–112

Weidmann P, de Chatel R, Ziegler WH, Flammer J, Reubi F (1978) Alpha- and beta-adrenergic blockade with oral administered labetalol in hypertension. Studies on blood volume, plasma renin and aldosterone and catecholamine excretion. Am J Cardiol 41:570–576

Wendt T, van der Does R, Schröder R, Landgraf H, Kober G (1987) Acute hemodynamic effects of the vasodilating and beta-blocking agent carvedilol in comparison to propranolol. J Cardiovasc Pharmacol 10 [Suppl 11]:S147–S150

Wendtland W, Pittner H (1983) Toxikologische Prüfung von Celiprolol, einem kardioselektiven β-Rezeptorenblocker. Arzneimittelforschung 33:41–49

Wesley AG, Hariparsad D, Pather M, Rocke DA (1983) Labetalol in tetanus. Anaesthesia 38:243–249

West MH, Wing LMH, Mulligan J, Walkley J, Grygiel JJ, Graham JR, Chalmers JP (1980) Comparison of labetalol, hydralazine and propranolol in the therapy of moderate hypertension. Med J Aust 1:224–225

Whitehead EM, McKaigue JP, Riddell JG, Shanks RG (1988) Beta-adrenoceptor antagonism and cardioselectivity of dilevalol in man. Br J Pharmacol 93 [Suppl]:C82 (abstr)

Wilcox PG, Ahmad D, Darke AC, Parsons J, Carruthers SG (1986) Respiratory and cardiac effects of metoprolol and bevantolol in patients with asthma. Clin Pharmacol Ther 39:29–34

Williams JG, De Voss K, Craswell PW (1978) Labetalol in the treatment of hypertensive renal patients. Med J Aust 1:225–228

Williams LC, Murphy MJ, Parsons V (1979) Labetalol in severe and resistant hypertension. Br J Clin Pharmacol 8 [Suppl]:143S–147S

Wilson DJ, Wallin JD, Vlachakis MD, Freis ED, Michelson EL, Longford HG, Flamenbaum W, Poland MP (1983) Intravenous labetalol in the treatment of severe hypertension and hypertensive emergencies. Am J Med 75 [Suppl 4A]:95–102

Wood AJ, Ferry DG, Bailey RR (1982) Elimination kinetics of labetalol in severe renal failure. Br J Clin Pharmacol 13 [Suppl]:81S–86S

Woods PB, Robinson ML (1981) An investigation of the comparative liposolubilities of beta-adrenergic blocking agents. J Pharm Pharmacol 33:172–173

Yamada K, Tojama J, Tanaka T (1986) Clinical effect and utility of nipradilol (K-351) in essential hypertension. Multicentre double-blind comparison with pindolol. Ther Res 4:1289–1320

Yasujima M, Goto Y, Yoshinaga K, Kumahara Y, Iimura O, Ishii M, Murakami E, Takeda T, Kokubu T, Arakawa K, Ikeda M (1988) Efficacy and tolerance of carvedilol in combination with a thiazide diuretic in the treatment of essential hypertension. An open study (short communication). Drugs 36 [Suppl 6]:118–123
Yeung CK, Thomas GW, Withworth JA, Kincaid-Smith P (1979) Comparison of labetalol, clonidine and diazoxide intravenously administered in severe hypertension. Med J Aust 2:499–500
Yoshimura M, Kojima J, Itoh T, Suzuki J (1985a) Pharmacokinetics of nipradilol (K-351), a new antihypertensive agent. I. Studies on interspecies variation in laboratory animals. J Pharmacobiodyn 8:738–750
Yoshimura M, Kojima J, Itoh T, Fujii M, Suzuki J (1985b) Pharmacokinetics of nipradilol (K-351) a new antihypertensive agent. II. Influence of the route of administration on bioavailability in dogs. J Pharmacobiodyn 8:503–512
Yoshimura M, Kojima J, Itoh T, Suzuki J, Tsutsui S, Kato K (1985c) Pharmacokinetics of nipradilol (K-351), a new antihypertensive agent, in human. Jpn Clin Pharmacol Ther 16:679–691
Yoshimura M, Kojima J, Itoh T, Suzuki J (1985d) Structural determination of dog and human urinary metabolites of nipradilol (K-351) a new antihypertensive agent. Chem Pharm Bull (Tokyo) 33:3456–3468
Zacest R, Gilmore E, Koch-Weser J (1972) Treatment of essential hypertension with combined vasdilation and beta-adrenergic blockade. N Engl J Med 286:617–622

CHAPTER 6

Centrally Acting Drugs (Clonidine, Methyldopa, Guanfacine)

W. KOBINGER and L. PICHLER

CONTENTS

1 History

A great number of drugs which act upon the CNS also lower blood pressure and heart rate, for example, some hypnotics and narcotic analgesics. These drugs, however, exert other central actions which are more prominent, and therefore the central hypotensive effect might be called nonspecific. The discovery of the antihypertensive action of clonidine and its central mode of action set a new standard for a class of drugs which might be called "specific central antihypertensives" (for reviews, VAN ZWIETEN 1975; SCHMITT 1977; KOBINGER 1978). Although clonidine has CNS side effects, its cardiovascular depressive effects are prominent; despite its peripheral cardiovascular effects, its central site of action is widely agreed to be primarily responsible for the hypotension. The history of reserpine illustrates the difficulty involved in specifying a multiply active drug as being mainly centrally or peripherally active (for review, KOBINGER 1984a). The class of clonidine-like hypotensive drugs was first defined by two criteria, namely a direct stimulation of peripheral α-adrenoceptors and a hypotensive effect of CNS origin (KOBINGER 1978). By means of these criteria a number of chemically different drugs were classified as members of the same group. Some of them are listed in Fig. 1, including guanfacine.

The antihypertensive effect of α-methyldopa can also be explained as clonidine-like using the criteria mentioned above. The active metabolite of α-methyl-

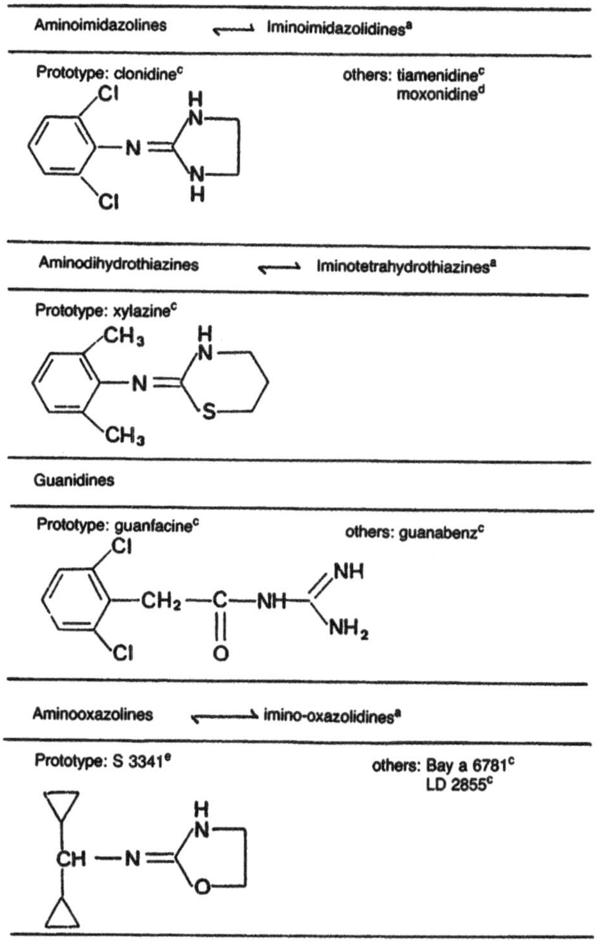

dopa is α-methylnoradrenaline. Originally it was assumed that this metabolite replaced the natural transmitter noradrenaline from peripheral sympathetic nerve endings, thereby impairing neurotransmission (false transmitter hypothesis: DAY and RAND 1964). Later, it was shown that α-methyldopa acts via its metabolite α-methylnoradrenaline by stimulating CNS α-adrenoceptors, much in the same way as clonidine (HENNING and VAN SWIETEN 1968; for review, VAN ZWIETEN 1975).

2 Chemistry

Figure 1 shows the chemical structure of the three drugs to be discussed and moreover shows a number of compounds which fit into the term clonidine-like drugs by the definition given in Sect. 1. These structures show similarities to the clonidine prototype. Thus, the first four substances have as a common structure an amidine moiety (JEN et al. 1972, 1975):

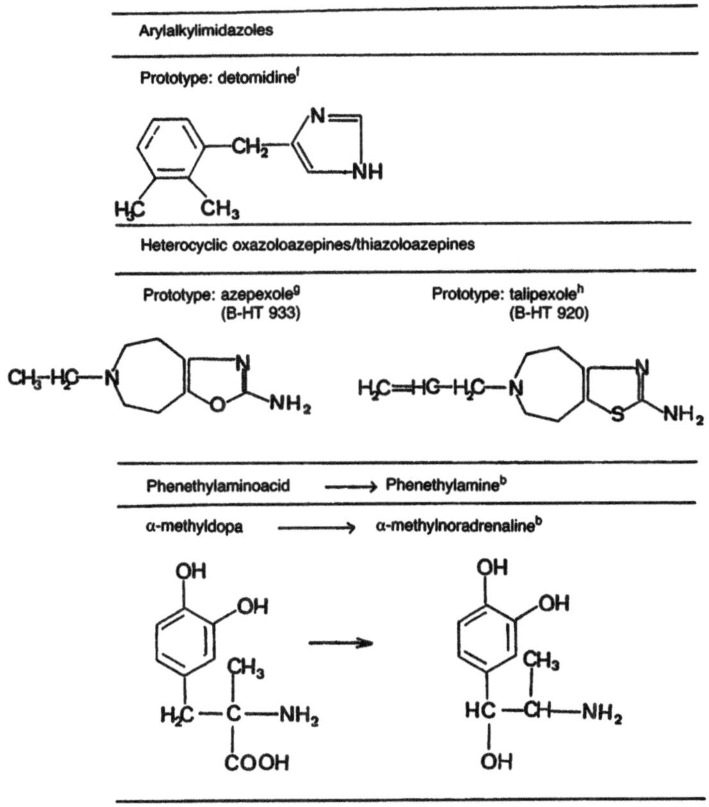

Fig. 1. Chemical structures of some clonidine-like drugs.
[a] Because of the possibility of tautomeric forms, a shift of the C=N double bond towards the bridge N results in the respective imino form. [b] The amine is the active principle. [c] KOBINGER 1978; [d] MANNHOLD 1987; [e] VAN ZWIETEN et al. 1986; [f] SAVOLA et al. 1985; [g] KOBINGER and PICHLER 1977; [h] PICHLER and KOBINGER 1981

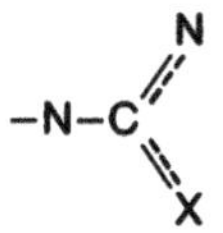

where X stands for C, N, O, or S. This includes cyclic guanidines, cyclic isoureas and isothioureas, as well as open-chain guanidines, e.g., guanfacine.

Others are chemically quite different, as for example, B-HT 920 and B-HT 933 as well as α-methylnoradrenaline, which is the active principle of α-methyldopa.

As will be described in Sect. 4.3, the mode of action of these drugs has been explained as stimulation of α-adrenoceptors. Therefore, attempts have been made by determination of several interatomic distances within a number of phenylethylamine and imidazolidine molecules to find common structures which fit into a hypothetical α-adrenoceptor model. These efforts have been successful for imidazolidines (WERMUTH et al. 1973). The crystal structure of azepexole (Fig. 1, B-HT 933) did not fit into the molecular model of the other clonidine-like drugs; however, common stereo-electronic properties were described which may explain the action on the α-adrenoceptor (HUMBLET et al. 1981).

On the other hand the spatial dimension requirements among biologically active arylalkylimidazoles were considered to be different from those of phenylethylamines (SAVOLA et al. 1986).

3 Pharmacokinetics, Metabolism

3.1 Clonidine

In humans, clonidine is excellently absorbed from the gastrointestinal tract; the bioavailability was calculated between 71% and 100% (DAVIES et al. 1977; ARNDTS 1983; ARNDTS et al. 1983). Elimination half-life in plasma was estimated between 7 and 11 h using gas chromatographic procedures (DAVIES et al. 1977; WING et al. 1977; FRISK-HOLMBERG et al. 1978). The introduction of a specific radioimmunoassay allowed the detection of pure clonidine, excluding any questionable metabolites, and the sensitivity of this method allowed us to follow the plasma concentrations for more than 72 h after reasonable therapeutic doses (ARNDTS 1983; ARNDTS et al. 1983). Using this method, half-life values of 20–25 h were reported for terminal elimination. The urinary excretion of unchanged clonidine averages about 62%, independent of the oral dose (varying between 0.075 and 2.1 mg). When clonidine was given in tablets 0.15 mg twice daily (12-h interval), steady state plasma concentrations were reached after day 4 with fluctuations between 0.8 and 1.1 ng/ml (ARNDTS et al. 1983), and there was no evidence of drug accumulation (WING et al. 1977).

Using [^{14}C]clonidine the total radioactivity excreted in urine was approximately 65% and in feces, 22% (REHBINDER and DECKERS 1969). Considering the high excretion rate of clonidine via the kidneys, it is not unexpected that excretion is retarded in patients with renal insufficiency. The disappearance rate of clonidine in plasma varies directly with creatinine clearance (HULTER et al. 1979). However, maintenance of blood pressure control could be achieved with appropriate dosing even in patients with end-stage renal disease, with clonidine plasma levels reaching as high as 30 ng/ml (LOWENTHAL et al. 1983).

The pharmacokinetic of clonidine in animals differs from that in humans insofar as elimination is much faster. Thus, the plasma half-life in rats, cats, dogs, and rabbits is between 1 and 2 h (JARROTT and SPECTOR 1978; PAALZOW and EDLUND 1979; REID et al. 1980), and tubular secretion of the drug has been shown in rats (CONWAY and JARROTT 1982). Tissue distribution of clonidine was studied in the rat: the kidney had the highest concentration followed by liver and spleen and then by small intestine and brain (CONWAY and JARROTT 1980). Obviously the drug does not accumulate selectively in the brain, the presumed site of action. Excretion of total radioactivity after oral [^{14}C]clonidine in rats and dogs amounted to approximately 66% and 80%, respectively, in the urine and to 33% and 18%, respectively, in feces (REHBINDER and DECKERS 1969).

There is no qualitative difference in the metabolic pattern of clonidine between humans, rats, and dogs (DARDA et al. 1978). The two main pathways of metabolism are hydroxylation of the phenyl ring to give *p*-hydroxyclonidine, and splitting of the imidazolidine ring to give dichlorophenylguanidine. The degree of metabolic degradation is different with these species, however, as humans and rats excrete mainly (approx. 55%–60%) unchanged clonidine in the urine, whereas dogs excrete mainly metabolites (approx. 94%; REHBINDER and DECKERS 1969; DARDA et al. 1978).

3.2 Guanfacine

After intravenous and oral application of single doses of [^{14}C]guanfacine in humans, the data regarding the parent compound reveal a bioavailability of approximately 100% in both cases and an elimination half-life of 18 and 21 h, respectively (KIECHEL 1980). A smaller mean plasma half-life or 12.2 (range 9.4–15.3 h) after an oral dose of 3 mg was reported by DOLLERY and DAVIES (1980) from normotensive volunteers. Excretion of total radioactivity in urine was 85%, including approximately 30% of the parent compound (KIECHEL 1980; SCHOLTYSIK et al. 1980).

Elimination seems to be much faster in animals than in humans as indicated in the review of KIECHEL (1980): in rats, no plasma concentrations could be measured 24 h after oral administration, and in rats and dogs only very low amounts were excreted in the urine after 24–48 h.

Metabolism of guanfacine in humans occurs at the aromatic nucleus only, starting with the formation of an epoxide intermediate (KIECHEL 1980). Thereafter, either hydroxylation at position 3 followed by conjugation as the *O*-glucuronide (35%) or sulphate (8%), or the formation of 3-mercapturic acid derivatives (17%). Essentially the same metabolites occur in rats and dogs; however, the ratio of parent compound to metabolites is smaller than in humans (BEVERIDGE et al. 1977, reviewed in KIECHEL 1980).

3.3 α-Methyldopa

After oral administration in humans, α-methyldopa is incompletely absorbed from the gastrointestinal tract. Following administration of 500 mg of ^{14}C-labelled α-methyldopa, only 43% of the radioactivity is recovered in the 48-h urine (STENBAECK et al. 1977). The parent drug appeared at a level of about 15%, and the maximal plasma concentration of unconjugated α-methyldopa was about 2.0 μg/ml, occurring 2 h after ingestion. When bioavailability was studied by comparison of plasma concentrations (area under the concentration-time curve) after oral and i.v. administration, it ranged between 9% and 18% (BARNETT et al. 1977). It must be considered, however, that bioavailability varies considerably from day to day due to interference with food; thus, a protein-rich meal seems to reduce both the rate and degree of bioavailability (for review, MYHRE et al. 1982).

Plasma elimination data from healthy volunteers have been reported recently by MYHRE et al. (1982). Based on chemical analysis of unconjugated α-methyldopa, a biphasic curve was observed: the half-life of the distribution phase was 0.21 h (range 0.16–0.26 h) and of the elimination phase, 1.28 h (range 1.02–1.69 h).

In patients with essential hypertension and normal renal function there was a good correlation between oral drug dose and plasma concentrations, but there was no correlation between plasma concentrations and the antihypertensive effect when patients with normal and impaired renal function were compared: patients with impaired renal function reacted much more sensitively (STENBAEK et al. 1971).

In contrast to the other drugs described in this section, the metabolism of α-methyldopa is not only of interest for the elimination of the drug but also provides the key to our understanding of its mode of action (Sect. 4.3). Some of

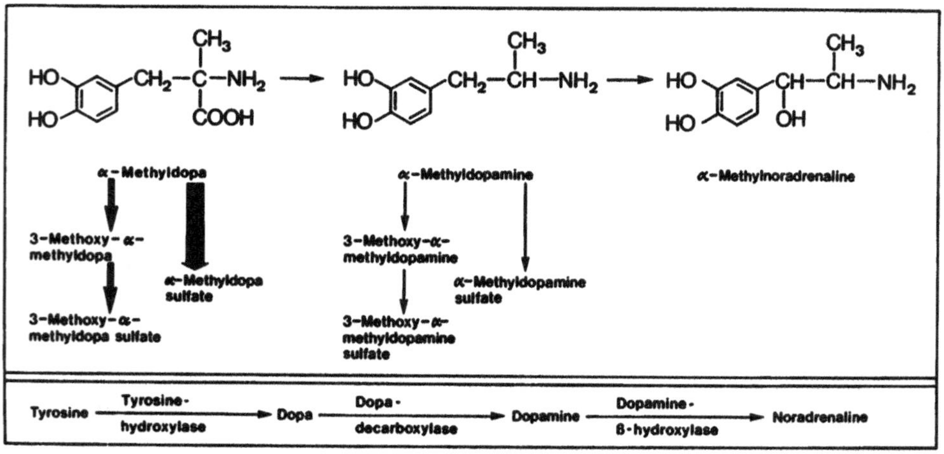

Fig. 2. *Upper part*, structure of α-methyldopa and of the metabolites of the "false transmitter pathway" (*horizontal arrows*); other metabolic pathways are indicated by *vertical arrows* (human, oral administration). *Lower part*, pathway of the natural transmitter and the enzymes involved

the metabolites are shown in Fig. 2. After oral administration 25%–50% of the total dose excreted by the kidneys are acid-labile conjugates, mainly *O*-sulfates of α-methyldopa (and α-methyldopamine), metabolites which after i.v. administration have only been observed in very small amounts. It therefore appears that these metabolites derive predominantly from a first pass effect of gastrointestinal absorption and/or enterohepatic circulation (SAAVEDRA et al. 1975; KWAN et al. 1976). Small amounts are excreted as 3-methoxy-α-methyldopa, 3-methoxy-α-methyldopamine, and their sulfate conjugates (see OATES et al. 1977).

A small but—as far as antihypertensive activity is concerned—important part of the metabolism of α-methyldopa is its conversion into α-methyldopamine and α-methylnoradrenaline. This can be seen from Fig. 2, and this figure also shows the last steps of the synthesis of the natural transmitter noradrenaline. After α-methyldopa has been taken up into peripheral adrenergic neurons and into the CNS, it undergoes biotransformation to α-methyldopamine and α-methylnoradrenaline, the latter displacing stoichiometrically the natural transmitter noradrenaline. α-Methylnoradrenaline accumulates in the storage granules of adrenergic neurons and is released by electrical stimulation instead of noradrenaline ("false transmitter"; CARLSSON and LINDQUIST 1962; MUSCHOLL and MAÎTRE 1963; DAY and RAND 1964; OATES et al. 1977).

4 Hemodynamic Effects, Pharmacodynamics, and Mechanism of Action

4.1 Hemodynamic Effects

4.1.1 Clonidine

A typical cardiovascular response pattern is elicited by rapid intravenous injection of clonidine (5–500 μg/kg) into anesthetized or conscious animals: an initial brief increase in blood pressure is followed by a gradual decrease; bradycardia and a decrease in cardiac output parallel the changes in blood pressure (Fig. 3). No pressor phase was observed after slow i.v. infusion (NAYLER et al. 1968), and no hypertension followed oral administration of therapeutic doses to humans. The extent of the initial pressure effect is negatively correlated with the initial blood pressure. In hypertensive patients clonidine produces a greater fall in blood pressure than in normotensive subjects (WING et al. 1977). The hypotension is due to a fall of both systolic and diastolic pressure by about the same degree (BENTLEY and LI 1968). The total peripheral vascular resistance is initially increased, falling to control levels during the hypotensive phase. In the experiment depicted in Fig. 3 the hypotension is solely due to decrease in cardiac output. Similar results were obtained in other animal experiments (LAUBIE and SCHMITT 1969; MAXWELL 1969) and in humans by GRABNER et al. (1966) and VORBURGER et al. (1968). However, there are also reports of a decrease in total peripheral resistance in animals (CONSTANTINE and MCSHANE 1968) and in humans (GRABNER et al. 1966; MUIR et al. 1969; ONESTI et al.

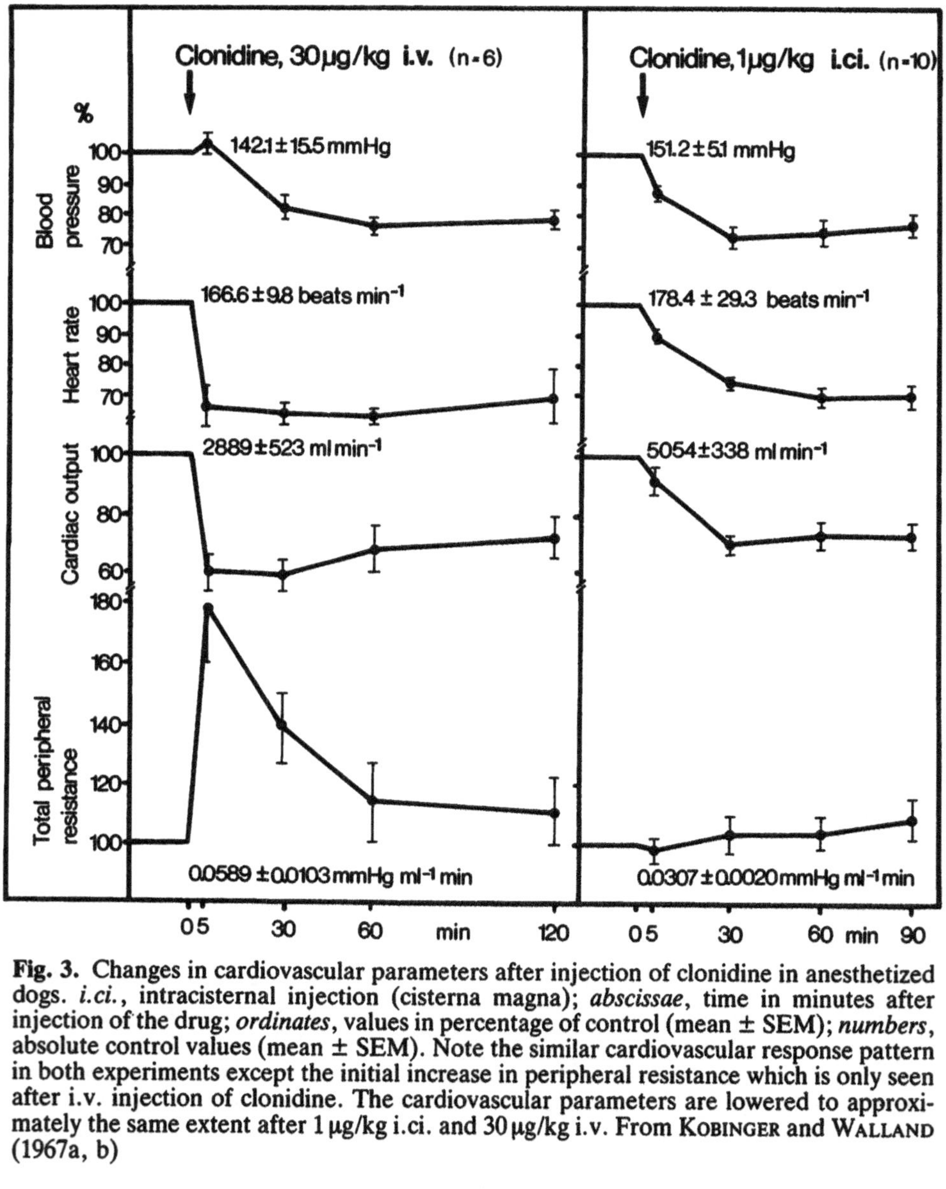

Fig. 3. Changes in cardiovascular parameters after injection of clonidine in anesthetized dogs. *i.ci.*, intracisternal injection (cisterna magna); *abscissae*, time in minutes after injection of the drug; *ordinates*, values in percentage of control (mean ± SEM); *numbers*, absolute control values (mean ± SEM). Note the similar cardiovascular response pattern in both experiments except the initial increase in peripheral resistance which is only seen after i.v. injection of clonidine. The cardiovascular parameters are lowered to approximately the same extent after 1 µg/kg i.ci. and 30 µg/kg i.v. From KOBINGER and WALLAND (1967a, b)

1969). There was no change in renal blood flow and glomerular filtration rate (ONESTI et al. 1969). During 12 weeks' treatment of hypertensive patients, clonidine in doses of 200 µg thrice daily reduced blood pressure, heart rate, and total peripheral resistance but did not significantly change cardiac output, renal blood flow, glomerular filtration rate, or blood volume (THANANOPAVARN et al. 1982). In humans, severe orthostatic side effects did not occur, and the clonidine-induced decrease in blood pressure was the same in the supine and erect positions (GRABNER et al. 1966; ONESTI et al. 1971; SCHWARTZ et al. 1973). The drug had little effect on the blood pressure response to a Valsalva maneuver and caused a slight decrease in the pressure response to immersion of one hand into ice cold water (DOLLERY et al. 1976). In animal experiments clonidine either decreased or did not decrease pressor reflexes, which are mediated mainly by the sympathetic nervous system; this is due to different states of anesthesia and to various degrees of reflex stimuli (see KOBINGER 1978).

4.1.2 Guanfacine

The cardiovascular reaction pattern for guanfacine is similar to that of clonidine (for review, SORKIN and HEEL 1986). After i.v. injection in anesthetized animals an initial blood pressure increase is followed by a secondary decrease, and the heart rate is reduced. In contrast to clonidine the pressure rise is more pronounced and of longer duration (SCHOLTYSIK et al. 1975; BARBER and REID 1982). Thus, in conscious rabbits the hypotensive effect started 1 h after injection as compared with approximately 3 min after clonidine. In these experiments i.v. injection of guanfacine, 300 μg/kg, lowered blood pressure to the same extent as clonidine, 30 μg/kg i.v., thus giving the relative potency of guanfacine as 0.1 when compared with clonidine (BARBER and REID 1982). The dose ratio of 1 : 10 was also reported by SAAMELI et al. (1982) for oral administration in hypertensive rats. OATES et al. (1978) described dose-response curves in anesthetized rats, in which the same maximal fall in blood pressure was obtained with guanfacine as with clonidine; the potency of guanfacine as compared with clonidine was 1/20 after i.v. and 1/10 after i.m. administration. In comparison with the hypotensive effect the vasopressor component of guanfacine seems to be more pronounced: in pithed rats the relative potency was 0.3 compared with clonidine (KLEINLOGEL et al. 1975). Guanfacine reduced the blood pressure of healthy volunteers. The potency as compared with clonidine was reported on a weight basis of 1/10 (DOLLERY and DAVIES 1980) and from 1/14 to 1/17 (systolic and diastolic, respectively; CHIERICHETTI et al. 1982). DOLLERY and DAVIS (1980) also compared the time course of the hypotensive effect of 3 mg guanfacine orally versus 0.3 mg clonidine orally. The main difference was the much slower onset of the effect of guanfacine: at 1.5 h the blood pressure was significantly lower after clonidine than after guanfacine; the lowest values were comparable for both drugs, and at other times the differences were not statistically significant. For both drugs blood pressure values at 24 h after ingestion remained below the control values, therefore, the statement that guanfacine acts longer than clonidine seems not justified (DOLLERY and DAVIES 1980).

Detailed data on the hemodynamic effects of guanfacine are available from human studies. During and immediately after i.v. administration of 4 mg guanfacine the blood pressure, peripheral resistance, and pulmonary artery pressure increase, and the heart rate and cardiac output decrease. Subsequently, blood pressure and peripheral resistance decrease, reaching a significant level after 24 h. Due to large individual differences, significant changes in the cardiac output were not found (MAGOMETSCHNIGG et al. 1980). Within 2 h after oral treatment a reduction of pulmonary arterial pressure, pulmonary capillary wedge pressure, and heart rate but no changes in systemic blood pressure, cardiac index, systemic and pulmonary vascular resistance were reported (FELDSTEIN et al. 1984). After chronic treatment (6 weeks, average dose 3.9 mg/day) of hypertensive patients the decrease in blood pressure was associated with a significant decrease in systemic vascular resistance without change in cardiac output (FELDSTEIN et al. 1984). In a 6-week, single-blind, crossover study with guanfacine (mean daily dose 3 mg) and guanethidine, lowering of blood pressure and heart rate but no orthostatic side effects were reported with guanfacine; guanethidine lowers blood pressure to the same extent but shows orthostatic hypotension in 11 of the 16 ambulant patients (SZÁM and KÁLLAY 1980).

4.1.3 α-Methyldopa

α-Methyldopa must be considered as a prodrug, and hypotensive activity can be observed only if the active metabolite appears at the sensitive site (CNS; Sect. 4.3.1). Therefore, hypotensive effects are not easily demonstrable in acute experiments in anesthetized normotensive animals (KRONEBERG 1962/63; TAUBERGER and KUHN 1971). In renal hypertensive rats a single s.c. injection of a high dose (300 mg/kg) of α-methldopa reduces blood pressure with a maximal effect after 4–8 h, returning to initial values within 24–48 h (WALDMEIER et al. 1975). In hypertensive patients α-methyldopa acutely decreases blood pressure, heart rate, and either total peripheral vascular resistance or cardiac output (for review, KIRKENDALL and WILSON 1962; SANNERSTEDT and CONWAY 1970). In long-term treatment of moderately severe hypertensive patients α-methyldopa at an average dose of 4.15 g/day was equieffective with clonidine (1.33 mg/day) in lowering blood pressure in the lying and standing positions as well as after exercise (CONOLLY et al. 1972). In long-term studies the decrease in blood pressure by α-methyldopa was reported to be associated with either reduction in peripheral vascular resistance or with reduction in cardiac index; renal vascular resistance and plasma renin activity were reduced whereas myocardial and cerebral blood flow were increased (for review, SCRIABINE 1980). Orthostatic reflexes as well as vascular changes to exercise were not severely impaired by α-methyldopa (REID and ELLIOTT 1984).

4.2 Pharmacodynamics

One property which is common to the three substances reviewed in this chapter is the stimulation of α-adrenoceptors at various sites. Therefore, this property will be summarized for all three substances. In the case of α-methyldopa its active metabolite, α-methylnoradrenaline, will be considered. Thus, the increase in blood pressure immediately following i.v. injection of clonidine, guanfacine (Sect. 4.1), and α-methylnoradrenaline (HOLTZ and PALM 1966) is due to stimulation of vascular α-adrenoceptors. The peripheral nature of the pressure effect of all three substances was demonstrated by the blood pressure increase in pithed rats, and this action was antagonized by α-adrenoceptor blocking substances (KOBINGER and PICHLER 1981, 1983a). All three substances were shown to contract the nictitating membrane of cats (AHLQUIST 1948; HOEFKE and KOBINGER 1966; SCHOLTYSIK et al. 1975), to contract isolated pulmonary artery strips, and to inhibit pendular movements of the rabbit intestine (for review, KOBINGER 1978). In some of those in vitro experiments as well as in isolated, perfused hind limbs of rats, clonidine acted as a partial antagonist at α-adrenoceptors (for review, KOBINGER 1978; KOBINGER et al. 1980). The direct effect upon postsynaptic α-adrenoceptors was proven by experiments in which endogenous noradrenaline stores were depleted by pretreatment with reserpine and/or α-methyl-*p*-tyrosine (an inhibitor of noradrenaline synthesis) for clonidine (for review, KOBINGER 1978), guanfacine (SCHOLTYSIK et al. 1975), and α-methyldopa (KRONEBERG and STOEPEL 1963). Other peripheral sympathomimetic effects have been described, mainly for clonidine, such as piloerection, contraction of the spleen, and contraction of the isolated vas deferens (reviews: SCHMITT 1977; KOBINGER 1978). A number of peripheral and central nervous effects have been described which are obviously due to stimulation of α-adrenoceptors as shown by the antagonism with α-adrenoceptor blockers. These include decrease in salivary secretion, sedation in various animal species, antinociceptive action, decrease in water intake, suppression of sudomotor-activity in the forepaws of cats, and facilitation of a spinal flexor reflex (clonidine: ANDÉN et al. 1970; PAALZOW and PAALZOW 1976; SCHMITT 1977; TIMMERMANS et al. 1981; KANIUCKI et al. 1984; WALLAND 1984; guanfacine: SCHOLTYSIK et al. 1975). Sedation was reported to be the most common side effect of α-methyldopa in humans (ALEXANDER and EVANS 1975). Other pharmacological effects were reported which may also be due to α-adrenoceptor stimulation such as a mydriatic effect, decrease in intraocular pressure, and decrease in gastric secretion (HOEFKE and KOBINGER 1966; INNEMEE and VAN ZWIETEN 1979; INNEMEE et al. 1979; HEY et al. 1985).

In isolated cardiac preparations stimulation of histamine H_2 receptors by clonidine increases spontaneous rate and contractility (CSONGRADY and KOBINGER 1974). Clonidine has been shown to exert local anesthetic effects in high concentrations (HOEFKE and KOBINGER 1966) and to induce endocrinological effects such as an increase in the level of growth hormone in plasma (for review, SCHMITT 1977), an effect which recently was used in patients with short stature as a screening test for the estimation of human growth hormone secretion (KELLER et al. 1983). Clonidine decreases renin secretion (Sect. 6).

4.3 Mode of Action: α-Adrenoceptor Stimulation within the Central Nervous System

It is widely accepted that the three drugs to be discussed act within the CNS by a mechanism which reduces sympathetic outflow from cardiovascular centers. On a molecular basis the effect is due to a direct stimulation of central nervous postsynaptic α-adrenoceptors, a property which all three substances have in common. Other mechanisms of action have been proposed, and they will be discussed at the end of this section. Clonidine has played a key role in the development of concepts concerning central blood pressure regulation and centrally acting antihypertensive drugs; therefore, most data have been published with respect to this drug (for historical reviews, STÄHLE 1982; KOBINGER 1984a).

4.3.1 Site of Action

The cardiovascular effects of clonidine, namely, a decrease in blood pressure, heart rate, and cardiac output, strongly indicate sympathoinhibition; the exclusion of peripheral adrenergic inhibitory effects then suggested the central origin of this effect (KOBINGER and WALLAND 1967a). Direct proof of the central site of attack comes from two sets of animal experiments (1) Small doses of clonidine (1 µg/kg) were injected into the cisterna magna and produced similar decreases in blood pressure, heart rate, and cardiac output to those produced by 10–30-fold higher doses administered i.v. (Fig. 3; KOBINGER 1967; KOBINGER and WALLAND 1967b). Analogous results were gained by SATTLER and VAN ZWIETEN (1967), who injected clonidine into the vertebral artery of cats. (2) Clonidine decreases the electrical discharges in preganglionic sympathetic nerves. This was first described by SCHMITT et al. (1967), HUKUHARA et al. (1968), and analyzed in detail by KLUPP et al. (1970).

Furthermore, it was shown that clonidine also increases vagal activities by an action within the CNS. Activation of the vagally mediated baroreceptor reflex by clonidine has already been described by ROBSON and KAPLAN (1969). Using the intracisternal injection technique KOBINGER and WALLAND (1971, 1972a) and WALLAND et al. (1974) localized this effect to the CNS. In these experiments in dogs, sympathetic cardiac effects were eliminated by pretreatment with a β-adrenoceptor blocking drug. Blood pressure increases were evoked by i.v. injections of angiotensin II or by inflation of an aortic cuff, and the resulting decreases in heart rate were recorded as the vagal reflex response. KORNER et al. (1974) then analyzed the facilitation of the baroreceptor reflex by clonidine in conscious rabbits, showing the participation of vagal activation as well as sympathoinhibition. This reciprocal reaction of both parts of the autonomic nervous system indicates that a complex response pattern with a physiological organization was triggered by the drug.

Infusion of guanfacine into the vertebral artery of anesthetized dogs (1 $\mu g\,kg^{-1}\,min^{-1}$ for 90 min) and injection into the lateral cerebral ventricle of anesthetized cats (3 µg/kg) cause reductions in blood pressure and heart rate, while the same dose given i.v. is ineffective. Intravenous administration of guanfacine induces a reduction in splanchnic nerve activity of cats and facilitation of the reflex bradycardia to blood pressure increases in anesthetized, β-adrenoceptor-blocked dogs (SCHOLTYSIK 1980; SCHOLTYSIK et al. 1975). For α-methyldopa a direct analysis of the central site of action was done by JAJU et al. (1966) and HENNING and VAN ZWIETEN (1967, 1968). The latter authors infused (L-α-methyldopa, 20 mg/kg) into the vertebral artery of anesthetized cats. A reduction in blood pressure followed which was slow in onset and lasted for 4–5 h. Intravenous infusion of the same dose was only slightly hypotensive. A decrease in spontaneous sympathetic nerve discharges was reported after repeated administration of the drug for several days to cats and rats (TAUBERGER and KUHN 1971; BAUM et al. 1972). Perfusion of the 3rd and 4th ventricle system of cats with α-methylnoradrenaline, α-methyldopamine, or α-methyldopa decreases blood pressure (HEISE and KRONEBERG 1972).

Attempts to localize the site of action of clonidine within the CNS reveal that the drug acts at various levels including regions of the forebrain, diencephalon, and spinal medulla; however, the most prominent site seems to be the oblongate medulla (for reviews, SCHMITT 1977; KOBINGER 1978). Sympathoinhibition as well as vagal activation by clonidine could be demonstrated after ablation of the brain of rats, cats, and dogs rostrally to the medulla (HUKUHARA et al. 1968; SCHMITT and SCHMITT 1969; KOBINGER and PICHLER 1975a, b).

Within the medulla the nucleus tractus solitarii has been claimed to be the main site of hypotensive action (SINHA et al. 1975; LIPSKI et al. 1976), but there are findings that contradict this idea: bilateral destruction did not significantly reduce the effect of clonidine upon blood pressure and heart rate (LAUBIE et al. 1976).

Another medullary site, the rostrolateral part of the ventral medulla (nucleus reticularis lateralis), has attracted the interest of mainly one research group, and the suggestion that clonidine attacks this site is based on experiments with topical applications and with its failure to act hypotensively after lesion of this region (BOUSQUET et al. 1975, 1981). However, other experiments with local destructions were reported which contradict these results (LAUBIE and SCHMITT 1977). Generally, results of local brain application must be interpreted cautiously with respect to non-specific effects. A number of substances such as nicotine, physostigmine, carbachol, pentobarbitone sodium, GABA, and others produce vasodepressor effects when applied to the ventral surface of the brain stem (GUERTZENSTEIN 1973; FELDBERG and GUERTZENSTEIN 1976). Clonidine has a potent local anesthetic (i.e., membrane stabilizing) effect (HOEFKE and KOBINGER 1966), and this property of the drug has been proposed by BOUSQUET et al. (1978) to explain the hypotensive effects of clonidine when applied to the ventral surface of the medulla. It is surprising, therefore, that the same group of researchers later proposed another mechanism of action for clonidine and applied several other drugs to the surface of the brain without excluding or referring to their membrane-stabilizing effect when applied locally (BOUSQUET et al. 1985; BOUSQUET and FELDMAN 1987).

In contrast to clonidine, guanfacine has no effect on blood pressure and heart rate when applied topically to the ventral surface of the medulla in cats. Microinjection of α-methylnoradrenaline into the nucleus tractus solitarii of rats induces hypotension (ZANDBERG and DEJONG 1977).

4.3.2 Mediator of the Effect: Central α-Adrenoceptors

In the minds of many researchers and physicians, stimulation of α-adrenoceptors is primarily associated with vasoconstriction and blood pressure rise. The idea that stimulation of α-adrenoceptors within the CNS may induce a decrease in blood pressure was therefore surprising, even though some experimental indications for such a hypothesis can be found in the older literature (HELLER 1933;

MCCUBBIN et al. 1960). Clonidine served as an important tool in the development of this idea, which was investigated along two lines as reviewed in the following two sections.

4.3.2.1 Effects of Clonidine, Guanfacine, and α-Methyldopa are Antagonized by α-Adrenoceptor Blocking Drugs

SCHMITT et al. (1971, 1973) reported that treatment with yohimbine or piperoxan prevented the decrease in sympathetic nerve activity caused by clonidine as measured by electrical discharges in the splanchnic and cardiac nerves of cats. At the same time KOBINGER and WALLAND (1971, 1972b) reported that the vagally mediated baroreceptor reflex which is enhanced by clonidine was reduced (antagonized) by subsequent i.v. or i.ci. injections of phentolamine or other α-adrenoceptor antagonists. In both these experimental designs no α-adrenoceptors are interposed between the CNS and the effector systems. Thus, the site of receptor interaction had to be localized to the CNS. Figure 4 shows the antagonism of the hypotensive effect of centrally administered clonidine by the α-adrenoceptor blocking agents piperoxan and yohimbine (SCHMITT et al. 1973). Many similar findings have been reported and are reviewed by SCHMITT (1977) and KOBINGER (1978).

The effect of guanfacine after intracerebroventricular application on blood pressure and heart rate in anesthetized cats was largely abolished by pre-injec-

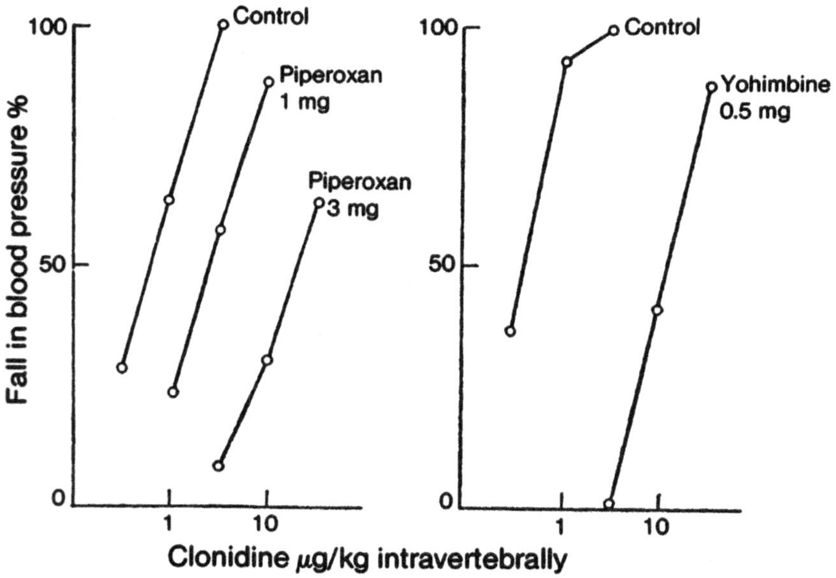

Fig. 4. Competitive antagonism of yohimbine and piperoxan on the decrease in blood pressure induced by intravertebral administration of clonidine in the dog. The decrease in blood pressure was induced by cumulative doses of clonidine into the vertebral artery. Piperoxan (*left*) and yohimbine (*right*) shift the dose-response curve to the right; this suggests a competitive antagonism. From SCHMITT et al. (1973)

tion intraventricularly of the α-adrenoceptor blocking drug phentolamine (SCHOLTYSIK et al. 1975). The decrease in blood pressure as induced by perfusion of the 3rd and 4th ventricle system of cats with α-methylnoradrenaline, α-methyldopamine or α-methyldopa was practically abolished by the additional infusion of yohimbine or phentolamine (HEISE and KRONEBERG 1972).

4.3.2.2 Cerebral Application of Various α-Adrenoceptor Stimulating Drugs

Cerebral application of various α-adrenoceptor stimulating drugs produces the same cardiovascular and autonomic nervous response pattern as clonidine, and this has been reviewed extensively by KOBINGER (1978, 1986).

4.3.3 α-Adrenoceptor Subtypes

4.3.3.1 Definition at Peripheral Sites

α-Adrenoceptor subtypes have been classified in two ways. First, on a morphological basis, α-adrenoceptors were described as either pre- or postsynaptic receptors (for reviews, LANGER 1977, 1981; STARKE 1977, 1981). The classic postsynaptic receptor is localized at the effector organ and mediates the response on muscular, secretory, or biochemical systems (Fig. 5). The presynaptic receptor is located on neuronal terminals or other sites of a neuron and modulates the release of the respective natural transmitter. In the case of adrenergic neurons the stimulation of presynaptic α-adrenoceptors, defined as autoreceptors, inhibits the release of catecholamines. The conclusion that pre- and post-

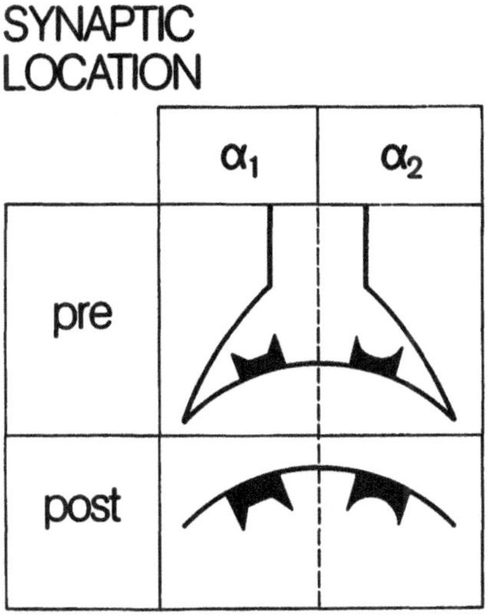

Fig. 5. α-Adrenoceptors at adrenergic neuron terminals (*pre*, presynaptic) and target tissues (*post*, postsynaptic). The classification into the subtypes pre- and postsynaptic is morphological. The classification α_1 and α_2 is pharmacological, based on different responses to different drugs (agonists and antagonists). As shown here, the subtypes α_1 as well as α_2 might be present pre- as well as postsynaptically. From KOBINGER (1981)

synaptic α-adrenoceptors are different is based on the different pre-/postsynaptic activity ratios of drugs, agonists as well as antagonists (Dubocovich and Langer 1974; Starke et al. 1975; Borowski et al. 1977; Doxey et al. 1977).

α-Adrenoceptors have also been classified on a pharmacologic basis (Fig. 5). The subclass α_2 is proposed when the relative potencies of clonidine, xylazine, and tramazoline are greater than those of phenylephrine and norphenylephrine. The α_1-receptor is defined by the reverse order of potency (Wikberg 1978, 1979; Berthelsen and Pettinger 1977; for review, Starke 1981).

Each of these subtypes (α_1 and α_2) might be present post- as well as presynaptically, and both pharmacological types have been observed together at the same morphological site (Docherty and McGrath 1980; Kobinger and Pichler 1980; Timmermans and van Zwieten 1980; Docherty 1984).

Evidence is primarily based on the "differential antagonism" of a given α-adrenoceptor blocker against different agonists. In pithed rats the blood pressure-increasing effects of clonidine and methoxamine were determined. The dose-response curve of clonidine was shifted by a given dose of yohimbine much more to the right along the abscissa than was the dose-response curve of methoxamine. Conversely, prazosin was a more effective antagonist against methoxamine than against clonidine (Kobinger and Pichler 1980). The best explanation of these results was the assumption of two receptor types at the postsynaptic vasoconstrictor effector site: one type, α_1, with high affinity for methoxamine and prazosin and another type, α_2, with high affinity for clonidine and yohimbine. Both receptor types mediate the same response, namely, vasoconstriction. This system has been used to determine α_1/α_2-selectivity for a number of α-adrenoceptor agonists using the α_1-selective antagonist prazosin and the α_2-selective antagonist rauwolscine. Details are given in the legend of Table 1. In this table the α_1/α_2-selectivity is expressed by the potency of rauwolscine (R) and prazosin (P), respectively, to antagonize the effect of agonists. It may be pointed out that the three substances on which this chapter is focused, namely clonidine, guanfacine, and α-methylnoradrenaline, have relatively low α_1/α_2 ratios (i.e., high α_2/α_1 ratios); clonidine has the highest α_1/α_2 ratio, approaching the ratio of the natural transmitter noradrenaline. From inspection of Fig. 5 and the great variety of agonists in Table 1 it appears as a logical concept that the response of a target system depends on: the α_1/α_2-selectivity of a given drug, and the α_1/α_2-adrenoceptor ratio in the target system (Kobinger and Pichler 1983a, b; Ahlquist and Kobinger 1984; Kobinger 1986).

4.3.3.2 Classification at Central Cardiovascular Sites

Presynaptic α-adrenoceptors within the CNS might be located on neuron endings and on cell bodies (somatodentritic receptors, autoreceptors) (Svensson et al. 1975; Starke 1979). There is no doubt that presynaptic α-adrenoceptors exist within the CNS and that their stimulation decreases adrenergic neuron activity. Thus, clonidine or oxymetazoline inhibits the liberation of noradrenaline from rat brain slices induced by electrical field stimulation (Farnebo and Hamberger

Table 1. α_1/α_2-Adrenoceptor selectivity and post/presynaptic α-adrenoceptor potency ratio of various agonists

Agonist	D_{10} (mg/kg i.v.)		Ratio $\frac{\alpha_1}{\alpha_2}$	Ratio[a] $\frac{\text{post}}{\text{pre}}$
	Rauwolscine	Prazosin	$\frac{D_{10R}}{D_{10P}}$	$\frac{ID_{50}}{PD_{30}}$
B-HT 920	1.25	100.0	0.012	0.09
Guanfacine	2.0	89.0	0.022	0.31
B-HT 933 (azepexole)	0.7	9.0	0.08	0.22
α-*m*-Noradrenaline	1.9	10.0	0.19	–
Xylazine	3.6	2.8	1.28	0.46
Clonidine	5.5	0.7	7.86	0.45
Noradrenaline	4.8	0.55	8.73	–
Adrenaline	3.7	0.12	30.83	–
Phenylephrine	9.5	0.06	158.33	–
Methoxamine	15.0	0.07	214.28	5.88

[a] Experimental data from KOBINGER and PICHLER (1980).
The blood pressure-increasing effect of the agonists was determined in pithed rats by means of dose-response curves. The α-adrenoceptor antagonists rauwolscine and prazosin shift the dose-response curves to the right. Those antagonist doses were evaluated that cause a tenfold shift of agonist dose-response curves to the right (D_{10}). The ratio D_{10} rauwolscine/D_{10} prazosin (D_{10R}/D_{10P}) was proposed as a measure of the α_1/α_2-selectivity for the agonists tested (ratio α_1/α_2). In these experiments, animals were treated with a β-adrenoceptor blocking agent. The post/presynaptic activity ratio (ratio post/pre) is expressed by the ratio ID_{50}/PD_{30}, where ID_{50} = dose that inhibited electrically induced tachycardia in pithed rats by 50% (presynaptic effect); PD_{30} = dose that increased blood pressure in spinal rats by 30 mmHg (postsynaptic effect). Both ratios are significantly correlated ($r = 0.998$; $P < 0.001$; $n = 6$). This is explained by an α-adrenoceptor ratio of approximately 1 at the postsynaptic site and a value of $\alpha_2 \gg \alpha_1$ at presynaptic sites (KOBINGER and PICHLER 1983b). From KOBINGER and PICHLER (1981, 1983a).

1971; STARKE and MONTEL 1973). Local application of clonidine inhibits the spontaneous firing rate of adrenergic cells in the locus coeruleus of rats (SVENSSON et al. 1975). Such findings stimulate the idea that the cardiovascular depressor effect of clonidine is caused by stimulation of these presynaptic α-adrenoceptors within cardiovascular regulatory centers. This was supported by the observation that agonists such as clonidine and antagonists such as yohimbine, which are preferentially active at peripheral presynatpic sites, are also active at central cardiovascular sites.

A presynaptic agonist decreases the release of endogenous adrenergic transmitter, and a pharmacological response can only be expected if the adrenergic neuron produces and liberates a certain level of the transmitter. In a series of experiments endogenous noradrenaline was depleted or reduced by pharmacological means, hypothesizing that a presynaptically acting α-adrenoceptor agonist would be ineffective thereafter. The following methods were used for depletion: intracisternal or intraventricular injection of 6-hydroxydopamine, which causes, after some days, a selective destruction of adrenergic neurons;

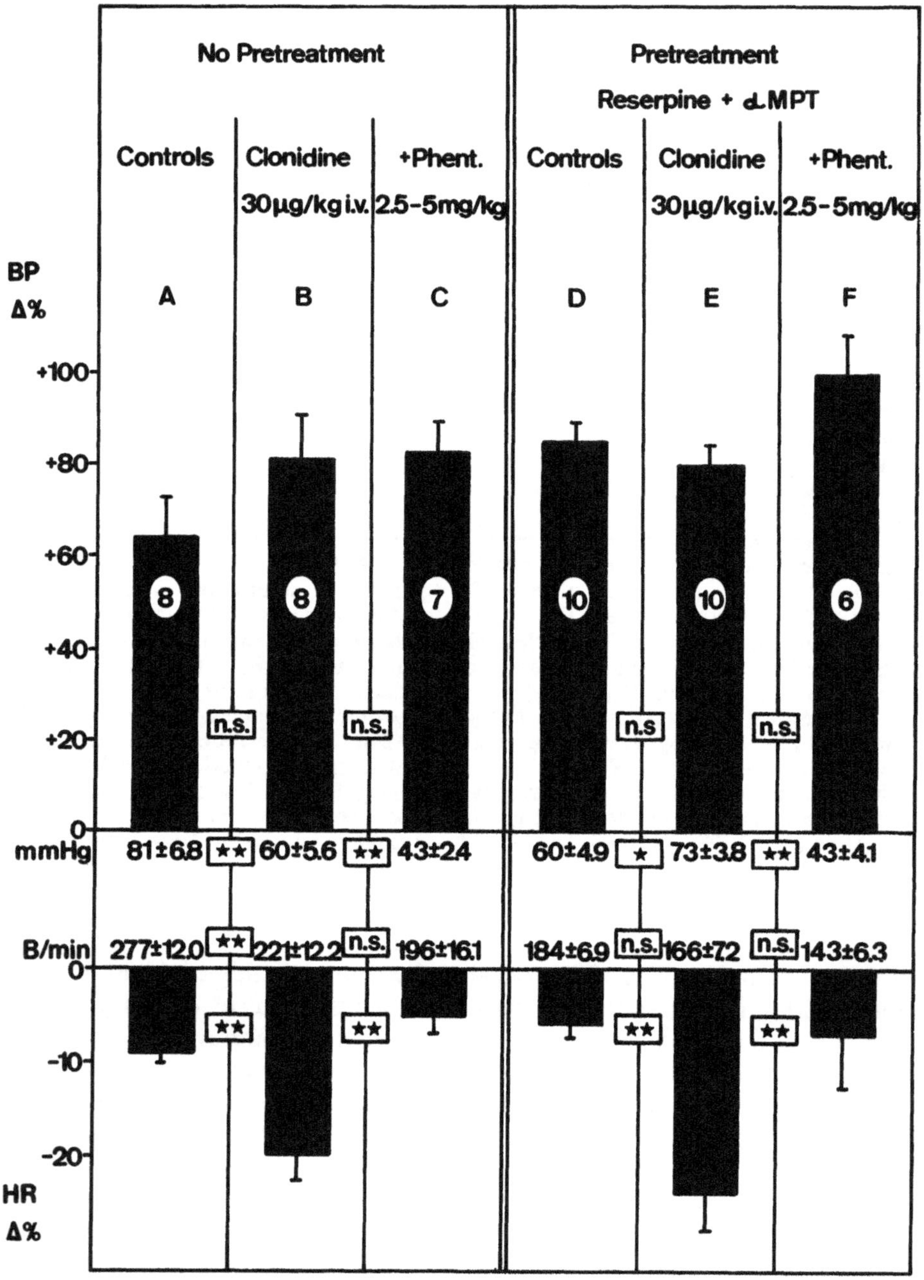

Fig. 6. Vagally mediated reflex bradycardia in decerebrate rats. To avoid influences of the sympathetic system upon the heart, the β-adrenoceptor blocking drug toliprolol (5 mg/kg s.c.) was given 30 min before starting the experiment. During control periods (*A*, *D*) angiotension II (0.03–0.25 µg/kg) was injected i.v., which resulted in a transient increase in blood pressure (*columns upwards*) accompanied by a reflex bradycardia (*columns downwards*). Thereafter, clonidine (30 µg/kg i.v.) was administered, and angiotensin II injections were repeated after 15–30 min (*B*, *E*). Approximately 30 min after

systemic injection of reserpine, which profoundly decreases catecholamine (and 5-hydroxytryptamine) stores; and systemic injection of α-methyl-*p*-tyrosine, which inhibits noradrenaline synthesis by inhibition of the enzyme tyrosine hydroxylase. Experiments with treatment by 6-hydroxydopamine led to contradictory results as the hypotensive and bradycardic effects of clonidine were reported to be abolished, markedly attenuated, or unaffected by this treatment (HAEUSLER and FINCH 1972; DOLLERY and REID 1973; FINCH 1975; REYNOLDSON et al. 1979). It must be pointed out that treatment with 6-hydroxydopamine only partially eliminates noradrenaline in the brain and leads to a nonspecific destruction of other, noncatecholaminergic neurons (for review, KOBINGER 1984b).

In dogs pretreated with reserpine, the vagally mediated baroreflex bradycardia is facilitated by clonidine, as it is in controls (KOBINGER and WALLAND 1973). Analogous results were obtained in rats pretreated with reserpine and in addition with α-methyl-*p*-tyrosine (Fig. 6; KOBINGER and PICHLER 1975a). Furthermore, the intracisternal injection of clonidine (1 μg/kg), oxymetazoline, the azepine derivatives B-HT 933 (azepexole) or B-HT 920 decreases splanchnic nerve discharges in reserpine plus α-methyl-*p*-tyrosine pretreated cats similar to controls (KOBINGER and PICHLER 1976; PICHLER et al. 1980; PICHLER and KOBINGER 1981). In dogs pretreated with reserpine and α-methyl-*p*-tyrosine, the intracisternal injection of B-HT 933 (azepexole) facilitates the vagally mediated baroreflex bradycardia, similar to controls (PICHLER et al. 1980).

Treatment with reserpine and with reserpine plus α-methyl-*p*-tyrosine efficiently depletes the brain of endogenous noradrenaline (to approx. 0.6%–2% of controls; for review, KOBINGER 1984b). Therefore, the ability of clonidine and other centrally active α-adrenoceptor agonists to elicit cardiovascular depression in these catecholamine-depleted animals similar to that seen in controls practically excludes the mode of action upon autoreceptors, and it strongly suggests an effect on postsynaptic α-adrenoceptors.

There are a number of arguments indicating that the α_2-type of adrenoceptor triggers cardiovascular depression within the CNS. All clonidine-like drugs are agonists with high α_2/α_1 (i.e., low α_1/α_2)-selectivity, and some of these are given in Table 1.

---

clonidine, the α-adrenoceptor blocking drug phentolamine (*Phent*, 2.5 or 5 mg/kg i.v.) was injected, and angiotension II injections were repeated 15–20 min later (*C*, *F*). *Reserpine* (7.5 mg/kg s.c.) was given 24 h, and α-methyl-*p*-tyrosine (*αMPT*, 250 mg/kg i.p.), 4 h prior to the experiment to inhibit storage and synthesis of noradrenaline (*D*–*F*). Resting values (i.e., immediately before angiotensin injection) for mean blood pressure (*BP*, mmHg) and heart rate (*HR*, beats (B)/min) are given at the *base of the columns*. Maximal changes of blood pressure and heart rate, as induced by the angiotensin injection, were expressed as percentages (Δ%) of the resting values and are given *by the columns*. All values are means ± SEM. Numbers of animals are indicated *within the columns*, significance of differences by *symbols between the groups* which have been compared (*t*-test): *n.s.*, not significant ($P > 0.05$); *star*, $P < 0.05$; *two stars*, $P < 0.01$. Note the reflex augmentation by clonidine and the antagonism of this effect by phentolamine; the results are the same in "intact" (*A*–*C*) as well as in catecholamine-depleted animals (*D*–*F*). From KOBINGER and PICHLER (1975a)

An interesting detail is the high α_2/α_1 ratio of α-methylnoradrenaline (Table 1), structurally more related to phenylephrine (which has a high α_1/α_2 ratio) then to any of the clonidine-like drugs. As pointed out in Sect. 3.3, this drug is the active metabolite of the antihypertensive agent α-methyldopa and within the CNS exerts effects similar to clonidine.

α_2-Adrenoceptors as mediators of the blood pressure-lowering effect of central antihypertensive drugs are also suggested by experiments with α-adrenoceptor antagonists. The α_2-selective drug rauwolscine is more effective in antagonizing the hypotensive effect of clonidine than the stereoisomer corynanthine, which is α_1-selective (TIMMERMANS et al. 1981). The antagonism by yohimbine of the hypotensive effect of α-methylnoradrenaline in perfusion experiments in the ventricle system of cats has been described in Sect. 4.3.2.1.

4.4 Mode of Action: Other Hypotheses

4.4.1 Clonidine and Guanfacine

There is one hypothesis which explains the antihypertensive effects by means of a sympathoinhibitory action at peripheral sites. It is based on many observations in animal experiments demonstrating the decrease in adrenergic transmitter release and/or adrenergic transmission by the drugs. This effect is due to a stimulation of presynaptic adrenergic receptors (autoreceptors) and has been described in Sect. 4.3.3. Inhibition is demonstrated after stimulation of various peripheral sympathetic nerves (e.g., cardiac accelerator nerves, lumbar sympathetic chain; SCHOLTYSIK et al. 1975; for review, STARKE 1981) and is seen at low but not at high stimulation frequencies (approximately <5 Hz).

The argument that this peripheral effect is not relevant for blood pressure lowering is delivered by animal experiments in which two imidazolines, oxymetazoline and St 91, which do not penetrate into the CNS, were compared with clonidine in cats. All three drugs exert similar effects on the spontaneous perfusion pressure (postsynaptic effect); they also inhibit the electrically induced increase in perfusion pressure in a hind limb (presynaptic effect). However, only clonidine lowers the systemic blood pressure (PICHLER and KOBINGER 1978). Moreover, it must be mentioned that from experiments in human volunteers the functional role of sympathoinhibition by stimulation of presynaptic α-adrenoceptors has been doubted (FITZGERALD et al. 1981; DEERING et al. 1987). It remains open whether this presynaptic mechanism contributes to the antihypertensive effect of the drugs in patients.

A number of hypotheses have been presented which try to explain the cardiovascular effects of these drugs by interference with endogenous mediator systems other than catecholamines at central sites. The involvement of central histamine H_2 receptors has been proposed on the basis of two arguments: clonidine stimulates peripheral H_2 receptors, albeit in high concentrations (KARPPANEN and WESTERMANN 1973; CSONGRADY and KOBINGER 1974), and observations that H_2 receptor antagonists inhibit the hypotensive effect of this drug (KARPPANEN et al. 1976; FINCH et al. 1978). This idea was contradicted by the results of MEDGETT and MCCULLOCH (1980) and MCCULLOCH et al. (1980), who showed that a number of clonidine analogues which effectively lower blood pressure have no H_2 receptor-stimulating properties. The latter view was confirmed by the finding that the effect of guanfacine is not antagonized by the H_2-blocker metiamide (for review, SCHOLTYSIK 1980).

Similar contradictory results have been reported with respect to involvement of opioid receptors, as morphine antagonists inhibited (FARSANG and KUNOS 1979) or did not affect (HEAD and DEJONG 1984) the actions of clonidine and α-methyldopa. The neuropeptide Y (NPY) is a cotransmitter of noradrenaline and adrenaline in brain stem catecholamine cell groups (HÖKFELT et al. 1983). It has been recently proposed that clonidine by stimulation of α_2-autoreceptors inhibits the release of NPY and thereby contributes to its own central actions (JARROTT et al. 1987).

Recently, two other mechanisms have been proposed to explain the central hypotensive effect of clonidine: inhibition of the pressor effect of an endogenous substance (clonidine-displacing substance; BOUSQUET et al. 1986) and stimulation of an imidazoline receptor rather than an α-adrenoceptor (BOUSQUET et al. 1985).

4.4.2 α-Methyldopa

For α-methyldopa the causal relationship between the lowering of blood pressure and an overall decrease in sympathetic nerve activity was demonstrated by MUSCHOLL and RAHN (1968), showing a parallel decrease in systolic blood pressure and renal excretion of noradrenaline. The hypothesis that this effect is due to inhibition of DOPA-decarboxylase was proven wrong (PORTER et al. 1961). A great number of papers were written on the subject of the "false transmitter hypothesis": α-methyldopa is converted into α-methylnoradrenaline, which is stored in and released from adrenergic nerve endings. This hypothesis is based on the assumption that α-methylnoradrenaline is a weaker vasoconstrictor than noradrenaline. However, it turns out to be untenable because under various experimental conditions stimulation of sympathetic nerves shows no or little diminution of the responses after treatment with α-methyldopa (for reviews, HOLTZ and PALM 1966; KOBINGER 1978), and α-methylnoradrenaline exerts the same pressor effect as noradrenaline (MUSCHOLL and MAÎTRE 1963). A contribution of this peripheral component to the antihypertensive effect of α-methyldopa, however, cannot be excluded completely.

5 Thereapeutic Use and Dosage

All three drugs lower blood pressure in essential hypertension, renal hypertension with various stages of renal insufficiency, and preeclamptic toxemia; they lower blood pressure in virtually all grades of hypotension without orthostasis at rest and after exercise (clonidine: Fig. 7; for reviews, ONESTI et al. 1971; MCMAHON 1984; REID and ELLIOTT 1984; SORKIN and HEEL 1986).

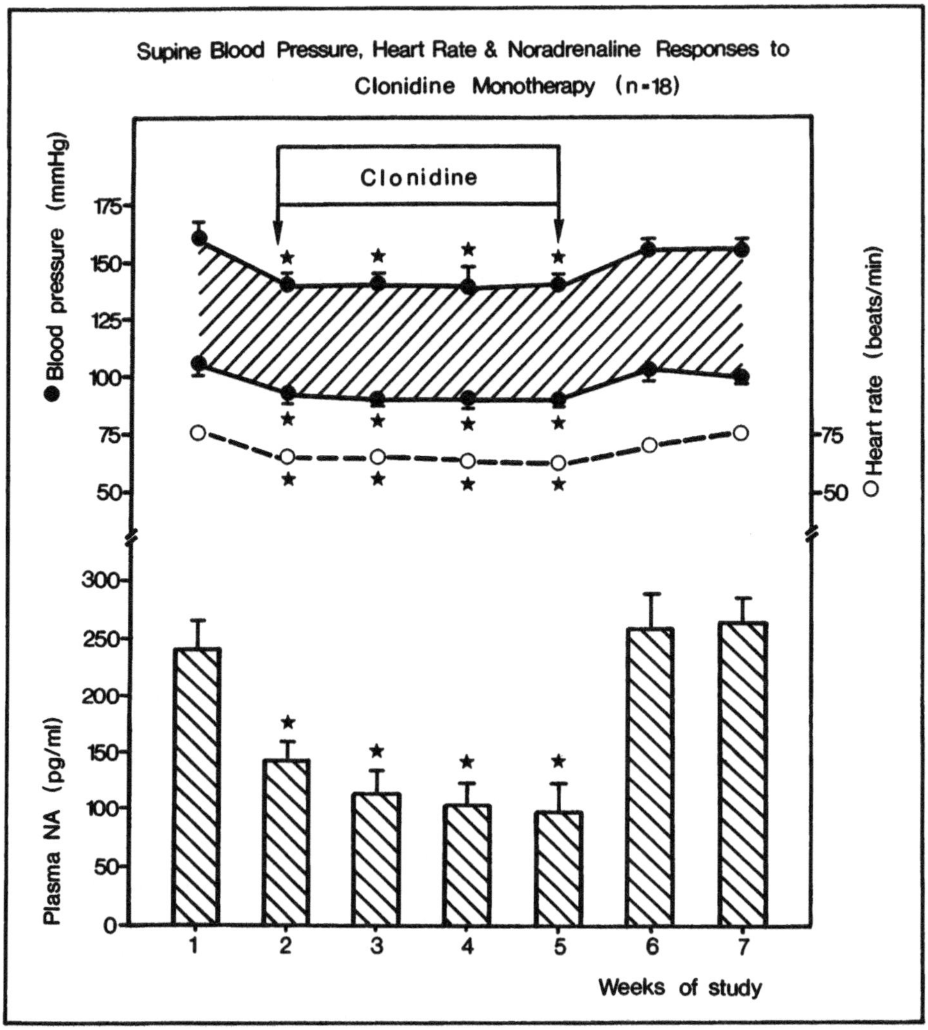

Fig. 7. Effect of clonidine monotherapy on supine blood pressure, heart rate, and plasma noradrenaline (mean ± SEM) in patients with untreated, essential hypertension ($n = 18$); treatment was started with clonidine 0.1 mg twice daily and—if diastolic blood pressure exceeded 90 mmHg—was increased in 0.2 mg increments per week up to a maximal dose of 0.6 mg per day. During the recovery period the drug was reduced slowly over a 3-day period. *Star*, significantly different from control. From BRAVO et al. (1985)

For clonidine, the successful treatment of hypertensive emergencies have been reported by the acute use of slow i.v. or by i.m. administration (single doses of 0.15–0.3 mg, BOCK et al. 1973; median dose of 0.3 mg, RUSS, et al. 1983).

The early clinical application of clonidine earned an image for the drug as mainly to be used in malignant hypertension, severe hypertension with complications, and at a late step in the schema of step-care therapy (SAMBHI 1983).

This resulted in the use of relatively high doses (SCHWARTZ et al. 1973) accompanied by a high degree of side effects. More recently, clonidine has been favored in the treatment of mild to moderate hypertension using small doses. Thus, treatment with oral doses of 0.0375–0.075 mg twice daily has a satisfactory hypotensive effect comparable to that of the β-blocker metoprolol in a dosage of 50 to 100 mg twice daily (71 patients, multicenter, double-blind study, 6 weeks' treatment period; KOLLOCH et al. 1985). SCHULTZ et al. (1981) report satisfactory effects of 200 μg or less twice daily and suggest the addition of another antihypertensive drug if this dosage regimen should be inadequate, rather than an increase in the dose of clonidine. This recommendation is consistent with the findings of WING et al. (1977), who showed that the hypotensive effect of clonidine is attenuated with high doses, when plasma concentrations are in excess of 1.5–2.0 ng/ml. THANANOPAVARN et al. (1983) used clonidine as monotherapy and titrated the drug from 0.05 mg twice daily to 0.2 mg thrice daily. Blood pressure decreased without major side effects. In 5 of the 15 patients the smallest dose was effective. Three patients required an additional small dose of a diuretic after 6 months of clonidine monotherapy.

For clonidine a transdermal therapeutic system (TTS) was developed which provides a rate-controlled, continuous administration of the drug by means of a skin patch; thereby, plasma concentrations of clonidine reach a steady state value in 2–3 days, remain steady for the duration of the wearing period, and show minimal fluctuations. Determined by the size of the patch the delivery rates are 100, 200, and 300 μg of clonidine per day (SHAW 1984).

Guanfacine shows a clinical efficacy similar to clonidine. In a single-blind, crossover study JÄÄTTELÄ (1980) reported a similar and statistically significant decrease in blood pressure in over half the group of patients with essential hypertension (WHO grade I or II) using a daily dose of 3–4 mg guanfacine or 0.3–0.45 mg clonidine. The drugs were administered either twice or thrice daily. JERIE (1980a) reported a mean daily dose of 3.4 mg of guanfacine used as monotherapy at the end of the 1st year of treatment, and 3.2 mg after 2 years. With the once daily and twice daily schedules the same antihypertensive effect was achieved as with the thrice daily one. For α-methyldopa REID and ELLIOTT (1984) noted that a twice daily regimen is recommended, with a starting dose of 250 mg twice daily and a maximum daily dose of 2 g.

6 Combination with Other Drugs

Beside monotherapy, centrally acting drugs can be used in combination with other hypotensive drugs in a step-care schedule. Combinations with saluretics (SCHWARTZ et al. 1973; MORGAN 1983; THANANOPAVARN et al. 1983; for reviews, KAPLAN 1975; SORKIN and HEEL 1986) have the advantage of reducing the tendency toward fluid retention which occurs with many antihypertensive drugs; on the other hand central antihypertensives reduce plasma renin activity which is activated by saluretics (HÖKFELT et al. 1970; WEBER et al. 1983; for reviews, HALUSHKA and KEISER 1974; SORKIN and HEEL 1986). There is also a rationale for combining these drugs with peripheral vasodilating substances such as hydralazine, calcium antagonists, and minoxidil: the centrally acting drugs suppress the sympathetic reflex overactivity induced by peripheral vasodilators (Velasco et al. 1978, 1983; Jerie 1980a; Seedat 1983).

From results with clonidine a combination with β-adrenoceptor blocking drugs seem possible (Pettinger et al. 1977; Weber et al. 1978) but is not always successful, and paradoxical hypertension has even been reported (Warren et al. 1979).

In surgical patients perioperative treatment with clonidine has been reported to reduce narcotic and anesthetic requirments, improve hemodynamics by avoiding up and down swings of blood pressure, reduce plasma catecholamines, and shorten the period of postoperative ventilation (Flacke et al. 1987; Longnecker 1987).

7 Drug Interactions

The central hypotensives, exerting sedative effects by themselves (Sect. 4.3.2.1), potentiate the effect of other CNS depressants in animal experiments (Delbarre and Schmitt 1971), and its clinical use has been described in the section above. Caution has to be taken with patients who combine these drugs with sedatives or alcohol. Antagonistic effects of α-adrenoceptor antagonists with affinity to the α_2-subgroup, such as yohimbine, phentolamine, and tolazoline, against cardiovascular actions of central antihypertensives have been described in Sect. 4.3.2.1. The antagonism of those drugs against the sedative effects will be described below (Sect. 8). Tolazoline has been recommended as an antidote against an overdose of clonidine (Bock et al. 1973; Schieber and Kaufman 1981). Tricyclic antidepressant drugs with α-adrenoceptor blocking potency have been reported to antagonize the antihypertensive action of clonidine in anesthetized cats (van Zwieten 1975); however, the clinical relevance of these interactions has been questioned (for review, Jarrott 1984).

With α-methyldopa, interactions can be expected from substances which interfere with the special metabolic pathway of this drug (Sect. 3.3). Treatment with the DOPA-decarboxylase inhibitor carbidopa, which penetrates poorly into the CNS, increases the hypotensive effect of α-methyldopa in rats (Scriabine et al. 1976). However, a clinically useful additional effect could not be observed in patients (Kersting et al. 1977). Hallucinosis has been reported after combined treatment with α-methyldopa and inhibitors of monoamine oxidase (Paykel 1966).

8 Side Effects, Toxicity, and Contraindications

The most common symptomatic side effects of the three central antihypertensives are sedation and dry mouth with marked reduction in salivary flow (Alexander and Evans 1975; Dollery et al. 1976; Reid et al. 1980; Sorkin and Heel 1986). Both effects are intimately connected with the mode of blood pressure-lowering effect via stimulation of α_2-adrenoceptors. This has been shown in animal experiments in which both sedation and evoked salivary secretion were antagonized by α_2-adrenoceptor blocking agents (Sect. 4.2). A tolerance develops towards both side effects during continuous treatment without a reduction of the hypotensive effect (WING et al. 1977; REID et al. 1980; SORKIN and HEEL 1986).

Sudden cessation of drug therapy can elicit a complex of symptoms which has been called the discontinuation syndrome, withdrawal syndrome, or rebound syndrome. Described and widely discussed first for clonidine, it later turned out also to occur after cessation of other antihypertensives of the centrally acting type and after treatment with β-adrenoceptor blockers or adrenergic neuron blockers (GOLDBERG et al. 1977; for reviews, GARBUS et al. 1979; HOUSTON 1981; WHITSETT 1983; SORKIN and HEEL 1986). The syndrome is characterized by symptoms of sympathetic overactivity, increase in blood pressure and heart rate, and behavioral effects such as anxiety, insomnia, and tremor, with elevated urinary catecholamine excretion. The symptoms begin to appear 18–21 h after the last dose with a duration of 1–5 days (GOLDBERG et al. 1977; for review, SORKIN and HEEL 1986). Incidence and severity of this syndrome is dose-dependent, and none of the studies reported an "overshoot hypertension" (blood pressure readings above those taken before therapy) with clonidine doses less than 1.2 mg/day (HOUSTON 1982; MCMAHON 1984). Incidences of the rebound phenomenon were more frequently reported for clonidine than for guanfacine and α-methyldopa (for reviews, HOUSTON 1981; REID and ELLIOTT 1984; SORKIN and HEEL 1986). In the treatment of mild to moderate hypertension an abrupt cessation of clonidine administration results in no instances in clinically significant symptoms or overshoot in blood pressure and heart rate (WHITSETT et al. 1978; WHITSETT 1983). It seems wise, however, to avoid abrupt cessation of any antihypertensive drug therapy.

A possible equivalent for the human rebound phenomenon has been described in rats which show episodes of blood pressure "up-swings" after cessation of a continuous infusion of clonidine, guanfacine, and α-methyldopa by means of an osmotic pump (THOOLEN et al. 1981, 1983).

Side effects which occur only occasionally, more trouble some than threatening, are gastrointestinal symptoms, vertigo, sleep disturbances, male sexual dysfunction, and headache (BOCK et al. 1973; JERIE 1980b; SCRIABINE 1980). α-Methyldopa has, in addition to those side effects which might be connected with its mode of action, some severe hypersensitivity reactions which might be specifically related to the molecule. A positive result of a direct Coombs antiglobulin test was found in 20%–30% of patients after 6–12 months of therapy and is reversible after cessation of treatment. A small percentage of the patients developed hemolytic anemia, signs of hepatoxicity, drug fever (for reviews, REID and ELLIOTT 1984; SCRIABINE 1980), and Parkinsonism (PEASTON 1964).

In light of 20 years' experience with clonidine in chronic oral treatment of hypertension the drug has been recommended as a non-toxic agent with no adverse changes in serum electrolytes, uric acid, blood sugar, serum lipid profile, or renal function (BOCK et al. 1973; SAMBHI 1983; DIEHM and MÖRL 1985; HOUSTON et al. 1987). Its percutaneous administration (TTS, Sect. 5) provokes cutaneous toxicity at the site of application. Slight and reversible skin reactions might occur following a few days of treatment; however, allergic contact dermatitis has been described at treatment periods of many weeks or even months. The symptoms consist of severe itching, spreading erythema, vesiculation, and/or infiltration. In those cases further transdermal clonidine application has to be avoided. A "flare up" phenomenon at a former contact area with clonidine TTS has been described after rechallenging with oral clonidine. The incidence of skin reactions seems to depend on geographical location and was reported to occur in between 15% and 43% of patients (GROTH et al. 1985; BOEKHORST and VAN TOL 1985). Skin toxicity studies show that contact sensitization occurred only by use of the clonidine TTS system and not by clonidine in petrolatum. It seems most likely that the sensitizing agent is a molecule formed by a clonidine-acetaldehyde reaction (MAIBACH 1985).

Contraindications for the use of α-methyldopa can be deduced from the toxic effects described above: hepatic deseases and hypersensitivity.

Summary

Two of the reviewed drugs, clonidine and guanfacine, have chemical structures related to each other; the third one, α-methyldopa, is completely different. Pharmacologically they have been classified as clonidine-like hypotensive drugs, as defined by two criteria: a direct stimulation of α-adrenoceptors and a hypotensive effect of central origin. The three drugs have in common their cardiovascular profile, i.e., a long-lasting decrease in blood pressure, heart rate, cardiac output, and/or peripheral vascular resistance due to a decrease in sympathetic and an increase in vagal activity. With rapid i.v. injection the pressure fall is preceded by a pressure rise, due to the stimulation of vascular α-adrenoceptors. They have in common a number of side effects also due to stimulation of α-adrenoceptors such as sedation and dryness of the mouth, and a "discontinuation syndrome" after rapid cessation of therapy. The degree and incidence of these side effects is reported to be different for the three drugs, clonidine being mentioned more frequently, which might be due to the pioneer role of this drug in the field. All three drugs lower blood pressure in virtually all grades of hypertension of various origins, without orthostasis at rest and after exercise. They differ in metabolism: clonidine and guanfacine have elimination half-lives of about 10 h or more, α-methyldopa of only about 1 h. α-Methyldopa acts as a prodrug which has to penetrate into the CNS and be converted to α-methylnoradrenaline, the active metabolite. Most evidence regarding mode of action is in favor of a direct stimulation of postsynaptic α_2-adrenoceptors within medullary cardiovascular centers; however, other mechanisms have also been proposed and are discussed here.

References

Ahlquist RP (1948) A study of the adrenotropic receptors. Am J Physiol 153:586–600

Ahlquist RP, Kobinger W (1984) Introduction. In: Kobinger W, Ahlquist RP (eds) Alpha and beta adrenoceptors and the cardiovascular system. Excerpta Medica, Amsterdam, p 1

Alexander WD, Evans JI (1975) Side effects of methyldopa. Br Med J 1:501

Andén N-E, Corrodi H, Fuxe K, Hökfelt B, Hökfelt T, Rydin C, Svensson T (1970) Evidence for a central noradrenaline receptor stimulation by clonidine. Life Sci 9: 513–523

Arndts D (1983) New aspects of the clinical pharmacology of clonidine. Chest 83: 397–400

Arndts D, Doevendans J, Kirsten R, Heintz B (1983) New aspects of the pharmacokinetics and pharmacodynamics of clonidine in man. Eur J Clin Pharmacol 24:21–30

Barber ND, Reid JL (1982) Comparison of the actions of centrally and peripherally administered clonidine and guanfacine in the rabbit: investigation of the differences. Br J Pharmacol 77:641–647

Barnett AJ, Bobik A, Carson V, Korman JS, McLean AJ (1977) Pharmacokinetics of methyldopa. Plasma levels following single intravenous, oral and multiple oral dosage in normotensive and hypertensive subjects. Clin Exp Pharmacol Physiol 4:331–339

Baum T, Shropshire AT, Varner LL (1972) Contribution of the central nervous system to the action of several antihypertensive agents (methyldopa, hydralazine and guanethidine). J Pharmacol Exp Ther 182:135–144

Bentley GA, Li DMF (1968) Studies of the new hypotensive drug St 155. Eur J Pharmacol 4:124–134

Berthelsen S, Pettinger WA (1977) A functional basis for classification of adrenergic receptors. Life Sci 21:595–606

Beveridge T, Kiechel JR, Meier J, Schreier E (1977) Guanfacine: ADME studies in animal and man. Sandoz internal document. Sandoz, Basel

Bock KD, Merguet P, Heimsoth VH (1973) Effect of clonidine on regional blood flow and its use in the treatment of hypertension. In: Onesti G, Kim KE, Moyer JH (eds) Hypertension: mechanisms and management. Grune and Stratton, New York, p 395

Boekhorst JC, Van Tol RGL (1985) Catapres transdermal therapeutic system (TTS) for longterm treatment of hypertension. In: Weber MA, Drayer JIM, Kolloch R (eds) Low dose oral and transdermal therapy of hypertension. Steinkopff, Darmstadt, p 106

Borowski E, Starke K, Ehrl H, Endo T (1977) A comparison of pre- and postsynaptic effects of α-adrenolytic drugs in the pulmonary artery of the rabbit. Neuroscience 2:285–296

Bousquet P, Feldman J (1987) The blood pressure effects of alpha-adrenoceptor antagonists injected in the medullary site of action of clonidine: the nucleus reticularis lateralis. Life Sci 40:1045–1052

Bousquet P, Feldman J. Velly I, Bloch R (1975) Role of the ventral surface of the brain stem in the hypotensive action of clonidine. Eur J Pharmacol 34:151–156

Bousquet P, Feldman J, Bloch R, Schwartz J (1978) Is the hypotensive effect obtained by application of drugs to the ventral surface of the brain stem due to a membrane stabilizing mechanism? A study with beta-blockers. Neuropharmacology 17:605–609

Bousquet P, Feldman J, Bloch R, Schwartz J (1981) The nucleus reticularis lateralis: a region highly sensitive to clonidine. Eur J Pharmacol 69:389–392

Bousquet P, Feldman J, Schwartz J (1985) The medullary cardiovascular effects of imidazolines and some GABA analogues: a review. J Auton Nerv Syst 14:263–270

Bousquet P, Feldman J, Atlas D (1986) An endogenous, non-catecholamine clonidine antagonist increases mean arterial blood pressure. Eur J Pharmacol 124:167–170

Bravo EL, Cressman MD, Pohl MA (1985) Cardiovascular and neurohumoral effects of long-term oral clonidine monotherapy in essential hypertensive patients. In: Weber MA, Drayer JIM, Kolloch R (eds) Low dose oral and transdermal therapy of hypertension. Steinkopff, Darmstadt, p 3

Carlsson A, Lindquist M (1962) In-vivo decarboxylation of α-methyl DOPA and α-methyl-metatyrosine. Acta Phys Scand 54:87–94

Chierichetti SM, Fiorella G, Vibelli C, Capitani M, Nami R, Gennari C (1982) Double-blind comparison between acute guanfacine and clonidine administrations on hypotensive activity and side effects in healthy volunteers and hypertensive patients. Curr Ther Res 31:588–600

Conolly ME, Briant RH, George CF, Dollery CT (1972) A crossover comparison of clonidine and methyldopa in hypertension. Eur J Clin Pharmacol 4:222–227

Constantine JW, McShane WK (1968) Analysis of the cardiovascular effects of 2-(2,6-dichlorophenylamino)-2-imidazoline hydrochloride (Catapres). Eur J Pharmacol 4: 109–123

Conway EL, Jarrott B (1980) Clonidine distribution in the rat: temporal relationship between tissue levels and blood pressure response. Br J Pharmacol 71:473–478

Conway EL, Jarrott B (1982) Tissue pharmacokinetics of clonidine in rats. J Pharmacokinet Biopharm 10:187–200

Csongrady A, Kobinger W (1974) Investigations into the positive inotropic effect of clonidine in isolated hearts. Naunyn Schmiedebergs Arch Pharmacol 282:123–128

Darda S, Förster H-J, Stähle H (1978) Metabolischer Abbau von Clonidin. Arzneimittelforschung 28:255–259

Davies DS, Wing LMH, Reid JL, Neill E, Tippett P, Dollery CT (1977) Pharmacokinetics and concentration-effect relationship of intravenous and oral clonidine. Clin Pharmacol Ther 21:593–601

Day MD, Rand MJ (1964) Some observations on the pharmacology of α-methyldopa. Br J Pharmacol 22:78–86

Deering AH, Riddell JG, Shanks RG, Harron DWG (1987) Baroreceptor function in man following peripheral $alpha_1$- and $alpha_2$-adrenoceptor stimulation. Eur J Clin Pharmacol 33:41–47

Delbarre B, Schmitt H (1971) Sedative effects of α-sympathomimetic drugs and their antagonism by adrenergic and cholinergic blocking drugs. Eur J Pharmacol 13:356–363

Diehm C, Mörl H (1985) Lipid metabolism and antihypertensive treatment. In: Weber MA, Drayer JIM, Kolloch R (eds) Low dose oral and transdermal therapy of hypertension. Steinkopff, Darmstadt, p 31

Docherty JR (1984) An investigation of presynaptic α-adrenoceptor subtypes in the pithed rat heart and in the rat isolated vas deferens. Br J Pharmacol 82:15–23

Docherty JR, McGrath JC (1980) A comparison of pre- and postjunctional potencies of several alpha-adrenoceptor agonists in the cardiovascular system and anococcygeus muscle of the rat. Evidence for two types of postjunctional alpha-adrenoceptor. Naunyn Schmiedebergs Arch Pharmacol 312:107–116

Dollery CT, Davies DS (1980) Centrally acting drugs in antihypertensive therapy. Br J Clin Pharmacol 10:5S–12S

Dollery CT, Reid JL (1973) Central noradrenergic neurons and the cardiovascular actions of clonidine in the rabbit. J Pharmacol 47:206–216

Dollery CT, Davies DS, Draffan GH, Dargie HJ, Dean CR, Reid JL, Clare RA, Murray S (1976) Clinical pharmacology and pharmacokinetics of clonidine. Clin Pharmacol Ther 19:11–17

Doxey JC, Smith CFC, Walker JM (1977) Selectivity of blocking agents for pre- and postsynaptic α-adrenoceptors. Br J Pharmacol 60:91–96

Dubocovich ML, Langer SZ (1974) Negative feed-back regulation of noradrenaline release by nerve stimulation in the perfused cat's spleen: differences in potency of phenoxybenzamine in blocking the pre- and postsynaptic adrenergic receptors. J Physiol 237:505–519

Farnebo L-O, Hamberger B (1971) Drug-induced changes in the release of ^{3}H-monoamines from field stimulated rat brain slices. Acta Physiol Scand [Suppl] 371:35–44

Farsang C, Kunos G (1979) Naloxone reverses the antihypertensive effect of clonidine. Br J Pharmacol 67:161–164

Feldberg W, Guertzenstein PG (1976) Vasodepressor effects obtained by drugs acting on the ventral surface of the brain stem. J Physiol (Lond) 258:337–355

Feldstein CA, Cohen AA, Sabaris RP, Burucúa JE (1984) Hemodynamic effects of

guanfacine in essential hypertension. Clin Ther 6: 325–334
Finch L (1975) The central hypotensive action of clonidine and Bay 1470 in cats and rats. Clin Sci Mol Med 48:273s–278s
Finch L, Harvey CA, Hicks PE, Owen DAA (1978) Clonidine-induced hypotension: further evidence for a central interaction with histamine H_2-receptor antagonists in the rat. Neuropharmacology 17:307–313
Fitzgerald GA, Watkins J, Dollery CT (1981) Regulation of norepinephrine release by peripheral α_2-receptor stimulation. Clin Pharmacol Ther 29:160–167
Flacke JW, Bloor BC, Flacke WE, Wong D, Dazza S, Stead SW, Laks H (1987) Reduced narcotic requirement by clonidine with improved hemodynamic and adrenergic stability in patients undergoing coronary bypass surgerv. Anesthesiology 67: 11–19
Frisk-Holmberg M, Edlund PO, Paalzow L (1978) Pharmacokinetics of clonidine and its relation to the hypotensive effect in patients. Br J Pharmacol 6:227–232
Garbus SB, Weber MA, Priest RT, Brewer DD, Hubbell FA (1979) The abrupt discontinuation of antihypertensive treatment. J Clin Pharmacol 19:476–486
Goldberg AD, Raftery EB, Wilkinson P (1977) Blood pressure and heart rate and withdrawal of antihypertensive drugs. Br Med J 1:1243–1246
Grabner G, Michalek P, Pokorny D, Vormittag E (1966) Klinische und experimentelle Untersuchungen mit der neuen blutdrucksenkenden Substanz 2-(2,6-dichlorphenylamino)-2-imidazolinhydrochlorid. Arzneimittelforschung 16:1174–1179
Groth H, Vetter H, Knüsel J, Baumgart P, Vetter W (1985) Transdermal clonidine in essential hypertension: problems during long-term treatment. In: Weber MA, Drayer JIM, Kolloch R (eds) Low dose oral and transdermal therapy of hypertension. Steinkopff, Darmstadt, p 60
Guertzenstein PG (1973) Blood pressure effects obtained by drugs applied to the ventral surface of the brain stem. J Physiol (Lond) 229:395–408
Haeusler G, Finch L (1972) On the nature of the central hypotensive effect of clonidine and α-methyldopa. Abstracts. Réunion Commune de la Deutsche Pharmakologische Gesellschaft et de l'Association Francaise des Pharmacologistes, Paris, p 16
Halushka PV, Keiser HR (1974) Effects of alpha methyldopa on mean blood pressure and plasma renin activity. Circ Res 35:458–463
Head GA, DeJong W (1984) Effects of naloxone on the cardiovascular responses to clonidine, α-methyldopa and 6-hydroxydopamine in conscious normotensive and spontaneously hypertensive rats. Clin Exp Hypertens A6:2051–2054
Heise A, Kroneberg G (1972) Alpha-sympathetic receptor stimulation in the brain and hypotensive action of α-methyl-DOPA. Eur J Pharmacol 17:315–317
Heller H (1933) Über die zentrale Blutdruckwirkung des Adrenalins. Naunyn Schmiedebergs Arch Exp Pathol Pharmakol 173:291–300
Henning M, Van Zwieten PA (1967) Central hypotensive effect of α-methyl-DOPA, J Pharm Pharmacol 19:403–405
Henning M, Van Zwieten PA (1968) Central hypotensive action of α-methyl-DOPA, J Pharm Pharmacol 20:409–417
Hey JA, Gherezghiher T, Koss MC (1985) Studies on the mechanism of clonidine-induced mydriasis in the rat. Naunyn Schmiedebergs Arch Pharmacol 328:258–263
Hoefke W, Kobinger W (1966) Pharmakologische Wirkung des 2-(2,6-dichlorphenylamino)-2-imidazolinhydrochlorids, einer neuen, antihypertensiven Substanz. Arzneimittelforschung 16:1038–1050
Holtz P, Palm D (1966) Brenzkatechinamine und andere sympathicomimetische Amine. Rev Physiol Biochem Pharmacol 58. Springer, Berlin Heidelberg New York
Hökfelt B, Hedeland H, Dymling J-F (1970) Studies on catecholamines, renin and aldosterone following catapresan® (2-(2,6-dichlorophenylamino)-2-imidazoline hydrochloride) in hypertensive patients. Eur J Pharmacol 10:389–397
Hökfelt T, Lundberg JM, Tatemoto K, Mutt V, Terenius L, Polak J, Bloom S, Saseh C, Elde R, Goldstein M (1983) Neuropeptide Y (NPY)- and FMRFamide neuropeptide-like immunoreactivities in catecholamine neurons of the rat medulla oblongata. Acta Physiol Scand 117:315–318
Houston MC (1981) Abrupt cessation of treatment in hypertension: consideration of clinical features, mechanisms, prevention and management of the discontinuation

syndrome. Am Heart J 102:415–430
Houston MC (1982) Clonidine hydrochloride. South Med J 75:713–721
Houston MC, Hays T, Nadeau J, Olafsson L, Burger C (1987) Effects of clonidine and atenolol monotherapy on serum lipids, lipoproteins, and glucose in mild primary hypertension. Clin Res 35:17A
Hulter HN, Licht JH, Ilnicki LP, Singh S (1979) Clinical efficacy and pharmacokinetics of clonidine in hemodialysis and renal insufficiency. J Lab Clin Med 94:223–231
Hukuhara T, Otsuka Y, Takeda R, Sakai F (1968) Die zentralen Wirkungen des 2-(2,6-dichlorphenylamino)-2-imidazolin-hydrochlorids. Arzneimittelforschung 18: 1147–1153
Humblet C, Marshall GR, Wermuth CG (1981) Computer-assisted molecular modeling applied to α_2-pre-synaptic adrenergic drugs. Abstracts. Chemical regulation of biological mechanisms, symposium, Cambridge
Innemee HC, Van Zwieten PA (1979) The central ocular hypotensive effect of clonidine. Naunyn Schmiedebergs Arch Pharmacol 307:R60
Innemee HC, Hermans AJM, Van Zwieten PA (1979) The influence of clonidine on intraocular pressure after topical application to the eyes of anaesthetized cats. Graefes Arch Clin Exp Ophthalmol 212:19–27
Jäättelä A (1980) Comparison of guanfacine and clonidine as antihypertensive agents. Br J Clin Pharmacol 10:67S–70S
Jaju BP, Tangri KK, Bhargava KP (1966) Central vasomotor effects of α-methyl-DOPA. Can J Physiol Pharmacol 44:687–690
Jarrott B (1984) Clonidine and related compounds. In: Doyle AE (ed) Clinical pharmacology of antihypertensive drugs. Elsevier Science, Amsterdam, p 113 (Handbook of hypertension, vol 5)
Jarrott B, Spector S (1978) Disposition of clonidine in rats as determined by radioimmunoassay. J Pharmacol Exp Ther 207:195–202
Jarrott B, Conway EL, Maccarrone C, Lewis SJ (1987) Clonidine: understanding its disposition, sites and mechanism of action. Clin Exp Pharmacol Physiol 14:471–479
Jen T, Dienel BV, Bowman H, Petta J, Helt A, Loev B (1972) Amidines. 2. A new class of antihypertensive agents. 1,2,3,5-tetrahydro imidazo (2,1-b) quinazolines. J Med Chem 15:727–731
Jen T, VanHoeven H, Groves W, McLean R, Loev B (1975) Amidines and related compounds. 6. Studies on structure-activity relationship of antihypertensive and antisecretory agents related to clonidine. J Med Chem 18:90–99
Jerie P (1980a) Clinical experience with guanfacine in long-term treatment of hypertension. Part I: efficacy and dosage. Br J Clin Pharmacol 10:37S–47S
Jerie P (1980b) Clinical experience with guanfacine in long-term treatment of hypertension. Part II: adverse reactions to guanfacine, Br J Clin Pharmacol 10:157S–164S
Kaniucki MD, Stefano FJE, Perec CJ (1984) Clonidine inhibits salivary secretion by activation of postsynaptic α_2-receptors. Naunyn Schmiedebergs Arch Pharmacol 326: 313–316
Kaplan NM (1975) Antihypertensive drugs in combination: effects of methyldopa on thiazide-induced changes in renal haemodynamics and plasma renin activity. Arch Intern Med 135:660–663
Karppanen HO, Westermann E (1973) Increased production of cyclic AMP in gastric tissue by stimulation of histamine$_2$ (H_2)-receptors. Naunyn Schmiedebergs Arch Pharmacol 279:83–87
Karppanen H, Paakkari I, Paakkari P, Huotari R, Orma A-L (1976) Possible involvement of central histamine H_2-receptors in the hypotensive effect of clonidine. Nature 259:587–588
Keller E, Sorger D, Willgerodt H (1983) Clonidine (Haemiton®) as a reliable stimulus of growth hormone secretion in patients with short stature. Exp Clin Endocrinol 81: 315–320
Kersting F, Reid JL, Dollery CT (1977) Clinical and cardiovascular effects of alpha methyldopa in combination with decarboxylase inhibitors. Clin Pharmacol Ther 21: 547–555
Kiechel JR (1980) Pharmacokinetics and metabolism of guanfacine in man: a review. Br

J Clin Pharmacol 10:25S–32S
Kirkendall WM, Wilson WR (1962) Pharmacodynamics and clinical use of guanethidine, bretylium and methyldopa. Am J Cardiol 9:107–115
Kleinlogel H, Scholtysik G, Sayers AC (1975) Effects of clonidine and BS 100–141 on the EEG sleep pattern in rats. Eur J Pharmacol 33:159–163
Klupp H, Knappen F, Otsuka Y, Streller J, Teichmann H (1970) Effects of clonidine on central sympathetic tone. Eur J Pharmacol 10:225–229
Kobinger W (1967) Über den Wirkungsmechanismus einer neuen antihypertensiven Substanz mit Imidazolinstruktur. Naunyn Schmiedebergs Arch Pharmacol 258: 48–58
Kobinger W (1978) Central α-adrenergic systems as targets for hypotensive drugs. Rev Physiol Biochem Pharmacol 81:39–100
Kobinger W (1981) The role of α-adrenoceptors in central nervous and peripheral vascular regulation. Jpn J Pharmacol 31 Suppl:13P–20P
Kobinger W (1984a) Central anti-hypertensives. In: Parnham MJ, Bruinvels J (eds) Haemodynamics, hormones & inflammation. Elsevier Science, Amsterdam, p 107 (Discoveries in pharmacology, vol 2)
Kobinger W (1984b) New concepts on α-adrenoceptors in pharmacology. J Pharmacol 15 (Suppl I):5–22
Kobinger W (1986) Drugs as tools in research on adrenoceptors. Naunyn Schmiedebergs Arch Pharmacol 332:113–123
Kobinger W, Pichler L (1975a) The central modulatory effect of clonidine on the cardiodepressor reflex after suppression of synthesis and storage of noradrenaline. Eur J Pharmacol 30:56–62
Kobinger W, Pichler L (1975b) Localization in the CNS of adrenoceptors which facilitate a cardioinhibitory reflex. Naunyn Schmiedebergs Arch Pharmacol 286:371–377
Kobinger W, Pichler L (1976) Centrally induced reduction in sympathetic tone—a postsynaptic α-adrenoceptor stimulating action of imidazolines. Eur J Pharmacol 40: 311–320
Kobinger W, Pichler L (1977) Pharmacological characterization of B-HT 933 (2-amino-6-ethyl-4,5,7,8-tetrahydro-6H-oxazolo-[5,4-d]-azepin-dihydrochloride) as a hypotensive agent of the "clonidine-type". Naunyn Schmiedebergs Arch Pharmacol 300: 39–46
Kobinger W, Pichler L (1980) Investigation into different types of post- and presynaptic α-adrenoceptors at cardiovascular sites in rats. Eur J Pharmacol 65:393–402
Kobinger W, Pichler L (1981) α_1- and α_2-Adrenoceptor subtypes: selectivity of various agonists and relative distribution of receptors as determined in rats. Eur J Pharmacol 73:313–321
Kobinger W, Pichler L (1983a) α_1/α_2 Selectivity ratio in a series of agonists and their relation to pre/postsynaptic activity ratios. Eur J Pharmacol 91:129–133
Kobinger W, Pichler L (1983b) Subgroups of α-adrenoceptors: selectivity of drugs and receptor importance in various target systems. In: Bock KD (ed) Catapresan® (Clonidin). Wege der Entwicklung eines Pharmakons. Arzneimittelforschung 28 (Suppl):83
Kobinger W, Walland A (1967a) Kreislaufuntersuchungen mit 2-(2,6-dichlorphenylamino)-2-imidazolin hydrochloride. Arzneimittelforschung 17:292–300
Kobinger W, Walland A (1967b) Investigations into the mechanism of the hypotensive effect of 2-(2,6-dichlorophenylamino)-2-imidazoline HCl. Eur J Pharmacol 2:155–162
Kobinger W, Walland A (1971) Involvement of adrenergic receptors in central vagus activity. Eur J Pharmacol 16:120–122
Kobinger W, Walland A (1972a) Evidence for a central activation of a vagal cardiodepressor reflex by clonidine. Eur J Pharmacol 19:203–209
Kobinger W, Walland A (1972b) Facilitation of vagal reflex bradycardia by an action of clonidine on central α-receptors. Eur J Pharmacol 19:210–217
Kobinger W, Walland A (1973) Modulating effect of central adrenergic neurones on a vagally mediated cardioinhibitory reflex. Eur J Pharmacol 22:344–350
Kobinger W, Lillie C, Pichler L (1980) Central cardiovascular α-adrenoceptors. Relation to peripheral receptors. Circ Res 46:I-21–I-25

Kolloch R, Finster H, Overlack A, Müller HM, Stumpe KO (1985) Low dose oral and transdermal application of clonidine in mild hypertension: hemodynamic and biochemical correlates. In: Weber MA, Drayer JIM, Kolloch R (eds) Low dose oral and transdermal therapy of hypertension. Steinkopff, Darmstadt, p 71
Korner PJ, Oliver JR, Sleight P, Chalmers JP, Robinson JS (1974) Effects of clonidine on the baroreceptor-heart rate reflex and on single aortic baroreceptor fibre discharge. Eur J Pharmacol 28:189–198
Kroneberg HG (1962/63) Pharmakologie der blutdrucksenkenden Arzneimittel. Verh Dtsch Ges Kreislaufforsch 28/29:172–184
Kroneberg G, Stoepel K (1963) Der Einfluß von α-Methyl-Dopa auf die Tyraminwirkung an mit Reserpin vorbehandelten Katzen. Experientia 19:252–253
Kwan KC, Foltz EL, Breault GO, Bear JE, Totaro JA (1976) Pharmacokinetics of methyldopa in man. J Pharmacol Exp Ther 198:264–277
Langer SZ (1977) Presynaptic receptors and their role in the regulation of transmitter release. Br J Pharmacol 60:481–497
Langer SZ (1981) Presynaptic regulation of the release of catecholamines. Pharmacol Rev 32:337–362
Laubie M, Schmitt H (1969) Effects hémodynamiques du St 155, 2-(2,6-dichlorophenylamino)-2-imidazoline hydrochloride, chez le chien hypertendu. Arch Int Pharmacodyn 179:23–25
Laubie M, Schmitt H (1977) Sites of action of clonidine: centrally mediated increase in vagal tone, centrally mediated hypotensive and sympathoinhibitory effects. Proc Brain Res 47:337–348
Laubie M, Schmitt H, Drouillat M (1976) Action of clonidine on the baroreceptor pathways and medullary sites mediating vagal bradycardia. Eur J Pharmacol 38:292–303
Lipski J, Przybylski J, Solnicka E (1976) Reduced hypotensive effect of clonidine after lesions of the nucleus tractus solitarii in rats. Eur J Pharmacol 38:19–22
Longnecker DE (1987) Alpine anesthesia: can pretreatment with clonidine decrease the peaks and valleys?, Anesthesiology 67:1–2
Lowenthal DT, Affrime MB, Meyer A, Kim KE, Falkner B, Sharif K (1983) Pharmacokinetics and pharmacodynamics of clonidine in varying states of renal function. Chest 83 (Suppl):386–390
Magometschnigg D, Hitzenberger G, Bonelli J (1980) Haemodynamic effects of guanfacine. Br J Clin Pharmacol 10:125S–131S
Maibach H (1985) Clonidine transdermal delivery system: cutaneous toxicity studies. In: Weber MA, Drayer JIM, Kolloch R (eds) Low dose oral and transdermal therapy of hypertension. Steinkopff, Darmstadt, p 55
Mannhold R (1987) Moxonidine hydrochloride. Drugs Future 12:553–555
Maxwell GM (1969) The effects of 2-(2,6-dichlorophenylamino)-2-imidazoline hydrochloride (catapres) upon the systemic and coronary haemodynamics and metabolism of intact dogs. Arch Int Pharmacodyn 181:7–14
McCubbin JW, Kaneko Y, Page IH (1960) Ability of serotonin and norepinephine to mimic the central effects of reserpine on vasomotor activity. Circ Res 8:849–858
McCulloch MW, Medgett IC, Rand MJ, Story DF (1980) Structure-activity relationship of imidazolidine derivatives related to clonidine at histamine H_2-receptors in guinea-pig isolated atria. Br J Pharmacol 69:397–405
McMahon FG (1984) Management of essential hypertension: the new low-dose era, 2nd edn. Futura, Mount Kisco NY
Medgett IC, McCulloch MW (1980) Receptor sites of action of clonidine: effects of clonidine and three structural isomers on prejunctional and postjunctional α-adrenoceptors and histamine H_2-receptors in guinea-pig isolated cardio-vascular tissues. J Pharm Pharmacol 32:137–138
Morgan T (1983) The use of centrally acting antihypertensive drugs in patients with renal disease. Chest 83 (Suppl):383–386
Muir AL, Burton JL, Lawrie DM (1969) Circulatory effects at rest and exercise of clonidine, an imidazoline derivative with hypotensive properties. Lancet II: 181–184
Muscholl E, Maître L (1963) Release by sympathetic stimulation of α-methyl-noradrenaline stored in the heart after administration of α-methyldopa. Experientia 19:

658–659
Muscholl E, Rahn KH (1968) Über den Nachweis und die Bedeutung von α-Methylnoradrenaline im Harn von Hypertonikern bei Verabreichung von α-Methyldopa. Pharmacol Clin 1:19–20
Myhre E, Rugstad HE, Hansen T (1982) Clinical pharmacokinetics of methyldopa. Clin Pharmacokinet 7:221–233
Nayler WG, Price JM, Swann JB, McInnes J, Race D, Lowe TE (1968) Effect of the hypotensive drug St 155 (Catapres) on the heart and peripheral circulation. J Pharmacol Exp Ther 164:45–59
Oates JA, Conolly ME, Prichard BNC, Shand DG, Schapel G (1977) The clinical pharmacology of antihypertensive drugs. In: Gross F (ed) Antihypertensive agents. Springer, Berlin Heidelberg NewYork, p. 571 (Handbook of experimental pharmacology, vol 39)
Oates HF, Stoker LM, McCarthy EP, Monaghan JC, Stokes GS (1978) Comparative haemodynamic effects of clonidine and guanfacine. Arch Int Pharmacodyn 231: 148–156
Onesti G, Schwartz AB, Kim KE, Schwartz CH, Brest AN (1969) Pharmacodynamic effects of a new antihypertensive drug, catapres (St 155). Circulation 39: 219–228
Onesti G, Schwartz AB, Kim KE, Paz-Martinez V, Schwartz CH (1971) Antihypertensive effect of clonidine. Circ Res 28 (Suppl 2):53–69
Paalzow G, Edlund PO (1979) Pharmacokinetics of clonidine in the rat and cat. J Pharmacokinet Biopharm 7:481–494
Paalzow G, Paalzow L (1976) Clonidine antinociceptive activity: effects of drugs influencing central monoaminergic and cholinergic mechanisms in the rat. Naunyn Schmiedebergs Arch Pharmacol 292:119–126
Paykel ES (1966) Hallucinosis on combined methyldopa and pargyline. Br Med J 1:803
Peaston MJT (1964) Parkinsonism associated with alpha methyldopa therapy. Br Med J 2:168
Pettinger WA, Mitchell HC, Guellner H-G (1977) Clonidine and the vasodilating beta blocker antihypertensive drug interaction. Clin Pharmacol Ther 22:164–171
Pichler L, Kobinger W (1978) Presynaptic activity at peripheral adrenergic sites and blood pressure effect of α-adrenoceptor stimulating drugs. Eur J Pharmacol 52: 287–295
Pichler L, Kobinger W (1981) Centrally mediated cardiovascular effects of B-HT 920 (6-allyl-2-amino-5,6,7,8-tetrahydro-4H-thiazolo-[4,5-d]-azepine dihydrochloride), a hypotensive agent of the "clonidine type". J Cardiovasc Pharmacol 3:269–277
Pichler L, Placheta P, Kobinger W (1980) Effect of azepexole (B-HT 933) on pre- and postsynaptic α-adrenoceptors at peripheral and central nervous sites. Eur J Pharmacol 65:233–241
Porter CC, Totaro JA, Leiby CM (1961) Some biochemical effects of α-methyl-3,4-dihydroxy-phenylalanine and related compounds in mice. J Pharmacol Exp Ther 134:139–145
Rehbinder D, Deckers W (1969) Untersuchungen zur Pharmakokinetik und zum Metabolismus des 2-(2,6-Dichlorphenylamino)-2-imidazolin-hydrochlorid (St 155). Arzneimittelforschung 19:169–176
Reid JL, Elliott HL (1984) Methyldopa. In: Doyle AE (ed) Clinical pharmacology of antihypertensive drugs. Elsevier Science, Amsterdam, p 92 (Handbook of hypertension, vol 5)
Reid JL, Barber ND, Davies DS (1980) The clinical pharmacology of clonidine: relationship between plasma concentration and pharmacological effect in animals and man. Arch Int Pharmacodyn (Suppl) 11–16
Reynoldson JA, Head GA, Korner PI (1979) Effect of 6-hydroxydopamine on blood pressure and heart rate responses to intracisternal clonidine in conscious rabbits. Eur J Pharmacol 55:257–262
Robson RD, Kaplan HR (1969) An involvement of St 155 (2-(2,6-dichlorophenylamino)-2-imidazoline hydrochloride (Catapres) in cholinergic mechanisms. Eur J Pharmacol 5:328–337
Russ GR, Whitworth JA, Kincaid-Smith P (1983) Comparison of intramuscular and

intravenous clonidine in severe hypertension. Med J Aust 2:229–231
Saameli K, Jerie P, Scholtysik G (1982) Guanfacine and other centrally acting drugs in antihypertensive therapy; pharmacological and clinical aspects. Clin Exp Hypertens A4:209–219
Saavedra JA, Reid JL, Jordan W, Rawlins MD, Dollery CT (1975) Plasma concentration of methyldopa and sulphate conjugates after oral administration of methyldopa and its ester. Eur J Pharmacol 8:381–386
Sambhi MP (1983) Clonidine monotherapy in mild hypertension. Chest 83 (Suppl): 427–430
Sannerstedt R, Conway J (1970) Hemodynamic and vascular responses to antihypertensive treatment with adrenergic blocking agents: a review. Am Heart J 79: 122–127
Sattler RW, Van Zwieten PA (1967) Acute hypotensive action of 2-(2,6-dichlorophenylamino)-2-imidazoline hydrochloride (St 155) after infusion into the cat's vertebral artery. Eur J Pharmacol 2:9–13
Savola J-M, Ruskoaho H, Puurunen J, Kärki NT (1985) Cardiovascular action of detomidine, a sedative and analgesic imidazole derivative with α-agonistic properties. Eur J Pharmacol 118:69–76
Savola J-M, Virtanen R, Karjalainen A, Ruskoaho H, Puurunen J, Kärki NT (1986) Reevaluation of drug-interaction with α-adrenoceptors *in vivo* and *in vitro* using imidazole derivatives. Life Sci 38:1409–1415
Schieber RA, Kaufman ND (1981) Use of tolazoline in massive clonidine poisoning. Am J Dis Child 135:77–78
Schmitt H (1977) The pharmacology of clonidine and related products. In: Gross F (ed) Antihypertensive agents. Springer, Berlin Heidelberg New York, p 299 (Handbook of experimental pharmacology, vol 39)
Schmitt H, Schmitt H (1969) Localization of the hypotensive effect of 2-(2,6-dichlorophenylamino)-2-imidazoline hydrochloride (St 155, Catapresan). Eur J Pharmacol 6:8–12
Schmitt H, Schmitt H, Boissier JR, Giudicelli JF (1967) Centrally mediated decrease in sympathetic tone induced by 2-(2,6-dichlorophenylamino)-2-imidazoline (St 155, Catapresan). Eur J Pharmacol 2:147–148
Schmitt H, Schmitt H, Fénard S (1971) Evidence for an α-sympathomimetic component in the effects of catapresan on vasomotor centres: antagonism by piperoxane. Eur J Pharmacol 14:98–100
Schmitt H, Schmitt H, Fénard S (1973) Action of α-adrenergic blocking drugs on the sympathetic centres and their interactions with the central sympathoinhibitory effect of clonidine. Arzneimittelforschung 23:40–45
Scholtysik G (1980) Pharmacology of guanfacine. Br J Clin Pharmacol 10:21S–24S
Scholtysik G, Lauener H, Eichenberger E, Bürki H, Salzmann R, Müller-Schweinitzer E, Waite R (1975) Pharmacological actions of the antihypertensive agent N-amidino-2-(2,6-dichlorophenyl) acetamide hydrochloride (BS 100–141). Arzneimittelforschung 25:1483–1491
Scholtysik G, Jerie P, Picard CW (1980) Guanfacine. In: Scriabine A (ed) Pharmacology of antihypertensive drugs. Raven Press, New York, p 79
Schultz HS, Chretien SD, Brewer DD, Eltorai MI, Weber MA (1981) Centrally acting antihypertensive agents: a comparison of lofexidine with clonidine. J Clin Pharmacol 21:65–71
Schwartz A, Banach S, Smith JS, Kim KE, Onesti G, Swartz CH (1973) Clinical efficacy of clonidine in hypertension. In: Onesti G, Kim KE, Moyer JH (eds) Hypertension: mechanisms and management. Grune and Stratton, New York, p 389
Scriabine A (1980) Methyldopa. In: Scriabine A (ed) Pharmacology of antihypertensive drugs. Raven Press, New York, p 43
Scriabine A, Ludden CT, Stone CA, Wurtman RJ, Watkins CJ (1976) Enhancement of the antihypertensive effect of methyldopa and other antihypertensive drugs by carbidopa in spontaneously hypertensive rats. Clin Sci Mol Med 51:407S–410S
Seedat YK (1983) Guanfacine alone and in combination therapy in the treatment of moderate and severe hypertension. Chest 83 (Suppl):403–404
Shaw JE (1984) Pharmacokinetics of nitroglycerin and clonidine delivered by the trans-

dermal route. Am Heart J 108:217–223
Sinha JN, Tangri KK, Bhargava KP, Schmitt H (1975) Central sites of sympathoinhibitory effects of clonidine and L-dopa. In: Milliez P, Safar M (eds) Recent advances in hypertension, vol 1. Société Aliéna, Reims, p 97
Sorkin EM, Heel RC (1986) Guanfacine. A review of its pharmacodynamic and pharmacokinetic properties, and therapeutic efficacy in the treatment of hypertension. Drugs 31:301–336
Stähle H (1982) Clonidine. In: Bindra JS, Lednicer D (eds) Chronicles of drug discovery, vol 1, Wiley, New York, p 87
Starke K (1977) Regulation of noradrenaline release by presynaptic receptor systems. Rev Physiol Biochem Pharmacol 77:1–124
Starke K (1979) Presynaptic modulation of catecholamine release in the central nervous system. Some open questions. In: Langer SZ, Starke K, Dubocovich ML (eds) Presynaptic receptors. Pergamon, Oxford, p 129 (Advances in the biosciences, vol 18)
Starke K (1981) α-Adrenoceptor subclassification. Rev Physiol Biochem Pharmacol 88: 199–236
Starke K, Montel H (1973) Involvement of α-receptors in clonidine-induced inhibition of transmitter release from central monoamine neurons. Neuropharmacology 12: 1073–1080
Starke K, Endo T, Taube HD (1975) Relative pre- and postsynaptic potencies of α-adrenoceptor agonists in the rabbit pulmonary artery. Naunyn Schmiedebergs Arch Pharmacol 291:55–78
Stenbaek O, Myhre E, Brodwall EK, Hansen T (1971) Hypotensive effect of methyldopa in renal failure associated with hypertension. Acta Med Scand 191:333–337
Stenbaek O, Myhre E, Rugstad HE, Arnold E, Hansen T (1977) Pharmacokinetics of methyldopa in normal man. J Clin Pharmacol Ther 12:117–123
Svensson TH, Bunney BS, Aghajanian GK (1975) Inhibition of both noradrenergic and serotonergic neurons in brain by the α-adrenergic agonist clonidine. Brain Res 92: 291–306
Szám I, Kállay K (1980) Comparative study of two antihypertensive agents: guanfacine and guanethidine. Br J Clin Pharmacol 10:85S–87S
Tauberger G, Kuhn P (1971) Untersuchungen der zentralnervösen sympathicusdämpfenden Wirkungen von α-Methyl-dopa. Naunyn Schmiedebergs Arch Pharmacol 268:33–43
Thananopavarn C, Golub MS, Eggena B, Barrett JD, Sambhi MP (1982) Clonidine, a centrally acting sympathetic inhibitor, as monotherapy for mild to moderate hypertension. Am J Cardiol 49:153–158
Thananopavarn C, Golub MS, Sambhi MP (1983) Clonidine in the elderly hypertensive. Monotherapy and therapy with a diuretic. Chest 83 (Suppl):410–411
Thoolen MJMC, Timmermans PBMWM, Van Zwieten PA (1981) Withdrawal syndrome after continuous infusion of clonidine in the normotensive rat. J Pharm Pharmacol 33:232–235
Thoolen MJMC, Hendricks JCA, Timmermans PBMWM, Van Zwieten PA (1983) Precipitation by yohimbine of the withdrawal syndromes of clonidine, guanfacine, and methyldopa in the spontaneously hypertensive rat. J Cardiovasc Pharmacol 5: 224–228
Timmermans PBMWM, Van Zwieten PA (1980) Postsynaptic α_1- and α_2-adrenoceptors in the circulatory system of the pithed rat: selective stimulation of the α_2-type by B-HT 933. Eur J Pharmacol 63:199–202
Timmermans PBMWM, Schoop AMC, Kwa HY, Van Zwieten PA (1981) Characterization of α-adrenoceptors participating in the central hypotensive and sedative effects of clonidine using yohimbine, rauwolscine and corynanthine. Eur J Pharmacol 70: 7–15
Van Zwieten PA (1975) Antihypertensive drugs with a central action. Prog Pharmacol 1:1–63
Van Zwieten PA, Thoolen MJMC, Jonkman FAM, Wilffert B, DeJonge A, Timmermans PBMWM (1986) Central and peripheral effects of S 3341 (N-dicyclopropylmethyl)-amino-2-oxazoline in animal models. Arch Int Pharmacodyn 279:130–149

Velasco M, Bertoncini H, Romero E, Urbina-Guintana A, Guevara J, Hernandez-Pieretti O (1978) Effect of clonidine on sympathetic nervous activity in hydralazine-treated hypertensive patients. Eur J Clin Pharmacol 13:317–320

Velasco M, Silva H, Morillo J, Urbina-Guintana A, Hernandez-Pieretti O, Angeli-Greaves M (1983) Cardiovascular hemodynamic interactions between clonidine and minoxidil in hypertensive patients. Chest 83 (Suppl):360–364

Vorburger C, Butikofer E, Reubi F (1968) Die akute Wirkung von St155 auf die cardiale und renale Haemodynamik. In: Heilmeyer L, Holtmeier H-J, Pfeiffer EF (eds) Hochdrucktherapie. Thieme, Stuttgart, p 86

Waldmeier P, Hedwall PR, Maître L (1975) On the role of α-methyldopamine in the antihypertensive effect of α-methyldopa. Naunyn Schmiedebergs Arch Pharmacol 289:303–314

Walland A (1984) Clonidine inhibits nicotinic effects in ganglia of the cholinergic-sympathetic system. Eur J Pharmacol 102:39–45

Walland A, Kobinger W, Csongrady A (1974) Action of clonidine on baroreceptor refelexes in conscious dogs. Eur J Pharmacol 26: 184–190

Warren SE, Ebert E, Swerdlin A-H, Steinberg SM, Stone R (1979) Clonidine and proprandol. Paradoxical hypertension. Arch Intern Med 139:253

Weber MA, Drayer JI, Hubbell A (1983) Effects on the reninangiotensin system of agents acting at central and peripheral adrenergic receptors. Chest 83 (Suppl): 374–377

Weber MA, Drayer JIM, Laragh JH (1978) The effects of clonidine and proprandol separately and in combination, on blood pressure and plasma renin activity in essential hypertension. J Clin Pharmacol 18:233–240

Wermuth CG, Schwartz J, Leclerc G, Garnier JP, Rout B (1973) Conformation de la clonidine et hypothèses sur son interaction avec un récepteur α-adrenergic. Chim Ther 1:115–116

Whitsett TL (1983) Abrupt cessation of treatment with centrally acting antihypertensive agents. A Review. Chest 83 (Suppl):400–402

Whitsett TL Chrysant SG, Dillard BL, Anton AH (1978) Abrupt cessation of clonidine administration: a prospective study. Am J Cardiol 41:1285–1290

Wikberg J (1978) Differentiation between pre- and postjunctional α-receptors in guinea pig ileum and rabbit aorta. Acta Physiol Scand 103:225–239

Wikberg JES (1979) The pharmacological classification of adrenergic α_1 and α_2 receptors and their mechanisms of action. Acta Physiol Scand 106 (Suppl 468):1–99

Wing LMH, Reid JL, Davies DS, Neill EAM, Tippett P, Dollery CT (1977) Pharmacokinetic and concentration-effect relationships of clonidine in essential hypertension. Eur J Clin Pharmacol 12:463–469

Zandberg A, DeJong W (1977) α-Methylnoradrenaline-induced hypotension in the nucleus tractus solitarii, of the rat: a localization study. Neuropharmacology 16: 219–222

CHAPTER 7

Rauwolfia Alkaloids (Reserpine)

L.G. HOWES and W.J. LOUIS

CONTENTS

1 Introduction

Reserpine (Fig. 1), an alkaloid derived from the roots of certain species of *Rauwolfia*, was isolated in 1952, and about 50 *Rauwolfia* alkaloids are known. Extracts of *Rauwolfia*, a plant genus belonging to the Apocynaceae family, were used by the Hindus for a variety of diseases including snake bites because of the resemblance of the roots to a snake (*Rauwolfia serpentina*). It was also used for the treatment of cardiovascular diseases, insomnia, and insanity (WEINER 1985). Reference to the medical use of *Rauwolfia* alkaloids appeared in the Western literature as early as 1563 (BEIN 1956). In 1931 SEN and BOSE reported in the *Indian Medical Journal* that the whole root could be used for the treatment of hypertension and psychosis. Widespread interest in their use for the treatment of hypertension, however, was aroused much later after VAKIL (1949) published his findings on the use of *Rauwolfia* alkaloids in the *British Heart Journal*.

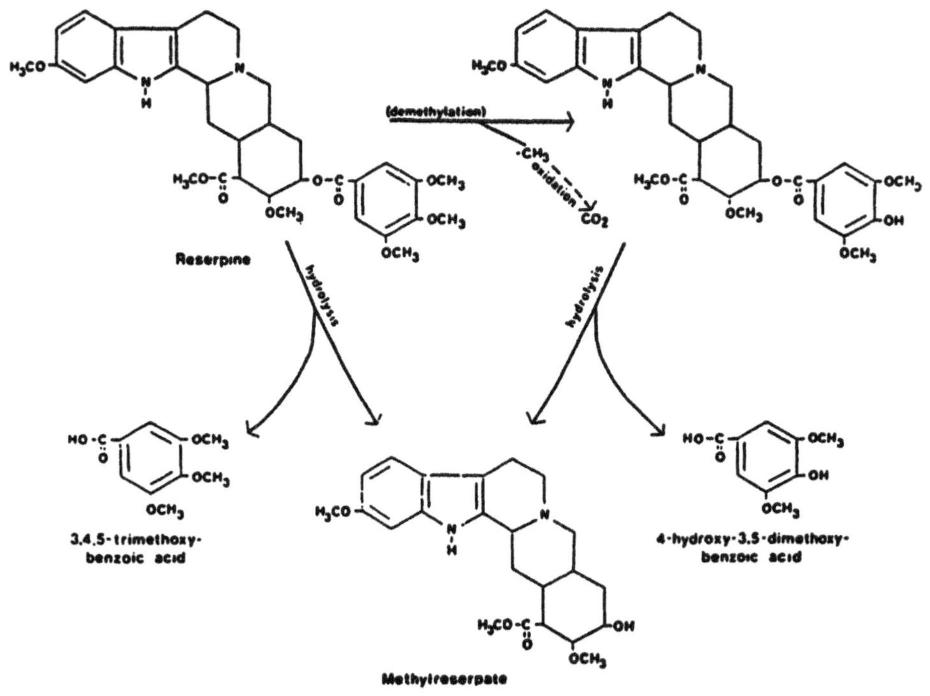

Fig. 1. Metabolism of reserpine

Parenteral usage became popular for hypertensive emergencies but has a tendency to produce excessive sedation.

In the Veteran's Administration Cooperative Study Group on Antihypertensive Drugs (1977) reserpine combined with hydrochlorothiazide was compared in a double-blind study with propranolol alone and in combination with either hydrochlorothiazide or hydralazine. The reserpine combination had the highest percentage of responders (88% of patients had diastolic blood pressures less than 90 mmHg) and a similar incidence of side effects to the other regimes.

Rauwolfia preparations were introduced in psychiatry as a sedative for the treatment of anxiety states and chronic psychoses. However, by the end of the 1960s reserpine had almost been withdrawn from psychiatric use as it had been replaced by more effective drugs, and it is now considered obsolete. In the treatment of hypertension reserpine is commonly used in combination, and there are numerous fixed-dose formulations available including reserpine and thiazide diuretics and reserpine with hydralazine. Reserpine has also been used effectively for the treatment of Raynaud's syndrome (Tindall et al. 1974; Meyers 1976; Coffman 1979; Nilsen and Jayson 1980 and Rosch et al. 1977), migraine (Graham 1970; Fog-moller et al. 1976; Nattero et al. 1976), and dyskinesias (Sato et al. 1971; Peters and Daly 1972; Duvoisin 1972; Villeneuve and Boszormenyi 1970). It has veterinary and farming uses, such as in poultry production where it can reduce the incidence of dissecting aneurysm in the aorta in domestic turkeys, which often have blood pressures of the order 204/144 mmHg (LAURENCE and BENNETT 1987).

In recent years the use of reserpine as an antihypertensive agent has diminished greatly because of concerns about side effects, particularly depression and breast cancer. Although several reports have suggested that there may be an association with breast cancer, other studies have failed to confirm it (see Sect. 4). Reserpine, however, is still used widely in certain countries such as the USSR and in the Indian subcontinent, and also remains an extremely valuable drug for research in laboratory pharmacology.

Space limits an extensive discussion of the pharmacology and actions of reserpine, and for a comprehensive examination of the earlier literature we recommend the earlier edition of this handbook (RAND and JUREVICS 1977). We have used the bibliography from this review to summarize the pre-1974 literature.

2 Mode of Action

The principle pharmacological action of reserpine is to deplete noradrenaline from peripheral sympathetic nerves and central noradrenergic neurons. Reserpine treatment has been shown to deplete sympathetic nerves of 95% or more of their noradrenaline content (LANGER and PINTO 1976; DUVAL et al. 1986). Reserpine interferes with catecholamine storage (see Sect. 2.1), but in contrast to false transmitters like α-methyl dopamine and α-methyl noradrenaline, the amount of reserpine present in tissues is too small to explain this depletion by *stochiometric* displacement. The resultant reduction in noradrenaline release leads to impaired function of central and peripheral noradrenergic neurons, which results in a lowering of blood pressure. However, reserpine also causes depletion of other transmitters and cotransmitters including 5-HT, dopamine, neuropeptide Y, and adrenaline from central and peripheral neurons in addition to possessing calcium channel-blocking activity. It is possible that these effects also contribute to the pharmacological and antihypertensive effects of the drug.

2.1 Neuronal and Extraneuronal Uptake

Reserpine depletes noradrenaline from central (HOLZBAUER and VOGT 1956; BRODIE et al. 1957) and peripheral (BERTLER 1956; HOLZBAUER and VOGT 1956; CARLSSON and HILLARP 1956; PAASONEN and KRAYER 1957, 1958; MUSCHOLL and VOGT 1958; BURN and RAND 1957, 1958a, b, 1959; WAUD et al. 1958; MUSCHOLL 1959; SJOSTRAND 1962; DE SCHAEPDRYVER 1960; DAHLSTROM 1967; BERKOWITZ et al. 1971) noradrenergic neurons by interfering with storage in catecholamine vesicles. It binds specifically to the catecholamine transporting system of noradrenaline storage vesicles and granules (NEAR and MAHLER 1983; CAUGHEY and KIRSHNER 1987; DEUPREE and WEAVER 1984), which is dependent upon the presence of Mg^{2+} and ATP (EULER and VON LISHAJKO 1963). WINKLER et al. (1981) suggested that although reserpine interferes with noradrenaline uptake, it does not interfere with ATP uptake in chromaffin granules. Reserpine also does not appear to interfere directly with extraneuronal uptake in vitro. However, MORTON (1985) reported that chronic treatment in rats results in a marked decrease in a cortisone-sensitive component of extraneuronal accumulation of [^{3}H]isoprenaline. MORTON (1985) concluded that extraneuronal uptake is dependent on a functional adrenergic innervation.

2.2 Binding Sites

Reserpine appears to bind to two distinct binding sites on membranes prepared from catecholamine storage granules, one with a maximum estimated number of binding sites (B_{max}) of 7 pmoles/mg of protein and a dissociation constant (K_d) of 0.7 n*M* (i.e., a high affinity, low capacity site) and one with a B_{max} of 60 pmoles/mg of protein and a K_d of 25 n*M* (i.e., a high capacity, low affinity site). This second binding site is probably equivalent to the binding site of tetrabenazine (another catecholamine-depleting drug), as the B_{max} and K_D for tetrabenazine binding is similar to that of reserpine, and tetrabenazine is capable of displacing reserpine from this lower affinity site but not from the high affinity site (SCHERMAN and HENRY 1984; GASNIER et al. 1987). Using the derivative, reserpic acid, CHAPLIN et al. (1985) demonstrated that this polar molecule which does not penetrate the chromaffin vesicle inhibits ATP-dependent noradrenaline uptake when added externally but not when trapped inside the chromaffin vesicle ghosts.

The binding of reserpine to the catecholamine transportation system is antagonized by Li^+ (RECHES et al. 1983), which inhibits reserpine effects on both noradrenaline and dopamine uptake. Studies with reserpine analogues have indicated that the catecholamine transportation of synaptic vesicles and granules possesses an amine binding site which binds the alkaloid ring system of reserpine rather than the trimethoxybenzoyl moiety (see Fig. 1). The binding site is probably hydrophobic, as the most potent reserpine analogues are hydrophobic derivatives (PARTI et al. 1987).

2.3 Noradrenaline Depletion

The depletion of noradrenaline from central and peripheral noradrenergic neurons leads to a failure of noradrenergic transmission, which results in widespread effects including a reduction in blood pressure. The noradrenaline-depleting action of reserpine is relatively slow in onset, reaching a maximum over a period of hours to days after a single doses depending upon the dose, the tissue that is innervated, the species, and the age of the animal. Reserpine does not have significant indirect sympathomimetic effects as the noradrenaline which it prevents from entering storage granules and vesicles is rapidly metabolized by monoamine oxidase to inactive metabolites (KOPIN and GORDON 1962, 1963). Indirect sympathomimetic effects of reserpine, however, can be demonstrated in the presence of monoamine oxidase inhibition (PLETSCHER et al. 1956; CHESSIN et al. 1957; GARATTINI et al. 1960b; BONACCORSI 1968; CASHIN 1972) or following spinal transection (DEJONGH and PROOSDIJ-HARTZEMA 1958; SCHNEIDER and RINEHARDT 1956; MAXWELL et al. 1957; SCHMITT and SCHMITT 1960) or ganglion blockade (MAXWELL et al. 1956; DOMINO and RECH 1957; BECK et al. 1957).

The rate of depletion of noradrenaline by reserpine is largely related to neuron activity and therefore to the rate of release of noradrenaline from neurons, (WAKADE 1980) and can be reduced by ganglionic blockade or spinal transection. Similarly, the dose required to achieve a particular degree of noradrenaline depletion within a given time period is greater for tissues with low levels of sympathetic nerve activity than for tissues with higher levels of sympathetic activity (WAKADE 1980). These observations probably largely explain the reported age, species, and tissue variations in susceptibility to reserpine-induced noradrenaline depletion.

Recovery of noradrenaline stores following reserpine treatment is slow and usually takes several weeks following a single dose or following cessation of chronic treatment (CARLSSON 1965; CARLSSON et al. 1957), suggesting that the binding of reserpine may be irreversible. Again, there is considerable age-, tissue-, and species-related variation (DAHLSTROM and HAGGENDAHL 1966a, b; CORRODI et al. 1971; CARLSSON et al. 1957; PAASONEN and KRAYER 1958; WAUD et al. 1958; KULKARNI and SHIDEMAN 1966; MUELLER and SHIDEMAN 1968). Functional recovery precedes the return to normal levels of noradrenaline storage and coincides with the partial recovery of the tissues' ability to take up and store noradrenaline (ANDEN et al. 1964; STJARNE 1964; IVERSEN et al. 1965; ANDEN and HENNING 1966; CARLSSON 1966; ALPERS and SHORE 1969; SUGRUE and SHORE 1971). However, it is likely that functional recovery of noradrenergic neurons is related more to the synthesis of new storage vesicles and granules within the cell body and their transport to the nerve terminal than to the reversal of reserpine binding (DAHLSTROM and HAGGENDAL 1966a,b).

2.4 Depletion of Transmitters Other Than Noradrenaline

2.4.1 Amines: 5-Hydroxytryptamine, Dopamine, and Adrenaline

Reserpine depletes 5-HT, dopamine, and adrenaline from central neurons by a similar mechanism to that which results in the loss of noradrenaline from noradrenergic neurons (SHASKAN and SNYDER 1970; DORRIS and SHORE 1971). In addition, reserpine depletes 5-HT from the intestines, stomach, platelets, kidney, lung, and spleen in a number of different species (BRODIE et al. 1955; PLETSCHER et al. 1955, 1956; ERSPAMER 1956; HARDISTRY et al. 1956; SANYAL and WEST 1958; GARATTINI et al. 1960a; KIM and SHORE 1963; THOMPSON and CAMPBELL 1967). However, the contribution that depletion of these amines makes to the pharmacological effects of reserpine has not been well-characterized.

Reserpine depletes adrenaline and noradrenaline from the adrenal gland with considerable interspecies variability (HOLZBAUER and VOGT 1956; CARLSSON and HILLARP 1956; PARRATT and WEST 1957; KRONEBERG and SCHUMANN 1957a,b, 1958; SCHUMANN 1958; COUPLAND 1958, 1959; DE SCHAEPDRYVER 1960; ERANKO and Hopsu 1958; Stjarne and Schapiro 1959; Callingham and Mann 1962). The rate of depletion of adrenal stores is generally slower than that of amine stores in the brain and other peripheral tissues (Callingham and Mann 1962), and higher doses of reserpine are required (Carlsson et al. 1957; Lee 1967).

2.4.2 Neuropeptide Y

Neuropeptide Y (NPY) is a putative peptide neurotransmitter which is colocalized with noradrenaline in many central and peripheral noradrenergic neurons (Maccarrone and Jarrott 1986). NPY is localized in storage vesicles in a similar manner to noradrenaline (Maccarrone and Jarrott 1986), although there is evidence that in some tissues NPY may be localized in storage vesicles that are distinct from those which store noradrenaline (Fried et al. 1985; Maccarrone and Jarrott 1987).

Reserpine treatment causes depletion of NPY from the adrenals, heart, kidney, blood vessels, and other peripheral tissues (Allen et al. 1986; Lundberg et al. 1985; Nagata et al. 1987) but not from brain regions (Schon et al. 1986), suggesting that most NPY in the brain is not located in catecholaminergic neurons. Reserpine-induced NPY depletion from peripheral tissues is generally not as great as catecholamine depletion (Morris et al. 1986), with the exception of the adrenals (Lundberg et al. 1986a). Accordingly, reserpine has a much greater inhibitory effect on the antegrade transport of noradrenaline in peripheral sympathetic nerves than NPY (Dahlstrom et al. 1987). Like the depletion of catecholamines, reserpine-induced depletion of NPY from peripheral sympathetic nerves and from the adrenals is dependent upon sympathetic nerve activity (Lundberg et al. 1986a; Franco-Cereceda et al. 1987).

In contrast to reserpine's effects on noradrenaline-mediated neurotransmission, reserpine-induced depletion of NPY results in an increase or maintenance of NPY release following nerve stimulation and an enhancement or maintenance of NPY-mediated responses (Lundberg et al. 1986b, 1987). It is possible that enhanced responsiveness to NPY following reserpine treatment may in part be due to an increased sensitivity of NPY receptors (Huidobro-toro 1985). The reserpine-induced reduction in NPY in the heart, spleen, and adrenal gland is markedly inhibited by clonidine, and this clonidine effect is inhibited by the adrenoceptor antagonists phenotolamine, prazosin, and yohimbine. In contrast, clonidine does not affect reserpine-induced noradrenaline depletion. These data suggest different mechanisms of storage of NPY and noradrenaline (Franco-Cereceda et al. 1987). This interpretation has received further support from reports that surgical sympathectomy results in substantially greater depletion of noradrenaline than NPY from the rat heart (Maccarrone and Jarrott 1987).

2.5 Adenosine Triphosphate

ATP is stored in the same terminal vesicles as noradrenaline (Lagercrantz 1976). However, Winkler et al. (1981) reported that reserpine depletes chromaffin granules of noradrenaline by more than 95% but does not interfere with

ATP uptake mechanisms or storage (KIRKPATRICK and BURNSTOCK 1987). WARLAND and BURNSTOCK (1987) demonstrated that ATP and noradrenaline are sympathetic cotransmitters in rabbit isolated ear artery and that ATP can act as a transmitter independently of noradrenaline in the vessel by acting on P_2 purinoceptors (WARLAND and BURNSTOCK 1987). In contrast to the noradrenergic system, the purinergic transmission does not appear to be affected by reserpine treatment.

2.6 Tyrosine Hydroxylase and Dopamine-β-Hydroxylase

Chronic reserpine administration induces a long-lasting increase in tyrosine hydroxylase activity and protein levels in central noradrenergic neurons, central adrenergic neurons, the adrenal gland, and sympathetic ganglia (THOENEN et al. 1969a, b; MUELLER et al. 1969a, b; AXELROD et al. 1970; BHAGAT et al. 1971; MOLINOFF et al. 1972; CHAMBA and RENAUD 1986; LABATUT et al. 1986). However, this may not result in increased noradrenaline synthesis because of blockade of dopamine uptake into storage vesicles where it is β-hydroxylated to form noradrenaline. In contrast, reserpine does not significantly increase tyrosine hydroxylase activity in dopaminergic neurons of the substantia nigra, although protein levels of the enzyme are increased (LABATUT et al. 1986). These effects are undoubtedly the result of removal of negative feedback inhibition as a consequence of reserpine-induced catecholamine depletion.

Unlike tyrosine hydroxylase, which is located in the cytosolic portion of catecholaminergic neurons, dopamine-β-hydroxylase is located solely within storage vesicles and granules. Thus dopamine must be taken up by these vesicles and granules prior to conversion to noradrenaline or adrenaline. In contrast to noradrenaline and adrenaline, dopamine can be formed in the soluble fraction of the cell.

Reserpine has a dose-dependent effect on the dopamine-β-hydroxylase activity of the adrenal glands (VIVEROS et al. 1969). Low doses produce marked depletion of catecholamines with little or no decrease in dopamine-β-hydroxylase activity, while high doses cause marked depletion of both. This suggests that high doses of reserpine cause destruction of catecholamine storage granules, possibly due to effects on membrane fluidity which appear to be distinct from the ability of the drug to block the catecholamine transport mechanism (PALM et al. 1970; BHISE et al. 1983).

2.7 Sympathetic Responses and Receptor Sensitivity

Reserpine reduces responses to postganglionic sympathetic nerve stimulation because of a failure of the nerves to release sufficient noradrenaline (BURN and RAND 1958b; MUSCHOLL and VOGT 1958; TRENDELENBLURG and GRAVENSTEIN 1958; KRAYER et al. 1962), although postsynaptic, Ca-channel-blocking effects of reserpine may play a minor role (see Sect. 2.11). Postsynaptic responses exhibit supersensitivity to noradrenaline, probably as a consequence of this failure of neurotransmission.

2.7.1 Sympathetic Transmission

The loss of peripheral sympathetic transmission has a latency period for onset and occurs some time after the onset of sedation, bradycardia, and a reduction in blood pressure, indicating that CNS effects of the drug appear relatively early and account for a substantial component of the drugs' hemodynamic effects. The degree of impairment of responses to sympathetic nerve transmission depends upon the extent of depletion of the noradrenaline stores (TRENDELENBURG 1961; FLEMING and TRENDELENBURG 1961; GAFFNEY et al. 1963; LEE 1967). Loss of noradrenergic transmission following reserpine treatment is not an universal finding, as in some tissues of certain species responses to electrical stimulation of peripheral noradrenergic nerves is maintained (TRENDELENBURG 1965; BARNETT and BENFORADO 1966; BLINKS 1966). It has been suggested that this is because of species and tissue differences in the sensitivity of different neuronal pools of noradrenaline, and that newly synthesized noradrenaline may be relatively resistant to reserpine-induced depletion (TRENDELENBURG 1965; DUVAL et al. 1986).

In the doses usually used to lower blood pressure in humans, peripheral symapthetic transmission, sympathetic reflexes, and sympathetic responses to indirectly acting sympathomimetic drugs appear to be intact (WHELAN and SKINNER 1963). This suggests that most of the antihypertensive effects of reserpine in humans are centrally mediated.

Recovery of sympathetic transmission after the end of reserpine treatment begins within several days—long before there is a substantial increase in tissue noradrenaline levels, but at a time when partial recovery of noradrenaline uptake by neurons can be demonstrated (ANDEN et al. 1964; STJARNE 1964; IVERSEN et al. 1965; ANDEN and HENNING 1966; CARLSSON 1966; ALPERS and SHORE 1969). Recovery of function is probably associated with the transfer of newly synthesized storage granules from the cell body to the nerve terminal rather than a reversal of reserpine binding to vesicles and granules (DAHLSTROM and HAGGENDAHL 1966a,b; HAGGENDAHL and DAHLSTROM 1970, 1972).

2.8 Postsynaptic Sensitivity

Reserpine treatment induces supersensitivity of postsynaptic responses of most tissues that have sympathetic innervation. The supersensitivity is not necessarily specific for adrenoceptor agonists and may affect responses to agonists which are selective for adrenoceptor subtypes in different ways. The nature of the supersensitivity following reserpine treatment appears to depend on the tissue and the species of animal studied and is probably in part determined by whether or not a particular adrenoceptor subtype is directly innervated and therefore likely to undergo denervation hypersensitivity. However, there is evidence that in some tissues a component of reserpine-induced hypersensitivity occurs independently of up-regulation of adrenoceptors or enhanced sensitivity of their second messenger systems. Thus, the response of vascular smooth muscle to noradrenaline, phenylephrine, 5-HT, and KC1 is increased by reserpine (BURN and

RAND 1958a,b; MACMILLAN et al. 1962; TAKENAKA 1963; BAUM 1963; FURCHGOTT et al. 1963; CARRIER and HOLLAND 1965; HUDGINS and FLEMING 1966; CARRIER and SHIBATA 1967; NASSERI et al. 1985; ABEL et al. 1981), while the response to angiotensin II appears to be unaltered (HAYASHI et al. 1980). The sensitivity of cardiac muscle to isoprenaline, noradrenaline, adrenaline, 5′-guanylylimido-diphosphate, forskolin (a direct stimulant of adenylate cyclase), and glucagon is increased following reserpine treatment (SPADARI et al. 1987; KHALIGHT et al. 1986; HAWTHORN et al. 1987; MEGHJI et al. 1978; TENNER et al. 1982; ROGERS and MCNEIL 1982; TORPHY et al. 1982; CROS and MCNEILL 1987), while responses to phenylephrine, histamine, or Gpp (NH)p remain unaltered (ROGERS and MC-NEILL 1982; TORPHY et al. 1982; CROS and MCNEIL 1987). These findings suggest that supersensitivity to β-mediated responses occurs which involves changes in the sensitivity of the cAMP second messenger system, while α_1-adrenoceptor and H_2-mediated responses are unchanged.

GRASSBY and BROADLEY (1986) reported that the increased sensitivity of cardiac muscle following reserpine is due to a selective increase in the sensitivity of β_1-receptor responses and that the sensitivity of β_2-receptor-mediated responses remains unchanged. It is uncertain whether the cardiac muscle response to Ca^{2+} is altered by reserpine, as there has been one report of increased sensitivity (TENNER and CARRIER 1978) and one report that it does not change (TORPHY et al. 1982).

Reserpine treatment increases the sensitivity of the vas deferens to phenylephrine, methacholine, isoprenaline, and KC1, suggesting that in this tissue the increased sensitivity may be relatively nonspecific (LOTT et al. 1982; NASSERI et al. 1985).

2.9 Modification of Postsynaptic Receptors

2.9.1 Adrenoceptors

Reserpine treatment causes an up-regulation of cardiac β-receptors (an increase in B_{max} with no change in K_d), while α_1-adrenoceptor binding remains unaltered (TENNER et al. 1982; CHESS-WILLIAMS et al. 1987; LATIFPOUR and MCNEILL 1984). However, some investigators have had difficulty demonstrating these changes in guinea pig heart (HAWTHORN and BROADLEY 1982; TORPHY et al. 1982). Reserpine treatment also increases the number of postsynaptic β-receptors in the frontal cortex (LEVIN and BIEGON 1984) as well as the number of dopamine-2-receptors in the striatum (TRAUB et al. 1986). Reserpine appears to increase the number of α_2-receptor binding sites in the vas deferens without altering α_1-adrenoceptor binding (WATANABE et al. 1982; COWAN et al. 1985). While reserpine does not appear to alter either the B_{max} or K_d of β-receptor binding in the rat parotid gland, the number of receptors in the high affinity state is increased (WELLSTEIN et al. 1984).

2.9.2 Serotonin Receptors

5-HT_2-receptors have been shown to have two affinity states for agonists (BATTAGLIA et al. 1987). Steady state levels and turnover of 5-HT_2-receptors are decreased in senescent rat brain, and these can be further reduced by chronic reserpine treatment (Battaglia et al. 1987). As these 5-HT_2 sites may play a role in the action of halucinogenic agents (Glennon et al. 1984) and antidepressants (Snyder and Petrouka 1982), it is of interest that they appear to be down-regulated by reserpine and tricyclic antidepressants (Clements-Jewery and Robson 1982), whereas these compounds increase dopamine receptors (Burt et al. 1977; Owen et al. 1980).

2.10 Effects of Reserpine on Receptor Transport With Neurons

Reserpine treatment reduces both the antegrade and retrograde transport of β-receptors in central noradrenergic neurons projecting to the frontal cortex. There is a rebound overshoot in the neuronal transport of these receptors during the recovery from reserpine therapy (Levin 1984; Levin and Biegon 1984). It is uncertain whether these effects on receptor transport are a consequence of noradrenaline depletion or a distinct pharmacological effect of reserpine.

2.11 Effects of Reserpine on Membrane Ca-Channels

Despite the evidence that reserpine treatment leads to a supersensitivity of postsynaptic responses, this may not be solely due to increased sensitivity of adrenoceptors or of their second messenger systems. There is evidence that reserpine possesses Ca-channel-blocking activity in some tissues. It is, however, unlikely that this activity contributes substantially to the hemodynamic effects of the drug. Reserpine decreases the Ca^{2+} content of vascular smooth muscle (Carrier and Shibata 1967) and displays voltage-dependent, Ca-channel-blocking activity (Casteels and Login 1983). In addition, chronic reserpine treatment increases the number of voltage-dependent Ca channels in vascular smooth muscle. Reserpine also blocks voltage-dependent Ca channels in the pituitary (Login et al. 1983) and inhibits calcium uptake by the vas deferens Grana et al. 1977) and by the endoplasmic reticulum of the submandibular gland (Hurley and Martinez 1987).

3 Pharmacodynamic Effects

3.1 Hemodynamic Effects

Reserpine administration results in a rapid reduction in heart rate, cardiac output, and peripheral resistance, resulting in a fall in blood pressure (Momatsu et al. 1977). These effects are principally due to a reduction in sympathetic activity, although enhanced vagal activity due to CNS actions of the drug may be involved. In the larger doses used in animal studies, failure of peripheral noradrenergic function is probably the major contribution to these hemodynamic effects (Green 1962). However, with the relatively small doses used as antihypertensive therapy in humans (0.125–0.5 mg/day), CNS effects of reserpine probably account for most of the antihypertensive effect as sympathetic reflexes are preserved and responses to peripherally acting sympathomimetic drugs are unaltered (WHELAN and SKINNER 1963). The antihypertensive effects of reserpine are maintained during chronic therapy (CHANNICK et al. 1981).

Reserpine is a very effective antihypertensive agent in humans, having the advantages of a long half-life (allowing once daily administration) and a relatively low cost. However, these are partially offset by the relatively high incidence of side effects compared with other antihypertensive agents (APPLEGATE et al. 1985; OGAWA et al. 1984; SEEDAT et al. 1984; LUXENBERG and FEIGENBAUM 1983).

4 Side Effects

Using the presently recommended very low doses (0.125–0.5 mg) of reserpine in combination with diuretics, a regimen arises that is relatively well-tolerated and comparable with other combination treatments, e.g., β-blockers and diuretics (Veterans Administration Study Group 1978). Reserpine monotherapy is not recommended any more. Many of the severe side effects have been reported with higher doses of the drug in earlier studies.

Most of the side effects of reserpine are due to an impairment or imbalance of autonomic nervous system function. Nasal stuffiness and conjunctival injection, probably due to a reduction in sympathetic tone, are common side effects which occur in about 40% of patients (SIGG 1968; SMIRK and DOYLE 1954). In addition, some patients may experience dryness of the mouth. Large doses of reserpine impair the function of most exocrine glands (MORTON et al. 1980; JIRAKALSOMCHOK and SCHNEYER 1987; BRANNON and SCOTT 1987), and chronically reserpinized rats have been used as an animal model of cystic fibrosis (WERLIN et al. 1983). However, this side effect is uncommon at the doses used to manage hypertension.

Depression and sedation are common side effects. In a review of 273 hypertensive patients 51 of 77 episodes of depression reported in 63 patients occurred with doses of 750 µg or more of reserpine daily. The average time of onset was 6.7 months after commencing therapy. Other related side effects include lethargy and nightmares, and a few patients show an increase in appetite and weight (MARTINDALE 1982).

Reserpine produces a number of relatively common gastrointestinal side effects that probably result from an imbalance of autonomic nervous system activity. These include stomach cramps, diarrhea, and an increase in gastric secretion that is responsible for an increased incidence of peptic ulcer (HAVERBACK et al. 1955; KLEIN 1968).

Reserpine produces substantial changes in pituitary and gonadal function in animals because of its effects on central dopaminergic and noradrenergic neurons and possibly because of direct effects on calcium metabolism in pituitary cells (LOGIN et al. 1983). Thus, reserpine depletes corticotropin-releasing factor from the median eminence of the hypothalamus (BHATTACHARYA and MARKS 1969) and ACTH from the anterior pituitary (MAHFOUZ and EZZ 1958; KITAY et al. 1959; SAFFRAN and VOGT 1960; MAICKEL et al. 1961). However, ACTH depletion only occurs with doses large enough to deplete brain catecholamine stores by greater than 50%. Similarly, the administration of reserpine to animals inhibits gonadotropin secretion and estrogen production, leading to effects on ovulation, reproduction, and puberty (Cranston 1958; Purshottam 1962; Hopkins and Pincus 1963; Brown 1966; Mayer et al. 1960; Khazan et al. 1960; Weiner and Ganong 1971). Reserpine impairs prolactin release in animals (Login et al. 1983), induces lactation (Kanematsu et al. 1983), and has mammotropic effects (Ben-David et al. 1968). The significance of these hormonal effects in humans are uncertain.

The administration of antihypertensive doses of reserpine to humans (0.25 mg–0.5 mg/day) has been shown to *increase* prolactin levels acutely (Asnis et al. 1981) but to have no effects on prolactin, luteinizing hormone, or sex steroid levels during chronic administration (Boyden et al. 1980). Chronic reserpine therapy is associated with a similar incidence of sexual dysfunction in humans as with hydrochlorothiazide therapy (Boyden et al. 1980). In contrast to the reported lack of chronic changes in prolactin levels in men, women receiving reserpine have prolactin levels that are 50% higher than controls. This increse would be expected to lead to a small increase in the incidence of breast cancer (Ross et al. 1984). Indeed, large doses of reserpine has been shown to be carcinogenic in rats and mice and to produce mainly mammary neoplasms in mice (Muradian, 1986). In 1974 the Boston Collaborative Drug Surveillance Program reported an apparently increased incidence of reserpine therapy in a group of 150 women recently diagnosed with breast cancer compared with matched medical controls. This study received support from Armstrong et al. (1974) but has been criticized by Heinonen et al. (1974), Garfinkel and Hammond (1974), Mack et al. (1975), O'Fallon et al. (1975), and Christopher et al. (1977).

Whether reserpine therapy increases the incidence of breast cancer in women in uncertain, but it is generally agreed that if an increased incidence exists, it is small (Labarthe and O'Fallon 1980; Curb et al. 1982). One of the problems is that the methodology of monitoring multiple unknown reactions often uses a 5% level of significance which means there is a 1 in 20 chance of coming up with a false positive. There is concern that both reserpine and Debendox (Fleming et al. 1981) are examples of false positives. One of the problems is that the sample size required to prove an association is often prohibitively large. If a new drug causes a modest increase (10%) in the incidence of a common disease (1 in 100 per annum), the number of patients that must be monitored to discover this is 250 000 (Stevens 1985).

5 Distribution and Metabolism

Following intraperitoneal injection into rats, [^{14}C]reserpine is rapidly concentrated in most tissues except fat and reaches maximum levels within 1 h. Maximum concentrations in the brain are achieved after about 20 min, and levels are undetectable in most tissues by 24 h (Sheppard et al. 1955, 1958).

However, the pharmacological effects of reserpine are not closely related temporally to tissue levels (SHEPPARD et al. 1957) as they are the result of the relatively small proportion of the drug that is highly bound to catecholamine storage granules and vesicles (MANARA et al. 1972).

Reserpine is absorbed from the gastrointestinal tract and is metabolized mainly by the liver and to an extent by the intestine. About 6% is excreted in the urine in the first 24 h and about 8% in the first 4 days (MAASS et al. 1969). Metabolism is mainly due to hydrolysis to methylreserpate and trimethoxybenzoic acid (see Fig. 1). However, there are marked species differences in the routes of metabolism of reserpine (SHEPPARD and TSIEN, 1955). Rat liver has the greatest ability for the oxidation of the 4-methoxy carbon of the 3,4,5-trimethoxybenzoic moiety of reserpine to carbon dioxide, but pigeon and rabbit livers are devoid of this activity. Guinea pig liver has the greatest ability for hydrolyzing reserpine to trimethoxybenzoic acid and methylreserpate; mouse, rabbit, and rat livers have a fair ability to hydrolyze reserpine, but dog and pigeon livers have practically none. In mouse liver, reserpine is hydrolyzed by an esterase of the microsomal fraction but may require initial oxidation by mixed function oxidase (STITZEL et al. 1972). The metabolites of reserpine are devoid of pharmacological activity and are excreted by the kidney, gut, and lung (SHEPPARD and TSIEN 1955). In humans the main excretory product is trimethoxybenzoic acid. Following the oral administration of a single dose of plasma levels of radioactive reserpine, plasma levels of reserpine show a biphasic decline with half-lives of 4.5 and 271 h. Radioactivity is detectable in urine and feces for 11–12 days, and in the feces it is largely present as unchanged reserpine (MAASS et al. 1969).

Summary

Derivatives of *Rauwolfia* alkaloids are best typified by the drug reserpine. Reserpine was one of the earliest drugs recognised to have antihypertensive activity. *Rauwolfia* alkaloids lower blood pressure by reducing the activity of central and peripheral noradrenergic neurons. This is the result of noradrenaline depletion because of a specific effect of blocking noradrenaline and dopamine uptake into the storage granules of noradrenergic neurons. Reserpine has similar effects on central dopaminergic and serotonergic neurons, the significance of which is not clear. At doses used for blood pressure reduction in humans, the major effect of the drug appears to be within the central nervous system. The clinical use of *Rauwolfia* has diminished in recent years because of the development of effective drugs with fewer side effects. However, reserpine remains an extremely useful drug for laboratory investigations of the physiology and pharmacology of catecholaminergic and serotonergic neurons.

References

Abel PW, U'rquilla PR, Goto K, Westfall DP, Robinson, RL, Fleming WW (1981) Chronic reserpine treatment alters sensitivity and membrane potential of the rabbit saphenous artery. J Pharmacol Exp Ther 217:430–439

Allen JM, Schon F, Yeats JC, Kelly JS, Bloom SR (1986) Effect of reserpine, phenoxybenzamine and cold stress on the neuropeptide Y content of the rat peripheral nervous system. Neuroscience 19:1251–1254

Alpers HS, Shore PA (1969) Specific binding of reserpine-association with norepinephrine depletion. Biochem Pharmacol 18:1363–1372

Anden NE, Henning M (1966) Adrenergic nerve function, noradrenaline level and noradrenaline uptake in cat nictitating membrane after reserpine treatment. Acta Physiol Scand 67:498–504

Anden NE, Magnusson T, Waldeck B (1964) Correlation between noradrenaline uptake and adrenergic nerve function after reserpine treatment. Life Sci 3:19–25

Applegate WB, Carper ER, Kahn SE, Westbrook L, Linton M, Baker MG, Runyan JW Jr (1985) Comparison of the use of reserpine versus alpha-methyldopa for second step treatment of hypertension in the elderly. J Am Geriatr Soc 33:109–115

Armstrong B, Stevens N, Doll R (1974) Retrospective study of the association between use of rauwolfia derivatives and breast cancer in English women. Lancet II:672–675

Asnis GM, Sachar EJ, Halbreich V, Ostrow LC, Nathan RS, Halpern FS (1981) The prolactin stimulating potency of reserpine in man. Psychiatry Res 5:39–45

Axelrod J, Mueller RA, Thoenen H (1970) Neuronal and hormonal control of tyrosine hydroxylase and phenylethanolamine N-methyltransferase activity. In: Schumann MJ, Kroneberg G (eds) New aspects of storage and release mechanisms of catecholamines. Springer, Berlin Heidelberg New York, pp 212–219

Barnett A, Benforado JM (1966) The nicotinic effects of choline esters and of nicotine in guinea pig atria. J Pharmacol Exp Ther 152:29–36

Battaglia G, Norman AB, Creese I (1987) Differential serotonin receptor recovery in mature and senescent rat brain after irreversible receptor modification: effect of chronic reserpine treatment. J Pharmacol Exp Ther 243:69–74

Baum T (1963) Vascular reactivity of reserpine-pretreated dogs. J Pharmacol Exp Ther 141:30–35

Beck L, Ybarra-Falcon L, Domino EF (1957) Hemodynamic responses to reserpine in unanesthetized dogs immobilized with neuromuscular blocking agents. J Pharmacol Exp Ther 119:133

Bein HJ (1956) The pharmacology of rauwolfia. Pharmacol Rev 8:435–483

Ben-David M, Khazen K, Khazan N, Sulman FG (1968) Correlation between depressant and mammotrophic effects in fifteen reserpine analogues. Arch Int Pharmacodyn 171:274–284

Berkowitz BA, Tarver JH, Spector S (1971) Norepinephrine in blood vessels: concentration, binding, uptake and depletion. J Pharmacol Exp Ther 117:119–126

Bertler A (1956) Effect of reserpine on the storage of catecholamines in brain and other tissues. Acta Physiol Scand 51:75–83

Bertler A, Carlsson A, Rosengren E (1956) Release by reserpine of catecholamines from rabbits' hearts. Naturwissenschaften 43:521

Bhagat B, Burke WJ, Davis JW (1971) Effect of reserpine on the activity of adrenal enzymes involved in the synthesis of adrenaline. Br J Pharmacol 43:819–827

Bhattacharya AN, Marks BH (1969) Reserpine and chlorpromazine induced changes in hypothalamo-hypophyseal-adrenal system in rats in the presence and absence of hypothermia. J Pharmacol Exp Ther 165:108–176

Bhise SB, Marwadi PR, Mathur SS, Srivastava RC (1983) Liquid membrane phenomenon in reserpine action. J Pharm Sci 72:599–601

Blinks JR (1966) Field stimulation as a means of effecting the graded release of autonomic transmitters in isolated heart muscle. J Pharmacol Exp Ther 151:221–235

Bonaccorsi A (1968) Studies on the hypertensive response elicited by reserpine or tetrabenazine in rats treated with amphetamine-like drugs. Eur J Pharmacol 3: 97–105

Boston Collaborative Drug Surveillance Program (1974) Reserpine and breast cancer. Lancet I:669–671
Boyden TM, Nugent CA, Ogihara T, Maeda T (1980) Reserpine, hydrochlorothiazide and pituitary-gonadol hormones in hypertensive subjects. Eur J Clin Pharmacol 17:329–332
Brannon PM, Scott D (1987) Impairment of pancreatic anion function by reserpine in vivo and in vitro. In Vitro Cell Dev Biol 23:429–435
Brodie BB, Pletscher A, Shore PA (1955) Evidence that serotonin has a role in brain function. Science 122:968
Brodie BB, Olin JS, Kuntzman RB, Shore PA (1957) Possible inter-relationship between release of brain norepinephrine and serotonin by reserpine. Science 125:1293–1294
Brown PS (1966) The effect of reserpine, 5-hydroxytryptamine and other drugs on induced ovulation in immature mice. J Endocrinol 35:161–168
Burn JH, Rand MJ (1957) Reserpine and noradrenaline in artery walls. Lancet II:1097
Burn JH, Rand MJ (1958a) Noradrenaline in artery walls and its dispersal by reserpine. Br Med J I:903–908
Burn JH, Rand MJ (1958b) The action of sympathomimetic amines in animals treated with reserpine. J Physiol (Lond) 144:314–336
Burn JH, Rand MJ (1959) The cause of the supersensitivity of smooth muscle to noradrenaline. J Physiol (Lond) 147:135–143
Burt DR, Creese I, Snyder SH (1977) Antischizophrenic drugs: chronic treatment elevates dopamine receptor binding in brain. Science 196:326–328
Callingham BA, Mann M (1962) Depletion and replacement of the adrenaline and noradrenaline contents of the rat adrenal gland, following treatment with reserpine. Br J Pharmacol 18:138–149
Carlsson A (1965) Pharmacological depletion of catecholamine stores. Pharmacol Rev 18:541–549
Carlsson A (1966) Physiological and pharmacological release of monoamines in the central nervous system. In: von Euler US, Rosell S, Uvnas B (eds) Mechanisms of release of biogenic amines. Pergamon, Oxford, pp 331–346
Carlsson A, Hillarp N-A (1956) Release of adenosine triphosphate along with adrenaline and noradrenaline following stimulation of adrenal medulla. Acta Physiol Scand 37:235–239
Carlsson A, Rosengren E, Bertler A, Nilsson J (1957) Effect of reserpine on the metabolism of catecholamines. In: Garattini S, Ghetti V (eds) Psychotropic drugs, vol 6. Elsevier, Amsterdam, pp 363–372
Carrier O Jr, Holland WC (1965) Supersensitivity in perfused isolated arteries after reserpine. J Pharmacol Exp Ther 149:212–218
Carrier O Jr, Shibata SA (1967) A possible role for tissue calcium in reserpine supersensitivity. J Pharmacol Exp Ther 155:42–49
Cashin CH (1972) Effect of sympathomimetic drugs in eliciting hypertensive response to reserpine in the rat, after pretreatment with monoamineoxidase inhibitors. Br J Pharmacol 44:203–209
Casteels R, Login IS (1983) Reserpine has a direct action as a calcium channel antagonist on mammalian smooth muscle cells. J Physiol 340:403–414
Caughey B, Kirshner N (1987) Effects of reserpine and tetrabenzine on catecholamine and ATP storage in cultured bovine adrenal medullary chromaffin cells. J Neurochem 49:563–573
Chamba G, Renaud B (1986) Increased tyrosine hydroxylase activity in central adrenaline neurons after reserpine treatment. Eur J Pharmacol 92:243–248
Channick BJ, Kessler WB, Marks AD, Adlin EV (1981) A comparison of chlorothalidone-reserpine and hydrochlorothiazide-methyldopa as step 2 therapy for hypertension. Clin Ther 4:175–183
Chaplin L, Cohen AH, Huettl P, Kennedy M, Njus D, Temperley SJ (1985) Reserpic acid as an inhibitor of norepinephrine transport into chromaffin vesicle ghosts. J Biol Chem 260:10981–10985
Chessin M, Kramer ER, Scott CC (1957) Modification of the pharmacology of reserpine and serotonin by iproniazid. J Pharmacol Exp Ther 119:453–460

Chess-Williams RG, Grassby PF, Broadley KJ, Sheridan DJ (1987) Cardiac alpha and beta adrenoceptor sensitivity and binding characteristics after long term reserpine treatment. Naunyn Schmiedebergs Arch Pharmacol 336:646–651
Christopher LJ, Crooks J, Davidson JF, Eskine ZG, Gallon SC, Moir DC, Weir RD (1977) A multicentre study of rauwolfia derivatives and breast cancer. Eur J Clin Pharmacol 11:409–417
Clements-Jewery S, Robson PA (1982) Intact 5HT neuroterminals are not required for 5HT2 receptor down regulation by amitriptyline. Neuropharmacology 21:725–727
Coffman JD (1979) Vasodilator drugs in peripheral vascular disease. N Engl J Med 300:713–717
Colpaert FC (1987) Pharmacological characteristics of tremor, rigidity and hypokinesia induced by reserpine in rat. Neuropharmacology 26:1431–1440
Corrodi H, Masuoka DT, Clark WG (1971) Effect of 6-hydroxydopamine on rat heart noradrenaline. Eur J Pharmacol 15:160–163
Coupland RE (1958) Strain sensitivity of albino rats to reserpine. Nature 181:930–931
Coupland RE (1959) The catecholamine content of the adrenal medulla of the rat following reserpine-induced depletion. J Endocrinol 18:154–161
Cowan FF Jr, Wong SK, Westfall DP, Fleming WW (1985) Effect of postganglionic denervation and pretreatment with reserpine on alpha-adrenoceptors of the guinea-pig vas deferens. Pharmacology 30:289–295
Cranston EM (1958) Effect of tranquilizers and other agents on sexual cycle of mice. Proc Soc Exp Biol Med 98:320–322.
Cros GH, McNeill JH (1987) Reserpine induced supersensitivity in adenylate cyclase preparations from guinea-pig heart. Eur J Pharmacol 139:97–101
Curb JD, Hardy RJ, Labarthe DR, Borhani NO, Taylor JO (1982) Reserpine and breast cancer in the hypertension detection and follow-up program. Hypertension 4: 307–311
Dahlstrom A (1967) The effect of reserpine and tetrabenazine on the accumulation of noradrenaline in the rat sciatic nerve after ligation. Acta Physiol Scand 69:167–179
Dahlstrom A, Haggendal J (1966a) Studies on the transport and lifespan of amine storage granules in a peripheral adrenergic neurone system. Acta Physiol Scand 67:278–288
Dahlstrom A, Haggendal J (1966b) Recovery of noradrenaline levels after reserpine compared with the life span of amine storage granules in rat and rabbit. J Pharm Pharmacol 18:750–752
Dahlstrom A, Booj S, Goldstein M, Larsson PA (1987) The synthesis of NPY and DβH is independently regulated in adrenergic nerves after reserpine. Neurochem Res 12: 221–225
De Jongh DL, van Proosdij-Hartzema EG (1958) Augmentation of blood pressure in rabbits by reserpine. Acta Physiol Pharmacol Neer 17:364–365
De Schaepdryver AF (1960) Hypertensive responses in reserpinized dogs. Flrcs Int Pharmacodyn 124:45–52
Deupree JD, Weaver JA (1984) Identification and characterization of the catecholamine transporter in bovine chromaffin granules using [^{3}H] reserpine. J Biol Chem 259: 10907–10912
Domino EF, Rech RH (1957) Observations on the initial hypertensive response to reserpine. J Pharmacol Exp Ther 121:171–182
Dorris RL, Shore PA (1971) Amine uptake and storage mechanisms in the corpus striatum of rat and rabbit. J Pharmacol Exp Ther 179:15–19
Duval N, Hicks PE, Langer SZ (1986) Reserpine resistant responses to nerve stimulation in the cat nictitating membrane involve the release of newly synthesized noradrenaline. Eur J Pharmacol 122:93–101
Duvoisin RC (1972) Reserpine for tardive dyskinesia. N Engl J Med 286:611
Eranko O, Hopsu V (1958) Effect of reserpine on the histochemistry and content of adenaline and noradrenaline in the adrenal medulla of the rat and the mouse. Endocrinology 62:15–23
Erspamer V (1956) Observations on the 5-hydroxytryptamine (Enteramine) release caused by reserpine in the rat. Experientia 12:63–64
Euler US, von Lishajko F (1963) Effect of reserpine on the uptake of catecholamines in

isolated nerve storage granules. Int J Neuropharmacol 2:127–134
Fleming DM, Knox JDE, Crombie DL (1981). Debendox in early pregnancy and fetal malformation. Br Med J 283:99–101
Fleming WW, Trendelenburg U (1961) The development of supersensitivity to norepinephrine after pretreatment with reserpine. J Pharmacol Exp Ther 133:41–51
Fog-Moller F, Bryndum B, Dalsgaard-Neilsen T et al. (1976). Therapeutic effect of reserpine on migraine syndrome: relationship to blood amine levels. Headache 15: 275–278
Franco-Cereceda A, Nagata M, Svensson TH, Lundberg JM (1987) Differential effects of clonidine and reserpine treatment on neuropeptide Y content in some sympathetically innervated tissues of the guinea pig. Eur J Pharmacol 142:267–723
Fried G, Terenius L, Hokfelt T, Goldstein M (1985) Evidence for differential localization of noradrenaline and neuropeptide Y (NPY) in neuronal storage vesicles from rat vas deferens. J Neurosci 5:450–458
Furchgott RF, Kirpekar SM, Rieker M, Schwab A (1963) Actions and interactions of norepinephrine, tyramine and cocaine on aortic strips of rabbit and left atria of guinea pig and cat. J Pharmacol Exp Ther 152:39–58
Gaffney TE, Chidsey CA, Braunwald E (1963) Study of the relationship between the neurotransmitter store and adrenergic nerve block induced by reserpine and guanethidine. Circ Res 12:264–269
Garattini S, Fresia P, Mortari A, Palma V (1960a) The pressor effect of reserpine after monoamine-oxidase inhibitors. Med Exp (Basel) 2:252–259
Garattini S, Kato R, Valzelli L (1960b) Effect of reserpine analogues on tissue serotonin. Experientia 16:120
Garfinkel L, Hammond EC (1974) Breast cancer and hypertension. Lancet II:1381
Gasnier B, Ellory JC, Henry JP (1987) Functional molecular mass of binding sites for [^{3}H] dihydrotetrabenazine and [^{3}H] reserpine and of dopamine beta hydroxylase and cytochrome b561 from chromofin granule membrane as determined by radiation inactivation. Eur J Biochem 165:73–78
Glennon RA, Titeler M, McKenney JD (1984) Evidence for 5HT2 involvement in the mechanism of action of hallucinogenic agents. Life Sci 35:2505–2512
Graham R (1970) Small blood vessels in migraine (letter). Lancet II:832
Grana E, Zonta F, Dondi P, Piccinini F, Favilli L (1977) Direct effect of reserpine. II. Response of the rat vas deferns to calcium. Farmaco [Sci] 32:897–904
Grassby PF, Broadley KJ (1986) Responses mediated via beta-1 adrenoceptors but not beta-2 receptors exhibit supersensitivity after chronic reserpine pretreatment. J Pharmacol Exp Ther 237:950–958
Green AF (1962) Antihypertensive drugs. Adv Pharmacol 1:161–225
Haggendal J, Dahlstrom A (1970) Uptake and retention of ^{3}H-noradrenaline in adrenergic nerve terminals after reserpine and axotomy. Eur J Pharmacol 10:411–415
Haggendal J, Dahlstrom A (1972) The recovery of the capacity for uptake-retention of ^{3}H noradrenaline in rat adrenergic nerves after reserpine. J Pharm Pharmacol 24:565–574
Hardistry RM, Ingram GIC, Stacey RS (1956) Reserpine and human platelet 5-hydroxytryptamine. Experientia 12:42
Haverback BJ, Stevenson TD, Sjoerdsma A, Terry LL (1955) The effects of reserpine and chlorpromazine on gastric secretion. Am J Med Sci 230:601–604
Hawthorn MH, Broadley KJ (1982) Beta adrenoceptor ligand binding and supersensitivity to isoprenaline of ventricular muscle after chronic reserpine pretreatment. Naunyn Schmiedebergs Arch Pharmacol 320:240–245
Hawthorn MH, Taylor DA, Fleming WW (1987) Characteristics of adoptive supersensitivity in the left atrium of the guinea-pig. J Pharmacol Exp Ther 241:453–457
Hayashi S, Miyazaki M, Toda N (1980) Responsiveness to vasoactive agents of cerebral and mesenteric arteries isolated from control and reserpine treated dogs. Br J Pharmacol 68:473–478
Heinonen OP, Shapiro S, Tuominen L, Turunen MI (1974) Reserpine use in relation to breast cancer. Lancet II:675–677
Bolzbauer M, Vogt M (1956) Depression by reserpine of the noradrenaline concentration

in the hypothalamus of the cat. J Neurochem 1:8–11
Hopkins TF, Pincus G (1963) Effects of reserpine on gonadotropin-induced ovulation in immature rats. Endocrinology 73:775–780
Hudgins PM, Fleming WW (1966) A relatively nonspecific supersensitivity in aortic strips resulting from pretreatment with reserpine. J Pharmacol Exp Ther 153:70–80
Huidobro-Toro JP (1985) Reserpine-induced potentiation of the inhibiting action of neuropeptide Y on the rat vas deferens neurotransmission. Neurosci Lett 59:247–252
Hurley TW, Martinez JR (1987) Differential effects of chronic reserpine exposure on Ca^{++} sequestering mechanisms in rat submandibular gland vesicles. Cell Calcium 8:353–363
Iversen LL, Glowinsky J, Axelrod J (1965) Uptake and storage of H^3-norepinephrine in the reserpine-pretreated rat heart. J Pharmacol Exp Ther 150:173–183
Jirakalsomchok D, Schneyer CA (1987) Effects of saliva from chronically reserpinized rat on Na and K transport in perfused main excretory duct of submandibular gland of normal rat. Proc Soc Exp Biol Med 185:392–395
Kanematsu S, Hillard J, Sawer CH (1963) Effect of reserpine on pituitary prolactin content and its hypothalamic site of action in the rabbit. Acta Endocrinol 44:467–474
Khalighi MR, Haque MA, Ziyai K, Firozian F, Parsaie H (1986) Influence of reserpine and guanethidine on the responses of the isolated rat ileum to catecholamines. Indian J Physiol Pharmacol 30:191–194
Khazan N, Sulman F, Winnik H (1960) Effect of reserpine on pituitary-gonadal axis. Proc Soc Exp Biol Med 105:201–204
Kim KS, Shore PA (1963) Mechanism of action of reserpine and insulin on gastric amines and gastric acid secretion, and the effect of monoamine oxidase inhibition. J Pharmacol Exp Ther 141:321–325
Kirkpatrick K, Burnstock G (1987) Sympathetic nerve-mediated release of ATP from the guinea-pig vas deferens is unafected by reserpine. Eur J Pharmacol 138:207–214
Kitay JI, Holub DA, Jailer JW (1959) "Inhibition" of pituitary ACTH release after administration of reserpine or epinephrine. Endocrinology 65:548–554
Klein F (1968) Hypotensive drugs. In: Meyler L, Herxheimer A (eds) Side effects of drugs. Exerpta Medica, Amsterdam, pp 202–211
Komatsu Y, Constanopoulos G, Gutkowska J, Rojo-Ortega JM, Genest J (1977) Effects of reserpine on water, cation, and norepinephrine contents of cardiovascular tissues of normotensive dogs. Can J Physiol Pharmacol 55:206–211
Kopin IJ, Gordon EK (1962) Metabolism of norepinephrine-H^3 released by tyramine and reserpine. J Pharmacol Exp Ther 138:351–359
Kopin IJ, Gordon EK (1963) Metabolism of administered and drug-released norepinephrine-H^3 in the rat. J Pharmacol Exp Ther 140:207–216
Krayer O, Alper MH, Paasonen MK (1962) Action of guanethidine and reserpine upon the isolated mammalian heart. J Pharmacol Exp Ther 135:164–173
Kroneberg G, Schumann HJ (1957a) Der EinfluB der Rauwolfia-Alkaloide Reserpin, Rescinnamin and Canescin auf den Katecholamin-Gehalt des Nebennierenmarks. Arzneimittelforschung 7:279–280
Kroneberg G, Schumann HJ (1957b) Die Wirkung des Reserpins auf den Hormongehalt des Nebennierenmarks. Naunyn Schmiedeberg Arch Exp Path Pharmak 231: 349–360
Kroneberg G, Schumann HJ (1958) Adrenalinsekretion und Adrenalinverarmung der Kanin-chennebennieren nach Reserpin. Naunyn-Schmiedeberg Arch Exp Pathol Pharmacol 234:133–146
Kulkarni AS, Shideman FE (1966) Sensitivities of the brains of infant and adult rats to the catecholamine-depleting actions of reserpine and tetrabenazine. J Pharmacol Exp Ther 153:428–433
Labarthe DR, O'Fallon WM (1980) Reserpine and breast cancer. A community based longitudinal study of 2,000 hypertensive women. JAMA 243:2304–2310
Labatut R, Buda M, Berod A (1986) Long term changes in rat brain tyrosine hydroxylase following reserpine treatment: a quantitative immunochemical analysis. J Neurochem 50:1375–1380
Lagercrantz H (1976) On the composition and function of large, dense-cored vesicles in

sympathetic nerves. Neuroscience 1:81–92
Langer SZ, Punto JE (1976) Possible involvement of a transmitter different from norepinephrine in the residual responses to nerve stimulation of the cat nictitating membrane after pretreatment with reserpine. J Pharmacol Exp Ther 196:697–713
Latifpour J, McNeill JH (1984) Reserpine induced changes in cardiac adrenoceptors. Can J Physiol Pharmacol 62:23–26
Laurence DR, Bennett PN (1987) Clinical pharmacology, 6th edn. Churchill Livingstone, Edinburgh, p 505
Lee FL (1967) The relation between norepinephrine content and response to sympathetic nerve stimulation of various organs of cats pretreated with reserpine. J Pharmacol Exp Ther 156:137–141
Levin BE (1984) Retrograde axonal transport of beta adrenoceptors in rat brain: effect of reserpine. Brain Res 300:103–112
Levin BE, Biegon A (1984) Reserpine and the role of axonal transport in the independent regulation of pre- and post synaptic beta-adrenoceptors. Brain Res 311: 39–50
Login IS, Cronin MJ, Lamberts SW, Valdenegro, CA, Macloed RM (1983) Reserpine inhibits rats anterior pituitary hormone secretion in vitro: effects of prolactin and ACTH and ultrastructural observations. Brain Res 260:99–106
Lott VJ, Cerino D, Kling P (1982) Characterization of the adrenoceptor activities of isoprenaline in the field stimulated rat vas deferens: selective supersensitivity to beta-2 mediated responses following reserpine treatment. J Auton Pharmacol 2:169–174
Lundberg JM, Savia A, Franco-Cereceda A, Hokfelt T (1985) Differential effects of reserpine and 6-hydroxydopamine on neuropeptide Y and noradrenaline in peripheral neurons. Naunyn Schmiedebergs Arch Pharmacol 328:331–340
Lundberg JM, Al-Safar A, Saria A, Theodorrson-Norheim E (1986a) Reserpine induced depletion of neuropeptide Y from cardiovascular nerves and adrenal gland due to enhanced release. Naunyn Schmiedebergs Arch Pharmacol 332:163–168
Lundberg JM, Rudehill A, Sollevi A, Theodorrson-Norheim E, Hamburger B (1986b) Frequency and reserpine dependent chemical coding of sympathetic transmission: differential release of noradrenaline and neuropeptide Y from pig spleen. Neurosci Lett 63:96–100
Lundberg JM, Pernow J, Fried G, Anggard A (1987) Neuropeptide Y and noradrenaline mechanisms in relation to reserpine induced impairment of sympathetic neurotransmission in the cat spleen. Acta Physiol Scand 131:1–10
Luxenberg J, Feigenbaum LZ (1983) The use of reserpine for elderly hypertensive patients. J Am Geriatr Soc 31:556–559
Maass AR, Jenkins B, Shen Y, Tannenbaum P (1969) Studies on absorption, excretion, and metabolism of 3H-reserpine in man. Clin Pharmacol Ther 10:366–371
Maccarrone C, Jarrott B (1986) Neuropeptide Y: a putative neurotransmitter. Neurochem Int 8:13–22
Maccarrone C, Jarrott B (1987) Differential effects of surgical sympathectomy on rat heart concentrations of neuropeptide Y-immunoreactivity and noradrenaline. J Auton Nerv Syst 21:101–107
Mack TM, Henderson BE, Vibeke R, Gerkins RN et al. (1975) Reserpine and breast cancer in a retirement community. N Engl J Med 292:1366–1371
Macmillan WH, Smith DJ, Jacobson JH (1962) Responses of normal, denervated and reserpine-treated arteries to sympathomimetic amines and nicotine in dogs. Br J Pharmacol 18:39–48
Mahfouz M, Ezz EA (1958) The effect of reserpine and chlorpromazine on the response of the rat to acute stress. J Pharmacol Exp Ther 123:39–42
Maickel RO, Westermann EO, Brodie BB (1961) Effects of reserpine and cold-exposure on pituitary-adrenocortical function in rats. J Pharmacol Exp Ther 134:167–175
Manara L, Mennini T, Carminati P (1972) Reduced binding of ^{3}H-reserpine to the hearts of 6-hydroxydopamine-pretreated rats. Eur J Pharmacol 17:183–185
Martindale (1982) Reynolds JEF (ed) Martindale. The Extrapharmacopea Pharmaceutical Press, London, p 163
Maxwell RA, Plummer AJ, Osborne MW, Ross SD (1956) Evidence for a peripheral

action of reserpine. J Pharmacol Exp Ther 116:42
Maxwell RA, Ross SD, Plummer AJ, Sigg EB (1957) A peripheral action of reserpine. J Pharmacol Exp Ther 119:69–77
Mayer G, Meunier JM, Thevenot-Duluc AJ (1960) Prolongation de la grossesse par retards de nitdation obtenus chez la ratte par administration de reserpine. Ann Endocrinol (Paris) 21:1–13
Meghji P, Tenner TE Jr, McNiell JH (1978) Reserpine induced supersensitivity to the inotropic and phosphorylase activating effects of glucagon in the perfused rat heart. Eur J Pharmacol 51:55–62
Meyers D (1976) Treatment of calcinosis circumscripta and Raynaud's phenomenon. Med J Aust 2:457
Molinoff PB, Brimijoin S, Axelrod (1972) Induction of dopamine-beta-hydroxylase and tyrosine hydroxylase in rat hearts and sympathetic ganglia. J Pharmacol Exp Ther 182:116–129
Morris JL, Murphy R, Furress JB, Costa M (1986) Partial depletion of neuropeptide Y from noradrenergic perivascular and cardiac axons by 6-hydroxydopamine and reserpine. Regul Pept 13:147–162
Morton AJ (1985) The effect of reserpine treatment on the extraneuronal uptake of ^{3}H-isoprenaline into rat atria. Br J Pharmacol 1:287–295
Morton D, Parker A, Estrada P, Martinez JR (1980) Exocrine pancreatic secretion in rats treated with reserpine after stimulation with pilocarpine, dopamine and caeralein. Pediatr Res 14:18–20
Mueller RA, Shideman FE (1968) A comparison of the absorption, distribution and metabolism of reserpine in infant and adult rats. J Pharmacol Exp Ther 163:91–97
Mueller RA, Thoenen H, Axelrod J (1969a) Compensatory increase in adrenal tyrosine hydroxylase activity after chemical sympathectomy. Science 163:468–469
Mueller RA, Thoenen H, Axelrod J (1969b) Increase in tyrosine hydroxylase activity after reserpine administration. J Pharmacol Exp Ther 169:74–79
Muradian RE (1986) Study of the potential carcinogenic activity of reserpine. Vopr Onkol 32:76–81
Muscholl E (1959) Die Konzentration von Noradrenalin und Adrenalin in den einzelnen Abschnitten des Herzens. Naunyn Schmiedeberg's Arch Exp Pathol Pharmacol 237:350–364
Muscholl E, Vogt M (1958) The action of reserpine on the peripheral sympathetic system. J Physiol (Lord) 141:132–155
Nagata M, Franco-Cereceda A, Saria A, Amann R, Lundberg JM (1987) Reserpine induced depletion of neuropeptide Y in the guinea pig: tissue specific effects and mechanisms of action. J Auton Nerv Syst 20:257–263
Nasseri A, Barakeh JF, Abel PW, Yoshida H (1985) Reserpine induced postjunctional supersensitivity in rat vas deferens and caudal artery without changes in alpha-adrenergic receptors. J Pharmacol Exp Ther 234:350–357
Nattero G, Lisino F, Brandi G et al. (1976) Reserpine for migraine prophylaxis. Headache 15:279–281
Near JA, Mahler JA (1983) Reserpine labels catecholamine transporter in synaptic vesicles from bovine caudate nucleus. FEBS Lett 158:31–35
Nilsen KH, Jayson MJV (1980) Cutaneous microcirculation in systemic sclerosis and response to intra-arterial reserpine. Br Med J 280:1408–1413
O'Fallon WM, Darwin RL, Leonard TK (1975) Raulwolfia derivatives and breast cancer. Lancet II:292–296
Ogawa K, Ban M, Ho T, Watanabe T, Kobayashi T, Yamazaki N, Suzaki Y (1984) Diltiazem for the treatment of essential hypertension: a double-blind controlled study with reserpine. Clin Ther 6:844–853
Owen F, Cross AJ, Waddington JL, Poulter M, Gamble SJ, Crow TJ (1980) Dopamine-mediated behaviour and ^{3}H-spiperone binding to striatal membranes in rats after nine months haloperidol administration. Life Sci 26:55–59
Paasonen MK, Krayer O (1957) Effect of reserpine upon the mammalian heart. Fed Proc 16:326–327
Paasonen MK, Krayer O (1958) The release of norepinephrine from the mammalian

heart by reserpine. J Pharmacol Exp Ther 123:153–160
Palm D, Grobecker H, Bak IJ (1970) Membrane effects of catecholamine releasing drugs. In: Schumann HJ, Kroneberg G (eds) New aspects of storage and release mechanisms of catcholamines. Springer, Berlin Heidelberg New York, pp 188–198
Parti R, Ozkan ED, Harnadek GJ, Njas D (1987) Inhibition of norepinephrine transport and reserpine binding by reserpine derivatives. J Neurochem 48:949–953
Peters HA, Daly RF (1972) Reserpine for tardive dyskinesia. N Engl J Med 286:106
Pletscher A, Shore PA, Brodie BB (1955) Serotonin release as a possible mechanism of reserpine action. Science 122:374–375
Pletscher A, Shore PA, Brodie BB (1956) Serotonin as a mediator of reserpine action in brain. J Pharmacol Exp Ther 116:84–89
Purshottam N (1962) Effects of tranquilizers on induced ovulation in mice. Am J Obstet Gynecol 83:1405–1409
Rand MJ, Jurevics H (1977) Pharmacology of Rauwolfia alkaloids. In: Gross F (ed) Antihypertensive agents. Springer, Berlin Heidelberg New York, pp 77–156
Reches A, Hassan MN, Jackson VR, Fahn S (1983) Lithium attenuates dopamine depleting effects of reserpine and tetrabenazine but not that of alphamethyl paratyrosine. Life Sci 33:157–160
Rogers RL, McNeill JH (1982) Effect of reserpine pretreatment on guinea pig ventricular performance and responsiveness to inotropic agents. J Pharmacol Exp Ther 221: 721–730
Rosch J, Porter JM, Gralino BJ (1977) Cryodynamic hand angiography in the diagnosis and management of Raynaud's Syndrome. Circulation 55:807–814
Ross RK, Paganini-Hill A, Krailo MD, Gerkins VR, Henderson BE, Pike MC (1984) Effects of reserpine on prolactin levels and incidence of breast cancer in postmenopausal women, Cancer Res 44:3106–3108
Saffran M, Vogt M (1960) Depletion of pituitary cortiocotrophin by reserpine and by a nitrogen mustard. Br J Pharmacol 15:165–169
Sanyal RK, West BG (1958) The relationship of histamine and 5-hydroxytryptamine to anaphylactic shock in different species. J Physiol (Lond) 144:525–531
Sato S, Daly R, Peters H (1971) Reserpine therapy of phenothiazide induced dyskinesia. Dis Nerv Syst 32:680–685
Scherman D, Henry JP (1984) Reserpine binding to bovine chromaffin granule membranes. Characterization and comparison with dihydrotetrabenazine binding. Mol Pharmacol 25:113–122
Schmitt H, Schmitt H (1960) Modifications des effects des amines sympathicomimetiques sur la pression arterielle et la membrane nictitante par la reserpine. Arch Int Pharmacodyn 125:30–47
Schneider JA, Rinehart RK (1956) Pharmacological interactions of serotonin and reserpine in dogs. J Pharmacol Exp Ther 116:51
Schon F, Allen JM, Yeats JC, Kent A, Kelly JS, Bloom SR (1986) The effect of 6-hydroxydopamine, reserpine and cold stress on the neuropeptide Y content of the rat central nervous system. Neuroscience 19:1247–1250
Schumann HJ (1958) Die Wirkung von Insulin und Reserpin auf den Adrenalin-und ATP-Gehalt der chromaffinen Granula des Nebennierenmarks. Naunyn Schmiedebergs Arch Exp Pathol Pharmacol 233:237–249
Seedat YK, Hoosen S, Bhigjee AI (1984) Reserpine plus hydroxychlorothiazide and sotalol plus hydrochlorothiazide in black and Indian hypertensive patients. S Afr Med J 65:915–917
Sen G, Bose KC (1931) Rauwolfia serpentina, a new Indian drug for insanity and high blood pressure. Indian Med World 2:194–201
Shaskan EG, Snyder SH (1970) Kinetics of serotonin accumulation into slices of rat brain: relationship to catecholamine uptake. J Pharmacol Exp Ther 175:404–418
Sheppard H, Tsien WH (1955) Metabolism of reserpine-C^{14}. II. Species differences as studied in vitro. Proc Soc Exp Biol Med 90:437–446
Sheppard H, Lucus RC, Tsien WH (1955) The metabolism of reserpine-C^{14}. Arch Int Pharmacodyn 103:256–269
Sheppard H, Tsien WH, Sigg EB, Lucas RH, Plummer AJ (1957) The metabolism of

reserpine-C^{14}. III. C^{14}-concentration vs time in the brains and other tissues of rats of guinea pigs. Arch Int Pharmacodyn 113:160–168

Sheppard H, Tsien WH, Plummer AJ, Pleets EA, Giletti BU, Shulert AR (1958) Brain reserpine levels following large and small doses of reserpine-H^3. Proc Soc Exp Biol Med 97:717–721

Sigg EB (1968) Autonomic side effects induced by psychotherapeutic agents. In: Psychopharmacology. A review of progress 1957–1967. Washington Public Health publication no. 1836, pp 581–588

Sjostrand NO (1962) Effect of reserpine and hypogastric denervation on the noradrenaline content of the vas deferens and the seminal vesicle of the guinea-pig. Acta Physiol Scand 56:376–380

Smirk FH, Doyle AE (1954) Hypotensive action of reserpine. Lancet I:1096–1097

Snyder SH, Petroatka SJ (1982) A possible role of serotonin receptors in antidepressant drug action. Pharmacopsychiatria 15:131–134

Spadari RC, Lamas JL, De Morreas S (1987) The effects of acute reserpine administration on the sensitivity of the isolated pacemaker from rat heart to isoprenaline and noradrenaline. J Pharm Pharmacol 39:662–664

Stevens MDB (1985) The detection of new adverse drug reactions. MacMillan, London pp 10–13

Stitzel RE, Wagner LA, Stawarz RJ (1972) Studies on the microsomal metabolism of ^{3}H-reserpine. J Pharmacol Exp Ther 182:500–506

Stjarne L (1964) Studies of catecholamine uptake storage and release mechanisms. Acta Physiol Scand 62 [Suppl 228]:1–97

Stjarne L, Schapiro S (1959) Effect of reserpine on secretion from the denervated adrenal medulla. Nature 184:2023–2024

Sugrue MF, Shore PA (1971) Further evidence for a sodium-dependent, optically specific and reserpine-sensitive amine carrier mechanism at the adrenergic neuron. J Pharmacol Exp Ther 177:389–397

Takenaka F (1963) Response of vascular strip preparations to noradrenaline and tyramine. Jpn J Pharmacol 13:274–281

Tenner TE Jr, Carrier O Jr (1978) Reserpine induced supersensitivity to the chronotropic and inotropic effects of calcium in rabbit atria. J Pharmacol Exp Ther 221:721–730

Tenner TE Jr, Mukherjee A, Hester RK (1982) Reserpine induced hypersensitivity and the proliferation of cardiac beta-adrenoceptors. Eur J Pharmacol 8:61–65

Thoenen H, Mueller RA, Axelrod (1969a) Transynaptic induction of adrenal tyrosine hydroxylase. J Pharmacol Exp Ther 169:249–254

Thoenen H, Mueller RA, Axelrod (1969b) Increased tyrosine hydroxylase activity after drug-induced alteration of sympathetic transmission. Nature 221:1264

Thompson JH, Campbell LB (1967) The effect of reserpine upon gastrointestinal serotonin in the Sprague-Dawley rat. Experientia 23:826–827

Tindall JP, Whalen RE, Burton EE (1974) Medical uses of intra-arterial injections of reserpine. Treatment of Raynaud's syndrome and of some vascular insufficiencies of the lower extremities. Arch Dermatol 110:233–237

Torphy TJ, Westfall DP, Fleming WW (1982) Effect of reserpine pretreatment on mechanical responsiveness and 124I idohydroxybenzylpindolol binding sites in the guinea-pig right atrium. J Pharmacol Exp Ther 223:332–341

Traub M, Reches A, Wagner HR, Fahn S (1986) Reserpine-induced up regulation of dopamine D_2 receptors in the rat striatum is enhanced by denervation but not by chronic receptor blockade. Neurosci Lett 70:245–249

Trendelenburg U (1961) Modification of the effect of tyramine by various agents and procedure. J Pharmacol Exp Ther 134:8–17

Trendelenburg U (1965) The effect of sympathetic nerve stimulation on isolated atria of guinea pigs and rabbits pretreated with reserpine. J Pharmacol Exp Ther 147: 313–318

Trendelenburg U, Gravenstein JS (1958) Effect of reserpine pretreatment on stimulation of the accelerans nerve of the dog. Science 128:901–903

Vakil RJ (1949) Clinical trial of *Rauwolfia serpentina* in essential hypertension. Br Heart J 11:350–355

Veterans Administration Cooperative Study Group on Antihypertensive Agents (1972) Propranolol in the treatment of hypertension. JAMA 237:2303–2310

Veterans Administration Study Group (1978) Evaluation of treatment in mild hypertension: VA-NHLBI feasibility trial. Plan and preliminary results of a two year feasibility trial for a multicenter intervention study to evaluate the benefits versus the disadvantages of treating mild hypertension. Prepared for the Veterans Administration-National Heart, Lung and Blood Institute Study Group for Evaluating Treatment in Mild Hypertension. Ann NY Acad Sci 304:267–292

Villeneuve A, Boszormenyi Z (1970) Treatment of drug induced dyskinesias. Lancet I:353–354

Viveros OH, Arqueros L, Kirshner N (1969) Mechanism of secretion from the adrenal medulla. V. Retention of storage vesicle membranes following release of adrenaline. Mol Pharmacol 5:342–349

Wakade AR (1980) A comparison of rates of depletion and recovery of noradrenaline stores of peripheral and central noradrenergic neurons after reserpine administration: importance of neuronal activity. Br J Pharmacol 68:93–98

Warland JI, Burnstock G (1987) Effects of reserpine and 6-hydroxydopamine on the adrenergic and purinergic components of symapthetic nerve responses of the rabbit saphenous artery. Br J Pharmacol 92:871–880

Watanabe Y, Lai RT, Maeda H, Yosdhida H (1982) Reserpine and sympathetic denervation cause an increase of post synaptic $alpha_2$ adrenoceptors. Eur J Pharmacol 80:105–108

Waud DR, Kottegoda SR, Krayer O (1958) Threshold dose and time course of norepinephrine depletion of mammalian heart by reserpine. J Pharmacol Exp Ther 124:340–346

Weiner N (1985) Norepinephrine, epinephrine and the sympathomimetic amines. In: Gilman AG, Goodman LS, Rall TW, Murad F II (eds) The pharmacological basis of therapeutics. McMillans, New York, p 130

Weiner RI, Ganong WF (1971) Effect of the depletion of brain catecholamines on puberty and the estrous cycle in the rat. Neuroendocrinology 8:125–135

Wellstein A, Jablonka B, Wiemer G, Palm D (1984) Increase in B_{max} values of beta adrenoceptor sites after chronic treatment with reserpine? Pol J Pharmacol Pharm 36:265–273

Werlin SL, Harb JM, Stefaniak J, Taylor T (1983) Pancreatic structure and function in immature reserpinized rat. Exp Mol Pathol 39:24–36

Whelan RF, Skinner SL (1963) Autonomic transmitter mechanisms. Br Med Bull 19: 120–124

Winkler H, Fischer-Colbrie R, Weber A (1981) Molecular organisation of vesicles storing transmitter: chromaffin granules as a model. In: Stjarne L, Hedqvist P, Lager-Crantz H, Wennmalm A (eds) Chemical neurotransmission 75 years. Academic, London, pp 57–68

CHAPTER 8

Guanethidine and Related Compounds

W.J. Louis and L.G. Howes

CONTENTS

1 Introduction

Guanethidine and related compounds have collectively been called adrenergic blocking drugs because their major pharmacological action is to prevent the release of noradrenaline from postganglionic neurons in response to sympathetic nerve stimulations. Guanethidine has other actions on catecholamine metabolism (see Sect. 2) and can cause significant tissue depletion of catecholamines. It does not, however, interfere with release of catecholamines from the adrenal medulla and does not produce parasympathetic blockade.

These drugs have been used as antihypertensive therapy for over 25 years, although their use has declined markedly in recent years in favor of drugs with fewer side effects. Guanethidine has also been used to treat glaucoma and bretylium has been used as an antiarrhythmic agent. As guanethidine is the most commonly used drug of this class, this review will concentration on its pharmacology. Discussion of the other commonly used adrenergic blocking drugs will be limited to aspects in which they differ from guanethidine. A list of adrenergic neuron blockers, whose chemical structures are illustrated in Fig. 1, is given here:

Quarternary ammonium derivatives
Bretylium
Guanidine derivatives

Guanethidine	Guanoxan
Bethanidine	Guanoclor
Debrisoquine	Guanabenz
Guanisoquin	

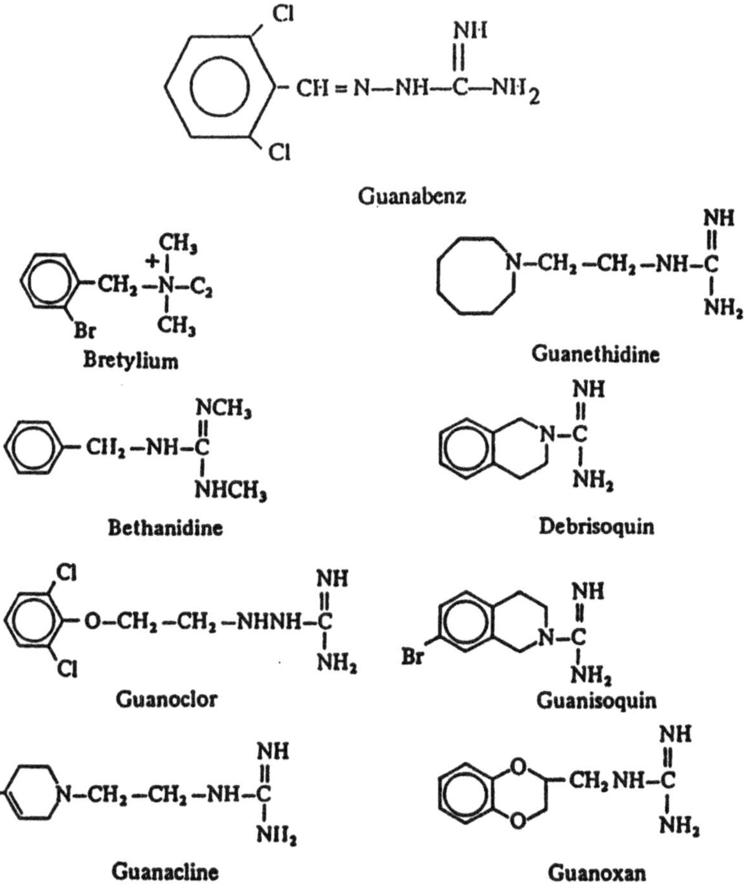

Fig. 1. Chemical structures of adrenergic neurone blockers

The development of adrenergic neuron blockers arose because of studies on two different groups of compounds. One group led to the development of the quarternary ammonium compounds such as bretylium, and the other led to the development of a group of related compounds with a strongly basic moiety, guanidine. The quarternary derivatives arose from studies of the derivatives of choline phenyl ethers on autonomic function (Brown and Hey 1956; Bein 1960; Hey and Willey 1954; Exley 1957, 1960; Boura et al. 1959, 1961; Boura and

GREEN 1959; COPP 1964). The development of guanidine derivatives began during experiments with the CNS stimulant methylphenidate, which was shown to block the sympathoexcitatory effects of indirectly acting sympathomimetics (MAXWELL et al. 1957, 1958).

The most striking feature that was common to these drugs was their ability to induce a long-lasting inhibition of noradrenaline release from sympathetic nerves that could not be explained by other mechanisms such as ganglion blockade.

2 Mode of Action of Guanethidine

There are five classically described effects of guanethidine on noradrenergic neurons (MAXWELL 1982):

(a) Inhibition of the release of neurotransmitter from noradrenergic neurons in response to action potentials.
(b) A transient indirect sympathomimetic effect due to enhanced release of noradrenaline stored in nerve terminals.
(c) Inhibition of neuronal uptake and storage of catecholamines by nerve terminals.
(d) A gradual depletion of noradrenaline stored in nerve terminals.
(e) Inhibition of noradrenaline release from nerve terminals by indirectly acting sympathomimetic drugs.

These observations can largely be explained by the chemical properties of the drug. Guanethidine is taken up and concentrated within noradrenergic neurons. While part of the uptake by nerve terminals appears to be nonspecific (SCHANKER and MORRISON 1965), the major mode of uptake is by the specific, high-affinity, energy-dependent amine pump (DENGLER et al. 1961; SCHANKER and MORRISON 1965). The specific neuronal uptake of guanethidine can be antagonized by other substrates and inhibitors of this uptake process (MITCHELL and OATES 1970). This property of the drug explains, in part, the pharmacological effects of inhibition of catecholamine uptake and storage and the transient sympathomimetic effects.

The high-affinity amine uptake pump is the same pump which is responsible for the uptake of noradrenaline into storage vesicles and granules (CHANG et al. 1964; OBIANWU et al. 1968; MAXWELL 1982), an effect which is prevented by reserpine (BRODIE et al. 1965). The resultant accumulation and storage of guanethidine in vesicles and granules partly explain the transient sympathomimetic effects of guanethidine and the ability of the drug to deplete noradrenaline from nerve terminals. None of these effects, however, explains the major mode of action by which guanethidine paralyzes sympathetic neurotransmission, as the ability to prevent noradrenaline release in response to nerve stimulation and sympathomimetic amines occurs long before there is any significant neuronal depletion of noradrenaline. It appears that once guanethidine is concentrated in sympathetic terminals, a distinct and poorly characterized chemical property of the drug prevents noradrenaline storage vesicles from fusing with the cell membrane and discharging their contents into the synaptic cleft.

Several mechanisms have been proposed to explain this effect (Maxwell 1982). Guanethidine (and other adrenergic neuron blockers) have a membrane stabilizing activity and weak local anesthetic effects (Hausler et al. 1968; Boura et al. 1960; Boura and Green 1965; Bein 1960). Guanethidine also possesses general inhibitory actions on nerve and muscle function at high concentrations (Mitchell and Oates 1970; Oates et al. 1971), and it is possible that sufficient concentrations are accumulated in noradrenergic storage vesicles to stabilize their membranes.

However, Rand and Wilson (1967) could not demonstrate a relationship between local anesthetic activity and adrenergic neuron blocking effects of a range of compounds, and Wilson (1970) reported that a compound (3-cyclohexylamino-*n*-propylguanidine) which is taken up by sympathetic nerve terminals and has local anesthetic activity is devoid of neuron blocking activity. Moreover, Misu et al. (1976) found that a compound (4-7-exomethylene-hexahydroisoindoline-ethyl-guanidine-hemisulphate) is a potent neuron blocker but lacks local anesthetic activity.

An alternate possibility is that guanethidine depresses noradrenaline release by limiting the access of calcium to sites in the sympathetic nerve terminal with which calcium interacts to cause noradrenaline release (Kirpekarsm et al. 1969). Support for this theory comes from the observation that tetraethylammonium and 4-aminopyridine which enhance noradrenaline release by increasing calcium entry into sympathetic nerves (Thoenen et al. 1967; Kirpekarsm et al. 1972, 1976; Kirpekarm et al. 1976) reverse the neuronal blockade induced by guanethidine (Kirpekarm et al. 1978).

In contrast, Stutzin et al. (1983) have suggested that guanethidine may block noradrenergic neurons by activating their calcium-activated potassium conductance (by releasing intracellular calcium), leading to a hyperpolarization of the synaptic membrane.

In large doses administered to animals guanethidine causes destruction of sympathetic neurons (Palmatier et al. 1987; Kidd et al. 1986), an effect which may be immune mediated (Manning et al. 1982, 1983). However, this effect is unrelated to the effect of guanethidine on neuronal transmission seen at lower doses. The related drug guanacline has been demonstrated to produce prolonged damage to sympathetic neurons in animals and in humans (Dawborn et al. 1969; Burnstock et al. 1971).

Guanethidine is a charged molecule at physiological pH and does not cross the blood-brain barrier to a significant extent (Boura et al. 1960; Boura and Green 1962; Kuntzman et al. 1962). However, guanethidine does affect neurons of the area postrema which is outside the blood-brain barrier (Newton et al. 1987). The pharmacological implications of this observation are uncertain.

2.1 Neuropeptide Y

Neuropeptide Y (NPY) is a putative peptide neurotransmitter which is colocalized with noradrenaline in many peripheral sympathetic nerves (for review, see

MACCARRONE and JARROTT 1986), although there is evidence that in some tissues NPY may be localized in storage vesicles that are distinct from those that store noradrenaline (FRIED et al. 1985).

Guanethidine abolishes the release of NPY in response to sympathetic nerve stimulation in the cat spleen (LUNDBERG et al. 1984). In addition, guanethidine inhibits the prolonged attenuation of cardiac vagal activity which normally follows sympathetic nerve stimulation and is believed to be mediated by NPY (POTTER 1987). There is no information concerning the effects of guanethidine on NPY release in other tissues.

2.2 Postsynaptic Responsiveness and Adrenoceptors

Acute and chronic guanethidine treatment increases the sensitivity of most tissues to directly acting sympathomimetic agents (BOURA and GREEN 1965). While part of this effect is probably due to competition for neuronal uptake between guanethidine released from the nerve terminal and the exogenous sympathomimetic amine, the enhanced sensitivity of post-synaptic receptors and effector mechanisms are probably involved, particularly during chronic therapy (KHAN and ASMAE 1968). Chronic guanethidine therapy has been shown to increase the number of β-adrenoceptors in rat heart (GLAUBIGER et al. 1978), but its effects on adrenoceptor numbers in other tissues is uncertain. It is likely that chronic guanethidine therapy induces hypersensitivity of effector mechanisms beyond the postsynaptic adrenoceptors, as the sensitivity to histamine, 5-HT, aminophylline, and calcium chloride is increased in a variety of tissues (GOKHALE et al. 1967).

3 Clinical Effects

3.1 Hemodynamic Effects

Acute intravenous injections of guanethidine in humans produce a short-lived pressor response with variable changes in heart rate (COHN et al. 1963). This is followed by a slight reduction in blood pressure, which is due to a reduction in cardiac output with no significant change in peripheral resistance. Titling the patient leads to a further reduction in blood pressure due to a reduction in peripheral resistance and a further fall in cardiac output (VILLARREAL et al. 1964). Following 1 week of treatment with guanethidine in hypertensive patients, blood pressure falls to a moderate degree in the supine position and to a more marked degree in the erect position. The heart rate is reduced, and sympathetic reflexes are impaired (RICHARDSON et al. 1960; SHAPIRO and KRIFCHER 1964; MASON and BRAUNWALD 1964). Long-term therapy with guanethidine has been associated with tolerance to its antihypertensive effects in humans and in some animal models of hypertension (RANKIN et al. 1984; DUNSTAN et al. 1972; Ronnov-Jennsen and HANSEN 1969). This may in part be due to fluid retention as weight gain and edema are common during guanethidine therapy (DOLLERY et al. 1960; LEISHMAN et al. 1959), and tolerance to its antihypertensive effects can be prevented in spontaneously hypertensive rats by angiotensin converting enzyme therapy. However, Safan et al. (1975) found that while plasma volume is significantly increased in hypertensive humans following 7 days of guanethidine therapy, PRA and aldosterone levels remain unchanged. During long-term guanethidine therapy, peripheral resistance falls, cardiac output returns to normal, and postural and exercise-induced hypotension persist (Chamberlain and Howard 1964; Villarreal et al. 1964; Prichard et al. 1968).

There is evidence that guanethidine can actually induce vasodilation in response to sympathetic nerve stimulation, an effect which may contribute to the reduction in peripheral resistance apparent during chronic administration (Angus et al. 1978). This does not appear to be due to a direct effect of guanethidine on vascular smooth muscle but may be mediated by enhanced histamine release (Angus et al. 1978) or increased sensitivity of vascular smooth muscle to histamine (Gokhale et al. 1967).

3.2 Other Clinical Effects

In addition to its use as an antihypertensive agent, guanethidine has proved to be a useful drug for lowering intraocular pressure in glaucoma (Bonomi et al. 1983; Castren and Pohjola 1962) and relieving painful and atrophic sympathetic dystrophies when administered by local intravenous injection (Hannington-Kiff 1977; Tabira et al. 1983).

Adrenergic neuron blockers possess antiarrhythmic activity. While this has been demonstrated for guanethidine (Leveque 1964; Raines et al. 1968; Ahmad and Achari 1968) and bethanadine (Leveque 1966), bretylium has been the subject of most of the research and clinical application in this area (Leveque 1965; Bacaner 1966, 1968a, b; Castaneda and Bacaner 1970; Day and Bacaner 1971; Bernstein and Koch-Weser 1972). The antiarrhythmic effects appear to be due to a direct effect on cardiac muscle in addition to adrenergic neuron blockade (Namm et al. 1975).

3.3 Effects on Atherogenesis

The effects of guanethidine on the development of atheroma is animal models has received very little attention. However, one study has reported that guanethidine antagonized the beneficial effects of exercise on plasma cholesterol and atheroma formation in cockerels fed an atherogenic diet (Orimilikwe et al. 1983).

4 Side Effects

The side effects of guanethidine are principally consequences of its action on peripheral sympathetic function. Postural and exercise-induced hypotension are common side effects that limit the usefulness of the drug (Green 1962; Maxwell 1962; Fawaz 1963; Prichard et al. 1968). Guanethidine produces loose stools or diarrhoea because of a predominance of parasympathetic tone to the gut. This effect may not be entirely due to adrenergic neuron blockade since the potent adrenergic neuron blocker bethanidine has been reported to produce significantly less diarrhoea than guanethidine (SMIRK 1963; BOURA and GREEN 1963). Sympathetic blockade by guanethidine may cause failure of ejaculation without loss of potency in men (DOLLERY et al. 1960; GREEN 1962; PRICHARD et al. 1968). Reduced sympathetic activity due to adrenergic neuron blockade may cause tenderness and swelling of the parotid glands (GREEN 1962).

4.1 Drug Interactions

Because of its multiple actions on catecholamine metabolism guanethidine may interact with a wide range of adrenergic agents including adrenaline and other sympathomimetic agents, antidepressants, monoamine oxidase inhibitors, and antipsychotics. It should not be given to patients with pheochromocytoma (REYNOLDS 1982; MAXWELL 1982).

5 Absorption, Distribution, and Metabolism

The absorption of guanethidine from the gastrointestinal tract is variable and incomplete, with a bioavailability of about 20%–40% (MCMARTIN et al. 1970; RAHN 1973; RAHN and GOLDBERG 1969) following acute dosing. Bioavailability during chronic dosing is unknown but may be less than for acute dosing because of the effects of guanethidine on intestinal motility (HENGSTMAN and FALKNER 1979).

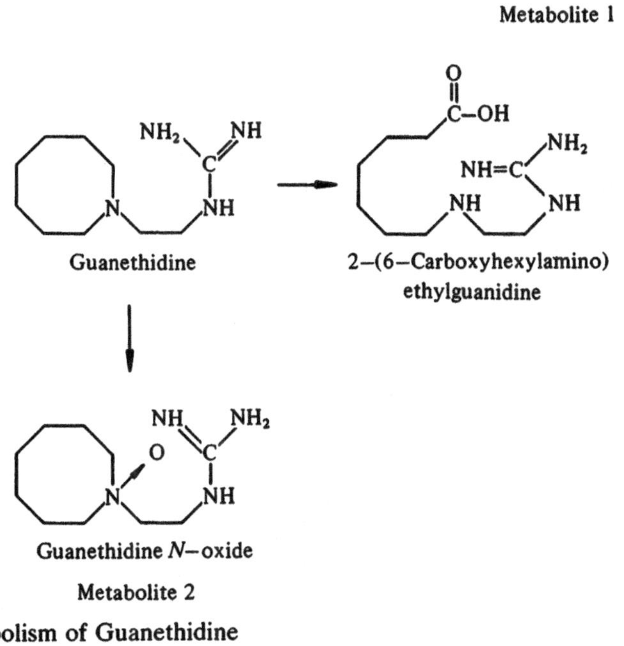

Fig. 2. Metabolism of Guanethidine

Following intravenous injection 60% of guanethidine is excreted unchanged in the urine (Rahn and Goldberg 1969). Guanethidine displays linear pharmacokinetics (Hengstmann and Falkner 1979). While early studies suggested that the eliminated half-life of guanethidine following acute administration was about 2 days (Rahn 1971), more recent studies following cessation of chronic administration suggest two phases of elimination, one with a half-life of about 1.5 days and a second with a half-life of 4.1–7.7 days (Hengstmann and Falkner 1979).

In studies of the excretion of radiolabelled guanethidine in humans, it has been demonstrated that 90% of the administered radioactivity can be recovered as either guanethidine or two major metabolites [guanethidine *N*-oxide and 2-(6-carboxyhexylamino) ethylguanidine] (Fig. 2; McMartin and Simpson 1971). The ratio of these metabolites to the parent drug is much higher after oral administration than after intramuscular injection, suggesting that guanethidine undergoes substantial first pass hepatic metabolism. Each of these metabolites possesses approximately 3% of the antihypertensive activity of guanethidine. The metabolism of guanethidine is inhibited by drugs that inhibit or compete for metabolism by hepatic mixed function oxidases (Mitchell et al. 1970).

6 Other Adrenergic Neuron Blockers

Of the other adrenergic blockers which have been developed bretylium, bethanidine, and debrisoquine have been most commonly used in humans. There are some differences in the pharmacology of these drugs compared with guanethidine, although none of these differences are major.

Debrisoquine appears to have relatively little ability to block neuronal uptake of noradrenaline (Moe et al. 1964). Bretylium, bethanidine, and debrisoquine are all less potent than guanethidine at depleting noradrenaline from sympathetic nerves (Boura et al. 1960; Boura and Green 1963, 1965; Moe et al. 1964), possibly because they possess weak monoamine oxidase inhibiting activity (Medina et al. 1969).

Bretylium, unlike guanethidine, blocks 5-hydroxytryptamine release in addition to blocking noradrenaline release (Schlicker and Gothert 1983). However, the clinical significance of this is unknown. Bethanidine has a similar antihypertensive potency to guanethidine in humans, but a shorter duration of action (Smirk 1963; Johnston et al. 1964; Mosler 1969). Debrisoquine undergoes extensive and rapid hepatic metabolism and therefore has a shorter duration of action than guanethidine (Medina et al. 1969; Allen et al. 1975).

Summary

Guanethidine and related compounds are classed as ganglion neuron blocking drugs because of their ability to impair noradrenaline release from sympathetic nerves. Although there are several factors which are responsible for this action, the primary one is the ability to prevent the release of noradrenaline from storage vesicles into the synaptic cleft. The result is a reduction in blood pressure which is much more marked in the erect than the supine position. This not infrequently produces symptoms of postural hypotension, a factor which has limited the clinical usefulness of the drugs in the management of hypertension. In addition, there is some evidence that secondary mechanisms such as fluid retention may lead to tolerance to their antihypertensive effects during chronic administration. Because of these factors and other side effects, the use of these drugs as antihypertensives has diminished in recent years as more effective drugs with fewer side effects have been developed.

References

Ahmad M, Achari G (1968) Anti-arrhythmic activity of guanethidine and methyldopa. J Indian Med Assoc 49:363–368

Allen JG, East PB, Francis RJ, Haigh JL (1975) Metabolism of debrisoquine sulfate. Identification of some urinary metabolites in rat and man. Drug Metab Dispos 3:332–337

Angus JA, Bobik A, Korner PI, Stoneham MT (1978) Guanethidine induced vasodilatation in the rabbit, mediated by endogenous histamine. Br J Clin Pharmacol 62:7–17

Bacaner M (1966) Bretylium tosylate for suppression of induced ventricular fibrillation. Am J Cardiol 17:528–534

Bacaner MB (1968a) Quantitative comparison of bretylium with other antifibrillatory drugs. Am J Cardiol 21:504–512

Bacaner MB (1968b) Treatment of ventricular fibrillation and other acute arrhythmias with bretylium tosylate. Am J Cardiol 21:530–543

Bein HJ (1960) Some pharmacological properties of guanethidine. In: Wolsten-Holme GEW, O'Connor M (eds) Adrenergic mechanisms. Ciba Foundation Symposium. Little, Brown, Boston

Bernstein JG, Koch-Weser J (1972) Effectiveness of bretylium tosylate against refractory ventricular arrhythmias. Circulation 45:1024–1034

Bonomi L, Perfetti S, Bulluci R, Massa F, Gamba GC (1983) Intraocular pressure lowering effect of low dosage combination of guanethidine and terbutaline in rabbit. Graefes Arch Clin Exp Opthalmol 220:197–199

Boura ALA, Green AF (1959) The actions of bretylium: adrenergic neurone blocking and other effects. Br J Pharmacol 14:536–548

Boura ALa, Green AF (1962) Comparison of bretylium and guanethidine: Tolerance and effects of adrenergic nerve function and responses to sympathomimetic amines. Br J Pharmacol 19:13–41

Boura ALA, Green AF (1963) Adrenergic neurone blockade and other acute effects caused by N-benzyl-N′N″-dimethylguanidine and its ortho-chloro deviate. Br J Pharmacol 20:36–55

Boura ALA, Green AF (1965) Adrenergic neuron blocking agents. Annu Rev Pharmacol 5:183–212

Boura ALA, Copp FC, Green AF (1959) New antiadrenergic compounds. Nature 184:70–71

Boura ALA, Copp FC, Duncombe WG, Green AF, McCoubrey A (1960) The selective accumulation of bretylium in sympathetic ganglia and their postganglionic nerves. Br J Pharmacol 15:265–270

Boura ALA, Copp FC, Green AF, Hodson HF, Ruffell GK, Sim MF, Walton E, Grivsky EM (1961) Adrenergic neuron blocking agents related to choline 2,6-xylyl ether bromide (TM 10), bretylium and guanethidine. Nature 191:1312–1313

Brodie BB, Chang CC, Costa E (1965) On the mechanism of action of guanethidine and bretylium. Br J Pharmacol 25:171–178

Brown BG, Hey P (1956) Choline phenyl ethers as inhibitors of amine oxidase. Br J

Pharmacol 11:58–65
Burnstock G, Doyle AE, Gannon BJ, Gerkens JF, Iwayama T, Mashford ML (1971) Prolonged hypotension and ultrastructural changes in sympathetic neurones following guanacline treatment. Eur J Pharmacol 13:175–187
Castaneda A, Bacaner M (1970) Effect of bretylium tosylate on the prevention and treatment of postoperative arrhythmias. Am J Cardiol 25:461–466
Castren JA, Pohjola S (1962) Guanethidine and aqueous humor dynamics. Acta Ophthalmol (Copenh) 40:348–361
Chamberlain DA, Howard J (1964) Guanethidine and methyldopa: a haemodynamic study. Br Heart J 26:528–536
Chang CC, Costa E, Brodie BB (1964) Reserpine-induced release of drugs from sympathetic nerve endings. Life Sci 3:839–844
Cohn JN, Liptak TE, Freis ED (1963) Hemodynamic effects of guanethidine in man. Circ Res 12:298–307
Copp FC (1964) Adrenergic neurone blocking agents. Adv Drug Res 1:161–189
Dawborn JK, Doyle AE, Ebringer A, Howqus J, Jerums G, Johnston CI, Mashford ML, Parkins JD (1969) Persistent postural hypotension due to guanacline. Pharmacol Clin 2:105
Day HW, Bacaner M (1971) Use of bretylium tosylate in the management of acute myocardial infarction. Am J Cardiol 27:177–189
Dengler HJ, Spiegel HE, Titus EO (1961) Uptake of tritium-labeled norepinephrine in brain and other tissues of cat in vitro. Science 133:1072–1073
Dollery CT, Emslie-Smith D, Milne MD (1960) Clinical and pharmacological studies with guanethidine in the treatment of hypertension. Lancet II:381–387
Dunstan HP, Tarazi R, Bravo L (1972) Dependence of arterial pressure on intravascular volume in treated hypertensive patients. N Engl J Med 286:861–866
Exley KA (1957) The blocking action of choline 2:6-xylyl ether bromide on adrenergic nerves. Br J Pharmacol 12:297–305
Exley KA (1960) The persistence of adrenergic nerve conduction after TM_{10} or bretylium in the cat. In: Wolsten-Holme GEW, O'Connor M (eds) Adrenergic mechanisms. Ciba Foundation Symposium. Little, Brown, Boston
Fawaz G (1963) Cardiovascular pharmacology. Annu Rev Pharmacol 3:57–90
Fried G, Terenicis L, Hockfelt T, Goldstein M (1985) Evidence for differential localization of noradrenaline and neuropeptide Y (NPY) in neuronal storage vesicles in rat vas deferens. J Neurosci 5:450–458
Glaubiger G, Tsai BS, Lefkowitz RJ, Weiss B, Johnson EM Jr (1978) Chronic guanethidine treatment increases cardiac beta-adrenergic receptors. Nature 273:240–242
Gokhale SD, Gulati OD, Kelkar VV (1967) Supersensitivity to catecholamines following guanethidine. Br J Pharmacol 30:445–462
Green AF (1962) Antihypertensive drugs. Adv Pharmacol 1:161–225
Hannington-Kiff JC (1977) Relief of Sudek's atrophy by regional intravenous guanethidine. Lancet I: 1132–1133
Hausler G, Thoenen H, Haefely W, Hurlimann A (1968) Durch Acetylcholin hervorgerufene antidrome Aktivitat im kardinalen Sympathicus und Noradrenalinfreisetzung unter Guanethidin. Helv Physiol Pharmacol Acta 26:352–354
Hengstmann JH, Falkner FC (1979) Disposition of guanethidine during chronic oral therapy. Eur J Clin Pharmacol 15:121–125
Hey P, Willey GL (1954) Choline 2:6-xylyl ether bromide; an active quaternary local anaesthetic. Br J Pharmacol 9:471–475
Johnston AW, Prichard BNC, Rosenheim ML (1964) The use of bethanidine in the treatment of hypertension. Lancet II:659–661
Khan I, Asmae R (1968) Effects of reserpine and guanethidine on the responses of the isolated rat fundus strip to substituted tryptamines and catecholamines. Life Sci 7:307–316
Kidd GJ, Heath JW, Dunkley PR (1986) Degeneration of myelinated sympathetic nerve fibres following treatment with guanethidine. J Neurocytol 15:561–572
Kirpekar M, Mirpekar SM, Prat JC (1976) Effect of 4-aminopyridine (4-AP) on release of norepinephrine (NE) from the perfused cat spleen by nerve stimulation (NS) and

potassium (K). Pharmacologist 18:208
Kirpekar M, Kirpekar SM, Prat JC (1978) Reversal of guanethidine blockade of sympathetic nerve terminals by tetraethylammonium and 4-aminopyridine. Br J Pharmacol 62:75–78.
Kirpekar SM, Wakade AR, Dixon W, Prat JC (1969) Effect of cocaine, phenoxybenzamine and calcium on the inhibition of norepinephrine output from the cat spleen by guanethidine. J Pharmacol Exp Ther 165:166–175
Kirpekar SM, Prat JC, Puig M, Wakade AR (1972) Modification of the evoked release of noradrenaline from the perfused cat spleen by various ions and agents. J Physiol 221:601–615
Kirpekar SM, Wakade AR, Prat JC (1976) Effect of tetraethylammonium and barium on the release of noradrenaline from the perfused cat spleen by nerve stimulation and potassium. Naunyn-Schmiedebergs Arch Pharmacol 294:23–29
Kuntzman R, Costa E, Gessa GL, Brodie BB (1962) Reserpine and guanethidine action on peripheral stores of catecholamines. Life Sci 1:65–74
Leishman AWD, Mathews HL, Smith AJ (1959) Guanethidine: hypotensive drug with prolonged action. Lancet II:1044–1048
Leveque PE (1964) Guanethidine as an anti-fibrillatory agent. Nature 203:1389
Leveque PE (1965) Anti-arrhythmic action of bretylium. Nature 207:203–204
Leveque PE (1966) Bethanidine: a new anti-fibrillatory agent. Arch Int Pharmacodyn 163:422–426
Lundberg JM, Anggard A, Theodorsson-Norheim E, Pernow J (1984) Guanethidine-sensitive release of neuropeptide Y-like immunoreactivity in cat spleen by sympathetic nerve stimulation. Neurosci Lett 52:175–180
Maccarrone C, Jarrott B (1986) Neuropeptide Y: a putative neurotransmitter. Neurochem Int 8:13–22
Manning PT, Russell JH, Johnson EM Jr (1982) Immunosuppressive agents prevent guanethidine-induced destruction of rat sympathetic neurons. Brain Res 241:131–143
Manning PT, Powers CW, Schmidt RE, Johnson EMJ (1983) Guanethidine-induced a destruction of peripheral sympathetic neurons occurs by an immune-mediated mechanism. J Neurosci 3:714–724
Mason DT, Braunwald E (1964) Effects of guanethidine, reserpine and methyldopa on reflex venous and arterial constriction in man. J Clin Invest 43:1449–1463
Maxwell RA (1962) Clinical and experimental pharmacology of sympathetic blocking agents. Conn Med 26:646–651
Maxwell RA (1982) Guanethidine after twenty years: a pharmacologists perspective. Br J Clin Pharmacol 13:35–44
Maxwell RA, Plummer AJ, Ross SD, Paytas JJ, Dennis AD (1957) Antihypertensive effects of the central nervous stimulant, methylphenidate. Arch Int Pharmacodyn 112:26–35
Maxwell RA, Plummer AJ, Ross SD, Daniel AI (1958) Studies concerning the cardiovascular actions of the central nervous stimulant, methylphenidate. J Pharmacol Exp Ther 123:22–27
McMartin C, Rondel RK, Vinter J, Allan BR, Humbersteon PM, Leishman AWD, Sandler G, Thirkettle JL (1970) The fate of guanethidine in two hypertensive patients. Clin Pharmacol Ther 11:423–431
McMartin C, Simpson P (1971) The absorption and metabolism of guanethidine in hypertensive patients requiring different doses of the drug. Clin Pharmacol Ther 11:423–430
Medina MA, Giachetti A, Shore PA (1969) On the physiological disposition and possible mechanism of the antihypertensive action of debrisoquin. Biochem Pharmacol 18: 891–901
Misu Y, Nishio H, Hosotani T, Hamano S (1976) A new Guanidine derivative: dissociation of the adrenergic neuron blocking activity from local anesthetic activity. Jpn J Pharmacol 26:367–375
Mitchell JR, Oates JA (1970) Guanethidine and related agents. I. Mechanism of the selective blockade of adrenergic neurons and its antagonism by drugs. J Pharmacol Exp Ther 172:100–107

Mitchell JR, Cavanaugh JH, Dingell JV, Oates JA (1970) Guanethidine and related agents. II. Metabolism by hepatic microsomes and its inhibition by drugs. J Pharmacol Exp Ther 172:108–114

Moe RA, Bates HM, Palkoski ZM, Banziger R (1964) Cardiovascular effects of 3,4-dihydro-2 (1H) isoquinoline carboxamidine (Declinax). Curr Ther Res 6:299–318

Mosler M (1969) Guanethidine and bethanidine in the management of hypertension. Am Heart J 77:423–426

Namm DH, Wang CM, El-Sayad S, Copp FC, Maxwell RA (1975) Effects of bretylium on rat cardiac muscle: electrophysiological effects and its uptake and binding in normal and immunosympathectomized rat hearts. J Pharmacol Exp Ther 193:194–208

Newton BW, Melvin JE, Hamill RW (1987) Central neurotoxic effects of guanethidine: altered serotonin and encephalin neurons within the area postrema. Brain Res 404: 157–161

Oates JA, Mitchell JR, Feagin OT, Kaufmann JS, Shand DG (1971) Distribution of guanidinium antihypertensives—mechanism of their selective action. Ann NY Acad Sci 179:302–309

Obianwu HO, Stitzel R, Lundborg P (1968) Subcellular distribution of [^{3}H] amphetamine and [^{3}H] guanethidine and their interaction with adrenergic neurons. J Pharm Pharmacol 20:585–594

Orimilikwe SO, Wong HY, David SN, Reinshagen JA (1983) Effect of exercise and guanethidine on plasma cholesterol and aortic atherosclerosis of atherogenic-fed cockerels. Artery 12:60–73

Palmatier MA, Schmidt RE, Plurad SB, Johnson EM Jr (1987) Sympathetic neuronal destruction in macaque monkeys by guanethidine and guanadine. Ann Neurol 21: 46–52

Potter EK (1987) Guanethidine blocks neuropeptide-Y like inhibitory action of sympathetic nerves of cardiac vagus. J Auton Nerv Syst 21:87–90

Prichard BNC, Johnston AW, Hill ID, Rosenheim ML (1968) Bethanidine, guanethidine, and methyldopa in treatment of hypertension: a within-patient comparison. Br Med J I:135–144

Rahn KH (1971) Plasmaspiegel and renale Ausschiedung von Guanethidin bei Hypertonikern. Arzneimittel forschung 21:1487–1492

Rahn KH (1973) The influence of renal function on plasma levels, urinary excretion, metabolism and antihypertensive effect of guanethidine (Ismelin). Clin Neurol 1: 14–18

Rahn KH, Goldberg LI (1969) Comparison of antihypertensive efficacy, intestinal absorption and excretion of guanethidine in hypertensive patients. Clin Pharmacol Ther 10:858–863

Raines A, Moros D, Levitt B (1968) The effect of guanethidine on ouabain-induced ventricular arrhythmia in the cat. Arch Int Pharmacodyn 174:373–377

Rand MJ, Wilson J (1967) The relationship between adrenergic neurone blocking activity and local anaesthetic activity in a series of guanidine derivatives. Eur J Pharmacol 1:200–209

Rankin GO, Haas GJ Jr (1984) Effects of captopril on the development of tolerance to guanethidine. Fed Proc 43:1342–1345

Rankin GO, Watkins BE, Sawutz DG (1984) Development of tolerance to guanethidine in three hypertensive rat models. Arch Int Pharmacodyn Ther 271:263–274

Reynolds JEF (1982) Martindale: the extrapharmacoepoeia. Pharmaceutical Press, London, p 146

Richardson DW, Wyso EM, Magee JH, Cavell GC (1960) Circulatory effects of guanethidine. Circulation 22:184–190

Ronnov-Jennsen V, Hansen J (1969) Blood volume and exchangable sodium during treatment of hypertension with guanethidine and hydrochlorothiazide. Acta Med Scand 186:255–263

Safan ME, Weiss YA, Corvol PL, Menard JE, London GM, Milliez PL (1975) Antihypertensive adrenergic blocking agents: effects on sodium balance, the renin-angiotensin system and hemodynamics. Clin Sci Mol Med 48 [Suppl 2]:93s–95s

Schanker LS, Morrison AS (1965) Physiological disposition of guanethidine in the rat and its uptake by heart slices. Int J Neuropharmacol 4:27–39

Shapiro AP, Krifcher E (1964) Pressor response to noxious stimuli in hypertensive patients. Effects of guanethidine sulfate and alpha methyldopa. Circulation 30: 671–678

Schlicker E, Gothert M (1983) Effects of bretylium and guanethidine on ^{3}H-noradrenaline and ^{3}H-serotonin release in rat brain cortex slices. Arch Int Pharmacodyn Ther 261:196–204

Smirk H (1963) The hypotensive action of B.W. 467C60. Lancet I:743–746

Stutzin A, Paravic F, Ormenno G, Orrego F (1983) Guanethidine effects on the guinea-pig vas deferens are antagonized by the blockers of calcium activated potassium conductance, apamin, methylene blue, and quinine. Mol Pharmacol 23:409–416

Tabira T, Shibasaki H, Kuroiwa Y (1983) Reflex sympathetic dystrophy (causalgia) treatment with guanethidine. Arch Neurol 40:430–432

Thoenen H, Haefely W, Staehelin H (1967) Potentiation by tetraethylammonium of the response of the cat spleen to postganglionic sympathetic nerve stimulation. J Pharmacol Exp Ther 157:532–540

Villarreal H, Exaire JE, Rubio V, Davila H (1964) Effect of guanethidine and bretylium tosylate on systemic and renal hemodynamics in essential hypertension. Am J Cardiol 14:633–640

Wilson J (1970) The uptake of adrenergic neurone blocking drugs. Br J Pharmacol 40: 159P–160P

CHAPTER 9

Calcium Antagonists

S. KAZDA and A. KNORR

CONTENTS

1 Chemistry

The calcium antagonists currently in clinical use belong to three structurally distinct chemical classes.

The first, verapamil (D-365), is 5-[(3,4-dimethoxyphenethyl)methylamino]-2-(3,4-dimethoxyphenyl)-2-isopropyl-valenenitrile (Appel 1962). The second class is composed of the 1,4-dihydropyridines, comprising nifedipine [BAY A 1040: 1,4-dihydro-2,6-dimethyl-4-(2-nitrophenyl)-3,5-pyridine-dicarboxylic acid dimethyl ester; Bossert and Vater 1971; Bossert et al. 1979], nicardipine [YC 93: 1,4-dihydro-2,6-dimethyl-4-(3-nitrophenyl)-3,5-pyridinedicarboxylic acid methyl 2-(*N*-benzyl-*N*-methyl amino) ethyl ester; Iwanami et al. 1979], as well as nitrendipine [BAY E 5009: 1,4-dihydro-2,6-dimethyl-4-(3-nitrophenyl)-3,5-pyridinedicarboxylic acid-3-ethyl-5-methyl ester; Meyer et al. 1981]. Because of the high therapeutic interest in dihydropyridine calcium antagonists, many more compounds of this chemical class are in development, or in the process of registration. Important examples of the latter are felodipine (H-154/82), nisoldipine (BAY K 5552), and isradipine (PN 200–110).

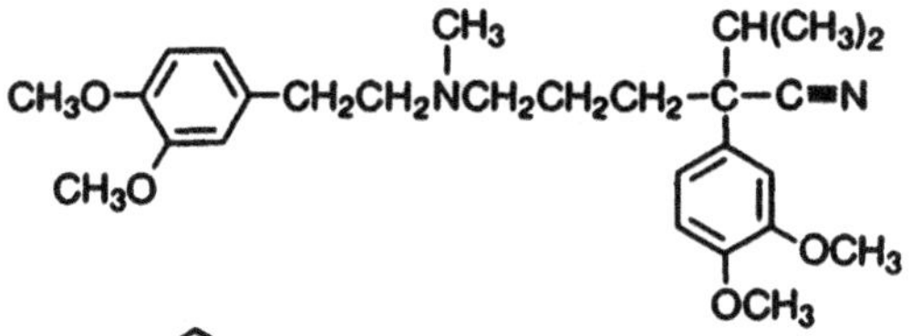

verapamil
(MW 454.59)

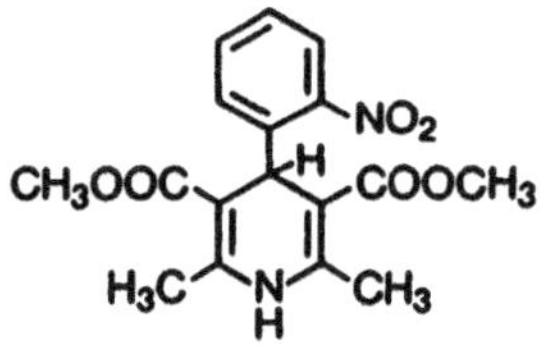

nifedipine
(MW 346.34)

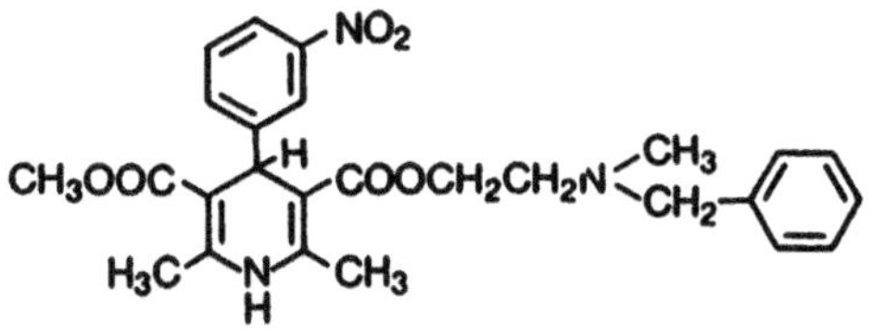

nicardipine
(MW 515.99)

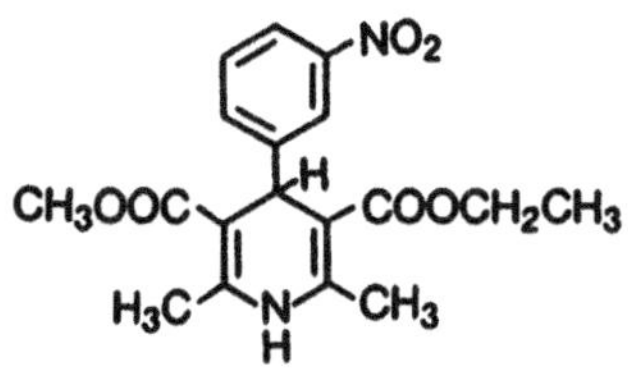

nitrendipine
(MW 360.37)

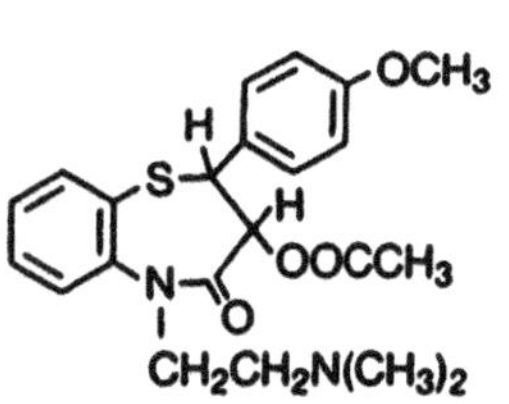

diltiazem
(MW 414.52)

Fig. 1. Chemical structures of calcium antagonists currently used in the treatment of hypertension

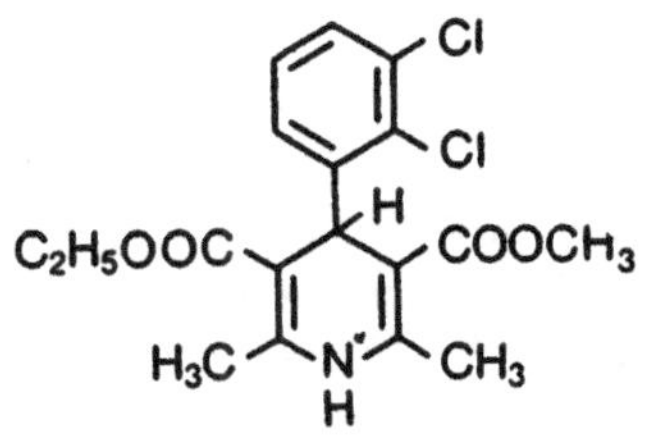

felodipine (MW 370.3)

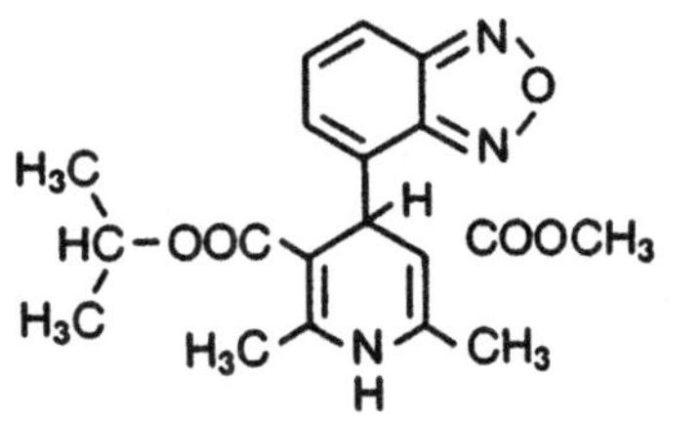

isradipine (MW 371.4)

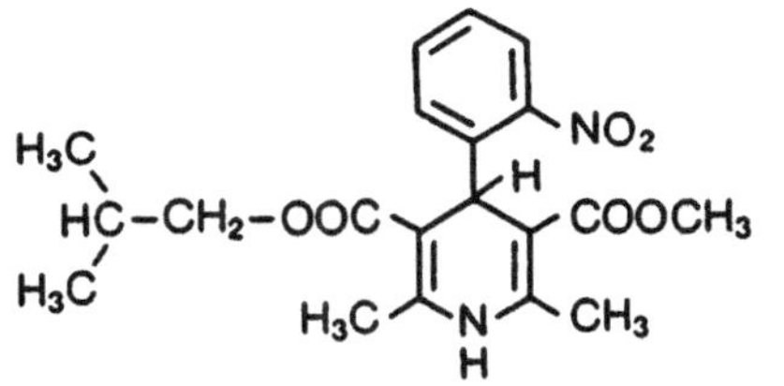

nisoldipine (MW 388.4)

Fig. 2. Chemical structures of some more recent calcium antagonists which are not yet available to general practice but are in the late stages of development

Diltiazem[3-(acetyloxy)-5-2-(dimethylamino)ethyl-2,3-dihydro-2-(4-methoxyphenyl)-1,5-benzothiazepin-4(5*H*)-one; Kugita et al. 1971] belongs to a third class, the benzothiazepines. It has two asymmetric carbons, the D-*cis* isomer being the active ingredient of pharmaceutical compositions.

The structural formulas and molecular weights of the calcium antagonists are given in Figs. 1 and 2. Except for nifedipine, which has no asymmetric carbon, all other compounds are chiral and therefore exist in stereoisomeric forms. Nifedipine and nitrendipine exhibit an extremely low water solubility.

For experimental use, these compounds are dissolved in lower alcohols such as polyethyleneglycol or otherwise in dimethyl sulfoxide. The hydrochloride salt of verapamil is water soluble (5%). The hydrochloride of nicardipine and especially that of diltiazem are also soluble in water. For nifedipine and less so nitrendipine and nicardipine, care should be taken to avoid exposure of solute to light, because of photo-oxidative degradation in solution. Sodium vapor light does not cause decomposition. The undissolved substances are much less light sensitive than the solute. Tablet contents are practically unaffected by photo-oxidation. The pKa of diltiazem is 7.7, that of verapamil is 8.7–9.2 (Hermann and Morselli 1985).

2 Pharmacology

2.1 Mechanisms of Action and Pharmacodynamics

The degree of contraction and relaxation of arterial smooth muscle is controlled by changes of the calcium concentration in the cytosol. The threshold for initiation of contraction is of the order of 10^{-7} *M*, and full contraction occurs at about a 10^{-5} *M* intracellular free calcium concentration. An increase in the intracellular concentration of calcium is detected by calmodulin (= *cal*cium-*modul*ating prote*in*). The calcium-calmodulin complex interacts with the myosin light chain kinase (MLCK) leading to phosphorylation of the myosin. Calcium-dependent myosin phosphorylation is the prerequisite for its interaction with actin and for shortening or tension development. Simultaneously, the phosphorylated myosin acts as an enzyme catalyzing the hydrolysis of ATP to ADP, thus supplying energy for the mechanical movement of the myofilaments and for cellular contraction (Fig. 3, right panel). Conversely, when the level of calcium is reduced, the MLCK is inactivated. Following the dissociation of calmodulin, the myosin is dephosphorylated to form a dormant state which causes the muscle to relax. Also, the energy supply through ATP hydrolysis ceases due to the decrease in cytosolic calcium concentration (Fig. 3, left panel) (WALSH and HARTSHORNE 1983).

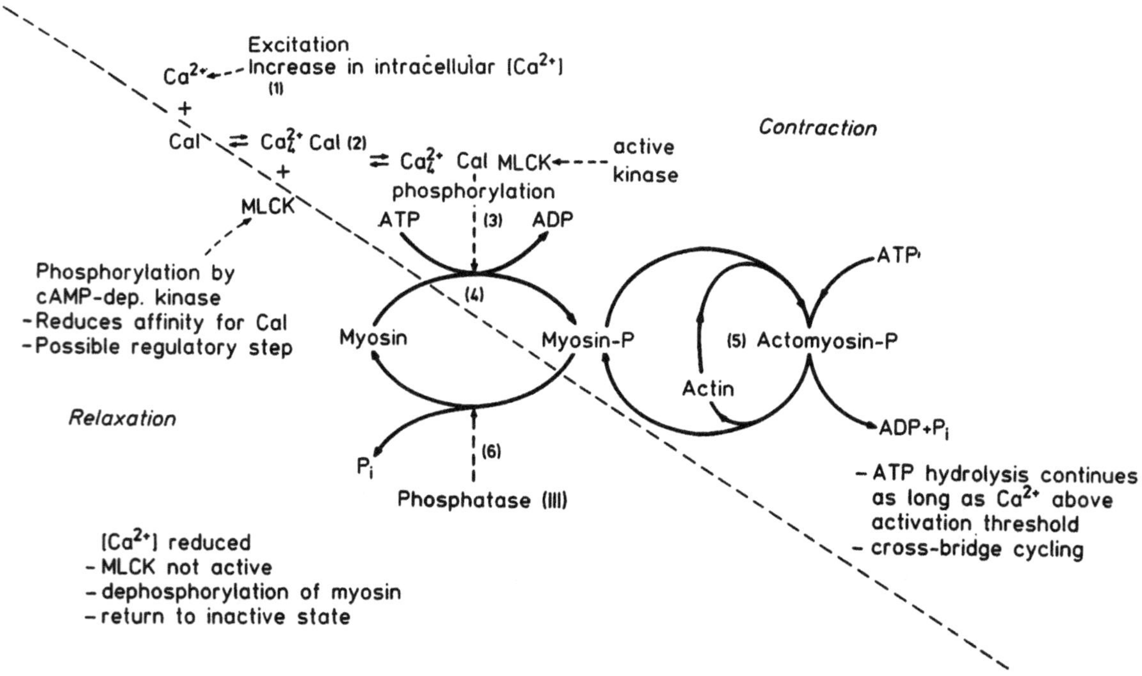

Fig. 3. Role of calcium ions and calmodulin in activation of contractile proteins. *Cal*, Calmodulin; *MLCK*, myosin light chain kinase. Outline of the phosphorylation theory of regulation in smooth muscle from WALSH and HARTSHORNE (1983), with kind permission of CRC Press

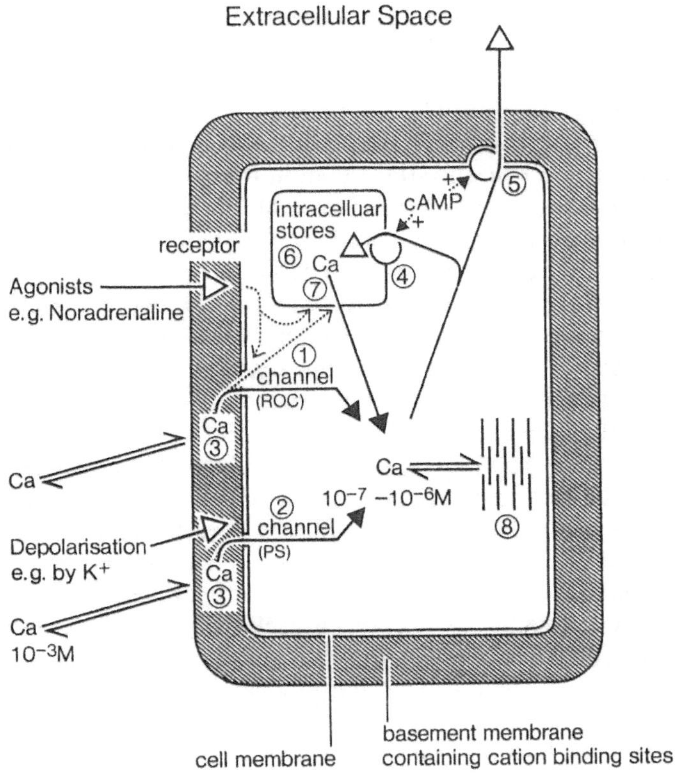

Fig. 4. Schematic representation of the calcium movements in vascular smooth muscle. Extracellular free calcium concentrations are of the order of 10^{-3} *M* and free cytoplasmic calcium, 10^{-7}–10^{-6} *M*. Excitation-induced inward calcium movements occur through receptor-operated channels (*ROC*) (*1*) or through potential-sensitive channels (*PS*) (*2*). Thus extracellular calcium (*3*) can enter the cell. To maintain homeostasis, leaks of calcium ions into the cell down their electrochemical gradient and excitation-induced calcium influxes through the channels are balanced by active calcium pumping into intracellular organelles (*4*) or back into the extracellular space (*5*). The intracellular sequestered calcium (*6*) is then available for release by agonist stimulation (*7*). When intracellular calcium concentrations are raised above 10^{-7}–10^{-6} *M*, a complex biochemical cascade causes contraction by activation of the actin-myosin complex (*8*). (From TOWART 1981, with kind permission of Thieme Verlag)

Cell calcium concentration is regulated by the activity of the cell membrane and sarcoplasmic reticulum. In the resting state the cell membrane has little permeability for calcium, thus maintaining the large transmembrane concentration gradient. Membrane excitation by depolarization induces calcium influx through potential-sensitive channels. Agonist-induced activation of membrane receptors leads to calcium influx through receptor-operated channels (BOLTON 1979). In turn, relaxation is induced by active calcium pumping into the extracellular space or the sarcoplasmic reticulum (Fig. 4).

Cell calcium abnormalities seem to be involved in the increased peripheral resistance in hypertension (HOLLOWAY and BOHR 1973). Stimulation by calcium ions induces greater tension in arterial smooth muscle of spontaneously hypertensive (SHR) than in normotensive rats (AOKI et al. 1974; LEDERBALLE PEDERSEN et al. 1977; PEDERSEN 1979; ASANO et al. 1986). In isolated mesenteric resistance vessels of SHR, tonic norepinephrine-induced contractions are found to occur at lower calcium concentrations than in those of normotensive Wistar Kyoto (WKY) rats (MULVANY and NYBORG 1980). In the same preparation a maximal dose of norepinephrine stimulated a much greater calcium influx in the resistance vessels of SHR than it did in WKY (CAUVIN and VAN BREEMEN 1986). BOHR and WEBB (1984) postulated that the calcium binding to smooth muscle membranes is deficient in hypertension, resulting in decreased membrane stabilization with increased cation permeability and sensitivity to vasoactive agents.

In the absence of calcium the contractile responses of smooth muscle cells are lost regardless of the mode of stimulation (BOHR 1964). Similar to calcium withdrawal, organic calcium antagonists completely inhibit contractions evoked by calcium in depolarized vascular (GODFRAIND and POLSTER 1968) or uterine (FLECKENSTEIN and GRÜN 1969) smooth muscle. Catecholamine-induced contractions are less sensitive to inhibition by calcium antagonists or to calcium withdrawal (GODFRAIND and KABA 1969). α-Sympathomimetic catecholamines and other receptor agonists also release intracellularly stored calcium in the process of activating contractions (Fig. 4). They are therefore inaccessible to the action of calcium antagonists (calcium entry blockers) (GODFRAIND and KABA 1972; VAN BREEMEN et al. 1982).

Calcium entry and vascular contraction may be blocked by the trivalent cation lanthanum (VAN BREEMEN et al. 1972) and other inorganic calcium antagonists by virtue of their ability to form a plug close to the outer orifice of the Ca channel (NAYLER 1987). In contrast, the organic calcium antagonists interact with chemically distinct and specific, but allosterically related receptor sites associated with the potentially sensitive Ca channel (BELLEMANN et al. 1981; BOLGER et al. 1982; HULTHEN et al. 1982a).

2.1.1 Site of Action

Three distinct drug receptor sites of the Ca channel have been postulated (Fig. 5) (GLOSSMANN et al. 1985): the 1,4 dihydropyridine, verapamil, and diltiazem receptor sites. Each exists in a low or high affinity state. The high and low affinity states were proposed as equivalent to the nonconducting (resting or inactivated) or conducting (open) states of the channel determined electrophysiologically in the intact cardiac membrane (GLOSSMANN et al. 1985).

It is believed that verapamil and the phenylalkylamines preferentially bind to a hydrophilic receptor site (open channel state). The hydrophobic 1,4-dihydropyridines bind primarily to receptor sites associated with the inactivated Ca channel, and this binding presumably tends to keep the channel in the inactivated state (TRIGGLE and JANIS 1987). State dependence of interaction may, to some extent, explain the different pharmacological profiles of the individual compounds. Moreover, some tissue specifity of the affinity to binding sites has been described in some ligands (GLOSSMANN et al. 1985). Tissue selectivity of the Ca channel ligands may also be due to the inhomogeneity of the Ca channels in various tissues.

The Ca channel may be pharmacologically modulated also in an opposite way. BAY K 8644 (SCHRAMM et al. 1983) and a couple of other dihydropyridine derivatives increase rather than decrease the transmembrane calcium influx with resulting increase of contraction of smooth and cardiac muscle (SCHRAMM and TOWART 1988). Recently, an extremely potent vasoconstrictor peptide has been isolated from vascular endothelial cells (YANAGISAWA et al. 1988a). The strong vasoconstriction produced by this 21-amino acid peptide ("endothelin") is also due to an enhancement of transmembrane calcium influx. It was proposed that endothelin is an endogenous agonist for the dihydropyridine-sensitive Ca channel (YANAGISAWA et al. 1988b).

The chemical nature of the Ca channel is presently under intensive investigation. The purified material from rabbit skeletal muscle transverse (T-) tubule membrane is reported to be composed of a large polypeptide of a molecular weight of 130000–170000 daltons, and one or two smaller polypeptides (30000 and 50000–56000) (BORSOTTO et al. 1984; CURTIS and CATTERALL 1984). The primary structure of the large polypeptide of the Ca channel has been predicted by cloning and sequence analysis of DNA complementary to its messenger RNA (TANABE et al. 1987).

Present knowledge of the tissue distribution of Ca channels cannot entirely explain the specific pharmacologic profile of the calcium antagonistic drugs. A great part of these investigations was done with heart, skeletal muscle, or brain,

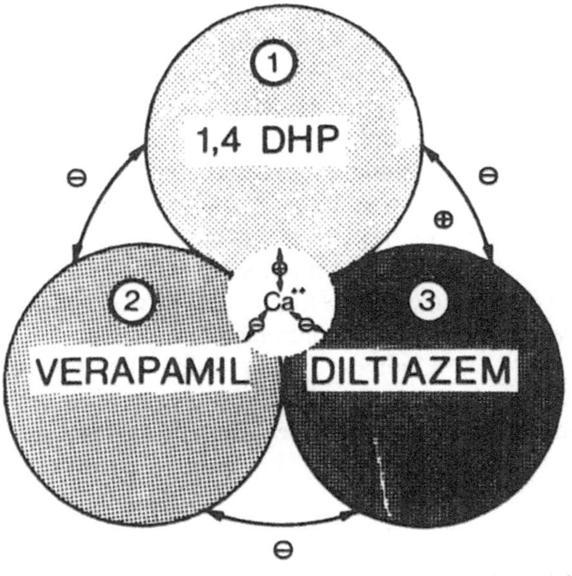

Fig. 5. The calcium channel. Interaction of receptor sites *1*, *2*, and *3* with Ca^{2+} binding sites. (From GLOSSMANN et al. 1985, with kind permission of Springer-Verlag)

which at present do not seem to be the primary target of the therapeutic effect of these drugs. Calcium antagonists probably bind to their receptor sites to varying degrees in all or most tissues. According to current concepts, this binding modulates the function of some Ca channels. Whether or not this binding leads to a detectable pharmacological effect is dependent on the state and type of Ca channel in the particular tissue.

Little is known about possible changes in the number or affinity of the calcium antagonist binding sites in hypertension. ISHII et al. (1983) found a greater number of [^{3}H]nitrendipine binding sites (B_{max}) in brain membranes of 10-week-old SHR in comparison with WKY; however, in heart membranes the maximal number of binding sites for WKY and SHR differ very little. CHATELAIN et al. (1984) found that in native heart membranes of 9-week-old SHR and WKY and of 24-week-old WKY, [^{3}H]nitrendipine binds to a single class of binding sites with high affinity and high capacity. By contrast, in heart membranes of 24-week-old SHR affinity (Kd) and B_{max} increase significantly. Feeding salt-sensitive Dahl-rats (S/JR) with a high salt diet for 3 weeks, resulting in the development of hypertension, did not affect the binding capacity for [^{3}H]nitrendipine in brain or heart membranes. Simultaneous treatment with nitrendipine prevented hypertension but caused augmentation of B_{max} values, mainly in the heart membranes. Receptor density also increased after 3 weeks of antihypertensive treatment with nitrendipine in salt-loaded SHR and SHR stroke prone (SP) (GARTHOFF and BELLEMANN 1987).

2.1.2 Effects on Isolated Cardiac Preparations

In principle, all specific calcium antagonists depress the force of myocardial contraction, inhibit sinus node pacemaker activity, and block the atrioventricular node excitability and impulse conduction with different relative potencies. Details of the cardiac mechanical and electrophysiological effects are summarized in several reviews, e.g., HENRY (1982) or SPERELAKIS (1987). The ratio between vascular, myocardial, and nodal effects is very different in each class of calcium antagonistic compounds. Figure 6 compares the relative effects on inotropism and SA node firing frequency. Verapamil is nearly equieffective in vasorelaxation and negative inotropism and chronotropism. The cardiac effects of nifedipine appear at much higher plasma concentrations than the vascular relaxation. This vascular selectivity is even more pronounced in some recent dihydropyridine derivatives such as nisoldipine (KAZDA et al. 1980), nitrendipine (SCRIABINE et al. 1984), or felodipine (LJUNG 1985). The relative potencies of diltiazem lie between those of verapamil and dihydropyridine derivatives so that its negative chronotropic and inotropic effects may be relevant hemodynamically (see Sect. 2.1.5).

2.1.3 Effects on Vascular Smooth Muscle

In several in vitro studies nifedipine led to more pronounced relaxation of calcium-induced contractions of isolated vessels from SHR than in muscle from WKY (LEDERBALLE PEDERSEN et al. 1977; AOKI et al. 1982a; HARRIS et al. 1984).

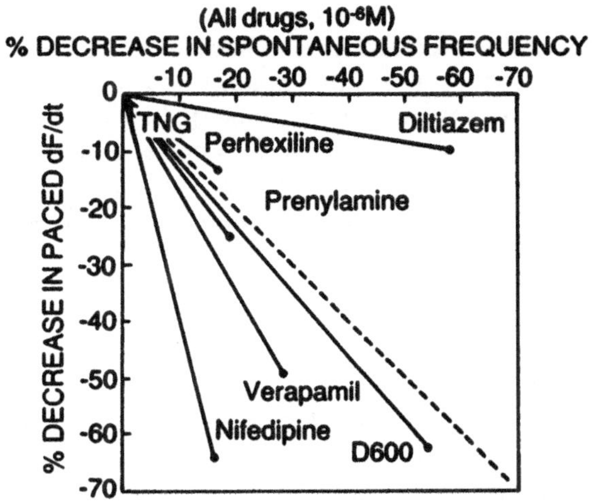

Fig. 6. Chronotropic and inotropic effects of vasodilators and calcium antagonists (HENRY et al. 1979, with kind permission of Excerpta Medica). *TNG*, trinitroglycerol; *D600*, gallopamil (methoxyverapamil), 1988 approved as antihypertensive drug. Responses of force development (*dF/dt*) during electrical pacing and of spontaneous rate (*frequency*) of isolated guinea pig atrium to selected vasodilators are shown

An increased sensitivity of the calcium-induced contraction of aortic strips to nifedipine is found also in renal and DOCA hypertensive rats. Nitroglycerin inhibits calcium-induced contractions in aorta from hypertensive rats with the same potency as in aorta from normotensive rats (CATTANEO et al. 1986). SHR femoral artery strips are more sensitive to the activation of the contractile response by the calcium agonistic dihydropyridine BAY K 8644 than by adrenoceptor stimulation with norepinephrine. BAY K 8644 is much less effective in eliciting the contractile response of the WKY femoral artery. The enhanced contractile responses of the SHR femoral artery to BAY K 8644 are antagonized competitively by both nifedipine and verapamil but not competitively by diltiazem. The contractile responses to norepinephrine via α-adrenoreceptors (in the presence of β-antagonist timolol) were not different between femoral arteries from SHR or WKY (ASANO et al. 1986).

Calcium antagonists affect differently vascular contractions elicited by selective stimulation of postsynaptic α_2- or α_1-adrenoceptors. In normotensive pithed rats, vasoconstriction induced by methoxamine (agonist of α_1-adrenoceptors) is refractory to calcium antagonists. In contrast, α_2-mediated vasoconstrictions (BHT 920 or xylazine) are dose-dependently antagonized by nifedipine, nisoldipine, verapamil, and other calcium entry blockers (VAN MEEL et al. 1981, 1983). Based on this finding it has been speculated that preferential interaction with α_2-mediated vasoconstriction might explain the vasorelaxant and possibly the antihypertensive effect of calcium antagonists (VAN ZWIETEN et al. 1982, 1983). However, preferential inhibition of α_2-mediated vasoconstriction is not specific for calcium antagonists. Sodium nitroprusside or hydralazine gives the same pattern of intereference with pressor response to methoxamine and BHT 920 in pithed normotensive rats (PEDRINELLI and TARAZI 1985). In hypertensive patients no evidence of preferential α_2-antagonism has been found. Verapamil antagonizes forearm vasoconstriction mediated by selective α_1- and α_2-agonists in a similar manner (PEDRINELLI et al. 1986a). In vitro contraction elicited by BHT 920 in aortic rings from SHRSP is more sensitive to the inhibition by nisoldipine than contraction in WKY vessels. Contractions produced by phenylephrine, which are rather refractory to nisoldipine in WKY vessels, are inhibited by higher concentrations of nisoldipine in vessels from SHR (KAZDA et al. 1985).

2.1.4 Effect on Blood Pressure

The acute hypotensive effect of calcium antagonists is more pronounced in hypertensive than in normotensive animals. In conscious SHR much lower doses of nifedipine are required for a similar decrease of blood pressure than in WKY. In contrast, the hypotensive effect of hydralazine is the same in SHR as in WKY (ISHII et al. 1980). Nitrendipine and hydralazine produce a similar fall in blood pressure in SHR, but in WKY hydralazine causes much greater hypotension than nitrendipine (KNORR and GARTHOFF 1984). In humans verapamil or nifedipine produce a much greater drop in blood pressure in patients with essential hypertension than in normotensive subjects (LEDERBALLE PEDERSEN et al. 1980; LEONETTI et al. 1982; MACGREGOR et al. 1982). In hypertensive subjects there is a significant correlation between pretreatment blood pressure and the percentage fall in blood pressure after nifedipine, indicating that the effectiveness of the drug increases with higher pretreatment levels of blood pressure (MACGREGOR 1986; MACGREGOR et al. 1983; Fig. 7). A similar correlation of effectiveness with pretreatment blood pressure values is found for verapamil (ERNE et al. 1983), nitrendipine, diltiazem, tiapamil, and isradipine (BÜHLER et al. 1985a,b). In contrast, no or even a reverse relationship between pretreatment blood pressure and fall of blood pressure is found after propranolol or captopril treatment (MACGREGOR et al. 1982; BÜHLER et al. 1985b).

The fall in mean blood pressure after verapamil or nifedipine is directly correlated with age, pretreatment mean blood pressure, and plasma noradrenaline concentration, but inversely correlated with plasma renin activity (PRA). These correlations were also significant for the decrease of diastolic blood pressure (BÜHLER et al. 1982a,b,c).

The correlation between the blood pressure response and the patient's age has not been confirmed unequivocally. In the later study of BÜHLER's group conducted with a large population of patients given different calcium antagonists, only a weak correlation was reported (KIOWSKI et al. 1985). In a recent study with nitrendipine no relationship was found between the blood pressure response and the patient's age: nitrendipine was similarly effective in elderly and younger patients (MEHTA et al. 1987). Reviewing several studies RAM (1987) concluded that calcium antagonists are effective in all age groups. The impressive antihypertensive response to these drugs in some elderly patients may be related to the level of their pretreatment blood pressure. The greatest fall in

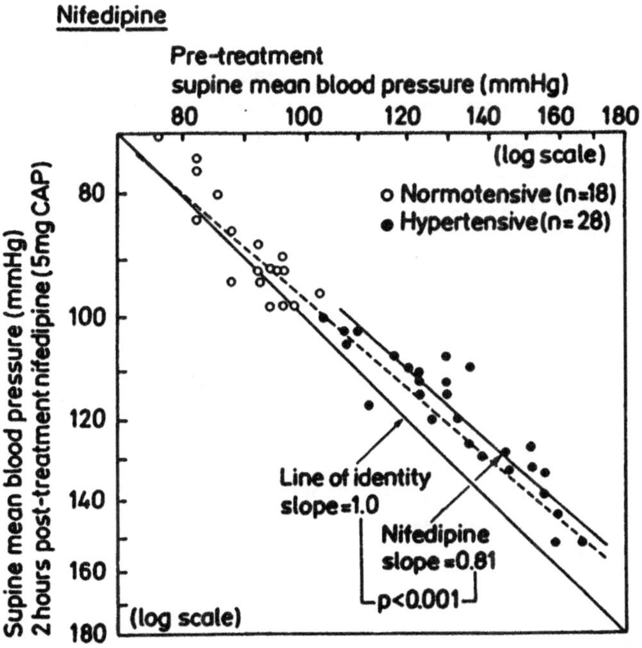

Fig. 7. Relationship between pretreatment supine mean blood pressure in 18 normotensive (*open circles*) and 28 hypertensive (*solid circles*) subjects against the supine mean blood pressure 2 h after a single capsule of nifedipine. The slope of the correlation line for the hypertensive subjects is significantly less than the line of identity, indicating that nifedipine becomes more effective, the higher the blood pressure. (From MacGregor 1986, with kind permission of Schattauer-Verlag)

blood pressure in patients with low PRA is found also after nifedipine (Erne et al. 1983), nitrendipine, diltiazem, tiapamil, and isradipine (Bühler et al. 1985a,b). This effect has been attributed to a greater calcium influx-dependent vasoconstriction in low renin patients possibly related to the activity of the sympathetic nervous system (Bühler et al. 1982a). This hypothesis was supported by direct measurements of the increase in forearm blood flow after verapamil by venous occlusion plethysmography performed independently by Bühler's group (Hulthén et al. 1982b) and by Robinson and colleagues (1982). An intraarterial infusion of verapamil causes greater vasodilation (increase in forearm blood flow) in hypertensive as compared with normotensive subjects. The nonspecific vasodilator sodium nitroprusside, which does not inhibit calcium influx, causes merely the same or even less increase in forearm flow in hypertensive than in normotensive subjects (Hulthen et al. 1982b; Robinson et al. 1982). The basal plasma norepinephrine level correlates positively with the increase in forearm flow following all doses of verapamil in hypertensive patients, but no correlations are found in normotensive ones. In hypertensive patients, there is also a negative correlation between basal PRA, plasma angiotensin II, and the vasodilatory response at higher dose levels of verapamil (Bühler et al. 1984). Subsequently, the same enhanced forearm vasodilation in hypertensives was described for nifedipine (ROBINSON 1983), nitrendipine (BÜHLER et al. 1985c), and nicardipine (HULTHÉN et al. 1985). The abnormal response to calcium antagonists in hypertension could not be accounted for by structural changes in the vessels but rather by a functional abnormality of vascular smooth muscle in primary hypertension (ROBINSON et al. 1982).

Based on the cellular mechanism of vascular action of calcium antagonists, these data were extrapolated into the theory of pathogenesis of human essential hypertension. From the preferred vasodilation in hypertensive patients by calcium antagonists as opposed to nonspecific vasodilator nitroprusside or α_1- or α_2-adrenoceptor antagonists, the deduction was made that the elevated peripheral resistance in hypertension is due to an enhanced calcium influx-dependent vasoconstriction. It is postulated that Ca channel blockers represent a pathophysiologically based antihypertensive treatment concept for the future (BÜHLER and HULTHÉN 1982; BÜHLER et al. 1982a,c, 1985a,b).

Further support for this hypothesis is found in measurements of the cytosolic concentration of ionized calcium in thrombocytes. The use of the easily accessible platelets as a possible representation of vascular smooth muscle seems justified by a number of similarities between these two cell types (e.g., calcium-dependent contraction-coupling mechanism, similar α_2-adrenoceptor cyclase system, etc.). Platelet calcium levels, as measured by the fluorescent dye technique using Quin 2, are significantly higher in patients with established or borderline hypertension than in normotensive subjects. There is a close correlation between platelet calcium levels and systolic, diastolic, and mean blood pressure in all three groups. Treatment for 8 weeks with verapamil, nifedipine, or nitrendipine results in a reduction in platelet calcium concentration parallel to the decrease in blood pressure. The treatment-induced changes in platelet calcium levels correlate with the change in systolic and diastolic blood pressures (ERNE et al. 1984). The difference in forearm blood flow due to treatment with nitrendipine correlates with the treatment-induced change in platelet free calcium concentration. It has been suggested that the platelet free calcium concentration may reflect the intracellular calcium concentration in vascular smooth muscle and thus that the reduction of intracellular calcium is the mechanism of the drug-induced decrease in peripheral resistance (BÜHLER et al. 1985c). However, this interpretation is complicated by the fact that a similar reduction of platelet calcium concentration is found in parallel with a decrease of blood pressure after treatment with either β-adrenoceptor antagonists (atenolol or oxprenolol) or the diuretic hydrochlorothiazide, which do not primarily reduce peripheral resistance.

The possibility that the increased intracellular calcium concentration in platelets is a consequence rather than a cause of elevated blood pressure could not be excluded (ERNE et al. 1984).

2.1.5 Hemodynamic Effects

Basically, the primary effect of all calcium antagonistic drugs is the decrease of vascular resistance due to vasodilation and, to some degree, a secondary baroreceptor-mediated reflex increase of sympathetic tone. In that sense their effects resemble those of other, nonspecific vasodilators (KOCH-WESER 1974). All calcium antagonists have direct negative inotropic and chronotropic effects. However, the hemodynamic profiles of the individual calcium antagonists differ substantially since they are composites of various direct and indirect cardiac and vascular actions. The net result of cardiac and circulatory effects is also dependent on the dose, frequency, route of administration, and the underlying status or pathology of the cardiovascular system. The voluminous literature on cardiac and hemodynamic actions of various calcium antagonists pertinent to heart diseases has been comparatively summarized in several reviews, e.g., STONE et al. (1980), HENRY (1982), SERRUYS et al. (1983) and SINGH and OPIE (1983). For practical purposes, only hemodynamic effects relevant to the treatment of hypertension will be discussed briefly in this chapter.

There is a more pronounced and rapid decrease in peripheral resistance after dihydropyridine derivatives than following verapamil and diltiazem. This may at least partially explain why heart rate and indices of cardiac contractility are consistently increased after one single dose of nifedipine and its analogues, but not necessarily after verapamil or diltiazem. Accordingly, plasma noradrenaline concentration increases parallel to the increase in heart rate after a 10 mg capsule of nifedipine (LEDERBALLE PEDERSEN et al. 1971; LEONETTI 1987a) but does not change after a 160 mg tablet of verapamil in hypertensive patients (LEONETTI 1987a). The transient increases in heart rate and in plasma noradrenaline concentration after nifedipine are less pronounced in hypertensive than in normotensive subjects (LEONETTI et al. 1982). These different effects on plasma catecholamines by the two calcium antagonists are also evident after 8 days treatment with verapamil (80 mg thrice daily) or nifedipine (10 mg thrice daily) (MUIESAN et al. 1981). Verapamil also induces reflex tachycardia when given as an intravenous bolus injection and causes an abrupt fall in blood pressure. After oral administration verapamil causes a slow reduction in vascular resistance and blood pressure without any increase in heart rate. Tachycardia is obviously related to the magnitude and velocity of onset of the vasodilation and reduction in blood pressure (GUAZZI 1983). Temporary tachycardia and increases in plasma norepinephrine after nifedipine, nitrendipine (VENTURA et al. 1983), and felodipine (SLUITER et al. 1985) are also coincident with the maximum decrease in blood pressure after the initial dose.

The reflex nature of the tachycardia after calcium antagonists has been confirmed by the observation that it is blunted by simultaneous administration of β-adrenoceptor antagonists in normotensive conscious (KIRCHHEIM and GROSS 1975) or anesthetized (ANGUS et al. 1976) dogs and normotensive human (LYDTIN et al. 1975) and hypertensive patients (AOKI et al. 1978; CLEMENT and DE PUE 1985). Whereas the increase in heart rate is diminished significantly by practolol or propranolol, the decrease of peripheral vascular resistance and blood pressure induced by nifepidine or verapamil remains unchanged. In conscious normotensive dogs equihypotensive intravenous doses of diltiazem (0.2 mg/kg), verapamil (0.25 mg/kg), or nifedipine (0.05 mg/kg) cause an increase in heart rate (28%, 75%, and 86%, respectively) which is attenuated by propranolol and abolished by propranolol plus atropine (NAKAYA et al. 1983).

The initial sympathetic response to the first dose of calcium antagonists in hypertensive patients becomes habituated during chronic treatment. Six weeks of therapy with nifedipine (20 mg thrice daily) result in a further decrease of blood pressure but not of systemic vascular resistance as compared with the initial effect of the first dose (10 mg capsule sublingually). Heart rate, cardiac index, and plasma norepinephrine level—although increased after the first dose—return towards pretreatment values after 6 weeks of therapy. The reduction of acutely increased sympathetic activity towards pretreatment values during long-term nifedipine therapy is associated with a further decrease in blood pressure (KIOWSKI et al. 1986). Similarly, the increased plasma norepinephrine concentration and heart rate found in the first days of treatment with nitrendipine (FOUAD et al. 1984; LUFT et al. 1985; PEDRINELLI et al. 1986b) are absent in patients given nitrendipine (10–20 mg twice daily) for up to 35 days (SIMON and SNYDER 1984; THANANOPAVARN et al. 1984a,b).

The lowered blood pressure combined with an unchanged heart rate after chronic treatment indicates resetting of the baroreflex. The sensitivity of the baroreflex-heart rate control remains unchanged (KIOWSKI et al. 1986) or is slightly increased (LITTLER et al. 1983) after long-term treatment with nifedipine. Nifedipine seems to reset baroreflex sensitivity through its effects on the pressor receptors in the carotid sinus and aortic arch (LITTLER et al. 1983). Similar baroreceptor "adaptation" has been observed after 4 weeks of treatment with diltiazem. The reflex increase in heart rate, cardiac index, and left ventricular ejection rate after the first dose of diltiazem is no longer observed after 4 weeks' treatment, whereas blood pressure and total peripheral resistance are reduced further (FROHLICH 1986).

The tachycardiac response to verapamil and diltiazem is obviously blunted also by their additional negative chronotropic action, which is not apparent in the dihydropyridines (MILLARD et al. 1982). In conscious hypertensive dogs the acute equieffective hypotension is followed by an initial increase in heart rate only after nifedipine, nitrendipine, and nisoldipine. A dose of diltiazem that produces the same decrease of blood pressure leads to only a slight increment in pulse rate. The dose-dependent hypotensive effect of verapamil is not regularly followed by tachycardia. In contrast, after the higher dose (30 mg/kg orally) three out of five dogs experienced long-lasting bradycardia during hypotension (KNORR and STOEPEL 1981; KNORR 1982).

The negative chronotropic effect of verapamil remains evident even after chronic treatment of hypertensive patients. It is compensated for by an increase in stroke volume, so that cardiac output is not changed by long-term treatment with verapamil (LUND-JOHANSEN 1984). After long-term treatment (mean: 11 months) of a similar group of hypertensive patients with nifedipine (20–40 mg tablet thrice daily), systolic, diastolic, and mean blood pressure are decreased due to a reduction of total peripheral resistance. Heart rate and cardiac index at rest or during exercise do not differ from pretreatment values (LUND-JOHANSEN and OMVIK 1983).

Although the arterial vasodilation by calcium antagonists is ubiquitious, there are substantial differences in the pattern of regional distribution of cardiac output between verapamil, diltiazem, and the dihydropyridine derivatives (HOF

1983). In this and numerous other studies a common feature of all calcium antagonists so far studied is the preferential increase in coronary blood flow independent of the species, techniques, and experimental design (for review, see SERRUYS et al. 1983). In contrast to the pronounced arterial (arteriolar) vasodilation, no hemodynamically significant venous relaxation has been found after calcium antagonists. This and the unimpaired sensitivity of arterial baroreflexes mentioned above may explain why orthostatic hypotension is not observed after calcium antagonists (MUIESAN et al. 1981; ZANCHETTI 1981; LITTLER et al. 1983; LUND-JOHANSEN and OMVIK 1986).

A decrease in total peripheral resistance is the predominant hemodynamic effect of all calcium antagonists. However, after acute and chronic administration in hypertension, their overall therapeutic effect differs qualitatively from that of other known arteriolar vasodilators (KAZDA et al. 1982a; ZANCHETTI 1981). Presumably, arterial vasodilation is only one facet of the antihypertensive effect of these drugs (GARTHOFF et al. 1983; KAZDA et al. 1983a,b).

Vasodilators such as hydralazine or minoxidil inevitably stimulate renin secretion (GOTTLIEB et al. 1972), probably by both sympathetic stimulation (ZANCHETTI 1977) and decrease of glomerular perfusion pressure (UEDA et al. 1968). Except for verapamil (MUIESAN et al. 1981) all antihypertensive calcium antagonists also provoke an immediate increment in PRA at their peak hypotensive effect. However, the increase in PRA after one single dose was short lasting and not detectable a few hours later in spite of a sustained blood pressure decrease (AOKI et al. 1978; LEONETTI et al. 1982). There was no difference in the renin increase between hypertensive and normotensive subjects after nifedipine (LEONETTI et al. 1982), nicardipine (CORUZZI et al. 1985; VAN SHAIK et al. 1984), or diltiazem (OYAMA 1978; FUNYU et al. 1981) despite the more pronounced hypotensive effect in hypertensive patients. In conscious normotensive rats nitrendipine acutely produces much less increase in PRA than hydralazine or minoxidil in equihypotensive doses (GARTHOFF et al. 1984).

In the long-term treatment of hypertensive patients the increased PRA normalizes after a few weeks on nifedipine (LEDERBALLE PEDERSEN et al. 1971) or nitrendipine (WEBER and DRAYER 1984) and remains normal for at least 1 year (WEBER 1987) in spite of the sustained decrease in blood pressure.

Changes in plasma or urinary aldosterone after calcium antagonists are not uniform. This may be caused by at least two factors. Nifedipine has been shown to inhibit specifically angiotensin II-induced aldosterone secretion in normal humans (MILLAR et al. 1982) and to lower plasma aldosterone in patients with primary aldosteronism (NADLER et al. 1985). On the other hand, all calcium antagonists have pronounced effects on the renal excretion of sodium which may be reflected in secondary changes in aldosterone secretion or excretion.

2.1.6 Renal Effects

The outstanding difference between calcium antagonists and nonspecific vasodilators is their contrasting effect on renal electrolyte and water excretion. The decrease of blood pressure by hydralazine, minoxidil, or diazoxide is associated with water and sodium retention, thereby partially offsetting their antihypertensive action (KOCH-WESER 1974). As early as 1972, KLÜTSCH et al. demonstrated that intravenous injection of nifedipine to hypertensive patients produces large falls in blood pressure but simultaneously increases sodium and water excretion by an increase in renal plasma flow and glomerular filtration.

Subsequently, the natriuretic effect of nifedipine was confirmed and found also in other calcium antagonists (GARTHOFF et al. 1983). Generally, the natriuretic effect has been demonstrated under various experimental or clinical conditions with all specific calcium antagonists. The extent and therapeutic relevance is different in the individual drugs, but usually none of them in therapeutic dosage induces sodium retention. This is the reason why calcium antagonists may be used for long-term therapy by themselves, and a combination with diuretics is not required. The diuretic effect seems to be greater in patients with high blood pressure than in normotensive controls (LEONETTI et al. 1982; MACGREGOR 1986).

The mechanism and site of the natriuretic effect of calcium antagonists is not definitively clarified as yet. All calcium antagonists have been shown to decrease renal vascular resistance.

In most animal studies so far published an increase of glomerular filtration rate (GFR) has been found, especially if it was impaired by exogenous vasoconstrictors. In contrast, in 9 out of 12 studies performed in conscious human subjects until 1985, GFR was not altered by calcium antagonists and increased in only 3 (for review, see LOUTZENHISER and EPSTEIN 1985). Interestingly, all three studies in human subjects demonstrating increases in GFR were performed with hypertensive patients (SAKURAI et al. 1972; VAN SHAIK et al. 1984; YOKOYAMA and KABURAGI 1983). It may appear that the ability of calcium antagonists to increase GFR is most apparent under experimental or clinical conditions in which basal renovascular tone is increased.

The vas afferens was postulated as a possible site of action. In microcirculatory studies in the hydronephrotic rat kidney, topically administered nitrendipine produces a dose-dependent preglomerular vasodilation independent of renal perfusion pressure (STEINHAUSEN et al. 1987).

Whether renal vasodilation is responsible for the increase in GFR and even for the occasionally large increase in natriuresis observed after some calcium antagonists remains questionable. Some other vasodilators (e.g., acetylcholine, prostaglandin E_2, papaverine, and others) increase renal blood flow without a corresponding rise in GFR or natriuresis (BAER and NAVAR 1973) or even reduce natriuresis, like hydralazine. The increase in sodium clearance correlates imperfectly with the reduction of renal vascular resistance in normotensive or hypertensive humans after acute administration of nifedipine. When a critical level of renal vasodilation is reached, sodium excretion does not increase further (LEDERBALLE PEDERSEN et al. 1986). A negative correlation between the reduction of supine diastolic blood pressure and the percentage changes in diuresis is found after felodipine (EDGAR et al. 1985). It seems that with higher degrees of vasodilation, the natriuretic effect of calcium antagonists is offset by the fall in blood pressure (LEDERBALLE PEDERSEN et al. 1986).

It is unlikely that the natriuretic effect is due to a suppression in aldosterone secretion or an interference with the action of aldosterone on distal tubular mechanisms. No decrease in the plasma aldosterone level (LEONETTI et al. 1982; BAUER et al. 1985) or in urinary excretion of aldosterone (THANANOPAVARN et al. 1984a) are found in connection with the increased natriuresis after nifedipine or nitrendipine in humans. In addition, a slight increase in potassium excretion parallels the strong natriuresis after acute administration of felodipine in rats and dogs (DI BONA 1985), and nicardipine, diltiazem, or verapamil in rats (ROSENKRANZ et al. 1984). In the latter study high doses of calcium antagonists cause an initial increase in plasma aldosterone concentration in parallel with a rather large increase of urinary sodium and volume excretion. Mild but definite kaliuresis with negative potassium balance persists over 7 days of treatment with felodipine (ZANCHETTI and LEONETTI 1985) or nitrendipine (THANANOPAVARN et al. 1984) in hypertensive patients. Occasionally, serum potassium has been reported to decrease slightly after prolonged treatment with nifedipine (LEDERBALLE PEDERSEN et al. 1971). In other studies no significant changes in potassium excretion after nifedipine (CHRISTENSEN et al. 1982; ZANCHETTI and LEONETTI 1985), nitrendipine (MORLEDGE et al. 1987), nicardipine (DI BONA 1987), or diltiazem (KINOSHITA et al. 1979) are found. Short-term treatment with nifedipine, nitrendipine, and diltiazem increases urinary excretion of sodium but not of potassium. Neither short- nor long-term treatment has any effect on the serum electrolytes level (BAUER et al. 1985).

There is ample evidence that calcium antagonists directly inhibit tubular sodium reabsorption. In a number of human studies natriuretic effects of various calcium antagonists without substantial alternations in renal plasma flow or GFR are well documented (for review, see LEONETTI and ZANCHETTI 1985).

In normotensive rats diltiazem, nifedipine, and nitrendipine increase urine flow and absolute and fractional sodium excretion without any change in GFR. The calcium excretion is increased, too. This obviously tubular effect—most pronounced with nitrendipine—is similar in both renally innervated and denervated rats (JOHNS 1984, 1985; JOHNS and MANITIUS 1987).

The renal effects seem to be more complicated in hypertensive animals. In micropuncture studies verapamil infused into tubules inhibits tubular fluid reabsorption in both two-kidney renal hypertensive and normotensive rats to a same degree. However, in the clearance study of the same researchers intravenous infusion of verapamil causes a greater increase in urine flow and in sodium and calcium excretion in hypertensive than in normotensive rats. Accordingly, GFR is increased only in the hypertensive animals (MACLAUGHLIN et al. 1985). Also, nifedipine elicits renal vasodilation with an increase in GFR and associated natriuresis and diuresis in SHR. However, the increase in absolute urinary sodium excretion is even greater, as reflected by a significant increase in fractional sodium excretion. This indicates that increases in filtered sodium load as well as relative decreases in net renal tubular sodium reabsorption contribute to the natriuresis in hypertensive animals (DI BONA 1987).

The site and mechanism of action on the tubular electrolyte absorption has not yet been clarified. Results of micropuncture or microperfusion studies on rat kidneys indicate an inhibition of electrolyte and fluid absorption in the proximal tubule by verapamil (MacLaughlin et al. 1985) and nitrendipine (Haeberle et al. 1987). In hypertensive patients a specific proximal tubular effect of nifedipine on sodium reabsorption has been proposed by Lederballe Pedersen et al. (1986) and Krussel et al. (1987). Close relationships between the increases in sodium and lithium clearance and sodium and uric acid clearance have been found after nifedipine. Both renal lithium and uric acid clearance are used as a specific tool for measurement of proximal tubular sodium reabsorption. On the other hand, an effect at a point beyond the distal nephron sodium-potassium exchange site has been anticipated. In recollection micropuncture experiments, an intravenous infusion of felodipine inhibits renal tubular reabsorption of water and sodium in the distal tubule and collecting duct; neither excretion nor reabsorption of potassium is affected. Proximal tubular and loop of Henle sodium, potassium, and water reabsorption are not affected by felodipine (Di Bona 1985, 1987).

The mechanism by which calcium antagonists may inhibit sodium reabsorption in the tubule is not known. Since verapamil seems to exert its effect on the contraluminal cell membrane, an interaction with the sodium-calcium countertransport system, in the proximal tubule has been proposed (MacLaughlin et al. 1985). Alternatively, an inhibition of the calcium-sensitive K channel as a possible explanation of the distal tubular effect of nisoldipine has been suggested by Giebisch et al. (1987).

At present it is not possible to evaluate exactly to what degree the natriuretic effects contribute to the long-term reduction of high blood pressure by calcium antagonists. As with diuretics it is difficult to demonstrate a long-term reduction in sodium balance. However, several direct or indirect findings in humans and animals indicate that the renal effect persists throughout therapy and is inherent to the therapeutic efficacy in hypertensive disease.

Treatment of hypertensive patients with felodipine increases sodium excretion on days 1 and 2, inducing a negative sodium balance averaging slightly more than 80 mmol; no further natriuretic effect is observed from day 3 onwards, but no rebound retention is observed either, so that a negative sodium balance of 80–100 mmol is maintained until the last (7th) day of felodipine administration (Zanchetti and Leonetti 1985). In some studies a small but significant loss of body weight persisting during long-term treatment with nifedipine and nitrendipine as an explanation of a long-term diuretic effect has been observed (Husted et al. 1982; MacGregor 1986). Probably after the initial strong natriuresis and diuresis the electrolyte and volume homeostasis is kept in a new, "healthy" steady state during chronic administration of these drugs. This might be the reason why no negative balance can be detected with chronic treatment despite persistent reduction of fluid volume (= body weight). This assumption arose from experiments with long-term treatment of hypertensive rats with nitrendipine and may be valid also for the long-term antihypertensive effect of diuretics (Kazda 1987). Support for this assumption can be found in a preliminary study with hypertensive patients (MacGregor et al. 1987). Six patients with essential

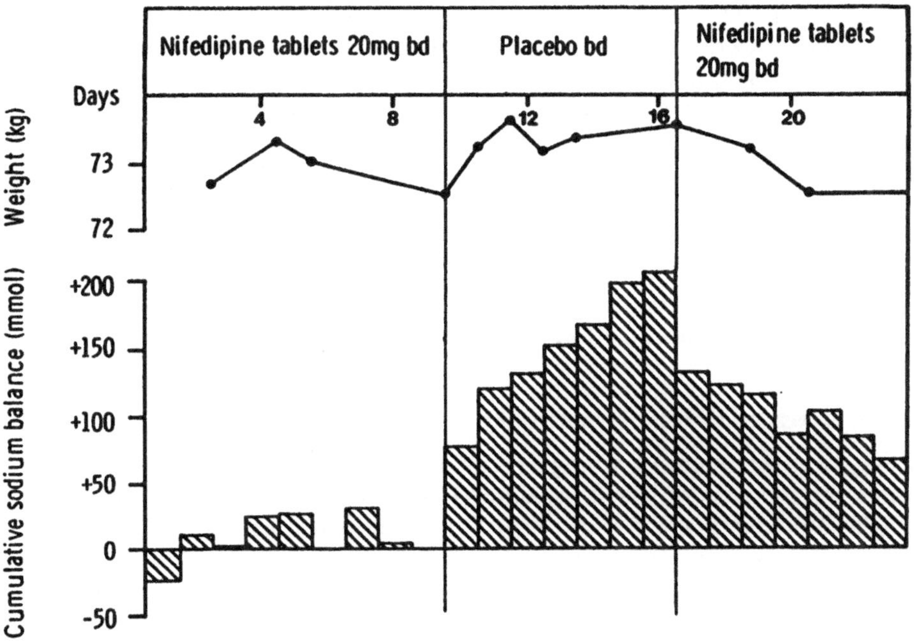

Fig. 8. Changes in cumulative sodium balance (*below*) and body weight (*above*) in a patient under long-term nifedipine treatment. The drug was withdrawn for 7 days, and then administration was resumed. (From MACGREGOR et al. 1987, with kind permission of Gower Academic Journals)

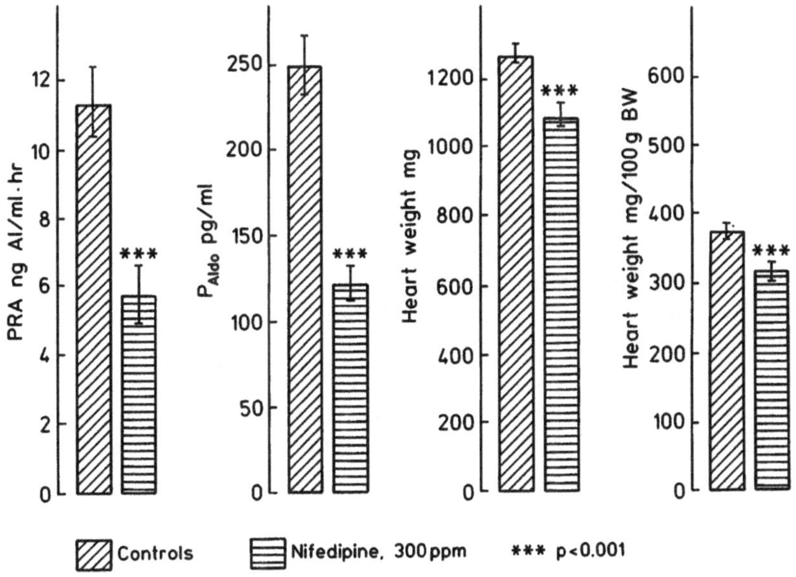

Fig. 9. Plasma renin activity (*PRA*), plasma aldosterone concentration (P_{Aldo}), *absolute* and *relative weight* of *heart* ventricle in spontaneously hypertensive rats after 60 weeks of nifedipine treatment (*vertically hatched*) compared with untreated controls (*hatched bars*). (From KAZDA et al. 1983b, with kind permission of Postgraduate Medical Journal)

hypertension who had been treated with nifedipine for at least 6 weeks (range 6–45 weeks) were placed on a constant dietary intake of 150 mmol sodium and 80 mmol potassium. After a control period on the diet, nifedipine was withdrawn and replaced with matching placebo tablets, single-blind, for 7 days. The 24-h mean urinary sodium excretion fell significantly on the first days after nifedipine withdrawal. The mean calculated positive sodium balance for 7 days of nifedipine withdrawal was 132 ± 39 mmol, which was associated with a significant increase in body weight (Fig. 8).

This study suggests that the acute natriuretic effect of nifedipine which changes the sodium balance is maintained over a long period of time and is similar to the natriuretic effect of thiazide diuretics.

2.1.7 Effects on Cardiac Hypertrophy

Long-term treatment of young SHR with calcium antagonists completely prevents the increase of blood pressure (FLECKENSTEIN et al. 1985; KAZDA et al. 1982b; VON WITZLEBEN et al. 1980), an effect which can be also achieved by hydralazine or minoxidil (SEN et al. 1977). However, these vasodilators aggravate the degree of cardiac hypertrophy and produce sustained increase in PRA despite effective control of high blood pressure (SEN et al. 1977; KAZDA et al. 1982a, b). In contrast, chronic treatment with nifedipine, nitrendipine (KAZDA et al. 1984; KAZDA and SCRIABINE 1986), or nisoldipine (STASCH et al. 1987a) provides normotension for nearly the entire life span and prevents cardiac hypertrophy. Moreover, PRA and plasma aldosterone concentrations are substantially reduced in the treated rats (GARTHOFF et al. 1983; Fig. 9). In 60-week-old control SHR heart failure develops as documented by a progressive decrease of systolic blood pressure and a drastic increase in plasma concentration of atrial natriuretic peptides (ANP). In SHR chronically treated with nitrendipine the increase in plasma ANP is not observed (KAZDA et al. 1987a). A reduction of cardiac mass has been achieved by treatment of adult, already hypertensive rats. In 22-week-old SHR therapeutic treatment with nitrendipine for 11 weeks results in a decrease of blood pressure, a regression of cardiac hypertrophy, and a reduction of PRA. Additionally, the elevated plasma ANP levels are reduced. In contrast, therapeutic treatment with minoxidil in the same regimen results in an aggravation of cardiac hypertrophy, an increase in PRA, and even an additional increase in plasma ANP despite the same degree of blood pressure reduction (Figs. 10, 11). Body weight was increased more in minoxidil-treated than in nitrendipine-treated or control rats, reflecting obviously the salt- and water-retaining effect of minoxidil. The aggravation of cardiac hypertrophy parallel to an additional increase in plasma ANP seems to result from the increased volume load by minoxidil. The volume status—and not blood pressure—is the important factor for changes in plasma ANP (KNORR et al. 1987; STASCH et al. 1987b). Conversely, regression of cardiac hypertrophy parallel to a decrease of elevated ANP is probably due to the persistent diuretic effect of nitrendipine resulting in a reduction of volume load. This assumption was confirmed in another experiment. Treatment with nisoldipine was started in the

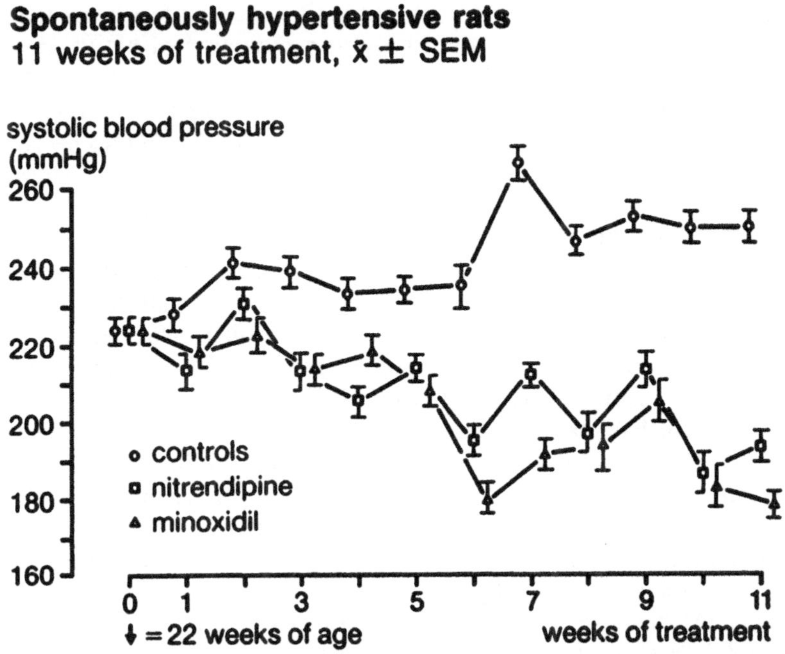

Fig. 10. Influence of long-term treatment with nitrendipine (*squares*) or minoxidil (*triangles*) on blood pressure of spontaneously hypertensive rats. (From KNORR et al. 1987, with kind permission of Elsevier Science Publishers)

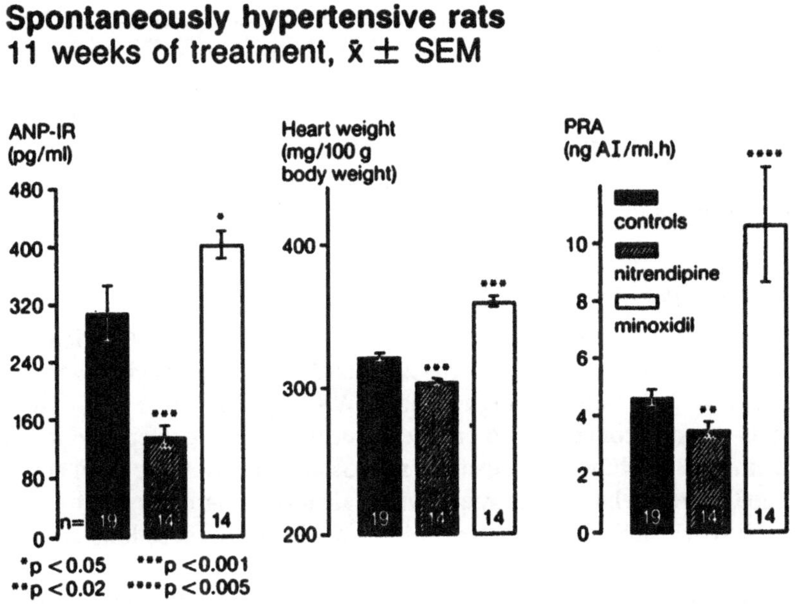

Fig. 11. Influence of 11 weeks' treatment of spontaneously hypertensive rats with nitrendipine (*hatched bars*) or minoxidil (*white bars*) on plasma ANP-immunoreactivity (*ANP-IR*), heart weights and plasma renin activity (*PRA*). (From KNORR et al. 1987, with kind permission of Elsevier Science Publishers)

end stage of hypertension in 60-week-old SHR with manifest heart failure. The 12 weeks of treatment resulted not only in a reduction of blood pressure but also in the regression of cardiac hypertrophy, of elevated plasma ANP, and of increased PRA. In all these experiments a positive correlation was found between the weight of heart ventricles and plasma ANP, whereas no correlation existed between systolic blood pressure and ANP in plasma (STASCH et al. 1987a).

The development of cardiac hypertrophy was prevented in young SHR treated from 4–16 weeks of age with diltiazem (NARITA et al. 1985). However, in a therapeutic administration to 20-week-old SHR with established hypertension the same dosage of diltiazem did not reduce cardiac mass despite significant reduction in blood pressure (NATSUMA et al. 1985). This finding is in distinct contrast to the results of the same group of investigators who found a clear-cut reduction of cardiac mass after nitrendipine (KOBRIN et al. 1984). Speculatively, the more pronounced renal effect of the dihydropyridine calcium antagonists may explain their beneficial effect in regression of cardiac hypertrophy by reduction of volume load in SHR. On the other hand, in some clinical trials a reduction of cardiac mass of hypertensive patients was described after 3–6 months treatment with nifedipine (MUIESAN et al. 1986; MOTZ et al. 1987), verapamil (MUIESAN et al. 1986; SCHMIEDER et al. 1987), or diltiazem but not propranolol (WEISS and BENT 1987). The same degree of reduction of cardiac mass was found after verapamil and nifedipine despite the different effects on sympathetic stimulation (MUIESAN et al. 1986).

In the hearts from adult SHR, treatment with nifedipine results in an improved capillary supply. Hearts from untreated SHR are characterized by greater and more variable intercapillary spacing than those from WKY at the age of 10 months. The treatment of SHR with nifedipine for 5 months results in a partial reduction of heart weight but in a complete normalization of morphometric indices characterizing capillary spacing, and in a significant decrease in myocyte to capillary ratio. Both the changes would be expected to improve the morphological conditions for oxygen transport within the tissue (TUREK et al. 1987).

2.1.8 Preservation of Vascular Integrity

In SHR the calcium content of the arterial wall (aorta, a. mesenterica superior) steadily rises until, at an age of 18–20 months, it may reach a value that is approximately 2–3 times as high as in a WKY of the same age. The excess calcium is mainly concentrated in the arterial media, preferably in vascular smooth muscle as shown by electron microscopic examination (FLECKENSTEIN et al. 1983). Prophylactic treatment with calcium antagonists kept both blood pressure and arterial calcium content at normal levels in these long-term experiments (FLECKENSTEIN et al. 1983, 1985).

Calcium overload seems to play a decisive role in the molecular pathway of cell damage and death (FLECKENSTEIN 1968, 1983). In Dahl sensitive (S) rats a high salt diet induces fulminant hypertension and a necrotizing vasculopathy with preferential localization in the kidney. Huge calcium deposits within

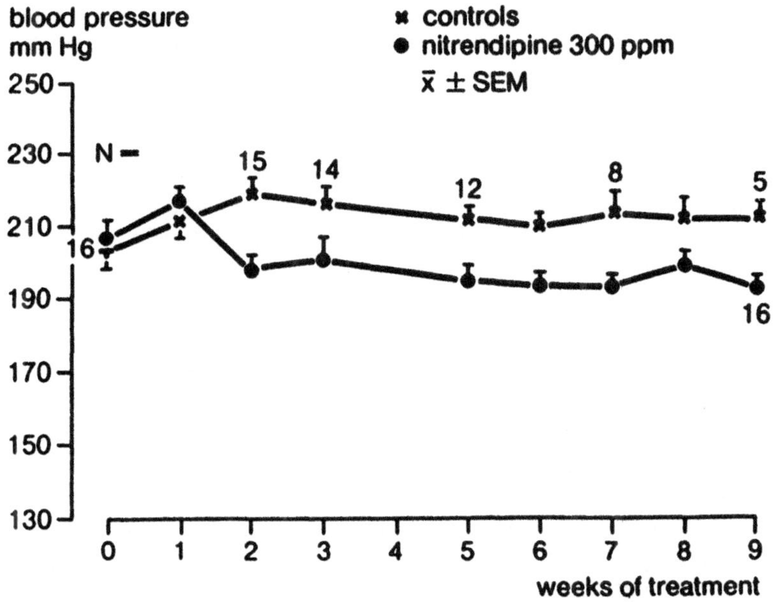

Fig. 12. High salt (8% NaCl) diet accelerated mortality in adult (5-month-old) male spontaneously hypertensive stroke prone rats without additional increase in blood pressure. Treatment with nitrendipine slightly decreased blood pressure but completely prevented mortality (*numbers above the curves* represent number of surviving animals). (From KAZDA et al. 1986a, with kind permission of Karger)

smooth muscle cells of renal arteries of hypertensive rats can be demonstrated by electron microscopy. Prophylactic treatment with nifedipine or nitrendipine prevents both hypertension and vascular damage and increases the survival rate in spite of a permanent feeding with a high salt diet (LUCKHAUS et al. 1982; KAZDA et al. 1983c; KAZDA 1986). Also, the subcellular calcium deposits are absent in the renal arteries of nifedipine-treated rats (KAZDA et al. 1987b). In Dahl S rats in which therapy with nifedipine was started in the already malignant stage of hypertension, blood pressure was normalized within a few weeks and the survival rate increased (GARTHOFF and KAZDA 1981). Moreover, the incidence and degree of morphological lesions were also improved by nifedipine treatment. Additionally, a reduplication of the internal elastic lamina with residual adventitial inflammatory cell reaction, distinct signs of healing processes of the previously existing arterial damage, were found after treatment with nifedipine (KAZDA et al. 1983b; LUCKHAUS et al. 1985).

It seems that tissue protection is not entirely dependent on the control of blood pressure by calcium antagonists. In adult SHRSP a dietary salt load accelerated the incidence of stroke with high mortality without additional increase in blood pressure. Treatment with nitrendipine in addition to 8% NaCl in the diet produced only a small decrease in blood pressure (Fig. 12). However, all the nitrendipine-treated animals survived, and the incidence and degree of arterial lesions were reduced. PRA was high in control rats despite the high salt diet, obviously reflecting ischemic renal damage. In nitrendipine-treated rats PRA remained low. The increase of plasma urea and creatinine was also prevented by nitrendipine treatment.

A high degree of protection in SHRSP is achieved by treatment with nimodipine, a calcium antagonist with a weak peripheral vascular effect. The high blood pressure is not decreased at all, but mortality and vascular lesions are reduced dramatically in nimodipine-treated animals (KAZDA et al. 1983c, d, 1986a). A similar protective and life-saving effect without influencing the high blood pressure in SHRSP is observed after bilateral parathyroidectomy. In these as well as in nimodipine-treated animals the tissue calcium content in the brain and kidneys remains normal. In the untreated, diseased rats the kidney calcium content is roughly 50% and the brain calcium, approximately 30% higher in comparison with that of age-matched WKY or young SHRSP (KAZDA et al. 1986b, 1987b). Clearly, specific calcium antagonists preserve tissue integrity in advanced hypertensive disease, primarily by preventing the harmful calcium overload and independently of the effect on blood pressure.

Calcium is implicated in many cell reactions thought to be important in the genesis and development of atherosclerosis. For several reasons it can be expected that compounds inhibiting the deposition of calcium in arterial walls will retard the development of atherosclerosis. In cholesterol-fed normotensive rabbits daily treatment with nifedipine (HENRY and BENTLEY 1981) or verapamil (ROULEAU et al. 1983) does not influence elevated plasma cholesterol and triglycerides but reduces the incidence and severity of aortic atherosclerotic plaques as well as cholesterol and calcium content in aortic tissue. The exact mechanism of the suppression of atherosclerosis by calcium antagonists is not known. Hemodynamic effects do not seem to be involved (BLUMLEIN et al. 1984). In cultured smooth muscle cells nifedipine depresses cholesteryl ester accumulation (ETINGIN and HAJJAR 1984). In primary culture of subendothelial intimal cells of human atherosclerotic aorta, verapamil causes a significant decrease in the intracellular content of phospholipids, triglycerides, and cholesteryl esters (OREKHOV et al. 1987). Nifedipine, verapamil, and diltiazem can inhibit the proliferation of cultured rat aortic smooth muscle cell whose growth has been stimulated either by serum or platelet derived growth factor (NILSSON et al. 1985). In addition, calcium antagonists may also affect smooth muscle migration (NAKAO et al. 1983) which may be important in suppressing the formation of atherosclerotic plaques (CHOBANIAN 1987).

It can be expected that this expanding research in the tissue protective and antiatherosclerotic effects of calcium antagonists will soon explain details of the mechanism of these actions as well as their therapeutic relevance in humans.

3 Pharmacokinetics and Metabolism

3.1 Verapamil

Verapamil is detected with high sensitivity in human plasma by gas chromatography/mass spectrometry (GC/MS) as described by SPIEGELHALDER and EICH-

ELBAUM (1977). More recently, high pressure liquid chromatography (HPLC) has allowed easy separation of the major metabolites from the mother compound (COLE et al. 1981).

Verapamil is absorbed rapidly and completely after oral administration. Peak plasma levels were observed after 1–2 h (SCHOMERUS et al. 1976; MCALLISTER and KIRSTEN 1982). Due to first pass metabolism the bioavailability of oral verapamil is only about 20%, and plasma concentrations vary among individuals (EICHELBAUM et al. 1979; MCALLISTER and KIRSTEN 1982). Plasma protein binding is around 90%. The volume of distribution of verapamil in humans is high, indicating wide distribution into various tissues (DOMINIC et al. 1981; MCALLISTER and KIRSTEN 1982; SCHOMERUS et al. 1976). In rats and dogs verapamil is found predominantly in heart, kidney, liver, and lung (HAMANN et al. 1983). Seventy percent of verapamil as polar metabolites is excreted renally, 15% with feces. Only up to 5% of verapamil is excreted as the unchanged compound (EICHELBAUM et al. 1979).

The elimination of verapamil after single administration does not follow simple first order kinetics. Norverapamil is the first metabolite to occur after oral administration. This product of *N*-demethylation of verapamil has some vasodilator activity in dogs (NEUGEBAUER 1978). In humans norverapamil occurs in approximately the same concentrations as the parent drug. *O*-demethylated metabolites of verapamil are active, but since they are quantitatively conjugated, they have no significant effect in vivo (Fig. 13). After multiple oral dosing the bioavailability of verapamil in patients has been found to be increased to about twice the value after a single dose. The same applies to its half-life. Steady

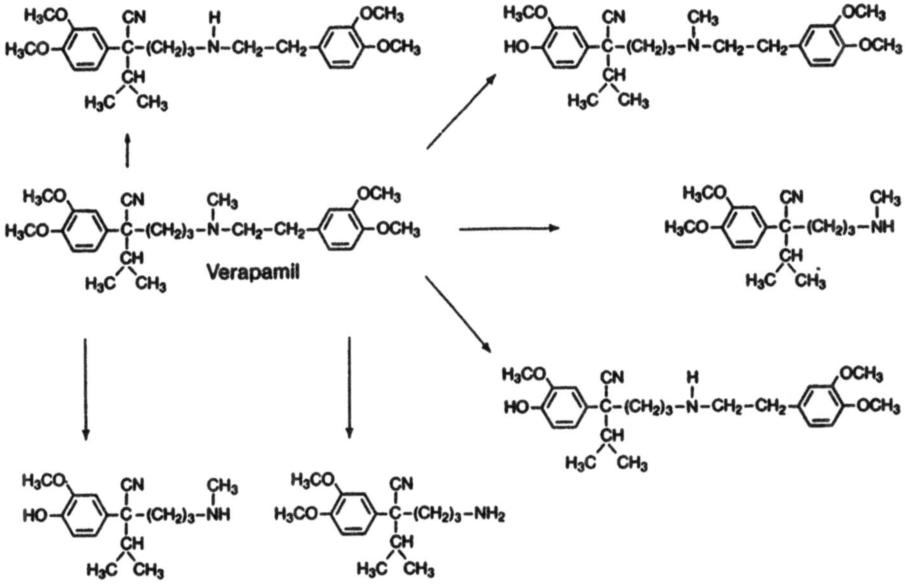

Fig. 13. Metabolism of verapamil (From EICHELBAUM et al. 1979, with kind permission of Williams & Wilkins, Baltimore)

state is reached within 3 days, approximately. The precise mechanism of the changes in pharmacokinetics is not yet quite clear. Both a partial saturation of hepatic enzyme systems (SHAND et al. 1981) and a reduction of the acutely increased hepatic blood flow with chronic administration of verapamil (MEREDITH et al. 1985) have been considered.

After oral administration the first pass metabolism of verapamil is stereoselective. Thus, (+)verapamil was found to have a 5 times higher peak plasma concentration, 2.5 times higher bioavailability, and a much slower oral clearance than (−)verapamil (VOGELSANG et al. 1984; HOON et al. 1986).

Various authors observed a great interindividual variability in systemic clearance of verapamil (HAMANN et al. 1984). In normal subjects the apparent terminal half-life varies between 3 and 5 h after p.o. administration with a tendency towards shorter half-lives after i.v. administration (MCALLISTER and KIRSTEN 1982; JOHNSTON et al. 1981). Administration of a slow-release formulation results in more stable plasma levels of verapamil, because the usual sharp initial rise in plasma concentration after each dosing is prevented (FOLLATH et al. 1986).

As terminal half-life is prolonged in patients with liver disease (SOMOGYI et al. 1981), intravenous doses of verapamil should be halved and oral doses should be reduced to one-fifth for them (HAMANN et al. 1984). Renal failure (MOOY et al. 1985) and hemodialysis (SHAN and WINER 1985) do not seem to affect the elimination of verapamil. Neither verapamil nor norverapamil were detected in the hemolysate. Chronic application might slow the elimination kinetics of verapamil, since a marked reduction in clearance, prolongation in plasma half-life, and a marked increase in AUC (area under the curve) were observed after the treatment of 12 hypertensive patients over a period of 4 weeks in a double-blind manner (ANDERSON et al. 1986; SCHWARTZ et al. 1985a). Also, advanced age may slow verapamil elimination (ABERNETHY et al. 1986).

Co-administration of digoxin or digitoxin with verapamil prolongs digoxin plasma half-life (KLEIN et al. 1982), yet just a slight rise in plasma digitoxin was observed in patients with cardiac insufficiency after multiple doses of verapamil (KUHLMANN and MARCIN 1985). Tuberculostatic therapy with rifampicin or its combinations with isoniazid or ethambutol are reported to reduce the oral bioavailability of verapamil (RAHN et al. 1985).

3.2 Dihydropyridines

3.2.1 Nifedipine

The specific and sensitive detection of nifedipine in biological samples is readily done by gas chromatography with electron capture detection, because no concentration of the samples is needed. A thorough description of this method is given by KUHLMANN et al. (1986). The light sensitivity of nifedipine calls for appropriate precautions when working with plasma. Whole blood, however, protects nifedipine from photo-oxidation (TUCKER et al. 1985).

After oral ingestion of a capsule, nifedipine is absorbed within 20–40 min, probably in the small intestine (RÄMSCH and SOMMER 1983). Nifedipine plasma levels have also been measured after sublingual and rectal (HORSTER 1975; RÄMSCH 1981) but not after transdermal application (KUHLMANN et al. 1986). Following more than 90% absorption, nifedipine undergoes first pass metabolism. Nevertheless, systemic bioavailability is high (50%–60%) (FOSTER et al. 1983; WALLER et al. 1984). The intestinal absorption of nifedipine is slowed after a meal with a high fat content. The time to peak plasma concentration is doubled from 1 to 1.9 h in comparison with a low-fat meal or the fasting state (REITBERG et al. 1987).

Plasma protein binding is 99%. The steady state distribution volume is 0.6–1.1 l/kg (KUHLMANN et al. 1986). After administration in capsules to healthy subjects, the plasma half-life of nifedipine is found to be approximately 4 h (FOSTER et al. 1983; KLEINBLOESEM et al. 1984a). Nifedipine tablets prolong plasma half-life to 5.9 h after single administration of 2 tablets containing 40 mg each (OCHS et al. 1984). In hypertensive patients even longer half-lives of about 10 h are reported by BANZET et al. (1983). Chronic administration does not appear to affect half-life (RÄMSCH and SOMMER 1983). After oral administration

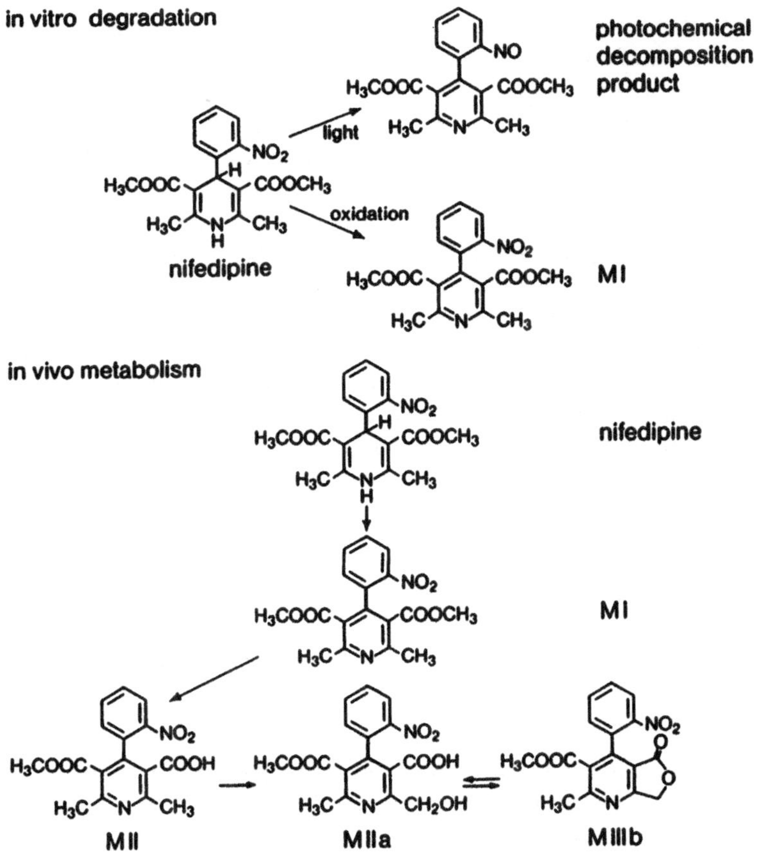

Fig. 14. Metabolism of nifedipine (From KUHLMANN et al. 1986, with kind permission of Schattauer-Verlag, Stuttgart)

of soft gelatine capsules with nifedipine solution (10 mg) peak plasma levels in the order of 75 μg/l were observed after 1 h. After a slow release tablet of 20 mg, a maximal level of only 20 μg/l was reached, but it was more sustained, causing a prolongation of plasma half-life up to 15 h (Kuhlmann et al. 1986).

Nifedipine is completely metabolized prior to excretion (Fig. 14). Thus, there is no renal clearance of the unchanged compound. It is first oxidized to yield the short-lived pyridine derivative (MI), which, in turn, is transformed into the monocarbonic acid (MII). After hydroxylation in the 2 or 6 position of the pyridine ring (MIII), formation of the lactone may occur under acidic conditions (Waller et al. 1984). None of the metabolites have calcium antagonistic activity. In urine, 70% of a dose is excreted as MII and MIII (Rämsch and Ziegler 1986). Practically no MI is found in the urine. A percentage of the metabolites is found as conjugates, and thus, biliary excretion is one more pathway of elimination of nifedipine. A genetic polymorphism of nifedipine-oxidizing microsomal enzymes was proposed by Kleinbloesem et al. (1984a,b) and Guengerich et al. (1986).

The pharmacokinetic behavior of nifedipine is unchanged by hemodialysis (Martre et al. 1985) and in terminal renal failure (Van Bortel et al. 1987) after oral administration. Creatinine clearance and free plasma nifedipine were inversely related after intravenous infusion, but not after oral application (Kleinbloesem et al. 1985a). However, in patients with liver dysfunction due to cirrhosis (Kleinbloesem et al. 1985b), the systemic bioavailability of nifedipine increases significantly, so that in such patients a reduction of the dose is advisable.

Unlike verapamil, nifedipine does not impair digoxin or digitoxin elimination (Kuhlmann and Marcin 1983; Kuhlmann et al. 1983, 1986). Co-administration of nifedipine with propranolol reduces nifedipine plasma concentrations and AUC, but other β-blockers, e.g., metoprolol or atenolol, have no such effects (Gangji et al. 1984; Kendall et al. 1984). Cimetidine, but not ranitidine, are reported to raise nifedipine plasma levels (Kirch et al. 1984a). Increases in phenytoin (Ahmad 1984), but occasional decreases in quinidine plasma concentration (Farringer et al. 1984; Green et al. 1983; Van Lith and Appelby 1985) with concomitant changes in the pharmacodynamics of these drugs are reported. Theophylline plasma levels are reported to rise in the presence of nifedipine (Parillo and Venditto 1984). More recently, however, when 16 patients chronically treated with theophylline were additionally treated with nifedipine for 2 weeks, no changes in plasma theophylline levels were observed (Christopher et al. 1987). The mechanisms of these interactions certainly warrant further investigation.

3.2.2 Nicardipine

Plasma concentrations of nicardipine hydrochloride have been determined by the use of tracer amounts of the compound labelled with ^{14}C in position 4 of the dihydropyridine ring (Graham et al. 1984). Generally, gas chromatography with electron capture detection is used (Higuchi et al. 1975).

After oral administration, nicardipine is found to be absorbed almost completely (86%) and rapidly. Maximal plasma concentration is obtained within from 20 min to 2 h (GRAHAM et al. 1984; DOW and GRAHAM 1986). Like other dihydropyridines, nicardipine is metabolized to a great extent during its first hepatic passage, but its systemic bioavailability increases disproportionately with increased dose. This may indicate a saturable presystemic elimination pathway, because the elimination kinetics is monoexponential (DOW and GRAHAM 1986). The considerable intersubject variability in plasma concentrations of nicardipine is probably due to this phenomenon.

Systemic bioavailability in humans is 6.5% after a dose of 10 mg and 30% after a dose of 40 mg (HIGUCHI and SHIOBARA 1980). When ingested after a meal, the peak plasma concentrations are found to be reduced by about one-third (GRAHAM et al. 1984). After i.v. application the initial half-life is 14 min, and terminal half-life is 4.75 h. The oral half-life after single doses of nicardipine is 45–97 min (HIGUCHI and SHIOBARA 1980). After chronic use, terminal half-life becomes 11.8 h (DOW and GRAHAM 1986).

Nicardipine is quantitatively metabolized in the liver, and no unchanged nicardipine is found in the urine, which is the primary route of excretion after oral administration (60%). Thirty-five percent of a dose is excreted fecally. After i.v. administration the difference is somewhat smaller (DOW and GRAHAM 1986).

Unlike nifedipine and nitrendipine, nicardipine yields a metabolite with one-tenth its vasodilator activity, which occurs at a proportion of 15% in human plasma (Clarke et al. 1984; RUSH et al. 1986). The metabolite still contains the dihydropyridine ring system and has a hydroxylated side chain. Other main plasma metabolites occurring in similar quantities are pyridine diesters and the corresponding acids, but they possess no calcium antagonist activity. The pharmacologically active dihydropyridine alcohol mentioned above and its pyridine analogue are the major urinary metabolites of nicardipine. Both are excreted as glucuronic acid conjugates.

According to a study by MARTINEZ et al. (1985), age has no influence on nicardipine pharmacokinetics. Otherwise, there is only sparse information about in vivo nicardipine pharmacokinetics. In patients with impaired renal function no evidence for potentially harmful drug accumulation was obtained (CLAIR et al. 1985). However, in that study the clearance of nicardipine was slowed by more than 50%. Hemodialysis had no influence.

Although desirable in a drug with important hepatic metabolism, no information is available on the pharmacokinetics of nicardipine in patients with liver disease. A single study assessing the influence of nicardipine on digoxin plasma levels (LESSEN and BELLINETTO 1983) reports a very slight increase of borderline significance. No pharmacokinetic interaction with enalapril was reported by DONNELLY et al. (1986). Information on interactions with H_2 antagonists is lacking.

3.2.3 Nitrendipine

Like nifedipine, its most recently released congener, nitrendipine is detected in plasma by gas chromatography with electron capture detection. Here nimodipine, another dihydropyridine, is employed as the internal standard.

Using ^{14}C- or ^{13}C-labelled nitrendipine in aqueous suspension, its pharmacokinetics and disposition were determined in healthy volunteers by KROL and colleagues (1987) and MIKUS and EICHELBAUM (1987). After oral ingestion of 20 mg of the agent in suspension, nitrendipine is 88% absorbed. Peak plasma concentrations were approx. 20 ng/ml after 1 h.

Due to its extensive presystemic metabolism, the bioavailability of nitrendipine in plasma is approximately 23%, (MIKUS and EICHELBAUM 1987) to 29% (RÄMSCH and SOMMER 1984). Plasma protein binding is high, between 97% and 99%. Nitrendipine has a high steady state distribution volume of 6.6 l/kg (RÄMSCH et al. 1986). In connection with this it has been postulated that nitrendipine is redistributed from some deep extravascular compartment to its receptor over a prolonger period of time (ARONOFF 1984).

Unlike nicardipine, the pharmacokinetics of nitrendipine are linear with increasing dose, thus indicating no saturable hepatic metabolism. These results were demonstrated in a crossover study in patients with essential hypertension (HANSSON et al. 1984). A good correlation of plasma levels with hemodynamic effects was also observed in this 3-week study; 85% of nitrendipine was excreted in urine and feces within 96 h after oral dosing (77% of this fraction is found in the urine, 8% in the stool). Practically no unmetabolized nitrendipine is excreted.

The first step in nitrendipine biotransformation is its inactivation by formation of the pyridine metabolite. Further steps include hydrolysis, hydroxylation, and glucuronide conjugation. This metabolism resembles that of nifedipine. Terminal half-lives of intravenous and oral solutions and of a tablet were on the order of 8 h (MIKUS and EICHELBAUM 1987).

In elderly subjects, peak plasma levels and AUC are increased (LETTIERI et al. 1987), probably because of its reduced hepatic elimination in those patients. However, another study employing elderly hypertensive patients failed to find any pharmacokinetic difference between young and old (KENDALL et al. 1987), neither after acute nor after multiple (8 days) dosing.

Renal failure did not interfere with single dose nitrendipine kinetics (ARONOFF 1984) in 18 patients. After 5 days of treatment peak plasma concentrations and AUC were similar in patients with normal and severely impaired renal function (VAN BORTEL et al. 1987). In a study with patients suffering from hepatic dysfunction due to liver cirrhosis who were treated with nitrendipine for 8 days, nitrendipine elimination was markedly suppressed. Maximum plasma levels were tripled, AUC was similarly increased, and elimination half-life was increased from 7 to 43 h. Therefore, in cases of hepatic impairment a reduction in dose should be considered (LASSETER et al. 1984).

The pharmacokinetic interaction of nitrendipine with various other drugs was studied by KIRCH et al. (1984b) after 1 week of co-administration. The β-adrenolytic drugs metoprolol, atenolol, and acebutolol, the H_2 antihistamine drugs cimetidine and ranitidine, as well as digoxin and digitoxin were co-administered with nitrendipine. No significant changes in nitrendipine plasma levels are observed in the presence of these drugs. Digoxin levels are reported increased by this group. However, the clinical relevance of this finding may be questioned, because in another study, steady state digoxin plasma levels were found completely unchanged in the presence of a dose of nitrendipine twice as high as that in the former study (ZIEGLER et al. 1987).

3.3 Diltiazem

Diltiazem concentration is measured in plasma either by gas chromatography with electron capture detection or with HPLC.

Diltiazem is over 90% absorbed after oral administration. Peak plasma levels are obtained after 2–4 h with doses of 30 or 60 mg (HERMANN and MORSELLI 1985; SMITH et al. 1983). After 120 mg, peak plasma concentrations were measured within less than 1 h (KÖLLE et al. 1983). Like verapamil, diltiazem is subjected to extensive first pass metabolism so that the bioavailaibility of diltiazem tablets is

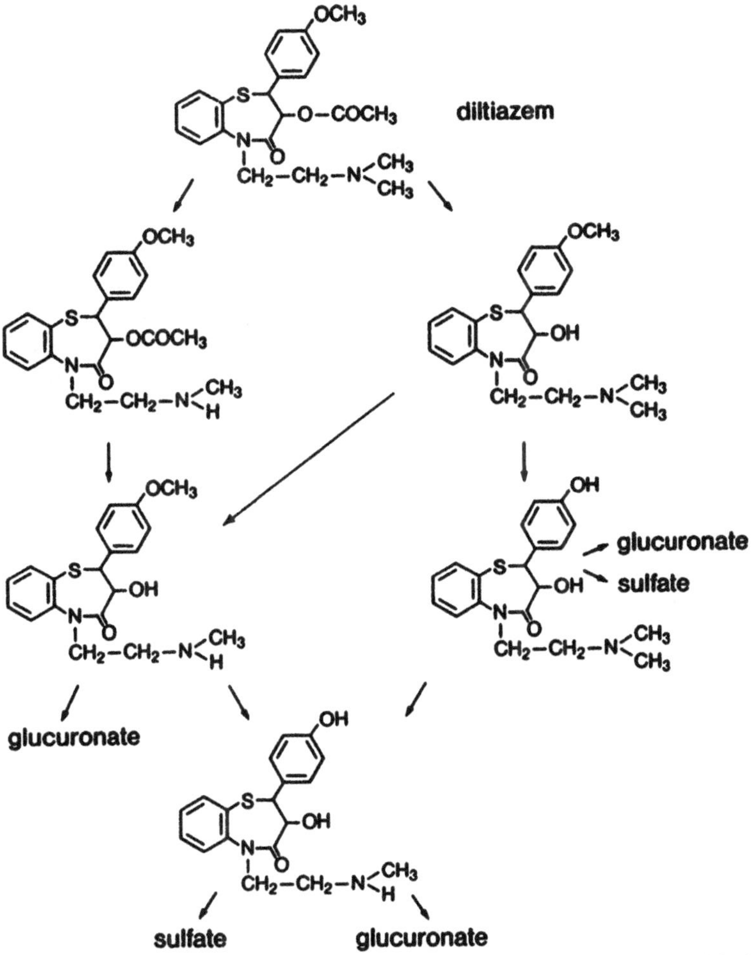

Fig. 15. Metabolism of diltiazem (From HERMANN and MORSELLI 1985, with kind permission of Munksgaard, Copenhagen)

between 30% and 40% (HERMANN and MORSELLI 1985) or 44% (KÖLLE et al. 1983) of the ingested dose after a single dosage. Diltiazem is bound about 80% to plasma proteins (MORSELLI et al. 1979; BLOEDOW et al. 1982). The volume of distribution was found to be 5 l/kg (KÖLLE et al. 1983).

Five percent of diltiazem is excreted renally as the unchanged compound. Biotransformation of diltiazem involves *O*-deacetylation as the major pathway yielding an active metabolite, deacetyldiltiazem (Fig. 15), which reaches plasma concentrations of about 30% of diltiazem (ROVEI et al. 1980; SMITH et al. 1983; SUGIHARA et al. 1984). SMITH et al. (1983) reported marked accumulation of diltiazem resulting in increases in AUC of more than 100% at steady state within 4 days of thrice daily dosing. This was ascribed to a potentially saturable first pass metabolism of diltiazem. The active metabolite deacetyldiltiazem was found to accumulate for a longer period of time; thus, its plasma level may exceed that of the parent compound (SMITH et al. 1983). Probably due to a high variability of first pass metabolism, MORSELLI et al. (1979) found a ten fold interindividual variation in plasma levels of diltiazem. After further phase I biotransformation, diltiazem metabolites are mostly conjugated and excreted mainly in the stool as glucuronides or sulfates. There is also evidence for some enterohepatic recirculation in rats (MESHI et al. 1971). The occurrence of high concentrations of diltiazem in mother's milk was reportd by OKADA et al. (1985).

Mean plasma elimination half-life after oral administration of tablets is 3–6 h (HERMANN and MORSELLI 1985) or 9.8 h when the terminal phase of a three-compartment model is used (KÖLLE et al. 1983). There is a significant reduction in the clearance of diltiazem in elderly patients (HERMANN and MORSELLI 1985; SCHWARTZ et al. 1985b), calling for a reduction in dosage for them.

Renal failure did not affect the elimination of diltiazem or deacetyldiltiazem after a single dose (POZET et al. 1983). However, in the light of the slow accumulation of deacetyldiltiazem, a repeated dose study might be advisable. No information is available on the disposition of diltiazem in patients with liver dysfunction.

Several authors have dealt with the interaction of diltiazem with digoxin kinetics. Most report increased plasma concentrations of digoxin (KUHLMANN et al. 1983; OYAMA et al. 1984; RAMEIS et al. 1984; THIERCELIN et al. 1983). Unwanted side effects are therefore possible, if these two agents are co-administered. Digitoxin pharmacokinetics are not affected by diltiazem (KUHLMANN and MARCIN 1983). Propranolol is displaced from plasma protein binding by diltiazem (PIEPER 1984), and additionally its hepatic extraction decreases (ETOH et al. 1983). It is also known that diltiazem reduces hepatic drug oxidation as shown by diminished antipyrine clearance in the presence of chronic diltiazem treatment (CARRUM et al. 1986). In patients treated with cimetidine, the maximal plasma concentration and AUC of diltiazem are increased. The same is true for the metabolite deacetyldiliazem. No statistically significant difference is observed with ranitidine (WINSHIP et al. 1985). Diazepam increases diltiazem plasma levels, but indometacin, phenylbutazone, phenytoin, and warfarin do not (MORSELLI et al. 1979). Chronic theophylline plasma levels are unaffected by a 2-week treatment with diltiazem (CHRISTOPHER et al. 1987).

4 Therapeutic Use and Dosage

First reports on the use of calcium antagonists in the treatment of human hypertension were published by Japanese and German investigators in the late 1960s and early 1970s (HAGINO 1968; BRITTINGER et al. 1970; MURAKAMI et al. 1972; KLUETSCH et al. 1972). During the next decade, there was little interest in these drugs for hypertension. The fall in blood pressure was viewed by many as a complication that was then increasingly found to be useful in patients with angina pectoris (MACGREGOR 1986). Systematic investigation of the therapeutic effects in hypertension began in the late 1970s, and now verapamil, nifedipine, and the analogues nitrendipine and nicardipine as well as diltiazem are approved for antihypertensive treatment in several countries.

4.1 Verapamil

The first, double-blind, placebo-controlled, therapeutic trial evaluating the antihypertensive efficacy of verapamil (LEWIS et al. 1978) involved 24 patients. They were given placebo, 80 mg, or 120 mg verapamil, each thrice daily for 1 month. A dose-dependent and significant reduction of both systolic and diastolic blood pressures was observed, with little postural effects. The only significant side effect was mild constipation.

Following this study, various researchers reported the therapeutic efficacy of verapamil in double-blind, placebo-controlled trials extending over periods of 10 days to 3 months (LEONETTI et al. 1981; DOYLE et al. 1981; MUIESAN et al. 1981, 1986; GOULD et al. 1982; HEDBÄCK and HERMANN 1983; CUBBEDU et al. 1986; MIDTBØ et al. 1982; CODY et al. 1986; SCHMIEDER et al. 1987). Doses of 80–160 mg administered thrice daily proved effective in a majority of patients. Even after 1 year of treatment with 80–160 mg verapamil thrice daily, in most cases plus thiazide diuretics (LEWIS et al. 1981), or 40–80 mg verapamil alone thrice daily (LUND-JOHANSEN 1985), patients were well controlled, and none developed tolerance.

In all studies heart rate is either unchanged or reduced, particularly during exercise (LUND-JOHANSEN 1985; GOULD et al. 1982). In comparison with β-adrenergic blocking drugs, verapamil produces less reduction in heart rate (LEONETTI et al. 1981; DOYLE et al. 1981) yet prolongs the P-R interval more (from 163.5 to 174.9 ms) than propranolol (from 160.3 to 164.4 ms) (CUBEDDU et al. 1986). The antihypertensive efficacy of verapamil is comparable with that of β-adrenergic blockers. Verapamil does not affect PRA, plasma catecholamines (DOYLE et al. 1981; MUIESAN et al. 1981), or body weight (LEONETTI et al. 1981) but, in contrast with β-adrenergic blockers, lowers total peripheral resistance.

In spite of its pronounced negative inotropic activity in pharmacological experiments, no depression of left ventricular function is found in patients (CODY et al. 1986; MUIESAN et al. 1986). Depressed heart rate during exercise is compensated for by an increase in stroke volume (LUND-JOHANSEN 1985).

In a 6-week, double-blind, crossover comparison with nifedipine in 28 patients with essential hypertension (WHO stage I-II), verapamil (160 mg thrice daily) lowered diastolic blood pressure more than nifedipine (20 mg slow-release tablet twice daily). However, systolic blood pressure was similarly reduced by both drugs. Verapamil, in contrast to nifedipine, produces significant heart rate reduction and slows atrioventricular conduction (P-R interval). In one patient sino-atrial block occurred after 7 days on verapamil after completion of the nifedipine period without complications. After withdrawal of verapamil, he recovered promptly (MIDTBØ et al. 1982).

In spite of the well-documented antihypertensive efficacy of verapamil, the inconvenience of a three to four times daily regimen potentially results in poor compliance. Therefore, a sustained-release (SR) formulation of verapamil has been made available, which allows once or twice daily administration, yet maintains therapeutic drug levels throughout the day in many patients (SCHÜTZ et al. 1982). After a 240-mg SR tablet a reduction to below 90 mmHg diastolic blood pressure was obtained in 14 of 17 patients after 2 weeks of treatment (POZENEL 1985). In a double-blind comparison of conventional verapamil (80–120 mg thrice daily) with SR tablets (240–360 mg once daily), similar reductions in blood pressure were achieved with both formulations. In spite of marked variations, serum concentrations were maintained over 24 h, but no correlation with blood pressure was seen. Of these patients 60% reached diastolic normotension while on SR tablets (ZACHARIAH et al. 1986). In another study (EDMONDS et al. 1987), 24-h antihypertensive action of verapamil SR was found in 12 out of 27 patients.

Of 97 ambulatory patients treated with SR tablets (240 mg once a day) 56 were satisfactorily controlled over a study period of 12 weeks, 25 needed a higher dose or addition of hydrochlorothiazide, and 5 patients withdrew due to adverse reactions (KÖNIG and ECKARDT 1984). In an open study conducted by BÜHLER et al. (1982c), 25 of 43 patients (WHO I-II) reached a diastolic blood pressure of 95 mmHg when treated with up to 240 mg of verapamil thrice daily. When compared intraindividually, the effects of verapamil, β-adrenergic blockers, and diuretics are similar.

Both verapamil and propranolol produce an uniform and comparable reduction in blood pressure throughout the whole day, together with a reduction in heart rate, which is greater with propranolol (Fig. 16) (HORNUNG et al. 1984).

FRISHMAN et al. (1982) and BRÜGMANN (1986) reported as a result of randomized, double-blind, crossover studies versus propranolol and of a randomized, double-blind study versus placebo on the successful treatment of patients with both essential hypertension and angina pectoris. In other studies verapamil proved to be more effective than β-blockers in black and white patients. Moreover, verapamil was equally effective in blacks and whites, whereas propranolol was more effective in whites than in blacks (CUBEDDU et al. 1986).

A dose of 120 mg twice daily of SR verapamil is equivalent to 80 mg thrice daily of conventional verapamil (COREA et al. 1983). Diuretics give a significant additional antihypertensive effect in 19 of 40 patients, who were not adequately controlled by 120 mg twice daily of SR verapamil alone (COREA et al. 1984). The successful use of additional diuretic therapy with verapamil is underlined by several reports (MACGREGOR et al. 1985a; MARLETTINI et al. 1986; RIBEIRO 1987).

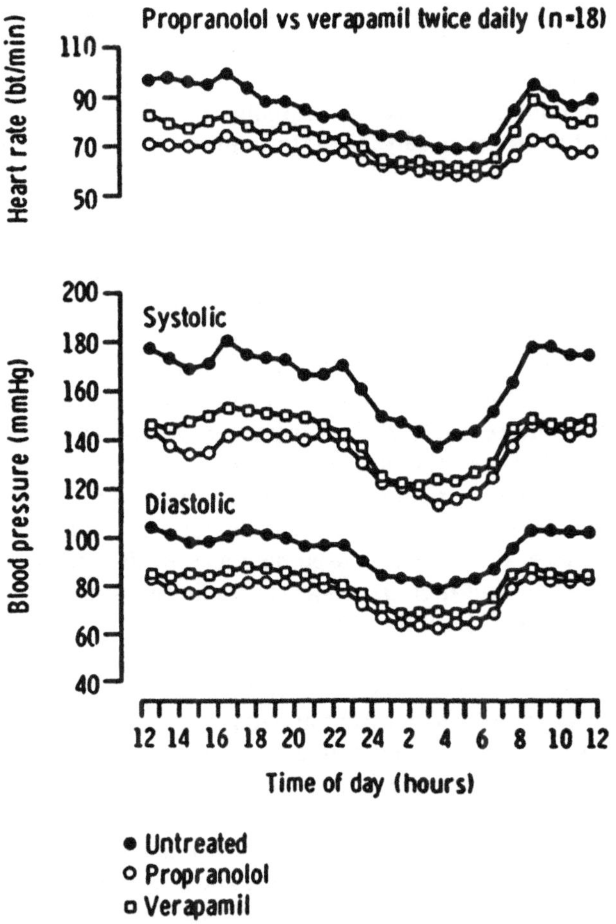

Fig. 16. Circadian variation of heart rate and systolic and diastolic blood pressure while untreated (*solid dots*), with propranolol twice daily (*white dots*), and with verapamil twice daily (*squares*). (From HORNUNG et al. 1984, with kind permission of CV Mosby, St. Louis)

The antihypertensive combination with angiotensin-converting-enzme inhibitors might prove particularly powerful, since 15 of 16 patients refractory to triple drug therapy (β-adrenergic blocker, diuretic, and vasodilator) and still inadequately controlled with verapamil or nitrendipine alone reached the therapeutic goal of 95 mmHg diastolic pressure when captopril was added (BROUWER et al. 1985a). This combination was more effective than that of captopril with a diuretic in the same patients. Similarly, when captopril alone failed to give satisfactory control of moderately severe hypertension in 18 patients, addition of 160 mg of verapamil twice daily after 4 weeks yielded a significant further reduction in blood pressure. When subsequently captopril was withdrawn, standing diastolic blood pressure was significantly higher after 4 weeks of verapamil alone (HEAGERTY and SWALES 1987).

The administration of verapamil to patients receiving β-adrenergic blocking drugs is reported to produce adverse cardiovascular reactions, but only few systemic investigations of this potential drug interaction have been performed in hypertensive patients. In 15 patients with angina pectoris who received high doses of propranolol or metoprolol, verapamil (40, 80, and 120 mg) produced a dose-dependent decrease in cardiac performance, cardiac index, stroke volume, and heart rate associated with increases in pulmonary capillary wedge and mean right atrial pressures. In contrast, repeat administration of 120 mg verapamil 24–30 h after withdrawal of β-blockade produced no significant cardiodepressant effects (PACKER et al. 1982). BÜHLER's group reviewed reports on the unwanted electrophysiologic and hemodynamic effects of single and combined therapy with β-blockers and verapamil, diltiazem, or nifedipine and summarized the scant experience of these drug combinations in patients with hypertension. Verapamil is more often associated with conduction problems (up to 9%) and dyspnea or heart failure (up to 8%). Intravenous verapamil is contraindicated in patients on β-blockers and the oral verapamil/β-blocker combination should not be used in patients with impaired left ventricular function and when conduction disturbances are likely to occur. In treating hypertensive patients without overt coronary artery disease, there is no argument against the use of the nifedipine/β-blocker combination, but there is a need for definitive studies of the verapamil/β-blocker combination (BROUWER et al. 1985b).

MCINNES et al. (1984) investigated the efficacy and safety of verapamil (120 mg three times a day) and propranolol (80 mg three times a day) alone or in combination in 11 patients with essential hypertension resistant to monotherapy. In this double-blind, placebo-controlled, crossover comparison, verapamil plus propranolol was highly effective in controlling blood pressure at rest and under exercise. The combination produces a significantly better response than either drug given separately, and the effects of the two drugs are additive. The drugs are generally well tolerated. All treatments cause prolongation of atrioventricular conduction, and this is more marked following verapamil plus propranolol. The only rhythm disturbances recorded on 24-h monitoring were two short episodes of second degree heart block in one patient during combination therapy. The heart rate was reduced in all active groups, and the lowest mean level occurred during combination therapy, but no dangerous disturbances were seen. Thus, preliminary results of this study are favorable, but more patients need to be studied to confirm that the combination is not only effective but safe (MCINNES et al. 1984). Until there are more data, the combination of verapamil plus β-blocker should be used with caution and only in patients without evidence of sick sinus syndrome or other atrioventricular conduction problems or heart failure (ROSENDORFF 1984; BROUWER et al. 1985b).

4.2 Nifedipine

The antihypertensive effect of this new coronary dilator was shown for the first time by KLUETSCH et al. and MURAKAMI et al. in 1972. Systematic investigation of nifedipine in the treatment of hypertension began in the late 1970s. In open (AOKI et al. 1976, 1978; COREA et al. 1979; GUAZZI et al. 1977; LEDERBALLE

Pedersen and Mikkelsen 1978), placebo-controlled (Beer et al. 1981), and double-blind (Thibonnier et al. 1980; Condorelli et al. 1982; Maranhao et al. 1983) studies, sublingual or oral administration of a 10-mg capsule causes a rapid and significant decrease in blood pressure in hypertensive patients. In normotensive subjects blood pressure does not change (Corea et al. 1979).

Daily treatment of mild to moderate hypertensive patients with a 10-mg capsule thrice daily (Corea et al. 1979; Giuntoli et al. 1981) or 10–20 mg thrice daily (Lederballe Pedersen and Mikkelsen 1978) results in a sustained decrease of blood pressure over 3–12 weeks. Hourly pressure readings in a placebo-controlled study show that the antihypertensive response to each "active" dose (10-mg capsule) lasts 8–12 h and that nifedipine every 6 h significantly reduces blood pressure throughout 24 h without postural hypotension (Olivari et al. 1979). In a double-blind, placebo-controlled study 1–3 capsules (10 mg) thrice daily result in a diastolic blood pressure below 90 mmHg in 75% (sitting) or 57% (standing) of 56 patients during 12 weeks of treatment (Pacheco et al. 1986). Development of drug resistance, sodium retention, plasma volume expansion, renin release, or angina pectoris were not observed in these studies. The blood pressure reduction when nifedipine was added to β-adrenoceptor blockade is of the same magnitude as that observed on nifedipine monotherapy in a double-blind study for 4 weeks. Side effects like heat sensations, palpitations, and headache are the reasons given for discontinuation in 4 of 18 patients on nifedipine alone. In contrast, none of the 9 patients on combined treatment dropped out (Lederballe Pedersen et al. 1980).

In 36 Japanese patients either monotherapy with a low oral dose of nifedipine (5 mg thrice daily) or its combination with a low dose of propranolol (10 mg thrice daily) and/or a low dose of thiazide controlled blood pressure during a 22-week study period. The plasma concentration of nifedipine was significantly correlated with the falls in systolic and diastolic blood pressure. No serious adverse or side effects necessitating discontinuation of nifedipine were observed (Aoki et al. 1982b).

In patients with arterial pressure inadequately controlled by the combination of a β-adrenoceptor antagonist and a diuretic (Bayley et al. 1982; Murphy et al. 1983; Dean and Kendall 1983) or clonidine with diuretic (Del Guercio and Gentile 1981), the addition of nifedipine (10–30 mg thrice daily) results in a further significant and dose-dependent reduction in blood pressure in both erect and supine positions in these double-blind trials. Heart rate, body weight, renal function, and plasma glucose are not altered. The only laboratory change is a fall in plasma potassium, probably due to an enhancement of the kaliuretic effect of thiazide by nifedipine (Murphy et al. 1983).

Nifedipine capsules taken sublingually or orally have a rapid and effective antihypertensive action. They are therefore well-suited for treating hypertensive emergencies. However, the effect is rather short and needs repeat administration. The slow release tablet developed later on with smooth onset and long duration of action has proved more convenient for the patient. In double-blind studies 20–80 mg lead to a significant smooth decrease in blood pressure with a duration of 10–12 h. The maximum effect is obtained after 90–180 min with nifedipine retard and after 30 min with nifedipine capsule. There is a linear relationship between the dose, AUC, and peak plasma levels of nifedipine (STREIFLER et al. 1985; CAPUCCHIO et al. 1986). In chronic treatment with 20 mg twice daily a normalization of blood pressure was achieved in 50% of patients after 3 weeks (THIBONNIER et al. 1985; DESIMONE et al. 1984) and 75% after 6–14 weeks (FAN et al. 1986; WING et al. 1986; ARIGO and CONSOLO 1987). A significant reduction of both systolic and diastolic blood pressure over 12 months was achieved in 9 of 10 patients treated with a 20-mg tablet once a day. Only one patient required twice daily administration. Creatinine clearance was greater and serum creatinine reduced after 12 months of treatment. The facial flushing which followed nifedipine capsule ingestion did not occur with the slow release tablet (VALDES et al. 1986). Heart rate, serum electrolytes, cholesterol, HDL cholesterol, blood glucose, and renal function were not changed after successful treatment of elderly patients for 8 weeks (LANDMARK and DALE 1985).

In patients resistant to combined β-blocker and diuretic therapy, the response rate to nifedipine capsules thrice daily was determined. All responders were then changed to sustained release tablets (20 mg twice daily), and subsequent control of arterial pressure was at least as good as it had been while taking the capsules. No patient reported any adverse effect (BAYLEY et al. 1982). In a continuous ambulatory intra-arterial blood pressure recording nifedipine tablets given twice daily provide 24-h control of blood pressure and maintain lower blood pressure during isometric and dynamic exercise. Once daily therapy produces a similar profile of blood pressure reduction for about 12 h after the morning dosage, but efficacy is diminished for the rest of the day (HORNUNG et al. 1983).

In a multicenter study most of the 1207 patients were treated for 6 months with 20 mg nifedipine twice daily as monotherapy (in 167 patients nifedipine was added to diuretics and in 62, to β-blockers). A good to very good response was achieved in 84% with regard to efficacy and in 85% with regard to tolerability (ZIEGLER and BACH 1986). In a 96-week trial nifedipine 20 mg twice daily as monotherapy significantly reduced supine and standing blood pressure in all 15 patients. The maximum antihypertensive effect was achieved after 48 weeks of treatment. Serum sodium was significantly reduced after 8 weeks which persisted until week 72. Serum potassium remained slightly reduced throughout the study. This observation indicates that nifedipine possesses a persistent saluretic and diuretic activity, which may contribute to the slow, progressive decline in blood pressure subsequent to the rapid initial fall due to vasodilation (LANDMARK 1986).

In double-blind studies nifedipine's effect is similar (ROSENTHAL 1983; DOUGLAS-JONES and MITCHELL 1984) or even more pronounced (WING et al. 1985) than that of thiazide diuretics or furosemide in long-term treatment.

Nifedipine produces an additive decrease of blood pressure in patients treated with diuretics (MACGREGOR et al. 1987). Also in patients uncontrolled by a diuretic alone (GAVRAS and GAVRAS 1985; OPSAHL et al. 1987) or by combined diuretic and β-blocker therapy (MYERS et al. 1986), the addition of 20 or 40 mg nifedipine twice daily results in a significant decrease of blood pressure compared with placebo. Target blood pressure was achieved in nearly all patients.

In contrast, it remains unclear whether diuretics have a further blood pressure-lowering effect when added to nifedipine, ROSENTHAL (1983), FERRARA et al. (1985), MAGAGNA et al. (1986), or MACGREGOR et al. (1985a,b, 1987a) found no additional decrease in blood pressure after addition of diuretics. HALLIN et al. (1983), POULTER et al. (1986), and NOTGHI et al. (1987) noted a greater effect with combined therapy than with either agent used singly. In patients who had persistent hypertension despite treatment with nifedipine 20 mg twice daily for 4 weeks, the addition of bendroflumethiazide resulted in a significant further decrease in blood pressure (ZEZULKA et al. 1987).

In comparison with β-adrenoceptor antagonists, nifedipine seems to produce an almost identical reduction in systolic and diastolic blood pressure at rest and after exercise (EGGERTSEN and HANSSON 1982; FRANZ and WIEWEL 1984; ZUSMANN et al. 1987). The addition of nifedipine enhances the antihypertensive effect of β-blockers (AOKI et al. 1978; COREA et al. 1980a; DANIELS and OPIE 1986; HUSTED et al. 1982; YAGIL et al. 1983) or allows the reduction of dose or frequency of administration (LEJEUNE et al. 1985).

In patients resistant to monotherapy with β-blockers blood pressure is well-controlled after addition of nifedipine (BAYLEY et al. 1982; OGILVIE 1985). The decrease of heart rate is usually of the same order as when β-blockers are given alone. The combination of a β-blocker with nifedipine may reduce the acute symptoms attributable to the vasodilation after nifedipine, especially when the rapid-release form (capsule) is used (HUSTED et al. 1982). Less impairment of physical performance is found with the combination than with β-blocker alone (KINDERMANN et al. 1987).

Combined treatment with the α- and β-blocking drug labetalol (200 mg twice daily) and nifedipine (20 mg twice daily) for 6 weeks produces a larger fall in blood pressure than either drug alone (OEHMAN et al. 1985). GUAZZI showed an additive effect of methyldopa with nifedipine and claimed some evidence that nifedipine was more effective with methyldopa than with a β-blocker (GUAZZI et al. 1980, 1983).

Promising therapeutic effects are reported from studies of combined use of nifedipine with angiotensin-converting-enzyme inhibitors, especially in patients not satisfactorily controlled by monotherapy. Nifedipine seems to be a better partner for combination with angiotensin-converting-enzyme inhibitors than diuretics, achieving better control of blood pressure and reducing unwanted side effects (BROUWER et al. 1985a; FERGUSON et al. 1986; GUAZZI et al. 1984; MACGREGOR et al. 1985a; MIMRAN and RIBSTEIN 1986).

High efficacy of nifedipine alone or in combinations is found in severe hypertension (diastolic blood pressure over 120 mmHg) (GUAZZI et al. 1980; IMAI et al. 1980; ISLES et al. 1986), in an acute hypertensive crisis (KAWAJIMA et al. 1978; MAGOMETSCHNIGG 1982; CLARY and SCHWEIZER 1987), or in patients with hypertensive acute pulmonary edema (COREA et al. 1980b). Both rapid- and slow-release formulations are effective. MACGREGOR (1986) suggested that nifedipine capsules should be reserved for patients with hypertensive encephalopathy or left ventricular failure, and to use nifedipine tablets, which are absorbed more slowly, in patients with severe hypertension.

Nifedipine seems to be particularly effective in controlling blood pressure in patients on dialysis for acute or chronic renal failure (ELIAHOU et al. 1982; KUSANO et al. 1982; KUBO et al. 1983), producing not only rapid reduction in blood pressure but also sustained control of hypertension.

4.3 Nicardipine

Nicardipine is a dihydropyridine calcium antagonist structurally related to nifedipine and, therefore, having a similar pharmacodynamic profile and therapeutic effects. Its antihypertensive efficacy is documented in open (LEE et al. 1986; MURRAY et al. 1986a,b) and double-blind, placebo-controlled (BROWN et al. 1985; CREYTENS and SAELEN 1986; FORRETTE et al. 1985) studies. In patients treated with 10, 20, 30, and 40 mg three times daily in a crossover trial, a target diastolic blood pressure (below 95 mmHg) was achieved after 30 mg three times daily in 32 of 33 patients (TAYLOR et al. 1985a). Blood pressure was satisfactorily controlled in 76% of patients, usually treated with 20 mg three times daily in several double-blind studies (BROWN et al. 1985; CREYTENS and SAELEN 1986; FORRETTE et al. 1985).

In a study with twice daily administration nicardipine doses were titrated from 30 to 60 mg. The blood pressure-lowering effect was lost 12 h after dosing in most patients (FRISHMAN et al. 1985a). Eight patients of 18 were withdrawn from a double-blind study (maximum dose of 60 mg twice daily) because of troublesome palpitations and headache (CHARLAP et al. 1986). Both reports conclude that nicardipine monotherapy in a twice daily regimen is ineffective in the treatment of hypertension.

The initial dose of nicardipine results in a strong increase in urine volume and sodium excretion. LITTLER et al. (1986) found a 100% increase in water excretion and 300% in sodium excretion but no changes in GFR. VAN SHAIK et al. (1984) found that the natriuretic effect in hypertension was due mainly to an increase in GFR and also to a slight distal tubular effect. On the 6th day of a 30 mg three times daily regimen, the renal vascular resistance and filtration fraction remained lowered whereas GFR was unchanged. Body weight was significantly decreased during 6 days' treatment, indicating the persistence of the diuretic effect (CHAIGNON et al. 1986). In a double-blind, placebo-controlled study of 30 patients over 6 weeks, nicardipine 30 mg thrice daily produced a reduction in blood pressure similar to verapamil 160 mg twice daily. Both treatments increase resting ejection fraction; nicardipine decreases whereas verapamil increases ejection time (AL KHAWAJA et al. 1986). Nicardipine 30 mg thrice daily was equally as effective as 20 mg twice daily nifedipine in 28 patients treated for 6 weeks (ARMSTRONG et al. 1987).

As indicated by a placebo-controlled, double-blind, multicenter trial involving 180 patients with essential hypertension with thrice daily administration of 30 mg nicardipine is at least as effective as twice daily administration of 25 mg hydrochlorothiazide. Addition of nicardipine in diuretic nonresponders lowers significantly supine blood pressure while additon of hydrochlorothiazide in nicardipine nonresponders does not (FAGAN et al. 1986). Nicardipine (30 mg thrice daily) produces a greater fall in blood pressure but also more side effects than cyclopenthiazide diuretic. However, in contrast to the diuretic, nicardipine does not affect serum potassium or uric acid, which would be a long-term cardiovascular risk factor (Murray et al. 1986c). Nicardipine in combination with chlorthalidone produces a similar percentage reduction in blood pressure (16%) as a combination of atenolol and chlorthalidone (20% and 18%, respectively). Adverse effects are significantly higher in the group treated with nicardipine and chlorthalidone (Douglas-Jones and Coxhead 1986).

The addition of nicardipine (5–20 mg three times daily) in 20 patients treated with 100 mg atenolol once daily produced a further significant decrease of blood pressure as compared with placebo. Side effects were minor and did not lead to discontinuation of treatment. No effect on atrioventricular conduction was observed (Kolloch et al. 1985).

In an open multicenter study with 1106 patients with mild to moderate hypertension, 65% were controlled with nicardipine alone (20 mg thrice daily or 20–40 mg twice daily); 78% of the 264 patients who required associated therapy (mostly, but not exclusively diuretics) achieved goal blood pressure (160/95 mmHg or lower). Some 49% had complications of hypertension or concomitant diseases (diabetes mellitus, coronary insufficiency, cardiac failure, cerebrovascular or chronic renal insufficiency, obstructive lung disease, or peripheral vascular disease), and none of the clinical symptoms of these conditions was aggravated during the 12 weeks of treatment (Leonetti 1987b).

In 12 patients inadequately controlled on enalapril monotherapy, the addition of nicardipine (30 mg thrice daily) resulted in a significant fall in supine and erect blood pressure. There was only a small and transient increase in heart rate (Donelly et al. 1986). When 12 hypertensive patients with impaired renal function were treated with 30 mg of nicardipine thrice daily, a significant fall in blood pressure and an increase in sodium, but not in potassium excretion were observed. Inulin or *para*-aminohippuric acid (PAH) clearance did not change (Lee et al. 1986). In 14 patients with severe renal failure receiving conservative (6) or hemodialysis (8) treatment, nicardipine (20 mg) induced a significant acute as well as chronic (20 mg thrice daily) improvement of systolic and diastolic blood pressure (Clair et al. 1985).

In numerous studies nicardipine has been used for acute intraoperative blood pressure control under anesthesia. Nicardipine hydrochloride is a water-soluble compound, which may easily be used for intravenous infusions. Usually an infusion rate of 0.32 mg/min or less is sufficient to produce a significant prompt decrease of blood pressure or to control hypertension associated with surgery. No serious complications except for mild tachycardia in a few cases have been reported (Chelly et al. 1987; Kishi et al. 1984; Momose et al. 1986; Tamai et al. 1986; Yoshiya et al. 1986). Nicardipine is superior to nitroglycerin or trimethaphan in controlling intraoperative hypertension (Momose 1985).

4.4 Nitrendipine

Nitrendipine differs from the other antihypertensive calcium antagonists in that it was developed solely for use in antihypertensive therapy. It has a sufficiently long duration of action to be administered on a once to twice daily schedule.

Its mid- and long-term efficacy in mild to moderate hypertension is documented in several double-blind studies (FAGAN et al. 1984; KIRKENDALL et al. 1987; MCMAHON et al. 1987; MOSER et al. 1984; ORÖ and RYMAN 1987; VITACOLONNA et al. 1986; WORTMANN et al. 1987; ZACHARIAH et al. 1987a,b), including two multicenter trials (B.M. MASSIE et al. 1987; MORLEDGE et al. 1987). In a double-blind, randomized, parallel comparison with the β-blocker acebutolol in 60 black Africans, nitrendipine was found slightly superior (M'BUYAMBA-KABANGU et al. 1987). In American blacks a 60%–70% rate of normalization of diastolic blood pressure was seen (DUSTAN 1987; WEINBERGER 1987), no difference being observed between blacks and whites (WEINBERGER 1987).

Nitrendipine was also found effective in elderly patients, in whom it was more active than acebutolol (BORZELLINO et al. 1987) or had a similar activity level to hydrochlorothiazide (GILES et al. 1987). Thus, isolated systolic hypertension in elderly patients may be treated successfully (FERREIRA-FILHO et al. 1987).

A more pronounced fall in blood pressure induced by nitrendipine was found by some authors in people of advanced age in comparison with younger patients (FRITSCHKA et al. 1984; KIOWSKI et al. 1985; MÜLLER et al. 1984; TOURKANTONIS et al. 1984) but denied by others (WEINBERGER 1987). There is, however, evidence from several studies of an inverse relationship between the drop in (diastolic) blood pressure after nitrendipine and the patient's baseline PRA (DUSTAN 1987; KIOWSKI et al. 1985; M'BUYAMBA-KABANGU 1987; MÜLLER et al. 1984; WEINBERGER 1987; ZACHARIAH et al. 1987a). Complete normalization of diastolic blood pressure is achieved at an overall rate of about 70% of patients treated.

Most patients are treated successfully with doses of 10 mg once daily up to 20 mg twice daily. Several studies suggest that a once daily regimen may frequently be sufficient to keep diastolic pressure within the normotensive range. In mild hypertension approximately 84% of patients were successfully treated this way (BRÜGMANN 1987; RÜDDEL et al. 1987; WANDEL et al. 1987; WORTMANN et al. 1987; CORSING et al. 1987; ZACHARIAH et al. 1987b). In a double-blind comparison of 10–20 mg once daily with 10 mg twice daily, 31 of 36 patients were successfully controlled, and no statistically significant difference was detected between the different regimens (VITACOLONNA et al. 1986).

No development of tolerance to the action of nitrendipine is observed after prolonged treatment over a year or more (FAULHABER et al. 1987; FRANCISCHETTI et al. 1987; TOURKANTONIS et al. 1984; TROST and WEIDMANN 1987). Nitrendipine either initially slightly increases PRA [less, however, than hydrochlorothiazide (MORLEDGE et al. 1987; WEINBERGER 1987)] or leaves it unchanged. Similarly, heart rate is increased slightly (less than 10 beats/min) in several studies, whereas in others it is not.

Acute and chronic administration of nitrendipine results in significant natriuresis and diuresis in hypertensive patients (LUFT et al. 1985; THANANOPAVARN et al. 1984a, b) as in normotensive volunteers (ENE et al. 1985). In the long-term, nitrendipine results in a resetting of the sodium and water balance and natriuresis ceases as observed with thiazide diuretics (SIMON and SNYDER 1984). Initial loss of serum potassium during the first week of nitrendipine was observed only in one study (THANANOPAVARN et al. 1984a, b).

Antihypertensive treatment with nitrendipine is at least as effective as that with hydrochlorothiazide (MORLEDGE et al. 1987; B.M. MASSIE et al. 1987; WEINBERGER 1987) or β-blockers (BORZELLINO et al. 1987; RÜDDEL et al. 1984; McMAHON et al. 1987; ZACHARIAH et al. 1987a,b) as shown in several, mostly double-blind, comparative trials. Nitrendipine may be more efficient than β-blockers in blacks (M'BUYAMBA-KABANGU et al. 1987; WEINBERGER 1987).

In a direct comparison, nitrendipine 20 mg once daily is as effective as enalapril 20 mg once daily but superior to captopril 50 mg twice daily in 30 patients (GENNARI et al. 1987).

Nitrendipine has less influence on PRA than hydrochlorothiazide (MORLEDGE et al. 1987; WEINBERGER 1987). It produces no change in glucose metabolism, serum cholesterol and triglycerides, potassium, or uric acid (FRANCISCHETTI et al. 1987; KIRKENDALL et al. 1987; JOHNSON et al. 1986). No impairment in glucose homeostasis was observed in 10 patients with hypertension and diabetes mellitus type II during more than 1 year of antihypertensive treatment with nitrendipine (TROST and WEIDMANN 1987).

Patients on hemodialysis responded well to treatment with nitrendipine over a period of a year or more (WANDEL et al. 1987).

Nitrendipine is combined with thiazide diuretics or β-blockers or both to yield satisfactory control of blood pressure in patients inadequately treated with nitrendipine alone (BURRIS et al. 1987; JAIN et al. 1984; ORÖ and RYMAN 1987; WEBER 1987). Likewise, patients with severe hypertension inadequately treated with combinations of diuretics and β-blockers or triple regimens may benefit from additional nitrendipine (HÖFFLER and STOEPEL 1984; KINDLER et al. 1987; RÖCKEL et al. 1987; SCHOENBERGER et al. 1987).

The antihypertensive effects of low doses (5 mg) of nitrendipine and enalapril are found to be additive (LANG et al. 1987).

Nitrendipine seems to preserve the physiologic response pattern to mental stress (MESSERLI et al. 1987) as well as acute and long-term physical exercise capacity in contrast to β-blockers (FRANZ and WIEWEL 1984; B.M. MASSIE et al. 1987; NANNAN et al. 1984), while retaining its antihypertensive effect.

In 13 patients with coexistent coronary artery disease and hypertension, nitrendipine lowered blood pressure and increased exercise tolerance and time to onset of angina pain by 25% (BRÜGMANN 1987). No impairment of cerebral blood flow was seen in 10 elderly patients after 4 weeks of 20 mg nitrendipine twice daily (CONEN et al. 1987), and no worsening of peripheral arterial occlusive disease was observed after 6 months of nitrendipine (MEYER et al. 1987).

Whereas no improvement in pulmonary arterial pressure was found in normotensive patients with chronic obstructive lung disease (MOLS et al. 1986), in 23 patients with concomitant hypertension resting pulmonary hemodynamics and oxygen transport were improved after 10–20 mg once daily (RUBIN et al. 1987). Pulmonary vascular resistance and pulmonary arterial pressure fell, whereas stroke volume and oxygen delivery rose by approximately 30%.

4.5 Diltiazem

Although the blood pressure lowering effect of diltiazem had already been recognized in 1971 (SATO et al. 1971), the consequent investigation of its antihypertensive efficacy began in the late 1970s and is still continuing. Most of the early trials were open studies conducted in Japan, generally with small numbers of patients (AOI et al. 1978; SAKAI 1978; TAKEMIYA and YAMAGUCHI 1978; YAMAKADO and TAGAWA 1978). Diltiazem (90–180 mg) was often added to the pre-existing antihypertensive regimen and produced an additional significant decrease in blood pressure over treatment periods of 1–6 months. Side effects such as flushing and headache were observed occasionally. A decade later, when Western scientists rediscovered this drug for hypertension, a series of open studies confirming the pioneering work of Japanese scientists was published in American journals (AMADEO et al. 1986; MOHANTY et al. 1985; MOSER et al. 1985; ROSATTI et al. 1984). Diltiazem was confirmed to be an effective antihypertensive agent when used alone.

At doses of 120–240 mg given twice daily diltiazem significantly lowers blood pressure in 60% of patients over 8 weeks. In the responders (12 of 18) a good control of blood pressure is sustained for 6 months. In patients with normal renal function, no overall effect on GFR, renal plasma flow, salt and water excretion, or body fluid composition was found after 8 weeks on diltiazem (SUNDERRAJAN et al. 1986). In individuals with a pretreatment GFR less than or equal to 80 ml min^{-1} 1.73 m^{-2}, diltiazem monotherapy showed both short-term and long-term improvement in GFR (62%) and effective renal plasma flow (34%). No long-term effect was seen on salt and water excretion or body fluid composition (SUNDERRAJAN et al. 1987).

The antihypertensive efficacy of diltiazem was confirmed in double-blind, placebo-controlled studies (IKEDA 1978; YORIFUGI et al. 1979; WALKER et al. 1984; NEUSS et al. 1987). After a titration period a dose of 180 mg twice daily was required in 85% of patients.

At that dose level average blood pressure in all positions is significantly reduced as compared with placebo. In a subsequent open-label study blood pressure remained well controlled over 8 months (POOL et al. 1985, 1986). Side effects such as headache, dizziness, and tinnitus were observed at a rate of 24% (NEUSS et al. 1987). BEER et al. (1986) found in a placebo-controlled study that 60 mg thrice daily of the usual diltiazem formulation produces a nearly identical decrease in blood pressure as 90 mg twice daily of a sustained release preparation in 90 patients with essential hypertension. Side effects such as angina, tremor, restlessness, and disturbed sleep were similar after both formulations.

In numerous double-blind comparisons with propranolol 60–84 mg per day or metoprolol 100–120 mg per day, it was shown that diltiazem monotherapy 60 mg four times a day (TRIMARCO et al. 1984), 90 mg twice daily (YAMAKADO et al. 1983; BERRINO et al. 1986; SZLACHCIC et al. 1987), and the sustained release preparation 60–180 mg twice daily (B.B. MASSIE et al. 1987) have a comparable antihypertensive effect. Heart rate is decreased after diltiazem in most studies but less than with the β-blocker. In a double-blind study of 40 patients, 60–180 mg diltiazem twice daily was equieffective in the control of blood pressure to propranolol 80–140 mg twice daily after a 6-month period. Diltiazem causes a significant reduction in left ventricular mass, whereas propranolol causes no changes (WEISS and BENT 1987). Little is known about the effect of combined therapy with diltiazem and β-blocker.

In a double-blind, parallel, 12-week trial, 90 mg diltiazem twice daily was equally as effective as 0.3 mg reserpine. The incidence of side effects in the diltiazem group was about half that in the reserpine group (12.3% and 27.1%, respectively) (OGAWA et al. 1984). In open (INOUYE et al. 1984; MOHANTY et al. 1987) as well as in double-blind (MOSER et al. 1985; SWARTZ 1987) studies diltiazem (120–180 mg twice daily) or hydrochlorothiazide (20–50 mg twice daily) produce a similar decrease in blood pressure for 8–26 weeks, achieving the goal blood pressure below 90 mmHg in 42% and 45% of patients, respectively (FRISHMAN et al. 1985b, 1987); 63% of patients who did not achieve the treatment goal in the double-blind study responded to diltiazem plus hydrochlorothiazide (FRISHMAN et al. 1985b). Vice versa, in patients who did not respond to diltiazem alone combined therapy with a thiazide diuretic resulted in better control of blood pressure (AKANABE et al. 1985; MAEDA et al. 1981; B.B. MASSIE et al. 1987; MOSER et al. 1985).

Little is known about the long-term effect of diltiazem in hypertensive patients. SAWAI (1983) reported that eight elderly patients who had taken dilitazem for approximately 5 years were well controlled in the sence of having achieved goal blood pressure without significant side effects.

In a double-blind parallel study of 47 patients with mild to moderate essential hypertension diltiazem (180–270 mg/day) was as equieffective as nifedipine capsule (30–60 mg/day) over a study period of 4 weeks each. The overall responder rate was 80%. Heart rate was unchanged after nifedipine and lowered after diltiazem. Pulmonary artery pressure was reduced only after nifedipine, not after diltiazem (YAMAKADO et al. 1985) treatment. Side effects were only mild and appeared in 6 of 24 patients on nifedipine and 5 of 23 on diltiazem. In no case was there a need to stop the treatment (KLEIN et al. 1983). Similar efficacy was found in a comparison of diltiazem (90 mg twice daily to 90 mg thrice daily) with slow release nifedipine tablets (20 mg twice daily to 20 mg thrice daily) in 40 patients treated in a double-blind manner over 8 weeks. Mild and transitory side effects were reported in 10 patients on diltiazem and 11 on nifedipine. No metabolic changes were found after each drug (SCHULTE et al. 1986).

Ditiazem (30–130 mg thrice daily) is equally as effective as nifedipine capsules (10–40 mg thrice daily) in controlling blood pressure in hypertensive patients with stable angina pectoris. Both drugs are equally effective in reducing anginal attacks, although nifedipine reduces the consumption of nitroglycerin more than diltiazem. Facial flushing and ankle edema are observed with nifedipine. One patient on diltiazem developed Mobitz type 1 heart block which resolved after withdrawal of the drug (FRISHMAN et al. 1985c).

5 Contraindications and Drug Interactions

5.1 Verapamil and Diltiazem

These two drugs are quite similar in their pharmacology and therefore have similar contraindications. Neither drug should be administered in the presence of cardiac rhythm disturbances such as second or third degree atrioventricular block, sick sinus syndrome, or sinoatrial block, or in cases of atrial flutter or fibrillation (e.g., Wolff-Parkinson-White syndrome). Patients with first degree atrioventricular block or sinus bradycardia must be treated with great caution. In patients with significant left ventricular dysfunction, decompensated heart failure, cardiogenic shock, or in the early post-infarct period, especially if complicated by concomitant bradycardia or hypotension, these calcium antagonists should not be used. Great caution is recommended if these drugs are used with β-blockers, antiarrhythmic drugs, and inhalation anesthetics, because of possible potentiation of cardiodepressive and negative chronotropic actions.

The plasma levels of concomitantly administered digoxin or carbamazepine may be increased. Therefore, neither drug should be used to treat digitalis intoxications. Cimetidine but not ranitidine may increase diltiazem plasma levels (Winship et al. 1985). The studies done with verapamil show controversial results (Somogyi and Muirhead 1987).

Diltiazem should, in addition, not be given in pregnancy, since it causes embryotoxicity in mice, rats, and rabbits at doses five- to ten-fold higher than the therapeutic dose (Quigley et al. 1985). The safety of verapamil in early pregnancy is not known. During lactation diltiazem should be avoided, because high concentrations of the drug are found to pass into the mother's milk (Okada et al. 1985).

Diltiazem should be used with caution in patients with hepatic dysfunction.

5.2 Nifedipine, Nicardipine, and Nitrendipine

One pharmacological property common to these dihydropyridine calcium antagonists is that of having little or no direct influence on cardiac excitation and conduction or on myocardial contractility at therapeutic doses. Their use in the presence of cardiac rhythm disturbances such as those mentioned in Sect. 5.1 is not restricted.

However, pregnancy is a contraindication for dihydropyridine calcium antagonists because high chronic doses of nifedipine are found to cause stillbirths or to be embryotoxic in animals. Some of these effects may be due to prolonged gestation because of uterine relaxation caused by excessive doses of the calcium antagonist. Nifedipine also passes into the mother's milk.

Caution should be exercised if these drugs are to be used in hypotensive states and in conjunction with other antihypertensives. There is, however, longstanding experience of successful use of nifedipine with β-blockers, diuretics, and ACE inhibitors. Use in cardiovascular shock is contraindicated.

Cimetidine but not ranitidine was reported by KIRCH et al. (1984a) and DYLEWICZ et al. (1986) to increase nifedipine plasma levels. On the other hand, KIRCH et al. (1984b) found no interaction of these H_2 blockers with nitrendipine. Information on the interaction of nicardipine with H_2 blockers is lacking.

6 Side Effects and Toxicity

It is problematic to compare the relative incidence of side effects for the calcium antagonists discussed in this chapter. On the one hand, their period of availability varies by decades between the oldest, verapamil, and the most recent, nitrendipine. On the other hand, all drugs are used to different degrees in hypertension and other cardiovascular disorders. The frequency with which side effects are reported is, in turn, related to the physician's and patient's perceptions of the severity of the disease treated, for example angina versus hypertension (see QUIGLEY et al. 1985). Side effects are rather frequent with calcium antagonists but are mostly benign, undisturbing, and reversible. On very rare occasions angina-like side effects have been observed. The overall rate of side effects for verapamil, diltiazem, and nifedipine was reported to be 8%–10%, 2%–10%, and 17% (TALBERT and BUSSEY 1983).

In a more recent, randomized, double-blind, placebo-controlled, crossover study, a direct clinical comparison was made between diltiazem and nifedipine in hypertensive patients with concomitant angina (FRISHMAN et al. 1985c). Whereas the number of patients reporting any side effects was similar with nifedipine and diltiazem, the cumulative number of side effects after diltiazem was only half that of nifedipine (15% vs. 28%, respectively). In this study, one patient was withdrawn while on diltiazem, because heart block developed. Despite the small number of patients employed, this direct comparison yielded side effect rates comparable to the figures given in the surveys mentioned above. In the following, the calcium antagonists will be discussed individually.

6.1 Verapamil

The patient's most prominent complaint during therapy with verapamil is constipation, which often responds to laxative treatment. Headaches, peripheral edema, facial flushing, and hypotension are noted occasionally. Atrioventricular block and bradycardia occur rarely. These effects are closely related to the effect of verapamil on impulse formation and conduction. Less drug-specific, but not uncommon complaints are nausea and anorexia (TALBERT and BUSSEY 1983). Although a meaningful quantification of overall occurrence of a drug's side effects is difficult, oral verapamil seems to be tolerated well in hypertension, unless used in patients with certain disturbances in cardiac function (see Sect. 5).

There are several reports on intoxication due to deliberate or accidental massive overdosing of verapamil (CRUMP et al. 1982; DA SILVA et al. 1979; DE FAIRE and LUNDMAN 1977; GELBKE et al. 1977; IMMONEN et al. 1981; KRÜGER 1984; MORONI et al. 1980; ORR et al. 1982; PASSAL and CRESPIN 1984; PERKINS

1978). Severe hypotension with loss of consciousness and cardiac rhythm disturbances are cardinal signs of verapamil intoxication. The majority of patients survive doses ranging up to 6.4 g (IMMONEN et al. 1981). Antidotes most frequently used are calcium gluconate and sympathomimetic drugs, especially dopamine. Also, prolonged electrical pacing is reported, since atrioventricular block and consequent bradycardia concomitant with profound hypotension are the most persistent signs of verapamil poisoning. Because of the difficulty of estimating the relative benefit of different antidotal drugs in cases of emergency, the results of a study in anesthetized rats by STRUBELT (1984) might be helpful. Best results were obtained with sympathomimetic drugs. Also $CaCl_2$ and plasma expanders had some beneficial effect.

6.2 Nifedipine

Side effects are reported by hypertensive patients treated with nifedipine at a frequency similar to verapamil, but the spectrum of complaints is somewhat different. Headaches, dizziness, vertigo, facial flushing, and a feeling of warmth are frequently reported, mainly at the onset of therapy. Local, especially ankle and pedal, edema is not uncommon and reflects local fluid extravasation following arteriolar dilatation rather than systemic fluid retention. This effect may be transient or might necessitate a reduction in dose. Reports on constipation or bradycardia are rare exceptions. Serious side effects, like deterioration of cardiac contractility in patients with compromised cardiac function or precipitation of atrioventricular nodal blockade, are very unusual with nifedipine. This is in accordance with the known differences in negative inotropic and chronotropic potency between verapamil, diltiazem, and nifedipine (in declining order of potency) relative to their vascular efficacy (HENRY 1980).

There are three reports on poisoning with nifedipine. All were voluntary overdosages and doses up to 900 mg were ingested (HERRINGTON et al. 1986; N.N. 1985; SCHIFFL et al. 1984). Main symptoms of poisoning are throbbing headaches and profound hypotension. Cardiac rhythm or atrioventricular node function and consciousness are not markedly impaired. Medical countermeasures taken were mainly gastric lavage, activated charcoal, and close observation of the patient's condition.

6.3 Nicardipine

The range of adverse reactions observed in patients treated with nicardipine is similar to that of nifedipine. Most complaints are related to peripheral vasodilation, including flushing, headache, and ankle edema. These effects are often only initial and reversible (SCHEIDT et al. 1985; TAYLOR et al. 1985b; for review, see SORKIN and CLISSOLD 1987).

Other side effects, like myalgia, skin rashes, gastrointestinal, and CNS-related symptoms like fatigue or dizziness are rare and in general do not call for cessation of nicardipine treatment (ASPLUND 1985; GELMAN et al. 1985; GHEOR-

GIADE et al. 1985; SCHEIDT et al. 1985; TAYLOR et al. 1985b). Because of the closely related pharmacological and side-effect profile, in cases of nicardipine intoxication similar countermeasures as for nifedipine are recommended.

6.4 Nitrendipine

Although the number of patients treated with nitrendipine is somewhat limited to date, it appears that the type of adverse reactions encountered are very similar to those with nifedipine tablets. In an open, multicenter trial involving 155 patients with essential hypertension who were treated with nitrendipine for a year (WEBER 1987), the prime complaints were transitory headache and peripheral edema. A few patients had tachycardia, palpitations, dizziness, sexual dysfunction, or skin rash. The total number of withdrawals because of adverse reactions was 8% in this study. Other authors report a similar spectrum of side effects (ESPER et al. 1984; FRITSCHKA et al. 1984; JAIN et al. 1984; TOURKANTONIS et al. 1984), but in a double-blind, placebo-controlled trial involving 135 patients in two parallel groups reported by MOSER et al. (1984), 30 patients of the placebo group complained about headache as opposed to only 10 in the treated group. Instead, there was an increased incidence of peripheral edema and polyuria in patients on nitrendipine. In a smaller (21 outpatients), double-blind, crossover comparison with nifedipine (ORÖ and RYMAN 1987), four patients complained about flush, edema, or headache after nifedipine, but none after nitrendipine. Whether there is a substantial improvement in the incidence of side effects over other dihydropyridines must await further studies.

6.5 Diltiazem

Having less negative inotropic and chronotropic activity than verapamil but more than the dihydropyridine calcium antagonists (HENRY 1980), the range of side effects with diltiazem resembles both drugs. Headache, peripheral edema, and dizziness are the most common complaints. Nausea, rash, and asthenia are also mentioned as relatively frequent events (QUIGLEY et al. 1985). However, the rate of unwanted reactions reported might be relatively low (KREBS 1983). Three placebo-controlled trials involving 63 (STRAUSS et al. 1982) or 57 (HOSSAK et al. 1982) patients with angina, and 77 patients with essential hypertension (POOL et al. 1986) indicate a very low incidence of adverse reaction. When in a double-blind trial 107 patients with essential hypertension were treated either with diltiazem or reserpine for 12 weeks, 27% of those on reserpine reported side effects, but only 12% on diltiazem (OGAWA et al. 1984). According to a survey of 3193 patients taking diltiazem (MCGRAW et al. 1982) the incidence of side effects was very low (2%). Occasionally, such effects may be serious conduction disorders like sinoatrial or atrioventricular block (HOSSAK 1982; IMAMURA et al. 1986). The likelihood of such conduction defects may increase during concomitant treatment with β-adrenoceptor blocking drugs (HOSSAK 1982; ISHIKAWA et al. 1983; HUNG et al. 1983).

Six instances of poisoning due to overdoses of up to 10.8 g of diltiazem have been reported (REY et al. 1983; BUFFET et al. 1984; GIBELIN et al. 1984; JEAN et al. 1985; MALCOLM et al. 1986; SNOVER and BOCCHINO 1986). None was fatal. Therapeutic measures taken included gastric lavage and electrical pacing. Atrioventricular block and deep hypotension with somnolence or unconsciousness are the prevalent features of poisoning, the first being the most persistent of the toxic symptoms.

Summary

Calcium antagonists are chemically heterogenous compounds all having a similar mechanism of action and therapeutic efficacy in hypertension. Their prominent effect is the inhibition of transmembrane calcium influx in activated vascular smooth muscle cells, resulting in a reduction of total peripheral vascular resistance. In contrast to other vasodilators, calcium antagonists increase sodium and water excretion by their direct renal effects. The relation of the renal effect to the peripheral vasodilation and the relative contribution of the diuretic action to the therapeutic efficacy may be different in the individual drugs.

The antihypertensive efficacy of calcium antagonists in monotherapy is comparable to that of thiazide diuretics or β-blockers. Metabolic abnormalities associated with diuretics are not observed with calcium antagonists. Unlike β-blockers, calcium antagonists are successfully used in patients with coexisting bronchopulmonary obstructive diseases and peripheral artery diseases.

The differences in relative potencies of vascular and cardiac effects and in pharmacokinetics determine the different use of individual calcium antagonists in specific patient populations.

Addition of calcium antagonists to other antihypertensives improves the therapeutic success in otherwise refractory hypertension. There are no major limitations for the combined use of calcium antagonists with other drugs; caution is required, however, in the combined use of verapamil and dilitiazem with β-blockers.

References

Abernethy DR, Schwartz JB, Todd EL, Luchi R, Suaer E (1986) Verapamil pharmacodynamics and disposition in young and elderly hypertensive patients. Altered electrocardiographic and hypertensive response. Ann Intern Med 105:329–336

Ahmad S (1984) Nifedipine-phenytoin interaction. J Am Coll Cardiol 3:1582

Akanabe H, Ishiguro M, Yagi Y, Ohshima S, Ohmae M, Mori M, Watanabe S, Yasue T (1985) Effect of diltiazem hydrochloride in essential hypertension. Int J Clin Pharmacol Ther Toxicol 23:63–69

Al Khawaja IM, Caruana MP, Lahiri A, Whittington JR, Lewis JG, Raftery EB (1986) Nicardipine and verapamil in essential hypertension. Br J Clin Pharmacol 22 (Suppl 3):S273–S282

Amadeo C, Kobrin I, Ventura HO, Messerli FH, Frohlich ED (1986) Immediate and short-term hemodynamic effects of diltiazem in patients with hypertension. Circulation 73:108–113

Anderson P, Bondessonon V, De Faire U (1986) Pharmacokinetics of verapamil in patients with hypertension. Eur J Clin Pharmacol 31:155–163

Angus JA, Dhumma-Upohorn P, Cobbin LB, Goodman AH (1976) Cardiovascular action of verapamil in the dog with particular reference to myocardial contractility and atrioventricular conduction. Cardiovasc Res 10:623–632
Aoi W, Suzuki S, Doi Y, Hashiba K (1978) Clinical use of diltiazem hydrochloride (Herbesser) in hypertension. Clin Rep 12:3589
Aoki K, Ikeda N, Yamashita K, Tazumi K, Sato I, Hotta K (1974) Cardiovascular contraction in spontaneously hypertensive rat: Ca^{2+} interaction of myofibrils and subcellular membrane of heart and arterial smooth muscle. Jpn Circ J 38:1115–1121
Aoki K, Yoshida T, Kato S, Tazumi K, Sato I, Takikawa K, Hotta K (1976) Hypotensive action and increased plasma renin activity by Ca^{2+} antagonist (nifedipine) in hypertensive patients. Jpn Heart J 17:479–484
Aoki K, Kondo S, Mochizuki A, Yoshida T, Kato S, Kato K, Takikawa K (1978) Antihypertensive effect of cardiovascular Ca^{2+}-antagonist in hypertensive patients in the absence and presence of beta-adrenergic blockade. Am Heart J 96:218–226
Aoki K, Kawaguchi Y, Sato K, Kondo S, Yamamoto M (1982a) Clinical and pharmacological properties of calcium antagonists in essential hypertension in humans and spontaneously hypertensive rats. J Cardiovasc Pharmacol 4 (Suppl 3):298–302
Aoki K, Sato K, Kawaguchi Y, Yamamoto M (1982b) Acute and long-term hypotensive effects and plasma concentrations of nifedipine in patients with essential hypertension. Eur J Clin Pharmacol 23:197–201
Appel W (1962) α-Isopropyl-α-[N-methyl-N-homoveratryl)-γ-amino-propyl]-3,4-dimethoxyphenylacetonitril, sein Nachweis in biologischem Material und sein Verhalten im Blut. Arzneimittelforschung 12:562–566
Armstrong C, Garnham J, Blackwood R (1987) Comparison of the efficacy of nicardipine, a new calcium channel blocker, with nifedipine in the treatment of mild to moderate essential hypertension. Postgrad Med J 63:463–466
Aronoff GR (1984) Pharmacokinetics of nitrendipine in patients with renal failure: comparison to normal subjects. J Cardiovasc Pharmacol 6:S974–S976
Arrigo F, Consolo F (1987) Long-term treatment of essential hypertension with slow-release nifedipine. Curr Ther Res Clin Exp 41:651–664
Asano M, Aoki M, Matsuda T (1986) Actions of calcium agonists and antagonists on femoral arteries of spontaneously hypertensive rats. In: Aoki I (ed) Essential hypertension. Calcium mechanisms and treatment. Springer, Berlin Heidelberg New York, pp 35–49
Asplund J (1985) Nicardipine hydrochloride in essential hypertension—a controlled study. Br J Clin Pharmacol 20 (Suppl 1):120S–124S
Baer PG, Navar LG (1973) Renal vasodilation and uncoupling of blood flow and filtration rate autoregulation. Kidney Int 4:12–21
Banzet O, Colin JN, Thibonnier M, Singlas E, Alexandre JM, Corvol PC (1983) Acute antihypertensive effect and pharmacokinetics of a tablet preparation of nifedipine. Eur J Clin Pharmacol 24:145–150
Bauer JH, Sunderrajan S, Reams G (1985) Effects of calcium entry blockers on renin-angiotensin-aldosterone system, renal function and hemodynamics, salt and water excretion and body fluid composition. Am J Cardiol 56:62H–67H
Bayley S, Dobbs RJ, Robinson BF (1982) Nifedipine in the treatment of hypertension: report of a double-blind controlled trial. Br J Clin Pharmacol 14:509–512
Beer M, Felder K, Presch HR (1986) Treatment of primary hypertension with diltiazem. A comparison of 2 dosage schemes. Therapiewoche 36:2432–2440
Beer N, Gallegos I, Cohen A, Klein N, Sonnenblick E, Frishman W (1981) Efficacy of sublingual nifedipine in the acute treatment of systemic hypertension. Chest 79: 571–574
Bellemann P, Ferry D, Lübbecke F, Glossmann H (1981) (^{3}H)-nitrendipine, a potent calcium antagonist, binds with high affinity to cardiac membranes. Arzneimittelforschung Drug Res 31:2064–2067
Berrino L, Fici F, Filippelli W, Lampa E, Marmo E, Marrazzo R (1986) Diltiazem and metoprolol in the therapy of hypertension: polygraphic assessment of systolic times during treatment. Br J Clin Pharmacol 21:104P
Bloedow DC, Piepho RW, Nies AS, Gal J (1982) Serum binding of diltiazem in humans.

J Clin Pharmacol 22:201–205

Blumlein SL, Sievers R, Kidd P, Parmley WW (1984) Mechanism of protection from atherosclerosis by verapamil in the cholesterol-fed rabbit. Am J Cardiol 54:884–889

Bohr D (1964) Electrolytes and smooth muscle contraction. Pharmacol Res 16:85–111

Bohr DR, Webb RC (1984) Vascular smooth muscle function and its changes in hypertension. Am J Med 77:3–17

Bolger GT, Gengo PJ, Luchowki EM, Siegel H, Triggle DJ, Janis RA (1982) High affinity binding of a calcium antagonist to smooth muscle and cardiac muscle. Biochem Biophys Res Commun 104:1604–1609

Bolton TB (1979) Mechanisms of action of transmitters and other substances on smooth muscle. Physiol Rev 59:606–718

Borsotto M, Barhanin J, Norman RI, Lazdunski M (1984) Purification of dihydropyridine receptor of the voltage-dependent Ca^{2+} channel from skeletal muscle transverse tubules using (+) (^{3}H) PN 200-110. Biochem Biophys Res Commun 122:1357–1366

Borzellino M, Homes G, Finizola A, Graterol S, Kobelt R, Rojas Z, Rodriguez JE, Rodriguez E, Finizola B (1987) Nitrendipine in elderly hypertensives. J Cardiovasc Pharmacol 9 (Suppl 4):S290–S294

Bossert F, Vater W (1971) Dihydropyridine, eine neue Gruppe stark wirksamer Koronartherapeutika. Naturwissenschaften 58:578

Bossert F, Horstmann H, Meyer H, Vater W (1979) The influence of the ester function on the vasodilating activity of 1,4-dihydro-2,6-dimethyl-4-nitrophenylpyridine-3,5-dicarboxylates. Azneimittelforschung Drug Res 29:226–229

Brittinger WD, Schwarzbeck A, Wittenmeier KW, Trittenhoff WD, Stegaru B, Huber W, Ewald RW, von Henning GE, Fabricius M, Strauch M (1970) Klinisch-experimentelle Untersuchungen über die blutdrucksenkende Wirkung von Verapamil. Dtsch Med Wochenschr 95:1871–1877

Brouwer RML, Bolli P, Erne P, Conen D, Kiowski W, Bühler FR (1985a) Antihypertensive treatment using calcium antagonists in combination with captopril rather than diuretics. J Cardiovasc Pharmacol 7:S88–S91

Brouwer RML, Follath F, Bühler FR (1985b) Review of the cardiovascular adversity of the calcium antagonist beta- blocker combination. Implications for antihypertensive therapy. J Cardiovasc Pharmacol 7 (Suppl 4):S38–S44

Brown ST, Freedman D, De Vault GA, Slay L (1985) Elderly multicenter study group. Safety, efficacy and pharmacokinetics of nicardipine in elderly hypertensive patients. Br J Clin Pharmacol 22 (Suppl):289S–295S

Brügmann U (1986) Calcium antagonists in hypertension and coronary heart disease. In: Rosenthal J (ed) Calcium antagonists and hypertension: current status. Excerpta Medica, Amsterdam, pp 209–219

Brügmann VE (1987) Acute antihypertensive and anti-ischemic effects of nitrendipine: results of a double-blined, randomized, crossover and placebo controlled study. J Cardiovasc Pharmacol 1 (Suppl 4):S197–S200

Bühler FR, Hulthén L (1982) Calcium channel blockers: a pathophysiologically based antihypertensive treatment concept for the future? Eur J Clin Invest 12:1–3

Bühler FR, Hulthén UL, Bolli P (1982a) Calcium channel inhibitors for identification of mechanisms and treatment of hypertension. J Cardiovasc Pharmacol 4 (Suppl 3): S267–S268

Bühler FR, Hulthén UL, Kiowsky W, Bolli P (1982b) Greater antihypertensive efficacy of the calcium channel inhibitor verapamil in older and low renin patients. Clin Sci 63:439S–442S

Bühler FR, Hulthén UL, Kiowksi W, Müller FB, Bolli P (1982c) The place of the calcium antagonist verapamil in antihypertensive therapy. J Cardiovasc Pharmacol 4 (Suppl 3):S350–S357

Bühler FR, Bolli P, Hulthén UL (1984) Calcium influx-dependent vasoconstrictor mechanisms in essential hypertension. In: Opie LH (ed) Calcium antagonists and cardiovascular disease. Raven, New York, pp 313–322

Bühler FR, Bolli P, Erne P, Kiowski W, Müller FB, Hulthén UL, Ji BH (1985a) Position of calcium antagonists in antihypertensive therapy. J Cardiovasc Pharmacol 7 (Suppl 4):S21–S27

Bühler FR, Bolli P, Kiowksi W, Müller FB, Erne P (1985b) Calcium antagonists for identification of mechanisms and treatment of patients with essential hypertension. In: Fleckenstein A, van Breemen C, Groß R, Hoffmeister F (eds) Cardiovascular effects of dihydropyridine-type calcium antagonists and agonists. Springer, Berlin Heidelberg New York, pp 445–457

Bühler FR, Bolli P, Erne P, Kiowski W, Müller FB, Hulthén UL (1985c) Adrenoceptors, calcium and vasoconstriction in normal and hypertensive humans. J Cardiovasc Pharmacol 7 (Suppl 6):S130–S136

Buffet M, Ostermann G, Raclot P, Bertault R, Rambourg MO, Jaussaud M (1984) Kinetics of diltiazem during voluntary overdose. Presse Med 13:1338

Burris JF, Mroczek WJ, Brobyn R, Kann J (1987) Long-term efficacy and safety of nitrendipine in severe hypertension. J Cardiovasc Pharmacol 9 (Suppl 4):S306–S310

Capuccio FP, Markandu ND, Tucker FA, MacGregor GA (1986) Dose-response and length of action of nifedipine capsules and tablets in patients with essential hypertension—a randomized crossover study. Eur J Clin Pharmacol 30:723–725

Carrum G, Egan JM, Abernethy DR (1986) Diltiazem treatment impairs hepatic drug oxidation: studies of antipyrine. Clin Pharmacol Ther 40:140–143

Cattaneo EA, Rinaldi GJ, Gende OA, Venosa RA, Cingolani HE (1986) Increased sensitivity to nifedipine of smooth muscle from hypertensive rats. J Cardiovasc Pharmacol 8:915–920

Cauvin C, van Breemen C (1986) Membrane Ca^{2+} permeability and calcium antagonistic effects in resistance vessels of spontaneously hypertensive rats. In: Aoki K (ed) Essential hypertension. Calcium mechanisms and treatment. Springer, Berling Heidelberg New York, pp 27–33

Chaignon M, Bellet M, Lucsko M, Rapoud C, Guedon J (1986) Acute and chronic effects of a new calcium inhibitor, nicardipine, on renal hemodynamics in hypertension. J Cardiovasc Pharmacol 8:892–897

Charlap S, Kimmel B, Laifer L, Weinberg P, Singer M, Lazar E, Saltzberg S, Dorsa F, Kafka K, Strom J (1986) Twice-daily nicardipine in the treatment of essential hypertension. J Clin Hypertens 2:271–277

Chatelain P, Demol D, Roba J (1984) Comparison of ^3H nitrendipine binding to heart membranes of normotensive and spontaneously hypertensive rats. J Cardiovasc Pharmacol 6:220–223

Chelly JE, Pool JL, Casar G, Turlapaty P, Laddu AR (1987) Treatment of postoperative hypertension with intravenous nicardipine. Clin Pharmacol Ther 41:209

Chobanian A (1987) Effects of calcium channel antagonists and other antihypertensive drugs on atherogenesis. J Hypertens 5 (Suppl 4) S43–S48

Christensen CK, Lederballe-Pedersen O, Mikkelsen E (1982) Renal effects of acute calcium blockade with nifedipine in hypertensive patients receiving beta-adrenoceptor blocking drugs. Clin Pharmacol Ther 32:572–576

Christopher MA, Harman E, Bell JA (1987) Measurement of steady-state theophylline concentrations before and during concurrent therapy with diltiazem or nifedipine. Drug Intell Clin Pharm 21:4A

Clair F, Bellet M, Guerret M, Druecke T, Grünfeld JP (1985) Hypotensive effect and pharmacokinetics of nicardipine in patients with severe renal failure. Curr Ther Res 38:74–82

Clarke B, Eglen RM, Patmore L, Whiting RL (1984) Cardioselective calcium entry blocking properties of a nicardipine metabolite. Br J Pharmacol 83:437P

Clary C, Schweizer E (1987) Treatment of MAOI hypertensive crisis with sublingual nifedipine. J Clin Psychol 48:249–250

Clement DL, DePue NY (1985) Effect of felodipine and metoprolol on muscle and skin arteries in hypertensive patients. Drugs 29 (Suppl 2):137–143

Cody RJ, Kubo SH, Covit AB, Müller FB, Lopez-Ovejero J, Laragh JH (1986) Exercise hemodynamics and oxygen delivery in human hypotension. Hypertension 8:3–10

Cole SCJ, Flanagan RJ, Johnston A, Holt DW (1981) Rapid high-performance liquid chromatographic method for the measurement of verapamil and norverapamil in blood plasma or serum. J Chromatogr 218:621–629

Condorelli M, Bonaduce D, Ferrara N, Petretta M, Caprio L (1982) Nifedipina en el

tratamiento de la hipertension esencial. Rev Esp Cardiol 35 (Suppl 2):7–12
Conen D, Gerber A, Orfei R, Müller J (1987) Long-term therapy with nitrendipine: effect on cerebral blood flow in elderly hypertensive patients. J Cardiovasc Pharmacol 9 (Suppl 4):S300–S302
Corea L, Miele N, Bentivoglio M, Boschetti E, Agabiti-Rosei E, Muiesan G (1979) Acute and chronic effects of nifedipine on plasma renin activity and plasma adrenaline and noradrenaline in controls and hypertensive patients. Clin Sci 57:115S–117S
Corea L, Alunni G, Bentivoglio M, Boschetti E, Cosmi F, Giaimo MD, Miele N, Motolese M (1980a) Acute and long-term effects of nifedipine on plasma renin activity and plasma catecholamines in controls and hypertensive patients before and after metoprolol. Acta Ther 6:177–189
Corea L, Bentivoglio M, Cosmi F, Alunni G, Prete G, Boschetti E (1980b) Plasma volume before and after treatment of hypertensive acute pulmonary edema with a vasodilating drug (nifedipine). Acta Ther 6:303–313
Corea L, Bentivoglio M, Verdecchia P, Bianchini C (1983) Long-term verapamil therapy in mild to moderate hypertension. Randomized study of normal and slow release formulation. Acta Ther 9:263–274
Corea L, Bentivoglio M, Verdecchia P, Provvidenza M (1984) Calcium antagonists and diuretics in arterial hypertension: a useful combination. In: Reid JL, Pickup AJ (eds) Calcium antagonists and the treatment of hypertension. Royal Society of Medicine, London, pp 23–30
Corsing C, Varchmin G, Stoepel K (1987) Once-daily nitrendipine: therapy in long-term patients with essential hypertension (mild to moderate), efficacy, and tolerance. J Cardiovasc Pharmacol 9 (Suppl 4):S136–S139
Coruzzi P, Biggi A, Musiari L, Ravanetti C, Novarini A (1985) Cadiovascular, baroreflex and humural responses in hypertensive patients during nicardipine therapy. Eur J Clin Pharmacol 29:371–374
Creytens G, Saelin A (1986) Comparative effects of nicardipine hydrochloride and hydrochlorothiazide in the treatment of mild to moderate hypertension: a double-blind parallel study. Br J Clin Pract 40:518–523
Crump BJ, Holt DW, Vale JA (1982) Lack of response to intravenous calcium in severe verapamil poisoning. Lancet (8304):939–940
Cubeddu LX, Aranda J, Singh B, Klein M, Brachfeld J, Freis E, Roman J, Eades T (1986) A comparison of verapamil and propranolol for the initial treatment of hypertension. JAMA 256:2214–2221
Curtis BM, Caterall WA (1984) Purification of the calcium antagonist receptor of the voltage sensitive calcium channel from skeletal muscle transverse tubules. Biochemistry 23:2113–2118
Daniels AR, Opie LH (1986) Atenolol plus nifedipine for mild to moderate systemic hypertension after fixed doses of either agent alone. Am J Cardiol 57:965–970
Da Silva OA, de Melo RA, Filho JPJ (1979) Verapamil acute self-poisoning. Clin Toxicol 14:361–367
Dean S, Kendall MJ (1983) Nifedipine in the treatment of difficult hypertension. Eur J Clin Pharmacol 24:1–5
De Faire U, Lundman T (1977) Attempted suicide with verapamil. Eur J Cardiol 6: 195–198
DelGuercio R, Gentile S (1981) Nifedipina et ipertensione arteriosa essenziale refrattaria a terapia ipotensiva: risultati di up'indagine preliminare in doppio cieco. Clin Ter 96:45–54
DeSimone G, Ferrara LA, DiLorenzo L, Lauria R, Fasano ML (1984) Effects of slow-release nifedipine on left ventricular mass and systolic function in mild to moderate hypertension. Curr Ther Res 36:537–544
DiBona GF (1985) Effects of felodipine on renal functions in animals. Drugs 29 (Suppl 2):168–175
DiBona GF (1987) Effects of vasodilator antihypertensive agents on renal function. J Cardiovasc Pharmacol 9 (Suppl 1):S14–S16
Dominic JA, Bourne DWA, Tan TG, Kirsten EB, McAllister RG (1981) The pharmacology of verapamil. III. Pharmacokinetics in normal subjects after intravenous

drug administration. J Cardiovasc Pharmacol 3:25–38
Donnelly R, Elliott HL, Reid SL (1986) Nicardipine combined with enalapril in patients with essential hypertension. Br J Clin Pharmacol 22 (Suppl 3):283S–287S
Douglas-Jones AP, Coxhead PF (1986) A general practice trial of antihypertensive therapy comparing a combination of nicardipine and chlorthalidone with atenolol and chlorthalidone. Br J Clin Pract 40:100–104
Douglas-Jones AP, Mitchell AD (1984) Comparison of nifedipine (retard formulation) and mefruside in the treatment of mild to moderate hypertension: a prospective randomized double-blind crossover study in general practice. Postgrad Med J 60: 529–532
Dow RJ, Graham DJM (1986) A review of the human metabolism and pharmacokinetics of nicardipine hydrochloride. Br J Pharmacol 22:1955–2025
Doyle AE, Anavekar SN, Oliver LE (1981) A clinical trial of verapamil in the treatment of hypertension. In: Zanchetti A, Krikler D (eds) Calcium antagonism in cardiovascular therapy: experience with verapamil. Excerpta Medica, Amsterdam, pp 252–258
Dustan H (1987) Nitrendipine in black U.S. patients. J Cardiovasc Pharmacol 9 (Suppl 4):S267–S271
Dylewicz P, Kirch W, Benesch L, Ohnhaus EE (1986) Nifedipine-H_2-receptor antagonist interaction in patients with coronary heart disease. In: Lichtlen PR (ed) New therapy of ischaemic heart disease and hypertension. 6th International Adalat Symposium, Geneva, 18–20 April 1985. Excerpta Medica, Amsterdam, pp 71–78
Edgar B, Bengtsson B, Emfeldt D, Lundborg P, Nyberg G, Rauer S, Rönn O (1985) Acute diuretic/natriuretic properties of felodipine in man. Drugs 29 (Suppl 2): 176–184
Edmonds D, Würth JP, Baumgart P, Vetter W, Vetter H (1987) Twenty-four-hour monitoring of blood pressure during calcium antagonist therapy. In: Fleckenstein A, Laragh JA (eds) Hypertension—the next decade: verapamil in focus. Churchill Livingstone, Edinburgh, pp 94–100
Eggertsen R, Hansson L (1982) Effects of treatment with nifedipine and metoprolol in essential hypertension. Eur J Clin Pharmacol 21:389–390
Eichelbaum M, Ende M, Remberg G, Schomerus M, Dengler HJ (1979) The metabolism of ^{14}C-D,L-verapamil in man. Drug Metab Dispos 7:145–148
Eliahou HE, Iaina A, Schneider R, Cohen D, Goldfarb D, Gross M (1982) Treatment of hypertension in dialysis and essential hypertension patients with nifedipine. Clin Exp Dial Apheresis 6:299–336
Ene MD, Williamson PJ, Roberts CJ, Waddell G (1985) The natriuresis following oral administration of the calcium antagonists—nifedipine and nitrendipine. Br J Clin Pharmacol 19:423–427
Erne P, Bolli P, Bertel O, Hulthén L, Kiowski W, Müller FB, Bühler F (1983) Factors influencing the hypotensive effects of calcium antagonists. Hypertension 5 (Suppl II):II97–II102
Erne P, Bolli P, Bürgisser E, Bühler FR (1984) Correlation of platelet calcium with blood pressure. N Engl J Med 310:1084–1088
Esper RJ, Esper RC, Baglivo HP, Castro JM, Rohwedder RW, Menna J (1984) Long-term effectiveness of BAY E 5009—nitrendipine—in the treatment of mild and moderate arterial hypertension. J Cardiovasc Pharmacol 6:S1096–S1099
Etingin OR, Hajjar DP (1984) Nifedipine increases arterial cholesterylester hydrolysis in vitro. Clin Res 32:163A
Etoh A, Kohno K, Shimizu T (1983) Studies on the drug interaction of diltiazem. II. Effect of co-administered diltiazem on the bioavailability of propranolol. J Pharm Soc Jpn 103:434–444
Fagan TC, Sternleib C, Vlachakis N, Deedwania PC, Metha JLC (1984) Efficacy and safety comparison of nitrendipine and hydralazine as antihypertensive monotherapy. J Cardiovasc Pharmacol 6:S1109–S1113
Fagan T, Brown R, Schnaper H, Smolens P, Montijo M, Michelsen E (1986) Nicardipine and hydrochlorothiazide in essential hypertension. Acta Pharmacol Toxicol 59 (Suppl 5):176

Fan F, Wright RA, Pacheco J, Horwitz L (1986) Use of nifedipine as 1st line therapy for mild hypertension. Clin Res 34:816A
Farringer JA, Green JA, O'Rourke RA, Linn WA, Clementi WA (1984) Nifedipine-induced alterations in serum quinidine concentrations. Am Heart J:1570–1572
Faulhaber HD, Gruner R, Rostock G, Naumann E, Hartrodt W (1987) Antihypertensive treatment with nitrendipine in mild and moderate arterial hypertension: long-term effects on plasma catecholamines and active renin. J Cardiovasc Pharmacol 9 (Suppl 4):S194–196
Ferguson RK, Vlasses PH, Michelson EL, Rush SE, Sawin HS, Langendorfer A, Lipschutz KH (1986) Enalapril and nifedipine, alone and combined, in essential hypertension. Chest 89 (Suppl):495S
Ferrara LA, DeSimone G, Mancini M, Fasano ML, Pasanisi F (1985) Changes in left ventricular mass during a double-blind study with chlorthalidone and slow-release nifedipine. Eur J Clin Pharmacol 27:525–528
Ferreira-Filho SR, Saragoca MA, Oliveira PC, Moriguti J, Ajzen H, Ramos OL (1987) Use of nitrendipine in the treatment of systolic hypertension in elderly patients. J Cardiovasc Pharmacol 9 (Suppl 4):S218–S220
Fleckenstein A (1968) Myokardstoffwechsel und Nekrose. In: Heilmeyer L, Holtmeier HS (eds) Herzinfarkt und Schock. Thieme, Stuttgart, pp 94–109
Fleckenstein A (1983) Calcium antagonism in heart and smooth muscle. Experimental facts and therapeutic prospects. Wiley, New York,
Fleckenstein A, Grün G (1969) Reversible blockade of excitation-contraction coupling in rat's uterine smooth muscle by means of organic calcium antagonists (iproveratril, D600, prenylamine). Pflugers Arch Gesamte Physiol 307:26
Fleckenstein A, Frey M, von Witzleben H (1983) Vascular calcium overload—a pathogenic factor in arteriosclerosis and its neutralization by calcium antagonists. In: Kaltenbach M, Neufeld HN (eds) New therapy of ischemic heart disease and hypertension. 5th International adalat symposium. Excerpta Medica, Amsterdam, pp 36–52
Fleckenstein A, Frey M, Zorn S, Fleckenstein-Grün G (1985) Experimental basis of the long-term therapy of arterial hypertension with calcium antagonists. Am J Cardiol 56:3H–14H
Follath F, Ha HR, Schütz E, Bühler F (1986) Pharmacokinetics of conventional and slow-release verapamil. Br J Clin Pharmacol 21 (Suppl 2):149S–153S
Forette F, Bellet M, Henry JF, Hervy MP, Poyard-Salmeron C, Bouchacourt P, Guerret M (1985) Effect of nicardipine in elderly hypertensive patients. Br J Clin Pharmacol 20 (Suppl 1):125S–129S
Foster TS, Hamann SR, Richards VR, Bryant PJ, Graves DA, McAllister RG (1983) Nifedipine kinetics and bioavailability after single intravenous oral doses in normal subjects. J Clin Pharmacol 23:161–171
Fouad FM, Pedrinelli R, Bravo EL, Textor SC, Tarazi RC (1984) Clinical and systemic hemodynamic effects of nitrendipine. Clin Pharmacol Ther 35:768–775
Francischetti EA, Oigman W, de Genellin A, Fagundes V, Sanjuliani AF, da Conceicao Cumha M (1987) Long-term therapy with nitrendipine; evaluation of its antihypertensive and metabolic effects. J Cardiovasc Pharmacol 9 (Suppl 4):S107–S112
Franz J-W, Wiewel D (1984) Antihypertensive effects on blood pressure at rest and during exercise of calcium antagonists, β-receptor blockers and their combination in hypertensive patients. J Cardiovasc Pharmacol 6:S1037–S1042
Frishman WH, Klein NA, Klein P, Strom JA, Tawil R, Strair R, Wong B, Roth S, LeJantel TH, Pollack S, Sonnenblick EH (1982) Comparison of oral propranolol and verapamil for combined systemic hypertension and angina pectoris. Am J Cardiol 50:1164–1172
Frishman W, Charlap S, Kimmel B, Lazar E, Weinberg P, Dorsa F (1985a) Ineffectiveness of twice-daily oral nicardipine in systemic hypertension. Clin Res 33:361A
Frishman WH, Kirkendall W, Lunn J, McCarron D, Moser M, Schnaper H, Smith LK, Sowers J, Swartz S, Zawada E (1985b) Diuretics versus calcium-channel blockers in systemic hypertension: a preliminary multicenter experience with hydrochlorothiazide and sustained-release diltiazem. Am J Cardiol 56:92H–96H
Frishman WH, Charlap S, Goldberger J, Kimmel B, Stroh J (1985c) Comparison of

diltiazem and nifedipine for both angina pectoris and systemic hypertension. Am J Cardiol 56:41H–46H

Frishman WH, Zawada ET Jr, Smith LK, Sowers J, Swartz SL, Kirkendall W, Lunn J, McCarron D, Moser M, Schnaper H (1987) Comparison of hydrochlorothiazide and sustained-release diltiazem for mild to moderate systemic hypertension. Am J Cardiol 59:615–623

Fritschka E, Distler A, Gotzen R, Thiede H-M, Philipp T (1984) Crossover comparison of nitrendipine with propranolol in patients with essential hypertension. J Cardiovasc Pharmacol 6:S1100–S1104

Frohlich ED (1986) Hemodynamic effects of diltiazem in the spontaneously hypertensive rat and in human hypertension. In: Aoki K (ed) Essential hypertension. Calcium mechanisms and treatment. Springer, Berlin Heidelberg New York, pp 191–218

Funyu T, Nigawara K, Ohno K, Hamada W, Yagihashi Y (1981) Effects of benzothiazepine derivative (CRD-401) on blood pressure, excretion of electrolytes, and plasma renin activity. Clin Ther 3:456–466

Gangji D, Juvent M, Niset G, Wathieu M, Degreve M, Bellens R, Poortmans J, Degre S, Fitzscimons TJ, Herchulez A (1984) Study of the influence of nifedipine on the pharmacokinetics and pharmacodynamics of propranolol, metoprolol and atenolol. Br J Clin Pharmacol 17:29S–35S

Garthoff B, Bellemann P (1987) Effect of salt loading and nitrendipine on dihydropyridine receptors in hypertensive rats. J Cardiovasc Pharmacol 10 (Suppl 10):36–39

Garthoff B, Kazda S (1981) Calcium antagonist nifedipine normalizes high blood pressure and prevents mortality in salt loaded DS substrain of Dahl rats. Eur J Pharmacol 74:111–113

Garthoff B, Kazda S, Knorr A, Thomas G (1983) Factors involved in the antihypertensive action of calcium antagonists. Hypertension 5 (Suppl II):II34–II38

Garthoff B, Kazda S, Knorr A, Luckhaus G, Stoepel K (1984) Pharmacology of a new antihypertensive calcium antagonist: nitrendipine. In: Scriabine A, Vanov S, Deck K (eds) Nitrendipine. Urban and Schwarzenberg, Baltimore, pp 11–24

Gavras I, Gavras H (1985) Nifedipine in the treatment of essential hypertension. J Clin Pharmacol 24:429–432

Gelbke HP, Schlicht HJ, Schmidt G (1977) Fatal poisoning with verapamil. Arch Toxicol 37:89–94

Gelman JS, Feldman RL, Scott E, Pepine CJ (1985) Nicardipine for angina pectoris at rest and coronary arterial spasm. Am J Cardiol 36:232–236

Gennari C, Nami R, Bianchini C, Pavese G (1987) Nitrendipine and the angiotensin converting enzyme inhibitors in the treatment of hypertension. J Cardiovasc Pharmacol 9 (Suppl 4):S245–S251

Gheorgiade M, St Clair C, St Clair J, Freeman D, Schwemer G (1985) Short- and long-term treatment of stable effort angina with nicardipine, a new calcium channel blocker: a double-blind placebo-controlled, randomized, repeated crossover study. Br J Clin Pharmacol 20 (Suppl 1):195S–205S

Gibelin P, Maccario M, Lapalus P, Morand P (1984) Intentional overdose with diltiazem. Presse Med 13:754

Giebisch G, Guckian VA, Klein-Robbenhaar G, Klein-Robbenhaar MT (1987) Renal clearance and micropuncture studies of nisoldipine effects in spontaneously hypertensive rats. J Cardiovasc Pharmacol 9 (Suppl 1):S24–S31

Giles TD, Sander GE, Roffidal LE, Thomas MG, Given MB, Quiroz AC (1987) A comparison of nitrendipine and hydrochlorothiazide on exercise in older patients with hypertension. J Cardiovasc Pharmacol 9 (Suppl 4):S190–S193

Giuntoli F, Guidi G, Scalabrino A, Galeone F, Pagliali E, Morini S, Binudelli A, Saba P (1981) Nifedipine as single drug therapy in hypertension. Curr Ther Res 30:447–452

Glossmann H, Ferry DR, Goll A, Striessnig J, Zernick G (1985) Calcium channels: introduction into their molecular pharmacology. In: Fleckenstein A, van Breemen C, Groß R, Hoffmeister A (eds) Cardiovascular effects of dihydropyridine-type calcium antagonists and agonists. Springer, Berlin Heidelberg New York, pp 113–139

Godfraind T, Kaba A (1969) Blockade or reversal of the contraction induced by calcium and adrenaline in depolarized arterial smooth muscle. Br J Pharmacol 35:549–560

Godfraind T, Kaba A (1972) The role of calcium in the actions of drugs on vascular smooth muscle. Arch Int Pharmacodyn Ther 196 (Suppl):35–49

Godfraind T, Polster P (1968) Etude comparative de médicaments inhibant la réponse contractile de vaisseaux isolés d'origine humaine ou animale. Therapie 23:1209–1230

Gottlieb TB, Katz FH, Chidsey CH (1972) Continued therapy with vasodilator drugs and beta adrenergic blockade in hypertension. A comparative study of mindoxidil and hydralazin. Circulation 45:571–582

Gould BA, Mann S, Kieso H, Subramanian VB, Raftery EB (1982) The 24-hour ambulatory blood pressure profile with verapamil. Circulation 65:22–27

Graham DJM, Dow RJ, Freedman D, Mroszczak E, Ling T (1984) Pharmacokinetics of nicardipine following oral and intravenous administration in man. Postgrad Med J 60 (Suppl 4):7–10

Green JA, Clementi WA, Porter C, Stigelman W (1983) Nifedipine-quinidine interaction. Clin Pharm 2:461–465

Guazzi MD (1983) Use of the calcium channel blocking agents in the treatment of systemic arterial hypertension. In: Stone PH, Antman EM (eds) Calcium channel blocking agents in the treatment of cardiovascular disorders. Futura, Mount Kisco NY, pp 377–402

Guazzi MD, Olivari MT, Polese A, Fiorentini C, Magrini T, Moruzzi P (1977) Nifedipine, a new antihypertensive with rapid action. Clin Pharmacol Ther 22:528–532

Guazzi MD, Fiorentini C, Olivari MT, Bartorelli A, Mecchi G, Polese A (1980) Short- and long-term efficacy of a calcium antagonistic agent (nifedipine) combined with methyldopa in the treatment of severe hypertension. Circulation 61:913–919

Guazzi MD, Polese A, Fiorentini C, Bartorelli A, Moruzzi P (1983) Treatment of hypertension with calcium antagonists. Hypertension 5:II85–II90

Guazzi MD, De Cesare N, Galli C, Salvioni A, Tramontana C, Tamborini G, Bartorelli A (1984) Calcium channel blockade with nifedipine and angiotensin converting enzyme inhibition with captopril in the therapy of patients with severe primary hypertension. Hypertension 70:279–284

Guengerich FB, Martin MV, Beane PH, Kremers P, Wolff T, Waxman DJ (1986) Characterization of rat and human liver microsomal cytochrome P-450 forms involved in nifedipine oxidation, a prototype for genetic polymorphism in oxidative drug metabolism. J Biol Chem 261:5051–5060

Haeberle DA, Kawata T, Davis JM (1987) The site of action of nitrendipine in the rat kidney. J Cardiovasc Pharmacol 9 (Suppl 1):S17–S23

Hagino K (1986) Application of proveratril in the pharmatherapy of hypertension. Jpn J Clin Exp Med 45:208–215

Hallin L, Andren L, Hansson L (1983) Controlled trial of nifedipine and bendroflumethiazide in hypertension. J Cardiovasc Pharmacol 5:1083–1085

Hamann SR, Todd GD, McAllister RG (1983) The pharmacology of verapamil. V. Tissue distribution of verapamil and norverapamil in rat and dog. Pharmacology 27:1–8

Hamann SR, Blovin RA. McAllister RG (1984) Clinical pharmacokinetics of verapamil. Clin Pharmacokinet 9:26–41

Hansson L, Andrén L, Orö L, Ryman T (1984) The antihypertensive effects and pharmacokinetics of nitrendipine in patients with essential hypertension. In: Scriabine A, Vanov S, Deck K (eds) Nitrendipine. Urban and Schwarzenberg, Baltimore, pp 423–433

Harris AL, Swamy VC, Triggle DJ (1984) Calcium reactivity and antagonism in portal veins from spontaneously hypertensive and normotensive rats. Can J Physiol Pharmacol 62:146–150

Heagerty AM, Swales JD (1987) The combination of verapamil and captopril in the treatment of essential hypertension. Pharmatherapeutica 5:21–25

Hedbäck B, Herrmann LS (1983) Antihypertensive effect of verapamil in patients with newly discovered mild to moderate essential hypertension. Acta Med Scand 681 (Suppl):129–135

Henry PD (1980) Comparative pharmacology of calcium antagonists: nifedipine, verapamil and diltiazem. Am J Cardiol 46:1047–1058

Henry PD (1982) Comparative cardiac pharmacology of calcium blockers. In: Flaim SF, Zelis R (eds) Calcium blockers. Mechanisms of action and clinical application. Urban and Schwarzenberg, Baltimore, pp 135–153

Henry PD, Bentley KI (1981) Suppression of atherogenesis in cholesterol-fed rabbit treated with nifedipine. J Clin Invest 68:1366–1369

Henry PD, Borda L, Shuchleib R (1979) Chronotropic and inotropic effects of vasodilators. In: Lichtlen PR, Kimura E, Taira N (eds) International Adalat panel discussion. New experimental and clinical results. Excerpta Medica, Amsterdam, pp 14–21

Hermann P, Morselli PL (1985) Pharmacokinetics of diltiazem and other calcium entry blockers. Acta Pharmacol Toxicol 57 (Suppl II):12–20

Herrington DM, Insley DM, Weinmann GG (1986) Nifedipine overdose. Am J Med 81:344–346

Higuchi S, Shiobara Y (1980) Comparative pharmacokinetics of nicardipine hydrochloride, a new vasodilator, in various species. Xenobiotica 10:447–454

Higuchi S, Sasaki H, Sado T (1975) Determination of a new cerebral vasodilator 2,6-dimethyl-4-(-3-nitrophenyl)-1,4-dihydropyridine-3,5-dicarboxylic acid 3-(2-N-benzyl-N-methylamino)-ethylester, 5-methylester hydrochloride (YC-93) in plasma by electron capture gas chromatography. J Chromatogr 110:301–307

Höffler D, Stoepel K (1984) Nitrendipine in hypertension that is difficult to control. J Cardiovasc Pharmacol 6:S1060–S1062

Hof RP (1983) Patterns of regional blood flow changes induced by five different calcium antagonists. Prog Pharmacol 5:71–82

Holloway ET, Bohr DF (1973) Reactivity of vascular smooth muscle in hypertensive rats. Circ Res 33:678–685

Hoon TJ, Baumann JL, Rodvold KA, Gallestegul J, Hariman RJ (1986) The pharmacodynamic and pharmacokinetic differences of the D- and L-isomers of verapamil: implications in the treatment of paroxysmal supraventricular tachycardia. Am Heart J 112:396–403

Hornung RS, Gould BA, Jones RI, Sonecha T, Raftery EB (1983) Nifedipine tablets for hypertension: a study using continuous ambulatory intra-arterial recording. Postgrad Med J 59 (Suppl 2):95–97

Hornung RS, Jones RI, Gould BA, Sonecha T, Raftery EB (1984) Propranolol versus verapamil for the treatment of essential hypertension. Am Heart J 108:554–560

Horster FA (1975) Pharmacokinetics of nifedipine-^{14}C in man. In: Lochner W, Braasch W, Kroneberg G (eds) 2nd international adalat symposium 1975. New therapy of ischemic heart disease. Springer, Berlin Heidelberg New York, pp 82–91

Hossak KF (1982) Conduction abnormalities due to diltiazem. N Engl J Med 307: 953–954

Hossak KF, Pool PE, Steele P, Crawford MH, DeMaria AN, Cohen LS, Ports TA (1982) Efficacy of diltiazem in angina on effort: a multicenter trial. Am J Cardiol 49:567–572

Hulthén UL, Landmann R, Bürgisser E, Bühler FR (1982a) High-affinity binding sites for [^{3}H] verapamil in cardiac membranes. J Cardiovasc Pharmacol 4 (Suppl 3): S291–S293

Hulthén UL, Bolli P, Amann FW, Kiowski W, Bühler FR (1982b) Enhanced vasodilation in essential hypertension by calcium channel blockade of verapamil. Hypertension 4 (Suppl 2):26–31

Hulthén UL, Bolli P, Bühler FR (1985) Vasodilatory effect of nicardipine and verapamil in the forearm of hypertension as compared to normotensive man. Br J Clin Pharmacol 20 (Suppl 1):62S–66S

Hung J, Lamb I, Connolly SJ, Jutzy KR, Goris ML, Schroeder JS (1983) The effect of diltiazem and propranolol, alone and in combination, on exercise performance and left ventricular function in patients with stable effort angina: double-blind, randomized, and placebo-controlled study. Circulation 68:560–567

Husted SE, Kraemmer NH, Christensen CK, Lederballe-Pedersen O (1982) Long-term therapy of arterial hypertension with nifedipine given alone or in combination with a beta-adrenoceptor blocking agent. Eur J Clin Pharmacol 22:101–103

Ikeda M (1978) Double-blind studies on diltiazem in essential hypertensive patients receiving thiazide therapy. In: Bing RJ (ed) New drug therapy with a calcium antagonist. Excerpta Medica, Amsterdam, pp 243–253

Imai Y, Abe K, Otsuka Y, Irokawa N, Yasujima M, Saito K, Sakurai Y, Chiba S, Ito T, Sato M, Haruyama T, Miura Y, Yoshinaga K (1980) Management of severe hypertensive with nifedipine in combination with clonidine or propranolol. Arzneimittelforschung Drug Res 30:674–678

Imamura T, Koiwaya Y, Nakamura M (1986) Sinoatrial block induced by oral diltiazem. Clin Cardiol 9:33–34

Immonen P, Linkola A, Waris E (1981) Three cases of severe verapamil poisoning. Int J Cardiol 1:101–105

Inouye IK, Massie BM, Benowitz N, Simpson P, Loge D (1984) Antihypertensive therapy with diltiazem and comparison with hydrochlorothiazide. Am J Cardiol 53:1588–1592

Ishii H, Itoh K, Nose T (1980) Different antihypertensive effects of nifedipine in conscious experimental hypertensive and normotensive rats. Eur J Pharmacol 64:21–29

Ishii K, Kano T, Kurobe Y, Amdo J (1983) Binding of ^{3}H—nitrendipine to heart and brain membranes from normotensive and spontaneously hypertensive rats. Eur J Pharmacol 88:277–278

Ishikawa T, Imamura T, Kiowaya Y, Tanaka K (1983) Atrioventricular dissociation and sinus arrest induced by oral diltiazem. N Engl J Med 309:1124–1125

Isles CG, Johnson AO, Milne FJ (1986) Slow release nifedipine and atenolol as initial treatment in blacks with malignant hypertension. Br J Pharmacol 21:377–383

Iwanami M, Shibanuma I, Fujimoto M, Kawai R, Tamazawa K, Takenaka T, Takahashi K, Murakami M (1979) Synthesis of new water-soluble dihydropyridine vasodilators. Chem Pharm Bull (Tokyo) 27:1426–1440

Jain AK, McMahon FG, Ryan JR, Marande R, Vlachakis N, Mroczek W (1984) Efficacy and safety of nitrendipine in patients with severe hypertension: a multiclinic study. J Cardiovasc Pharmacol 6:S1053–S1059

Jean P, Hayek Lanthois M, Hermann P (1985) Acute poisoning with diltiazem: report of a case. Clin Toxicol 23:447–448

Johns EJ (1984) The effect of acute administration of diltiazem and nifedipine on the function of denervated rat kidney. Br J Pharmacol 82 (Suppl):328 P

Johns EJ (1985) The influence of diltiazem and nifedipine on renal function in the rat. Br J Pharmacol 84:707–713

Johns EJ, Manitius J (1987) The renal actions of nitrendipine and its influence on the neural regulation of calcium and sodium reabsorption in the rat. J Cardiovasc Pharmacol 9 (Suppl 1):S49–S56

Johnson BF, Romero L, Marwaka R (1986) Hemodynamic and metabolic effects of the calcium channel blocking agent nitrendipine. Clin Pharmacol Ther 39:389–394

Johnston A, Burgess CD, Hamer J (1981) Systemic availability of oral verapamil and effect on PR interval in man. Br J Clin Pharmacol 12:397–400

Kawajima I, Ueda K, Kamata C, Matsushita S, Karamoto K, Marakawi M, Hada Y (1978) A study on the effects of nifedipine in hypertensive crises and severe hypertension. Jpn Heart J 19:455–467

Kazda S (1986) Effects of nitrendipine on vascular integrity. Am J Cardiol 58:31D–34D

Kazda S (1987) Discussion. J Cardiovasc Pharmacol 9 (Suppl 4):95

Kazda S, Scriabine A (1986) Pharmacology of nifedipine. In: Krebs R (ed) Treatment of cardiovascular diseases by Adalat^R (nifedipine). Schattauer, Stuttgart, pp 43–92

Kazda S, Garthoff B, Meyer H, Schloßmann K, Stoepel K, Towart R, Vater W, Wehinger E (1980) Pharmacology of a new calcium antagonistic compound, isobutyl methyl 1,4 dihydro-2,6-dimethyl-4-(2 nitrophenyl)-3,5-pyridine carboxylate (nisoldipine, BAY K 5552). Arzneimittelforschung Drug Res 30:2144–2162

Kazda S, Garthoff B, Thomas G (1982a) Antihypertensive effect of calcium antagonists in rats differs from that of vasodilators. Clin Sci 63:S363–S365

Kazda S, Garthoff B, Thomas G (1982b) Antihypertensive effect of a calcium antagonistic drug: regression of hypertensive cardiac hypertrophy by nifedipine. Drug Dev Res 2:313–323

Kazda S, Garthoff B, Knorr A (1983a) Nitrendipine and other calcium entry blockers

(calcium antagonists) in hypertension. Fed Proc 42:196–200
Kazda S, Garthoff B, Luckhaus G (1983b) Calcium antagonists in hypertensive disease: experimental evidence for a new therapeutic concept. Postgrad Med J 59 (Suppl 2): 78–83
Kazda S, Garthoff B, Luckhaus G (1983c) Calcium antagonists prevent brain damage in stroke-prone spontaneously hypertensive rats independent of their effect on blood pressure. J Cereb Blood Flow Metab 3 (Suppl 1):S526–S527
Kazda S, Knorr A, Towart R (1983d) Common properties and differences between various calcium antagonists. Prog Pharmacol 5:83–116
Kazda S, Garthoff B, Luckhaus G (1984) Mode of antihypertensive action of nitrendipine. J Cardiovasc Pharmacol 6 (Suppl 7):S956–S962
Kazda S, Garthoff B, Knorr A (1985) Interference of the calcium antagonist nisoldipine with the abnormal response of vessels from hypertensive rats to α-adrenergic stimulation. J Cardiovasc Pharmacol 7 (Suppl 6):S61–S65
Kazda S, Garthoff B, Luckkaus G (1986a) Calcium and malignant hypertension in animal experiments: effects of experimental manipulation of calcium influx. Am J Nephrol 6 (Suppl 1):145–150
Kazda S, Garthoff B, Hirth C, Preis W, Stasch JP (1986b) Parathyroidectomy mimics the protective effect of the calcium antagonist nimodipine in salt loaded stroke-prone spontaneously hypertensive rats. J Hypertens 4 (Suppl 3):S483–S485
Kazda S, Stasch JP, Hirth C (1987a) Nitrendipine in experimental hypertension: effects on cardiac hypertrophy, heart failure and atrial natriuretic peptides. J Cardiovasc Pharmacol 9 (Suppl 4):590–595
Kazda S, Grunt M, Hirth C, Preis W, Stasch J-P (1987b) Calcium antagonism and protection of tissues from calcium damage. J Hypertens 5 (Suppl 4):S37–S42
Kendall MJ, Jack DB, Laugher SJ, Lobo J, Smith SR (1984) Lack of a pharmacokinetic interaction between nifedipine and the β-adrenoceptor blockers metoprolol and atenolol. Br J Clin Pharmacol 18:331–335
Kendall MJ, Lobo J, Jack DB, Main ANH (1987) The influence of age on the pharmacokinetics of nitrendipine. J Cardiovasc Pharmacol 9 (Suppl 4):S96–S100
Kindermann W, Widmann W, Rieder TH, Kullmer TH (1987) Physical fitness during antihypertensive treatment: results of combined treatment with a calcium antagonist and a beta blocker. Fortschr Med 105:75–81
Kindler J, Planz G, Giani G, Clasen W, Homburg A, Kierdorf H (1987) Comparison of nitrendipine and dihydralazine in a triple combination therapy in moderate and severe arterial hypertension. J Cardiovasc Pharmacol 9 (Suppl 4): S256–S262
Kinoshita M, Kusakawa R, Shimono Y, Motomura M, Tomonaga G, Hoshino T (1979) The effect of diltiazem hydrochloride upon sodium diuresis and renal function in congestive heart failure. Arzneimittelforschung Drug Res 29:676–681
Kiowski W, Bühler FR, Fadayomi MO, Erne P, Müller FB, Hulthén UL, Bolli P (1985) Age, race, blood pressure and renin predictors for antihypertensive treatment with calcium antagonists. Am J Cardiol 56:81H–85H
Kiowski W, Erne P, Bertel O, Bolli P, Bühler F (1986) Acute and chronic sympathetic reflex activation and antihypertensive response to nifedipine. J Am Coll Cardiol 7:344–348
Kirch W, Hoensch H, Ohnhaus EE, Janisch HD (1984a) Ranitidin-Nifedipine-Interaktion. Dtsch Med Wochenschr 109:1223
Kirch W, Hutt HJ, Heidemann H, Rämsch K, Janisch HD, Ohnhaus EE (1984b) Drug interactions with nitrendipine. J Cardiovasc Pharmacol 6:S982–S985
Kirchheim H, Gross R (1975) Hemodynamic effects of Adalat in unanestethized dog. In: Lochner W, Braasch W, Kroneberg G (eds) 2nd International adalat symposium 1975. New therapy of ischemic heart disease. Springer, Berlin Heidelberg New York, pp 82–91
Kirkendall WM, Adlin V, Canzanello V, Cubberley R, Haider B, MacCarthy P, Mroczek W, Nelson E, Schoenberger J, Solomon R (1987) Comparative study of the safety and effectiveness of nitrendipine, atenolol and hydrochlorothiazide in combination in the treatment of hypertension. J Cardiovasc Pharmacol 9 (Suppl 4) S232–S237
Kishi Y, Okumura F, Furuya H (1984) Haemodynamic effects of nicardipine hydrochlo-

ride. Studies during its use to control acute hypertension in anaesthetized patients. Br J Anaesth 56:1003–1007

Klein HO, Lang R, Weiss E, Desegni E, Libhaber C, Fuerrero J, Kaphinsky E (1982) The influence of verapamil on serum digoxin concentrations. Circulation 65:998–1003

Klein W, Brandt D, Vrecko K, Härringer M (1983) Role of calcium antagonists in the treatment of essential hypertension. Circ Res 52 (Suppl I):174–181

Kleinbloesem CH, van Brummelen P, Faber H, Danhoff M, Vermeulen NPE, Breimer DD (1984a) Variability in nifedipine pharmacokinetics and dynamics: a new oxidation polymorphism in man. Biochem Pharmacol 33:3721–3724.

Kleinbloesem CH, van Brummelen P, van der Linde JA, Voogd PJ, Breimer DD (1984b) Nifedipine: kinetics and dynamics in healthy subjects. Clin Pharmacol Ther 35:742–749

Kleinbloesem CH, van Brummelen P, van Harten J, Danhoff M, Breimer DD (1985a) Nifedipine: influence of renal function on pharmacokinetic/hemodynamic relationship. Clin Pharmacol Ther 37:563–574

Kleinbloesem CH, van Harten J, Wilson JPH, van Brummelen P, Danhof M, Breimer DD (1985b) Nifedipine: kinetics and haemodynamic effects in patients with liver cirrhosis after i.v. and oral administration. PhD thesis of CH Kleinbloesem, University of Leiden, Netherlands

Kluetsch K, Schmidt P, Grosswendt J (1972) Der Einfluß von BAY A 1040 auf die Nierenfunktionen des Hypertonikers. Arzneimittelforschung Drug Res 22:377–380

Knorr A (1982) Nisoldipine (BAY K K 5552), a new calcium antagonist. Antihypertensive effect in conscious, unrestrained renal hypertensive dogs. Arch Int Pharmacodyn 260:141–150

Knorr A, Garthoff B (1984) Differential influence of the calcium antagonist nitrendipine and the vasodilator hydralazine on normal and elevated blood pressure. Arch Int Pharmacodyn Ther 269:396–322

Knorr A, Stoepel K (1981) Effect of a new calcium antagonist, nitrendipine on blood pressure and heart rate of conscious, unrestrained dogs. Arzneimittelforschung Drug Res 31:2062–2064

Knorr A, Hirth C, Stasch JP, Kazda S, Luckhaus G (1987) Antihypertensive and tissue protective effects of nitrendipine. In: Rand MJ, Raper C (eds) Pharmacology. Elsevier Science, Amsterdam pp 517–522

Kobrin I, Sesoko S, Pegram BL, Frohlich ED (1984) Reduced cardiac mass by nitrendipine is dissociated from systemic or regional hemodynamic changes in rats. Cardiovasc Res 18:158–162

Koch-Weser J (1974) Vasodilating drugs in the treatment of hypertension. Arch Intern Med 133:1017–1019

Kölle EV, Ochs HR, Vollmer KO (1983) Pharmacokinetic model of Diltiazem. Arzneimittelforschung Drug Res 33:972–977

König B, Eckardt A (1984) Isoptin^{R} -RR bei ambulanten Patienten mit essentieller Hypertonie. Therapiewoche 34:7009–7015

Kolloch R, Stumpe KO, Overlack A (1985) Blood pressure, heart rate and AV-conduction responses to nicardipine in hypertensive patients receiving atenolol. Br J Clin Pharmacol 20 (Suppl 1):130S–134S

Krebs R (1983) Adverse reactions with calcium antagonists. Hypertension 5 (Suppl II): 125–129

Krol GJ, Lettieri JT, Yeh SC, Burkholder DE, Birkett JP (1987) Disposition and pharmacokinetics of ^{14}C-nitrendipine in healthy volunteers. J Cardiovasc Pharmacol 9 (Suppl 4):S122–S128

Krüger P (1984) Suicide attempts with isoptin (verapamil). 2 Case reports. Therapiewoche 34:2483–2491

Krussel LR, Christensen CK, Pedersen OL (1987) Acute natriuretic effect of nifedipine in hypertensive patients and normotensive controls—a proximal tubular effect? Eur J Clin Pharmacol 32:121–126

Kubo K, Shiraishi K, Muto H, Suzuki T, Sugino N (1983) Treatment of hypertension in haemodialysis patients with nifedipine. Hypertension 5 (Suppl II):109–112

Kugita H, Inoue H, Ikezaki M, Konda M, Takeo S (1971) Synthesis of 1,5-benzothiazipine derivatives. III. Chem Pharm Bull (Tokyo) 19:595–602

Kuhlmann J, Marcin S (1983) Lack of significant effect of nifedipine and diltiazem on the pharmacokinetic of digitoxin. Proc IInd world conference on clinical pharmacology and therapeutics, Washington DC, 31 July–5 August 1983, p 136 (abstract 792)

Kuhlmann J, Marcin S (1985) Effects of verapamil on pharmacokinetics and pharmacodynamics of digitoxin in patients. Am Heart J 110:1245–1250

Kuhlmann J, Marcin S, Frank KH (1983) Effects of nifedipine and diltiazem on the pharmacokinetics of digoxin. Naunyn Schmiedebergs Arch Pharmacol 324 (Suppl): R81

Kuhlmann J, Graefe K-H, Rämsch K-D, Ziegler R (1986) Clinical pharmacology, Chapter V. In: Krebs R (ed) Treatment of cardiovascular diseases by Adalat[R] (nifedipine). Schattauer, Stuttgart, pp 93–144

Kusano E, Asono Y, Takeda K, Matsumoto Y, Ebihara A, Hosoda S (1982) Hypotensive effect of nifedipine in hypertensive patients with chronic renal failure. Arzneimittelforschung 32:1575–1580

Landmark K (1986) Antihypertensive and diuretic effects of long-term nifedipine therapy. In: Lichtlen P (ed) 6th International Adalat[R] symposium. New Therapy of ischaemic heart disease and hypertension. Excerpta Medica, Amsterdam, pp 521–527

Landmark K, Dale J (1985) Antihypertensive, haemodynamic and metabolic effects of nifedipine slow-release tablets in elderly patients. Acta Med Scand 218:389–396

Lang R, Degenhardt, Ollenschläger G, Barth A (1987) Effect of a low-dose combination nitrendipine/enalapril in less-severe degrees of hypertension. J Cardiovasc Pharmacol 1 (Suppl 4):S254–S255

Lasseter KC, Shamblen EC, Murdoch AA, Burkholder DE, Krol GJ, Taylor RJ, Vanov SK (1984) Steady-state pharmacokinetics of nitrendipine in hepatic insufficiency. J Cardiovasc Pharmacol 6:S977–S981

Lederballe Pedersen O, Mikkelsen E, Christensen NJ, Kornerup HJ, Pedersen EB (1971) Effect of nifedipine on plasma renin, aldosterone and catecholamines in arterial hypertension. Eur J Clin Pharmacol 15:235–245

Lederballe Pedersen O, Mikkelsen E, Anderson KE (1977) Increased Ca^{2+}-dependency in aorta and portal vein of the spontaneously hypertensive rat—increased sensitivity to nifedipine. Acta Pharmacol Toxicol 41 (Suppl 4):61–65

Lederballe Pedersen O, Mikkelsen E (1978) Acute and chronic effects of nifedipine in arterial hypertension. Eur J Clin Pharmacol 14:375–381

Lederballe Pedersen O, Christensen CK, Mikkelsen E, Rämsch KD (1980) Relationship between the antihypertensive effect and steady-state plasma concentration of nifedipine given alone or in combination with a beta-adrenoceptor blocking agent. Eur J Clin Pharmacol 18:287–293

Lederballe Pedersen O, Krusell LR, Christensen CK, Jespersen LT, Thomsen K (1986) Effects of calcium antagonists in essential hypertension with special reference to renal function. In: Aoki K (ed) Essential hypertension. Calcium mechanisms and treatment. Springer, Berlin Heidelberg New York Tokyo, pp 149–160

Lee SM, Williams R, Warnock D, Emmett M, Wolbach RA (1986) The effect of nicardipine in hypertensive subjects with impaired renal function. Br J Clin Pharmacol 22 (Suppl):297S–306S

Lejeune P, Gunselmann W, Hennies L, Hess K, Rittgerodt K, Winn K, Gferer G, Schreiber U (1985) Effects of BAY L 5240, a fixed combination of low-dose nifedipine and acebutolol on hypertension: comparison with standard dose nifedipine. Eur J Clin Pharmacol 28:17–21

Leonetti G (1987a) Calcium antagonists: clinical pharmacology. In: Fleckenstein A, Laragh JH (eds) Hypertension—the next decade: verapamil in focus. Churchill Livingstone, Edingburgh, pp 67–80

Leonetti G (1987b) Antihypertensive efficacy of nicardipine, in monotherapy and association, in mild to moderate hypertensives with and without concomitant disease: interim report of Italian multicentre study. J Hypertens 5 (Suppl 5):S575–S577

Leonetti G, Zanchetti A (1985) Renal effects of calcium antagonists in hypertensive patients. J Hypertens 3 (Suppl 3):535–539

Leonetti G, Pasotti C, Ferrari GP, Zanchetti A (1981) Double-blind comparison of the antihypertensive effects of verapamil and propranolol. In: Zanchetti A, Krikler D (eds) Calcium antagonism in cardiovascular therapy: experience with verapamil. Excerpta Medica, Amsterdam, pp 260–267

Leonetti G, Cuspidi C, Sampieri L, Terzoli L, Zanchetti A (1982) Comparison of cardiovascular, renal, and humoral effects of acute administration of few calcium channel blockers in normotensive and hypertensive subjects. J Cardiovasc Pharmacol 4:S319–S324

Lessem J, Bellinetto A (1983) Interaction between digoxin and the calcium antagonists nicardipine and tiapamil. Clin Ther 5:595–602

Lettieri J, Krol G, Yeh S, Ryan J, Jain A, McMahon FG, Burkholder D, Birkett JP (1987) Pharmacokinetics of nitrendipine in elderly and young healthy volunteers. J Cardiovasc Pharmacol 9 (Suppl 4):S142–S147

Lewis GRJ, Morley KD, Lewis BM, Bones RJ (1978) The treatment of hypertension with verapamil. NZ Med J 87:351–354

Lewis GRJ, Stewart DJ, Lewis BM, Bones PJ, Morley KD, Janus ED (1981) The antihypertensive effect of oral verapamil—acute and long-term administrations and its effects on the high-density lipoprotein values in pharma. In: Zanchetti A, Krikler D (1981) Calcium antagonism in cardiovascular therapy: experience with verapamil. Excerpta Medica, Amsterdam Oxford Princeton, pp 270–277

Littler WA, Watson RDS, Stallard TJ, McLeay RAB (1983) The effect of nifedipine on arterial pressure and reflex cardiac control. Postgrad Med J 59 (Suppl 2) 109–113

Littler WA, Young MA, Smith SA (1986) The acute and chronic effects of nicardipine on blood pressure, heart rate, neurocirculatory reflexes and renal function in hypertensive patients. Br J Clin Pharmacol 22 (Suppl 3):239S–241S

Ljung B (1985) Vascular selectivity of felodipine. Drugs 29 (Suppl 2):46–58

Loutzenhiser R, Epstein M (1985) Effect of calcium antagonists on renal hemodynamics. Am J Physiol 249:F619–F629

Luckhaus G, Garthoff B, Kazda S (1982) Prevention of hypertensive vasculopathy by nifedipine in salt loaded Dahl rats. Arzneimittelforschung Drug Res 32:1421–1425

Luckhaus G, Nash G, Garthoff B, Kazda S, Feller W (1985) Healing of malignant hypertensive arteriopathy in Dahl rats by nifedipine. Arzneimittelforschung Drug Res 35:115–121

Luft FC, Aronoff GR, Sloan RS, Fineberg NS, Weinberger MH (1985) Calcium channel blockade with nitrendipine: effects on sodium homeostasis, the renin-angiotensin system and the sympathetic nervous system in humans. Hypertension 7:438–442

Lund-Johansen P (1984) Hemodynamic effects of antihypertensive agents. In: Doyle AE (ed) Clinical pharmacology of antihypertensive drugs. Elsevier Science, Amsterdam, pp 39–66 (Handbook of hypertension, vol 5)

Lund-Johansen P (1985) Hemodynamic effects of calcium channel blockers at rest and during exercise in essential hypertension. Am J Med 79 (Suppl 4A):11–18

Lund-Johansen P, Omvik P (1983) Hemodynamic effects of nifedipine in essential hypertension at rest and during exercise. J Hypertens 1:159–163

Lund-Johansen P, Omvik P (1986) Hemodynamic changes in essential hypertension and the hemodynamic effects of calcium antagonists. In: Aoki K (ed) Essential hypertension. Calcium mechanisms and treatment. Springer, Berlin Heidelberg New York Tokyo, pp 199–211

Lydtin H, Lohmöller G, Lohmöller R, Schmitz H, Walter I (1975) Hemodynamic studies on adalat in healthy volunteers and in patients. In: Lochner W, Braasch W, Kroneberg G (eds) 2nd International adalat symposium. New therapy of ischemic heart disease. Springer, Berlin Heidelberg New York, pp 112–123

MacGregor GA (1986) Hypertension. In: Krebs R (ed) Treatment of cardiovascular diseases by Adalat[R] (nifedipine). Schattauer, Stuttgart, pp 231–258

MacGregor GA, Rottelar C, MarKandu D, Smith SJ, Sagnella GA (1982) Contrasting effects of nifedipine, captopril and propranolol in normotensive and hypertensive subjects. J Cardiovasc Pharmacol 4 (Suppl 3):S358–S362

MacGregor GA, Markandu ND, Rottelar C, Smith SJ, Sagnella GA (1983) The acute response to nifedipine is related to pretreatment blood pressure. Postgrad Med J 59 (Suppl 2):91–94

MacGregor GA, Markandu ND, Smith SJ, Sagnella GA (1985a) Captopril: contrasting effects of adding hydrochlorothiazide, propranolol, or nifedipine. J Cardiovasc Pharmacol 7 (Suppl 1):82–87
MacGregor GA, Markandu ND, Smith SJ, Sagnella GA (1985b) Does nifedipine reveal a functional abnormality of arteriolar smooth muscle cell in essential hypertension—the effect of altering sodium balance. J Cardiovasc Pharmacol 7 (Suppl 6):178–181
MacGregor GA, Pevahouse J, Capuccio FP, Markandu ND (1987) Nifedipine, diuretics and sodium balance. J Hypertens 5 (Suppl 4):S127–S131
MacLaughlin M, de Mello Aires M, Malnic G (1985) Verapamil effect on renal function of normotensive and hypertensive rats. Renal Physiol 8:112–119
Maeda K, Takasugi T, Tsukano Y, Tanaka Y, Shiota K (1981) Clinical study on the hypotensive effect of diltiazem. Int J Clin Pharmacol Ther Toxicol 19:47–55
Magagna A, Abdel-Haq B, Pedrinelli R, Salvetti A (1986) Does chlorthalidone increase the hypotensive effect of nifedipine? J Hypertens 4 (Suppl 5):S519–S521
Magometschnigg D (1982) Zur Therapie der hypertensiven Krisen. Dtsch Med Wochenschr 107:1423–1428
Malcolm N, Callegari P, Goldberg J, Strauss H, Caille G, Vezina M (1986) Massive diltiazem overdose: clinical and pharmacokinetic observations. Drug Intell Clin Pharm 20:888
Maranhao MF, Constantini CR, Souza NS, Rojas RI (1983) Eficacia antihypertensiva da nifedipina. Avalacao clinica e ergometrica. Arq Bras Cardiol 41:417–419
Marlettini MG, Salomone T, Agostini D, Trisolino G, Trabatti M, Musiani M, De Novellis M (1986) Long-term treatment of primary hypertension with verapamil. Curr Ther Res 39:59–65
Martinez JJ, Markus EF, Ling T, Freedman D, Massey I, Garg D, Kessler K, Jallad N, Weidler DJ (1985) Nicardipine pharmacokinetics in the elderly. J Clin Pharmacol 25:468
Martre H, Sari R, Taburet AM, Jacobs C, Singlas E (1985) Haemodialysis does not affect the pharmacokinetics of nifedipine. Br J Clin Pharmacol 20:155–158
Massie BB, McCarthy ER, Ramanathan KB, Weiss RS, Anderson M, Eidelson BA (1987) Diltiazem and propranolol in mild to moderate essential hypertension as monotherapy or with hydrochlorothiazide. Ann Intern Med 107:150–157
Massie BM, Tubau J, Szlachcic J, Byyny R, Giles TD, Conradi E (1987) Nitrendipine vs hydrochlorothiazide in essential hypertension: effects during exercise. J Cardiovasc Pharmacol 9 (Suppl 4):S276–S279
M'Buyamba-Kabangu JR, Fagard R, Lijnen P, Amery A (1987) Nitrendipine and acebutolol in hypertensive african blacks. J Cardiovasc Pharmacol 9 (Suppl 4): S263–S266
McAllister RG, Kirsten EB (1982) The pharmacology of verapamil. IV. Kinetic and dynamic effects after single intravenous and oral doses. Clin Pharmacol Ther 31: 418–426
McGraw BF, Walker SD, Hemberger JA, Gitamer SL, Nakama M (1982) Clinical experience with diltiazem in Japan. Pharmacotherapy 2:156–161
McInnes GT, Findlay I, Murray GD, Dargie HJ (1984) Calcium antagonists and beta-blockers. In: Reid JL, Pickup AJ (eds) Calcium antagonists and the treatment of hypertension. Royal Society of Medicine, London, pp 69–75
McMahon FG, Brobyn R, Kann J, Levy B, Margolis R, Reeves R, Sperling DC, Sweet D, Zachariah PK, Zager P, Zellner SR (1987) A double-blind comparative study of nitrendipine and propranolol in the treatment of hypertension. J Cardiovasc Pharmacol 9 (Suppl 4):S228–S231
Mehta J, Lopez LM, Deedwania PC, Fagan TC, Sternlich CM, Vlachakis ND, Birkett JP, Schwartz LA (1987) Similar efficacy of nitrendipine in young and elderly hypertensive patients. Am J Cardiol 60:1096–1100
Meredith PA, Elliott HL, Pavanisi F, Kellman AW, Sumner BJ, Reid JL (1985) Verapamil pharmacokinetics and apparent hepatic and renal blood flow. Br J Clin Pharmacol 20:101–106
Meshi T, Sugihara J, Sato Y (1971) Metabolic fate of d-cis-3-acetoxy-5- 2-(dimethylamino)-ethyl-2,3-dihydro-2-(p-methoxyphenyl)-1,5-benzothiazepin-4(5H)-one hydro-

chloride (CRD-401). Chem Pharm Bull (Tokyo) 19:1546–1556
Messerli FH, Schmieder RE, Ventura HO, Frohlich ED (1987) The effects of nitrendipine on systemic hemodynamics in essential hypertension. J Cardiovasc Pharmacol 9 (Suppl 4):S178–S181
Meyer H, Bossert F, Wehinger E, Stoepel K, Vater W (1981) Synthesis and comparative pharmacological studies of 1,4-dihydro-2,6-dimethyl-4-(3-nitrophenyl)pyridine-3,5-dicarboxylates with non-identical ester functions. Arzneimittelforschung Drug Res 31:407–409
Meyer P, Rudofsky G, Nobbe F (1987) Effect of the new calcium channel blocker nitrendipine in hypertensive patients with concomitant arterial occlusive disease. J Cardiovasc Pharmacol 9 (Suppl 4):S311–S312
Midtbø K, Heds O, van der Meer J (1982) Verapamil compared with nifedipine in the treatment of essential hypertension. J Cardiovasc Pharmacol 4 (Suppl 3):S363–S367
Mikus G, Eichelbaum M (1987) Pharmacokinetics, bioavailability, metabolism, and hemodynamic effects of the calcium channel antagonist nitrendipine. J Cardiovasc Pharmacol 9 (Suppl 4):S140–S141
Millar JA, Struthers AD, Beastall GH, Reid JL (1982) Effect of nifedipine on blood pressure and adrenocortical response to trophic stimuli in humans. J Cardiovasc Pharmacol 4:S330–S334
Millard RW, Lathrop DA, Grupp G, Ashraf M, Grupp JL, Schwartz A (1982) Differential cardiovascular effects of calcium channel blocking agents: potential mechanism. Am J Cardiol 49:499–506
Mimran A, Ribstein J (1986) Effect of nifedipine in hypertension not controlled by converting enzyme inhibitor and diuretic. Postgrad Med J 62 (Suppl I):135–138
Mohanty PK, Sowers JR, McNamura C, Welch B, Beck F (1985) Effects of diltiazem on hormonal and hemodynamic responses to lower body negative pressure and tilt in patients with mild to moderate systemic hypertension. Am J Cardiol 56:28H–33H
Mohanty PK, Sowers JR, Thames MD (1987) Effects of hydrochlorothiazide and diltiazem on reflex vasoconstriction in hypertension. Hypertension 10:35–42
Mols P, Naeije R, Hallemans R, Melat G, Lejeune P (1986) Central and regional haemodynamic effects of nitrendipine in normotensive patients with chronic obstructive lung disease. J Cardiovasc Pharmacol 8:77–81
Momose T (1985) Control of intraoperative hypertension with calcium entry blocker (nicardipine)—comparison with nitroglycerin and trimethaphon. Acta Anaesthesiol Scand 29 (Suppl 80):81
Momose T, Ito K, Takeya H (1986) Result of randomized comparative clinical study of nicardipine hydrochloride and trimethaphan camsylate on control of blood pressure during surgery. Jpn J Anaesthesiol 35:540–550
Mooy J, Schols M, van Baak M, van Hoof M, Muytjens A, Rahn KH (1985) Pharmacokinetics of verapamil in patients with renal failure. Eur J Clin Pharmacol 28:405–410
Morledge J, Brown RD, Byyny R et al. (1987) Comparative study of the effects of nitrendipine and hydrochlorothiazide in hypertensive patients. J Cardiovasc Pharmacol 9 (Suppl 4):S224–S227
Moroni F, Mannaioni PF, Dolara A, Ciaccheri M (1980) Calcium gluconate and hypertonic sodium chloride in a case of massive verapamil poisoning. Clin Toxicol 17: 395–400
Morselli PL, Rovei V, Mitchard M, Durand A, Gomeni R, Larriband J (1979) Pharmacokinetics and metabolism of diltiazem in man (observations on healthy volunteers and angina pectoris patients). In: Bing RJ (ed) New drug therapy with calcium antagonists. Diltiazem Hakone symposium 1978. Excerpta Medica, Amsterdam, pp 152–168
Moser M, Lunn J, Nash DT, Burris JF, Winer N, Simon G, Vlachakis ND (1984) Nitrendipine in the treatment of mild to moderate hypertension. J Cardiovasc Pharmacol 6:S1085–S1089
Moser M, Lunn J, Materson BJ (1985) Comparative effects of diltiazem and hydrochlorothiazide in blacks with systemic hypertension. Am J Cardiol 56:101H–104H
Motz W, Klepzig M, Strauer BE (1987) Regression of cardiac hypertrophy: experimental

and clinical results. J Cardiovasc Pharmacol 10 (Suppl 6):S148–S152
Muiesan G, Agabiti-Rosei E, Alicandri C, Beschi M, Castellano M, Corea L, Fariello R, Romanelli G, Passini C, Plato L (1981) Influence of verapamil on catecholamines, renin and aldosterone in essential hypertensive patients. In:Zanchetti A, Krikler DM (eds) Calcium antagonism in cardiovascular therapy: experience with verapamil. Excerpta Medica, Amsterdam, pp 238–249
Muiesan G, Agabiti-Rosei E, Romanelli G, Muiesan ML, Castellano M, Beschi M (1986) Adrenergic activity and left ventricular functions during treatment of essential hypertension with calcium antagonists. Am J Cardiol 57:44D–49D
Müller FB, Bolli P, Erne P, Block LH, Kiowski W, Bühler FR (1984) Antihypertensive therapy with the long-acting calcium antagonist nitrendipine. J Cardiovasc Pharmacol 6:S1073–S1076
Mulvany MJ, Nyborg N (1980) An increased sensitivity of mesenteric resistance vessels in young and adult spontaneously hypertensive rats. Br J Pharmacol 71:585–596
Murakami M, Murakami N, Takekoshi N (1972) Antihypertensive effect of 4-(2′nitrophenyl)-2,6-dimethyl, 1,4-dihydropyridine-3,5 dicarbonic acid dimethylester (nifedipine, BAY A 1040) a new coronary dilator. Jpn Heart J 13:128–135
Murphy MB, Scriven AJI, Dollery CT (1983) Efficacy of nifedipine as a step 3 antihypertensive drug. Hypertension 5 (Suppl II):II–118–II–121
Murray TS, East BW, Robertson JIS (1986a) Nicardipine vs propranolol in the treatment of essential hypertension: effect on total body elemental composition. Br J Clin Pharmacol 22 (Suppl):259S–265S
Murray TS, Langan J, Coxhead PF, Levinson N (1986b) Long-term effects of nicardipine in the treatment of essential hypertension. Br J Clin Pharmacol 22 (Suppl):249S–257S
Murray TS, Langan JJ, Coxhead PF (1986c) A trial comparing nicardipine and cyclopenthiazide-K in a group of general practice patients with mild to moderate hypertension. Br J Pharmacol 22 (Suppl 3):243S–247S
Myers MG, Leenen FH, Burns R, Frenkel DC (1986) Nifedipine tablet vs hydralazine in patients with persisting hypertension who receive combined diuretic and beta-blocker therapy. Clin Pharmacol Ther 39:409–413
Nadler JL, Hsueh W, Horton R (1985) Therapeutic effect of calcium channel blockade in primary aldosteronism. J Clin Endocrinol Metab 60:896–899
Nakao J, Ito H, Oyama T, Chang WC, Murota SC (1983) Calcium dependence of aortic smooth muscle cell migration induced by 12-1-hydroxy-5,8,10,14-eicosatetraeonic acid effects of A 23187, nicardipine and trifluoperazine. Athereosclerosis 46:309–319
Nakaya H, Schwartz A, Millard RW (1983) Reflex chronotropic and inotropic effects of calcium channel-blocking agents in conscious dogs. Circ Res 52:302–311
Nannan ME, Melin JA, Vanbutsele RJ, Lavenne F, Detry JMR (1984) Acute and long-term effects of nitrendipine on resting and exercise hemodynamics in essential hypertension. J Cardiovasc Pharmacol 6:S1043–S1048
Narita H, Nagao T, Inamasu M, Iwasaki HO, Morita T (1985) Effects of diltiazem on developing blood pressure and accompanying cardiac and vascular hypertrophy in SHR (in Japanese). Nippon Yakurigaku Zasshi 86:165–174
Natsuma T, Gallo AJ, Pegram BL, Frohlich ED (1985) Hemodynamic effects of prolonged treatment with diltiazem in conscious normotensive and spontaneously hypertensive rats. Clin Exp Hypertens [A] A7:1471–1479
Nayler WG (1987) The pharmacology of the calcium antagonists. In: Fleckenstein A, Laragh JH (eds) Hypertension—the next decade: verapamil in focus. Churchill Livingstone, Edinburgh, pp 53–66
Neugebauer G (1978) Comparative cardiovascular actions of verapamil and its major metabolite in the anesthetized dog. Cardiovasc Res 12:247–254
Neuss J, Philipp H, Pichler H (1987) Diltiazem 90 mg in the therapy of mild to moderate hypertension. Therapiewoche 37:899–903
Nilsson J, Sjolung M, Palmberg L, von Euler AM, Jonzon B, Thyberg J (1985) The calcium antagonist nifedipine inhibits arterial smooth muscle proliferation. Atherosclerosis 58:109–122
N.N. (1985) Nifedipine overdose-profound hypotension. Reactions 118:9
Notghi A, Fiskerstrand CE, Burnet ME, Anderton JL (1987) Effect of nifedipine and

mefruside on renal function and platelet function in hypertensive patients. Curr Med Res Opin 10:441–449
Ochs HR, Rämsch KD, Verburg-Ochs B, Greenblatt DJ, Gerloff J (1984) Nifedipine: kinetics and dynamics after single oral doses. Klin Wochenschr 62:427–429
Oehmann KP, Weiner L, von Schenck H, Karlberg BE (1985) Antihypertensive and metabolic effects of nifedipine and labetalol alone and in combination in primary hypertension. Eur J Clin Pharmacol 29:149–154
Ogawa K, Ban M, Ito T, Watanabe T, Kobayashi T, Yamazaki N, Suzuki Y (1984) Diltiazem for treatment of essential hypertension: a double-blind controlled study with reserpine. Clin Ther 6:844–853
Ogilvie RI (1985) Effect of nifedipine and propranolol on blood flow, venous compliance and blood pressure in essential hypertension. Can Med Assoc J 132:1137–1141
Okada M, Inove H, Nakamura Y, Kishimoto M, Suzuki T (1985) Excretion of diltiazem in human milk. N Engl J Med 312:992–993
Olivari MT, Bartorelli C, Polese A, Fiorentini C, Moruzzi P, Guazzi MD (1979) Treatment of hypertension with nifedipine, a calcium antagonistic agent. Circulation 59:1056–1060
Opsahl JA, Abraham PA, Halstenson CE, Keane WF (1987) Antihypertensive and humoral effects of nifedipine in essential hypertension uncontrolled by hydrochlorothiazide alone (Abstract P III B8). Clin Pharmacol Ther 41:218
Orekhov AN, Tertov VV, Khasimov KA, Kudryashov SS, Smirnov VN (1987) Evidence of antiatherosclerotic action of verapamil from direct effects on arterial cells. Am J Cardiol 59:495–496
Orö L, Ryman T (1987) Combination of nitrendipine with metoprolol and a comparison with nifedipine in patients insufficiently treated with the β-blocker alone. J Cardiovasc Pharmacol 9 (Suppl 4):S238–S244
Orr GM, Bodanksy HJ, Dymond DS, Taylor M (1982) Fatal verapamil overdose. Lancet ii (8309):1218–1219
Oyama Y (1978) Hemodynamics and electrophysiologic evaluations of diltiazem hydrochloride: a clinical study. In: Bing RJ (ed) New drug therapy with a calcium antagonist. Excerpta Medica, Amsterdam, pp 169–189
Oyama Y, Fujii S, Kanda K, Akino E, Kawasaki H, Nagata M, Goto K (1984) Digoxin-diltiazem interaction. Am J Cardiol 53:1480–1481
Pacheco JP, Fan F, Wright RA, Corkadel LK, Howitz LD (1986) Monotherapy of mild hypertension with nifedipine. Am J Med 81 (Suppl 6A):20–24
Packer M, Meller J, Medina N, Yushak M, Smith H, Holt J, Guererro J, Todd QD, McAllister RG, Gorlin R (1982) Hemodynamic consequences of combined beta-adrenergic and slow calcium channel blockade in man. Circulation 65:660–668
Perkins CM (1978) Serious verapamil poisoning: treatment with intravenous calcium gluconate. Br Med J 6145:1127
Parrillo SJ, Venditto M (1984) Elevated theophylline blood levels from institution of nifedipine therapy. Ann Emerg Med:216–217
Passal DB, Crespin FH (1984) Verapamil poisoning in an infant. Pedriatrics 73:543–545
Pedersen O (1979) Role of extracellular calcium in isometric contractions of the SHR aorta. Influence of age and antihypertensive treatment. Arch Int Pharmacodyn 239: 208–220
Pedrinelli R, Tarazi RC (1985) Calcium entry blockade and alpha-adrenergic responsiveness in vivo. J Cardiovasc Pharmacol 7 (Suppl 6):S199–S209
Pedrinelli R, Taddei S, Graziadei L, Panarace G, Salvetti A (1986a) Verapamil antagonizes forearm vasoconstriction mediated by selective $alpha_1$- and $alpha_2$-agonists in hypertensive patients. J Hypertens 4 (Suppl 5):S451–S454
Pedrinelli R, Fouad FM, Tarazi RC, Bravo EL, Textor SC (1986b) Nitrendipine, a calcium-entry blocker. Renal and humoral effects in human arterial hypertension. Arch Intern Med 146:62–65
Pieper JA (1984) Serum protein binding interactions between propranolol and calcium channel blockers. Drug Intell Clin Pharm 18:492
Pool PE, Seagren SC, Salel AF (1985) Effects of diltiazem on serum lipids, exercise

performance and blood pressure: randomized, double-blind, placebo-controlled evaluation for systemic hypertension. Am J Cardiol 56:86H–91H
Pool PE, Massie BM, Venkataraman K, Hirsch AT, Samant DR, Seagren SC, Gaw J, Salal AF, Tubau JF (1986) Diltiazem as monotherapy for systemic hypertension: a multicenter, randomized, placebo-controlled trial. Am J Cardiol 57:212–217
Poulter N, Thompson AV, Sever PS (1986) Do diuretics enhance the hypotensive effect of nifedipine? A double-blind crossover trial in black hypertensive patients. J Hypertens 4:792–793
Pozenel H (1985) Die antihypertensive Wirkung von Verapamil. Ergebnisse mit einer neuen Retardform zur Einmaldosierung. Fortschr Med 23:639–642
Pozet N, Brazier JL, Hadj Aissa A, Khenfer D, Faucon G, Apoil E, Traeger J (1983) Pharmacokinetics of diltiazem in severe renal failure. Eur J Clin Pharmacol 24: 635–638
Quigley MA, White KL, McGraw BF (1985) Interpretation and application of worldwide safety data on diltiazem. Acta Pharmacol Toxicol (Copenh) 57 (Suppl 2):61–73
Rahn KH, May J, Bohm R, van der Vet A (1985) Reduction of bioavailability of verapamil by rifampicin. N Engl J Med 312:920–921
Ram CVS Calcium antagonists as antihypertensive agents are effective in all age groups. J Hypertens 5 (Suppl 4):S115–S118
Rameis H, Magometschnigg D, Ganzinger U (1984) The diltiazem-digoxin interaction. Clin Pharmacol Ther 36:183–189
Rämsch KD (1981) Zur Pharmakokinetik von Nifedipin. Schwerpunkt Med 4:55–61
Rämsch KD, Sommer J (1983) Pharmacokinetics and metabolism of nifedipine. Hypertension 5 (Suppl II):18–24
Rämsch KD, Sommer J (1984) Pharmacokinetics and metabolism of nitrendipine. In: Scriabine A, Vanov S, Deck K (eds) Nitrendipine. Urban and Schwarzenberg, Baltimore, pp 409–422
Rämsch KD, Ziegler R (1986) Plasma concentrations of various nifedipine formulations in healthy volunteers. In: Lichtlen PR (ed) New therapy of ischaemic heart disease and hypertension. 6th International adalat symposium, 18–20 April 1985, Geneva. Excerpta Medica, Amsterdam, pp 23–32
Rämsch KD, Graefe KH, Scherling D, Sommer J, Ziegler R (1986) Pharmacokinetics and metabolism of calcium-blocking agents nifedipine, nitrendipine, and nimodipine. Am J Nephrol 6 (Suppl 1):73–80
Reitberg DP, Love SJ, Quercia GT, Zinny MA (1987) Effect of food on nifedipine pharmacokinetics. Clin Pharmacol Ther 42:72–75
Rey JL, Lecuyer D, Bernasconi P, Quiret JC (1983) Deliberate intoxication with diltiazem with sinus deficiency and atrial ventricular block. Presse Med 12:1873–1874
Ribeiro JM (1987) The long-term use of slow release verapamil either alone or associated with a diuretic in systemic arterial hypertension. In: Fleckenstein A, Laragh JH (eds) Hypertension—the next decade: verapamil in focus. Churchill Livingston, Edinburgh, pp 317–320
Robinson BF (1983) The response of forearm resistance vessels to dilator agents in patients with primary hypertension: use of nifedipine in long-term therapy. Postgrad Med J 59 (Suppl 2):104–108
Robinson BF, Dobbs BJ, Bayley S (1982) Response of forearm resistance vessels to verapamil and sodium nitroprusside in normotensive and hypertensive men: evidence for a functional abnormality of vascular smooth muscle in primary hypertension. Clin Sci 63:33–42
Röckel A, Meairs S, Abdelhamid S, Fiegel P, Walb D (1987) Treatment of "therapy-resistant" hypertension with nitrendipine. J Cardiovasc Pharmacol 9 (Suppl 4): S303–S305
Rosatti F, Cella PL, Fici F, Rossi F, Chieppa S, Marmo E (1984) Diltiazem in the therapy of arterial hypertension: polygraphic assessment of left ventricular performance. Curr Ther Res 36:701–711
Rosendorff C (1984) Calcium channel blockers and hypertension. In: Opie LH (ed) Calcium antagonists and cardiovascular disease. Raven, New York, pp 323–331

Rosenkranz RP, McClelland DL, Roszkowski AP (1984) Effects of nicardipine, nifedipine, verapamil, and diltiazem on urine volume, sodium and potassium excretion and plasma aldosterone levels in the rat. Proc West Pharmacol Soc 27:67–72

Rosenthal J (1983) Antihypertensive effects of nifedipine, mefruside and a combination of both substances in patients with essential hypertension. In: Kaltenbach M, Neufeld HN (eds) 5th International Adalat[R] symposium. New therapy of ischaemic heart disease and hypertension. Excerpta Medica, Amsterdam, pp 175–181

Rouleau JL, Parmley WW, Stevens J, Coffelt JW, Sievers R, Mahley RW, Havel RJ (1983) Verapamil suppresses atherosclerosis in cholesterol-fed rabbits. J Am Coll Cardiol 1:1453–1460

Rovei V, Gomeni R, Mitchard M, Larribaud J, Blatrix C, Thebault JJ, Morselli PL (1980) Pharmacokinetics and metabolism of diltiazem in man. Acta Cardiol (Brux) 35:35–45

Rubin JM, Rubin LJ, Mason T, Light RW, Deedwania P, Weber KT (1987) Effects of nitrendipine on hemodynamics and oxygen transports in patients with pulmonary hypertension secondary to chronic obstructive pulmonary disease. J Cardiovasc Pharmacol 9 (Suppl 4):S313–S316

Rüddel H, Schmieder R, Langewitz W, Neus J, Wagner O, von Eiff AW (1984) Efficacy of nitrendipine as baseline antihypertensive therapy. J Cardiovasc Pharmacol 6: S1049–S1052

Rüddel H, Neus J, Langewitz W, von Eiff AW (1987) Impact of different medication schedules of nitrendipine on clinical casual blood pressure, 24 h ambulatory blood pressure, and blood pressure during exercise. J Cardiovasc Pharmacol 9 (Suppl 4): S161–S163

Rush WR, Alexander O, Hall DJ, Cairncross L, Dow RJ, Graham DJG (1986) The metabolism of nicardipine hydrochloride in healthy male volunteers. Xenobiotica 16:341–349

Sakai K (1978) Long-term Herbesser therapy in hypertension. Mod Clin Med 20:1053

Sakurai T, Kurita T, Nagano S, Sonoda T (1972) Antihypertensive vasodilating and sodium diuretic actions of D-cis isomers of benzothiazepine derivative (CRD-401). Acta Urol Jpn 18:695–701

Sato M, Nagao T, Yamaguchi J, Nakajima H, Kiyomoto A (1971) Pharmacological studies of a new 1,5-benzothiazepine derivative (CRD-401). Cardiovascular action. Arzneimittelforschung 21:1338–1343

Sawai K (1983) Effects of long-term administration of diltiazem hydrochloride in hypertensive patients. Clin Ther 5:422–435

Scheidt S, LeWinter MM, Hermanovich J, Venkataraman K, Freedman D (1985) Nicardipine for stable angina pectoris. Br J Clin Pharmacol 20 (Suppl 1):S178–S182

Schiffl H, Ziupa J, Schollmeyer P (1984) Clinical features and management of nifedipine overdosage in a patient with renal insufficiency. Clin Toxicol 22:387–395

Schmieder RE, Messerli FH, Garavaglia GE, Nunez BD (1987) Cardiovascular effects of verapamil in patients with essential hypertension. Circulation 75:1030–1036

Schoenberger JA, Glasser SP, Ram CVS, McMahon SG, Vanov SK, Leibowitz DA (1987) Comparison of nitrendipine combined with low-dose hydrochlorothiazide to hydrochlorothiazide alone in mild to moderate essential hypertension. J Cardiovasc Pharmacol 6:S1105–S1108

Schomerus M, Spiegelhalder B, Stieren B, Eichelbaum M (1976) Physiological disposition of verapamil in man. Cardiovasc Res 10:1–8

Schramm M, Towart R (1988) Calcium channels as drug receptors In: Baker PF (ed) Calcium in drug actions. Springer, Berlin Heidelberg New York, pp 89–114 (Handbook of experimental pharmacology, vol 83)

Schramm M, Thomas G, Towart R, Franckowiak G (1983) Novel dihydropyridines with positive inotropic action through activation of Ca channels. Nature 303:535–537

Schütz E, Riemha H, Bühler FR, Follath F (1982) Serum concentrations and antihypertensive effects of slow-releasing verapamil. J Cardiovasc Pharmacol 4 (Suppl 3): S346–S349

Schulte KL, Meyer-Sabellek WA, Haertenberger A, Thiede HM, Roecker L, Distler A, Gotzen R (1986) Antihypertensive and metabolic effects of diltiazem and nifedipine.

Hypertension 8:859–865
Schwartz JB, Abernethy DR, Egan JM, Mitchel JR (1985a) Differing pharmacokinetic and dynamic responses of diltiazem in the elderly. Circulation 72:50
Schwartz JB, Abernethy DR, Taylor AA, Mitchell JR (1985b) An investigation of the cause of accumulation of verapamil during regular dosing in patients. Br J Clin Pharmacol 19:512–516
Scriabine A, Garthoff B, Kazda S, Rämsch KD, Schlüter G, Stoepel K (1984) Nitrendipine. In: Scriabine A (ed) New drugs annual: cardiovascular drugs. Raven, New York, pp 37–49
Sen S, Tarazi RC, Bumpus FM (1977) Cardiac hypertrophy and antihypertensive therapy. Cardiovasc Res 11:427–433
Serruys PW, Vanhaleweyk GLJ, Hugenholtz PG (1983) The hemodynamic effects of the calcium channel blocking agents. In: Stone PH, Antman EM (eds) Calcium channel blocking agents in the treatment of cardiovascular disorders. Futura, Mount Kisco NY, pp 203–240
Shah GM, Winer RL (1985) Verapamil kinetics during maintenance hemodialysis. Am J Nephrol 5:338–341
Shand DG, Hammill SC, Aanonsen L, Pritchett ELC (1981) Reduced verapamil clearance during long-term oral administration. Clin Pharmacol Ther 30:701–703
Simon G, Snyder DK (1984) Altered pressor responses in long-term nitrendipine treatment. Clin Pharmacol Ther 36:315–319
Singh BN, Opie LH (1983) Calciumantagonists. In: Opie LH (ed) Drugs for the heart. Grune and Straton, Orlando FL pp 39–64
Sluiter HE, Huysmans FTM, Thien TA, van Lier HJJ, Koener RAP (1985) Hemodynamic, humoral and diuretic effects of felodipine in healthy normotensive volunteers. Drugs 29 (Suppl 2):26–35
Smith MS, Verghese CP, Shand DG, Pritchett ELC (1983) Pharmacokinetic and pharmacodynamic effects of diltiazem. Am J Cardiol 51:1369–1374
Snover SW, Bocchino V (1986) Massive diltiazem overdose. Ann Emerg Med 15: 1221–1224
Somogyi A, Muirhead M (1987) Pharmacokinetic interaction of cimetidine. Clin Pharmacokinet 12:321–326
Somogyi A, Albrecht M, Kleines G, Schäfer K, Eichelbaum M (1981) Pharmacokinetics, bioavailability and ECG response of verapamil in patients with liver cirrhosis. Br J Clin Pharmacol 12:51–60
Sorkin EM, Clissold SP (1987) Nicardipine: a review of its pharmacodynamic and pharmacokinetic properties and therapeutic efficacy, in the treatment of angina pectoris, hypertension and related cardiovascular disorders. Drugs 33:296–345
Sperelakis N (1987) Electrophysiology of calcium antagonists. J Moll Cell Cardiol 19 (Suppl II):19–47
Spiegelhalder B, Eichelbaum M (1977) Determination of verapamil in human plasma by mass fragmentography using stable isotope-labelled verapamil as internal standard. Arzneimittelforschung 27:94–97
Stasch JP, Kazda S, Hirth C, Morich F (1987a) Role of nisoldipine on blood pressure, cardiac hypertrophy, and atrial natriuretic peptides in spontaneously hypertensive rats. Hypertension 10:303–307
Stasch JP, Kazda S, Hirth C (1987b) The different effects of a calcium antagonist and a sodium retaining vasodilator on blood pressure, cardiac hypertrophy and atrial natriuretic peptides in adult spontaneously hypertensive rats. J Hypertens 5 (Suppl 5):S211–S213
Steinhausen M, Flemming JT, Holz FG, Parekh N (1987) Nitrendipine and the pressure-dependent vasodilation of vessels in the hydronephrotic kidney. J Cardiovasc Pharmacol 9 (Suppl 1):S39–S47
Stone PH, Antman EM, Müller JE, Braunwald E (1980) Calcium channel blocking agents in the treatment of cardiovascular disorders. Part II. Hemodynamic effects and clinical applications. Ann Intern Med 93:886–904
Strauss WE, McIntyre KM, Parisi AF, Shapiro W (1982) Safety and efficacy of diltiazem hydrochloride for the treatment of stable angina pectoris: report of a cooperative

clinical trial. Am J Cardiol 49:560–566
Streifler JY, Zylber-Katz E, Rosenfeld JF (1985) Dose of nifedipine tablets with its plasma concentration in patients with essential hypertension. Int J Clin Pharmacol Ther Toxicol 23:657–661
Strubelt O (1984) Antidotal treatment of the acute cardiovascular toxicity of verapamil. Acta Pharmacol Toxicol 55:231–237
Sugihara J, Sugawara Y, Ando H, Harigaya S, Etoh S, Kohno K (1984) Studies on the metabolism of diltiazem in man. J Pharmacabiodyn 7:24–32
Sunderrajan S, Reams G, Bauer JH (1986) Renal effects of diltiazem in primary hypertension. Hypertension 8:238–242
Sunderrajan S, Reams G, Bauer JH (1987) Long-term renal effects of diltiazem in essential hypertension. Am Heart J 114:383–388
Swartz SL (1987) Endocrine and vascular responses in hypertensive patients to long-term treatment with diltiazem. J Cardiovasc Pharmacol 9:391–395
Szlachcic J, Hirsch AT, Tubau JF, Vollmer C, Henderson S, Massie BM (1987) Diltiazem versus propranolol in essential hypertension: responses of rest and exercise blood pressure and effects on exercise capacity. Am J Cardiol 59:393–399
Takemiya T, Yamaguchi H (1978) Hypotensive effect of diltiazem hydrochloride (Herbesser): evaluation in 20 clinical cases. Mod Clin Med 20:1235–1240
Talbert RL, Bussey HJ (1983) Update on calcium channel blocking agents. Clin Pharm 2:403–416
Tamai S, Mori K, Ishii S (1986) A comparison between nicardipine hydrochloride (YC-93) and trimethaphan camsylate for treatment of acute hypertension during surgery. A double blind study in 12 institutions. Jpn J Anesthesiol 35:528–539
Tanabe I, Takeshima H, Mikami A, Flockerzi V, Takahashi H, Kangawa K, Kojima M, Matsuo H, Hirose T, Numa S (1987) Primary structure of the receptor for calcium channel blockers from skeletal muscle. Nature 328:313–316
Taylor SH, Frais MA, Lee P, Verma SP, Jackson N (1985a) Antihypertensive dose-response effects of nicardipine in stable essential hypertension. Br J Clin Pharmacol 20 (Suppl 1):135S–138S
Taylor SH, Frais MA, Lee P, Verma SP, Jackson N (1985b) A study of the long-term efficacy and tolerability of oral nicardipine in hypertensive patients. Br J Clin Pharmacol 20 (Suppl 1):139S–142S
Thananopavarn C, Golul MS, Eggena P, Barrett JD, Samblu MP (1984a) Renal effects of nitrendipine monotherapy in essential hypertension. J Cardiovasc Pharmacol 6 (Suppl 7):S1032–S1036
Thananopavarn C, Samblu MP, Golul MS, Eggena P, Barrett JD (1984b) Saluretic and diuretic effects of nitrendipine during antihypertensive monotherapy. Clin Pharmacol Ther 35:279
Thibonnier M, Bonnet F, Corvol P (1980) Antihypertensive effect of fractionated sublingual administration of nifedipine in moderate essential hypertension. Eur J Clin Pharmacol 17:161–164
Thibonnier M, Sassano P, Corvol P (1985) Evaluation de l'effet antihypertenseur des formes capsules et comprimés de nifedipine dans l'hypertension moderée. Arch Mal Coeur 78:25–28
Thiercelin JF, Hermann P, Warrington S, Thénot JP, Morselli PL (1983) Interaction study between digoxin and calcium antagonists: verapamil and diltiazem. In: Lemberger L, Reidenberg MM (eds) Proceedings IInd world conference on clinical pharmacology and therapeutics, Washington DC, 31 July–5 August, 1983, p 47
Tourkantonis A, Lasaridis A, Settas L (1984) Clinical experience with long-term nitrendipine treatment in essential hypertension. J Cardiovasc Pharmacol 6:S1090–S1095
Towart R (1986) New pharmacological aspects of calcium antagonism. In: Rafflenbeul W, Lichtlen PR, Balcon R (eds) Unstable angina pectoris. Thieme, Stuttgart, pp 70–79
Triggle DJ, Janis RA (1987) Calcium channel ligands. Ann Rev Pharmacol Toxicol 27:347–369
Trimarco B, DeLuca N, Ricciardelli B, Volpe M, Veniero A, Cuocolo A, Cicala M (1984) Diltiazem in the treatment of mild or moderate essential hypertension.

Comparison with metoprolol in a crossover double-blind trial. J Clin Pharmacol 24:218–227
Trost BN, Weidmann P (1987) Nitrendipine in patients with hypertension and diabetes mellitus. J Cardiovasc Pharmacol 9 (Suppl 4):S280–S285
Tucker FA, Minty PS, MacGregor GA (1985) Study of nifedipine photodecomposition in plasma and whole blood using capillary gas-liquid chromatography. J Chromatogr 342:193–198
Turek Z, Kubat K, Kazda S, Hoofd L, Rakusan K (1987) Improved myocardial capillarisation in spontaneously hypertensive rats treated with nifedipine. Cardiovasc Res 21:725–729
Ueda H, Yagi S, Kaneko Y (1968) Hydralazine and plasma renin activity. Arch Intern Med 122:387–391
Valdés G, Montero J, Tobar M, Chacón C (1986) Comparison of the effect of capsule and retard preparations of nifedipine in hypertensive patients. In: Lichtlen PR (ed) 6th International Adalat^R symposium. New Therapy of ischaemic heart disease and hypertension. Excerpta Medica, Amsterdam, pp 313–317
Van Bortel LM, Boehm RO, Mooy JM, Schiffers PM, Thijssen HH (1987) Plasma levels of nifedipine and nitrendipine in terminal kidney insufficiency. Ned Tijdschr Geneeskd 131:1369
Van Breemen C, Farinas BR, Gerba P, McNaughton ED (1972) Excitation-contraction coupling in rat aorta studies by the lanthanum method for measuring calcium influx. Circ Res 30:44–45
Van Breemen C, Mangel A, Fahim M, Meisheri K (1982) Selectivity of calcium antagonistic action in vascular smooth muscle. Am J Cardiol 49:507–510
Van Lith RM, Appelby DH (1985) Quinidine-nifedipine interaction. Drug Intell Clin Pharm 19:820–831
Van Meel JCA, De Jonge A, Kalkman HO, Wilffert B, Timmermans PBMWM, van Zwieten PA (1981) Organic and inorganic calcium antagonists reduce vasoconstriction in vivo mediated by postsynaptic alpha$_2$-adrenoceptors. Naunyn Schmiedebergs Arch Pharmacol 316:288–293
Van Meel JCA, Towart R, Kazda S, Timmermans PBMWM, van Zwieten PA (1983) Correlation between the inhibitory activity of calcium entry blockers on vascular smooth muscle contraction in vitro after K^+-depolarization and in vivo after alpha$_2$-adrenoceptor stimulation. Naunyn Schmiedebergs Arch Pharmacol 322:34–37
Van Shaik BAM, van Nistelrooy AEJ, Geyskes GG (1984) Antihypertensive and renal effects of nicardipine. Br J Clin Pharmacol 18:57–63
Van Zwieten PA, van Meel JCA, Timmermans PBMWM (1982) Calcium antagonists and alpha$_2$-adrenoceptors: possible role of extracellular calcium ions in alpha$_2$-mediated vasoconstriction. J Cardiovasc Pharmacol 4 (Suppl 3):S273–S279
Van Zwieten PA, van Meel JCA, Timmermans PBMWM (1983) Pharmacology of calcium entry blockers: interaction with vascular alpha-adrenoceptors. Hypertension 5 (Suppl II):8–17
Ventura HO, Messerli FH, Oigmann W, Dunn FG, Reisin E (1983) Immediate hemodynamic effects of a new calcium channel blocking agent (nitrendipine) in essential hypertension. Am J Cardiol 51:783–786
Vitacolonna E, Guagnano MT, Capasi F, Sensis S (1986) Nitrendipine treatment of mild to moderate hypertension. Curr Ther Res 39:414–420
Vogelsang B, Echizen H, Schmidt E, Eichelmann M (1984) Stereoselective first-pass metabolism of highly cleared drugs: study of the bioavailability of L- and D-verapamil examined with a stable isotope technique. Br J Clin Pharmacol 18:733–740
Von Witzleben H, Frey M, Keidel J, Fleckenstein A (1980) Normalization of blood pressure in spontaneously hypertensive rats by long-term oral treatment with verapamil and nifedipine (Abstract). Pflugers Arch 384 (Suppl):R9
Walker SD, Skalland ML, Galbraith H, Lewis J, Balfour D, Brown S, Edin A (1984) Antihypertensive effects of diltiazem: a single blind multicentre study. Chest 86:305
Waller DG, Renwick AG, Gruchy BS, George CF (1984) The first pass metabolism of nifedipine in man. Br J Clin Pharmacol 18:951–954
Walsh MP, Hartshorne DJ (1983) Calmodulin. In: Stephens NL (ed) Biochemistry of

smooth muscle, vol II.CRC, Boca Raton, pp 2–84
Wandel E, Weber M, Zschiedrich H, Marx M, Köhler H (1987) Single-dose effect of nitrendipine on blood pressure of hemodialysis patients with hypertension. J Cardiovasc Pharmacol 9 (Suppl 4):S295–S299
Weber MA (1987) A one-year experience with the calcium channel blocking agent, nitrendipine, in patients with essential hypertension: report of a multicenter study. J Cardiovasc Pharmacol 9 (Suppl 4):S182–S189
Weber MA, Drayer JIM (1984) The calcium channel blocker nitrendipine in single- and multiple-agent regimens: preliminary report of a multicenter study. J Cardiovasc Pharmacol 6 (Suppl 7):S1077–S1084
Weinberger MH (1987) The role of age, race, and plasma renin activity in influencing the blood pressure response to nitrendipine or hydrochlorothiazide. J Cardiovasc Pharmacol 9 (Suppl 4):S272–S275
Weiss RJ, Bent B (1987) Diltiazem-induced left ventricular mass regression in hypertensive patients. J Clin Hypertens 3:135–143
Wing LM, Chalmers JP, West MJ, Bune AJC (1985) Slow-release nifedipine as a single or additional agent in the treatment of hypertension—placebo controlled crossover study. Clin Exp Hypertens [A] A 7:1173–1185
Wing LHM, Chalmers JP, West MJ, Bune AJC (1986) Double-blind randomized crossover study of slow-release nifedipine in patients with essential hypertension. In: Lichtlen P (ed) 6th International Adalat[R] symposium. New therapy of ischaemic heart disease and hypertension. Excerpta Medica, Amsterdam, pp 492–494
Winship LC, McKenney JM, Wright JT, Wood JH, Goodmann RP (1985) The effect of ranitidine and cimetidine on single-dose diltiazem pharmacokinetics. Pharmacotherapy 5:16–19
Wortmann A, Schmidt M, Bachmann K (1987) Antihypertensive action of nitrendipine once daily. Schweiz Rundsch Med Prax 76:469–472
Yagil Y, Kobrin I, Stessmann J, Ghanem J, Leibel B, Ben-Ischay D (1983) Effectiveness of combined nifedipine and propranolol treatment in hypertension. Hypertension 5 (Suppl II):II–113–II–117
Yamakado T, Oonishi N, Kondo S, Noziri A, Nakano T, Takezawa H (1983) Effects of diltiazem on cardiovascular responses during exercise in systemic hypertension and comparison with propranolol. Am J Cardiol 52:1023–1027
Yamakado T, Oonishi N, Nakano T, Takezawa H (1985) Effects of nifedipine and diltiazem on hemodynamic responses at rest and during exercise in hypertensive patients. Jpn Circ J 49:415–421
Yamakado M, Tagawa T (1978) Hypotensive effect of diltiazem HCl (Herbesser). Mod Clin Med 20:1877–1881
Yanagisawa M, Kurihara H, Kimura S, Tomobe Y, Kobayashi M, Mitsui Y, Yazaki Y, Goto K, Masaki T (1988a) A novel potent vasoconstrictor peptide produced by vascular endothelial cells. Nature 332:411–415
Yanagisawa M, Kurihara H, Kimura S, Goto K, Masaki T (1988b) Endothelium-derived novel vasoconstrictor peptide endothelin: a possible endogenous agonist for voltage-dependent Ca^{2+} channel. In: Morad M, Nayler W, Kazda S, Schramm M (eds) The calcium channel: structure, function and implications. Springer, Berlin Heidelberg New York, pp 575–585
Yokoyama S, Kaburagi T (1983) Clinical effects of intravenous nifedipine on renal function. J Cardiovasc Pharmacol 5:67–71
Yorifugi S, Kawai Y, Arami S (1979) Hypotensive effect of diltiazem hydrochloride (Herbesser tablets) in patients with essential hypertension. J Adult Dis 9:893–907
Yoshiya I, Mori K, Miyazaki M (1986) Antihypertensive effects of nicardipine hydrochloride (YC-93) on patients with hypertension during neuroleptanesthesia. Jpn J Anesthesiol 35:520–527
Zachariah PK, Sheps SG, Schirger A (1986) Efficacy of sustained-release verapamil: automatic ambulatory blood pressure monitoring. J Clin Hypertens 3:S133–S142
Zachariah PK, Schwartz GL, Ritter SG, Strong CG (1987a) Plasma predictors of calcium channel blocker efficacy in hypertension. J Cardiovasc Pharmacol 9 (Suppl 4): S148–S153

Zachariah PK, Sheps SG, Schwartz GL, Ilstrup DM, Schirger A, Ritter SG (1987b) Continuous blood pressure monitoring—nitrendipine antihypertensive response. J Cardiovasc Pharmacol 9 (Suppl 4):S154–S160

Zanchetti A (1977) Neural regulation of renin release: experimental evidence and clinical implications in arterial hypertension. Circulation 56:691–698

Zanchetti A (1981) Perspectives in antihypertensive treatment. In: Zanchetti A, Krikler D (eds) Calcium antagonism in cardiovascular therapy: experience with verapamil. Excerpta Medica, Amsterdam, pp 292–300

Zanchetti A, Leonetti G (1985) Natriuretic effect of calcium antagonists. J Cardiovasc Pharmacol 7 (Suppl 4):S33–S37

Zezulka AV, Gill JS, Beevers DG (1987) The effect of bendroflumethiazide added to nifedipine in patients with hypertension. J Clin Pharmacol 27:41–45

Ziegler WJ, Bach D (1986) Efficacy of nifedipine retard tablets as antihypertensive treatment and interactions with concomitant medication. Results of a prospective multicentre study in Switzerland. In: Lichtlen P (ed) 6th International Adalat[R] symposium. New therapy of ischaemic heart disease and hypertension. Excerpta Medica, Amsterdam, pp 328–336

Ziegler R, Wingender W, Boehme K, Raemsch K, Kuhlmann J (1987) Study of pharmacokinetic and pharmacodynamic interaction between nitrendipine and digoxin. J Cardiovasc Pharmacol 9 (Suppl 4):S101–S106

Zusman R, Christensen D, Federman E, Kochar MS, MacCarron D (1987) Comparison of nifedipine and propranolol used in combination with diuretics for the treatment of hypertension. Am J Med 82 (Suppl 3B):37–41

CHAPTER 10

Converting Enzyme Inhibitors

T. UNGER, P. GOHLKE, and M.-G. GRUBER

CONTENTS

1 Development of Converting Enzyme Inhibitors

1.1 Converting Enzyme

Converting enzyme (CE; EC 3.4.15.1) is an exopeptidase which catalyzes the hydrolytic removal of carboxyterminal dipeptide residues from polypeptide substrates. This enzyme is involved in blood pressure regulation in a unique manner. First, it catalyzes the conversion of the inactive decapeptide angiotensin I (ANG I) to the octapeptide, angiotensin II (ANG II) (SKEGGS et al. 1956), which constitutes one of the most powerful vasoconstricting, salt-retaining, and, thus, blood pressure-increasing agents of the organism. In additon, CE inactivates the vasodilatory and natriuretic nonapeptide bradykinin, since it is identical with the enzyme kininase II (ERDÖS 1975). Thus, CE helps to increase blood pressure by its dual action: generation of a vasopressor and salt-retaining principle (ANG II) and degradation of a vasodepressor and salt-excreting principle (bradykinin) (Fig. 1). As it is known that the renin-angiotensin system (RAS) plays an important, sometimes a key, role in the pathogenesis of human high blood pressure disease (VECSEI et al. 1978; SWALES 1979), it could be expected that inhibitors of CE would become useful antihypertensive agents.

CE was first isolated from horse serum in 1956 (SKEGGS et al.) and was long believed to be active predominantly in the circulating blood. Only some 10 years later, when synthetic ANG I was available, did it become apparent that the source of ANG II, the biologically active effector peptide of the RAS, was the lung vascular bed and that the contribution of CE in the blood to ANG II generation was rather small.

Shortly afterwards, CE was detected in the kidney and in various blood vessels and was subsequently recognized as an ubiquitously occurring enzyme of the vascular endothelium.

Besides being localized in the luminal plasma membrane of the entire vascular endothelium, CE has also been found in epithelial cells of the kidney (tubular brush border), gastrointestinal tract, testis, and also epithelial and neuronal structures of the brain. In most tissues CE is membrane-bound, while being present in a soluble form in the body fluids (for review, see ERDÖS 1975; ERDÖS and SKIDGEL 1987; SKIDGEL et al. 1988). CE is a single chain glycoprotein. Its molecular weight was reported to be about 140 000 dalton when determined by SDS gel electrophoresis (LANZILLO and FANBURG 1976) and 112 000 dalton when determined by neutron scattering (BAUDIN et al. 1988). CE is chloride-dependent and contains zinc ions (DAS and SOFFER 1975; RIORDAN et al. 1986). Most recently, cDNAs encoding mouse and rabbit CE have been isolated (BERNSTEIN et al. 1988; ROY et al. 1988), showing that different CE isoenzymes in lung and testis are encoded by two distinct mRNAs (ROY et al. 1988). The complete amino acid sequence of human CE has been disclosed by molecular cloning of the enzyme (ALHENC-GELAS et al. 1988).

CE degrades not only ANG I and bradykinin but also a number of other peptide substrates including Substance P and Luteinizing Hormone Releasing Hormone (LHRH) (see reviews cites above). The substrate specificity, kinetic

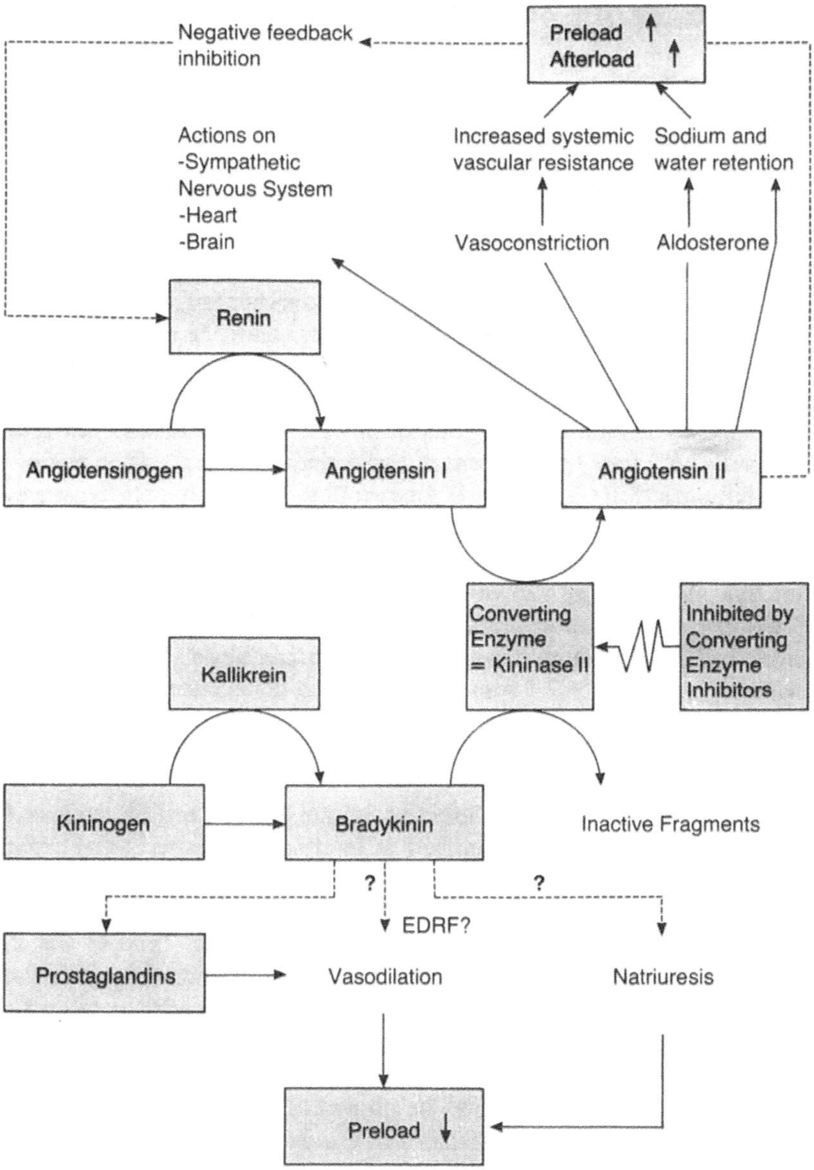

Fig. 1. The renin-angiotensin-aldosterone and kallikrein-kinin-prostaglandin systems and their effects on cardiovascular homeostasis

characteristics, and catalytic mechanism of CE have been described by BÜNNING et al. (1983), BÜNNING (1983), and RIORDAN et al. (1986).

1.2 Development of Orally Active Converting Enzyme Inhibitors

The first specific converting enzyme inhibitors (CEI) were isolated from snake venom by FERREIRA et al. (1970) and, independently, by ONDETTI et al. (1971).

These substances were peptides with five to nine amino acid residues, all of them highly specific in inhibiting ANG I conversion and in potentiating the actions of bradykinin. A nonapeptide, teprotide (SQ 20881), turned out to be the most potent and stable of all these peptide inhibitors and to be an effective drug for the treatment of human hypertension (GAVRAS et al. 1974).

Since this peptide inhibitor was not orally active but had to be applied by the intravenous route, teprotide could not be considered as a drug for the treatment of chronic diseases like hypertension. It became apparent that nonpeptide CEI had to be developed which could be administered orally without loss of activity. The development of these substances as achieved by CUSHMAN et al. (1977) and ONDETTI et al. (1977) is one of the fine examples of a logical and elegant approach to the synthesis of a new drug [see also FERREIRA (1985) on the history of the CEI development].

1.2.1 Synthesis of Captopril

The ignition spark for the development of an orally active CEI was the realization that CE — although different from other carboxypeptidases which release amino acids but not dipeptides from the C-terminal end of peptide substrates — has some similarities to another Zn^{2+}-containing metalloprotein, namely carboxypeptidase A, from pancreatic tissue. By analogy to the well-characterized active site of this enzyme, a hypothetical model of the active site of CE was developed (ONDETTI et al. 1977; CUSHMAN et al. 1979) which in its present form (BÜNNING 1987) is shown in Fig. 2.

It was postulated that the active site should contain a positively charged group like the amino acid arginine in the case of carboxypeptidase A to form ionic bonds with the negatively charged terminal carboxyl groups of the substrate. A tightly bound Zn^{2+} ion polarizes the carbonyl group of the peptide bond cleaved by the enzyme. A (x-H) group was assumed to interact with the

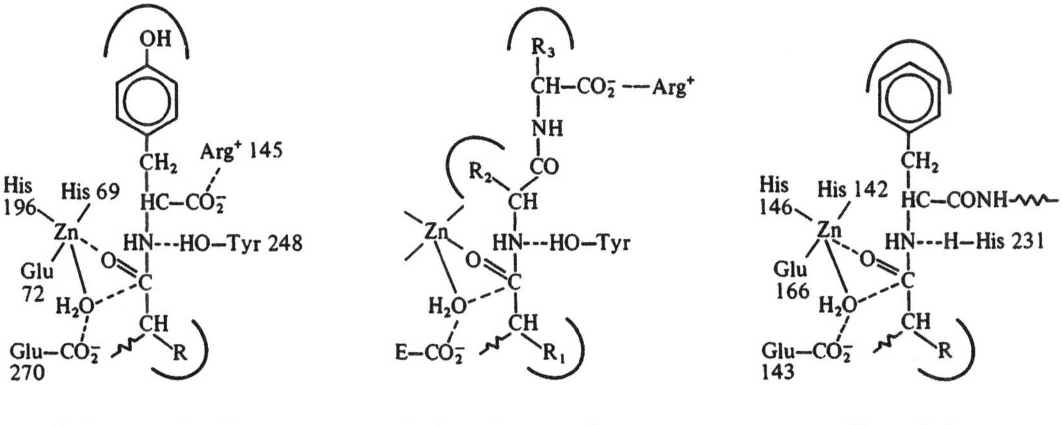

Fig. 2. Comparison of the hypothetical active sites of converting enzyme with those proposed for carboxypeptidase A and thermolysin. (From BÜNNING 1984)

	Structure	Designation	Activity (μg/ml)				
			Angiotensin-converting enzyme of rabbit lung	Excised guinea pig ileum			
			(IC_{50})	AI (IC_{50})	AII (IC_{50})	Ach IC_{50}	BK (AC_{50})
1	<Glu–Trp–Pro–Arg–Pro–Gln–Ile–Pro–Pro	(SQ20.881)	1.0	0.068	>32	>32	0.0017
2	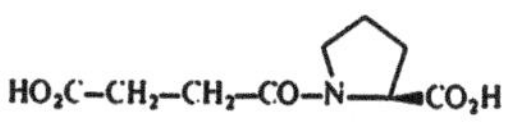		135	94	>100	>100	8.0
3	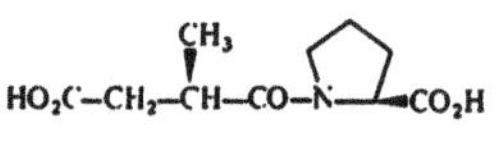	(SQ13.297)	12	13	>100	>100	0.2
4	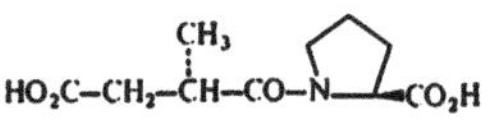		340	>100	>100	>100	15
5	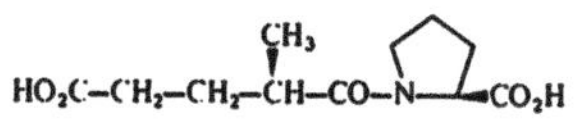		1.0	4.6	>100	>100	1.0
6	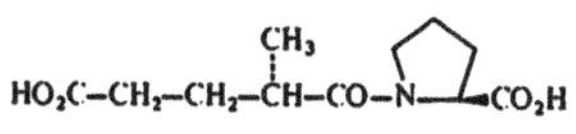		230	>100	>100	>100	4.7
7	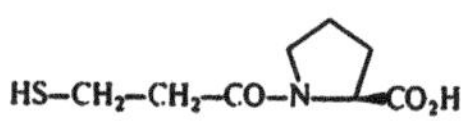	(SQ13.863)	0.04	0.06	>100	>100	0.005
8	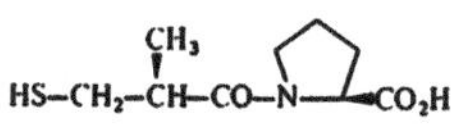	(SQ14.225)	0.005	0.005	>100	>100	0.0007
9	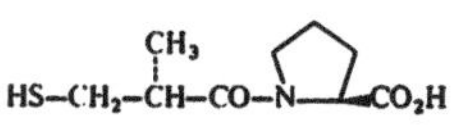		0.50	1.7	>100	>100	3.1

Fig. 3. Activities in vitro of inhibitors of converting enzyme. IC_{50}, concentration of compound producing 50 percent inhibition of enzyme activity or agonist effect; AC_{50}, concentration of compound producing 50 percent augmentation of agonist effect; *AI*, angiotensin I; *AII*, angiotensin II; *BK*, bradykinin; *Ach*, acetylcholine. (From ONDETTI et al. 1977)

C-terminal amide bond, most likely by hydrogen bonding. The side chains R_1 and R_2 of the peptide substrate were expected to interact with the corresponding pockets of the enzyme's active site.

Although this model was purely hypothetical in the beginning, it has been increasingly substantiated by the subsequent verification of the presence of Zn^{2+} (DAS and SOFFER 1975) in CE and evidence of arginine, tyrosine, and glutamic acid residues at the active site of the enzyme (BÜNNING et al. 1978).

The search for a synthetic CEI was greatly stimulated by the finding of Byers and Wolfenden that D-2-benzylsuccinic acid was a potent competitive inhibitor of carboxypeptidase A (BYERS and WOLFENDEN 1972). It was suggested that this was due to specific interaction of the compound with the three constituents

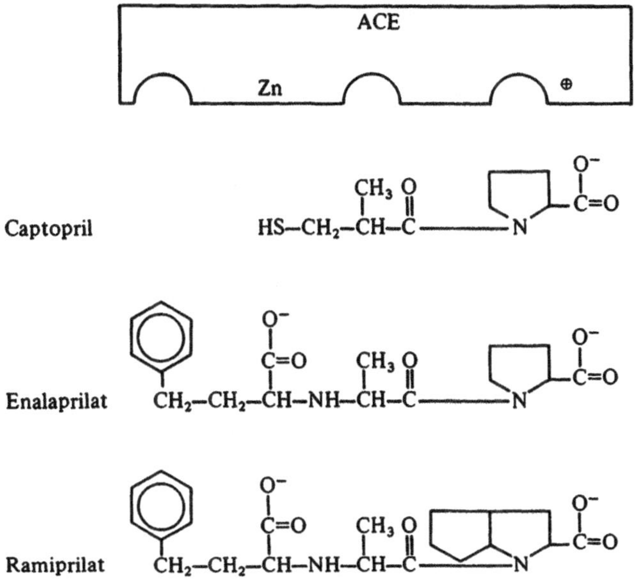

Fig. 4. Hypothetical model for the binding of captopril, enalaprilat, and ramiprilat to the active site of converting enzyme. (From BÜNNING 1987)

of the enzyme's active site, the positively charged group, the "hydrophobic pocket", and the zinc ion.

By analogy to the carboxypeptidase A inhibitor, the compound succinyl-proline was synthesized as the first synthetic competitive CE inhibitor. A succinyl derivative of an amino acid rather than a succinic acid was chosen because the distance between the cationic carboxylic binding site and the Zn^{2+} atom had to be greater than in carboxypeptidase A by about the length of one amino acid residue. Proline was chosen as the amino acid for a number of reasons including the finding that all naturally occurring peptide inhibitors of CE have proline as their C-terminal residue and that, among many peptide analogues tested, those with the C-terminal sequence Ala-Pro were most inhibitory to CE (ONDETTI et al. 1977; CUSHMAN et al. 1979). This prototype of the nonpeptide CEI was, although specific, by far not as active as the most powerful peptide inhibitor of converting enzyme, teprotide.

The further steps in the development of a synthetic CEI were therefore designed to augment the inhibitory potency. As can be seen in Fig. 3, the most favorable results were obtained by introducing a 2-D-methyl group and by replacing the succinyl-carboxyl group by a mercapto group. This led to a dramatic improvement of the inhibitory potency without loss of specificity and to the development of the compound D-3-mercapto-2-methyl propanoyl-1-proline (SQ14225 or captopril), which is highly specific and has an inhibitory potency as high as the most potent stable peptide inhibitor of converting enzyme, teprotide (Fig. 3) (ONDETTI et al. 1977). Figure 4 shows in a hypothetical model how

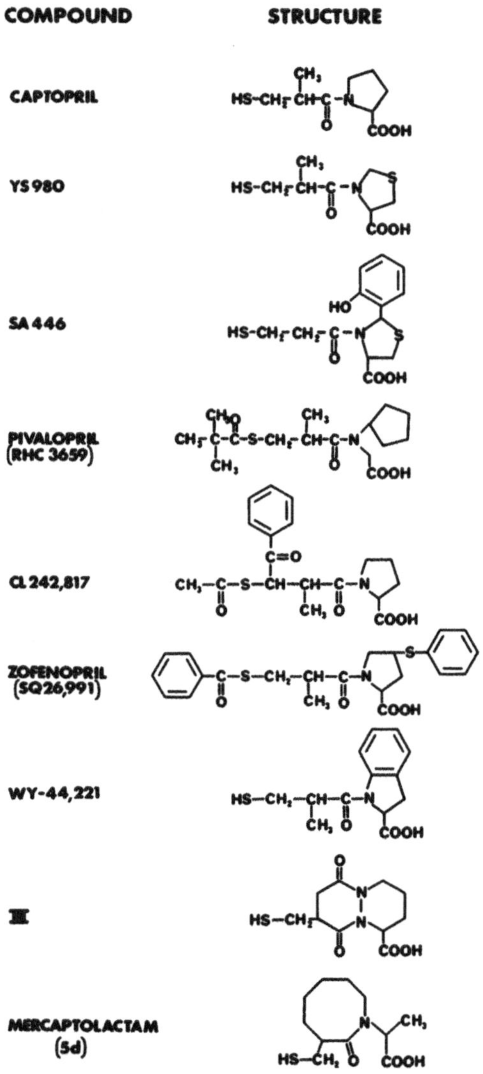

Fig. 5. The structures of converting enzyme inhibitors that contain sulfur. (From COHEN 1985)

captopril and the later developed CEI enalaprilat and ramiprilat bind to the active site of CE.

1.2.2 Other Captopril-Related Converting Enzyme Inhibitors

Further synthesis was directed towards compounds structurally related to captopril and led to CEI such as YS980 (FUNAE et al. 1980; UNGER et al. 1981a), SA 446 (ISO et al. 1981; UNGER et al. 1982a; TAKATA et al. 1982), pivalopril (RHC 3659-(s)) (WOLF et al. 1984; BURNIER et al. 1981), CL 242 817 (LAI et al. 1983), and zofenopril (SQ 26 991) (DEAN et al. 1984).

Table 1. Activities of converting enzyme (CE) inhibitors in vitro against purified CE from rabbit lung from UNGER et al. (1982b)

Tissue (rat)	IC_{50}(n*M*) Enalaprilat	Captopril
Plasma	12	120
Lung	28	140
Brain	30	175
Kidney	72	1050
Adrenal gland	29	240

The affinity of these sulfur-containing compounds for CE is similar to or lower than that of captopril. However, differences between these compounds exist with respect to their lipophilicity. SA 446, for instance, is an extremely lipophilic compound (UNGER et al. 1982a) which, therefore, has the propensity to penetrate biological barriers such as the blood-brain barrier more easily than other, less lipophilic compounds of this group.

A more recent development of a sulfur-containing CEI is WY-44221 which is 10–20 times more potent than captopril (STANTON et al. 1983; LAPPE et al. 1984) (Fig. 5).

1.2.3 Synthesis of Pro-Drug Converting Enzyme Inhibitors

Captopril was initially used at relatively high doses in clinical studies. Some of the side effects emerging from these studies such as skin rashes, loss of taste, and disturbances of the hematopoietic system were attributed to the sulfhydryl moiety of the compound, because of the similarity of these effects to those produced by penicillamine, another therapeutically used sulfhydryl-containing molecule (see also Sect. 11). Although, on subsequent reduced dosage, the occurrence of side effects including those mentioned above was greatly reduced, further synthetic efforts were directed towards CEI without the sulfhydryl moiety. The first potent non-sulfhydryl-containing CEI was enalapril/enalaprilat (MK 421/MK 422), a substituted *N*-carboxymethyl-dipeptide (PATCHETT et al. 1980; SWEET et al. 1981a). The affinity of enalaprilat, the dicarboxylic acid of this compound, for CE is about 5–10 times higher than that of captopril (UNGER et al. 1982b; SWEET 1983) (Table 1 and Fig. 6). However, since the bioavailability of enalaprilat is very low (BIOLLAZ et al. 1981; SWEET 1983), enalapril, an ethyl-ester of the compound, was developed as a pro-drug form. Enalapril, while having a very low activity against CE, is fairly well absorbed from the gut and subsequently hydrolyzed to the active diacid form by esterases in the liver, blood, and other tissues (ULM et al. 1982; UNGER et al. 1982b; COHEN and KURZ 1983).

Enalapril became the prototype for the development of structurally related pro-drug CEI (Fig. 7) such as indolapril (CI 907) (SYBERTZ et al. 1983; KAPLAN et al. 1984) and quinapril (CI-906) (KAPLAN et al. 1984). Further bicyclic pro-drug CEI with high affinity for CE include cilazapril (Ro 31-2848) (ATTWOOD

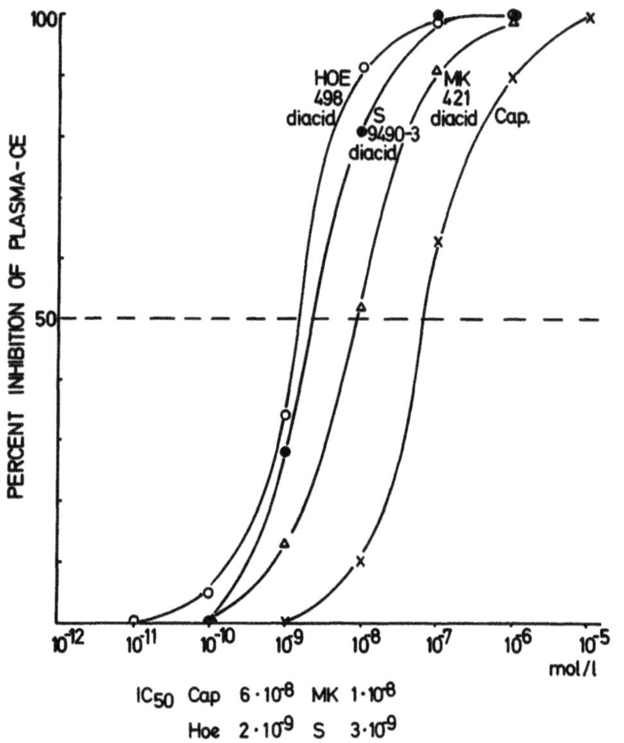

Fig. 6. In vitro inhibition of converting enzyme (*CE*) in rat plasma by ramiprilat (*Hoe 498 diacid*), perindoprilat (*S 9490–3 diacid*), enalaprilat (*MK 421 diacid*), and captopril (*Cap*) (From UNGER et al. 1986a)

et al. 1984; NATOFF et al. 1985), benazepril (CGS 14 824A) (PARSONS et al. 1983), and ramipril (Hoe 498) (BECKER et al. 1984; SCHÖLKENS et al. 1984a). Compared with enalapril, ramipril has a greater bioavailability and a higher potency against CE in plasma and tissues upon oral administration (BECKER et al. 1984; UNGER et al. 1984a; Table 2). As will be outlined below, the CE inhibitory mechanism of ramiprilat, the active diacid parent compound of ramipril, is characterized by a longer dissociation half-life of the enzyme-inhibitor complex when compared with enalaprilat (BÜNNING 1987), resulting in a more prolonged inhibitory action.

Further bicyclic pro-drug CEI lacking the phenethylamine side chain include pentopril (CGS 13945) (CHEN et al. 1984), substance 20 (HAYASHI et al. 1983), and perindopril (VINCENT et al. 1982; LAUBIE et al. 1984). Perindopril (S 9490-3) (Fig. 8) is the most active compound of this group. Its bioavailability and the affinity of its active diacid compound for CE are similar to ramipril and ramiprilat, respectively (UNGER et al. 1986a) (Table 2, Fig. 6).

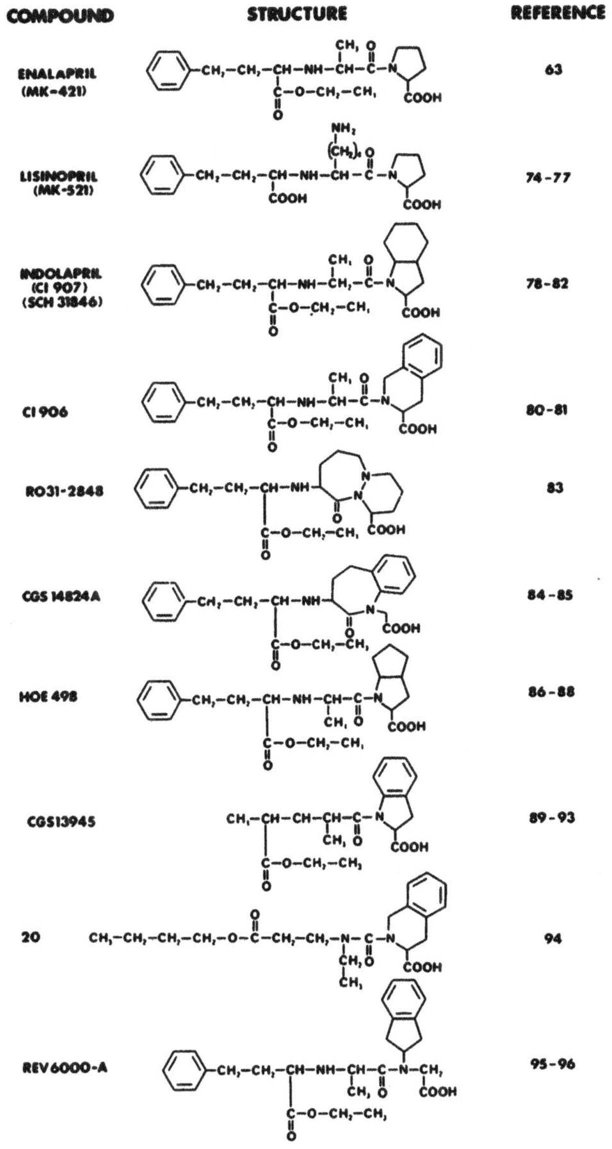

Fig. 7. The structures of converting enzyme inhibitors that do not contain sulfur or sulfhydryl moieties. (From COHEN 1985)

1.2.4 Non-Prodrug Nonsulfhydryl Converting Enzyme Inhibitors

Non-prodrug CEI without a sulfhydryl group have also been developed. The compounds indalapril [Rev 6000 A(SS)] (MANN et al. 1984) and lisinopril (MK 521) (BIOLLAZ et al. 1981; ULM et al. 1982) belong to this group. Indalapril has a nonrigid, bicyclic ring structure. In contrast to all the other CEI described so far, its proline nitrogen is not included in a ring structure (Fig. 7).

Table 2. Pharmacodynamic properties of converting enzyme inhibitors

Generic name	Captopril	Cilazapril	Enalapril	Lisinopril	Perindopril	Ramipril
Sulfhydryl containing	yes	no[34]	no	no	no	no
Pro-drug	no[3]	yes[34]	yes[1,2]	no	yes[23]	yes[22,24,25]
Active metabolite	–	cilazaprilat[34]	enalaprilat[1,2]	–	perindo-prilat	diacid of ramipril[22,24,25]
Liver metabolized	yes[3] (to a variety of metabolites)	yes[35] (to cilaza-prilat-also occurs in blood)	yes[1,4] (to active drug)	no	yes (to active drug)	yes[3] (to active drug and 3 further metabolites)
Parent drug immediately active intravenously	yes	no[34,35]	no[4,5]	yes		no[22]
Bioavailability	70%[6]	N.D.	40%[1,8] (as enalaprilat)	25%[7]	N.D.	54.65%[26]
Effect of food	35% reduction in fed state[6]	N.D.	nil[10]	nil[9]	N.D.	N.D.
Time to peak blood level after oral dose:						
Parent drug	0.5–1.5h[11]	1.8±0.2h[36]	1h[4]	7h[4]	8h[28]	0.3–1h[27]
Metabolite		1.3h[37] (mean 2.1h) 3.2±0.5h[36]	4h[4]			1.5–3h[24]
Effective plasma half-life	2h[12]	1.5h[35,37] 7.5±0.7h[36]	11h[8]	12.6h[7]	N.D.	10.8±1.3h[26] (very variable estimates range 11–27h[29])
Binding to plasma proteins						
Parent drug	30%[6,14]	N.D.	–	3%–10%[15]	N.D.	73%±2%[26]
Metabolite	–	N.D.	up to 50%[13]	–		56%±2%[26]

Route of elimination	renal (including metabolites)	renal[35] (80%–99%)	renal (as enalaprilat)	renal[4]	N.D.	metabolite cleared mainly through kidneys[22]
Mode of elimination	glomerular filtration[6] and tubular secretion[33]	N.D.	glomerular filtration and tubular secretion[4]	glomerular filtration[4]	N.D.	precise renal route not known
In vitro IC^{50} for ACE						
Parent drug	$2.6\times10^{-8}M$[15] (pig plasma) $3.5\times10^{-8}M$[30] (rabbit lung)	N.D.	$2.4-12\times10^{-7}M$[15] (pig plasma) $4.1\times10^{-7}M$[30] (rabbit lung)	$1.7\times10^{-9}M$[15] (pig plasma)	$3\times10^{-6}M$[31]	$2.6\times10^{-8}M$[30] (rabbit lung)
Metabolite		$1.93\times10^{-9}M$[38] (rabbit lung) $0.6\times10^{-9}M$[38] (human plasma)	$5.2\times10^{-9}M$[30] (rabbit lung)	–	$2.4\times10^{-9}M$[31]	$4.2\times10^{-9}M$[30] (rabbit lung)
In vitro potency relative to captopril (where captopril = 1)						
Parent drug	1.0[15]	N.D.	0.02–0.1[15] (pig plasma)	15.0[15] (pig plasma)	0.01	0.7[30] (rabbit lung)
Metabolite	–	3.6[38] (rabbit lung) 25.7[38] (human plasma)	6.7[30] (rabbit lung)	–	14.6	8.3[30] (rabbit lung)
In vitro potency (ED_{50}) against pressor response to angiotensin I						
Parent drug	60.5μg/kg i.v.[30]	approx. 1 mg p.o.[39]	27μg/kg i.v.[30]	2.3μg/kg i.v.	5.9μg/kg i.v.[31]	2.7μg/kg i.v.[30]
Metabolite	–		8.7 μg/kg i.v.[30]	–	2.6 μg/kg i.v.[31]	4.6 μg/kg i.v.[30]
In vivo potency relative to captopril (where capto-						

Table 2. (con't)

Generic name	Captopril	Cilazapril	Enalapril	Lisinopril	Perindopril	Ramipril
pril = 1)						
Parent drug	1.0	no comp. data	2.2	26.3	10.3	2.2
Metabolite	–		7.0	−23.3	13.1	
Time to onset of action after oral dose	0.5h[11]	1h[36]	2–4h[16,17]	2h[4]	1–2h[28]	1–2h[32]
Daily dosage:						
a) hypertension	once[40] to thrice daily[6]	once daily[35] (if dose >1 mg/day)	once daily[8]	once daily[15,20]	once daily[24,32]	
b) heart failure	twice to thrice daily[6]	N.D.	once to twice daily[19]	once daily[21]	N.D.	N.D.

This table was adapted from the table "ACE Inhibitor Pharmacology" provided by ICI Pharmaceuticals, Macclesfield, UK.

[1] Tocco et al. (1981)
[2] Unger et al. (1982b)
[3] Kripalani et al. (1980)
[4] Ulm et al. (1982)
[5] Nakashima and Nishijima (1982)
[6] Heel et al. (1980)
[7] Beerman et al. (1986)
[8] Davies et al. (1984a)
[9] Mojaverian et al. (1986)
[10] Ferguson et al. (1986)
[11] Case et al. (1978)
[12] Duchin et al. (1982)
[13] Davies et al. (1984a)
[14] McKinstry et al. (1978)
[15] Lisinopril—Data on file ICI Pharmaceuticals
[16] Biollaz et al. (1981)
[17] Ferguson et al. (1982b)
[18] Bergstrand et al. (1982)
[19] Todd and Heel (1986)
[20] Gomez et al. (1985)
[21] Warner et al. (1986)
[22] Witte et al. (1984a)
[23] Lees and Reid (1985)
[24] Manheim et al. (1985)
[25] Witte et al. (1984b)
[26] Eckert et al. (1984)
[27] Mannhold (1985)
[28] Bussien et al. (1986)
[29] Kondo et al. (1986)
[30] Becker et al. (1984)
[31] Laubie et al. (1984)
[32] Stumpe et al. (1986)
[33] Kubo and Cody (1985)
[34] Ajavyi et al. (1986)
[35] Sanchez et al. (1988)
[36] Shionori et al. (1988)
[37] Francis et al. (1987)
[38] Natoff et al. (1985)
[39] Belz et al. (1987)
[40] Schönberger and Wilson (1986)

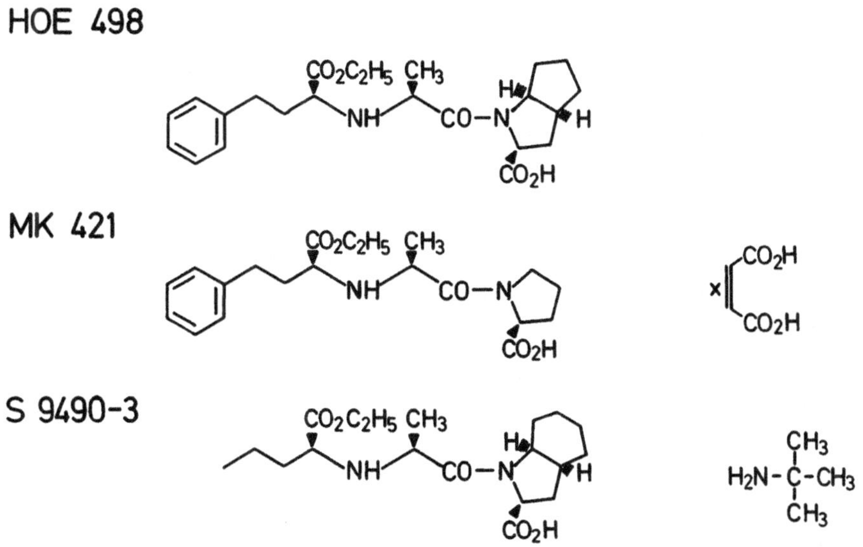

Fig. 8. Chemical structure of perindopril (*S 9490–3*) in comparison with ramipril (*Hoe 498*) and enalapril (*MK 421*)

Lisinopril is structurally closely related to and has an affinity for CE similar to enalprilat. The potential advantage of lisinopril over enalapril resides in the fact that, despite being a dicarboxylic acid, it does not have to be hydrolyzed to the active compound in the organism.

Another synthetic approach to develop nonsulfhydryl CEI resulted in the replacement of the sulfhydryl group by a phosphorous group. (Fig. 9). Fosenopril (SQ 28 555) is a pro-drug CEI with a CE inhibitory potency in vitro similar to captopril but with a longer duration of action than captopril following oral administration (POWELL et al. 1984).

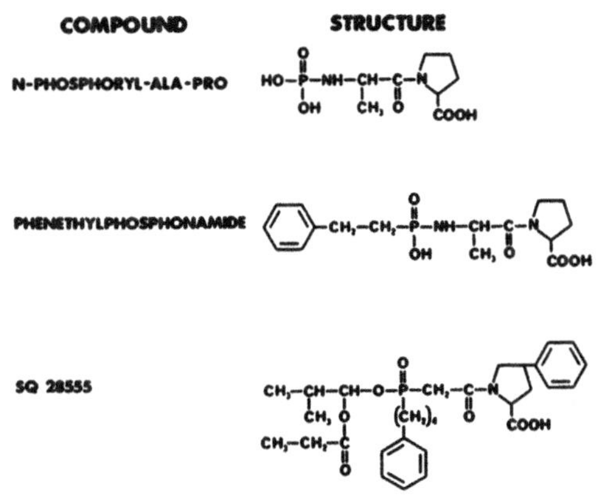

Fig. 9. The structure of converting enzyme inhibitors that contain phosphorus. (From COHEN 1985)

For further details on the development of CEI see reviews by CUSHMAN and ONDETTI (1980), COHEN (1985), and WYNRATT and PATCHETT (1985).

2 Pharmacokinetic Properties of Converting Enzyme Inhibitors

In general, CEI do not seem to differ greatly from each other with respect to their pharmacodynamic actions. However, their pharmacokinetic properties, including rate and degree of absorption, protein binding, tissue distribution, metabolism, and site of excretion, may vary to a large extent. These kinetic differences can have an impact on the choice of drug in a given clinical situation.

Table 2 summarizes the clinically relevant pharmacokinetic data of some CEI, which have already been introduced into clinical practice or await their introduction in the near future.

2.1 Captopril

The pharmacokinetics of captopril have been reviewed by MIGDALOF et al. (1984) and by DRUMMER and JARROTT (1986).

2.1.1 Absorption

Captopril is rapidly and reasonably well absorbed in all species tested including humans. Table 3 compares the T_{max} and C_{max} values of unchanged captopril and total radioactivity after oral administration of radiolabelled captopril in five

Table 3. Blood levels of radioactivity and unchanged captopril after oral administration (from MIGDALOF et al. 1984)

		Total radioactivity		Unchanged captopril	
Species	Dose (mg/kg)	T_{max} (h)	C_{max} (μg/ml)	T_{max} (h)	C_{max} (μg/ml)
Mouse (gavage)	50	0.5	40.8	0.5	21.5
Rat (gavage)	30	0.8	9.2	0.6	5.0
Monkey	2.5	1.0	0.8	0.8	0.4
(gavage)	25	2.0	11.2	ND[a]	ND
	450	4.9	138	5.3	94
Dog	2.5	1.3	1.9	1.0	1.2
(capsule)	25	1.2	22.6	ND	ND
	200	2.0	158	1.5[a]	93[a]
Man (tablet)	(100 mg)	1.0	1.58	0.9	0.8

NDs not determined.
[a] Estimated value; insufficient number of samples were analyzed for unchanged captopril.

species including humans. Studies in rodents suggested that ingestion of food can reduce absorption and bioavailability of captopril to some extent (SINGHVI et al. 1982), although this does not appear to have an impact on the clinical effectiveness of the drug in humans.

2.1.2 Distribution

Upon intravenous bolus administration, captopril and/or its metabolites are distributed to most of the tissues of the rat. In initial studies using radioactively labelled captopril, no radioactivity was found in the brain, suggesting that captopril does not penetrate the blood-brain barrier (see UNGER et al. 1984c). However, in subsequent investigations, inhibition of CE in structures of the central nervous system was observed in animals and in humans upon systemic administration of the drug (see Sect. 10), so that some degree of penetration of captopril from the blood to the brain has to be assumed. Access of captopril to other tissues such as the blood vessel wall, heart, and kidney is discussed in the respective sections on tissue CE inhibition.

Captopril was detected (as radioactivity) in the fetuses and amniotic fluid of rats after a single dose (ITA et al. 1982). However, in human umbilical cord blood captopril concentrations were very low, despite the presence of the drug in maternal venous blood and uterine blood at the time of delivery (see DRUMMER and JARROTT 1986). Penetration of captopril into the milk of lactating women appears to be limited, since less than 0.1% of the plasma peak concentration of captopril was found (DRUMMER and JARROTT 1986).

2.1.3 Protein Binding and Metabolism

Captopril forms reversible disulfide bonds with albumin and other proteins. Metabolites in the blood include a disulfide dimer and mixed disulfides of captopril with L-cysteine and glutathione. In whole blood and plasma, captopril is readily converted to its disulfide dimer and other oxidative metabolites. Evidence for a dynamic equilibrium in vivo between captopril and its metabolites in the blood has been presented. Biotransformation occurs predominantly at the sulfur atom of the sulfhydryl group. Consequently, the products of biotransformation recovered from the urine of various species include the disulfide dimer, mixed disulfides, *S*-methyl captopril, and the *S*-methyl sulfoxide of captopril (see reviews cited above).

2.1.4 Route of Elimination

Captopril and its metabolites are predominantly excreted by the kidneys. In a study in rhesus monkeys, 70% of a single 450 mg/kg dose of [^{14}C]captopril was excreted in the urine within 96 h, 45% was unchanged captopril, 38% captopril disulfide, and 6% *S*-methyl captopril. In rats, the relative amount of unchanged captopril in urine was found to be higher than in humans, monkeys, and dogs, but qualitatively the urinary excretion patterns of captopril and its metabolites are similar in all four species (MIGDALOF et al. 1984).

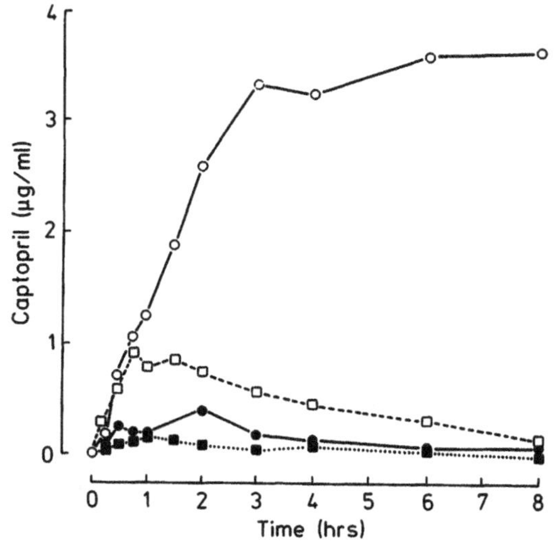

Fig. 10. Mean plasma levels of captopril in uremic patients (○) and in subjects with normal renal function (●), and mean plasma levels of total captopril disulfides in uremic patients (□) and in subjects with normal renal function (■) and after a single 50 mg oral dose of captopril. Total disulfides are expressed as captopril equivalents following reduction of the disulfides. (From DRUMMER and JARROTT 1986)

Studies in dogs and monkeys revealed that the renal excretory mechanism of captopril involves glomerular filtration as well as tubular excretion (MIGDALOF et al. 1984; see Table 2).

In patients with chronic renal failure a large increase in the blood levels of total captopril disulfides was observed over the first 8 h after a single oral dose of captopril, and the apparent half-life of these metabolites was prolonged to 36 h (DRUMMER and JARROTT 1986) (Fig. 10).

In other studies, variable effects of chronic renal failure on the elimination half-life and peak plasma levels of captopril and its metabolites were reported. However, there is no doubt that significant reduction in the urinary excretion rate and increases in $t_{1/2}$ occur at creatinine clearances below 20 ml/min, and there seems to be a linear relationship between the individual overall elimination rate constants of captopril and endogenous creatinine clearances (DRUMMER and JARROTT 1986).

2.2 Enalapril

The pharmacokinetics of enalapril/enalaprilat have been reviewed by ULM (1983) and TODD and HEEL (1986).

2.2.1 Absorption

Enalaprilat, the active diacid compound of enalapril, is poorly absorbed in all species tested including rat, dog, monkey, and humans. Absorption of MK422 was estimated at 5% in rats, 12% in dogs, and less than 10% in humans (ULM 1983).

Administration of the drug as its monoethyl ester (enalapril) significantly improved absorption to 39% in rats, 64% in dogs, and 53%–74% in humans (ULM 1983; TODD and HEEL 1986).

Enalapril is promptly bioactivated by esterases to the active diacid compound. In the rat, this hydrolytic activation takes place predominantly in the blood. However, other organs including the kidney, liver and, to a minor extent, brain also contain esterases to hydrolyze enalapril (UNGER et al. 1982b; ULM 1983; TODD and HEEL 1986; GOHLKE et al. 1989). In dogs, monkeys, and humans, the liver appears to be the predominant site of the hydrolytic activation of enalapril (ULM 1983).

As shown in Table 2, peak blood levels of the pro-drug can be observed after about 1 h, while the active diacid drug peaks later, about 3–4 h after oral administration of the pro-drug. Detectable levels of enalaprilat can still be found after 72–96 h (see TODD and HEEL 1986). The prolonged terminal phase is probably due to binding of enalaprilat to circulating CE (SWEET and ULM 1984). Food intake does not appear to have a significant influence on the drug absorption from the gut (SWANSON et al. 1984).

2.2.2 Distribution

Enalaprilat is less than 50% bound to protein in human plasma (DAVIES et al. 1984a) (Table 2). As outlined in the respective sections on CE inhibition in tissues, there is evidence that enalapril/enalaprilat will bind to and inhibit CE in various tissues. However, recent studies on the penetration of orally applied CE inhibitors into the CSF of rats suggest that, due to their low lipophilicity, enalapril/enalaprilat penetrate biological barriers less easily than more lipophilic CE inhibitors (GOHLKE et al. 1989).

Data on whether enalapril or enalaprilat enter into breast milk or transfer across the placenta are currently not available.

2.2.3 Metabolism

Besides being hydrolyzed to enalaprilat, there seems to be no significant further metabolism of enalapril in humans (DRUMMER et al. 1988). The hydrolytic conversion of enalapril to enalaprilat was calculated to be about 60% efficient in healthy subjects (DAVIES et al. 1984a) and was reported to be slower in patients with cirrhosis (TODD and HEEL 1986).

2.2.4 Route of Elimination

Enalapril and enalaprilat are excreted unchanged in the urine and feces. Following an oral dose of 10 mg in healthy subjects, 33% of the dose was recovered in feces (6% as enalapril and 27% as enalaprilat) and 61% in the urine (18% as enalapril and 43% as enalaprilat) within 72 h (ULM 1983). Some degree of biliary excretion of enalaprilat was reported in rats and dogs (see TODD and HEEL

1986). Whether biliary excretion occurs in humans is not known at present. The renal excretion mechanism involves both glomerular filtration (enalapril, enalaprilat) and tubular secretion (enalapril) (Table 2).

In patients with chronic renal failure, the impairment of the excretion of enalapril/enalaprilat follows a similar pattern as has been demonstrated with captopril, with increased peak serum concentrations and decreased urinary excretion rates. These changes were observed in patients with a glomerular filtration rate of <20–30 ml/min per 1.73 m^2 and/or with a creatinine clearance of less than 40 ml/min (see TODD and HEEL 1986). Dosage reduction according to impairment of renal function is required in these patients. Reduced renal function associated with age does not seem to contribute significantly to the greater antihypertensive efficacy of enalapril observed in a group of elderly versus young subjects (see TODD and HEEL 1986).

Pharmacokinetic data of cilazapril, lisinopril, perindopril, and ramipril can be obtained from Table 2 and from the literature cited in the legend to this table.

3 Inhibitory Mechanism of Converting Enzyme Inhibitors

Comparative enzyme kinetic studies have been performed with captopril, enalaprilat, and ramiprilat. They have classified these drugs as competitive enzyme inhibitors. The binding of these inhibitors to CE follows a two-step mechanism, with rapid formation of an enzyme inhibitor complex (EI) which then undergoes a slow isomerization process (EI*) (SHAPIRO and RIORDAN 1984a,b; BÜNNING 1984, 1987):

$$E + I \underset{k_2}{\overset{k_1}{\rightleftharpoons}} EI \underset{k_4}{\overset{\text{slow}}{\overset{k_3}{\rightleftharpoons}}} EI^*$$

Since a prolonged time interval is necessary to establish the equilibrium between CE and inhibitor, these compounds have been classified as slow and tight-binding inhibitors.

The inhibition constants for ramiprilat, enalaprilat, and captopril are shown in Table 4. Binding to CE is extremely tight, so that special kinetic procedures had to be employed to measure the respective inhibition constants. The tighter binding of enalaprilat and ramiprilat compared with captopril is reflected in the

Table 4. Equilibrium and rate constants for the inhibition of angiotensin-converting enzyme by ramiprilat, captopril, and enalaprilat

Inhibitor	K_i^* (pmol/l)	K_i (nmol/l)	K_3 (s^{-1})	K_4 (s^{-1})
Ramiprilat	7	10.8	2.8×10^{-2}	1.8×10^{-5}
Captopril	330	47	5.6×10^{-2}	4.0×10^{-4}
Enalaprilat	30	9.2	1.9×10^{-2}	1.1×10^{-4}

Values were obtained from SHAPIRO and Riordan (1984a,b) and BÜNNING (1987).

longer lifespan of the enzyme-inhibitor complex. The half-life for the dissociation of the enzyme inhibitor complex as estimated from the k_4 values of Table 4 is 29 min for captopril, 105 min for enalaprilat, and 640 min for ramiprilat.

These enzymekinetic data help to explain the differences with respect to potency and duration of action between captopril, enalaprilat, and ramiprilat.

4 Mechanism of Antihypertensive Action of Converting Enzyme Inhibitors

The reduction of circulating ANG II levels in the blood, leading to a diminution of the effects of the peptide on vascular tone, aldosterone release, and renal sodium handling, constitutes a principal mechanism of the antihypertensive action of CEI.

Inhibition of CE in the vascular endothelium of the lung and — to a minor extent — in the vascular endothelia of other organs and in the blood plasma accounts for the reduction in circulating ANG II levels.

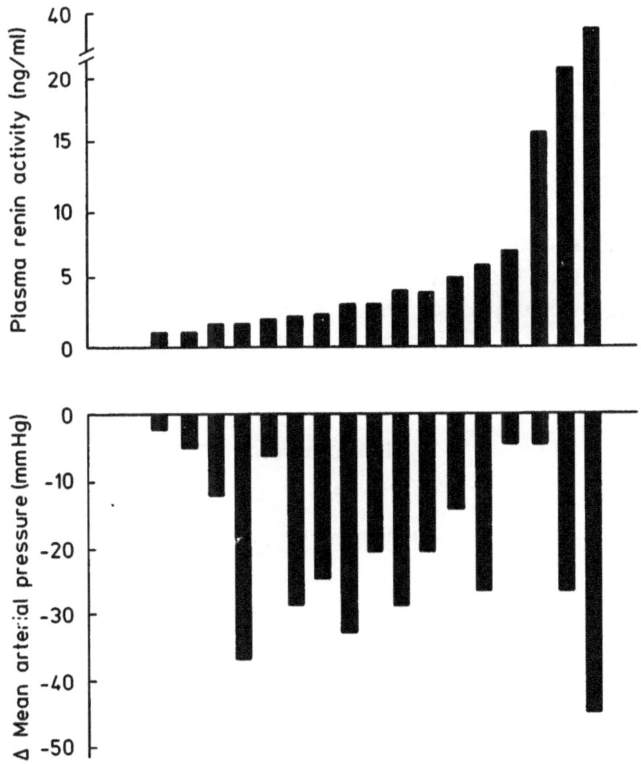

Fig. 11. Relation between pretreatment basal plasma renin activity (ranked in order of elevation) and decreases in mean arterial pressure in individual patients following 3 days of treatment with captopril on a dietary sodium intake of 100 mEq/day. (From BRAVO and TARAZI 1979)

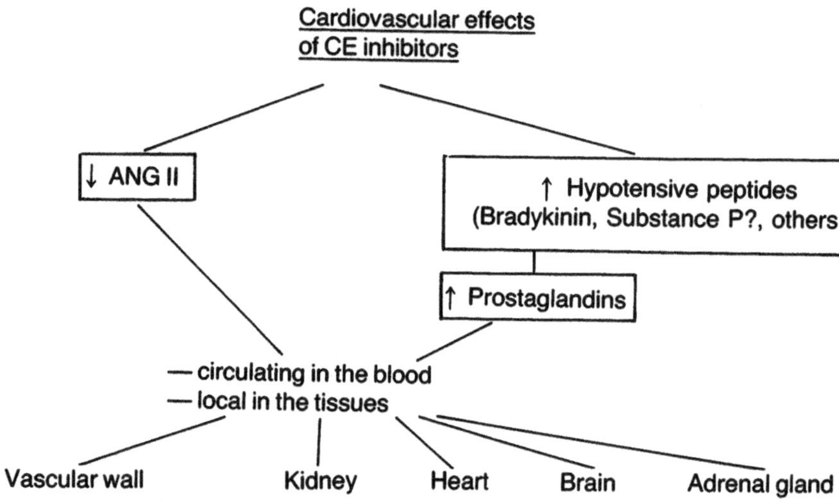

Fig. 12. Cardiovascular actions of converting enzyme (*CE*) inhibitors. *ANG II*, angiotensin II

However, accumulated evidence from studies in animals with various types of experimental hypertension, as well as from clinical studies showing that blood pressure could be lowered by CEI irrespective of whether the plasma RAS was stimulated or not (Fig. 11), has cast some doubt on the initial idea that the antihypertensive actions of CEI can be explained exclusively on the basis of reduced circulating ANG II levels. Therefore, additional pharmacodynamic effects of these drugs have to be considered.

Because CE is identical with the bradykinin degrading enzyme, kininase II, CE inhibitors could, theoretically, potentiate the direct, EDRF-, or prostaglandin-mediated vasodepressor effects of endogenous kinins (see Table 6).

Moreover, actions of CE inhibitors possibly unrelated to CE inhibition, such as alterations of vascular smooth muscle permeability to sodium (ITO et al.

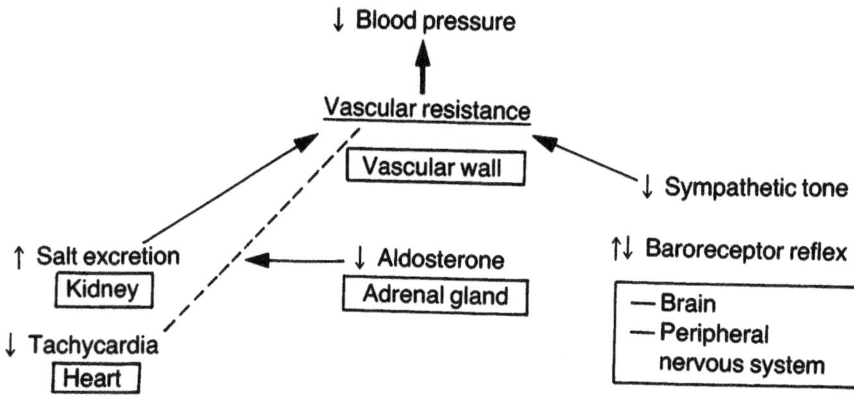

Fig. 13. Antihypertensive actions of converting enzyme inhibitors

1981), may play a role, although there is little evidence for such a mechanism.

An additional aspect of the mechanism of action of CEI, which has become a focus of scientific interest in recent years, is the inhibition of CE in various tissues involved in cardiovascular regulation, such as the heart, blood vessel wall, kidney, and brain (Fig. 12). Evidence for a contribution of tissue CE inhibition to the cardiovascular actions of CEI is discussed in later sections.

Finally, CEI have been demonstrated to interfere with sympathetic transmission, most likely by antagonizing the facilitating action of ANG II on presynaptic transmitter release, and to improve the function of the baroreceptor reflex. These features of the CEI are also discussed in a separate section.

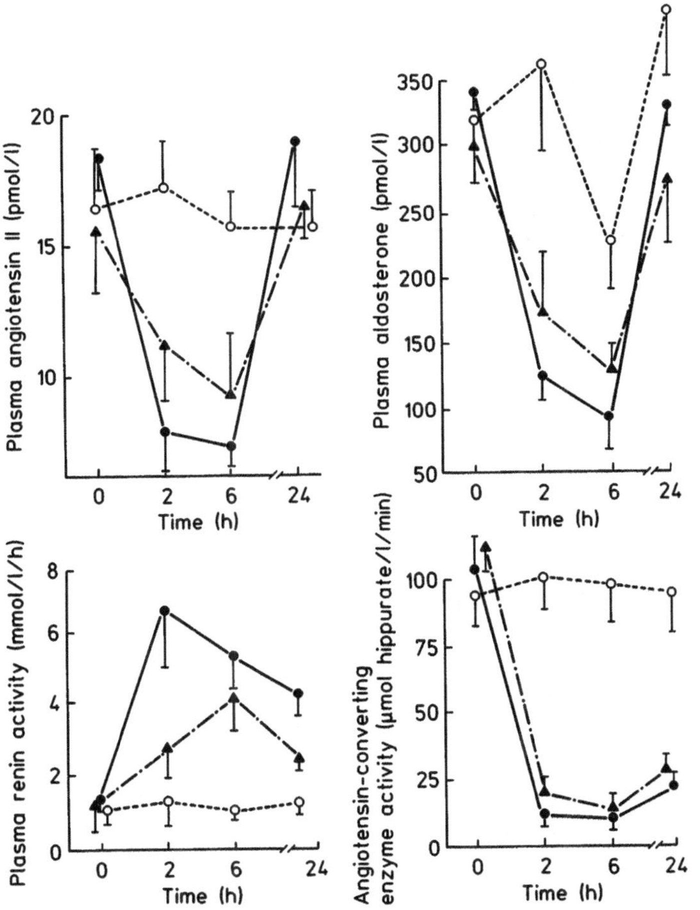

Fig. 14. Mean changes (± SEM) in plasma angiotensin II and aldosterone concentrations and in plasma renin and converting enzyme activities after single dose of placebo (○), 5 mg enalapril (△), and 20 mg enalapril (●) in nine normotensive subjects. Placebo caused no significant change except for the fall at 6 h in plasma aldosterone ($P < 0.02$). Compared with placebo, enalapril caused significant falls at 2 and 6 h in plasma angiotensin II ($P < 0.001$) and aldosterone ($P < 0.02$). Plasma renin activity rose significantly with enalapril and remained high 24 h after dosing ($P < 0.005$). CE activity was significantly reduced by enalapril at 2, 6, and 24 h ($P < 0.001$). (From MacGregor et al. 1981)

Figure 13 summarizes the various ANG II-related actions of CEI which can be brought about by a reduction of the circulating levels of the peptide but which could also be due to diminished local ANG II generation in the tissues indicated.

4.1 Evidence for and Against the Plasma Renin-Angiotensin System

Most of the early pharmacological and clinical studies in CEI focussed on acute effects of the drugs on blood pressure and parameters of the RAS. In these studies it has been repeatedly demonstrated that, upon CE administration, the expected changes of blood parameters of the RAS did occur: ANG II was lowered, ANG I increased, CE activity inhibited, renin activity increased due to the withdrawal of the negative feedback inhibition by ANG II, aldosterone levels in plasma or urine decreased, as were the plasma concentrations of the high molecular substrate for renin, angiotensinogen, due to enhanced comsumption (Fig. 14; see also references in Table 5).

In addition, the pressor responses to intravenous ANG I, but not ANG II, were blunted, a frequently employed test to estimate the degree of CE inhibition in lung vascular endothelium and plasma in vivo (BRUNNER et al. 1985a).

Moreover, in some instances of acute treatment, a close temporal association between serum levels of CEI, inhibition of plasma CE, and decrease in blood pressure was observed (Fig. 15) (JOHNSTON et al. 1983).

However, a careful analysis, especially of cases under chronic treatment, revealed that the antihypertensive actions of CEI were either not always accompanied by the expected changes in the parameters of the plasma RAS or that inhibition of the plasma RAS alone could not explain the blood pressure lowering effects of these drugs.

A few samples are given below. In addition, the data summarized in Table 5 illustrate the frequently observed discrepancies between changes in blood pressure and parameters of the plasma RAS under CEI treatment (see references 6–14 of Table 5).

THURSTON and SWALES (1978) reported that in salt-depleted rats the nonapeptide SQ 20881 lowered blood pressure even in the presence of ANG II receptor blockade with the compeptitive ANG II receptor antagonist saralasin.

SWEET et al. (1981b) observed a two-phasic depressor effect following oral administration of captopril and enalapril in spontaneously hypertensive rats (SHR) and renal hypertensive rats. Only the initial depressor response corresponded to the inhibition of the ANG I pressor responses. The resultant sustained blood pressure decrease occurred after the ANG I pressor responses had returned to normal (i.e., in the absence of CE inhibition in plasma and lung endothelium).

In stroke-prone spontaneously hypertensive rats (SHRSP), using SA 446 and captopril, we observed that after 4 weeks of oral treatment with 50 mg/kg per day the captopril-treated rats showed a reduction of the ANG I pressor responses of 52%, while the SA 446-treated rats showed a reduction of 18%. Blood pressure, however, was lowered to a similar extent in both groups. In

Table 5. Effects of converting enzyme inhibitor treatment on the plasma renin–angiotensin–aldosterone system. CEI, converting enzyme inhibitor; MAP, mean arterial blood pressure; CEA, converting enzyme activity; ANG, angiotensin; PRA, plasma renin activity; ALDO, aldosterone; ANG'ogen, angiotensiongen; SHR, spontaneously hypertensive rat; SHRSP, stroke prone spontaneously hypertensive rat; RVH, renovascular hypertension; CRF, chronic renal failure; d, day; w, Week; m, month; AI, angiotensin I.

Species	Type of hypertension	CEI	Dose (mg/kg)	Time	MAP (mmHg)	CEA (nmol/ml per min)	ANG II (pg/ml)	ANG I (pg/ml)	PRA (ngANGI/ ml per h)	ALDO (ng/dl)	ANG'ogen (pmol/ml)	Reference
Rat	SHRSP	Perindopril	0	3d	185[a]	94.3		607	1.09[b]		312	1
			0.1		150*	78.0*		1140	2.45*		301	
			1		120*	39.6*		1610*	2.18*		248*	
			3		100*	18.0*		2008*	4.09*		210*	
			10		100*	4.5*		1670*	5.37*		146*	
			0	2w	185	83		565	1.84		272	
			0.1		155*	64.1*		1050*	4.67*		295	
			1		120*	29.6*		1380	4.82*		229	
			3		100*	16.3*		1410	6.32*		151*	
			10		90*	2.8*		2090*	6.49*		57*	
			0	4w	195	75.9		190	1.91		258	
			0.1		170	85.7		380	3.83*		253	
			1		130*	52.2*		420	4.98*		179*	
			3		110*	18.1*		420	6.59*		86*	
			10		85*	3.0*		1000*	6.52*		26*	
		Control	–	2w	197		9.4 5.9[d]	109				
		perindopril	1		110	30%[c]	3.4 3.5	445				
		enalapril	30		105	70%	3.8 4.6	679				
		ramipril	1		115	55%	6.2 2.1	276				
Human	Normotensive	Enalapril	20	d1/0h	114/78[c]	1.55	12.5 7.6[d]	30	1.0	9		2
				d1/4h	105/71	0.01*	6.3* 2.0*	165*	7.1*	4.2*		
				d4/0h	109/76	0.2*	13.3 7.5	81	4.9*	8.6		
				d4/4h	100/70	0.005*	8.4* 3.1*	462*	12.4*	4.0*		

Table 5. (con't)

Species	Type of hypertension	CEI	Dose (mg/kg)	Time	MAP (mmHg)	CEA (nmol/ml per min)	ANG II (pg/ml)	ANG I (pg/ml)	PRA (ngANGI/ml per h)	ALDO (ng/dl)	ANG'ogen (pmol/ml)	Reference
Human	Primary hypertension (normal Na⁺)	Enalapril	10	0h	111.6	29.7	12.9	557	3.3[b]	10.9	3	3
				8h	98.3*	14.7*	8.7*	1138*	12.4*	8.2*		
	primary hypertension (low Na⁺)	Enalapril	10	0h	102.3	29.2	29.5	385	5.9	12.5		
				8h	86.5*	14.6*	12.0*	1347*	30.8*	9.1*		
Human	Hypertension	Control	–	–	128	96.7	24		2.76	18.1		4
		enalapril	25	24h	118	35	18		4.2	17		
			20	24h	108*	15.1*	13.7*		7.56*	7.8*		
Human	Normotensive	Enalapril	5	0h	121/70[c]	110	16.7		1.5	10.8		5
				2h	117/62	20*	11.5*		3.6*	6.3*		
				6h	108*/62*	15*	8.5*		5.2*	4.7*		
				24h	115/66	25*	17.3		3.1*	9.9		
			20	0h	121/70	105	18.8		1.7*	12.2		
				2h	114*/61*	10*	4.7*		8.4*	4.5*		
				6h	112*/62*	10*	3.1*		6.5*	3.2*		
				24h	121/67	20*	19.5		5.3*	12.1		
Rat	Normotensive	Enalapril	0	0h	111	215	9.9[d]		5.6			6
			10	3h	86*	<15*	9.7		26.5*			
			30	3h	81*	<15*	2.3*		21.3*			
			30	1w	87*	<15*	28.9*		9.9			
			30	2m	85*	<15*	43.1*		9.4			
Rat	SHRSP	Control	–	2w	180[a]	110	120	337	1.5[b]		320	7
		ramipril	10		115*	18*	89*	740*	4.9*		220*	

		enalapril	10		160*	80*	78*	519	3.2		350*	
		Control	–	4w	205	95	115	194	1.5		200	
		ramipril	10		115*	10*	78*	493*	4.2*		120*	
		enalapril	10		170*	65*	89*	480*	1.9		210	
Rat	SHR	Captopril	10	0h	182	147.6						8
				0.25h	182	13.8*						
				1h	165*							
				3h	164*							
				24h	163*	155						
		Enalapril	1	0h	180	147.6						
				0.25h		26.5*						
				1h	172*	2.1*						
				3h	166*	3.3*						
				24h	172*	150						
Rat	SHRSP	Captopril		0w	185[a]		84		0.9[b]		310	9
				2w	160*		63*		1.9		213*	
				4w	142*		86		5.9*		204*	
		SA446		0w	180		84		1.0		295	
				2w	175*		63*		1.0		243*	
				4w	155*		84		2.6		231*	
Human	Normotensive	Placebo	–	0h	85.9	21.5	11.2	11.1	26	6.2		10
				4h	89.8	21.5	7.7	8.8	24	6.4		
				12h	90.9	21.7	9.4	10.4	32	5.4		
				24h	85.5	21.5	11.7	12.0	36	8.7		
		Ramipril	5	0h	88.6	21.2	13.5	12.1	30[f,b]	8.2		
				4h	88.8*	2.0*	4.9*	32.7*	60*	4.6*		
				12h	86.2*	5.2*	6.5	34.1*	73*	3.8		
				24h	83.8*	8.3*	10.2	29.8*	57*	7.1*		
			20	0h	89.9	21.2	12.6	11.3	32	7.6		
				4h	83.2*	0.8*	3.0*	65.5*	151*	4.1*		

Table 5. (con't)

Species	Type of hypertension	CEI	Dose (mg/kg)	Time	MAP (mmHg)	CEA (nmol/ml per min)	ANG II (pg/ml)	ANG I (pg/ml)	PRA (ngANGI/ml per h)	ALDO (ng/dl)	ANG'ogen (pmol/ml)	Reference
				12h	88.8	4.2*	7.0	55.8*	114*	4.0		
				24h	84.9*	7.3*	11.2	39.2*	77*	7.5		
			50	0h	88.7	20.8	12.9	10.2	28	7.7		
				4h	84.9*	0.5*	2.9*	114.1*	210*	6.2		
				12h	86.9*	1.7*	4.5	87.5*	180*	3.4*		
				24h	83.8	4.7*	9.8	44.6*	105*	8.6		
Human	Primary hypertension (normal PRA)	Captopril	100	0h	165/104[c]				0.79			11
				2h	159/101				4.38			
				6h	146*/98*				2.36			
	Primary hypertension (low PRA)	Captopril	100	0h	182/115				0.21			
				2h	177/109				0.31			
				6h	170*/104				0.21			
	RVH	Captopril	100	0h	222/122				2.94			
				2h	186*/106*				11.93*			
				6h	200/112				10.11*			
	All	Captopril	100	0h		36.9			0.9	10.5		
				2h		16.9*			4.5*	5.5*		
				6h		26.0*			3.5*	6.5*		
Human	Primary hypertension	Enalapril	2,5[g]	0h	134[g]	100[g]			2	16		12
				4h	129	19*			8	10.0*		
				24h	131	30*			6	2		
			5	0h	128	38**			3	16		
				4h	124	<5*			16*	9.0*		
				24h	123	21*			4	13		

			10	0h	123**	32**		3	18	
				4h	116*	<5*		25*	5.0*	
				24h	121	15*		8	15	
			20	0h	119**	22**		4	16	
				4h	112*	<5*		23*	7.0*	
				24h	122	10*		15*	11	
		Enalapril	20	0h	181/112[c]	95	21	2	15	
				4h	140*/92*	<5*	7.0*	17	5.0*	
				24h	152*/101*	11*	11.5	10	8.5	
				1m	153*/100*	6*	11.5	11	13	
				3m	138*/90*	<5*	16	20*	12.5	
				6m	142*/96*	5*	28	26*	14	
Human	Anephric	Captopril	100	0min	128/72[c]			1.6[h]		13
				30min	118/63*	51%[c]		1.6		
				60min	115/59*	63%		1.2		
				90min	112/57*	72%		1.1		
				24h	107/54*	70%		2.1		
Human	RVH	Control	–	–	180/117[l]	70[l]		24[l]	18[l]	14
		captopril	200 (2x)	4–6d	132/91	20		51	7	
				109d[i]	150/88	85		38	30	
				109d[k]	127/88	27		65	14	
	Primary hypertension	Control	–	–	172/116	72		5	20	
		captopril	200 (2x)	4–6d	143*/92*	23		15	12	
		Captopril +diuretics	200 (2x)	42d[i]	138/93*	61		20	30	
				42d[k]	131/87*	18		40	9	
	CRF	Control	–	–	195/121	84		3	23	

Table 5. (con't)

Species	Type of hypertension	CEI	Dose (mg/kg)	Time	MAP (mmHg)	CEA (nmol/ml per min)	ANG II (pg/ml)	ANG I (pg/ml)	PRA (ngANGI/ml per h)	ALDO (ng/dl)	ANG'ogen (pmol/ml)	Reference
		captopril	200 (2x)	4–6d	156/104	12			13	8		
		Captopril +diuretics	200 (2x)	57d[i]	133/87	26			25	25		
				57d[k]	121/84	15			30	19		

[a] Systolic blood pressure
[b] Plasma renin concentration
[c] % inhibition
[d] HPLC controlled
[e] Systolic/diastolic
[f] mU/l
[g] Successive treatment with increasing dose: * significant versus time 0 of dose; ** significant versus time 0 of study
[h] μU/ml—plasma active renin
[i] 1 h before captopril
[k] 1 h after captopril
[l] Significances not provided

[1] UNGER et al. (1986a)
[2] NUSSBERGER et al. (1986)
[3] JACKSON et al. (1984)
[4] GAVRAS et al. (1981)
[5] MACGREGOR et al. (1981a)
[6] MENTO and WILKES (1987)
[7] UNGER et al. (1984a)
[8] COHEN and KURZ (1982)
[9] UNGER et al. (1982a)
[10] MANHEM et al. (1985)
[11] LECHI et al. (1985)
[12] BIOLLAZ et al. (1982)
[13] MAN IN'T VELD et al. 1980
[14] WAEBER et al. (1980)

Additional references: JACKSON et al. (1988), EISEN et al. (1987), NAKATA et al. (1987), NORMAN et al. (1987), NAMBU et al. (1986), PHILLIPS and KIMURA (1986), CORVOL et al. (1984), WILKES (1984), LAUBIE et al. (1984), HOWLETT and LONGMAN (1983), JOHNSTON et al. (1980), NUSSBERGER et al. (1988), MERSEY et al. (1987), DCLEEUW and BIRKENHÄGER (1986), NUSSBERGER et al. (1985), FOUAD et al. (1984), JOHNSTON et al. (1984), GIVEN et al. (1984), MOOKHERJEE et al. (1983), SHOBACK et al. (1983b), FERGUSON et al. (1982a), MILLAR et al. (1982), MACGREGOR et al. (1981b), MILLAR et al. (1981), BRUNNER et al. (1981), ATKINSON et al. (1980), SWARTZ et al. (1980), MORTON et al. (1980), SWARTZ et al. (1979), JOHNSTON et al. (1979), BRAVO and TARAZI (1979).

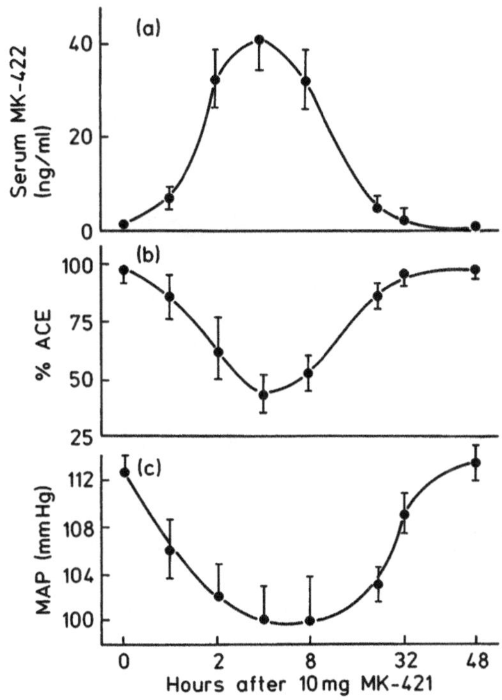

Fig. 15. **a** *MK-422* (enalaprilat) levels, **b** percentage converting enzyme (*%ACE*) activity, and **c** mean arterial blood pressure (*MAP*) after 10 mg enalapril for 12 patients with essential hypertension. (From Johnston et al. 1983)

addition, only the captopril-treated SHRSP showed the characteristic signs of plasma RAS inhibition at this time.

Crantz et al. (1980) were unable to correlate reductions of circulating ANG II with the antihypertensive effects of SQ 20881 and captopril in patients with primary hypertension and normal renin.

Boomsma et al. (1981) observed that in hypertensive patients upon withdrawal from chronic treatment with captopril, the inhibited plasma CE activity quickly returned to normal or supranormal levels, yet blood pressure remained lowered for days. Similar results were obtained in our laboratory in experiments using enalapril, ramipril, and perindopril in SHR (Fig. 16) (Unger et al. 1985, 1986a). In addition, the prolonged posttreatment blood pressure reduction was associated with a persistent tissue CE inhibition in the aorta, mesenteric vasculature, and kidney (see also Sect. 9).

Schalekamp et al. (1982) reported that sometimes the short-term, but never the long-term, effects of CEI monotherapy on systemic arterial pressure were positively correlated with pretreatment renin levels. The conclusion that a mechanism independent of circulating renin may contribute to CEI antihypertensive effects is supported by their results in nephrectomized patients on maintenance hemodialysis, in whom a decrease in systemic arterial pressure was

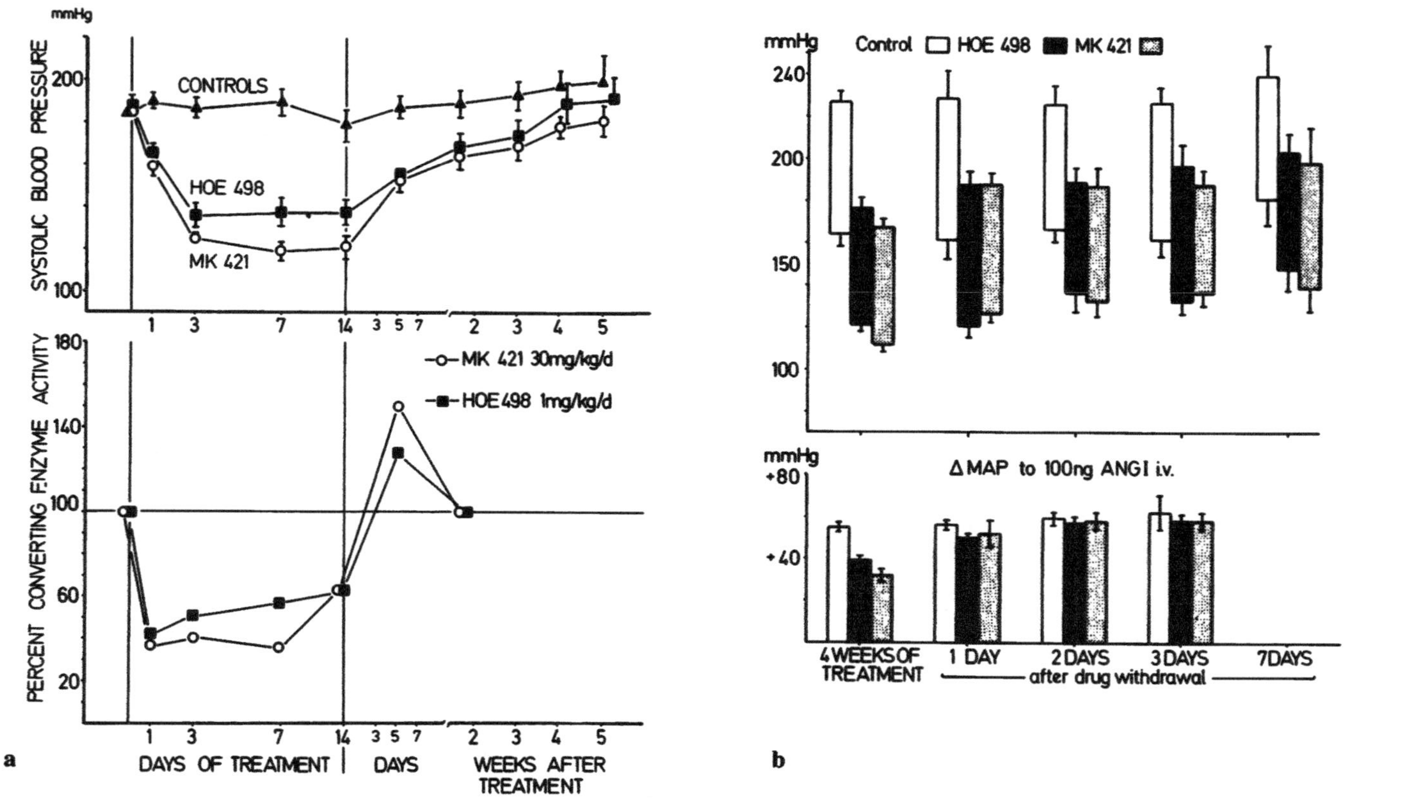

Fig. 16.a Systolic blood pressure and plasma converting enzyme (CE) activity during and after oral treatment with ramipril (*Hoe 498*) and enalapril (*MK 421*) in SHRSP. CE was inhibited during treatment ($P < 0.001$) and increased 5 days after drug discontinuation ($P < 0.001$). Blood pressure was significantly lowered in both treatment groups for 2 weeks after discontinuation of treatment (from UNGER et al. 1985). **b** Recovery of systolic blood pressure (*upper panel*) and pressor responses to angiotensin I (*ANG I*) 100 ng i.v. (*lower panel*) following 4 weeks of oral treatment with ramipril (*Hoe 498*, 3 mg/kg per day) and enalapril (*MK 421*, 30 mg/kg per day) in spontaneoulsy hypertensive, strokeprone rats. Blood pressure was significantly lowered ($P < 0.05$–0.01) during the whole post-treatment observation period whereas the pressor responses to ANG I were inhibited only on the morning after the last night of treatment ($P < 0.01$) (From UNGER et al. 1985)

shown after treatment with captopril. This effect was seen only after the subjects had been fluid-depleted by ultrafiltration. The well-known potentiation of the antihypertensive effects of captopril by the use of diuretics may therefore be independent, at least in part, of the diuretic-induced stimulation of the hormonal plasma RAS.

In addition, numerous clinical studies have now confirmed that under chronic treatment conditions CEI are equally effective in patients with high renin levels as in patients with normal or low renin levels (see reviews by HEEL et al. 1980; VIDT et al. 1982; EDWARDS and PADFIELD 1985; TODD and HEEL 1986), although the acute effects of CEI after the first dose are usually more marked in patients with high renin, especially those pretreated with diuretics or those with renal artery stenosis.

In summary, there is no doubt that the inhibition of the plasma RAS plays an important role for the acute antihypertensive effects of CEI upon the initiation of treatment. Under chronic treatment conditions, however, the plasma RAS appears to become less important, and additional antihypertensive mechanisms may be involved. Among those, a local inhibition of CE in various blood pressure controlling organs has been suggested by several investigators (COHEN and KURZ 1982; UNGER et al. 1986b; DZAU 1987b; LINZ and SCHÖLKENS 1987). The evidence for such a tissue-related mechanism of action is discussed below.

4.2 Role of Endogenous Kinins

Whereas the inhibtion of ANG II generation in plasma or tissue is generally acknowledged to be important for the antihypertensive actions of CEI, the relevance of a possible potentiation of endogenous kinins by these drugs has not yet been defined clearly. A number of publications on this topic are summarized in Table 6. This table also contains conclusions of the authors as to the importance of a kinin-dependent mechanism for the action of the CEI used in their respective model of hypertension. Since the effects of CEI on prostaglandin generation are closely linked to the kinin system, studies on CEI-induced changes in prostaglandins levels as well as the effect of pharmacological inhibition of prostaglandin synthesis on the actions of CEI are included in this table.

A possible contribution of kinins to the beneficial effects of CEI on the heart is discussed in Sect. 8).

5 Hemodynamic Effects of Converting Enzyme Inhibitors

5.1 Effects on Blood Pressure

5.1.1 In Normotensive Animals and Humans

In normotensive, sodium-replete rats CEI administration usually has little effect on blood pressure (see reviews by HEEL et al. 1980; TODD and HEEL 1986), while in normotensive, sodium-replete dogs dose-related reductions of blood pressure have been observed after a single oral dose of captopril and other CEI (HARRIS et al. 1978). In normotensive, sodium-depleted animals (with a stimulated

Table 6. Effects of converting enzyme inhibitors on endogenous kinins and prostaglandins

Species	Hypertension model	Drug tested	Blood pressure (mmHg)	Plasma Bradykinin (BK)	Urinary kallikrein	Hemodynamic effects	Prostaglandins	Conclusions	Reference
segment human basilar artery		Captopril $5\times10^{-6}M$				No change in concentration effect of BK (relaxation)		CE in basilar artery does cleave BK.	WHALLEY et al. 1987
SD rat female normotensive		*Exp. 1: in vivo* Ramipril a) 2.5×10^{-6}, b) 2.5×10^{-7}, c) 2.5×10^{-9} Mol/kg p.o., 60 min later aorta dissected *Exp. 2: in vitro* Ramiprilat incubation of aorta portions at a) $10^{-9}M$, b) $10^{-6}M$, c) $10^{-4}M$ *Exp. 3:* Aprotinin 40,000 U/kg s.c. 60 min before protocol 2					*6keto-PGF1$_\alpha$ in Medium:* [$pmol\cdot mg^{-1}\cdot 30mm^{-1}$] *Exp. 1:* 0:63.9±4.7 a) 82.7±5.5 b) 80.3±4.9 c) 62.5±7.3 *Exp. 2:* 0:68.6±3.6 a) 75.3±7.3 b) 82.3±5.6 c) 93.9±6.0 *Exp. 3:* Control: 82.3±5 +aprotinin: 51.5±5	Ramipril stimulates PGI 2 synthesis; Since aprotinin inhibits PGI increase, this stimulation of PG synthesis seems to be dependent on an intact kallikrein-kinin system	SCHERF et al. 1986
SHRsp WKY				*Dose response (SBP) to BK* (ED_{50})	*4w:* 1a:34.6 1b:38.1 [µg BK/min/ 24 h volume]			Urinary kallikrein excretion	UNGER et al. 1981a

		Group 1a: SHR YS980 50mg/kg per day, ×12w *Group 1b:* Control SHR *Group 2a:* WKY, YS980 *Group 2b:* Control WKY	*1a:* 0w:137±3 12w:150±6 *1b:* 0w:134±2 12w:208±3 *2a:* 0w: 99±2 12w:106±3 *2b:* 0w:102±1 12w:121±5	*1a:* 74 ng *1b:* 660 ng *2a:* 60 ng *2b:*1400 ng	2a:38.9 2b:32.4 *8w:* 1a:45.8 1b:48.1 2a:39.6 2b:45.5 *12w:* 1a:53.5 1b:60.6 2a:70.9 2b:62.2	unchanged by YS980. Thus, renal kallikrein cannot be crucial for chronic YS980 and captopril effects	
Wistar rat (Na^+-depleted) Wistar rat, (normal Na^+diet)	normotensive 2K-1C	a) BK 400ng/kg i.v., b) Rabbit-anti-BK Ab (KAb) or normal rabbit globulin (NR) c) Captopril 0 or 100 mg/kg i.v. d) BK i.v.	*BK effect:* BK:−27 NR+CEI +BK:−45 KAb+CEI +BK:−8 *Normotensive rats:* NAb+C:−25 NR+C:−32 *2K-1C rats:* KAb:±0 NR:±0 KAb+C:−21 NR+C:−5			Local role of kinins not excluded or supported. Antibodies do not reach distal nephron or CNS: block only circulating kinins. Acute captopril effect: in 2K-1C due to increased kinins, in normal rats due to ANGII	Carretero et al. 1981

Table 6. (con't)

Species	Hypertension model	Drug tested	Blood pressure (mmHg)	Plasma Bradykinin (BK)	Urinary kallikrein	Hemodynamic effects	Prostaglandins	Conclusions	Reference
SD rat female	normotensive	Captopril 1.7 μg/min; BK 0.1 μg/min or vehicle i.v. ×7 days On days 1,2, 6,7: stilbestrol 500 μg/kg s.c.	Day 1: C: −10 B: − 8, C: lasted 7 days B: lasted 3 days	*Uterine BK binding sites:* (fmol/mg protein) Day 2: Control: 700 C: 555 B: 536 Day 7: Control: 632 C: 465 B: 640				Negative feedback of BK on number of binding sites. No sustained hypotensive effect of BK: circulating BK alone cannot contribute to chronic captopril effect	YASUJIMA et al. 1982
SD Rat male	normotensive	*Exp. A:* Enalapril 0,1,10 mg/kg p.o. twice daily, 2 or 4 days. *Exp. B:* Enalapril 0 or 10 mg/kg twice daily for 4 days			*Exp. B:* (μg/24h) *Control:* day0: 26±2.5 day4: 30±3.7 *Enalapril:* day0: 31±5.7 day4: 44±8.3		*Exp. A:* Urinary PGE_2 (ng/8h): 4 day control: 15±5.1 4 day Enalapril: 10±2.5	Prostaglandins don't seem to be mediating enalapril-induced renin release (Exp. A). No evidence for stimulation of renin secretion by kinins: no increase in urinary kallikrein in rats with elevated PRA after enalapril (Exp. B)	SCHIFFRIN et al. 1984

Wistar rat, male	2K-1C	*Group 1:* Enalapril (E) 1 mg/kg i.v. single dose; after 30–90 min BK-antagonist (B) 0, 40μg/min i.v. for 10 min	*Group 1:* 168±6 +E:127±5 +B:+12±3	30% of blood pressure decrease after enalapril due to BK, 70% due to ANG II. No correlation between baseline blood pressure or enalapril effect and response to BK-antagonist	Benetos et al. 1986a
		Group 2: Saralasin (S) 10μg/kg per min cont'ed i.v., after 30 min BK-antagonist as in group 1, day2 same as group 1	*Group 2:* 181±6 +S:156±7 +B:0 day2:as in group 1		
		Group 3: Na-nitro-prusside (N) 10μg/min to titrate blood pressure then BK-antagonist as in group 1	*Group 3:* 183±7 +N:128±8 +B:0		
Wistar rat, male	normotensive	*Group 1:* BK-antagonist 2x 1 mg in aorta, injections 5 min apart	*Group 1:* 117±4 1st injection: +12 (n:6) −29 (n:4) 2nd injection: +15 (n:6) +12 (n:4)	BK plays role in maintenance of normal blood pressure. Magnitude of BK-antagonist effect not affected by	Benetos et al. 1986b

Table 6. (con't)

Species	Hypertension model	Drug tested	Blood pressure (mmHg)	Plasma Bradykinin (BK)	Urinary kallikrein	Hemodynamic effects	Prostaglandins	Conclusions	Reference
		Group 2: 5%dextrose (D) 0.2 ml; 5 min later BK-antagonist (B) 1 mg *Group 3:* Ramipril (R) 1 mg/kg, 45 min later BK-antagonist as group 1	*Group 2:* 117±4 D:+3 B:+16 *Group 3:* 120±5 Ramipril −13 R:+11 B:+17					ramipril. Forms of hypertension due to BK deficiency?	
SD rat	normotensive hypertensive with aortic ligation between renal arteries	*Group 1:* (normotensive) BK 100,200, 400 ng/kg i.v. boluses 5 min apart Then BK-antagonist i.v. cont'ed, After 5 min BK injection repeated. 30 min later enalaprilat 60μg/kg, BK+BK-antagonist repeated as above	*Group 1:* (BK 400ng) 113±3 BK:−25 E+BK:−35 BKa+BK:−12 E+BK+BKa: −17					Aortic ligation model of hypertension leads to expected high kinin levels by tissue damage. Hypotensive effect of CEI blunted by BK antagonist. No increase in plasma kinins after CEI	CARBONELL et al. 1988

		Groups 2/3: (hypertensive) Saline or BK-antagonist cont'ed i.v. for 15 min after 5 min enalaprilat 60μg/kg i.v.	*Group 2:* 180±7 Saline: ±0 Enalaprilat after 5 min: 136 30 min: 150 *Group 3:* 177±3 BK-antagonist: ±0 E 5 min: 155 E30 min: 170			
		Group 4: (hypertensive) enalaprilat 60μg/kg i.v.	*Group 4:* −42	[pg/ml] Control: 41±10 E: 68±20		
Rabbit (intact and anephric)	normotensive	*Exp. 1:* (intact and anephric) – BK 1 μg/kg i.v. – Captopril 1 mg/kg i.v. – 5 min later BK – Indometha-acin 2.5 μg/kg i.v. – BK	*Exp. 1:* *Intact:* 101±6 BK: −20 Cap+BK: −55 Cap+BK+I: −45 *Anephric:* 101±5 BK: −32 Cap+BK: −45 Cap+BK+I: −40		BK effect in normotensive rabbits sustained 20 min, in anephric rabbits 2 min. Captopril caused 850% enhancement of BK effect in normal rabbits, 256% in anephric rabbits.	Murthy et al. 1978

Table 6. (con't)

Species	Hypertension model	Drug tested	Blood pressure (mmHg)	Plasma Brady-kinin (BK)	Urinary kallikrein	Hemodynamic effects	Prostaglandins	Conclusions	Reference
		Exp. 3: (anephric) – BK 1 μg/kg – Saline 5 ml – BK – Captopril – BK	*Exp. 3:* Sal+BK:+0 Cap:+0 Cap+BK: enhanced BK effect					Increased contribution of renal prostaglandins to hypotensive BK effect after captopril	
Dog Pentobar-bitone anesthesia, artificial ventilation	normotensive	*Group 1:* Captopril 1.5 mg/kg i.v.	*Group 1:* 126±5 to 109±6	*Group 1:* [ng/ml] renal venous and arterial BK unchanged	*Group 1:* [ng/min] Increased kinin excretion: 280 to 410	*Group 1:* [ml/min] RBF:192±40 to 247±46 RVR:0.8±0.5		Important role of BK in renal hemodynamics after CE inhibition with captopril. Short-term effect of CEI is in part mediated by KK-system	CLAPPISON et al. 1981
		Group 2: Saline 10 ml i.v.	*Group 2:* ±0	*Group 2:* [ng/ml] renal venous and arterial BK unchanged	*Group 2:* [ng] no change in kinin excretion	*Group 2:* RBF, RVR, no change			
		Group 3: ANGII-antagonist 0.25 mg/kg per min i.v. for 30 min, then captopril 1.5 mg/kg i.v.	*Group 3:* 130 to 120		*Group 3:* transient increase kallikrein, small increase in kinin excretion	*Group 3:* [ml^{-5}/min] RBF: 180 to 210 RVR: decreased 22%			
humans, healthy	normotensive	Placebo or captopril 25 mg p.o. or	no change with any drug			Skin weal thickness: captopril same		Captopril: short half-life. Low dose of	FERNER et al. 1987

		enalapril 10 mg p.o. single dose, BK 0,1,3,10 µg intradermally in arm				as placebo enalapril ca. 150% of control at 2.5 or 5h after injection of all doses		Enalapril: decrease in intradermal BK metabolism, also systemic BK effects (flushing, cough)	
humans, low or normal renin. Divided into low and normal kallikrein subgroups (LKH,NKH) by urinary estimate	mild hypertension	Captopril 50 mg p.o. ×1	*LKH:* 0 min:117±4 40 min:112±4 60 min:111±4 2 h:116 *NKH:* 0 min:113±5 40 min:106±5 60 min:105±4 2 h:103±4		*LKH:* 172±60pkat/h to 180±58 *NKH:* 405±126pkat/h to 540±157			Blunted effect of captopril in the LKH subgroup, significant blood pressure fall in NKH subgroup. Significant correlation between blood pressure fall and pretreatment kallikrein excretion; data support hypothesis that renal KK-system has role in acute CEI effect	MADEDDU et al. 1987
18 patients, diet: Na 10mEq/day, K 80 mEq/day, no other drugs	mild moderate hypertension	*Period A:* Placebo 5 days *Period B:* *Group 1:* Captopril	*Group 1:* A:118±1	*Urinary* *kinins* (ng/h) *Group 1:* A:630±109	[KAU]= Kallikrein activity units *Group 1:* A:445±125		*Urinary* PGE_2: *Group 1:* (ng/day) A:65±14 B:83±9	Urinary kinins unaffected by captopril; indomethacin reduced both	QUILLEY et al. 1987

Table 6. (con't)

Species	Hypertension model	Drug tested	Blood pressure (mmHg)	Plasma Brady-kinin (BK)	Urinary kallikrein	Hemodynamic effects	Prostaglandins	Conclusions	Reference
		25 mg p.o. thrice daily, if needed 50 mg p.o. thrice daily 3 more days *Group 2:* Indomethacin 50 mg thrice daily *Period C:* *Group 1:* Cap+I for 3 days *Group 2:* I+Cap for 3 or 6 days *Period D:* Captopril 25 or 50 mg (as needed) for 3 days	B:102±1 C:−5 (SBP) D:0 *Group 2:* A:120 B:0 C:−6/8 D:0	B:586±105 C:358±115 D:585±85 *Group 2:* A:663±130 B:391±92 C:651±159 D:788±233	B:157±49 C:211±90 D:340±90 *Group 2:* A:339±88 B:245±61 C:211±45 D:349±67		C:57±30 D:61±22 *Group 2:* A:188±68 B: 66±29 C:0 D:50% of A *Urinary* PGF_2 (ng/day) *Group 1:* A:195±60 B:183±63 C:120±41 D:176±54 *Group 2:* A:307±84 B:107±22 C,D:0	kinin and kallikrein. Questionable role of prostaglandins in activation of KK-system. Indomethacin attenuates hypotensive effect of captopril: evidence for role of prostaglandins. No evidence for role of kinins in captopril effect	
humans	primary hypertension n:4 reno-vascular n:1	Alacepril 25 mg p.o. ×1, then alacepril 25 mg p.o. twice daily (primary HT) / 12.5 mg twice daily (renal HT) ×7 days	0h:119.3 1h:104.5 2h:100.8 4h:102.3 8d:106.8	[10g/ml] 0h: 8.7±2.1 1h:17.0±5.4 2h:17.3±3.3 4h:42.6±9.8 8d:16.0±5.1				Significant negative correlation between blood pressure and kinin levels	Tanaka et al. 1987

humans, ramipril group divided in low and normal renin subgroup	primary hypertension	*Group 1:* Captopril 50 mg p.o.	*Group 1:* 0h:126 2h:110	(pg/ml) *Group 1:* 0h:8 1h:16 3h:118 4h:14	(ng/min) *Group 1:* 0h:68 4h:58 2h:12	All CEI lead to significant BP decreases and kinin increases. Negative correlation between blood pressure and BK changes. Results suggest that CEI effects are due to ANG II decrease and BK increase. Hypotensive effect of ramipril due to ANG II decrease and kinin increase in normal-renin group, while due to kinin increase but not to ANG II decrease in low-renin group	IIMURA et al. 1986
		Group 2: Alacepril 25 mg p.o. 4h:100	*Group 2:* 0h:119 2h:100 2h:16	*Group 2:* 0h:8 1h:16 4h:40			
		Group 3: Ramipril 5 mg p.o.	*Group 3:* Low-renin: 0h:120 4h:105 Normal-renin: 0h:121 4h:103	*Group 3:* Low-renin: 0h:22 4h:70 Normal-renin: 0h:10 4h:38			
		Group 4: Captopril 75 mg p.o. for 14 days	*Group 4:* 0d:135 14d:116	*Group 4:* 0d:11 pg/ml 14d:17 pg/ml	*Group 4:* 0d:86 14d:80		

CE, conventing enzyme; SD, Sprague-Dawley; SHR, spontaneously hypertensive rat; WKY, Wistar-Kyoto; W, week; 2K-1C, two-kidney-one-clip; ANG, angiotensin; CNS, central nervous system; RBF, renal blood flow; SBP, systolic blood pressure; d, day. BK, brady kinin; KK syst, kallikrein-kinin-system. RVR, renal vascular resistance; pKat, catalytic activity of kallikrein in a standardized commercial test; diss, dissected.

plasma RAS) CEI generally lower blood pressure by maximally 20%–30% upon acute or chronic administration (see reviews cited above).

In healthy, salt-replete, normotensive subjects, single oral doses of enalapril (5–40 mg) or ramipril (10 mg) moderately reduced blood pressure for up to 36 h (see TODD and HEEL 1986; THUILLEZ et al. 1987). As could be expected from animal studies, the blood pressure lowering effect was more pronounced in salt-depleted subjects with a stimulated RAS. Age seems to play a role, since HOCKINGS et al. (1985) observed a greater fall in blood pressure in elderly compared with younger subjects upon acute oral treatment with enalapril despite similar plasma CE inhibition. This difference could not be attributed to the prevailing degree of plasma RAS stimulation, since elderly people usually have lower plasma renin than young individuals, nor was it due to reduced renal elimination of the drug in the elderly.

However, upon long-term administration blood pressure was shown to be reduced to a similar extent in the young and in the elderly (ARR et al. 1985; MONCLOA et al. 1985).

5.1.2 In Hypertensive Animals

The antihypertensive effects of CEI have been established in a number of animal models of hypertension following single-dose as well as repeated-dose administration of the drugs. Generally, upon acute treatment blood pressure reduction was more rapid and more pronounced in renin-dependent forms of hypertension, while under chronic treatment this difference between low or normal and high renin types of hypertension tends to disappear. The various CEI proved to be of similar efficacy when given at appropriate doses, although — depending on their respective inhibitory activity against CE — their antihypertensive potency following equidose treatment and the duration of action at equipotent doses may vary.

5.1.2.1 Renin-Dependent Models of Hypertension

Captopril given at daily oral doses ranging from 6–45 mg/kg reduced blood pressure in 2-kidney-1-clip hypertensive rats by 20%–40% (see HEEL et al. 1980) and prolonged survival in these animals (HOROVITZ et al. 1979). The latter effect was even more apparent when captopril was combined with a diuretic, hydrochlorothiazide, which by itself does not influence survival. Similar antihypertensive actions as with captopril were reported with enalapril and other more recently developed CEI such as ramipril, cilazapril, and indolapril (SWEET et al. 1981 a,b; SCHÖLKENS et al. 1984a; NATOFF et al. 1985; RYAN et al. 1984). For instance, blood pressure was normalized in 2-kidney-1 clip hypertension by ramipril given at a daily oral dose of 1 mg/kg (SCHÖLKENS et al. 1984a).

5.1.2.2 Nonrenin-Dependent Hypertension

CEI were also shown to be antihypertensive in models of renal or renovascular hypertension that are not associated with a stimulated plasma RAS, such as

1-kidney-1-clip hypertension in rats and dogs (BENGIS et al. 1978; SWEET et al. 1981 a; SELIG et al. 1983) or wrapped kidney hypertension in dogs (SCHÖLKENS et al. 1984a). Whether or not CEI lower blood pressure in animal models of mineralocorticoid hypertension such as DOCA-salt hypertension is still a matter of controversy (see HEEL et al. 1980), although most investigators would agree that this type of hypertension is least responsive to CEI treatment.

5.1.2.3 Genetic Hypertension

SHR or SHRSP are by far the most extensively studied animal model of hypertension with respect to the antihypertensive actions of CEI. This type of genetic hypertension in the rat is considered the most appropriate animal model for primary hypertension in humans. The plasma RAS may be stimulated in some substrains, but more often it is suppressed in these animals (RASCHER et al. 1982). In SHR, captopril given at a single intravenous dose of 2 mg/kg was shown to produce a gradual and progressive decrease in blood pressure of maximally 42 mmHg within 3 h of drug injection (HUTCHINSON et al. 1980). In adult SHR or SHRSP repeated oral doses in the range of 6–200 mg/kg given over days or months were shown to produce marked antihypertensive effects without, however, actually bringing blood pressure down to normal levels. In long-term studies captopril proved to be most effective at oral doses between 50–100 mg/kg per day (e.g., ANTONACCIO et al. 1979; UNGER et al. 1982a) to produce a sustained decrease in blood pressure between 40 and 65 mmHg (Fig. 17). Doses of captopril between 30–100 mg/kg per day were shown to prevent

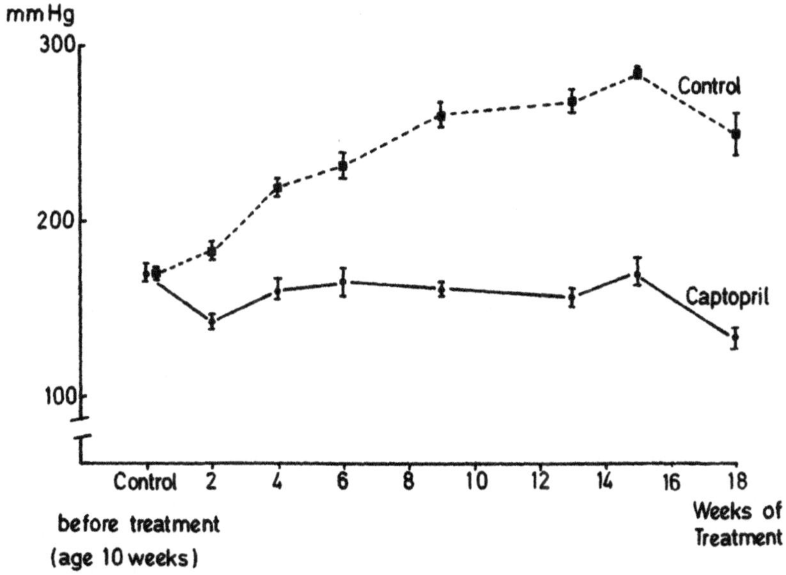

Fig. 17. Systolic blood pressure during chronic oral treatment with captopril (50 mg/kg per day) in stroke-prone, spontaneously hypertensive rats

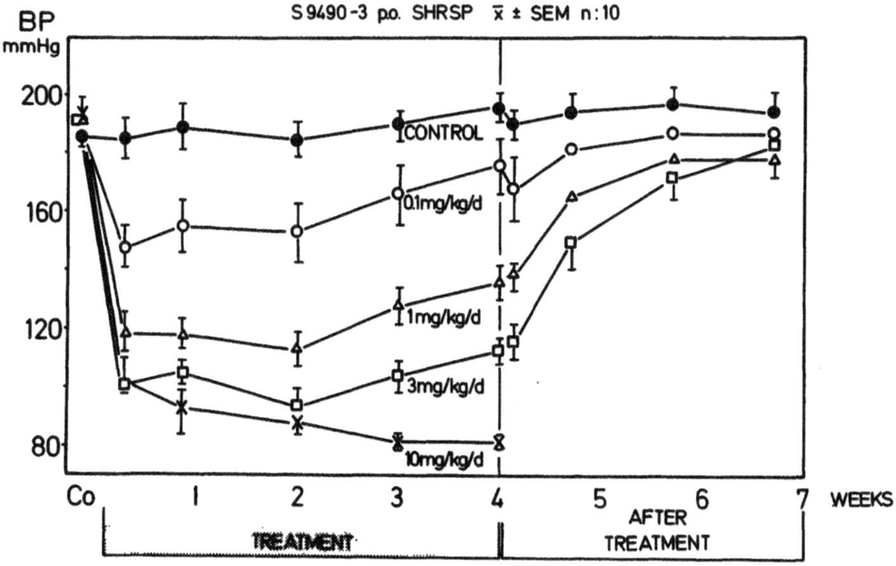

Fig. 18. Effect of chronic oral treatment with perindopril on systolic blood pressure (*BP*) in stroke-prone, spontaneously hypertensive rats (*SHRSP*) (n=10 per group). When compared with untreated, control SHRSP, blood pressure was significantly reduced ($P <$ 0.001) in the groups treated with 1, 3, and 10 mg/kg daily throughout. In the group treated with 0.1 mg/kg daily, the decrease in blood pressure was significant ($P <$ 0.05–0.001) up to the 2nd week of treatment. Upon drug withdrawal, blood pressure was still significantly lowered for 2 weeks in the groups treated with 1 and 3 mg/kg daily ($P <$ 0.05–0.001) (From UNGER et al. 1986a)

the development of hypertension in SHR and SHRSP (see HEEL et al. 1980; HENRICHS et al. 1980).

Some authors have reported that bilateral nephrectomy markedly reduces the antihypertensive actions of captopril in SHR, pointing to a critical role of the kidney for the effects of CEI on blood pressure, while in other studies the antihypertensive action of captopril persisted after removal of the kidneys (see HEEL et al. 1980).

Other sulfhydryl-containing CEI such as SA 446 were shown to exert their antihypertensive actions in SHR at similar doses to captopril (UNGER et al. 1982a), while enalapril, ramipril, perindopril, indolapril, or cilazapril were active at lower doses (see BAUM et al. 1983; UNGER et al. 1984a, 1986a; SCHÖLKENS et al. 1984a; NATOFF et al. 1985; TODD and HEEL 1986).

For instance, in SHR, long-term oral administration of ramipril for 30 days resulted in dose-dependent decreases in blood pressure with a threshold antihypertensive effect of 0.01 mg/kg per day (SCHÖLKENS et al. 1984a). In SHRSP the threshold antihypertensive dose for ramipril and perindopril was below 0.1 mg/kg per day. Normalization of blood pressure was obtained within a dose range of 1–10 mg/kg per day (UNGER et al. 1984a, 1986a). (Fig. 18).

5.1.3 In Hypertensive Patients

The antihypertensive efficacy of captopril and enalapril in hypertensive patients was demonstrated in a multitude of open and placebo-controlled trials. Excellent reviews on this topic have been provided by HEEL et al. (1980), VIDT et al. (1982), EDWARDS and PADFIELD (1985), DAVIES et al. (1984b), BRUNNER et al. (1985a,b), TODD and HEEL (1986), and the reader is referred to these articles for detailed information. Therapeutic trials in hypertensive patients with the CEI lisinopril, perindopril, and ramipril are compiled in several publications, e.g., Journal of Cardiovascular Pharmacology (Vol. 9 [Suppl. 3], 1987) for lisinopril, and American Journal of Cardiology (Vol. 59 (10), 1987) for ramipril. A detailed discussion of these numerous studies is beyond the scope of this chapter.

Table 2 provides some information on the antihypertensive potency of several CEI and on currently recommended dosing regimens. It is noteworthy that the antihypertensive doses of captopril have been constantly reduced over the years, so that today's recommended doses as shown in Table 2 are almost tenfold lower than those used upon its clinical introduction. Moreover, whereas previously it was thought that captopril has to be administered in three daily doses, there are recent reports suggesting that a once daily regimen may suffice to achieve persistent 24-h blood pressure reductions (SCHÖENBERGER and WILSON 1986; DE CESARIS et al. 1987).

Enalapril and the other clinically used CEI were introduced at much lower doses than captopril, partly due to their higher antihypertensive potency as determined in preclinical and phase I clinical pharmacology studies (e.g., SWEET et al. 1981a; SCHÖLKENS et al. 1984a; RYAN et al. 1984; BRUNNER et al. 1985b; UNGER et al. 1986a; HOLCK et al. 1986) and partly due to lessons learned from previous experience with captopril, particularly with respect to the increased incidence of side effects during high-dose treatment.

Adequate blood pressure control can be achieved with all CEI tested thus far in about 50%–70% of patients on CEI monotherapy. Addition of a diuretic (loop or thiazide diuretic) usually provides adequate blood pressure control in the remainder (Fig. 19).

There is little difference in the antihypertensive efficacy of the various CEI when adequately dosed (e.g., enalapril 10 mg once daily, captopril 50 mg o.d., lisinopril 20 mg o.d.). Enalapril, for instance, was shown to be as effective as propranolol, metoprolol, and hydrochlorothiazide in mild to moderate primary hypertension. In moderate to severe hypertension, enalapril proved to be as effective as atenolol and captopril (see TODD and HEEL 1986). When combined with a diuretic, both the CEI and the diuretic may be reduced to doses lower than normally employed as monotherapy. This can be explained by their synergistic action. The latter stimulate the plasma RAS and, hence, render blood pressure controls more dependent on the RAS. Under these conditions, inhibitors of the RAS can be expected to be more effective in lowering blood pressure. On the other hand, diuretics may also interact with CEI by mechanisms unrelated to the plasma RAS, as suggested by a study of SCHALEKAMP et al. (1982) cited above.

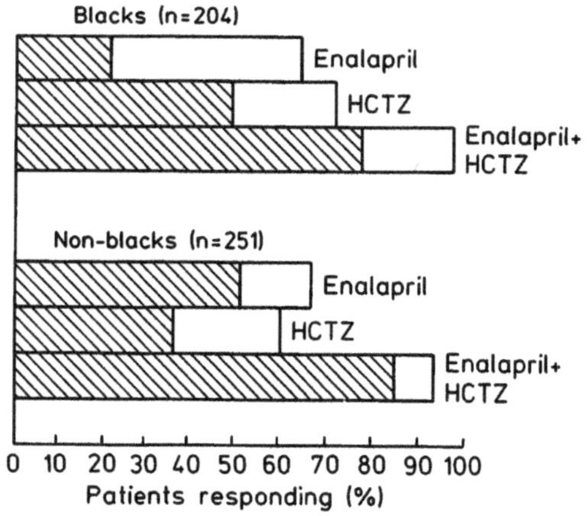

Fig. 19. Percentage of black and nonblack patients with mild to moderate essential hypertension achieving an excellent (▨= supine diastolic pressure ≤ 90 mmHg) and good (□= supine diastolic pressure decrease ≥ 10 mmHg versus placebo, but not reaching ≤ 90 mmHg) response after 8 weeks' treatment with titrated dosages of enalapril 20 to 40 mg/day, hydrochlorothiazide (*HCTZ*) 50 to 100 mg/day, or their combination. (After VIDT 1984)

Patients with secondary hypertension due to mineralocorticoid excess were reported to respond least to CEI treatment (BRUNNER et al. 1980), especially if the underlying disease is an adrenal adenoma (EDWARDS and PADFIELD 1985), whereas secondary hypertension of renal origin can be excellently controlled with CEI, provided that the appropriate precautions are taken (see Sect. 2 and 7).

5.2 Effects on Vascular Resistance

5.2.1 In Hypertensive Animals

In a series of studies, RICHER et al. (1983, 1987) investigated the effects of different CEI on general and regional hemodynamics in anesthetized SHR using the microsphere technique. Following 8 days of oral treatment with equidepressor doses of captopril (100 mg/kg daily), enalapril (25 mg/kg daily), perindopril, trandolapril, and ramipril (each at 5 mg/kg daily), total peripheral resistance was significantly decreased to a similar extent with all CEI. Heart rate was slightly decreased or unchanged, and the cardiac index showed a tendency to increase in all groups, although this effect was statistically not significant. Regional vascular resistances were reduced in the following order: renal > splenic = liver > skin > total peripheral > muscle = brain (Fig. 20). Despite the reduced perfusion pressure, captopril, trandolapril, and ramipril significantly increased renal blood flow. Splenic, hepatic, and cutaneous blood flow were also increased in some cases.

The authors have recently confirmed these results in an acute study using a different technique (pulsed Doppler flow) (RICHER et al. 1989). Again, the

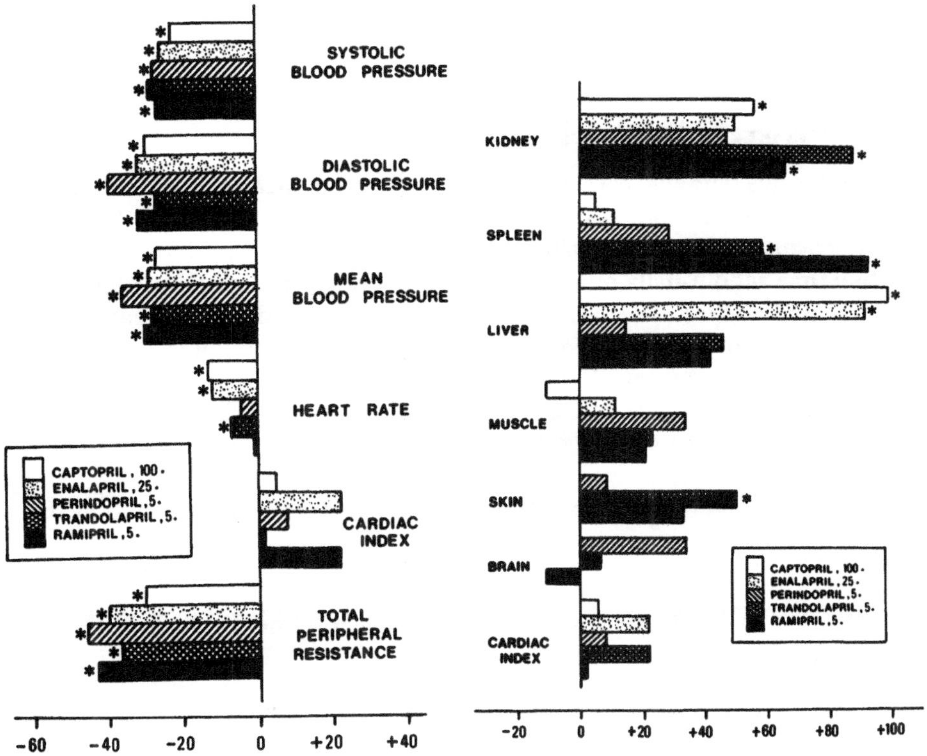

Fig. 20. Percentage of variations from corresponding control groups of the hemodynamic parameters induced by five converting enzyme inhibitors. In the kidney, spleen, liver, muscle, skin, brain regional blood flow was measured. *Asterisk*, significant difference from corresponding control value ($P < 0.05$). (From RICHER et al. 1987)

increase in renal blood flow was the most impressive regional hemodynamic change with all CEI. Captopril was somewhat different from the other CEI studied, in that it reduced renal resistance most markedly while, on the other hand, increasing hindlimb resistance at low doses.

5.2.2 In Humans

In humans as in experimental animals a decrease in total peripheral resistance associated with unchanged cardiac output and heart rate is usually observed following acute and chronic CEI treatment. For instance, in patients with primary hypertension, chronic treatment with enalapril at doses between 10 and 80 mg/day for up to 12 weeks was reported to reduce total peripheral resistance by 21%–34% (see TODD and HEEL 1986). Patients with high pretreatment total peripheral resistance may profit particularly from combined treatment with CEI and diuretics (LUND-JOHANSEN and OMVIK 1984). In hypertensive patients, forearm vascular resistance was repeatedly shown to be reduced upon CEI treatment (see TODD and HEEL 1986; WEBB and COLLIER 1986). These findings, among others, gave rise to the conclusion that CEI reduce vascular tone in large arteries in addition to resistance vessels (see Sect. 9).

5.3 Effects on Cardiac Function

In hypertensive patients, cardiac function parameters such as heart rate, cardiac output, ejection fraction, stroke volume, left ventricular fractional shortening, left ventricular end-systolic wall stress, or pre-ejection period/left ventricular ejection time ratio usually remain unchanged during chronic CEI treatment (see reviews cited above). The lack of reflex tachycardia under CEI treatment has been attributed to a resetting of the baroreceptor reflex without change in reflex sensitivity (GUIDICELLI et al. 1985). However, baroreceptor reflex sensitivity may also be altered following CEI administration, and this effect may contribute to the overall pattern of cardiovascular changes induced by CEI (see Sect. 6 and 10).

Further information on the cardiac actions of CEI is provided in Sect. 8.

6 Interference with Neurogenic Vasoconstriction and Autonomic Reflexes

ANG II exerts its effect on blood pressure not only by a direct vasoconstrictor action or by renal salt retention but also by a facilitatory action on the sympathetic nervous system (for review see ZIMMERMAN 1981).

NAKAMURA et al. (1986) showed that ANG II can be released from isolated mesenteric arteries upon β-adrenergic stimulation with isoproterenol. Further

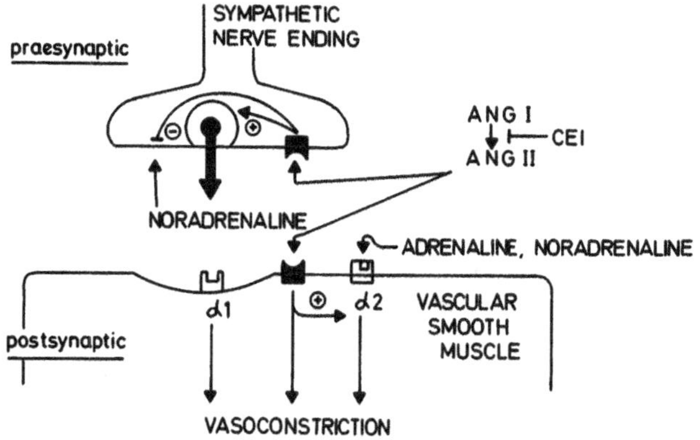

Fig. 21. Pre- and postsynaptic facilitatory action of angiotensin (*ANG*) II on neurogenic vasoconstriction. ⊕, potentiating effect; ⊖, inhibitory effect; α_1, α_1-adrenoceptors; α_2, α_2-adrenoceptors. By inhibiting ANG II generation, converting enzyme inhibitors (*CEI*) reduce the direct vasoconstrictor action of ANG II via vascular ANG II receptors and the vasoconstrictor action mediated by the sympathetic nerves

results by the same authors together with those by KAWASAKI et al. (1984) and GÖTHERT and KOLLECKER (1986) suggested that in isolated rat mesenteric vessels, the β-adrenoceptor-mediated enhancement of vascular noradrenergic transmission was brought about by a stimulation of local vascular ANG II synthesis, since this effect was blocked by CEI.

Several investigators have, therefore, studied the question whether CEI could interfere with the effects of ANG II on neurogenic vasoconstriction and by this mechanism exert some of their antihypertensive actions (Fig. 21).

6.1 Studies in Isolated Vessel Preparations

RUBIN et al. (1978) reported that captopril at a concentration of 5×10^{-4} mol/l had little or no effect on the contractile response to noradrenaline (NA) in excised vascular tissue of large arteries and veins.

On the other hand, OKUNO et al. (1979) found that captopril diminished the contraction in response to NA in isolated rat mesenteric vessels, starting at a concentration of 5 μg/ml (1.5×10^{-5} mol/l). Complete inhibition occurred at 81 μg/ml (4×10^{-3} mol/l). This inhibitory effect was not altered by the presence of ANG II or bradykinin in the perfusate, and the peptide CEI teprotide at 1–243 μg/ml was without effect. Thus, captopril appears to exert a postsynaptic inhibition of the NA pressor action unrelated to ANG II and to the inhibition of CE.

COLLIS and KEDDIE (1981) expanded on these results, again using the model of isolated rat mesenteric arteries. Their findings were somewhat more complex: Captopril, added to the perfusate at concentrations of 2×10^{-6} up to 1×10^{-5} mol/l, had no effect on the rise in perfusion pressure in response to sympathetic nerve stimulation or exogenous NA. However, at concentrations ranging from 10^{-4} to 3×10^{-4} mol/l, both responses were attenuated. Exogenous ANG I and ANG II did not have a direct vasoconstrictor effect but potentiated the responses to nerve stimulation. Captopril at low concentrations of 6.7×10^{-8} to 2×10^{-6} mol/l antagonized this potentiating effect of ANG I, while the ANG II receptor antagonist saralasin antagonized the potentiating effects of both ANG I and ANG II. The authors concluded that low captopril concentrations block the local vascular conversion of ANG I into ANG II and may by this means reduce sympathetic vasoconstrictor tone, whereas high concentrations of captopril antagonize the responses to NA and nerve stimulation independently of peptide hormones, probably by a direct action on vascular smooth muscle cells. However, these high concentrations are unlikely to be reached in vivo during antihypertensive treatment.

In a more recent in vitro and ex vivo study, ATKINSON et al. (1987) investigated the effect of captopril on sympathetically mediated vasoconstriction in tail arteries isolated from SHR. Perfusion of these arteries with captopril ($10^{-7}\times10^{-4}$ mol/l) had no effect on basal perfusion pressure or on vasoconstriction induced by exogenous NA or sympathetic nerve stimulation. In addition, in isolated tail arteries removed from captopril-treated SHR (4 mg/kg i.v. for 2 weeks or 20 mg/kg i.v. for 4 days) the responses to sympathetic nerve stimulation and ex-

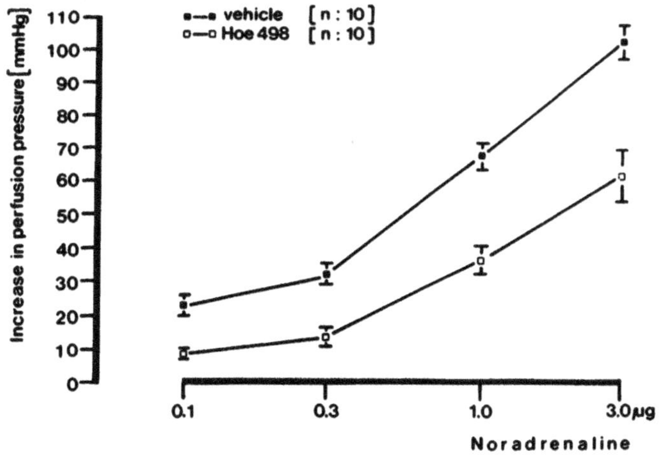

Fig. 22. Influence of single oral pretreatment with ramipril (*Hoe 498*; 1 mg/kg) on vasoconstrictor responses to *noradrenaline* in isolated perfused rat superior mesenteric vascular beds (ex vivo). (From SCHÖLKENS et al. 1984b)

ogenous NA were the same as in controls. The authors concluded that captopril had no direct postsynaptic effect in the isolated tail artery preparation.

In contrast, SCHÖLKENS et al. (1984b) demonstrated that in isolated vascular preparations (pulmonary artery from guinea pigs, thoracic aorta from rabbits, and rat mesentry) CEI attenuated the vasoconstrictor responses to ANG I but not ANG II and, at the same time, reduced the vasoconstrictor responses to NA but not to potassium chloride. An important aspect of this study resides in the fact that local ANG II generation and sympathetic neurotransmission were inhibited not only by CE inhibition in vitro but also by oral CE pretreatment prior to removal of vascular tissue (ex vivo) (Fig. 22).

6.2 Studies in Isolated Rat Kidneys

CHIBA et al. (1982) compared the effect of two captopril concentrations [0.05 and 5 μg/ml (2.5×10^{-7} and 2.5×10^{-5} mol/l)] on vascular reactivity in the same isolated kidney preparation. Both concentrations blocked the vasoconstrictor response to exogenous ANG I, but only at the higher concentration were the vasoconstrictor responses to NA reduced. However, this concentration also attenuated the pressor responses to ANG II and to lysine-vasopressin but not to PGE_2. Indomethacin was without effect on the inhibitory action of captopril. The authors concluded that captopril decreased vascular reactivity by a mechanism unrelated to CE inhibition and unrelated to a prostaglandin-dependent mechanism. However, it is important to note that the captopril concentration of 2.5×10^{-5} mol/l used in this study is still above peak plasma levels of the drug that can be expected after ingestion of the highest presently recommended oral captopril doses in humans. The inhibitory effect of the lower concentration (0.25×10^{-6} mol/l) on the vasoconstrictor responses to ANG I demonstrates that a local conversion of ANG I to ANG II takes place in the kidney which corresponds to the above-mentioned findings in mesenteric vessels. This local ANG II generation can be prevented by doses of the CEI which are therapeutically used in humans.

6.3 Studies in Pithed Rats

Another experimental approach to study CEI interaction with neurogenic vasoconstriction is the use of the pithed rat, i.e. an animal model in which connections between the central and peripheral nervous system are mechanically destroyed. This model has the advantage of coming closer to in vivo conditions than isolated organ preparations.

Antonaccio and Kerwin (1980) reported that in pithed SHR the oral application of captopril in doses of 10 and 100 mg was without effect on pressor responses to i.v.-administered ANG II and NA but reduced the pressor responses to electrical sympathetic outflow stimulation. Interestingly, the inhibitor did not affect the increases in heart rate to sympathetic stimulation. They concluded that captopril produces a presynaptic inhibition of NA release selectively in the vascular system, probably due to inhibition of ANG II formation in the vasculature. This finding gains importance through the fact that the oral captopril doses used in this study have repeatedly been found to lower blood pressure in SHR. A selective inhibition of local ANG II generation within the vasculature was suspected, since nephrectomy, i.e., removal of the main source of systemic renin, did not affect the inhibition of the sympathetic response by captopril, and since captopril had no inhibitory effect on cardiac responses to sympathetic stimulation.

In studies by Hatton and Clough (1982), captopril was injected i.v. at 0.1 and 1 mg/kg, doses which could give rise to an initial maximal blood concentration of approximately 5×10^{-6} and 5×10^{-5} mol/l. Both doses of captopril reduced the vasoconstrictor responses to sympathetic nerve stimulation and exogenous NA, and intravenous infusion of a suppressor dose of ANG II reversed this inhibitory effect of captopril. The ANG II receptor antagonist saralasin was also found to reduce the vasoconstrictor responses to sympathetic nerve stimulation and exogenous. NA. Bradykinin infusion had no effect on the responses to either stimulus. Following bilateral nephrectomy circulating renin activity was undetectable. Saralasin no longer inhibited the responses to either stimulus, whereas captopril, at the higher dose, still maintained some inhibitory action on the responses to NA.

These data suggested that captopril, at doses which are therapeutically used, can act through a CE-dependent mechanism by reducing the facilitatory effect of ANG II on neurogenic vasoconstriction. Interestingly, the plasma levels of ANG II required to restore the potentiation of adrenergic vasoconstriction were below the levels that cause direct vasoconstriction.

In subsequent experiments using SHR and two strains of normotensive rats (Clough et al. 1982), captopril (30 mg/kg p. o.) lowered blood pressure in those two strains (SHR and Alderly Park Wistar rats) which proved to be sensitive to the adrenergic facilitating actions of ANG II, but not in Wistar-Kyoto rats, which are comparatively insensitive. In the above-cited, more recent study in SHR by Atkinson et al. (1987), i.v. treatment with captopril both at 4 mg/kg for 2 weeks and at 20 mg/kg for 4 days attenuated the responses to exogenous NA and sympathetic nerve stimulation when the animals were studied in the pithed state at the end of the respective treatment periods. This effect was not dependent on the hypertensive effect of the drug, which was only seen after the higher captopril dose.

Dominiak et al. (1987a) found that upon 2-week oral treatment with CEI basal blood pressure in SHR was lowered compared with untreated controls when the animals were studied in the pithed state, and the blood pressure increases to spinal cord stimulation were attenuated. However, in contrast to acute CEI administration, the NA and adrenaline release in response to spinal cord stimulation was unchanged, suggesting that the acute sympatho-inhibitory effects of CEI are blunted during long-term treatment.

6.4 Studies in Intact Animals

Kohlmann et al. (1984) compared the effects of oral 2-week treatment with equidepressor doses of enalapril (4 mg/kg daily) and hydralazine (20 mg/kg daily) on plasma and tissue catecholamines in normotensive rats. In contrast to hydralazine, enalapril did not elevate plasma NA and adrenaline levels. Furthermore, enalapril decreased the NA turnover in the brain stem and the heart. Thus, the stimulation of the sympathetic system in response to the blood pressure decrease was attenuated and the tissue sympathetic activity even reduced in enalapril-treated animals.

On the other hand, Dominiak et al. (1987b) did not observe any changes in catecholamine synthesis or storage in the adrenal medulla and heart of SHR following 2-week oral treatment with captopril, enalapril, or ramipril.

Results by Richer et al. (1983) with perindopril support the notion that CEI act in part through interference with the sympathetic nervous system. The authors demonstrated pre- and postjunctional sympatho-inhibitory effects of the drug after 1-week oral treatment at an oral dose of 5 mg/kg daily in SHR.

Further support to this idea comes from experiments by Moursi et al. (1987), who demonstrated that intravenous ramiprilat significantly lowered blood pressure in rats under ganglionic blockade, when blood pressure was maintained by intravenous NA infusion (Fig. 23). When blood pressure was maintained by intravenous ANG II or when ANG II was added at suppressor doses to the NA infusion, ramipril failed to lower blood pressure.

6.5 Studies in Humans

Imai et al. (1982) reported on results that were quite compatible with those attained in the rat. In healthy volunteers a single antihypertensive dose of captopril (50 mg) was given orally. It significantly attenuated the pressor responses to i.v. infusions of NA and vasopressin, while leaving the reflex slowing

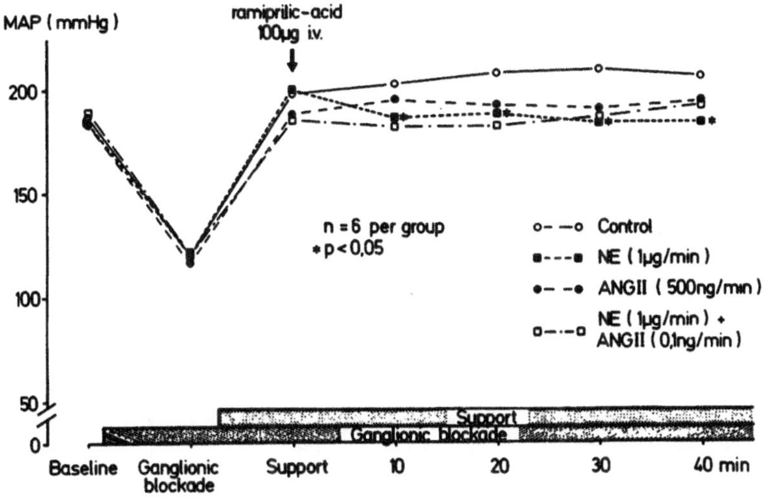

Fig. 23. Influence of ramiprilat on noradrenaline-, ANG II-, and noradrenaline plus suppressor ANG II-supported blood pressure in conscious rats following ganglionic blockade. (From MOURSI et al. 1987)

of the heart to these two pressor agents unchanged. Also, the CEI augmented the pressor responses to i.v. ANG II. On the other hand, a subpressor dose of ANG II reversed the effects of captopril on the blood pressure responses to NA and vasopressin. Subdepressor infusions of bradykinin had no effect on the responses to NA, and blockade of prostaglandin synthesis by indomethacin did not influence the inhibition of the NA pressor responses by captopril.

The results suggest that the interference of the CEI with NA-induced vasoconstriction was due primarily to a depletion of endogenous ANG II, while the potentiation of bradykinin as well as prostaglandin-mediated effects did not seem to play a role. The fact that captopril reduced the pressor actions of two different pressor agents, NA and vasopressin, was interpreted by the authors as possibly being due to the reported ability of ANG II to induce a nonsepecific sensitization to pressure substances of vascular smooth muscle cells (DAY and MOORE 1976). Furthermore, the finding of unchanged reflex bradycardia in the presence of reduced pressor responses to NA and vasopressin indicates that captopril produces a potentiation of the autonomic reflexes, as was suggested earlier from animal experiments by CONWAY et al. (1981).

MITCHELL et al. (1983) found decreased plasma NA concentrations after 3 months of antihypertensive captopril treatment in hyperadrenergic patients and in eunoradrenergic hypertensive patients. The authors concluded that this compound had a dampening effect on the sympathetic nervous system. The observation of decreased sympathetic activity following chronic CEI treatment is not shared by all investigators (e.g., MILLAR et al. 1982). However, there is general agreement that if CEI attenuate the activity of the sympathetic nervous system, this does not occur at the expense of physiological sympathetic reflexes (e.g. NIARCHOS et al. 1982).

In summary, the results of several experimental and clinical studies suggest that CEI act in part through sympatho-inhibition, most probably by attenuating presynaptic NA release and postsynaptic NA action. When present in high concentrations, CEI appear to exert additional direct sympatholytic actions. These are, however, clinically irrelevant, since such high concentrations will never be reached during antihypertensive therapy with CEI. Indices of sympathetic activity, such as plasma NA concentrations and heart rate, are usually unchanged under antihypertensive CEI treatment. Since other vasodilating drugs, e.g., dihydralazine, nifedipine, or prazosin, invariably induce sympathetic reflex responses, the lack of sympathetic stimulation under CEI can be ascribed to the sympatho-inhibitory properties of these drugs. Finally, the CEI-induced sympatho-inhibition is usually more prominent under acute than under chronic treatment conditions.

For further discussion of the interference of CEI with the sympathetic nervous system see also Sects. 8,9,10.

7 Renal Effects of Converting Enzyme Inhibitors

7.1 Intrarenal Actions of Angiotensin II

Glomerular and possibly also tubular structures of the kidney host ANG II receptors. They are mainly localized in the mesangium (OSBORNE et al. 1975; SKORECKI et al. 1983). An ANG II-induced contraction of the glomeruli that has been demonstrated in vitro (AUSIELLO et al. 1980) still awaits confirmation by in vivo studies. ANG II constricts pre- and, particularly, postglomerular arterioles (EDWARDS 1983; DAVALOS et al. 1978; NAVAR et al. 1982; STEINHAUSEN et al. 1986). Experiments from in vitro studies and indirect evidence in vivo suggest that ANG II also enhances sodium reabsorption in the proximal tubules and, in addition, contributes to the tubuloglomerular feedback mechanism, regulating glomerular filtration in the individual nephron (SCHUSTER et al. 1984; DE LEEUW et al. 1983). Inhibition of these intrarenal actions of ANG II form part of the mechanism of action of CEI.

7.2 Renal Effects in Normotensive Individuals

7.2.1 Renal Perfusion and Glomerular Filtration Rate

In animal studies with anesthetized dogs or rats, acute or chronic administration of captopril was frequently shown to increase renal blood flow and to decrease renal vascular resistance (see HEEL et al. 1980). An increase in renal plasma flow during captopril treatment was also observed in humans, although the effect seems to be rather small and variable (see HEEL et al. 1980). In animals and humans salt depletion (with subsequent stimulation of the RAS) generally enhances the effects of captopril on renal blood flow (see BRUNNER et al. 1987). Similar results have been obtained with enalapril, which has regularly been shown to increase renal plasma or blood flow and to decrease renal vascular resistance in normotensive volunteers and in normotensive patients with congestive heart failure (see TODD and HEEL 1986).

In normotensive sodium-replete animals and humans CEI treatment normally does not effect the GFR (see HEEL et al. 1980; TODD and HEEL 1986; BRUNNER et al. 1987), although under conditions of sodium depletion, decreases in GFR have been observed (see HEEL et al. 1980).

7.2.2 Renal Salt Excretion

Natriuresis is a frequently observed initial feature of CEI treatment in experimental animals and in humans (see reviews cited above). Although it was thought in the beginning that this effect is mainly due to a reduced ANG II-mediated aldosterone secretion, more recent findings point to a direct interference with actions of ANG II on renal sodium transport (for review, see BRUNNER et al. 1987; RITZ and MANN 1987). Experiments in dogs revealed that the maintenance of sodium balance under the extremes of sodium loading and sodium depletion can be profoundly influenced by CEI treatment (see BRUNNER et al. 1987).

7.3 Renal Effects in Renovascular Hypertension

The effects of CEI on renal function in renovascular hypertension have been a matter of great interest, both from experimental and clinical points of view.

When — due to renal artery stenosis — the renal perfusion pressure is reduced to levels of 70–80 mmHg, renal perfusion and GFR can only be maintained by renal autoregulation. Most likely, the underlying mechanism of this autoregulation is a progressive increase in the vascular resistance of the efferent glomerular arterioles. ANG II appears to be the predominant mediator of the efferent vasoconstriction (HALL et al. 1977a,b). Therefore, it is understandable that in cases of bilateral renal artery stenosis or unilateral kidney, the integrity of the RAS can become critical for the maintenance of renal function (for review, see ANDERSON and WOODS 1987). Under these conditions, significant, though usually reversible, decreases in renal plasma flow and GFR associated with increased serum creatinine conentration have been observed under CEI therapy with captopril and enalapril (for review, see JOHNSTON and JACKSON 1987). These effects were more pronounced in states of hypovolemia due to concomitant or prior treatment with diuretics (MURPHY et al. 1984; see also Sect. 11).

7.4 Renal Effects in Primary Hypertension

Similar to normotensive animals and humans, CEI were frequently reported to increase renal plasma flow and GFR in genetic hypertension in rats and in primary hypertension in patients (RICHER et al. 1987; HOLLENBERG et al. 1979; HOLLENBERG 1985; TODD and HEEL 1986).

RICHER et al. (1987) investigated the effects of five CEI (captopril, enalapril, perindopril, trandolapril, and ramipril) on general and regional hemodynamics

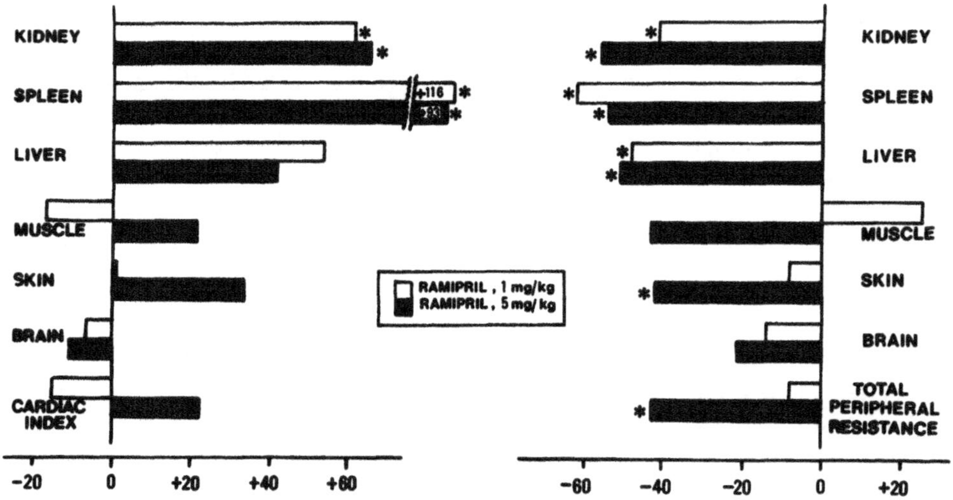

Fig. 24. Percentage of variations from corresponding control group of the regional blood flow and vascular resistance induced by two different doses of ramipril. *Asterisk*, significant difference from corresponding control value ($P < 0.05$). From RICHER et al. 1987)

in SHR. Following 1 week of treatment with equidepressor does of all five drugs, renal blood flow was most prominently increased despite the decrease in perfusion pressure, and renal vasodilatation was even observed at doses that lacked any effect on total peripheral resistance (Fig. 24).

In a subgroup of patients with primary hypertension, treatment with CEI restored the impaired renal responsiveness to increased salt intake and ANG II infusions (SHOBACK et al. 1983a). It was suggested that the functional renal disturbance in these "nonmodulators" is due to increased local concentrations of ANG II in the kidney.

7.5 Renal Effects in Hypertension Associated with Disturbed Renal Function

In patients with impaired renal functions due to hypertension or renal parenchymal disease, CEI in general do not seem to increase serum creatinine, if there is no simultaneous volume depletion (e.g., by diuretics). There are even reports indicating that in patients with mild to moderate impairment of renal functions, GFR may improve and serum creatinine may slightly decrease under chronic CEI treatment (JENKINS et al. 1985; BAUER and JONES 1984; BAUER and REAMS 1985), although the increase in GFR has not been confirmed by other groups (COOPER et al. 1985; MCFATE SMITH et al. 1984a).

In some patients with renal failure (MURPHY et al. 1984) and with congestive heart failure (FUNCK-BRENTANO et al. 1986; CODY 1985; DICARLO et al. 1983), a deterioration of renal function was observed under CEI treatment. This effect appears to be a class effect of CEI and can be explained by the importance of the RAS for adaptation to salt depletion (BLYTHE 1983) and to cardiac failure (DZAU et al. 1981). The initial deterioration of renal function in patients with congestive heart failure is usually reversible and can be controlled by careful, individual dosing and avoidance of volume depletion (MURJAIS et al. 1984; PIERPONT et al. 1981; CONSENSUS Study 1987).

On the other hand, renal function may also improve under CEI treatment. In experimental models of renal failure such as extensive ablation of kidney mass (ANDERSON et al. 1985), streptosotoxin-induced diabetes mellitus (ZATZ et al. 1986), or immunologically induced glomerular damage (BRENNER 1983), glomerular hydraulic pressure increases together with proteinuria and glomerulosclerosis. These changes appear to be partly attributable to intrarenal actions of ANG II (HOSTETTER et al. 1982) and usually go along with elevated systemic blood pressure. Treatment with CEI proved to be superior to other antihypertensive agents such as *Rauwolfia* alkaloids, vasodilators, diuretics, or calcium channel blockers in that all drugs equally lowered systemic blood pressure, but only CEI lowered the intraglomerular pressure and, consequently, reduced albuminuria and retarded the progressive loss of renal function (MEYER et al. 1985; RAJI et al. 1985; ANDERSON et al. 1985; MEGGS et al. 1988). These experimental findings from animal studies, although still awaiting confirmation in humans, raise the hope that CEI may have beneficial long-term effects on renal function in patients with glomerulosclerosis of various origins.

7.6 Antihypertensive Treatment with Converting Enzyme Inhibitors in Patients with Diabetic Nephropathy

Diabetes mellitus is frequently diagnosed in patients with arterial hypertension. In these patients, a deterioration of glucose metabolism secondary to antihypertensive treatment has to be carefully avoided.

Many β-blocking agents as well as thiazide diuretics are known to exert a negative influence on glucose and lipid metabolism (STRUTHERS 1985). Under antihypertensive CEI treatment, a worsening of glucose tolerance could not be detected in patients with non-insulin-dependent diabetes mellitus (MATTHEWS et al. 1986).

There is experimental evidence indicating that the insulin sensitivity of patients with non-insulin-dependent diabetes mellitus could be transiently increased under CEI treatment (RETT et al. 1988). The clinical significance of these findings is presently under investigation.

Since diabetic nephropathy is the most important life-limiting factor for patients with diabetes mellitus (HOSTETTER et al. 1982), many studies have focussed on the influence of antihypertensive treatment on diabetic nephropathy. It could be shown that in patients with diabetic nephropathy the annual decline of the creatinine clearance was diminished and renal plasma flow was increased under antihypertensive treatment with CEI (BJÖRCK et al. 1986). Other studies noted a reduction of albuminuria (HOMMEL et al. 1986; TAGUMA et al. 1985). This finding was attributed to a CEI-induced decrease of glomerular filtration pressure (MANN and RITZ 1988).

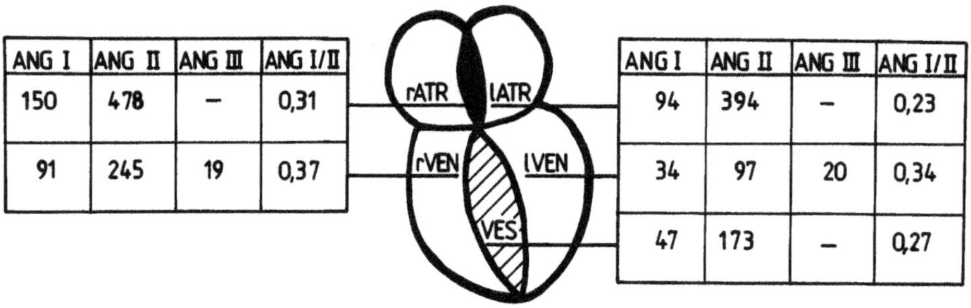

Fig. 25. Angiotensin concentrations in monkey cardiac tissue

There are also studies showing that the use of captopril in hypertensive patients with insulin-dependent or with non-insulin-dependent diabetes mellitus did not exert a negative effect on GFR, renal plasma flow, and sodium, chloride, and calcium excretion. A decrease was only found for renal phosphate and potassium clearance (GAMBARO et al. 1985).

8 Cardiac Actions of Converting Enzyme Inhibitors

8.1 Local Renin-Angiotensin System in the Heart

Evidence for a local RAS in the heart has not only been obtained by the isolation and biochemical characterization of the various components of the system from heart tissue but also more recently by the demonstration of renin and angiotensinogen mRNA in the cardiac tissue of rats and mice (DZAU et al. 1986; CAMPBELL 1987; LINDPAINTNER et al. 1988).

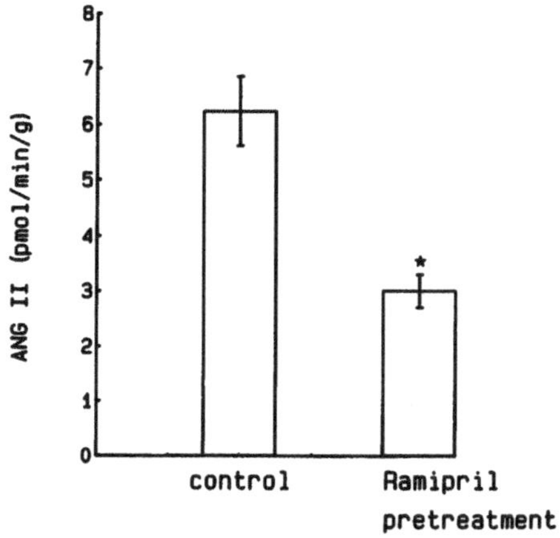

Fig. 26. Effect of ramipril pretreatment (1 mg/kg p.o.) on angiotensin II concentration in the effluate of isolated working rat hearts perfused with angiotensin I (1×10^{-7} mol/l) (ex vivo).*, $P < 0.05$, n=20. (From SCHÖLKENS et al. 1988a)

The myocardial levels of ANG peptides were measured in rhesus monkeys (Fig. 25). ANG II was higher in the atria than in the ventricles and higher in the left than in the right atrium (GANTEN et al. 1985). Perfusion of isolated rat hearts with renin led to a concentration-dependent release of ANG I and II, an perfusion with ANG I to a release of ANG II. The ANG II release could be prevented by addition of CEI to the perfusate (LINDPAINTNER et al. 1988). The rate of conversion of ANG I to ANG II in untreated hearts was found to be 7%, corresponding to a production of ANG II at a rate of 0.8 pmol/min (LINDPAINTNER et al. 1987).

Inhibition of cardiac ANG II generation by CEI was also demonstrated in ex vivo experiments. Isolated hearts from CEI-pretreated rats had reduced ANG II levels in the effluate when perfused with ANG I (Fig. 26) (LINZ et al. 1986b). Direct measurements of CE activity in heart tissue led further support to a local cardiac ANG II generation. Acute and chronic oral antihypertensive treatment of SHR with enalapril, ramipril, or perindopril inhibited the CE activity in cardiac tissue; this effect was demonstrable as early as 15 min after oral CEI administration (UNGER et al. 1984a, b, 1986a).

8.2 Cardiac Effects of Angiotensin II

ANG II can exert pronounced effects on the heart. In addition to its marked vasoconstrictor effects on coronary arteries (HEEG et al. 1965), exogenously administered ANG II is known to be an effective inotropic agent, enhancing myocardial contractility by both direct myotropic and indirect mechanisms. With the use of isolated preparations, ANG II has been found, with rare exceptions (FREER et al. 1976), to exert a positive inotropic influence on myocardial function. A major focus of investigative efforts in this area has been the separation of direct and indirect positive inotropism of ANG II, the latter being primarily due to its effects on sympathetic nervous function. When sympathetic facilitation was carefully avoided or excluded, dose-dependent direct positive inotropic effects of angiotensin II have been shown in isolated atria and papillary muscle strips of rabbits (FREER et al. 1978), dogs (KOBAYASHI et al. 1978), cats (DEMPSEY et al. 1971; KOCH-WESER 1964), and guinea pigs (HEEG and MENO 1965).

The precise mechanism by which the myotropic effects of ANG II are mediated is not known, but the recent identification of myocardial ANG II binding sites (WRIGHT et al. 1984) may suggest modulation of intracellular calcium via the phosphatidyl inositol system after ANG II receptor stimulation. In addition, ANG II may influence the heart by facilitating cardiac sympathetic nerve action, thus contributing to its inotropic actions (see LINDPAINTNER et al. 1988).

8.3 Functional Aspects of Cardiac Converting Enzyme Inhibition

Possible pathophysiological and clinical implications of an inhibition of local CE in the heart were investigated in several experimental studies using models of myocardial ischemia and cardiac hypertrophy. Ex vivo and in vitro studies with captopril revealed that CEI can protect isolated perfused rat hearts from reper-

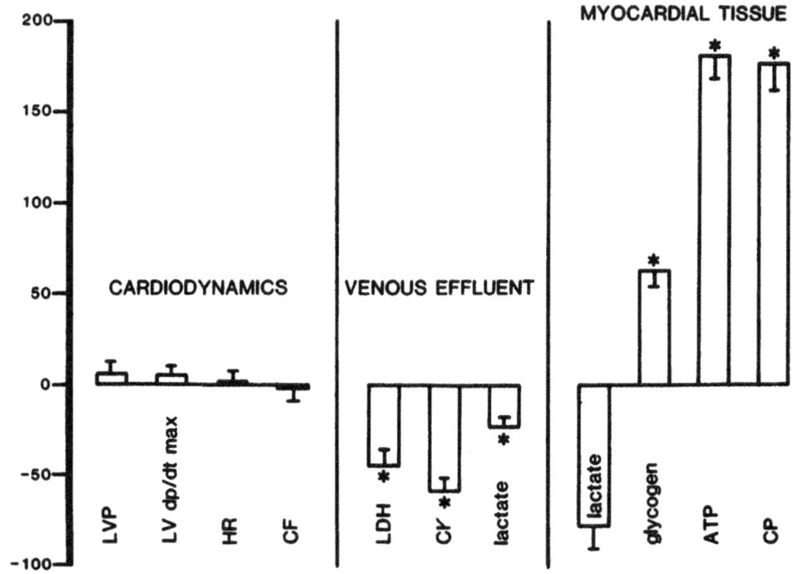

Fig. 27. Effect of a local CE inhibition with ramiprilat (2.58×10^{-5} mol/l) in isolated working rat hearts (±%, * $P < 0.05$). *Left*, cardiodynamics: *LVP*, left ventricular pressure; *dp/dt max*, maximal myocardial force of contraction; *HR*, heart rate; *CF*, coronary flow. *Middle*, coronary venous effluate: *LDH*, lactate dehydrogenase; *CK*, creatine kinase. *Right*, myocardial tissue: *CP*, creatine phosphate. (From SCHÖLKENS et al. 1988a)

fusion arrhythmia (VAN GILST et al. 1984), which, on the other hand, was exaggerated by ANG I and ANG II. Furthermore, CEI treatment abolished the arrhythmogenic effects of ANG I but did not affect those of ANG II (LINZ et al. 1986a; 1987; DE GRAEFF et al. 1986). In addition, CEI-pretreated hearts released markedly less lactate dehydrogenase, creatinine kinase, and lactate, while the myocardial concentrations of glycogen, ATP, and creatinine phosphate were elevated. CEI also improved cardiac function in this model as evidenced by enhanced left ventricular pressure, contractility, and coronary flow (LINZ et al. 1986a; SCHÖLKENS et al. 1988a) (Fig. 27).

8.3.1 Role of Bradykinin

Interestingly, similar enzymatic and metabolic effects as with CEI were obtained with bradykinin in the perfusate at concentrations too low to have any cardiodynamic actions (Fig. 28) (LINZ and SCHÖLKENS et al. 1987; SCHÖLKENS e al. 1987, 1988a). The specificity of these bradykinin-induced effects was underlined by the finding that the cardioprotective actions of bradykinin and of CEI were obliterated by a bradykinin antagonist (SCHÖLKENS et al. 1988b).

Thus, the beneficial actions of CEI in the heart could be mediated not only by a suppression of local ANG II generation but also by a potentiation of local kinin actions. Bradykinin has been shown to increase coronary flow, capillary flow, and glucose uptake in isolated hearts and cardiac myocytes (RÖSEN et al.

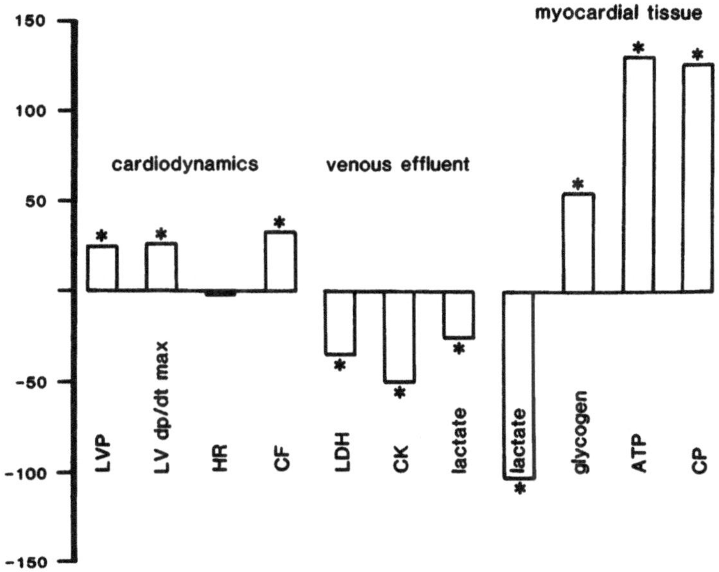

Fig. 28. Effect of bradykinin perfusion (1×10^{-10} mol/l) in isolated working rat hearts ($\pm$%, * $P < 0.05$). For abbreviations, see Fig. 24. (From SCHÖLKENS et al. 1988a)

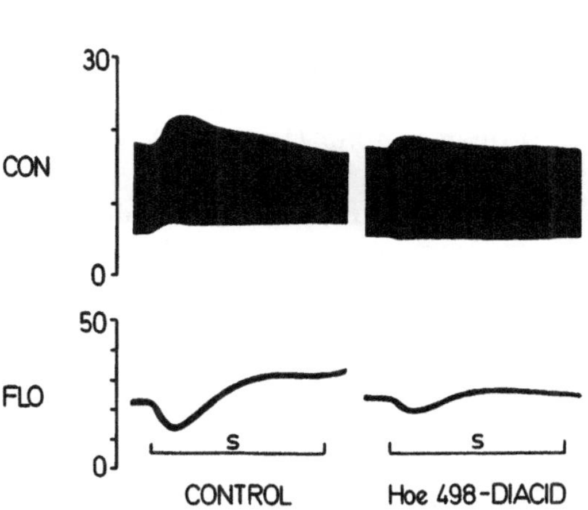

Fig. 29. Influence of ramiprilat (*Hoe 498-DIACID*) (10 μg/ml per min) on the effects of sympathetic nerve stimulation in isolated rabbit hearts. *s*, stimulation period; *HR*, heart rate (bpm); *CON*, force of contraction; *FLO*, coronary flow (ml/min). (From XIANG et al. 1985)

1983; SCHRÖR et al. 1979). Moreover, a bradykinin-induced stimulation of cardiac prostacyclin biosynthesis (MIKI et al. 1984; VAN GILST et al. 1987), tissue plasminogen activator (RAISH et al. 1985), and EDRF release (PALMER et al. 1987) all have to be taken into account as mechanisms by which bradykinin potentiation could contribute to the cardiac actions of CEI.

8.3.2 Sympathetic Transmission

Inhibition of sympathetic transmission in the heart has to be considered as an additional factor involved in the cardiac actions of CEI. In isolated hearts, CEI (captopril, enalapril, ramipril) were shown to reduce NA overflow upon ischemia (DE GRAEFF et al. 1986; CARLSSON and ABRAHAMSSON 1988) and to antagonize the effects of sympathetic nerve stimulation on coronary flow and contractility (Fig. 29) (XIANG et al. 1985). These inhibitory actions on cardiac sympathetic transmission might be related to the reduced local ANG II synthesis (see LINDPAINTNER et al. 1988; and Sect. 6).

8.4 Effects of Converting Enzyme Inhibitors on Cardiac Hypertrophy

CEI can also prevent or reduce hypertension-induced cardiac hypertrophy. Regression of left ventricular hypertrophy by CEI was demonstrated in normal rats (FREEMAN et al. 1987) and in different forms of experimental hypertension in rats such as Dahl salt-sensitive rats (FERNANDEZ et al. 1984) and SHR (CLOZEL and HEFTI 1988). A significant decrease in left ventricular mass following prolonged (3–7 months) treatment with CEI has also been observed in hypertensive patients (DUNN et al. 1984; NAKASHIMA et al. 1984).

When rats with experimentally induced aortic stenosis were treated for several weeks with equi-antihypertensive doses of ramipril, the calcium antagonist nifedipine, and the vasodilator dihydralazine, cardiac hypertrophy developed in the nifedipine- and dihydralazine- treated animals but not in the ramipril-treated animals. In parallel, the plasma ANG II concentrations were only reduced in the CEI-treated group (LINZ et al. 1988; SCHÖLKENS et al. 1988a).

In a similar study using the same experimental model of hypertension, left ventricular hypertrophy was significantly blunted by quinapril (KROMER and Riegger 1988).

In view of the documented cell proliferative effects of ANG II (see Sect. 9), these findings suggest that CEI prevent cardiac hypertrophy not only through their antihypertensive actions, i.e., by afterload reduction, but more specifically by reducing systemic or local ANG II synthesis, thereby eliminating a factor contributing to cell proliferation. The pathophysiological role of ANG II as a growth factor (JACKSON et al. 1988) leading to cardiac and vascular hypertrophy in hypertension needs to be elucidated, and further research efforts have to be directed to the question as to how effectively and specifically the cell proliferative actions of ANG II can be antagonized by CEI.

8.5 Effects of Converting Enzyme Inhibitors in Congestive Heart Failure

CEI have been successfully introduced clinically into the treatment of congestive heart failure. Indeed, the addition of enalapril to conventional drug therapy significantly reduced mortality in advanced stages (IV NYHA) of the disease (CONSENSUS STUDY 1987). The beneficial effect of CEI in these patients cannot be explained on the basis of afterload reduction alone. It rather appears that direct cardiac actions (as discussed above) play an important role. The therapeutic efficacy of captopril in congestive heart failure has been reviewed by ROMANKIEWICZ et al. (1983). For more recent reviews on the use of CEI in congestive heart failure see PACKER (1985, 1987), CLELAND and DARGIE (1987), CAPTOPRIL MULTICENTER RESEARCH GROUP I (1983, 1985), DZAU (1987a), PFEFFER and PFEFFER (1988), RYDEN (1988), and LEE and PACKER (1986).

9 Contribution of Converting Enzyme Inhibition in the Vascular Wall to the Antihypertensive Actions

The idea that vascular renin may contribute locally to blood pressure regulation and hypertension independently of the plasma RAS (ROSENTHAL et al. 1969; GANTEN et al. 1970; THURSTON and SWALES 1977; THURSTON et al. 1979) has gained substantial support in recent years by the biochemical demonstration of the presence in the vascular wall of the components of the RAS and of the genetic material required for local angiotensin production (DARBY et al. 1985; CAMPBELL and HABENER 1986; DZAU 1987b; SWALES and HEAGERTY 1987).

Locally generated vascular angiotensin could be involved in a variety of hemodynamic functions, including direct or sympathetically mediated vasoconstriction and vascular spasm, but could also modulate the vascular angiotensin receptors and, hence, the response to circulating angiotensin. In addition, local angiotensin might induce cell proliferation and contribute to inflammatory vascular responses as well as edema formation (see DZAU 1987b).

9.1 Converting Enzyme in the Vascular Wall

9.1.1 Localization of Vascular Converting Enzyme

CE has been demonstrated in vascular tissue of large and small arteries and in veins of humans and various animal species by using methods to measure enzyme activity or, more recently, by immunofluorescence or radioinhibitor binding assays (MIYAZAKI et al. 1984; JACKSON et al. 1986; WILSON et al. 1987). In the majority of these studies, the enzyme was found predominantly in the endothelial layer, but it may also occur in the adventitia (WILSON et al. 1987; OKUNISHI et al. 1987). A study by VELLETRI and BEAN (1982), demonstrating that a substantial portion of the enzyme activity was localized within the tunica media of rat aorta, suggested that ANG II could be generated in vascular smooth muscle. The observation by SAYE et al. (1984) that ANG I contracts endothelium-denuded rings of rabbit aorta, equally suggests a conversion of

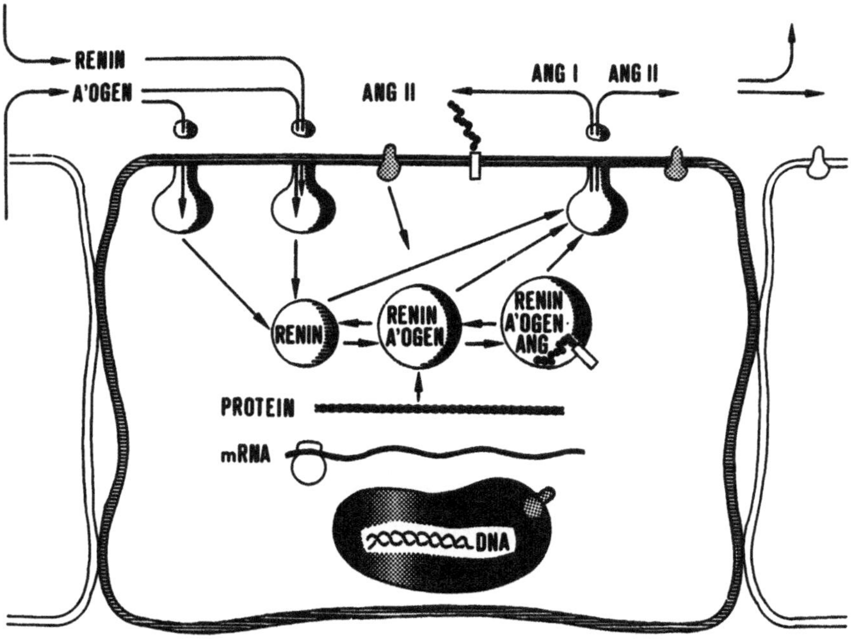

Fig. 30. Proposed model for intracellular renin-angiotensin synthesis and release

ANG I to ANG II in extra-endothelial layers of the vascular wall. Other investigators, however, have not been able to detect appreciable amounts of the enzyme in the medial layer of blood vessels (WILSON et al. 1987; OKUNISHI et al. 1987).

Thus, localization studies and the above cited evidence for angiotensinogen and renin production in endothelial cells point to the endothelium as the major site of vascular ANG II synthesis (Fig. 30).

9.1.2 Specificity of Vascular Converting Enzyme

CE can degrade a number of vasoactive peptides in addition to ANG I (SKIDGEL et al. 1988), and the CE-dependent metabolism of these peptides may have as much an impact on vascular tone and vascular function as the ANG II-generating capacity of the enzyme. In addition, there is growing evidence that CE is not the only enzyme to generate ANG II in the vascular wall (for review, see UNGER et al. 1988 b). Thus, inhibition of vascular CE by CEI may not abolish total ANG II-synthesizing capacity in some vascular territories in which the homeostasis of the local RAS can be maintained to some extent by non-CE, ANG II-generating enzymes. This may explain the observation in nephrectomized rabbits that after single-dose, oral CEI treatment with ramipril (10 mg/kg), ANG II — though at reduced concentrations — was still measurable in the aortic wall (GANTEN et al. 1985).

9.2 Effects of Converting Enzyme Inhibitors on Vascular Converting Enzyme Activity

9.2.1 Inhibition of Vascular Converting Enzyme

Indirect evidence for vascular CE inhibition following systemic CEI treatment was presented in earlier studies performed in rats with renal hypertension. In these experiments, the slow decrease in vascular renin-like activity after bilateral nephrectomy correlated better with the slow decline in blood pressure and the depressor responses to blockers of the RAS than the rapid fall in plasma renin activity (for review see SWALES and HEAGERTY 1987). In further experiments, it was demonstrated that chronic oral antihypertensive treatment of SHR with captopril increased renin concentrations in the vascular wall of the aorta (ASSAD and ANTONACCIO 1982; UNGER et al. 1982c) and that this increase could be dissociated from the increase of plasma renin of renal origin (ASSAD and ANTONACCIO 1982).

Direct evidence for an inhibition of CE in the vascular wall following oral treatment with CEI was subsequently provided by several groups. In a series of experiments in SHR, COHEN and KURZ (1982) and COHEN et al. (1983b) demonstrated that acute oral treatment with captopril and enalapril at antihypertensive doses dramatically reduced CE activity in the aorta, mesenteric, and carotid artery as well as in the vena cava, mesenteric, and jugular vein. In contrast to the CE inhibition in the blood, that in the arterial walls persisted for more than 24 h.

A prolonged inhibition of CE activity in the aortic wall but not in the blood serum following repeated intraperitoneal injections of captopril was also observed by VELLETRI and BEAN (1982). Differences in the extent and duration of aortic CE inhibition following acute oral administration of CEI in rats were observed in our laboratory when comparing ramipril and enalapril at antihypertensive doses which had similar inhibitory effects on plasma CE activity (1 mg/kg and 30 mg/kg, respectively). Ramipril produced a more than 90% inhibition of the aortic enzyme which lasted for more than 48 h, while enalapril produced a less pronounced CE inhibition of shorter duration (UNGER et al. 1984a).

Similar findings were reported by CHEVILLARD et al. (1988), who compared the CE-inhibitory actions of trandolapril and enalapril in blood serum and various tissues including the aorta following single, oral, subdepressor doses (3–300 μg/kg) of the two compounds in normotensive rats. At doses that equally inhibited serum CE activity, trandolapril inhibited aortic CE to a greater extent than enalapril. At 24 h after dosing, aortic CE was still inhibited by approximately 40% in the enalapril group, with a tendency back to control values, whereas aortic CE continued to be maximally (>90%) inhibited in the trandolapril group.

In addition, chronic oral treatment with enalapril, ramipril, and perindopril markedly inhibited the enzyme in the aortic and mesenteric wall (UNGER et al. 1984a,b, 1986b). Again, differences between the CEI with respect to vascular CE inhibition were observed in these studies, with ramipril being more potent than perindopril and enalapril.

9.2.2 Antihypertensive Actions of Converting Enzyme Inhibitors and Vascular Converting Enzyme Inhibition

Attempts to design in vivo studies to relate the CE inhibition in the vascular wall to the antihypertensive effects of CEI proved to be extremely difficult, especially to separate clearly the effect of these drugs on tissue CE from those on the plasma RAS. One experimental approach, the elimination of the plasma RAS by bilateral nephrectomy, has already been mentioned. Studies using this approach provided evidence that a stimulated RAS in the vascular wall may contribute to the maintenance of elevated blood pressure and that the vascular RAS is sensitive to specific RAS inhibitor treatment (SWALES and HEAGERTY 1987).

Additional results have shown that oral treatment with CEI can reduce not only vascular CE activity but also vascular ANG II concentrations independently of the plasma RAS (GANTEN et al. 1985). A single oral dose of ramipril (10 mg/kg) was given to rabbits that had been bilaterally nephrectomized 20 h previously to eliminate circulating renin as a confounding factor. At 4 h after treatment, tissue ANG II concentrations were found to be significantly reduced in the vascular wall of the aorta when compared with vehicle-treated controls.

In a second approach to answer the question how tissue CE inhibition relates to the antihypertensive effects of CEI, the CEI-induced changes in blood pressure were correlated with the degree of RAS inhibition in plasma versus tissue.

NAKATA et al. (1987) treated SHR and two-kidney, one-clip renal hypertensive rats (RHR) orally with SA 446 for 1 week and found that the maximum decrease in blood pressure was correlated with the maximum CE inhibition in the aorta but not in the brain, lung, heart, or blood.

NAMBU et al. (1986) investigated the tissue distribution of [^{14}C]-captopril and [^{14}C]alacepril, a captopril-related drug, following a single oral dose in RHR. They found that the tissue distribution of both drugs correlated well with the local CE inhibition in serum, lung, aorta, and kidneys. Although the extent and duration of the antihypertensive effects of the inhibitors could not be directly related to CE inhibition in the specific tissues, the differences in the pharmacological profile of the drugs were more strongly associated with the respective total CE inhibition in serum and tissues than with the individual CE inhibition there.

In a third experimental approach the drugs were withdrawn following more or less extended periods of treatment, and the persistent posttreatment blood pressure reduction was related to posttreatment changes in the plasma RAS or tissue CE. SHRSP were treated orally for several weeks with enalapril (30 mg/kg daily) and ramipril (3 mg/kg daily). Blood pressure was normalized, and plasma and tissue CEs in various organs were inhibited during treatment. Upon withdrawal of the drugs, the reduced pressor responses to intravenous ANG I and the reduced CE activity in the blood plasma were restored to normal within 1 day, while blood pressure remained decreased for an additional 2 weeks, and the CE inhibition persisted in the kidney and the aortic and mesenteric vascular wall (UNGER et al. 1984a, 1985) (Fig. 31). These findings demonstrated that the

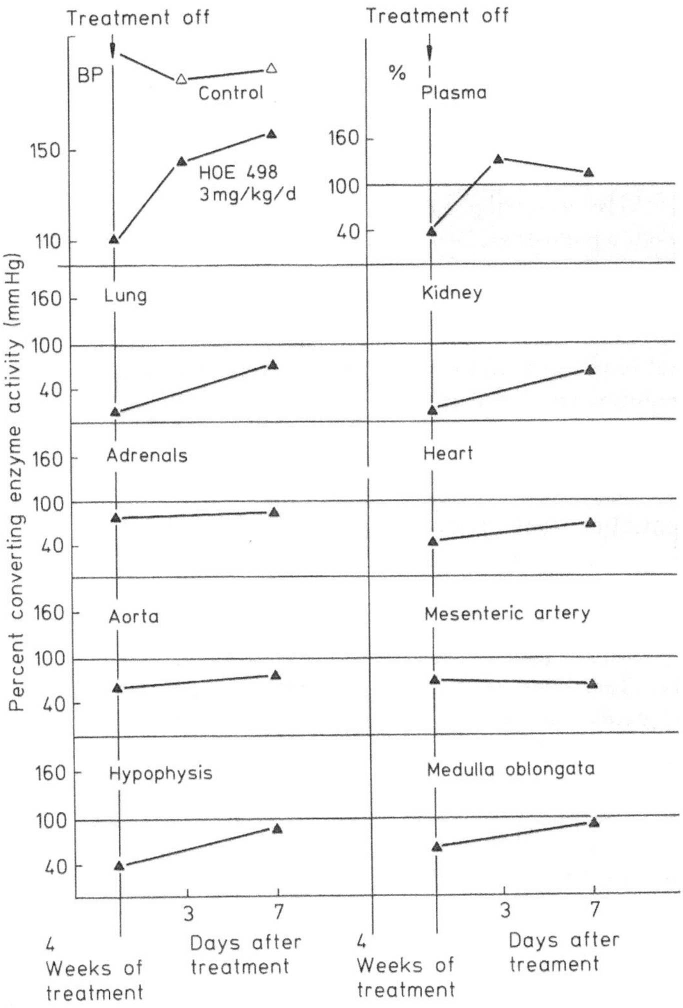

Fig. 31. Systolic blood pressure and plasma and tissue converting enzyme activity in stroke-prone, spontaneously hypertensive rats after 4 weeks of oral treatment with ramipril (*Hoe 498*) and 1 week after drug withdrawal. Converting enzyme activity values are given as percentage of the values in the respective untreated control group. (From UNGER et al. 1984b)

prolonged antihypertensive action of the CEI was unrelated to CE inhibition in the plasma and lung endothelium but was associated with a persistent CE inhibition in the kidney and the aortic and mesenteric vascular wall.

In similar experiments, LONGMAN and HOWLETT (1986) studied the relationship between the blood pressure lowering activity of CEI and inhibition of plasma and tissue CE in sodium-deficient, normotensive rats. Tissue CE activity in the aorta, mesenteric bed, and lung was inhibited for up to 96 h after cessation of a 3-week course of treatment, while the reduction of blood pressure and the inhibition of plasma CE lasted for only 48 h posttreatment. Although it appears from these data that blood pressure follows inhibition of the plasma RAS rather than vascular wall CE, it should be pointed out that, due to sodium depletion prior to treatment, the plasma RAS was stimulated in these animals; hence, its importance in blood pressure control may have increased.

Most recently, NAKAMURA et al. (1988) reported on vascular tissue CE inhibition in SHR following a single oral dose of cilazapril (0.3 and 3 mg/kg). They observed a persistent, 24-h inhibition of CE in the aortic, carotid, brachial, and femoral arteries and veins and in the pulmonary vein, while the inhibition in the mesenteric and renal vessels and in the pulmonary, subclavian, and circle of Willis arteries lasted less than 24 h postdosing. The decrease in blood pressure was maximal between 4 and 6 h and still significant 24 h after treatment. As in the other studies described above, the marked inhibition of CE in the larger arteries and veins represents a consistent feature of systemic CEI treatment. This raises the possibility that the vascular changes induced by these drugs may not only be related to vascular resistance controlled by the small arteries but also to the distensibility of the larger vessels.

9.3 Significance of Converting Enzyme Inhibition in Large Arteries

The large conduit arteries such as the aorta, the coronary, carotid, and renal arteries have long been underestimated with respect to their participation in blood flow regulation. Recent evidence indicates that these vessels, through their conduit and buffering functions, play an important role in blood pressure control and within pathophysiological events in many cardiovascular disorders. An increasing number of experimental and clinical studies suggest that the therapeutic benefit of CEI in hypertension and congestive heart failure can be partially explained by their effects on vascular compliance and distensibility of the large arteries. This aspect of vascular converting enzyme inhibitor action has recently been reviewed by DZAU and SAFAR (1988), and the reader is referred to this review for more detailed information. The authors conclude with the notion that increases in arterial caliber and distensibility may both contribute to the cardiovascular effects of CEI, promoting regression of cardiac hypertrophy, reducing hypertensive vascular injury, and preventing congestive heart failure.

9.4 Functional Aspects of Vascular Converting Enzyme Inhibition

As outlined above, locally generated ANG II may exert a number of different actions to influence vascular tone and distensibility. These include a direct vasoconstriction by stimulation of angiotensin receptors on the smooth muscle cells of the vascular media (OLIVER and SCIACCA 1984), facilitation of adrenergic transmission leading to vasoconstriction by an increased vascular tone (MALIK and NASJLETTI 1976; ZIMMERMANN 1981), and stimulation of Na^+ and Ca^{2+} transport systems across the cell membrane, as recently demonstrated in cultured vascular smooth muscle cells (KURIYAMA et al. 1988). In addition, ANG II may even exert vasodilatory actions through stimulation of endothelial prostacyclin synthesis (Toda 1984), although the functional significance of this effect is still unclear.

Evidence pointing to a pathophysiological role of a stimulated vascular RAS in hypertension has been provided by several groups. In addition to the studies cited above, which report on a stimulated vascular RAS in SHR and animals with hypertension of renal origin, Okamura et al. (1986) demonstrated not only increased vascular CE activity but also an enhanced vasoconstrictor response to ANG I in arteries isolated from two-kidney, one-clip hypertensive rats. Interestingly, both enalapril and an ANG II receptor antagonist lowered blood pressure in these animals, despite the fact that the plasma RAS was not stimulated. This finding adds support to the idea that vascular rather than plasma RAS stimulation helps to maintain high blood pressure in some forms of hypertension.

Results indicating that local vascular ANG II generation can also be reduced by CEI in humans have been obtained by Webb and Collier (1986). The authors reported that during an infusion of ramiprilat, the active parent diacid of ramipril, into the brachial artery of hypertensive patients and normotensive individuals, the intrabrachially infused doses of ANG I had to be increased by a factor of 20 to obtain the same vasoconstriction as before ramipril, while the vasoconstrictor responses to ANG II were not affected by the drug.

9.4.1 Effects Unrelated to Vascular Angiotensin II

Although the data discussed above suggest that CEI may antagonize the vascular RAS when acting locally, it should be kept in mind that interference of these drugs with vascular CE may not only lead to reduced vascular ANG II synthesis but may also have an impact on other local peptide systems such as kinins and might even alter vascular texture by mechanisms unrelated to CE inhibition. The following examples may suffice to illustrate these potentially important aspects of local CEI action.

Scherf et al. (1986) reported on a stimulation of prostacyclin synthesis in isolated aortic preparations from rats treated orally with ramipril ex vivo; and in aortic tissue exposed to ramiprilat in vitro. Since aprotinin, a kallikrein inhibitor, attenuated the effect of ramiprilat, the increase in prostacyclin production was interpreted to be due to a CEI-induced accumulation of vascular kinins (see also Table 6).

On the other hand, Oshima et al. (1983) observed a decrease in aortic prolylhydroxylase, the rate-limiting enzyme of collagen synthesis, following prolonged oral treatment of SHR with antihypertensive doses of captopril. Since the authors were unable to demonstrate this effect after single-dose, oral captopril administration in SHR and also when aortic tissue from untreated normotensive rats was exposed to captopril in vitro, they concluded that the reduction in prolylhydoxylase could not ascribed to the antihypertensive rather than to a direct vascular action of the CEI.

Table 7. Cross-sectional area (μm^2) of arterial media at different sites of the arterial tree (mean values $\times 10^3 \pm$ SEM). (From HENRICHS et al. 1980)

	Thoracic aorta	Abdominal aorta	Renal artery	Intrarenal arteries				Peripheral renal arteries
				1st division	2nd division	3rd division	4th division	
Treated SH rats	346 ± 28	298 ± 18	65 ± 17	21 ± 4	14 ± 3	4.4 ± 0.8	1.7 ± 0.3	0.7 ± 0.2
Untreated SH rats	633 ± 101	433 ± 61	103 ± 20	40 ± 6	26 ± 5	8.3 ± 2.3	4.1 ± 1.2	1.3 ± 0.4
Control WK rats	378 ± 31	335 ± 11	71 ± 13	20 ± 2	12 ± 1	5.2 ± 0.8	1.6 ± 0.1	0.8 ± 0.3

9.4.2 Effects on Vascular Hypertrophy

In previous morphometric experiments designed to investigate the effects of antihypertensive treatment on vascular hypertrophy, we made the observation that in normotensive, 6-month-old SHRSP, whose mothers had been treated with an antihypertensive dose of captopril during pregnancy and who had been kept on captopril until killing, the renal arteries, their branches, and their resistance vessels did not exhibit any signs of media hypertrophy (HENRICHS et al. 1980) (Table 7). As in the study by OSHIMA et al. (1983), the lack of development of vascular hypertrophy could be explained hemodynamically, i.e., by the failure of these animals to develop hypertension, but it is also possible that captopril exerted some direct actions on the vascular texture.

Thus, it remains to be demonstrated in further, more detailed experiments, whether or not chronic CEI treatment alters vascular texture independently of hemodynamic changes and whether this alteration is due to the CE inhibition (e.g., suppressed proliferative actions of ANG II) or to an unspecific effect of these drugs unrelated to CE inhibition.

10 Centrally Mediated Antihypertensive Actions of Converting Enzyme Inhibitors

The presence of a complete intrinsic brain RAS is now firmly established (for review, see GANTEN et al. 1984; PHILLIPS 1987; UNGER et al. 1988). Brain angiotensin appears to participate in central cardiovascular and osmotic control by influencing hormone release from the pituitary gland, sympathetic activity, and autonomic reflexes. Changes of some of the components of the brain RAS have been found in SHR which are compatible with the idea that a stimulated brain RAS contributes to the maintenance of hypertension (see reviews cited above). Whether or not the action of CEI includes a CNS-related component has been vigorously debated over the past 10 years and is still far from being settled (for review, see PHILLIPS 1983; UNGER et al. 1984c; TODD and HEEL 1986).

10.1 Effects of Local Administration of Converting Enzyme Inhibitors

Since the original observation by SOLOMON et al. (1974) that administration of the Bottrops jararaca venom peptides SQ 20475 and teprotide intracerebroventricularly (i.c.v.) attenuated the pressor responses to i.c.v. injected ANG I in anesthetized cats, it has been repeatedly demonstrated by numerous pharmacological and biochemical studies that CEI, when applied locally to the brain, reduce the activity of brain CE (for review see UNGER et al. 1984c).

Changes in angiotensin peptide concentrations in brain tissue consistent with CE inhibition were observed upon i.c.v. treatment with CEI. Following i.c.v. injections of captopril in nephrectomized rats, ANG I was significantly increased in the hypothalamus, while ANG II showed a tendency towards decrease (GAN-

TEN et al. 1983). Following i.c.v. injections of ramiprilat, the active moiety of ramipril, ANG II was reported to be lowered in the brainstem of SHR (PHILLIPS and KIMURA 1986).

However, the effects of a CE inhibition in the brain comprise more than a reduction of ANG II, since CE acts on several peptide substrates which are all present in the brain, including kinins, substance P, LHRH, and opioid peptides (see SKIDGEL et al. 1988). Thus, when CEI act on CE in the brain a number of angiotensin-unrelated actions of the enzyme may be equally affected in addition to ANG II generation.

10.1.1 Blood Pressure Lowering Action of Intracerebroventricularly Administered Converting Enzyme Inhibitors

Administration of the CE inhibitor captopril into the CSF lowered blood pressure in SHR (SCHÖLKENS et al. 1979; STAMLER et al. 1980; HUTCHINSON et al. 1980; SUZUKI et al. 1981; OKUNO et al. 1983) as well as in renal hypertensive rats (SUZUKI et al. 1981) and in DOCA-salt hypertensive rats (POCHIERO et al. 1983). Relatively high doses (up to 2 mg/kg) of captopril were used in some of these studies. Since CEI pass easily from the CSF into the blood (UNGER et al. 1981b), peripheral antihypertensive mechanisms could not be excluded, despite the fact that the same doses, if tested intravenously, produced much smaller antihypertensive effects.

When captopril was injected i.c.v. at a low dose of 5 μg in SHRSP, blood pressure was significantly lowered for about 20 min and the centrally induced hypertensive actions could be dissociated from the blockade of the enzyme in the periphery (UNGER et al. 1981b) (Fig. 32). A high i.c.v. dose of captopril (500 μg) produced a much greater fall in blood pressure. In this case, the CE inhibition was not confined to the CNS but was also observed in the periphery. Nevertheless, the antihypertensive action outlasted by far the peripheral CE blockade: At 4 h after the i.c.v. injection of captopril the pressor responses to intravenous ANG I were almost completely restored, while blood pressure was still maximally decreased. As in previous studies, the same doses of captopril were much less antihypertensive when given intravenously and did not lower blood pressure in normotensive WKY following administration by either route.

PHILLIPS and KIMURA (1986) confirmed these findings by using enalaprilat and ramiprilat in a similar protocol. On the other hand, BAUM et al. (1983) and GAUL et al. (1984) reported that i.c.v. administration of captopril and enalaprilat in SHR reduced the pressor responses to i.c.v. ANG I but did not lower blood pressure.

In further studies, the effects of long-term i.c.v. infusions of captopril were investigated. OKUNO et al. (1983) infused captopril i.c.v. at a rate of 1.25 μg/h into young SHR from the 7th to 11th week of age. This treatment led to a marked attenuation of the development of hypertension. When the same dose of captopril was infused intravenously, hypertension progressed as in vehicle-treated rats. Since central captopril administration did not alter the plasma vasopressin concentration or the resting activity of the peripheral sympathetic

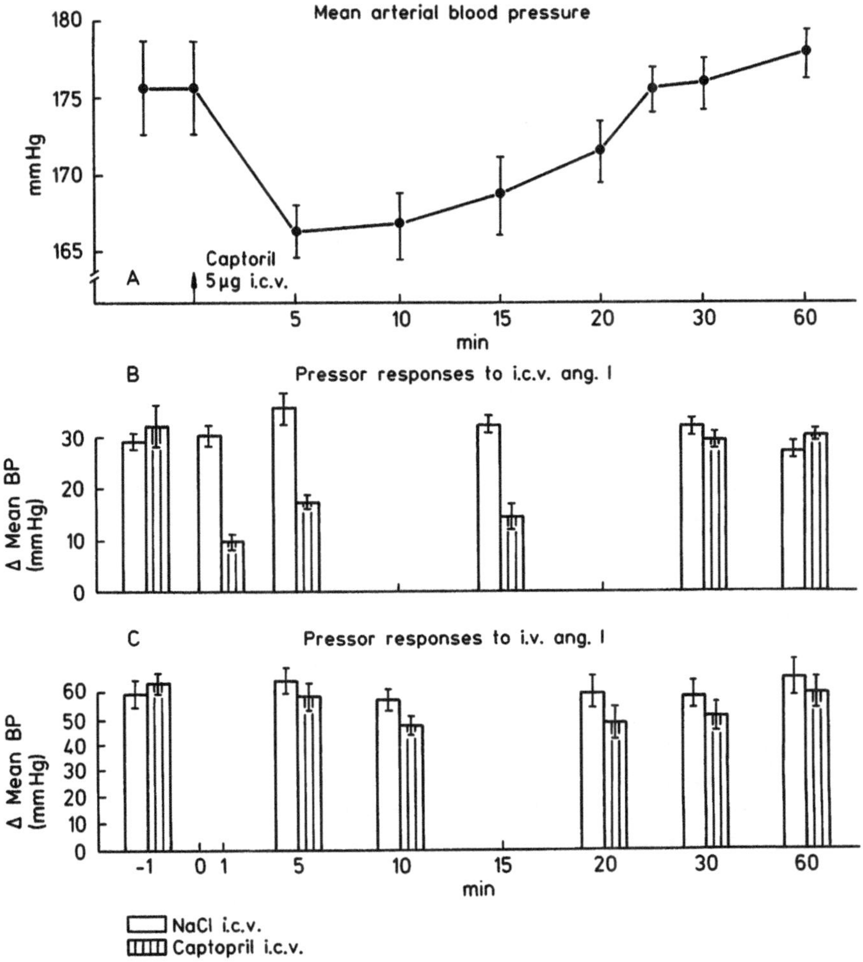

Fig. 32A–C. Decrease of blood pressure (**A**) and central (**B**) and peripheral (**C**) pressor responses to angiotensin I (*Ang I*) following injection of captopril (5 μg) into the lateral brain ventricle (i.c.v.) in stroke-prone, spontaneously hypertensive rats. (From UNGER et al. 1981b)

nervous system as assessed by measurements of plasma NA, the authors concluded that its central antihypertensive action was due neither to an inhibition of vasopressin release nor to a reduction of sympathetic tone but rather to some unidentified mechanism.

Subsequent studies (BERECEK et al. 1983) showed that a 4-week-long i.c.v. infusion of captopril (1.25 μg/h) in young SHR not only decreased blood pressure but attenuated the increases in regional vascular resistance in response to intravenous phenylephrine and vasopressin. In addition, the heart rate baroreceptor reflex appeared to be sensitized. Again, when given i.v., captopril was without effect on these parameters. In further studies there authors demonstrated that electrical posterior hypothalamic stimulation, intravenous NA administration, and sympathetic nerve stimulation resulted in smaller increases in blood pressure and renal mesenteric vascular resistance in SHR treated for 4 weeks with i.c.v.-administered captopril than in vehicle-treated rats (BERECEK et al. 1987).

Results by TAKEDA et al. (1986) and from our laboratory (MOURSI et al. 1987) have confirmed the baroreceptor reflex sensitizing effect of centrally administered CEI such as captopril and ramiprilat in SHR.

Thus, results from the majority of studies testing the effects of i.c.v.-administered CEI in various animal models of hypertension are compatible with a centrally induced antihypertensive action of these drugs. The blood pressure lowering mechanisms are still not fully understood but may include a sensitization of the baroreceptor reflex, as well as an alteration of vascular reactivity.

10.2 Effects of Systemically Administered Converting Enzyme Inhibitors on Brain Converting Enzyme

One of the most controversial topics concerning the central actions of CEI has been whether these drugs gain access to the CNS and inhibit CE in the brain upon systemic administration.

When antihypertensive doses of captopril or enalapril were given acutely by the intravenous or oral route, they could scarcely be detected in the brain or in the CSF, and the pressor responses to i.c.v.-administered ANG I were usually unaltered (UNGER et al. 1984a). These findings suggested that following acute peripheral administration, captopril and enalapril did not penetrate the blood brain barrier in sufficient quantity to inhibit CE in the brain tissue or CSF.

In addition, some authors observed thirst and salt appetite in rats treated systemically with CEI (LEDINGHAM and SIMPSON 1981; SCHIFFRIN and GENEST 1982; DI NICOLANTONIO et al. 1983; MINSKER et al. 1984). This effect seemed to be related to the salt status of the animals (LEDINGHAM and SIMPSON 1981).

In a series of experiments in rats, EVERED et al. (1980) and EVERED and Robinson (1983) demonstrated that acute subcutaneous low-dose treatment with captopril (0.1–1.0 mg/kg) inhibited the pressor responses to intravenous ANG I and enhanced the drinking response to various stimuli, including hypovolemia and water deprivation, but not to i.c.v.-injected ANG I. In contrast, subcutaneous pretreatment with higher (antihypertensive) doses of captopril (5–100 mg/kg) blocked drinking in response to i.c.v.-injected renin and ANG I but did not enhance the drinking response to hypovolemia and water deprivation. A similar observation was made in our laboratory: Captopril given at a single oral dose of 20 mg/kg significantly attenuated drinking to i.c.v.-injected renin without affecting the response to i.c.v.-administered ANG II (UNGER et al. 1984c).

Further evidence for an inhibition of CE in the brain following acute or chronic systemic administration of various CEI was provided by ex vivo studies measuring CE activity biochemically in brain tissue from CEI-treated rats. COHEN and KURZ (1982) reported a substantial CE inhibition in brain cortex homogenates from SHR following a single dose of captopril (10 mg/kg). Enalapril given at equidepressor doses (0.3–1 mg/kg) did not inhibit brain CE, but at doses between 10–30 mg/kg, brain CE activity was inhibited by 30%–40% for 24 h. An almost identical inhibition of the CE activity in the brain cortex following a single oral dose of enalapril (30 mg/kg) was observed in our laboratory, while an equi-antihypertensive dose of the CE inhibitor ramipril (1 mg/kg) produced a slightly greater inhibition (UNGER et al. 1984a).

In chronic studies in SHRSP using enalapril, ramipril, and perindopril, we observed a significant CE inhibition in the brain cortex with all CEI, while only ramipril reduced the activity of the enzyme in other brain areas (UNGER et al. 1984b, 1986a). In additional studies we tested the in vivo inhibition of central CE following chronic oral antihypertensive treatment with different CEI. We found that in ramipril- and SA 446-treated groups the pressor responses to i.c.v.-administered ANG I were significantly reduced, while in captopril- and enalapril-treated animals these responses remained unchanged (UNGER et al. 1982a, 1984b).

A recent report by NAKATA et al. (1987) confirmed the inhibitory action of SA446 on brain CE following 1 week of oral treatment in SHR, WKY, and RHR.

The differences among the various CEI with respect to their inhibitory action on brain CE upon systemic administration may partly reside in the fact that the access to brain structures inside the blood-brain barrier depends on the lipid solubility of a given component. For instance, SA 466 is structurally and pharmacologically closely related to captopril (UNGER et al. 1982a). However, due to its much higher lipid solubility, this compound can probably penetrate the blood-brain barrier more easily and thus inhibit brain CE more readily than captopril, as evidenced in our studies.

GOHLKE et al. (1989) have demonstrated that ramipril and the more lipid soluble Hoe 288 both inhibit CE in the CSF following acute oral administration of doses between 10–30 mg/kg (ramipril) and 1–30 mg (Hoe 288). In contrast, enalapril, the least lipophilic CEI used in this study, did not significantly inhibit CE in the CSF (Fig. 33). Penetration of CEI through the blood-brain barrier could thus be related to the lipid solubility of the drugs.

An additional factor governing the access of prodrug-CEI such as enalapril, ramipril, or perindopril to structures inside the blood-brain barrier may be the degree and site of metabolic activation of these drugs following oral application. Rat brain, for instance, appears to have only a limited capacity to hydrolyze prodrug-CEI to the active diacid compounds (UNGER et al. 1982b; COHEN and KURZ 1983; GOHLKE et al. 1989). Therefore, the degree to which brain CE is inhibited by a prodrug CEI appears to depend on how much of the respective diacid compound can enter the brain from the blood. Recently, an inhibition of CE in human cerebrospinal fluid following a single oral dose of captopril (75 mg) was reported by GEPPETTI et al. (1987).

Apart from the CE activity, other components of the brain RAS were also analyzed after systemic treatment with CEI. In SHRSP, increased concentrations of renin were measured in the medulla oblongata, hypothalamus, and

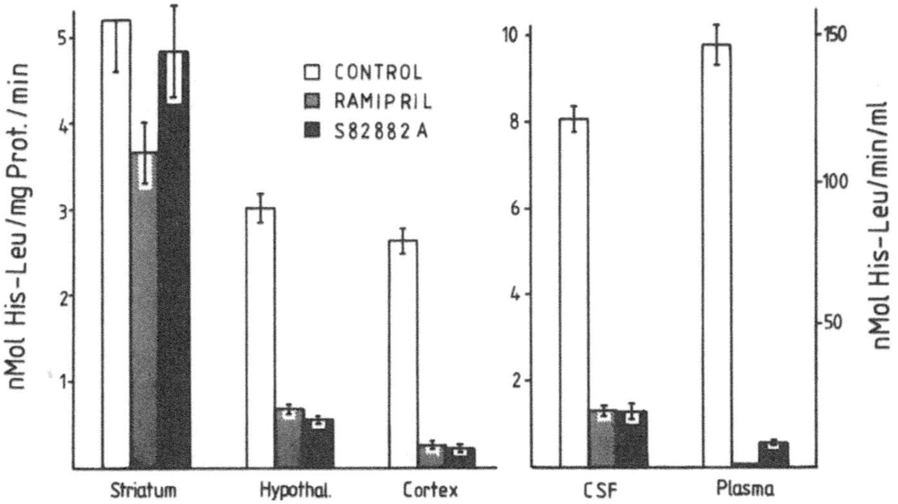

Fig. 33. Inhibition of converting enzyme in different brain areas, cerebrospinal fluid (*CSF*), and blood plasma following 1 week of oral treatment with *ramipril* or Hoe 288 (*S82882 A*) in normotensive rats. Both drugs were given by gavage once daily at a dose of 10 mg/kg

neurohypophysis following prolonged oral treatment with captopril (UNGER et al. 1982c). FELIX and SCHELLING (1982) reported on increased renin concentrations in the septal area and the anterior hypothalamus in SHRSP and WKY after chronic oral captopril treatment. At the same time angiotensinogen was reduced in the CSF. If one assumes that the regulatory mechanisms between ANG II, renin, and angiotensiogen in the brain are similar to those in the periphery, the above findings would be compatible with a reduced ANG II generation in brain tissue.

Direct measurements of ANG II concentrations in the brain following systemic CEI treatment were performed more recently. Bilaterally nephrectomized rabbits were treated with a single oral dose of 10 mg/kg ramipril. Four hours later the animals were killed and ANG II concentrations were measured in various organs including the brain. ANG II was significantly lowered in the medulla oblongata but was increased in the hypothalamus of the ramipril-treated animals (GANTEN et al. 1985).

In SHR, intravenous administration of ramiprilat (50 μg/kg) produced a significant increase of ANG II in the hypothalamus (PHILLIPS and KIMURA 1986). A cross-reaction with ANG III was unlikely in these experiments since the ANG II measurements were controlled by HPLC, so that the ANG II radioimmunoassay used would only measure true ANG II peptides.

It appears from these findings that acute systemic administration of CEI leads to a differential inhibition of the CE in the brain. If the inhibitors gain access more readily to other brain structures than to the hypothalamus, the initial result may indeed be an increased ANG II generation in the hypothalamus due to the enhanced supply of blood-borne ANG I. The acute natriuretic actions of these compounds could be explained by such a mechanism, since brain ANG II can exert powerful natriuretic actions (UNGER et al. 1989). On the other hand, if one assumes that endogenous ANG II acts on the cardiovascular centers of the brainstem to attenuate the baroreceptor reflex, a CEI-induced reduction of the ANG II biosynthesis in the brainstem could lead to the sensitization of the baroreceptor reflex discussed above.

In summary, there is substantial evidence from ex vivo and in vivo studies indicating that brain CE can be inhibited following acute and chronic systemic treatment with CEI. Measurements of CE activity and ANG II concentrations in brain homogenates have revealed that systemically administered CEI do not uniformly inhibit the enzyme throughout the brain. Increased ANG II concentrations induced by acute oral or intravenous application of these drugs have been observed in the hypothalamus, which could account for some of the initial effects of these drugs on electrolyte and body fluid balance. The effects of chronic antihypertensive treatment with CEI on brain ANG II concentrations have not yet been analyzed.

The question as to whether the observed CE inhibition in the brain contributes to the cardiovascular actions of CEI cannot be answered definitively as yet. CEI have repeatedly been reported to sensitize the baroreceptor reflex, and this component of their actions may be related to an inhibition of ANG II biosynthesis in the brain.

Finally, we do not know at present whether or not these drugs really have to penetrate the blood-brain barrier to exert their inhibitory actions on the brain RAS. SAKAGUCHI et al. (1988) have recently demonstrated that acute oral treatment with lisinopril significantly reduced CE activity in circumventricular brain structures outside the blood-brain barrier, including the subfornical organ (SFO) and the organum vasculosum of the lamina terminalis (OVLT), but not in brain areas inside the blood-brain barrier. In view of the direct ANG II-containing projections from the circumventricular structures to other brain regions (LIND et al. 1984), it is conceivable that an inhibition of CE in forebrain and brain stem structures outside the blood-brain barrier could reduce the CE-dependent supply of endogenous ANG II for these pathways and by this mechanism antagonize an inadequately high activity of the brain RAS in pathological states such as hypertension.

11 Side Effects of Converting Enzyme Inhibitors

CEI are generally well-tolerated drugs. Side effects observed frequently under antihypertensive treatment such as tachycardia, impotence, bronchospasm, sedation, memory impairment, orthostatic hypotension, or adverse effects on laboratory values are either extremely rare or nonexistent. However, there has been some concern about a number of side effects which, although occurring very rarely, may have serious consequences. These include bone marrow depression, angioneurotic edema, and deterioration of renal function. More common and less dangerous side effects are hypotension, rash, taste disturbance, and dry cough. In the first years of the clinical use of CEI, the incidence of untoward effects was reported to be much higher than in more recent studies. This discrepancy can be explained by the fact that with increasing experience it became more and more evident that the desired therapeutic actions could be achieved with drug doses far below those employed initially.

Captopril, the first CEI in clinical use, was initially used in patients with severe, therapy-resistant hypertension often associated with multiorgan failure at doses up to 600 mg daily (recommendation today: 50 mg daily in one or two divided dosages). These circumstances have to be taken into account when analyzing the pattern, incidence, and severity of the side effects reported during this early period of drug use. When the spectrum of patients treated shifted towards patients with uncomplicated hypertension and less organ damage, and the doses were reduced, some of the previously reported side effects disappeared completely, and the incidence of the others declined, in some cases dramatically.

11.1 Captopril

The most important adverse effects seen with captopril are hypotension (large and unexpected falls in blood pressure, frequently after the first dose), skin rash, taste disturbance, cough, impairment of renal function, and very rarely neutropenia and angioneurotic edema. The incidence and the pattern of side effects during the first years of captopril use in clinical practice has been reviewed by HEEL et al. (1980) and VIDT et al. (1982). Table 8, taken from a more recent review by EDWARDS and PADFIELD (1985), summarizes the most common side effects of captopril observed during treatment of nearly 5000 patients in the General Use Study. In this study, 4,220 patients with moderate to severe, 107 with mild, and 522 with renovascular hypertension were treated for 1–12 months. The dose did not exceed 150 mg/day.

11.1.1 Neutropenia

Among the adverse effects listed above, neutropenia is considered the most worrying one. According to COOPER (1983), the frequency of neutropenia was 0.02% in patients with normal renal function but increased to 0.04% in patients with impaired renal function and even to 7.2% in patients with renal failure and additional collagen disease. Neutropenia usually occurred within 3 months of treatment and frequently resolved quickly upon drug withdrawal. However, in many of these instances neutropenia may not have been related to captopril alone but also to concurrent treatment with other drugs (EDWARDS and PADFIELD) 1985). Also, it should be kept in mind that the above figures reflect the treatment situation during the first years of clinical use, when captopril was administered at doses up to ten times higher than those recommended today.

Table 8. Side effects of captopril treatment (n = 4849) (From EDWARDS and PADFIELD 1985)

	Occurrence
Rash	6.0%
Taste disturbance	3.1%
Neutropenia	0.04%
Proteinuria (>1 g / 24 h)	0.6%
Headache	2.9%
Lassitude/fatigue	2.7%
Hypotension	2.5%

11.1.2 Renal Side Effects

The most prominent renal side effect of captopril was proteinuria (>1 g/24 h). This effect disappeared or substantially decreased in most patients whether or not the drug was continued (EDWARDS and PADFIELD 1985). A nephrotic syndrome has been described in patients taking high-dose captopril, and histologically a membranous glomerulopathy has been demonstrated which may or may not have been drug-related (CAPTOPRIL COLLABORATION STUDY GROUP 1982). Hyperkalemia may also occur in patients with renal failure (WARREN and O'CONNOR 1980), most likely due to the inhibitory action of captopril on aldosterone release. Since a reduction of plasma aldosterone concentration is a general feature of CEI, these drugs should not be used in conjunction with potassium-sparing diuretics such as spironolactone, amiloride, or triamterene.

11.1.3 Angioneurotic Edema

Angioneurotic edema together with urticaria constitute a rare (estimated incidence 0.03%–0.07%; see WERNZE 1988) but potentially dangerous side effect of captopril and other CEI, that has been appreciated relatively late after the introduction of these drugs into clinical practice. WOOD and MANN (1987) reported on 6 patients with angio-edema treated by captopril and 13 patients treated by enalapril observed in the United Kingdom from the introduction of the drugs in May 1981 and January 1985, respectively, until January 1986. The reaction occurred after the first dose or within days of the beginning of treatment. Resolution was rapid upon drug withdrawal. In a few cases there was a positive rechallenge. The onset of the reaction was too rapid to be accounted for by stimulation of a specific immune response.

In patients with hereditary angioneurotic edema, a hereditary defect of a C_1-esterase inhibitor leads to episodical increases in bradykinin synthesis due to kallikrein activation. Since patients with CEI-induced angio-edema responded to treatment with a C_1-esterase inhibitor, impaired kinin degradation was suspected to be a causative factor for this side effect of CEI (WERNZE 1988), but direct evidence for such a mechanism has not yet been presented.

11.1.4 Fetal Abnormalities

There are a few reports from animal studies together with a clinical case (DUMINY and BURGER 1981) on fetal abnormalities or fetal deaths associated with the use of captopril during pregnancy (BROUGHTON-PIPKIN et al. 1980; KEITH et al. 1982). Therefore, treatment of hypertension with captopril (or other CEI) during pregnancy should be avoided.

11.1.5 Significance of the Mercapto Group

A number of the untoward effects of captopril reported during the first new years of its use were thought to be attributable to the mercapto group (sulfhydryl group) of the captopril molecule, in analogy to other sulfhydryl-containing drugs such as penicillamine. Part of the incentive to develop new non-sulfhydryl CEI stems from the idea that avoiding the mercapto group in the molecule would eliminate some of the side effects of the drug. This approach has yielded a great number of new non-sulfhydryl-containing CEI. However, since the pattern of side effects with these new CEI remained essentially the same, the potential of the mercapto group in producing side effects of CEI has to be questioned.

On a more theoretical basis, it also appears unlikely that the mercapto group in the captopril molecule should produce similar effects to the mercapto group of penicillamine. Thus, because of the vicinity of the sulfhydryl group to an amino group in the penicillamine molecule, this compound is a powerful metalchelating agent and can undergo facile reactions with aldehydes to yield stable cyclic derivatives. Thanks to this property, penicillamine can inhibit collagen cross-linking, causing a disease state similar to lathyrism. Captoril lacks this specific molecular arrangement between the mercapto and an amino group. In addition, it does not have two methyl groups vicinal to the mercapto group that seems to be critical for the lathyrogenic effect of penicillamine. Thus, although captopril and penicillamine both have a sulfhydryl group in common, this does not mean that this group in the captopril molecule should give rise to the same side effects as in the penicillamine molecule.

11.1.6 Incidence of Side Effects in Postmarketing Studies

Postmarking studies on captopril have been performed in the United Kingdom, New Zealand, Japan, and Switzerland. In the British study (CHALMERS et al. 1987) on 13,295 hypertensive patients, captopril was withdrawn in 7.17% because of adverse reactions. These include malaise/lassitude (1.55%), gastrointestinal upset (1.07%), rash (0.81%), dizziness/vertigo (0.75%), headache (0.61%), hypotension (0.34%), altered taste (0.33%), anxiety/tachycardia (0.27%), irritable throat/cough (0.20%), and others (1.24%). Seventeen patients (0.13%) were withdrawn as a result of deteriorating renal function. Of these, two-thirds had pre-existing renal disease, while in the remainder, there was no baseline information on renal function available. No death was thought to be linked to captopril treatment.

In the New Zealand study (EDWARDS et al. 1987), in 4% of 4,124 hypertensive patients under captopril (range 20–300 mg/day, about 60% treated with 75–150 mg/day during the years 1981–84) adverse events were reported, the majority being cutaneous (1%) and gastrointestinal (0.7%). Interestingly, a specific taste survey revealed a high incidence of taste disturbance in the control population, although taste loss was significantly higher for the captopril-treated group. In 3 patients treatment was withdrawn (1 pruritus, 2 rash).

In the report by OMAE et al. (1987) data were reviewed from phase III and phase IV clinical studies on captopril performed in Japan. While captopril in the phase III study (1,304 patients, doses between 15–300 mg/day) was associated with an incidence of 3.8% rash, 0.5% dysgeusia, and 0.3% hypotension, the respective incidences were decreased in the phase IV study (6,775 patients, 25–150 mg/day) to 0.5% (rash), 0.1% (dysgeusia), and 0.2% (hypotension).

In the Swiss study (SANER and BRUNNER 1988) data on adverse effects under captopril (≤75 mg/day) were reported from 1,241 hypertensive patients. Captopril was withdrawn because of subjective side effects in 7.7%. These included unspecific symptoms such as dizziness, headache, fatigue, sleep disturbance (overall incidence 8.6%), gastrointestinal disturbances (6.6%), cardiovascular symptoms (3.1%), and cutaneous reactions (1.7%). Taste disturbance (0.24%) and dry cough (0.16%) were relatively rare as was (orthostatic) hypotension (0.6%). Captopril-related changes in parameters of renal function such as serum creatinine, urinary protein, or serum potassium were not observed. A small decrease in total leucocyte count by 228/mm^3 occurred, which was considered to be clinically not relevant.

11.2 Enalapril

11.2.1. Pattern and Incidence of Side Effects

The overall pattern and the incidence of adverse effects under enalapril therapy are very similar to those reported for captopril (see above) and are probably common for all CEI. The side effects of enalapril were reviewed in 1984 by McFATE SMITH et al. (1984a,b). At that time point, data from about 1,000 patients who had received enalapril for 1 year and about 600, for more than 2 years were analyzed. No deaths were attributable to the drug. The most frequent side effects in patients with hypertension were headache (3.0%–3.8%, depending on doses between 10–40 mg/day), dizziness (2.6%–4.0%), fatigue (1.5%–2.5%), diarrhea (0.5%–1.3%), nausea (0.8%–1.2%), rash (0.3%–1.4%), cough (0.5%–0.8%), and hypotension (0.4%–1.1%). With the exception of cough, which seems to be consistently related to CEI, and of rash, these adverse effects can be observed with similar frequencies under placebo treatment. A relationship between the dose of enalapril and the incidence of these side effects could not be established. The withdrawal rate for patients receiving enalapril (including those receiving an additional diuretic) was 3.3%, compared with 4% under placebo and 5.6% receiving other antihypertensive drugs in control groups. Other side effects reported in this review were neutropenia (isolated white cell counts less than 3000/mm^3) in 16 of 3094 patients (0.5%). In 11 of these patients the white cell count returned to normal values on continuation of enalapril treatment. Underlying infections or diseases such as scleroderma may have contributed to the reduction in white cell counts in some of the patients. Transient loss of taste was reported in 2 patients, dysgeusia in 10 patients, and 1 patient presented with a hyperesthesia of the oral mucosa. In most cases these effects were reversible with continued treatment.

A very similar picture emerges from another report (DAVIES et al. 1984b) which included almost 2000 patients under enalapril monotherapy and 880 patients under enalapril plus other antihypertensives. In addition to the above-reported side effects, proteinuria (urinary protein values above 1.0 g/24 h or 0.5 g/12 h) was observed in 0.66% of the patients with hypertension and in 1 patient cut of 134 with congestive heart failure under enalapril monotherapy. In the latter patient the relationship to enalapril monotherapy. In the latter patient the relationship to enalapril was doubtful; in the hypertensive patients values returned to normal during continued therapy. No cases of nephrotic syndrome or membranous glomerulonephritis were reported with enalapril. The occurrence of angioneurotic edema under enalapril treatment has been mentioned above.

11.2.2 Side Effects in Postmarketing Studies

A most recently published postmarketing surveillance of enalapril using the method of prescription-event monitoring included a 1-year analysis of 12543 patients (INMAN et al. 1988). The frequencies of side effects reported in this study are summarized in Table 9. They were in the range of those reported before except for the frequency of drug-persistent cough which was higher in this report, probably because doctors are now more alerted to this adverse effect than previously. Altogether, 1098 patients (8%) died. In 10 of 39 patients who died of renal failure, enalapril appeared to have contributed to a decline in renal function and subsequent death. Characteristics of these patients included old age, high dose, co-treatment with potassium-sparing diuretics, preexisting renal disease, or the addition of nonsteroidal antiinflammatory drugs (SPEIRS et al. 1988). No death was encountered in patients with uncomplicated hypertension.

11.2.3 Death Rate with Enalapril

Generally, the death rate under enalapril therapy is not higher than in non-enalapril-treated populations of similar age and health conditions. About two-thirds of the fatal events reported worldwide during enalapril therapy occurred in patients with severe congestive heart failure, in whom the drug was often used among many others as ultima ratio and despite existing contraindications and/or arrhythmias. The remainder occurred in patients with severe kidney disease. In addition, one patient thus far has died of an angioneurotic edema, and two patients have died of severe leucopenia. On the other hand, the addition of enalapril to conventional drug therapy has recently been shown to improve life

Table 9. Numbers of patients experiencing events of special interest (From INMAN et al. 1988)

Selected individual event	No. during 12 months of observation	% of patients (n = 12543)
Skin:		
Angioedema	27	0.2
Photosensitivity	15	0.1
Urticaria	32	0.3
Other acute events	298	2.4
Central nervous system and eye:		
Syncope	155	1.2
Dizziness	483	3.9
Headache	310	2.5
Convulsions	22	0.2
Paresthesia	126	1.0
Taste disturbance	25	0.2
Conjunctivitis	67	0.5
Cardiovascular:		
Hypotension	218	1.7
Tachycardia	194	1.5
Respiratory:		
Cough	360	2.9
Renal:		
Renal failure	82	0.7
Miscellaneous:		
Cramp	96	0.8
Diarrhea	236	1.9
Nausea and vomiting	326	2.6

expectancy significantly in patients with severe (stadium IV, NYHA) congestive heart failure (CONSENSUS STUDY 1987).

11.3 Other Converting Enzyme Inhibitors

Experience as to the incidence and the pattern of adverse effects with other CEI is by far less advanced than with captopril and enalapril. However, it appears from the data reported so far that the side effects observed during treatment with the CEI developed more recently are not different from those known for captopril and enalapril (e.g. WITTE and WALTER 1987). For further information on the safety profiles of captopril, enalapril, and lisinopril, see a recent report by WARNER and RUSH (1988).

In summary, common and/or important side effects of CEI include headache, cough, angioneurotic oedema, azotemia, and hypotension. The incidence of these events has steadily declined over the years with the reduction of doses recommended. Profound first-dose hypotension has been reported in patients with hypertension and, particularly, in patients with congestive heart failure (HODSMAN et al. 1983). This event is most often association with previous volume depletion by aggressive treatment with diuretics, hyponatremia, as well as severe and secondary forms of hypertension. Commencing therapy at low doses (captopril 6.25 mg, enalapril 2.5 mg) and withdrawal of diuretics a few days before CEI treatment minimizes the risk of first-dose hypotension. Special care concerning dosage has to be taken in patients with renal disease as outlined in the section on renal effects of CEI. Evidence from animal studies and from a clinical case suggesting a causal relationship between fetal abnormalities and captopril treatment preclude the use of CEI during pregnancy.

References

Ajayi AA, Elliott HL, Reid JL (1986) The pharmacodynamics and dose-response relationships of the angiotensin converting enzyme inhibitor, cilazapril, in essential hypertension. Br J Clin Pharmacol 22:167–175

Alhenc-Gelas F, Soubrier F, Hubert C, Allegrini J, John M, Tregaer G, Corvol P (1988) Molecular cloning and complete aminoacid sequence of human angiotensin I-converting enzyme. Hypertension 12 (abstract 29):340

Anderson S, Meyer TW, Rennke HG, Brenner BM (1985) Control of glomerular injury in rats with reduced renal mass. J Clin Invest 76:612–619

Anderson WP, Woods RL (1987) Intrarenal effects of angiotensin II in renal artery stenosis. Kidney Int 31 [Suppl 20]:S-157–S-167

Antonaccio MJ, Kervin L (1980) Evidence for prejunctional inhibition of norepinephrine release by captopril in spontaneously hypertensive rats. Eur J Pharmacol 68:209–212

Antonaccio MJ, Rubin B, Horovitz ZP, Laffan RJ, Goldberg ME, High JP, Harris DN, Zaidi I (1979) Effects of chronic treatment with captopril (SQ 14225), an orally active inhibitor of angiotensin I-converting enzyme, in spontaneously hypertensive rats. Jpn J Pharmacol 29:285–294

Arr SM, Woollard ML, Fairhurst G, Pippen C, Rao SK, Cooper WD (1985) Safety and efficacy of enalapril in essential hypertension in elderly. Br J Clin Pharmacol 20: 279P–280P

Assad MM, Antonaccio MJ (1982) Vascular wall renin in spontaneously hypertensive rats. Hypertension 4:487–493

Atkinson AB, Morton JJ, Brown JJ, Davies DL, Fraser R, Kelly P, Leckie AF, Lever AF, Robertson JIS (1980) Captopril in clinical hypertension: Changes in components of renin-angiotensin system and in body composition in relation to fall in blood pressure with a note on measurement of angiotensin II during converting enzyme inhibition. Br Heart J 44:290–296

Atkinson J, Sonnay M, Sautel M, Abdel-Kader F (1987) Chronic treatment of the spontaneously hypertensive rat with captopril attenuates responses to noradrenaline in vivo but not in vitro. Naunyn-Schmiedeberg's Arch Pharmacol 335:624–628

Attwood MR, Francis RJ, Hassall CH, Krohn A, Lawton G et al. (1984) New potent inhibitors of angiotensin converting enzyme. FEBS Lett 165:201–206

Ausiello DA, Kreisberg, JI, Roy G, Karnovsky MJ (1980) Concentration of cultured rat glomerular cells of apparant mesangial origin after stimulation with angiotensin II and arginine vasopressin. J Clin Invest 65:754–760

Baudin B, Timmins PA, Drouet L, Legrand Y, Baumann FC (1988) Molecular weight and shape of angiotensin-I converting enzyme. A neutron scattering study. Biochem Biophys Res Commun 154 (3):1144–1150

Bauer JH, Jones LB (1984) Comparative studies: enalapril versus hydrochlorothiazide as first-step therapy for the treatment of primary hypertension. Am J Kidney Dis 4: 55–62

Bauer JH, Reams GP (1985) Hemodynamic and renal function in essential hypertension during treatment with enalapril. Am J Med 79 [Suppl 3C]:10–13

Baum T, Becker FT, Sybertz EJ (1983) Attenuation of pressor responses to intracerebroventricular angiotensin I by angiotensin converting enzyme inhibitors and their effects

on systemic blood pressure in conscious rats. Life Sci 32:1297–1303
Becker RHA, Schölkens BA, Metzger M, Schulze KJ (1984) Pharmacological properties of the new orally active angiotensin converting emzyme inhibitor 2-(N-((S)-1-ethoxycarbonyl-3-phenylpropyl)-L-alanyl)-(1S, 3S, 5S)-2-azabicyclo(3.3.0)octane-3-carboxylic acid (HOE498). Drug Res 34 (II):1411–1416
Beerman B, Gomez HJ, Till AE, Junggren I-L (1986) Pharmacokinetics of lisinopril in healthy volunteers. Acta Pharmacol Toxicol [Suppl V] (abstract 130)
Belz GG, Essig J, Wellstein A (1987) Hemodynamic responses to angiotensin I in normal volunteers and the antagonism by the angiotensin-converting enzyme inhibitor cilazapril. J Cardiovasc Pharmacol 9:219–224
Benetos A, Gavras H, Stewart JM, Vavrek RJ, Hatinoglou A, Gavras I (1986a) Vasodepressor role of endogenous bradykinin assessed by a bradykinin antagonist. Hypertension 8:971–974
Benetos A, Gavras I, Gavras H (1986b) Hypertensive effect of bradykinin antagonist in normotensive rats. Hypertension 8:1089–1092
Bengis RG, Coleman TG, Young DB, McCaare (1978) Long-term blockade of angiotensin formation in various normotensive and hypertensive rat models using converting enzyme inhibitor (SQ 14 225). Circ Res 43 [Suppl I]:45–53
Berecek KH, Okuno T, Nagahama S, Oparil S (1983) Altered vascular reactivity and baroreflex sensitivity induced by chronic central administration of captopril in the spontaneously hypertensive rat. Hypertension 5:689–700
Berecek KH, Kirk KA, Nagahama S, Oparil S (1987) Sympathetic function in spontaneously hypertensive rats after chronic administration of captopril. Am J Physiol 252:H796–H806
Bergstrand R, Johansson S, Vedin A, Wilhelmsson C (1982) Comparison of once-a-day and twice-a-day dosage regimens of enalapril (MK-421) in patients with mild hypertension. Proc Br Pharm Soc 14:136p (abstr)
Bernstein KE, Martin BM, Bernstein EA, Linton J, Striker L, Striker G (1988) The isolation of angiotensin-converting enzyme cDNA. J Biol Chem 263:11021–11024
Biollaz J, Burnier M, Turini GA, Brunner DB, Porchet M et al. (1981) Three new long-acting converting-enzyme inhibitors: relationship between plasma converting-enzyme activity and response to angiotensin I. Clin Pharmacol Ther 29:665–670
Biollaz J, Brunner HR, Gavras I, Waeber B, Gavras H (1982) Antihypertensive therapy with MK 421:angiotensin II-renin relationships to evaluate efficacy of converting enzyme blockade. J Cardiovasc Pharmacol 4:966–972
Björck S, Nyberg G, Mulec H, Granerus G, Herlitz H, Aurell M (1986) Beneficial effects of angiotensin converting enzyme inhibition on renal function in patients with diabetic nephropathy. Br Med J 293:471–474
Blythe WB (1983) Captopril and renal autoregulation. N Engl J Med 308:390–391
Boomsma F, De Bruyn JHB, Derkx FHM Schalekamp MADH (1981) Opposite effects of captopril on angiotensin I-converting enzyme "activity" and "concentration"; relation between enzyme inhibition and long-term blood pressure response. Clin Sci 60:491–498
Boutrouy et al. (1984) Captopril administration in pregnancy impairs fetal angiotensin converting enzyme activity and neonatal adaptation. Lancet ii;935–936
Bravo El, Tarazi RC (1979) Converting enzyme inhibition with an orally active compound in hypertensive man. Hypertension 1:39–46
Brenner BM (1983) Hemodynamically mediated glomerular injury and the progressive nature of kidney disease. Kidney Int 23:647–655
Broughton-Pipkin F, Turner SR, Symonds EM (1980) Possible risk with captopril in pregnancy: some animal data. Lancet ii:1256
Brunner DB, Desponds G, Biollaz J, Keller I, Ferber F, Gavras H, Brunner HR, Schelling JL (1981) Effect of a new angiotensin converting enzyme inhibitor MK 421 and its lysine analogue on the components of the renin system in healthy subjects. Br J Clin Pharmacol 11:461–467
Brunner HR, Gavras H, Waeber B, Textor SL, Turini GA, Wauters JP (1980) Clinical use of an orally acting converting enzyme inhibitor: captopril. Hypertension 2: 558–566

Brunner HR, Nussberger J, Waeber B (1985a) The present molecules of converting enzyme inhibitors. J Cardiovasc Pharmacol 7:S2–S11
Brunner HR, Nussberger J, Waeber B (1985b) Effects of angiotensin converting enzyme inhibition: a clinical point of view. J Cardiovasc Pharmacol 7 [Suppl 4]:S73–S81
Brunner HR, Waeber B, Nussberger J (1987) Angiotensin converting enzyme inhibition and the normal kidney. Kidney Int 31 [Suppl 20]:S-104–S-107
Burnier M, Turini GA, Brunner HR, Porchet M, Kruithof D, Vukovich RA, Gavras H (1981) RHC 3659: a new orally active angiotensin converting enzyme inhibitor in normal volunteers. Br J Clin Pharmacol 12:893–899
Bünning P (1983) The catalytic mechanism of angiotensin converting enzyme. Clin Exp Hypertens [A] 5:1263–1275
Bünning P (1984) Inhibition of angiotensin converting enzyme by Hoe 498 diacid—comparison with captopril and enalaprilat. Drug Res 34 (II):1406–1410
Bünning P (1987) Kinetic properties of the angiotensin converting enzyme inhibitor ramiprilat. J Cardiovasc Pharmacol 10 [Suppl 7]:S31–S35
Bünning P, Holmquist B, Riordan JF (1978) Functional residues at the active site of angiotensin converting enzyme. Biochem Biophys Res Commun 83:1442–1449
Bünning P, Holmquist B, Riordan JF (1983) Substrate specificity and kinetic characteristics of angiotensin converting enzyme. Biochemistry 22:103–110
Bussien J-P, D'Amore TF, Perret L, Porchet M, Nussberger J, Waeber B, Brunner HR (1986) Single and repeated dosing of the converting enzyme inhibitor perindopril to normal subjects. Clin Pharmacol Ther 39:554–558
Byers LD, Wolfenden R (1972) A potent reversible inhibitor of carboxypeptidase A. J Biol Chem 247:606–608
Campbell DJ (1987) Tissue renin-angiotensin system: sites of angiotensin formation. J Cardiovasc Pharmacol 10 [Suppl 7]:S1–S8
Campbell DJ, Habener JF (1986) Angiotensinogen gene is expressed and differentially regulated in multiple tissues of the rat. J Clin Invest 78:31–39
Captopril Collaborative Study Group (1982) Does captopril cause renal damage in hypertensive patients? Lancet i:988–990
Captopril Multicenter Research Group I (1983) A placebo-controlled trial of captopril in refractory chronic congestive heart failure. J Am Coll Cardiol 2:755–763
Captopril Multicenter Research Group I (1985) A cooperative multicenter study of captopril in refractory chronic congestive heart failure: Hemodynamic effects and long-term response. Am Heart J 110:439–447
Carbonell LF, Carretero OA, Stewart JM, Scicli AG (1988) Effect of a kinin antagonist on the acute antihypertensive activity of enalaprilat in severe hypertension. Hypertension 11:239–243
Carlsson L, Abrahamsson T (1988) Ramiprilat alternates local ischemia-induced release of noradrenaline (NA) via a reduction in angiotensin II generation and bradykinin degradation. J Mol Cell Cardiol 20 [Suppl V]: S69 (abstr)
Carretero OA, Miyazaki S, Scicli AG (1981) Role of kinins in the acute antihypertensive effect of the converting enzyme inhibitor, captopril. Hypertension 3:18–22
Case DB, Atlas SA, Laragh JH, Sealey JE, Sullivan PA, McKinstry DN (1978) Clinical experience with blockade of the renin-angiotensin-aldosterone system by an oral converting enzyme inhibitor (SQ 14225, captopril) in hypertensive patients. Prog Cardiovasc Dis 21:195–206
Chalmers D, Dombey SL, Lawson DH (1987) Post marketing surveillance of captopril (for hypertension): a preliminary report. Br J Clin Pharmacol 24:343–349
Chen DS, Watkins BE, Ku EC, Dorson RA, Burell RD Jr (1984) Pharmacological profiles of two new angiotensin-converting enzyme (ACE) inhibitors: CGS 13945 and CGS 13934. Drug Dev Res 4:167–178
Chevillard C, Brown NL, Mathieu M-N, Laliberte F, Worcel M (1988) Differential effects of oral trandolapril and enalapril on rat tissue angiotensin-converting enzyme. Eur J Pharmacol 147:23–28
Chiba S, Quilley CP McGiff JC (1982) Decreased vascular responsiveness produced by angiotensin-converting enzyme inhibitors in the rat isolated kidney. Hypertension 4:1180–1185

Clappison BH, Anderson WP, Johnston CI (1981) Renal hemodynamic and renal kinins after angiotensin-converting enzyme inhibition. Kidney Int 20:615–620
Cleland JGF, Dargie HJ (1987) Heart failure, renal function, and angiotensin converting enzyme inhibitors. Kidney Int 31 [Suppl 20]:S-220–S-228
Cleland JGF, Dargie HJ, McAlpine H, Ball SG, Morton JJ, Robertson JIS, Ford I (1985) Severe hypotension after first dose of enalapril in heart failure. Br Med J 291: 1309–1312
Clough DP, Collis MG, Hatton R, Keddie JR, Collis MG (1982) Hypotensive action of captopril in spontaneously hypertensive and normotensive rats. Interference with neurogenic vasoconstriction. Hypertension 4:764–772
Clozel J-P, Hefti F (1988) Cilazapril prevents the development of cardiac hypertrophy and the decrease of coronary vascular reserve in spontaneously hypertensive rats. J Cardiovasc Pharmacol 11:568–572
Cody RJ (1985) Clinical and hemodynamic experience with enalapril in congestive heart failure. Am J Cardiol 55:36–44
Cohen ML (1985) Synthetic and fermentation-derived angiotensin-converting enzyme inhibitors. Annu Rev Pharmacol Toxicol 25:307–323
Cohen ML, Kurz KD (1982) Angiotensin-converting enzyme inhibition in tissues from spontaneously hypertensive rats after treatment with captopril or MK-421. J Exp Pharmacol Ther 220:63–69
Cohen ML, Kurz K (1983) Captopril and MK 421; stability on storage, distribution to the central nervous system, and onset of activity. Fed Proc 42:171
Cohen ML, Kurz KD, Schenck KW (1983a) Tissue angiotensin converting enzyme inhibition as an index of the disposition of enalapril (MK-421) and metabolite MK-422. J Pharmacol Exp Ther 226:192–196
Cohen ML, Wiley KS, Kurz KD (1983b) Effect of acute oral administration of captopril and MK-421 on vascular angiotensin converting enzyme activity in the spontaneously hypertensive rat. Life Sci 32:565–569
Collis MG, Keddie JR (1981) Captopril attenuates adrenergic vasoconstriction in rat mesenteric arteries by angiotensin-dependent and -independent mechanisms. Clin Sci 61:281–286
Corsersus Trial Study Group (1987) Effects of enalapril on mortality in severe congestive heart failure. N Engl J Med 316:1429–1435
Conway J, Hatton R, Clough DP (1981) Angiotensin interaction with homeostatic reflexes. In: Horovitz ZP (ed) Angiotensin converting enzyme inhibitors, mechanisms of action and clinical implications. Urban and Schwarzenberg, Baltimore, pp 81–87
Cooper RA (1983) Captopril-associated neutropenia. Arch Intern Med 143:659–660
Cooper WD, Doyle G, Donohoe J, Laher A, Ledingham J (1985) Enalapril in the treatment of hypertension associated with impaired renal function. Br J Clin Pharmacol 20:280–281
Corvol P, Michel JB, Evin G, Gardes J, Bensala-Alaoui A, Menard J (1984) The role of the renin-angiotensin system in blood pressure regulation in normotensive animals and man. J Hypertens 2 [Suppl 2]:25–30
Crantz FR, Swartz SL, Hollenberg NK, Moore ThJ, Dluhy RG, Williams GH (1980) Differences in response to the peptidyldipeptide hydrolase inhibitor SQ 20881 and SQ 14225 in normal-renin essential hypertension. Hypertension 2:604–609
Cushman DW, Ondetti MA (1980) Inhibitors of angiotensin-converting enzyme. Prog Med Chem 17:42–104
Cushman DW, Cheung HS, Sabo EF, Ondetti MA (1977) Design of potent competitive inhibitors of angiotensin-converting enzyme. Carboxyalkanoyl and mercaptoalkanoyl amino acids. Biochemistry 16:5484–5491
Cushman DW, Cheung HS, Sabo EF, Ondetti MA (1979) Development of specific inhibitors of angiotensin I converting enzyme (kininase II). Fed Proc 38:2778–2782
Darby I, Aldred P, Crawford RJ, Fernley RT, Niall HD, Penschow JD, Ryan GB, Coghlan JP (1985) Gene expression in vessels of the bovine renal cortex. J Hypertens 3:9–12
Das M, Soffer RL (1975) Pulmonary angiotensin-converting enzyme. Structural and catalytic properties. J Biol Chem 250:6762–6768

Davalos M, Frega NS, Saker B, Leaf A (1978) Effect of exogenous and endogenous angiotensin II in the isolated perfused rat kidney. Am J Physiol 235:605–610
Davies RO, Gomez HJ, Irvin JD, Walker JF, Moncloa F (1984a) An overview of the clinical pharmacology of enalapril. Br J Clin Pharmacol 18 [Suppl 2]:215S–229S
Davies RO, Irvin JD, Kramsch DK, Walker JF, Moncloa F (1984b) Enalapril worldwide experience. Am J Med 77(2A):23–35
Day MD, Moore AF (1976) Interaction of angiotensin II with noradrenaline and other spasmogens on rabbit isolated artic stripe. Arch Int Pharmacodyn Ther 219:29
Dean AV, Kripalani KJ, Migdalof BH (1984) Disposition of SQ 26,991 (zofenopril) and SQ 26,900, new angiotensin converting enzyme (ACE) inhibitors in rats. Fed Proc 43:349
De Cesaris R, Ranieri G, Salzano EV, Liberatore SM (1987) once daily therapy with angiotensin converting enzyme inhibitors in mild hypertension: a comparison of captopril and enalapril. J Hypertens 5 [Suppl 5]:S595–S597
De Graeff PA, Van Gilst WH, De Langen CDJ, Kingma JH, Wesseling H (1986) Concentration-dependent protection by captopril against ischemic-perfusion injury in the isolated rat heart. Arch Int Pharmacodyn Ther 280:181–193.
DeLeeuw D, Navis GI, Donker AJM, De Jong PE (1983) The angiotensin converting enzyme inhibitor enalapril and the effects on renal function. J Hypertens 1:93–97
DeLeeuw PW, Birkenhäger WH (1986) Changes in the pathophysiologic profile of blood pressure determinants during short-term enalapril administration. J Cardiovasc Pharmacol 8 [Suppl 1]:S26–S29
Dempsey PJ, McCallum ZT, Kent KM, Cooper T (1971) Direct myocardial effects of angiotensin II. Am J Physiol 220:477
Devlin RG, Fleiss PM (1981) Captopril in human blood and breast milk. J Clin Pharmacol 21:110–113
DiCarlo I, Chatterjee K, Parmley WW, Swedberg K, Atherton B (1983) Enalapril: a new angiotensin-converting enzyme inhibitor in chronic heart failure: acute and chronic hemodynamic evaluations. Am J Cardiol 2:865–871
Di Nicolantonio R, Mendelsohn FAO, Hutchinson JS (1983) Central angiotensin converting enzyme—blockade and thirst. Pharmacol Biochem Behav 18:731
Dominiak P, Elfarth A, Türck D (1987a) Biosynthesis of catecholamines and sympathetic outflow in spontaneously hypertensive rats (SHR) after chronic treatment with CE blocking agents. J Cardiovasc Pharmacol 10 [Suppl 7]:S122–S124
Dominiak P, Elfarth A, Türck D (1987b) Effects of chronic treatment with ramipril, a new ACE blocking agent, on presynaptic sympathetic nervous system of SHR. Clin Exp Hypertens [A] 9 (2,3):369–373
Drummer OH, Jarrott B (1986) The disposition and metabolism of captopril. Med Res Rev 6 (1):75–97
Drummer OH, Kourtis S, Jakovidis D (1988) Biotransformation studies of di-acid angiotensin converting enzyme inhibitors. Drug Res 38:647–650
Drummer PH, Miach P, Jarrott B (1983) S-methylation of captopril: Demonstration of captopril thiol methyltranferase activity in human erythrocytes and enzyme distribution in rat tissues. Biochem Pharmacol 32:1557–1562
Duchin KL, Singhvi SM, Willard DA, Migdalof BH, McKinstry DN (1982) Captopril kinetics. Clin Pharmacol Ther 31:452–458
Duminy PC, Burger P du T (1981) Fetal abnormality associated with the use of captopril during pregnancy. SA Med J 60:805.
Dunn FG, Oigman W, Ventura HO, Messerli FH, Kobrin I et al. (1984) Enalapril improves systemic and renal hemodynamics and allows regression of left ventricular mass in essential hypertension. Am J Cardiol 53:105–108
Dzau VJ (1987a) Renal effects of angiotensin-converting enzyme inhibition in cardiac failure. Am J Kidney Dis 10:74–80
Dzau VJ (1987b) Vascular angiotensin pathways: a new therapeutic target. J Cardiovasc Pharmacol 10 [Suppl 7]:S9–S16
Dzau VJ, Safar ME (1988) Large conduit arteries in hypertension: role of the vascular renin-angiotensin system. Circulation 77:947p¨–954
Dzau VJ, Colucci WS, Hollenberg NK, Williams GH (1981) Relation of the renin-angio-

tensin-aldosterone system to clinical state in congestive heart failure. 63:645–651
Dzau VJ, Ingelfinger JR, Pratt RE (1986) Regulation of tissue renin and angiotensin gene expressions. J Cardiovasc Pharmacol 8 [Suppl 10]:S11–S16
Eckert HG, Badian MJ, Gantz D, Kellner H-M, Volz M (1984) Pharmacokinetics and biotransformation of 2-(N-((S)-1-ethoxycarbonyl-3-phenylpropyl)-L-alanyl)-(1S, 3S, 5S)-2-azabicyclo(3.3.0)octane-3-carboxylic acid (HOE498) in rat, dog and man. Drug Res 34:1435–1447
Edwards CRW, Padfield PL (1985) Angiotensin-converting enzyme inhibitors: past, present, and bright future. Lancet i:30–34
Edwards IR, Coulter DM, Beasley DMG, MacIntosh D (1987) Captopril: 4 years of post marketing surveillance of all patients in New Zealand. Br J Clin Pharmacol 23: 529–536
Edwards RM (1983) Segmental effects of norepinephrine and angiotensin II on isolated renal vessels. Am J Physiol 244:526–534
Eisen V, Munday MR, Slater JDH (1987) Effects of angiotensin I converting enzyme inhibition and calcium channel blockade on plasma levels of active and inactive renin in conscious rabbits. Biochem Pharmacol 36:2331–2335
Erdös EG (1975) Angiotensin I converting enzyme. Circ Res 36 (2):247–254
Erdös EG, Skidgel RA (1987) The angiotensin I-converting enzyme. Lab Invest 56: 345–348
Evered MD, Robinson MM (1983) Effects of captopril on salt appetite in sodium-replete rats and rats treated with desoxycorticosterone acetate (DOCA). J Pharmacol Exp Ther 2:416
Evered MD, Robinson MM, Richardson MA (1980) Captopril given intracerebroventricularly, subcutaneously or by gavage inhibits angiotensin-converting enzyme activity in the rat brain. Eur J Pharmacol 68:443
Felix D, Schelling P (1982) Angiotensin-converting enzyme blockade by captopril changes angiotensin II receptors and angiotensinogen concentrations in the brain of SHRSPand WKY rats. Neurosci Lett 34:45
Ferguson RK, Vlasses PH, Swanson BN, Mojaverian P, Hichens M, Irvin JD, Huber PB (1982a) Effects of enalapril, a new converting enzyme inhibitor, in hypertension. Clin Pharmacol Ther 32:48–53
Ferguson RK, Irvin JD, Swanson BN, Viasses PH, Bergqvist PA, Till AE, Feinberg JA (1983) Food does not alter the absorption of enalapril maleate (MK-421) as measured by the disposition of its active metabolite. Clin Pharmacol Ther 33:254
Ferguson RK, Vlasses PH, Irvin JD, Swanson BN, Lee RB (1982b) A comparative pilot study of enalapril, a new converting enzyme inhibitor and hydrochlorothiazide in essential hypertension. J Clin Pharmacol 22:281–289
Fernandez PG, Snedden W, Idikio H, Fernandez D, Kin BK, Triggle CR (1984) The reversal of left ventricular hypertrophy with control of blood pressure in experimental hypertension. Scand J Clin Lab Invest 44:711–716
Ferner RE, Simpson JM, Rawlins MD (1987) Effects of intradermal bradykinin after inhibition of angiotensin converting enzyme. Br Med J 294:1119–1120
Ferreira SH (1985) History of the development of inhibitors of angiotensin I conversion. Drugs 30 [Suppl I]:1–5
Ferreira SH, Bartelt DC, Greene LJ (1970) Isolation of bradykinin-potentiating peptides from Bothrops jararaca venom. Biochemistry 9:2583–2593
Fiocchi R, Lijnen R, Eagard R, Staessen J, Amery A, Van Assche F, Spitz B, Rademaker M (1984) Lancet ii:1153
Fouad FM, Tarazi RC, Bravo EL, Textor SC (1984) Hemodynamic and antihypertensive effects of the new oral angiotensin-converting-enzyme inhibitor MK-421 (enalapril). Hypertension 6:167–174
Francis RJ, Brown AN, Kler L, Fasanella-D'Amore T, Nussberger J, Waeber B, Brunner HR (1987) Pharmacokinetics of the converting enzyme inhibitor cilazapril in normal volunteers and the relationship to enzyme inhibition: development of a mathematical model. J Cardiovasc Pharmacol 9:32–38
Frankling SS, Smith RD (1985) Comparison of effects of enalapril plus hydrochlorothiazide versus standard triple therapy on renal function in renovascular hypertension.

Am J Med 79 [Suppl 3C]:14–23
Freeman GL, Little WC, Haywood JR (1987) Reduction of left ventricular mass in normal rats by captopril. Cardiovasc Res 21:323–327
Freer RJ, Pappano AJ, Peach MJ, Bing KT, McLean MJ, Vogel S, Sperelakis N (1976) Mechanisms for the positive inotropic effect of angiotensin II on isolated cardiac muscle. Circ Res 39:178
Funae Y, Komori T, Sasaki D, Yamamoto K (1980) Inhibitor of angiotensin I converting enzyme: (4R)-3—(2S)-3-mercapto-2-methylpropanoyl—4-thiazolidinecarboxylic acid (YS-980) Biochem Pharmacol 29:1543–1547
Funck-Brentano C, Chatellier G, Alexandre JM (1986) Reversible renal failure after combined treatment with enalapril and furosemide in a patient with congestive heart failure. Br Heart J 55:596–598
Gambaro G, Morbiato F, Cicerello E, Del Turco M, Sartori L, D'Angelo A, Crepaldi G (1985) Captopril in the treatment of hypertension in type I and type II diabetic patients. J Hypertens 3 [Suppl 2]:S149–S151
Ganten D, Hayduk K, Brecht HM, Boucher R, Genest (1970) Evidence of renin release or production in splanchnic territory. Nature 226:551–552
Ganten D, Hermann K, Bayer C, Unger T, Lang RE (1983) Angiotensin synthesis in the brain and increased turnover in hypertensive rats. Science 221:869–870
Ganten D, Lang RE, Lehmann E, Unger T (1984) Brain angiotensin: on the way to becoming a well-studied neuropeptide system. Biochem Pharmacol 33 (22):3523–3528
Ganten D, Balz W, Hense HW, Schölkens BA, Horstmann G, Lang GE, Unger T (1985) Characterization and regulation of angiotensin (ANG) peptides in tissue of rabbit and primates. J Hypertens 3 [Suppl]:S552–S553 (abstr)
Gaul SL, Martin GE, Sweet CS (1984) Comparative effects of enalapril, enalaprilic acid and captopril in blocking angiotensin I-induced pressor and dipsogenic responses in spontaneously hypertensive rats. Clin Exp Hypertens [A] (6):1187
Gavras H, Brunner HR, Laragh JH, Sealey JE, Gavras I, Vukovich RA (1974) An angiotensin-converting enzyme inhibitor to identify and treat vasoconstrictor and volume factors in hypertensive patients. N Engl J Med 291:817–821
Gavras H, Waeber B, Gavras I, Biollaz J, Brunner HR, Davies RO (1981) Antihypertensive effects of the new oral angiotensin converting enzyme inhibitor "MK-421". Lancet ii:543–547
Geppetti P, Spillantini MG, Frilli S, Pietrini U, Fanciullacci M, Sicuteri F (1987) Acute oral captopril inhibits angiotensin converting enzyme activity in human cerebrospinal fluid. J Hypertens 5:151
Giudicelli JF, Berdeaux A, Edouard A, Richer C, Jacolot D (1985) The effect of enalapril on baroreceptor mediated reflex function in normotensive subjects. Br J Clin Pharmacol 20:211–218
Given BD, Taylor T, Hollenberg NK, Williams GH (1984) Duration of action and short-term hormonal responses to enalapril (MK421) in normal subjects. J Cardiovasc Pharmacol 6:436–441
Gohlke P, Urbach H, Schölkens BA, Unger T (1989) Inhibition of converting enzyme in the cerebrospinal fluid of rats after oral treatment with converting enzyme inhibitors. J Pharmacol Exp Ther 249:609–616
Gomez HJ, Smornovsky J, Kristianson K, Cirillo VJ, Wilhelmsson CE, Berglund G (1985) Lisinopril dose response in mild to moderate hypertension. Clin Pharmacol Ther 37:198 (abstr C48)
Göthert M, Kollecker P (1986) Subendothelial β_2-adrenoceptors in the rat vena cava: facilitation of the release via local stimulation of angiotensin II synthesis. Naunyn-Schmiedeberg's Arch Pharmacol 334:156–165
Hall JE, Guyton AC, Cowley AW Jr (1977a) Dissociation of renal blood flow and filtration autoregulation by renin depletion. Am J Physiol 232:215–221
Hall JE, Guyton AC, Jackson TE, Coleman TG, Lohmeier TE, Tippodo WC (1977b) Control of glomerular filtration rate by renin angiotensin system. Am J Physiol 233:366–372
Harris DN, Heran CI, Goldenberg HJ, High JP, Laffen RJ, Rubin B, Antonaccio MJ, Goldberg ME (1978) Effects of SQ 14.225, an orally active inhibitor of angiotensin-

converting enzyme on blood pressure, heart rate and plasma renin activity of conscious normotensive dogs. Eur J Pharmacol 51:345–349

Hatton R, Clough DP (1982) Captopril interferes with neurogenic vasoconstriction in the pithed rat by angiotensin-dependent mechanisms. J Cardiovasc Pharmacol 4:116–123

Hayashi K, Nunami KI, Sakai K, Ozaki Y, Kato J et al. (1983) Studies on angiotensin converting enzyme inhibitors. II. Synthesis and angiotensin converting enzyme inhibitory activities of carboxyethylcarbamoy-1,2,3,4-tetrahydroisoquinoline-3-carboxylic acid derivatives. Chem Pharm Bull (Tokyo) 31:3553–3561

Heeg E, Meng K (1965) Die Wirkung des Bradykinins, Angiotensins und Vasopressins auf Vorhof, Papillarmuskel, und isoliert durchströmte Herzpräparate des Meerschweinchens. Naunyn Schmiedeberg's Arch Pharmacol 250:35

Heel RC, Brogden RN, Speight TM, Avery GS (1980) Captopril: a preliminary review of its pharmacological properties and therapeutic efficiency. Drugs 20:409–452

Henrichs KJ, Unger T, Berecek KH, Ganten D (1980) Is arterial media hypertrophy in spontaneously hypertensive rats a consequence of or a cause for hypertension. Clin Sci 59:331s–333s

Hirakata, H, Onoyama K, Iseki K, Omae T, Fujimi S, Hawahara Y (1981) Captopril (SQ 142259) clearance during hemodialysis treatment. Clin Nephrol 16:321–323

Hockings N, Ajayi LAA, Hughes DM, Lees KR, Reid JL (1985) Effects of age on the pharmacodynamic responses to the angiotensin converting enzyme inhibitors enalapril and enalaprilat. Br J Clin Pharmacol 19:140P

Hodsman GP, Isles CG, Murray GD, Usherwood TP, Webb DJ, Robertson JIS (1983) Factors related to first dose hypotensive effect of captopril: prediction and treatment. Br Med J 286:832–834

Holck M, Fischli W, Hefti F, Gerold M (1986) Cardiovascular effects of the new angiotensin-converting-enzyme inhibitor, cilazapril, in anesthetized and conscious dogs. J Cardiovasc Pharmcol 8:99–108

Hollenberg NK (1985) Angiotensin-converting enzyme inhibition: renal aspects. J Cardiovasc Pharmacol 7:S40–S44

Hollenberg NK, Swartz SL, Pasau DR (1979) Increased glomerular filtration rate following converting enzyme inhibition in essential hypertension. N Engl J Med 301:9–12

Hommel E, Parving H-H, Mathiesen E, Edsberg B, Damkjaer Nielsen M, Giese J (1986) Effect of captopril on kidney function in insulin-dependent diabetic patients with nephropathy. Br Med J 193:467–470

Horovitz ZP, Antonaccio MJ, Rubin B, Panasevich RE (1979) Influence of various antihypersive agents on lifespan of renal hypertensive rats. Br J Clin Pharmacol 7 [Suppl 2]:243S–248S

Hostetter TH, Rennke HG, Brenner BM (1982) The cause for intrarenal hypertension in the initiation and progression of diabetic and other glomerulapathies. Am J Med 72: 375–380

Howlett DR, Longman SD (1983) Effects of chronic enalapril (MK-421) treatment on the renin-angiotensin system in the sodium deficient rat. Br J Pharmacol 79:323P

Hutchinson JS, Mendelsohn FAO, Doyle AE (1980) Blood pressure responses of conscious normotensive and spontaneously hypertensive rats to intracerebroventricular and peripheral administration of captopril. Hypertension 2:546

Iimura O, Shimamoto K, Tanaka S, Hosoda S, Nishitani T, Ando T, Masuda A (1986) The mechanism of the hypotensive effect of captopril (converting enzyme inhibitor) with special reference to the kallikrein-kinin and renin-angiotensin system. Jpn J Med 25:34–39

Imai Y, Abe K, Seino M, Haruyama T, Tajiama J, Sato M, Goto T, Hiwatari M, Kasai Y, Yoshinaga K, Sekino H (1982) Attenuation of pressor response to norepinephrine and vasopressin by captopril in human subjects. Hypertension 4:444–451

Inmann WHW, Rawson NSB, Wilton LV, Pearce GL, Speirs CJ (1988) Postmarketing surveillance of enalapril. I: Results of prescription-event monitoring. Br Med J 297: 826–829

Iso T, Yamauchi H, Suda H, Nakata K, Nishimura K et al. (1981) A new potent inhibitor of converting enzyme: (2R,4R)-2-(2-hydroxyphenyl)-3-(3-mercaptopropionyl)-4-thiazolidinecarboxylic acid (SA446). Jpn J Pharmacol 31:875–882

Ita CE, Singhvi SM, Heald AF, Migdalof BH (1982) Distribution of captopril to foetuses and milk of rats. Xenobiotica 12:627-632

Ito K, Koike H, Miyamoto M, Ozaki H, Kishimotot T, Urakawa N (1981) Longterm effects of captopril on cellular sodium content and mechanical properties of aortic smooth muscle from spontaneously hypertensive rats. J Pharmacol Exp Ther 219: 520–525

Iwai N, Matsunaga M, Kita T, Tei M, Kawai C (1987) Regulation of angiotensin converting enzyme activity in cultured human vascular endothelial cells. Biochem Biophys Res Commun 149:1179–1185

Jackson B, Cubela R, Johnston CI (1984) Effect of dietary sodium on angiotensin-converting enzyme (ACE) inhibition and the acute hypotensive effect of enalapril (MK-421) in essential hypertension. J Hypertens 2:371–377

Jackson B, Cubela R, Johnston C (1986) Angiotensin converting enzymè (ACE), characterization by ^{125}I-MK351A binding studies of plasma and tissue ACE during variation of salt status in the rat. J Hypertens 4:759–765

Jackson B, Cubela RB, Johnston CI (1988) Inhibition of tissue angiotensin converting enzyme by perindopril: in vivo assessment in the rat using radioinhibitor binding displacement. J Pharmacol Exp Ther 245 (3):950–955

Jackson TR, Blair LAC, Marshall J, Goedert M, Hanley MR (1988) The *Mas* oncogene encodes an angiotensin receptor. Nature 335:437–440

Jenkins AC, Dreslinski GR, Tadros SS, Groel JT, Fand R, Herczeg SA (1985) Captopril in hypertension: seven years later. J Cardiovasc Pharmacol 7:96–101

Johnson H, Drummer OH (1988) Hydrolysis of angiotensin I by peptidase in homogenates of rat lung and aorta. Biochem Pharmacol 37:1131–1136

Johnston CI, Jackson B (1987) Overview: angiotensin converting enzyme inhibition in renovascular hypertension. Kidney Int 31 [Suppl 20]:S-154–S-156

Johnston CI, McGrath BP, Millar JA, Matthews PGF (1979) Long-term effects of captopril (SQ14 225) on blood pressure and hormone levels in essential hypertension. Lancet ii:493–496

Johnston CI, Millar JA, Casley DJ, McGrath BP, Matthews PG (1980) Hormonal responses to angiotensin blockade. Circ Res 46 [Suppl I]:I-128–I-134

Johnston CI, Jackson B, McGrath B, Matthews G, Arnolda L (1983) Relationship of antihypertensive effect of enalapril to serum MK-422 levels and angiotensin converting enzyme inhibition. J Hypertens 1 [Suppl 1]:71–75

Johnston CI, Jackson B, Cubela R, Arnolda L (1984) Mechanism of hypotensive action of angiotensin converting enzyme inhibitors. Clin Exp Hypertens [A] 6:551–561

Juul B, Aalkjaer C, Mulvany MJ (1987) Contractile effects of tetradecapeptide renin substrate on rat femoral resistance vessels. J Hypertens 5 [Suppl 2]:S7–S10

Kaplan HR, Cohen DM, Essenburg AD, Major TC, Mertz TE et al. (1984) CI-906 and CI-907: New orally active nonsulfhydryl angiotensin-converting enzyme inhibitors. Fed Proc 43:1326–1329

Kawasaki H, Cline WH Jr, Su C (1984) Involvment of the vascular renin-angiotensin system in beta adrenergic receptor-mediated facilitation of vascular neurotransmission in spontaneously hypertensive rats. J Pharmacol Exp Ther 231:23–32

Keith IM, Will JA, Weir EK (1982) Captopril: associated with fetal death and pulmonary vascular changes in the rabbit (41446). Proc Soc Exp Biol Med 170:378–383

Kifor I, Dzau VJ (1987) Endothelial renin-angiotensin pathway: Evidence for intracellular synthesis and secretion of angiotensins. Circ Res 60:422–428

Kobayashi M, Furkawa Y, Chiba S (1978) Positive chronotropic and inotropic effects of angiotensin II in the dog heart. Eur J Pharmacol 50:17

Koch-Weser J (1964) Myocardial actions of angiotensin. Circ Res 14:337

Kohlmann O, Bresnahan M, Gavras H (1984) Central and peripheral indices of sympathetic activity after blood pressure lowering with enalapril (MK-421) or hydralazine in normotensive rats. Hypertension 6 [Suppl I]:I1–I6

Kondo K, Saruta T, Shimura M, Toyodera K (1986) Tolerability, pharmacodynamics and kinetics of HOE498 after single administration of 4 step rise increased doses (placebo, 1.25 mg, 2.5 mg and 5 mg) in healthy male subjects. Jpn J Pharmacol Ther 14: 315–337

Kripalani KJ, McKinstry DN, Singhvi SM, Willard DA, Vukovich RA, Migdalof BH (1980) Disposition of captopril in normal subjects. Clin Pharmacol Ther 27:636–641
Kromer EP, Riegger AJ (1988) Effects of long-term angiotensin converting enzyme inhibition on myocardial hypertrophy in experimental aortic stenosis in the rat. Am J Cardiol 62:161–163
Kubo SH, Cody RJ (1985) Clinical pharmacology of the angiotensin converting enzyme inhibitors: a review. Clin Pharmacokinet 10:377–391
Kuriyama S, Nakamura A, Hopp L, Fine BP, Kino M, Cragoe E Jr, Aviv A (1988) Angiotensin II effect on $^{22}Na^{+}$ transport in vascular smooth muscle cells. J Cardiovasc Pharmacol 11:139–146
Lai FM, Cervoni P, Tanikella T, Shepherd C, Quirk G et al. (1983) Some in vitro and in vivo studies of a new angiotensin I-converting enzyme inhibitor (S-(R*,S*)-1-((3-Acetylthio)-3-benzoyl-2-methylpropionyl)-L-proline) (CL 242,817) in comparison with captopril. Drug Dev Res 3:261–269
Lanzillo JJ, Fanburg BL (1976) The estimation and comparison of molecular weight of angiotensin I converting enzyme by sodium dodecyl sulfate-polyacrylamide gel electrophoresis. Biochim Biophys Acta 439:125–132
Lanzillo JJ, Dasarathy Y, Stevens J, Fanburg BL (1986) Conversion of angiotensin I to angiotensin II by a latent endothelial cell petidyl dipeptidase that is not angiotensin-converting enzyme. Biochem Biophys Res Commun 134:770–776
Lappe RW, Kocmund S, Todt JA, Wendt RL (1984) Effects of Wy-44,221, a new angiotensin converting enzyme inhibitor, on regional vascular resistance in the conscious SHR. Fed Proc 43:554
Laubie M, Schiavi P, Vincent M, Schmitt H (1984) Inhibition of angiotensin I-converting enzyme with S-9490: biochemical effects, interspecies differences, and role of sodium diet in haemodynamic effects. J Cardiovasc Pharmacol 6:1076–1082
Lechi A, Covi, G, Capuzzo MG, Lechi C, Minuz P, Delva P, Scuro LA (1982) A discrepancy between the effects of a single oral dose of captopril on blood pressure, plasma renin activity, and serum angiotensin-converting enzyme levels. Int J Clin Pharmacol Ther Toxicol 21:569–574
Ledingham JM, Simpson FO (1981) Effect of captopril on blood pressure, total body sodium and fluid consumption of genetically hypertensive (GH) and normotensive (N) rats. Clin Exp Hypertens 3:1239
Lee WH, Packer M (1986) Prognostic importance of serum sodium concentration and its modification by converting enzyme inhibition in patients with severe chronic heart failure. Circulation 73:257–267
Lees KR, Reid JL (1985) Single and multiple administration of an angiotensin converting enzyme inhibitor, S-9490-3 in normotensive subjects. Br J Clin Pharmacol 19: 132P–133P
Lilly LS, Pratt RE, Alexander RW (1984) Renin expression by vascular endothelial cells in culture. Circ Res 57:312–318
Lind RW, Swanson LW, Ganten D (1984) Angiotensin II immunoreactivity in the neutral afferents and efferents of the subfornical organ of the rat. Brain Res 321:209–215
Lindpaintner K, Wilhelm MJ, Jin M, Unger T, Lang RE, Schölkens BA, Ganten D (1987) Tissue renin-angiotensin systems: Focus on the heart. J Hypertens 5 [Suppl 2]: S33–S38
Lindpaintner K, Jin M, Wilhelm MJ, Suzuki F, Linz W, Schölkens BA, Ganten D (1988) Intracardiac generation of angiotensin and its physiologic role. Circulation 77 [Suppl I]:I–18
Linz W, Schölkens BA (1987) Influence of local converting enzyme inhibition on angiotensin and bradykinin effects in ischemic rat hearts. J Cardiovasc Pharmacol 10 [Suppl 7]:S75–S82
Linz W, Schölkens BA, Han YF (1986a) Beneficial effects of the converting enzyme inhibitor, ramipril, in ischemic rat hearts. J Cardiovasc Pharmacol 8 [Suppl 10]: S91–S99
Linz W, Schölkens BA, Jin M, Wilhelm M, Ganten D (1986b) The heart as a target of converting enzyme inhibitors: studies in ischaemic isolated working rat hearts. J Hypertens 4 [Suppl 6]:S477–S479

Linz W, Schölkens BA, Donaubauer HH, Ganten D (1988) Effects of ramipril, nifedipine and dihydralazine on cardiac hypertrophy in rats. Clin Exp Hypertens [A] 10 (4):711 (abstr)
Lisinopril—Data on file—ICI Pharmaceuticals, Macclesfield, UK
Longmann SD, Howlett DR (1986) Angiotensin-converting enzyme responses following enalapril in the sodium deficient rat. Eur J Pharmacol 123:379–386
Lund-Johansen P, Omvik P (1984) Long-term haemodynamic effects of enalapril (alone and in combination with hydrochlorothiazide) at rest and during exercise in essential hypertension. J Hypertens 2 [Suppl 2]:49–56
MacGregor GA, Markandu ND, Bayliss J, Roulston JE, Squires M, Morton JJ (1981a) Non-sulfhydryl-containing angiotensin-converting enzyme inhibitor (Mk421): evidence for role of renin system in normotensive subjects. Br Med J 283:401–403
MacGregor GA, Markandu ND, Roulston JE, Jones JC, Morton JJ (1981b) Maintenance of blood pressure by the renin-angiotensin system in normal man. Nature 291: 329–331
Madeddu P, Oppes M, Rubattu S, Dessi'-Fugheri P, Glorioso N, Soro A, Rappelli A (1987) Role of renal kallikrein in modulating the antihypertensive effect of a single oral dose of captopril in normal- and low-renin essential hypertensives. J Hypertens 5:645–648
Malik KU, Nasjletti A (1976) Facilitation of adrenergic transmission by locally generated angiotensin II in rat mesenteric arteries. Circ Res 38:26–30
Manheim PJO, Ball SG, Morton J, Murray GD, Leckie BJ, Fraser R, Robertson JIS (1985) A dose-response study of HOE498, a new non sulphhydryl converting enzyme inhibitor, on blood pressure, pulse rate and the renin angiotensin aldosterone system in normal man. Br J Clin Pharmacol 20:27–35
Man In't Veld AJ, Schicht IM, Derkx, FHM, De Bruyn JHB, Schalekamp MADH (1980) Effects of an angiotensin-converting enzyme inhibitor (captopril) on blood pressure in anephric subjects. Br Med J 6210:288–290
Mann J, Ritz E (1988) Renin-Angiotensinsystem beim diabetischen Patienten. Klin Wochenschr 66:883–891
Mann WS, Samuels AI, Bauer K, Schwab A, Wolf PS et al. (1984) Indalapril (I), a new non-sulfur containing ACE inhibitor: pharmacological characterization in rats and dogs. Fed Proc 43:958
Mannhold R (1985) Ramipril. Drugs Future 10:400–404
Mathews DM, Wathen CG, Bell D, Collier A, Muir AL, Clarke BF (1986) The effect of captopril on blood pressure and glucose tolerance in hypertensive non-insulin dependent diabetes. Postgrad Med J 62 (Suppl 1):73–75
McFate Smith W, Davies RP, Gabriel MA, Kramsch DM, Moncloa F (1984a) Tolerance and safety of enalapril. Br J Clin Pharmacol 18 [Suppl]:249–253
McFate Smith W, Kulaga SF, Moncloa F, Pingeon R, Walker JF (1984b) Overall tolerance and safety of enalapril. J Hypertens 2 [Suppl 2]:113–117
McKinstry DN, Singhvi SM, Kripalani KH, Dreyfus J, Willard DA, Vukovich RA (1978) Disposition and cardiovascular-endocrine effects of an orally active angiotensin-converting enzyme inhibitor, SQ 14225, in normal subjects. Clin Pharmacol Ther 23: 121–122
Meggs LG, Garrick R, Chander P, Ben-Ari J, Ganemon D, Goodman AI (1988) Amelioration of systemic hypertension by converting enzyme inhibition in the venol ablation model. Am J Hypertens 1:190–192
Mento PF, Wilkes BM (1987) Plasma angiotensins and blood pressure during converting enzyme inhibition. Hypertension 9 [Suppl III]:III-42–III-48
Mersey JH, Ceballos L, Swartz S (1987) Inhibition of captopril-induced renin release by angiotensin II. J Cardiovasc Pharmacol 10:575–579
Meyer TW, Anderson S, Rennke HG, Brenner BM (1985) Converting enzyme inhibitor therapy limits progressive glomerular injury in rats with renal insufficiency. Am J Med 79 [Suppl 3C]:31–36
Migdalof HM, Antonaccio MJ, McKinstry DN, Singhvi SM, Lan S-J, Egli P, Kripalani KJ (1984) Captopril: pharmacology, metabolism, and disposition. Drug Metab Rev 15 (4):841–869

Millar JA, McGrath BP, Matthews PG, Johnston CI (1981) Acute effects of captopril on blood pressure and circulating hormone levels in salt-replete and depleted normal subjects and essential hypertensive patients. Clin Sci 61:75–83
Millar JA, Derkx FHM, McLean K, Reid JL (1982) Pharmacodynamics of converting enzyme inhibition: the cardiovascular, endocrine amd autonomic effects of MK421 (enalapril) and MK521. Br J Clin Pharmacol 14:347–355
Miki M, Ogawa K, Hirata M, Kitaguchi H, Funahara Y (1984) Prostacyclin release from the coronary vascular wall by vasoactive substances. Thromb Res 35:665–679
Minsker DH, Bagdon WJ, Robertson RT, Bokelman DL (1984) Two inhibitors of angiotensin-converting enzyme, enalapril and captopril, increase salt appetite of rats. J Toxicol Environ Health 14:715
Mitchell HC, Pettinger WA, Gianotti L, Reed G, Kirk L, Kuhnert LV, Matthews C, Anderson R (1983) Further studies on the hypernoradrenergic state of treated hypertensives: effect of captopril. Clin Exp Hypertens [A] 5 (10):1611–1627
Miyazaki M, Okunishi H, Mishimura K, Toda N (1984) Vascular angiotensin-converting enzyme activity in man and other species. Clin Sci 66:39–45
Miyazaki M, Okunishi H, Okamura T, Toda N (1987) Elevated vascular angiotensin converting enzyme in chronic two-kidney, one-clip hypertension in the dog. J Hypertens 5:155–160
Mizuno K, Shigetomi S, Matsui J, Fukuchi S (1981) Effect of sodium intake on the brain and the aortic angiotensin-converting enzyme activity in spontaneously hypertensive rats. Jpn Heart J 22:839–845
Mojaverian P, Rocci ML, Viasses PH, Hoholick C, Clementi RA, Ferguson RK (1986) Effect of food on the bioavailability of lisinopril, a nonsulfhydryl angiotensin-converting enzyme inhibitor. J Pharmacol Sci 75:395–397
Moncloa F, Sromovsky JA, Walker JF, Davies RO (1985) Enalapril in hypertension and congestive heart failure. Overall review of efficacy and safety. Drugs 30 [Suppl I]: 82–89
Mookherjee S, Anderson GH Jr, Eich R, Hill N, Smulyan H, Streeten DHP, Vardan S, Warner R (1983) Acute effects of captopril on cardiopulmonary hemodynamics and renin-angiotensin-aldosterone and bradykinin profile in hypertension. Am Heart J 105:106–112
Morton JJ, Tree M, Casals-Stenzel J (1980) The effect of captopril on blood pressure and angiotensin I, II and III in sodium-depleted dogs: problems associated with the measurement of angiotensin II after inhibition of converting enzyme. Clin Sci 58: 445–450
Moursi M, El-Dakhakany M, Schölkens BA, Unger T (1987) Interference with the autonomic nervous system by the converting enzyme inhibitor ramipril in conscious spontaneously hypertensive rats. J Cardiovasc Pharmacol 10 [Suppl 7]:S125–128
Murjais Sk, Fonad FM, Textor SC (1984) Transient renal dysfunction during initial inhibition of converting enzyme in congestive heart failure. Br Heart J 52:63–71
Murphy BF, Whithworth JA, Kincaid-Smith (1984) Renal insufficiency with combination of converting enzyme inhibitors and diuretics. Br Med J 288:844–845
Murthy VS, Waldron TL, Goldberg ME (1978) The mechanism of bradykinin potentiation after inhibition of angiotensin-converting enzyme by SQ 14,225 in conscious rabbits: Circ Res 45:588–592
Nagai R, Ohuchi Y, Yazali Y, Takayama Y, Seki A (1984) Initial dose of enalapril maleate (MK-421) in renovascular hypertension. Curr Therap Res Clin Exp 35: 860–862
Nakamura M, Jackson EK, Inagami T (1986) Beta adrenoceptor mediated release of angiotensin II from mesenteric arteries. Am J Physiol 250:H144–H148
Nakamura Y, Nakamura K, Matsukura T (1988) Vascular angiotensin converting enzyme activity in spontaneously hypertensive rats and its inhibition with cilazapril. J Hypertens 6:105–110
Nakashima M, Nishijima K (1982) Effect in healthy subjects of a new nonthiol-containing angiotensin-converting enzyme inhibitor, enalapril maleate (MK-421). Clin Sci 63: 183S–185S
Nakashima Y, Fouad FM, Tarazi RC (1984) Regression of left ventricular hypertrophy

from systemic hypertension by enalapril. Am J Cardiol 53:1044–1049
Nakata K, Nishimura K, Takada T, Ikuse T, Yamauchi H, Iso T (1987) Effects of an angiotensin-converting enzyme (ACE) inhibitor, SA446, on tissue ACE activity in normotensive, spontaneously hypertensive, and renal hypertensive rats. J Cardiovasc Pharmacol 9:305–310
Nambu K, Matsumoto K, Takeyama K, Hosoki, Miyazaki H, Hashimoto M (1986) Tissue levels, tissue angiotensin converting enzyme inhibition and antihypertensive effect of the novel antihypertensive agent alacepril in renal hypertensive rats. Drug Res 36 (1):47–51
Natoff IL, Nixon JS, Francis RJ, Klevans LR, Brewster M, Budd J, Patel AT, Wenger J, Worth E (1985) Biological properties of the angiotensin-converting enzyme inhibitor cilazapril. J Cardiovasc Pharmacol 7:569–580
Navar LG, Jirakulsomchok D, Bell PD, Thomas CE, Huang WC (1982) Influence of converting enzyme inhibition on renal hemodynamics and glomerular dynamics in sodium restricted dogs. Hypertension 4:56–58
Niarchos AP, Pickering TG, Morganti A, Laragh JH (1982) Plasma catecholamines and cardiovascular responses during converting enzyme inhibition in normotensive and hypertensive man. Clin Exp Hypertens [A] 4 (4,5):761–789
Norman JA, Lehmann M, Goodman FR, Carclay BW, Zimmerman MB (1987) Central and peripheral inhibition of angiotensin converting enzyme (ACE) in the SHR: Correlation with the antihypertensive activity of ACE inhibitors. Clin Exp Hypertens [A] 9 (2,3):461–468
Nussberger J, Brunner DB, Waeber B, Brunner HR (1985) True versus immunoreactive angiotensin II in human plasma. Hypertension 7 [Suppl I]:I-1–I-7
Nussberger J, Brunner DB, Waeber B, Burnner HR (1986) Specific measurement of angiotensin metabolites and in vitro generated angiotensin II in plasma. Hypertension 8:476–482
Nussberger J, Waeber G, Waeber B, Bidville J, Brunner HR (1988) Plasma angiotensin-(1–8) octapeptide measurement to assess acute angiotensin-converting enzyme inhibition with captopril administered parenterally to normal subjects. J Cardiovasc Pharmacol 11:716–721
Okabe T, Yamagata K, Fujisawa M, Takaku F, Hidaka H, Umezawa Y (1987) Induction by fibroblast growth factor of angiotensin converting enzyme in vascular endothelial cells in vitro. Biochem Biophys Res Commun 145:1211–1216
Okamura T, Miyazaki M, Inagami T, Toda N (1986) Vascular renin-angiotensin system in two-kidney, one clip hypertensive rats. Hypertension 8:560–565
Okunishi H, Miyazaki M, Toda N (1984) Evidence for a putatively new angiotensin II-generating enzyme in the vascular wall. J Hypertens 2:277–284
Okunishi H, Miyazaki M, Okamura T, Toda N (1987) Different distribution of two types of angiotensin II-generating enzymes in the aortic wall. Biochem Biophys Res Commun 149:1186–1192
Okuno T, Kondo K, Konishi K, Saruta T, Kato E (1979) SQ14225 attenuates the vascular response to norepinephrine in the rat mesenteric arteries. Life Sci 25:1343–1350
Okuno T, Nagahama S, Lindheimer MD, Oparil S (1983) Attenuation of the development of spontaneous hypertension in rats in chronic central administration of captopril. Hypertension 5:653
Oliver JA, Sciacca RR (1984) Local generation of angiotensin II as a mechanism of regulation of peripheral vascular tone in the rat. J Clin Invest 74:1247–1251
Omae T, Kawano Y, Yoshida K (1987) Side effects and metabolic effects of converting enzyme inhibitors. Clin Exp Hypertens [A] 9 (2,3):635–642
Ondetti MA, Williams NJ, Sabo EF, Pluscec J, Weaver ER, Kocy O (1971) Angiotensin-converting enzyme inhibitors from the venom of Bothrops jararaca. Isolation, elucidation of structure, and synthesis. Biochemistry 10:4033–4039
Ondetti MA, Rubin B, Cushman DW (1977) Design of specific inhibitors of angiotensin-converting enzyme: new class of orally active antihypertensive agents. Science 196: 441–444
Osborne M, Droz P, Meyer P, Morel F (1975) Angiotensin II: renal localisation in glomerular mesangial cells by autoradiography. Kidney Int 8:245–254

Oshima T, Matsushita Y, Miyamoto M, Koike H (1983) Effects of long-term blockade of angiotensin converting enzyme with captopril on blood pressure and aortic prolyl hydroxylase activity in spontaneously hypertensive rats. Eur J Pharmacol 91:283–286
Packer M (1985) Converting-enzyme inhibition of severe chronic heart failure: views from a skeptic. Int J Cardiol 7:111–120
Packer M (1987) Converting-enzyme inhibition in the management of severe chronic congestive heart failure: physiological concepts. J Cardiovasc Pharmacol 10 [Suppl 7]:S83–S87
Palmer RMJ, Ferrige AG, Moncada S (1987) Nitric oxide release accounts for the biological activity of endothelium-derived relaxing factor. Nature 327:524–526
Parsons WH, Davidson JL, Taub D, Aster SD, Thorsett ED, Patchett AA (1983) Benzolactams. A new class of converting enzyme inhibitors. Biochem Biophys Res Commun 117:108–113
Patchett AA, Harris E, Tristram EW, Wyvratt MJ, Wu MT et al. (1980) A new class of angiotensin-converting enzyme inhibitors. Nature 288:280–283
Pfeffer JM, Pfeffer MA (1988) Angiotensin converting-enzyme inhibition and ventricular remodeling in heart failure. Am J Med 84 [Suppl 3A]:37–44
Phillips MI (1983) New evidence for brain angiotensin and for its role in hypertension. Fed Proc 42:2667
Phillips MI (1987) Functions of angiotensin in the central nervous system. Annu Rev Physiol 49:413–435.
Phillips MI, Kimura B (1986) Converting enzyme inhibitors and brain angiotensin. J Cardiovasc Pharmacol 8 [Suppl 10]:S82–S90
Pierpont GL, Francis GS, Cohn JN (1981) Effect of captopril on renal failure in patients with congestive heart failure. Br J Heart Dis 46:522–527
Pochiero M, Nicoletta P, Losi E, Bianchi A, Caputi AP (1983) Cardiovascular responses to conscious doca-salt hypertensive rats to acute intracerebroventricular and intravenous administration of captopril. Pharmacol Res Commun 2:173
Powell JR, De Forrest JM, Cushman DW, Rubin B, Petrillo EW (1984) Antihypertensive effects of a new angiotensin-converting enzyme (ACE) inhibitor, SQ 28,555. Fed Proc 43:P733.
Quilley J, Duchin KL, Hudes EM, McGiff JC (1987) The antihypertensive effect of captopril in essential hypertension: relationship to prostaglandins and the kallikrein-kinin system. J Hypertens 5:121–128
Raish RJ, Smith DS, Owen WG (1985) Secretion of plasminogen activator by the isolated perfused rat heart in response to vasoactive agents. Thromb Haemost 54:170
Raji L, Chiou X-C, Owens R, Wrigley B (1985) Therapeutic implications of hypertension-induced glomerular injury. Am J Med 79 [Suppl 3C]:37–41
Rascher W, Clough D, Ganten D (eds) (1982) Hypertensive mechanisms. Schattauer, Stuttgart
Rassier ME, Li T, Zimmerman BG (1986) Analysis of influence of extra- and intrarenally formed angiotensin II on renal blood flow. J Cardiovasc Pharmacol 8 [Suppl 10]: S106–S110
Re R, Fallon JT, Dzau VJ, Quay SC, Haber E (1982) Renin synthesis by canine aortic smooth muscle cells in culture. Life Sci 30:99–106
Rett K, Lotz N, Wicklmayr M, Fink E, Jauch K-N, Günther B, Dietze G (1988) Verbesserte Insulinwirkung durch ACE-Hemmung beim Typ-II-Diabetiker. Dtsch Med Wochenschr 113:243–249
Richer C, Dousseau M-P, Giudicelli J-F (1983) Effects of captopril and enalapril on regional vascular resistance and reactivity in spontaneously hypertensive rats. Hypertension 5:312–320
Richer C, Dousseau M-P, Giudicelli J-F (1986) Systemic and regional pre- and post-junctional sympathoinhibitory effect of perindopril in spontaneously hypertensive rats. J Hypertens 4 [Suppl 3]:S513–S516
Richer C, Dousseau M-P, Giudicelli J-F (1987) Systemic and regional hemodynamic profile of five angiotensin I converting enzyme inhibitors in the spontaneously hypertensive rat. Am J Cardiol 59:12D–17D
Richer C, Dousseau M-P, Giudicelli J-F (1989) Differential systemic and regional hemo-

dynamic profiles of four angiotensin I converting enzyme inhibitors in the rat. Cardiovasc Drugs Ther (in press)
Riordan JF, Harper JW, Martin M (1986) The catalytic mechanism of angiotensin converting enzyme and related zinc enzymes. J Cardiovasc Pharmacol 8 [Suppl 10]: S29–S34
Ritz E, Mann J (1987) Renale Effekte von Konversioenzymhemmern. In: Brunner HG, Lehmann K (eds) Enalapril in der Behandlung der Hypertonie. Thieme, Stuttgart, pp 25–33
Romankiewicz JA, Brogden RN, Heel RC, Speight TM, Avery GS (1983) Captopril: an update review of its pharmacological properties and therapeutic efficacy in congestive heart failure. Drugs 25:6–40
Rösen P, Eckel J, Rainauer H (1983) Influence of bradykinin on glucose uptake and metabolism studied in isolated cardiac myocytes and isolated perfused rat hearts. Hoppe-Seyler's Z Physiol Chem 364:1431–1438
Rosenthal J, Boucher R, Rojo Ortega JM, Genest J (1969) Renin activity in aortic tissue of rats. Can J Physiol Pharmacol 47:53
Roy SN, Kusari J, Soffer RL, Lai CY, Sen GC (1988) Isolation of cDNA of rabbit angiotensin converting enzyme: identification of two distinct mRNAS for the pulmonary and the testicular isoenzymes. Biochem Biophys Res Commun 155 (2):678–684
Rubin B, Laffan RJ, Kotler DG, O'Keefe EH, De Maio DA (1978) SQ14225 (D-3-mercapto-2methylpropanol-L-proline), a novel orally active inhibitor of angiotensin I-converting enzyme. J Pharmacol Exp Ther 204:271–280.
Ryan MJ, Boucher DM, Cohen DM, Essenburg AD, Major TC, Mertz TE, Olszewski BJ, Randolph AE, Singer RM, Kaplan HR (1984) Antihypertensive effects of CI-907 (Indolapril): a novel nonsulfhydryl angiotensin converting enzyme inhibitor. J Pharmacol Exp Ther 228:312–318
Ryden L (1988) When and how to use angiotensin-converting enzyme inhibition in congestive heart failure. Am J Cardiol 62:75A–80A
Sakaguchi K, Chai SY, Jackson B, Johnston CI, Mendelsohn FAO (1988) Differential changes in tissue angiotensin converting enzyme activity after lisinopril administration demonstrated by quantitative in vitro autoradiography. Hypertension 11: 230–238
Sanchez RA, Traballi CA, Barclay CA, Gilbert HB, Muscara M, Giannone C, Moledo LI (1988) Antihypertensive, enzymatic and hormonal activity of cilazapril, a new angiotensin-converting enzyme inhibitor in patients with mild to moderate essential hypertension. J Cardiovasc Pharmacol 11:230–234
Saner H, Brunner HR (1988) Antihypertensive Wirksamkeit und Verträglichkeit von Captopril: Ergebnisse einer schweizer Feldstudie. Therapiewoche Schweiz 2:157–165
Saye JA, Singer HA, Peach MJ (1984) Role of endothelium in conversion of angiotensin I to angiotensin II in rabbit aorta. Hypertension 6:216–221
Schalekamp MADH, Wenting GJ, De Bruyn JHB, Man in t'Veld AJ, Derkx FHM (1982) Hemodynamics of captopril in essential and renovascular hypertension: correlation with plasma renin. In: ACE inhibition in hypertension: from principle to practice, symposium Dallas, Nov 1981. Biomed Inf Corp, New York, pp 19–39
Scherf H, Pietsch R, Landsberg G, Kramer HJ, Düsing R (1986) Converting enzyme inhibitor ramipril stimulates prostacyclin synthesis by isolated rat aorta: evidence for a kinin-dependent mechanism. Klin Wochenschr 64:742–745
Schiffrin EL, Genest J (1982) Mechanism of captopril-induced drinking. Am J Physiol 11:R136
Schiffrin EL, Gutowska J, Thibault G, Genest J (1984) Effect of enalapril (MK-421), an orally active angiotensin I converting enzyme inhibitor, on blood pressure, active and inactive plasma renin, urinary prostaglandin E_2, and kallikrein excretion in conscious rats. Can J Physiol Pharmacol 62:116–123
Schmidt M, Giesen-Crouse EM, Krieger JP, Welsch C, Imbs JL (1986) Effect of angiotensin converting enzyme inhibitors on the vasoconstrictor action of angiotensin I on isolated rat kidney. J Cardiovasc Pharmacol 8 [Suppl 10]:S100–S105
Schölkens BA, Steinbach R, Jung W (1979) Intracerebroventricular injection of an angiotensin I converting enzyme inhibitor (SQ 14225) in animals with experimental

hypertension (abstr). Naunyn-Schmiedeberg's Arch Pharmacol 307 [Suppl]:R46
Schölkens BA, Becker RHA, Kaiser J (1984a) Cardiovascular and antihypertensive activities of the novel non-sulfhydryl converting enzyme inhibitor 2-(N-((S)-1-Ethoxycarbonyl-3-phenylpropyl)-L-alanyl)-(1S,3S,5S)-2-azabicyclo(3.3.0)octane-3-carboxylic acid (HOE 498). Drug Res 34 (II):1417–1425
Schölkens BA, Xiang JZ, Tilly H (1984b) Influence of the converting enzyme inhibitors Hoe 498, enalapril and captopril on vascular reactivity of isolated arterial preparations. Clin Exp Hypertens [A] 6 (10,11):1807–1813
Schölkens BA, Linz W, Lindpaintner K, Ganten D (1987) Angiotensin deteriorates but bradykinin improves cardiac function following ischaemia in isolated rat hearts. J Hypertens 5 [Suppl 5]:S7–S9
Schölkens BA, Becker RHA, Linz W (1988a) Pharmakologische Beeinflussung des Konversionsenzyms: Lokale und systemische Effekte an Herz und Gefäßen. Z Kardiol 77 [Suppl 3]:13–21
Schölkens BA, Linz W, König W (1988b) Effects of the angiotensin converting enzyme inhibitor ramipril in isolated ischaemic rat heart are abolished by a bradykinin-antagonist. J Hypertens 6 [Suppl 4]:S25–S28
Schoenberger JA, Wilson DJ (1986) Once-daily treatment of essential hypertension with captopril. J Clin Hypertens 4:379–387
Schrör K, Metz U, Krebs K (1979) The bradykinin-induced coronary vasodilation. Evidence for an additional prostaglandin-independent mechanism. Naunyn-Schmiedeberg's Arch Pharmacol 307:213–221
Schuster VL, Kokko JP, Jacobsen HR (1984) Angiotensin II directly stimulates sodium transport in rabbit proximal convoluted tubules. J Clin Invest 73:507–515
Selig SE, Anderson WP, Korner PI, Casley DJ (1983) The role of angiotensin II in the development of hypertension and in the maintenance of glomerular filtration rate during 48 hours of renal artery stenosis in conscious dogs. J Hypertens 1:153–158
Shapiro R, Riordan JF (1984a) Inhibition of angiotensin converting enzyme: mechanism and substrate dependence. Biochemistry 23:5225–5233
Shapiro R, Riordan JF (1984b) Inhibition of angiotensin converting enzyme: dependence on chloride. Biochemistry 23:5234–5240
Shionori H, Gotoh E, Takagi N, Takeda K, Yabana M, Kaneko Y (1988) Antihypertensive effects and pharmacokinetics of single and consecutive doses of cilazapril in hypertensive patients with normal and impaired renal function. J Cardiovasc Pharmacol 11:242–249
Shoback DM, Williams GH, Moore TJ, Dluhy RG, Podolsky S, Hollenberg NK (1983a) Defect in the sodium modulated tissue responsiveness to angiotensin II in essential hypertension. J Clin Invest 72:2115–2124
Shoback DM, Williams GH, Swartz SI, Davies RO, Hollenberg NK (1983b) Time course and effect of sodium intake on vascular and hormonal responses to enalapril (MK421) in normal subjects. J Cardiovasc Pharmacol 5:1010–1018
Silas JH, Klenka Z, Solomon SA, Bone JM (1983) Captopril induced reversible renal failure: a marker of renal artery stenosis affecting a solitary kidney. Br Med J 286:1702–1703
Singhvi SM, McKinstry DN, Shaw JM, Willard DA, Migdalof BH (1982) Effect of food on the bioavailability of captopril in healthy subjects. J Clin Pharmacol 22:135–140
Skeggs LT, Kahn JR, Shumway NP (1956) The preparation and function of the hypertension-converting enzyme. J Exp Med 103:295–299
Skidgel RA, Defendini R, Erdös EG (1988) Angiotensin I converting enzyme and its role in neuropeptide metabolism. In: Turner AJ (ed) Neuropeptides and their petidases. Ellis Horwood, Chichester, pp 165–188
Skorecki KL, Ballermann BJ, Rennke HG, Brenner BM (1983) Angiotenin II receptor regulation in isolated glomeruli. Fed Proc 42:3064–3070
Solomon T, Cavera AI, Buckley JP (1974) Inhibition of central effects of angiotensin I and II. J Pharm Sci 63:511
Speirs CJ, Dollery CT, Inman WHW, Rawson NSB, Wilton LV (1988) Postmarketing surveillance of enalapril. II: Investigation of the potential role of enalapril in deaths with renal failure. Br Med J 297:830–832

Stamler JF, Brody MJ, Phillips MI (1980) The central and peripheral effects of captopril (SQ 14,225) on the arterial pressure of the spontaneously hypertensive rat. Brain Res 186:499
Stanton JL, Gruenfeld N, Babiarz JE, Ackerman MH, Friedmann RC et al. (1983) Angiotensin converting enzyme inhibitors: N-substituted monocyclic and bicyclic amino acid derivatives. J Med Chem 26:1267–1276
Steinhausen M, Kücherer H, Parekh N, Weis S, Wiegman DL, Wilhelm KR (1986) Angiotensin II control of the renal microcirculation; effect of blockade by saralasin. Kidney Int 30:56–61
Struthers AD (1985) The choice of antihypertensive therapy in the diabetic patient. Postgrad Med J 61:563–569
Stumpe KO, Overlack A, Kolloch R, Schatz J, Witte PJ, Pahnke K (1986) Effecfs of the new angiotensin-converting enzyme inhibitor, a ramipril, in patients with essential hypertension. Klin Wochenschr 64:558–562
Suzuki H, Kondo K, Hand M, Saruta T (1981) Role of the brain isorenin-angiotensin system in experimental hypertension in rats. Clin Sci 61:175
Swales JD (1979) Renin-angiotensin system in hypertension. Pharmacol Ther 7:173–201
Swales JD, Heagerty AM (1987) Vascular renin-angiotensin system: the unanswered questions. J Hypertens 5:S1–S5
Swanson BN, Vlasses PH, Ferguson RK, Berquist PA, Till AE et al. (1984) Influence of food on the bioavailability of enalapril. J Pharm Sci 73:1655–1657
Swartz SL, Williams GH, Hollenberg NK, Moore TJ, Dluhy RG (1979) Converting enzyme inhibition in essential hypertension: the hypotensive response does not reflect only reduced angiotensin II formation. Hypertension 1:106–11
Swartz SL, Williams GH, Hollenberg NK, Crantz FR, More TJ, Levine L, Sasahara AA, Dluhy RG (1980) Endocrine profile in the long-term phase of converting-enzyme inhibition. Clin Pharmacol Ther 28:449–508
Sweet CS (1983) Pharmacological properties of the converting enzyme inhibitor, enalapril maleate (MK-421). Fed Proc 42:167–170
Sweet CS, Ulm EH (1984) Enalapril. In: Scriabine A (ed) New drugs annual: cardiovascular drugs, vol 2: Raven, New York, pp 1–17
Sweet CS, Gross DM, Arbegast PT, Gaul SL, Britt PM et al. (1981a) Antihypertensive activity of N-((S)-(ethoxycarbonyl)-3-phenylpropyl))-L-Ala-a-Pro (MK-421), an orally active converting enzyme inhibitor. J Pharmacol Exp Ther 216:558–566
Sweet CS, Arbegast PT, Gaul SL, Blaine EH, Gross DM (1981b) Relationship between angiotensin I blockade and antihypertensive properties of single doses of MK-421 and captopril in spontaneous and renal hypertensive rats. Eur J Pharmacol 76:167–176
Sybertz EJ, Baum T, Ahn HS, Nelson S, Eynon E et al. (1983) Angiotensin-converting enzyme inhibitory activity of SCH 31846, a new non-sulfhydryl inhibitor. J Cardiovasc Pharmacol 5:643–654
Taguma Y, Kitamoto Y, Futaki G, Ueda H, Monma H, Ishizaki M, Takahashi H, Sekino H, Sasaki Y (1985) Effect of captopril on heavy proteinuria in azotemic diabetics. N Engl J Med 313:1617–1620
Takata Y, DiNicolantonio R, Hutchinson JS, Mendelsohn FAO, Doyle AE (1982) In vivo comparison of three orally active inhibitors of angiotensin-converting enzyme. Am J Cardiol 49:1502–1504
Takeda K, Ashizawa H, Oguro M, Nakamura Y, Fukuyama M, Lee LC, Inoue A, Sasaki S, Yoshimury M, Nakagawa M, Ijichi H (1986) Acute effects of captopril on the baroreflex of normotensive and spontaneously hypertensive rats. Jpn Heart J 4:511
Tanaka S, Shimamoto K, Ando T, Nakahashi Y, Ura N, Hosoda S, Ishida H, Yamaji I, Yokoyama T, Masuda A, Iimura O (1987) Role of renin-angiotensin and kallikrein-kinin systems on the mechanism of the hypotensive effects of converting enzyme inhibitor, alacepril. Clin Exp Hypertens 8 (2,3):605–609
Textor SC, Novick AE, Steinmuller DR, Streem SB (1983) Renal failure limiting antihypertensive therapy as an indication for renal revascularization. Arch Intern Med 143:2208–2211
Thuillez C, Richer C, Guidicelli J-F (1987) Pharmacokinetics, converting enzyme inhibition and peripheral arterial hemodynamics of ramipril in healthy volunteers. Am J

Cardiol 59:38D–44D
Thurston H, Swales JD (1977) Blood pressure response of nephrectomized hypertensive rats to converting enzyme inhibition: evidence for persistent vascular renin activity. Clin Sci Mol Med 52:299–304
Thurston H, Swales JD (1978) Converting enzyme inhibitor and saralasin infusion in rats. Evidence for an additional vasodepressor property of converting enzyme inhibitor. Circ Res 42:588–592
Thurston H, Swales JD, Bing RF, Hurst BC, Marks ES (1979) Vascular renin-like activity and blood pressure maintenance in the rat: studies of the effect of changes in sodium balance, hypertension and nephrectomy. Hypertension 1:643–649
Tillman DM, Malatino LS, Cumming AMM (1984) Enalapril in hypertension with renal artery stenosis: long-term follow-up and effects on renal function. J Hypertens 2 [Suppl 2]:93–100
Tocco DJ, Deluna FA, Duncan EW, Vassil TC, Ulm H (1981) The physiological disposition and metabolism of enalapril maleate in laboratory animals. Drug Metab Dispos 10:15–19
Toda N (1984) Endothelium-dependent relation induced by angiotensin II and histamine in isolated arteries of dog. Br J Pharmacol 81:301–307
Todd PA, Heel RC (1986) Enalapril: a review of its pharmacodynamic and pharmacokinetic properties, and therapeutic use in hypertension and congestive heart failure. Drugs 31:198–248
Ulm EH (1983) Enalapril maleate (MK-421), a potent nonsulfhydryl angiotensin-converting enzyme inhibitor: absorption disposition, and metabolism in man. Drug Metab Rev 14 (1):99–110
Ulm EH, Hichens M, Gomez HJ, Till AE, Hand E, Vassil TC, Biollaz J, Brunner HR, Schelling JL (1982) Enalapril maleate and a lysine analogue (MK-521) disposition in man. Br J Clin Pharmacol 14:357–362
Unger T, Rockhold RW, Bönner G, Rascher W, Schaz K, Speck G, Schömig A, Ganten D (1981a) Antihypertensive effects of the novel converting-enzyme inhibitor YS 980 in spontaneously hypertensive rats. Clin Exp Hypertens 3 (1):121–140
Unger T, Kaufmann-Bühler I, Schölkens B, Ganten D (1981b) Brain converting enzyme inhibition: a possible mechanism for the antihypertensive action of captopril in spontaneously hypertensive rats. Eur J Pharmacol 70:467–478
Unger T, Yukimura T, Marin-Grez M, Lang RE, Rascher W et al. (1982a) SA446, a new orally active converting enzyme inhibitor: antihypertensive action and comparison with captopril in stroke-prone spontaneously hypertensive rats. Eur J Pharmacol 78:411–420
Unger T, Schüll B, Rascher W, Lang RE, Ganten D (1982b) Selective activation of the converting enzyme inhibitor MK-421 and comparison of its active diacid form with captopril in different tissues of the rat. Biochem Pharmacol 19:3063–3070
Unger T, Hübner D, Schüll B, Lang RE, Rascher W, Rettig R, Ganten D (1982c) Effect of chronic oral captopril treatment on tissue renin concentration and converting enzyme activity in stroke-prone spontaneously hypertensive rats. In: Rascher W, Clough D, Ganten D (eds) Hypertensive mechanisms. Schattauer, Stuttgart 768–773
Unger T, Ganten D, Lang RE, Schölkens BA (1984a) Is tissue converting enzyme inhibition a determinant of the anithypertensive efficacy of converting enzyme inhibitors? Studies with the two different compounds, Hoe498 and MK421, in spontaneously hypertensive rats. J Cardiovasc Pharmacol 6:872–880
Unger T, Fleck T, Ganten D, Lang RE, Rettig R (1984b) 2-(N)-(S)-1-ethoxycarbonyl-3-phenylpropyl-L-alamyl)-(1S,3S,5S)-2-azabicyclo (3.3.0)octane-3-carboxylic acid (Hoe 498):antihypertensive action and persistent inhibition of tissue converting enzyme activity in spontaneously hypertensive rats. Drug Res 34 (II):1426–1430
Unger T, Ganten D, Lang RE, Schölkens BA (1984c) Central actions of converting enzyme inhibitors in animal experiments. In: van Zwieten PA, Schonbaum (eds) Inhibitors of converting enzyme. Progress in pharmacology vol 5/3. Fischer Stuttgart, pp 51–68
Unger T, Ganten D, Lang RE, Schölkens BA (1985) Persistent tissue converting enzyme inhibition following chronic treatment with Hoe 498 and MK 421 in spontaneously

hypertensive rats. J Cardiovasc Pharmacol 7:36–41
Unger T, Moursi M, Ganten D, Hermann H, Lang RE (1986a) Antihypertensive action of the converting enzyme inhibitor perindopril (S9490–3) in spontaneously hypertensive rats: comparison with enalapril (MK421) and ramipril (HOE 498). J Cardiovasc Pharmacol 8:276–285
Unger T, Ganten D, Lang RE (1986b) Tissue converting enzyme and cardiovascular actions of converting enzyme inhibitors. J Cardiovasc Pharmacol 8 [Suppl 10]:S75–S81
Unger T, Badoer E, Ganten D, Lang RE, Rettig R (1988) Brain angiotensin: pathways and pharmacology. Circulation 77 [Suppl I]:I40–I54
Unger T, Gohlke P, Ganten D, Lang RE (1989a) Converting enzyme inhibitors and their effects on the renin-angiotensin system of the blood vessel wall. J Cardiovasc Pharmacol 13 (Suppl 3):S8–S16
Unger T, Horst PJ, Bauer M, Demmert G, Rettig R, Rohmeiss P (1989b) Natriuretic actrion of central angiotensin II in conscious rats. Brain Res 486:33–38.
Van Gilst WH, De Graeff PA, Kingma JH, Wesseling H, De Langen CDJ (1984) Captopril reduces purine loss and reperfusion arrhythmias in the rat heart after coronary artery occlusion. Eur J Pharmacol 100:113–117
Van Gilst WH, Van Wijngaarden J, Scholtens E, De Graeff PA, De Langen CDJ, Wesseling H (1987) Captopril-induced increase in coronary flow: an SH-dependent effect on arachidonic acid metabolism? J Cardiovasc Pharmacol 9 [Suppl 2]:S31–S36
Vecsei P, Hackenthal E, Ganten D (1978) The renin-angiotensin-aldosterone system. Past, present and future. Klin Wochenschr 56 [Suppl I]:5–21
Velletri P, Bean BL (1982) The effect of captopril on rat aortic angiotensin-converting enzyme. J Cardiovasc Pharmacol 4:315–325
Vidt DG (1984) A controlled multiclinic study to compare the antihypertensive effects of MK-421, Hydrochlorothiazide, and MK-421 combined with hydrochlorothiazide in patients with mild to moderate essential hypertension. J Hypertens 2 [Suppl 2]:81–88
Vidt DG, Bravo EL, Fouad FM (1982) Drug therapy: captopril. New Engl J Med 306: 214–219
Vincent M, Remond G, Portevin B, Serkiz B, Laubie M (1982) Stereoselective synthesis of a new perhydroindol derivative of chiral iminodiacid, a potent inhibitor of angiotensin converting enzyme. Tetrahedron Lett 23:1677–1680
Vinci JM, Horwitz D, Zusman RM, Pisano JJ, Catt KJ, Keiser HR (1979) The effect of converting enzyme inhibition with SQ20,881 on plasma and urinary kinins, prostaglandin E, and angiotensin II in hypertensive man. Hypertension 1:416–426
Waeber B, Brunner HR, Brunner DB, Curtet A-L, Turini GA, Gavras H (1980) Discrepancy between antihypertensive effect and angiotensin converting enzyme inhibition by captopril. Hypertension 2:236–242
Warner NJ, Rush JE (1988) Safety profiles of the angiotensin-converting enzyme inhibitors. Drugs 35 [Suppl 5]:89–97
Warner NJ, Blumberg AF, Bolognese JA, Gomez HJ, Brunner-Ferber F (1986) Lisinopril dose and duration of effect in patients with congestive heart failure (abstr) Acta Pharmacol Toxicol 66 [Suppl V]:132
Warren SE, O'Connor DT (1980) Hyperkalemia resulting from captopril administration. JAMA 244:2551
Webb DJ, Collier JG (1986) Vascular angiotensin conversion in humans. J Cardiovasc Pharmacol 8 [Suppl 10]:S40–S44
Wenting GJ, Tan Tjiong HL, Derkx FHM, DeBruyn JHM, Man in't Veld AJ, Schalekamp MADH (1984) Split renal function after captopril in unilateral renal artery stenosis. Br Med J 288:886–890
Wernze H (1988) Angioneurotisches Odem unter ACE-Hemmern: Häufigkeit, klinische Charakteristik, Auslösemechanismen. Z Kardiol [Suppl 3]:61–64
Whalley ET, Amure YO, Lye RH (1987) Analysis of the mechanism of action of bradykinin on human basilar artery in vitro. Naunyn Schmiedeberg's Arch Pharmacol 335: 433–437
Wilkes BM (1984) Evidence for a vasodepressor effect of the angiotensin-converting enzyme inhibitor, MK421 (enalapril), independent of blockade of angiotensin II formation. J Cardiovasc Pharmacol 6:1036–1042

Wilson SK, Lynch DR, Snyder SH (1987) Angiotensin-converting enzyme labelled with-^{3}H-Captopril. Tissue localization and changes in different models of hypertension in the rat. J Clin Invest 80:841–851

Witte PU, Irmisch R, Hajdu P, Metzger H (1984a) Pharmacokinetics and pharmacodynamics of a novel orally active angiotensin converting enzyme inhibitor (HOE498) in healthy subjects. Eur J Clin Pharmacol 27:577–581

Witte PU, Metzger H, Eckert HG, Irmisch R (1984b) Tolerance and pharmacokinetics of the angiotensin converting enzyme inhibitor 2-(N-((S)-1-ethoxycarbonyl-3-phenylpropyl)-L-alanyl)-(1S, 3S, 5S)-2-azabicyclo(3.3.0)octane-3-carboxylic acid (HOE498) in healthy volunteers. Arzneimittelforschung 34:1448–1451

Witte PU, Walter U (1987) Comparative double-blind study of ramipril and captopril in mild to moderate essential hypertension. Am J Cardiol 59:115D–120D

Wolf PS, Mann WS, Suh JT, Loev B, Smith RD (1984) Angiotensin-converting enzyme inhibitory and antihypertensive activities of pivalopril (RHC 3659-(s)). Fed Proc 43:1322–1325

Wood SM, Mann RD (1987) Angio-oedema and urticaria associated with angiotensin converting enzyme inhibitors. Br Med J 294:91–92

Wright GB, Alexander RW, Eckstein LS, Gimbrone MA Jr (1984) Characterization of rabbit ventricular myocardial receptors for angiotensin II: Evidence of two sites with different affinities and specifities. Mol Pharmacol 25:213

Wyhratt MJ, Patchett AA (1985) Recent development in the design of angiotensin-converting enzyme inhibitors. Med Res Rev 5 (4):483–581

Xiang J, Linz W, Becker H, Ganten D, Lang RE, Schölkens BA, Unger T (1985) Effects of converting enzyme inhibitors: ramipril and enalapril on peptide action and sympathetic neurotransmission in the isolated heart. Eur J Pharmacol 113:215–223

Yasujima M, Matthews G, Johnston CI (1982) Decreased uterine bradykinin receptors during captopril infusion in rats. Am J Cardiol 49:1518–1520

Zatz R, Dunn BR, Meyer TW, Anderson S, Rennke HG, Brenner BM (1986) Prevention of diabetic glomerulopathy by pharmacological amelioration of glomerular capillary hypertension. J Clin Invest 77:1925–1930

Zimmerman BG (1981) Adrenergic facilitation by angiotensin: does it serve a physiological function? Clin Sci 60:343–348

CHAPTER 11

Renin Inhibitors

R. HENNING, A. WAGNER, and B.A. SCHÖLKENS

CONTENTS

1 Brief History of Development

The very high utility of inhibitors of angiotensin converting enzyme (ACE) for the amelioration of all forms of hypertension has made them drugs of choice for basic treatment. Many researchers have now focussed their interest on renin inhibitors with the hope that interference with the renin-angiotensin system at the level of this highly specific enzyme will give rise to antihypertensive agents with a low incidence of side effects.

Results of the early efforts have been compiled in a number of excellent reviews and perspective articles (ANTONACCIO and CUSHMAN 1981; ANTONACCIO and WRIGHT 1987; BURTON et al. 1982b; BOGER 1987; CORVOL and MÉNARD 1986; CORVOL et al. 1983; GANTEN et al. 1984; GREENLEE 1988; HABER 1979, 1980, 1983a, 1984a–c, 1985a,b, 1986; HABER et al. 1983, 1987; HOFBAUER and WOOD 1984, 1985; HOFBAUER et al. 1985; KOKUBU and HIWADA 1987; KAY 1985; ONDETTI and CUSHMAN 1982; RICH 1986; TREE et al. 1985; WOOD et al. 1987c; WAEBER et al. 1986). The design of inhibitors started with the determination of the *N*-terminal 14-amino acid sequence of angiotensinogen by SKEGGS et al.

(1968). Pioneering studies on subsite variations in the minimum substrate were done by BURTON et al. (1980). Backbone variations, initially performed by SZELKE et al. (1982, 1983, 1985) and BOGER et al. (1983) led to the discovery of the first highly potent inhibitors. The inhibitor design was greatly aided by the revelation of the inhibitory mechanism of pepstatin A, a general inhibitor of aspartyl proteases found by UMEZAWA et al. (1970).

The early inhibitors were still peptides of relatively high molecular weight with little stability to proteases. Their high lipophilicity caused problems with solubility and bile excretion. Efforts in recent years have concentrated on improvement in these parameters in order to obtain an orally effective inhibitor which might be useful clinically as an antihypertensive drug. The concepts of the design and their results will be discussed below in some detail. Numbers refer to chemical formulae in the tables.

2 Chemistry

It has become common practice to classify the available inhibitors according to their gross chemical structure into the following subclasses (ANTONACCIO and WRIGHT 1987; GANTEN et al. 1984; GREENLEE 1988; ONDETTI and CUSHMAN 1982; RICH 1986): (1) renin antibodies; (2) substrate analogues; (3) transition state analogues; (4) prosegment peptides. These subclasses are discussed separately.

Molecular modeling has contributed a lot to inhibitor design; Sect. 2.5 is therefore devoted to the results of these studies.

2.1 Renin Antibodies

Although their therapeutic use as antihypertensives is highly questionable, antibodies against purified renins have been valuable pharmacological tools. Polyclonal antibodies against canine renin (DZAU 1985; DZAU et al. 1980, 1982) as well as Fab fragments (DZAU 1985; DZAU et al. 1983, 1984) have been produced and shown to have a hypotensive effect in sodium-depleted dogs. Recently, monoclonal antibodies of very high affinity against canine as well as human renin have become available (DZAU 1985; DZAU et al. 1983; GALEN et al. 1984; HOFBAUER et al. 1985; HOFBAUER and WOOD 1985; WOOD et al. 1986). The antibodies raised against human renin are effective in primate models (see Sect. 4).

2.2 Substrate Analogues

Inhibitors of this type were produced by shortening of the *N*-terminal sequence of angiotensinogen (*1*) (Table 1).

The minimal substrate with the native octapeptide structure (*2*) (SKEGGS et al. 1968) is both a substrate and a competitive inhibitor (POULSEN et al. 1973). Tetrapeptides (like *3*) corresponding to residues 10–13 of angiotensinogen are renin-stable competitive inhibitors, albeit in the millimolar range (KOKUBU et al. 1973). Systematic variation of amino acid residues led to a decapeptide (*4*),

Table 1. Substrate analogues

Inhibitor	Structure	IC_{50} (n*M*)
	6 7 8 9 10 11 12 13 P_5 P_4 P_3 P_2 P_1 P_1' P_2' P_3'	
N-terminal sequence of angiotensinogen (human) (*1*)	Asp–Arg–Val–Tyr–Ile–His–Pro–Phe–His–Leu–Val–Ile–His–Asn–...	
Minimal substrate (*2*)	His–Pro–Phe–His–Leu–Val–Ile–His	(313000)
(*3*)	Leu–Leu–Val–Phe–OMe	(670000)
RIP (*4*)	Pro–His–Pro–Phe–His–Phe–Phe–Val–Tyr–Lys	(2000)
RI-103 (*5*)	Phe–(4-I) Phe–Val–Tyr–Lys	(2000)

IC_{50} values in parentheses are obtained with purified kidney enzyme; IC_{50}, concentration at which 50% of the enzyme is inhibited.

which is termed RIP (renin inhibitory peptide; BURTON et al. 1980; CODY et al. 1980). The pentapeptide RI-103 (*5*) is claimed to be equally effective (BURTON et al. 1983).

2.3 Transition State Analogues

The transition state analogue concept developed by WOLFENDEN (1976) has been extremely useful in enzyme inhibitor design in various fields. It is based on the assumption that the enzyme acts as a catalyst by tight binding to the respective transition state, thereby lowering the free energy of activation. The transition state of a reaction is defined as the state of maximum energy though which all molecules participating in the reaction have to pass on their way from starting material to product. Molecules resembling the transition state of the catalyzed reaction should therefore be bound tightly to the active site of the enzyme. For the class of aspartyl proteases, to which renin belongs, a number of possibilities can be envisaged to mimic the pivotal tetrahedral intermediate *B* that is produced during hydrolysis of the peptide bond in substrate *A*:

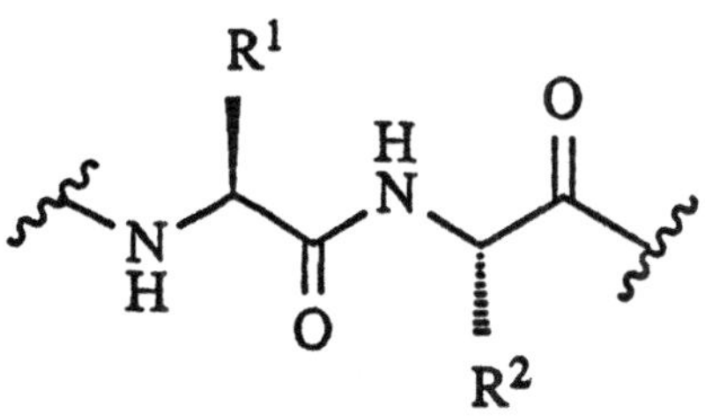

A

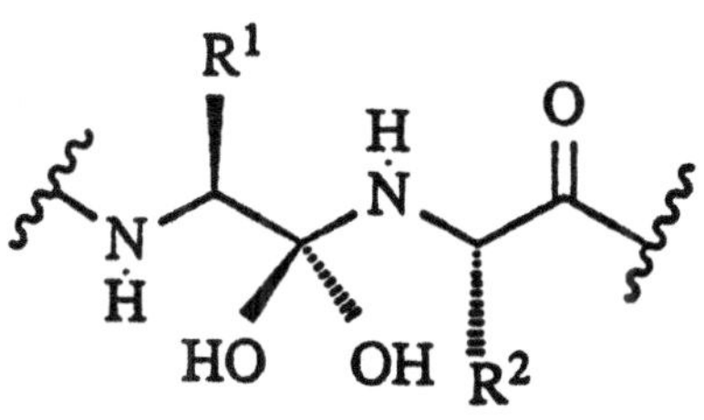

B

Most of these mimics, which are termed isosteres, have been utilized in renin inhibitor design. Enzyme specificity is a consequence of incorporating these mimics into peptides with specific P_n and P_n' residues.

2.3.1 Reduced Peptide Isosteres

In these compounds, the scissile amide bond in the substrate is replaced by an amino methylene unit (*C*).

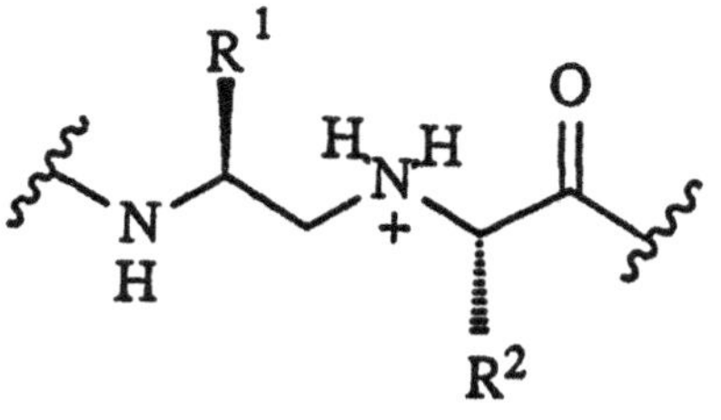

C

Tight binding of inhibitors of this type is expected to result from electrostatic interaction of the basic amine with the active site aspartates. Compound H-142 (*6*), which is related to RIP and which resulted from this approach, is a highly potent and specific inhibitor of human renin (IC_{50} = 10 n*M*, Table 2; SZELKE et al. 1983; LECKIE et al. 1985). On the contrary, H-77 (*7*), which contains a reduced Leu-Leu unit, is a specific inhibitor of canine and porcine renin (SZELKE et al. 1982), also active in vivo (see Sect. 4). Other groups have also pursued this approach and have reported potent inhibitors (*8*, PLATTNER et al. 1986; *9*, EPPS et al. 1988).

2.3.2 Inhibitors Containing Statine or Modified Statines

As already mentioned, pepstatin A, a naturally occurring aspartic protease inhibitor discovered by UMEZAWA et al. (1970), is a fairly weak inhibitor of renin (BOGER et al. 1983; SCHÖLKENS and JUNG 1974). It contains the unusual amino

Table 2. Reduced peptide isosteres

Inhibitor	Structure	IC_{50} (n*M*)
	6 7 8 9 10 11 12 13	
	P_5 P_4 P_3 P_2 P_1 P_1' P_2' P_3'	
Minimal substrate (*2*)	His–Pro–Phe–His–Leu–Val–Ile–His	
H-142 (*6*)	Pro–His–Pro–Phe–His–Leu $\overset{R}{-}$ Val–Ile–His–Lys	10
H-77 (*7*)	D-His–Pro–Phe–His–Leu $\overset{R}{-}$ Leu–Val–Tyr	
(*8*)	BOC–Phe–His–Cal $\overset{R}{-}$ Val–NH-2-methylbutyl	(8.6)
(*9*)	Ac–D-Ftr–Pro–Phe–His–Phe $\overset{R}{-}$ Phe–Val–Tyr–NH_2	

R over a peptide bond denotes a reduced peptide bond (CH_2NH).
Values in parentheses are obtained on purified kidney enzyme, all others on human plasma enzyme.
Cal, cyclohexylalanine; Ftr, *N*-formyl-tryptophan; BOC, tert. butyloxycarbonyl; Ac, acetyl.

acid statine (*D*) [4-(*S*)-amino-3(*S*)-hydroxy-6-methyl-heptanoic acid], which is proposed to act as a transition state mimic by means of the 3(*S*)-hydroxyl group (MARCINISZYN et al. 1976; RICH 1986), replacing a water molecule bound between the aspartates in the active site:

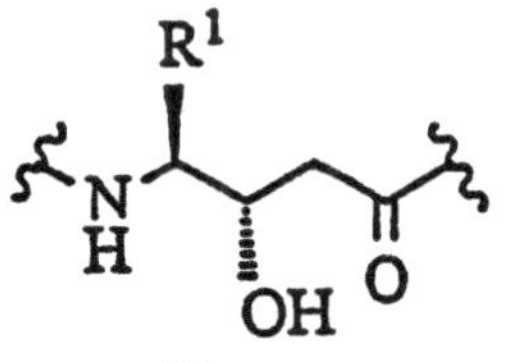

D

R^1 = isobutyl: statine
R^1 = phenyl: AHPPA
R^1 = cyclohexyl: ACHPA

A number of analogues still containing the natural Sta-Ala-Sta unit have been prepared; the most potent ones are *10* (IC_{50} = 5.8 μ*M*, EID et al. 1981) and *11* (IC_{50} = 28 n*M*, GUÉGAN et al. 1986; DIAZ 1987) (Table 3). Taking into account the high sequence specificity of renin, compounds with statine built into the human angiotensinogen sequence have been prepared. Results suggest that statine is able to replace Leu^{10}-Val^{11} of the natural sequence, as compounds *12* (SCRIP, statine containing renin inhibitory peptide; BOGER et al. 1983), *13* (CGP-29,287; WOOD et al. 1985), and *14* (ES-305; KOKUBU et al. 1986) are potent inhibitors with IC_{50} values in the nanomolar range.

Remarkable is the replacement of Phe^8 by a *bis*(naphthylmethyl)acetyl moiety and further shortening of the *C*- and *N*-terminal ends, leading to a relatively low molecular weight tripeptide (*14*). Molecular modeling studies (see Sect. 2.5) suggest that the isobutyl side chain of statine can be replaced by larger residues. This results in the synthesis of inhibitors containing 4(*S*)-amino-5-phenyl-3(*S*)-hydroxypentanoic acid (AHPPA) and 4(*S*)-amino-5-cyclohexyl-3(*S*)-hydroxypentanoic acid (ACHPA) with further increased *in vitro* potencies. Examples are *15* (ACRIP; BOGER et al. 1985a), which corresponds to SCRIP, and the tripeptide *16* (SHAM et al. 1986). Further *C*- and *N*-terminal variations lead to compounds like *17* (ES-6864; KOKUBU et al. 1988) and *18* (BREIPOHL et al. 1987) with IC_{50} values in the nanomolar range. SR 43845 (*19*) was even described to have an IC_{50} value of $\leq 10^{-11}$ *M* (NISATO et al. 1987a). Inhibitors of renin containing AHPPA, the ahpatinins (*20*), have recently been isolated from the culture broth of a *Streptomyces* species (OMURA et al. 1986).

2.3.3 Hydroxymethylene Isosteres and Related Inhibitors

In this class of inhibitors, the scissile peptide bond is replaced by a -CH(OH)-CH_2 unit (*E*). The hydroxyl group serves the same function as in the statine series. Due to geometric similarities, P_1 and P_1'side chains are located very near to the position of the natural substrate.

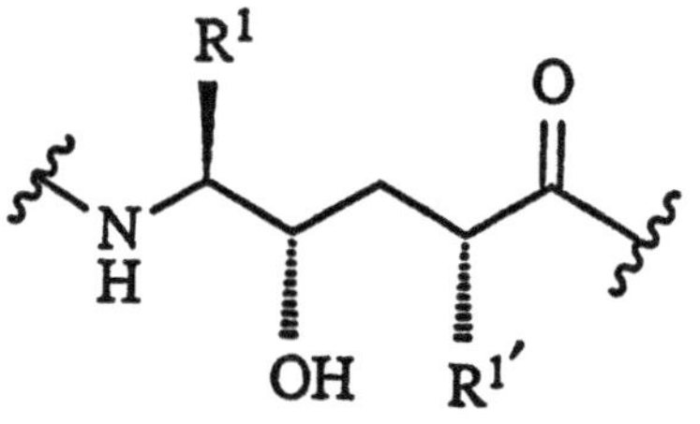

E

Table 3. Inhibitors containing statine or modified statines

Inhibitor	Structure	IC_{50} (n*M*)
	6 7 8 9 10 11 12 13	
	P_5 P_4 P_3 P_2 P_1 P_1' P_2' P_3'	
Minimal substrate (*2*)	His–Pro–Phe–His–Leu–Val– Ile –His	
Pepstatin A	Iva–Val–Val——Sta——Ala–Sta	22 000
(*10*)	Iva–Val–Val——Sta——Ala–Sta–Glu	(5 800)
SR 42,128 (*11*)	Iva–Phe–Nle——Sta——Ala–Sta	28
SCRIP (*12*)	Iva–His–Pro–Phe–His——Sta——Leu–Phe–NH_2	16
CGP-29,287 (*13*)	Z–Arg–Arg–Pro–Phe–His——Sta—— Ile –His–Lys(BOC)OMe	10
ES-305 (*14*)	BNMA–His——Sta——NH–2-methylbutyl	9.2
ACRIP (*15*)	Iva–His–Pro–Phe–His–ACHPA–Leu–Phe–NH_2	0.17
(*16*)	BOC–Phe–His–ACHPA–NH–2-methylbutyl	(4)
ES-6864 (*17*)	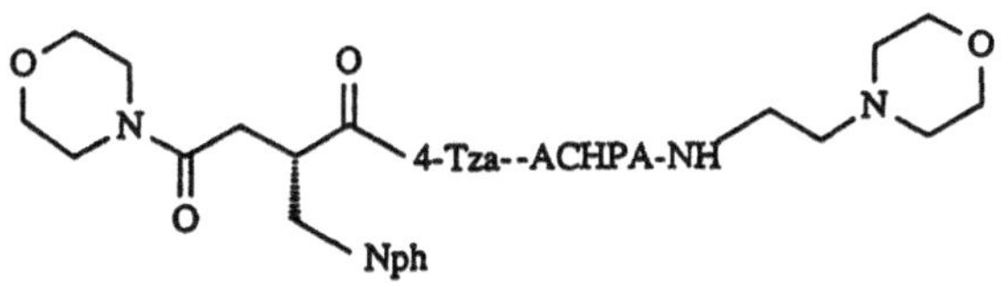	6.9
(*18*)	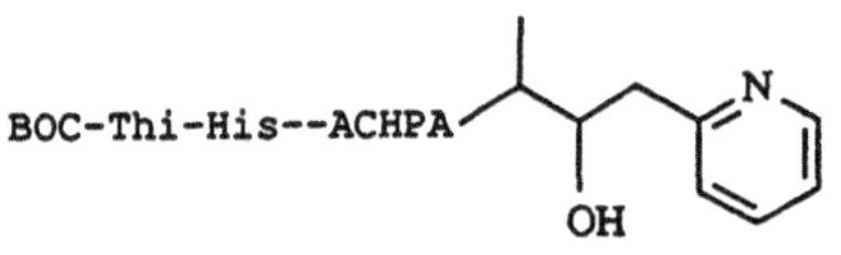	(1)
SR 43845 (*19*)	3–Pyr–$(CH_2)_2$–CO–Phe–His–ACHPA–Ile–NH–C$(CH_2OH)_2CH_3$	≤0.01
Ahpatinin G (*20*)	Iva–Val–Val–AHPPA– Ala–AHPPA	

All values in parentheses are measured with purified kidney renin, all others on human plasma enzyme
4-Tza, 4-thiazolylalanine;
BNMA, *bis*(1-naphthyl-methyl)acetyl; Nph, 1-naphthyl;
Thi, 3-(2-thienyl)alanine; Iva, isovaleroyl;
Z, benzyloxycarbonyl; Pyr, pyridyl; ACHPA, 4(*S*)-amino-5-cyclohexyl-3(*S*)-hydroxy-pentanoic acid.

Introduction of this transition state mimic into the octapeptide derived from human angiotensinogen leads to the very potent inhibitor H-261 (*21*; SZELKE et al. 1983) (Table 4). This stimulated efforts in a number of groups, leading to highly potent compounds such as U-71,038 (*22*; THAISRIVONGS et al. 1986a), *23* (THAISRIVONGS et al. 1987c), *24* (SAWYER et al. 1988b), *25* (KEMPF et al. 1987), *26* (TENBRINK et al. 1988), and CGP-38,560A (*27*; BÜHLMAYER et al. 1988; BRUNNER et al. 1988). In these derivatives, binding contributions of residues away from the central unit have been probed. As these inhibitors have progressively less peptidal character and become smaller in size, they also constitute progress en route to orally active inhibitors (see Sect. 4).

Some recent work has shown that in hydroxymethylene isosteres, the *C*-terminal end can be truncated to a large extent. This observation is based on the results of KOKUBU et al. (1984) and FEHRENTZ et al. (1985b), who have shown that aldehydes, ending with the carbonyl function of the scissile bond, are moderately potent inhibitors (for example, *28*). Extension in such a way that a residue for occupation of the P_1'-binding site is provided again yields potent inhibitors such as *29* (BOLIS et al. 1987), *30* (DELLARIA et al. 1987), and *31* (LULY et al. 1988), in which the P_1'-residue is connected via sulfur. Also, the retro-inverso analogue *32* (ROSENBERG et al. 1987), the norstatine analogue KRI-1230 (*33*; IIZUKA et al. 1988a,b), and imidazole analogue *34* (DEFORREST et al. 1988) fall into this category. HANSON et al. (1985) have shown that glycols like *35* containing an additional hydroxyl group are active inhibitors; extension of this principle led to the preparation of compounds *36* (THAISRIVONGS et al. 1987b) and A 64,662 (*37*; KLEINERT et al. 1988a,b; BRUNNER et al. 1988).

2.3.4 Miscellaneous Inhibitors

The ability of aldehydes such as *28* to act as inhibitors rests in their capacity to add water to form hydrates, which then mimic the transition state. The same is probably true for ketone isosteres such as *38* (LECKIE et al. 1985) and for α,α-difluoroketone and trifluoroketone analogues like *39* (THAISRIVONGS et al. 1986b; FEARON et al. 1987) (Table 5). Two different peptide-mimic features have been built into the same molecule, giving rise to amino alcohols like *40* (FREE et al. 1985; DANN et al. 1986) and statine analogues like *41* (BOCK et al. 1985).

Replacement of the hydroxyl group of statine by an amino group leads to a loss in potency (*42*; ARROWSMITH et al. 1986). The same is true for the difluorostatine series (*43*; THAISRIVONGS et al. 1987a).

The use of peptide bond mimics, in which binding interactions with the active site aspartates are impossible, such as a methylenethio group (SMITH et al. 1988) or an E-olefin (JOHNSON 1984) gives rise to only weak inhibitors.

2.4 Prosegment Peptides

The synthesis of prosegment peptides as renin inhibitors is based on the assumption that in inactive prorenin, the storage form of the enzyme in the kidney, the prosegment is folded back into the active site, thereby acting as an

Table 4. Hydroxymethylene isosteres and related inhibitors

Inhibitor	Structure	IC_{50} (n*M*)
	6 7 8 9 10 11 12 13	
	P_5 P_4 P_3 P_2 P_1 P'_1 P'_2 P'_3	
Minimal substrate (*2*)	His–Pro–Phe—His–Leu—Val–Ile–His	
H 261 (*21*)	BOC–His–Pro–Phe—His–Leu$^{\underline{OH}}$Val–Ile–His	(0.7)
U-71,038 (*22*)	BOC–Pro–Phe$_{\overline{Me}}$His–Leu$^{\underline{OH}}$Val–Ile–AMP	(0.39)
(*23*)	BOC–α–Me–Pro–Phe—His–Leu$^{\underline{OH}}$Val–Ile–AMP	(2)
(*24*)	Ac–Ftr–Pro–Phe—His–Leu$^{\underline{OH}}$Val–NH_2	(0.31)
(*25*)	BOC–Phe—His–Leu$^{\underline{OH}}$Dha–NH–isopentyl	(1.5)
(*26*)	BOC–Phe–ProΨ[CH_2O]Phe—His–Leu$^{\underline{OH}}$Val–Ile–AMP	(1.6)
CGP 38,560A (*27*)	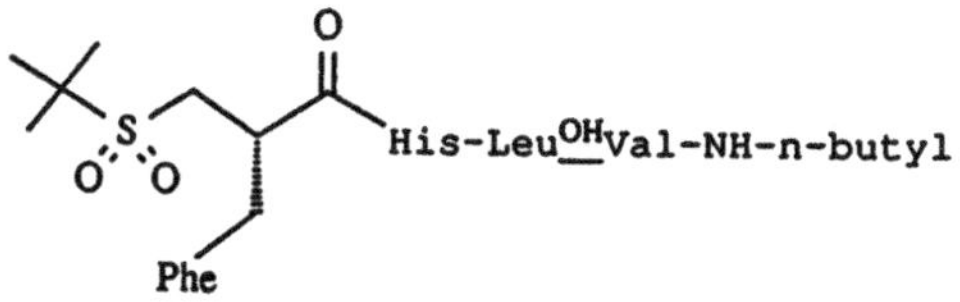	1
RRM-188 (*28*)	Z–Nal–His–Leu–al	(80)
	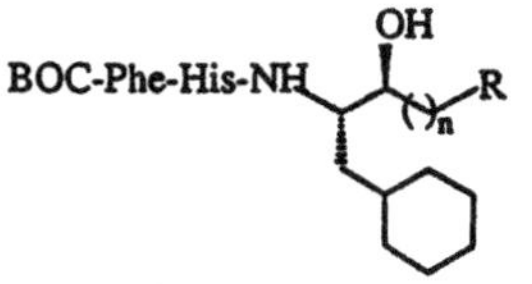	
(*29*)	R = SO_2–isopropyl	(7.6)
(*30*)	R = SO_2–cyclohexyl	(2.5)
(*31*)	R = S–isopropyl	(4)
(*32*)	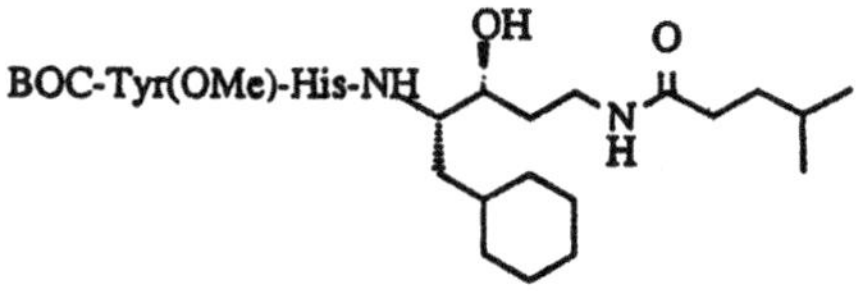	4
KRI-1230 (*33*)	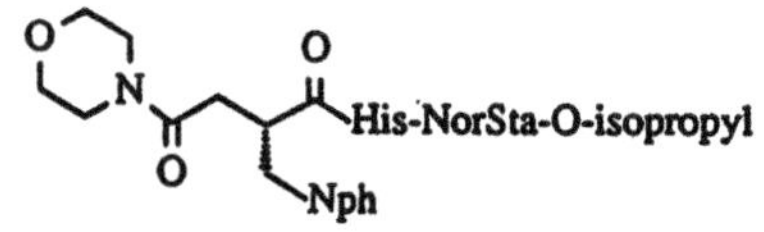	7.8
(*34*)	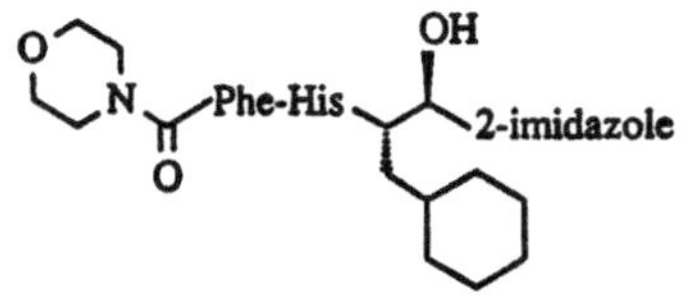	~10

Table 4. (Cont.)

Inhibitor	Structure	IC_{50} (n*M*)
(*35*)	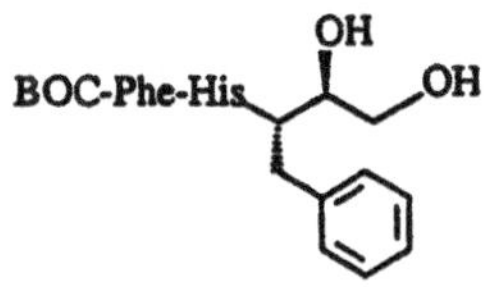	2600
(*36*)	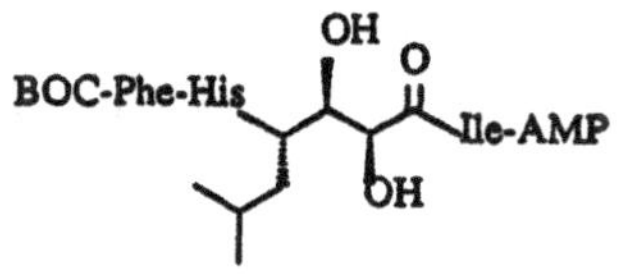	(0.35)
A 64,662 (*37*)	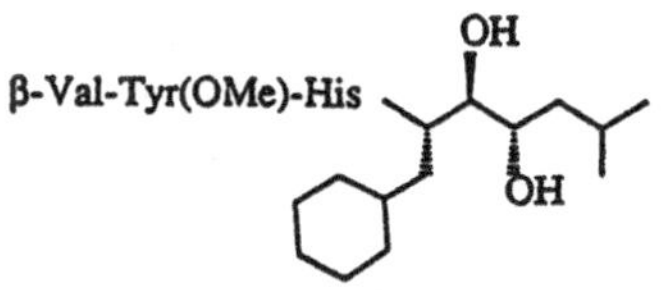	(0.6)

All values in parentheses are measured with purified enzyme, the others with human plasma.
OH over a peptide bond denotes a hydroxymethylene isostere [$CH_2CH(OH)$]; Me under a peptide bond denotes an *N*-methylated bond.
AMP, 2-aminomethyl pyridine; Nal, 3-(1-naphthyl)alanine; Dha, dehydroalanine; Leu-al, 2-amino-4-methyl-pentanal (Leucinal); NorSta, 3-amino-2-hydroxy-5-methyl-hexanoic acid (norstatine); see Tables 2, 3 also.

internal inhibitor. The most potent inhibitor based on this concept is tert. butyloxycarbonyl-Leu-Lys-Arg-Met-Pro-OMe with a K_I of 16.6 μ*M* (CUMIN et al. 1985).

2.5 Molecular Modeling

The crystal structure of human renin of recombinant origin has only recently become available and has not been used for modeling studies yet (MORRIS 1988; JAMES et al. 1988). All studies so far were done using computer models of renin that are based on the crystal structures of other aspartyl proteases, in which the appropriate amino acids are replaced, and minimum energy conformations are obtained by molecular dynamics calculations (AKAHANE et al. 1985a,b; BLUNDELL et al. 1983, 1987; CARLSON et al. 1984, 1985, 1987; JAMES and SIELECKI 1983; PLATTNER et al. 1986). Comparison of the structure of human renin with the models suggests a close similarity in the region of the active site with larger deviations distant from it; the results obtained with the models are therefore quite valid.

Table 5. Miscellaneous inhibitors

Inhibitor	Structure	IC_{50} (n*M*)
	6 7 8 9 10 11 12 13	
	P_5 P_4 P_3 P_2 P_1 P_1' P_2' P_3'	
Minimal substrate (*2*)	His–Pro–Phe–His –Leu–Val– Ile– His	
(*38*)	BOC–His–Pro–Phe–His –Leu$\overset{K}{-}$Val– Ile–AMP	6
(*39*)	BOC–Phe–His –(F_2–Sto)– Ile–AMP	1.4
(*40*)	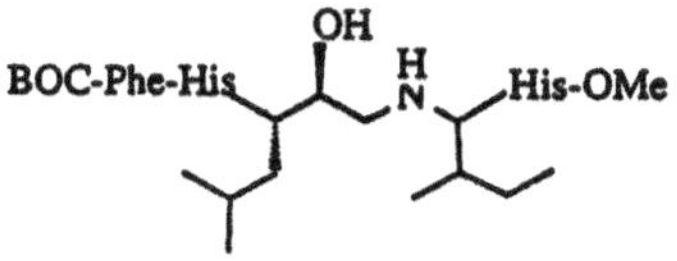	(31)
(*41*)	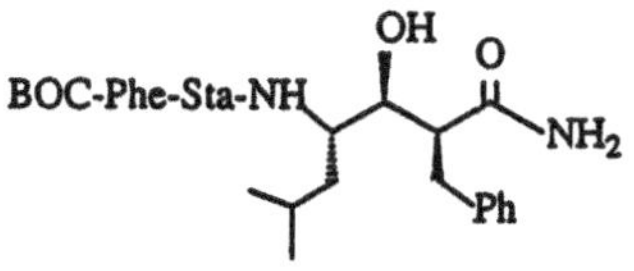	(60)
(*42*)	His–Pro–Phe–His–Asta–Val–Ile– Phe	(60)
(*43*)	BOC–Phe–His –(F_2) Asta– Ile–AMP	

All values in parentheses are obtained with purified kidney enzyme, all others with human plasma.
^{K} over a peptide bond denotes a ketone isostere (CH_2CO).
F_2-Sto, 2,2-difluorostatone; Asta, 3-amino-3-deoxystatine; (F_2)Asta, 2,2-difluoro-3-amino-3-deoxystatine; Sta, statine; Ph, phenyl; see Tables 2–4 also.

The X-ray structures of pepsin (ANDREEVA et al. 1984), penicillopepsin (JAMES and SIELECKI 1983), and endothiapepsin (PEARL and BLUNDELL 1984) serve as a basis for the models. Structures of these enzymes with various inhibitors bound have also become available (BOTT et al. 1982; FOUNDLING et al. 1987a,b; HALLETT et al. 1985; JAMES and SIELECKI 1983), giving valuable information about binding modes and geometries of the inhibitors.

Modelling studies were performed using NMR on enzyme-free inhibitors (ROY et al. 1987) as well as conformational (LIEPINA et al. 1984) and Free-Wilson calculations (NISATO et al. 1987b). The most important predictions derived from the models are the higher potency of ACHPA-containing inhibitors and the plausibleness of statine as a dipeptide mimic (BOGER 1985a,b, 1986). Construction of conformationally restricted analogues were also suggested (BOGER 1985a,b, 1986; SHAM et al. 1988; THAISRIVONGS et al. 1988). Many groups routinely use the models to evaluate whether newly synthesized inhibitors are accommodated well by the active site (DELLARIA et al. 1987; EPPS et al. 1988; HUI et al. 1987; SAWYER et al. 1988a,b; TENBRINK et al. 1988; THAISRIVONGS et al. 1987b,c, 1988).

3 Pharmacokinetics and Metabolism

Due to their peptidic nature, the early inhibitors are absorbed orally to a negligable extent and are cleaved rapidly by peptidases, thus giving a very short duration of action even upon intravenous administration. Good stability towards peptidases in vitro has been shown for a number of inhibitors (Bolis et al. 1987; Boger et al. 1985b; Dellaria et al. 1987; Hiwada et al. 1988; Iizuka et al. 1988b). Amide bonds involving statine have been shown to be metabolically stable. Other amide bonds in the molecule have been stabilized by using either unnatural amino acids or by modification such as by *N*-methylation (Thaisrivongs 1986c). In general, reduction in the number of peptide bonds seems to lead to increased stability towards hydrolysis.

Another important issue in this context is the prevalence of biliary excretion due to the relatively high lipophilicity and molecular weight of the inhibitors, leading to rapid elimination from the circulation. For instance, the compound Iva-His-D-Pro-Phe-His-Sta-Leu-benzylamide appears undegraded in bile to the extent of 63% after i.v. administration to dogs (Boger et al. 1985b). Although there is precedence that molecular weight is not the sole determinant for biliary excretion (e.g., cyclosporine, erythromycin), the borderline for predominant elimination via this pathway is estimated to be approximately 500 daltons. All inhibitors described so far have molecular weights higher than this value.

In most cases their excretion pathways have not been investigated. Probably, fine tuning of the molecular properties of new inhibitors will have to be applied to resolve this problem. Quite frequently, a difference of inhibitory potency of varying magnitude is observed between plasma and purified renin assays (Bock et al. 1987; Cumin et al. 1985; Evans et al. 1985). A reasonable explanation might be tight binding of the inhibitor to plasma components, reducing the capability to interact with renin. Again, for most inhibitors, the possible significance of such an effect has not been investigated.

4 Mechanism of Action, Pharmacodynamics, and Hemodynamic Effects

4.1 Biochemical Studies

In order to be suitable as an antihypertensive agent, a new inhibitor has to be specific for human renin, as opposed to other aspartic proteinases. This specificity has been demonstrated for a number of compounds (Hiwada et al. 1988; Iizuka et al. 1988a,b; Kokubu et al. 1984, 1985, 1986; Luly et al. 1987; Sham et al. 1988). Enzymes that have been included in these investigations are renins from other species (dog, pig, rat, goat, and monkey), porcine pepsin, cathepsin D, trypsin, chymotrypsin, kininase II, and glandular kallikrein.

Detailed biochemical studies on the association of inhibitors with the enzyme have been performed by two groups. Kati et al. (1987) could show for compound *22* that a minimal two-step mechanism is followed. A loosely bound enzyme-inhibitor complex is formed first with a inhibitory constant K_I of 12 nM, which is followed by rearrangement to another more tightly bound (64-fold) complex with an overall K_I of 0.19 nM. Inhibition was shown to be competitive. On a molecular basis, one can speculate that the inhibitor is first bound to the open active site cleft; after this event, the flap region of the enzyme rotates and contributes further strong binding interactions.

CUMIN et al. (1987a,b) utilized tritium-labeled SR 42,128 (*11*) and found a distinct pH dependence of binding. Moreover, at pH 7.4, the inhibitor binds specifically to human renin, whereas at lower pH values, affinities for renin, cathepsin D, pepsin, and gastricsin are in the same range.

4.2 Pharmacological Studies

Pharmacological investigations of renin inhibitors have posed great problems due to the lack of animal models that can be used in routine testing. The rat must be excluded, since rat renin is completely insensitive to inhibitors designed for the human enzyme. There have been attempts to infuse rats with exogenous renin followed by inhibitor (GARDES et al. 1980; PALS et al. 1986; THAISRIVONGS et al. 1987c), but this approach is not very viable. The blood pressure of normal animals is fairly insensitive to renin inhibition (SERRE et al. 1987; KLEINERT et al. 1988b). At least tenfold higher doses have to be applied in order to obtain similar effects as under sodium restriction (see below). Usually animal models are employed, wherein the renin-angiotensin system has been stimulated by some kind of prior intervention. The most common method is sodium depletion by pretreatment with a loop diuretic which has been applied to dogs (BLAINE et al. 1984, 1985; BOGER et al. 1985a; LECKIE et al. 1983; OLDHAM et al. 1984; SMITH et al. 1987) and various monkey species (baboon, cynomolgus, rhesus, marmoset). Either conscious or anesthetized animals are used (BOLIS et al. 1987; DELLARIA et al. 1987; DECLAVIERE et al. 1985a,b; DIAZ 1987; HANSON et al. 1987; HIWADA et al. 1988; IIZUKA et al. 1988a,b; KLEINERT et al. 1988a,b; KOKUKU et al. 1988; LULY et al. 1988; PLATTNER et al. 1986; PAPAIOANNOU et al. 1985a; SERRE et al. 1987; SZELKE et al. 1985; TAKAORI et al. 1987; THAISRIVONGS et al. 1986a; TREE et al. 1983; WOOD et al. 1987a,b).

4.2.1 Intravenous Application

Due to problems already described, administration of the early inhibitors has only been possible by the intravenous route, either by infusion or bolus. With antibodies against canine renin and their respective Fab fragments, complete blockade of the enzyme and a significant fall in blood pressure were observed in anesthetized, sodium-depleted dogs (DZAU 1985), whereas no effect was seen in sodium-replete dogs. The fall in blood pressure correlates with PRA. Systemic and hemodynamic effects were compared with the ACE inhibitor teprotide (DZAU et al. 1983). Blood pressure reduction is comparable for both treatments, but teprotide causes a greater renal vasodilation. Similar results are obtained in sodium-depleted marmosets with polyclonal (MICHEL et al. 1984) and monoclonal antibodies (HOFBAUER et al. 1985; HOFBAUER and WOOD 1985) against human kidney renin.

First results with peptide-based inhibitors are described in reviews by BOGER et al. (1985a) and HOFBAUER and WOOD (1985). In essence, effective inhibition of PRA is observed. In sodium-depleted animals, a fall in blood pressure is usually seen. Due to metabolic instability and rapid biliary excretion, the duration of action is usually quite short (< 1 h). Recently, however, progress has been made towards longer-acting inhibitors. In marmosets, CGP 29,287 (13) causes a fall in blood pressure lasting for 1–3 h following bolus i.v. applications of 0.1–10 mg/kg. The longer duration of action in this fairly large peptide has been ascribed to the *C*- and *N*-terminal blockade with large residues, rendering the compound fairly stable to degradation (WOOD et al. 1985). SR 42128 (*11*) causes inhibition of PRA and a hypotensive response after doses of 5–10 mg/kg i.v. (bolus) lasting for 2–3 h in anesthetized and conscious baboons (DE-CLAVIERE et al. 1985a; DIAZ 1987; SERRE et al. 1987). A single dose of 5 mg/kg of U-71,038 (*22*) in conscious cynomolgus monkeys, infused over a 17-min period, led to a reduction of PRA and hypotension lasting for 3 h (PALS et al. 1986; THAISRIVONGS et al. 1986a). With 1 mg/kg i.v. of SR 43845 (*19*) a complete blockade of PRA can be obtained in the same model, which lasts for > 5 h. A 30-mm drop in blood pressure is also seen, which lasts only for 3 h, however (NISATO et al. 1987a). Finally, the low dose of 0.1 mg/kg i.v. of A64,662 (37) completely inhibits PRA in anesthetized, salt-depleted cynomolgus monkeys for 30 min, accompanied by a modest fall in blood pressure (KLEINERT et al. 1988a,b). Increases in dose to 1 and 10 mg/kg prolong the PRA suppression and strongly intensify the hypotensive response. In salt-replete monkeys 0.1 mg/kg is also sufficient to block PRA completely but without an effect on blood pressure. Dose increase also produces hypotension in these animals despite no further marked effect on PRA. Furthermore, 1 and 10 mg/kg of this compound given i.v. to anephric monkeys (having no detectable PRA) produce a fall in blood pressure (KLEINERT et al. 1988b). Another report describes the chronic administration of inhibitor *13*, which was given at doses up to 30 mg/kg per day i.p. with osmotic minipumps to sodium-depleted marmosets. At the highest dose, a persistent hypotensive response was observed. PRA was initially reduced by 93% but returned to pretreatment levels on day 14 (WOOD et al. 1987a). These last results may be interpreted by the assumption that complete inhibition of PRA is a prerequisite for and correlated with the onset of blood pressure effects, but it is not sufficient per se. Other factors, not thoroughly investigated yet, like the inhibition of renin or renin-like activity in tissues, for instance, the vascular wall, may be important determinants (CAMPBELL 1985, 1987; DZAU 1986; WOOD et al. 1988). This assumption is corroborated by the finding that the renin gene is expressed in several extrarenal tissues (SAMANI et al. 1988).

4.2.2 Oral Application

Progress has also been made in the development of inhibitors that show activity after application by the oral route in sodium-restricted animals. With the high dose of 100 mg/kg, CGP 29,287 (*13*) reduces PRA and blood pressure for longer than 1 h in the marmoset (Wood et al. 1985). U-71,038 (*22*, 50 mg/kg) causes PRA inhibition and a hypotensive response lasting for at least 5 h (PALS et al. 1986). For KRI-1230 (*33*), a drop in PRA and blood pressure after an oral dose of 30 mg/kg last for 6 h with a slow onset in the conscious marmoset (IIZUKA et al. 1988a,b). The long duration of action compared with i.v. application may be explained either by slow resorption or alternatively by enterohepatic circulation, which seems plausible for this very lipophilic compound. An oral dose of 31.5 mg/kg of compound *34* causes an 80% reduction in PRA and a 15-mm drop in blood pressure in salt-depleted cynomolgue monkeys (DEFORREST et al. 1988). Compound A 64662 (*37*) demonstrates intraduodenal activity at 10 mg/kg in salt-depleted, anesthetized cynomolgus monkeys. A blood pressure fall of approximately 15% accompanied by a 95% inhibition of PRA is observed. Both effects last for 2–3 h. A slight reflex tachycardia is also seen (KLEINERT et al. 1988a). SR 43845 (*19*, 30 mg/kg) given orally to conscious marmosets gives rise to a significant blood pressure reduction for 1.5 h and nearly complete inhibition of PRA, lasting for at least 5 h (NISATO et al. 1987a). ES-6864 (*17*) at a dose of 30 mg/kg in the same model leads to a 20-mm fall in blood pressure, lasting for more than 10 h (HIWADA et al. 1988; KOKUBU et al. 1988). The blood pressure reduction outlasts inhibition of PRA, which returns to baseline after 6 h. An involvement of tissue renin activity may again cause this effect. Another possibility is the participation of unidentified metabolites. Plasma concentrations of intact ES-6864 were measured after the 30 mg/kg dose; a peak concentration of 1.2 µg/ml at 1 h after application was observed, descreasing rapidly in a first phase, following by a slow decay between 3 and 8 h.

The predictive value of results obtained in sodium-depleted animals for the efficacy of inhibitors of renin in human essential hypertension is still highly questionable. Some groups have therefore made attempts to develop animal models that resemble the pathological situation more closely. Pentapaptide RI-78 [Phe(4-Cl)-Phe-Val-Tyr-Lys-NH_2] was applied in an acute renal hypertensive monkey model; a reduction in blood pressure could be observed (TAKAORI et al. 1987). By ligation of the minor branch of one renal artery, chronic renal hypertension is established in marmosets. In this model, PRA is only slightly increased initially and decreases thereafter. CGP 29287 (*13*) lowers blood pressure at 1 mg/kg i.p. to the same extent as enalaprilat 2 mg/kg (NEISIUS and WOOD 1987).

When comparing oral doses necessary to produce an antihypertensive response with in vitro potency, one arrives at the conclusion that even the best compounds described to date have a fairly low bioavailability. In order to achieve improvements in oral absorption, much work still has to be done on chemical modifications and possibly on pharmaceutical formulation [e.g., coapplication of absorption promoters (FIX et al. 1986; LEE 1986)].

The relative effectivity o renin inhibitors and ACE inhibitors in hypertension treatment remains an open question. Some comparative studies have been performed in sodium-depleted animals. The maximum change in blood pressure observed with H-142 or CGP 29287 on the one hand and with the ACE inhibitors teprotide, captopril, and enalapril on the other hand is comparable (Hofbauer et al. 1985). ACRIP (*15*) and enalaprilat were compared in one-kidney dogs before and after constriction of a renal artery (Smith et al. 1987). ACRIP was infused at 0.003–0.1 mg/kg per min i.v., enalaprilat was given in the same doses as a bolus. Maximum effects were seen 3 days after clamping. Blood pressure was reduced to the same extent with both drugs; also, a comparable reduction in glomerular filtration rate and renal plasma flow was observed. Upon pretreatment with H-142 followed by teprotide, no additional hypotensive effect of the ACE inhibitor was seen. The same is also true for the inverse sequence of treatments (Hofbauer et al. 1985). Thus, at least under the conditions of sodium restriction, renin inhibitors and ACE inhibitors seem to be equieffective.

5 Administration in Humans

Only very limited studies have been performed in humans with renin inhibitors so far. RIP (*4*) was given to healthy, salt-depleted volunteers in increasing doses of 0.05 to 1 mg/kg per min for 10 min. A significant hypotensive response was seen at 0.5 mg/kg per min in the upright and 1 mg/kg per min in the supine position. In a low renin patient with essential hypertension, RIP at 1 mg/kg per min caused a precipitous fall in blood pressure and heart rate. H-142 (*6*) was also investigated in volunteers. Infusions of 1 and 2.5 mg/kg per min were applied for 30 min (Webb et al. 1983, 1985, 1987). PRA was markedly reduced, and a dose-dependent, highly significant drop in diastolic, but not in systolic, blood pressure was observed.

Recently, two other inhibitors, A 64662 (*37*) and CGP 38560A (*27*), have been administered intravenously to healthy volunteers (Brunner et al. 1988). A dose-dependent reduction in PRA and plasma angiotensin II levels is observed with both compounds. Blood pressure is not affected. The angiotensin II levels are comparable to the situation after acute ACE inhibition. As with H-142, active and total renin measured by a direct assay increase in response to both agents. Long-term studies will have to be performed in order to show that the rise in active renin caused by feedback release can be overcome by the inhibition.

With the available data, it is much too early to speculate on the long-term antihypertensive efficacy in hypertensive humans. Possible advantages or disadvantages compared with ACE inhibition will also have to be investigated thoroughly in humans. The possibility exists, however, that renin inhibitors will emerge as a valuable addition to the armentarium for the treatment of hypertension.

Summary

With the advent of angiotensin converting enzyme (ACE) inhibitors, pharmacological intervention in the renin-angiotensin system has become an accepted method for the control of hypertension. Inhibitors of renin have been pursued intensely as tools of increased specificity. The design and synthesis of such inhibitors has been achieved; they are highly potent *in vitro* and show interesting pharmacological activity in *in vivo* models. However, compounds with oral activity sufficient for clinical use as antihypertensive agents are not available yet. They are the goal of future work in this field and will enable clinical researchers to verify the relative merits of renin inhibitors versus ACE inhibitors in hypertension treatment.

References

Akahane K, Nakagawa S, Umeyama H (1985a) Three-dimensional structure of human renin and renin inhibitors. New approach to drug design. J Pharmacobiodyn 8:S174

Akahane K, Umeyama H, Nakagawa S, Moriguchi I, Hirose S, Iizuka K, Murakami K (1985b) Three-dimensional structure of human renin. Hypertension 7:3–12

Andreeva NS, Zdanov AS, Gustchina AE, Fedorov AA (1984) Structure of ethanol-inhibited porcine pepsin at 2-Å resolution and binding of the methyl ester of phenylalanyl-diiodotyrosin to the enzyme. J Biol Chem 259:11353–11365

Antonaccio MJ, Cushman DW (1981) Drugs inhibiting the renin-angiotensin system. Fed Proc 40:2275–2284

Antonaccio MJ, Wright JJ (1987) Enzyme inhibitors of the renin-angiotensin system. Prog Drug Res 31:161–191

Arrowsmith R, Carter K, Dann JG, Davies DE, Harris J, Morton JA, Lister P, et al. (1986) Novel renin inhibitors: synthesis of aminostatine and comparison with statine-containing analogues. J Chem Soc Chem Commun:755–757

Blaine EH, Schorn TW, Boger J (1984) Statine-containing renin inhibitor. Dissociation of blood pressure lowering and renin inhibition in sodium-deficient dogs. Hypertension [Suppl 1] 6:111–118

Blaine EH, Nelson BJ, Seymour AA, Schorn TW, Sweet CS, Slater EE, Nussberger J, Boger J (1985) Comparison of renin and converting enzyme inhibition in sodium-deficient dogs. Hypertension [Suppl 1] 7:I66–I71

Blundell T, Sibanda BL, Pearl L (1983) Three-dimensional structure, specificity and catalytic mechanism of renin. Nature 304:273–275

Blundell TL, Cooper J, Foundling SI, Jones DM, Atrash B, Szelke M (1987) On the rational design of renin inhibitors: X-ray studies of aspartic proteinases complexed with transition-state analogues. Biochemistry 26:5585–5590

Bock MG, DiPardo RM, Evans BE, Rittle KE, Boger JS, Freidinger RM, Veber DF (1985) Dipeptide analogues. Synthesis of a potent renin inhibitor. J Chem Soc Chem Commun 109–110

Bock MG, DiPardo RM, Evans BF, Rittle KE, Boger J, Poe M, LaMont BI, et al. (1987) Renin inhibitors. Statine-containing tetrapeptides with varied hydrophobic carboxy termini. J Med Chem 30:1853–1857

Boger J (1985a) Renin inhibitors. Design of angiotensin transition-state analogs containing statine. In: Kostka V (ed) Aspartic proteinases and their inhibitors. Springer, Berlin Heidelberg New York, pp 401–420

Boger J (1985b) Renin inhibition. Annu Rep Med Chem 20:257–266

Boger J (1986) Renin inhibitors: Drug design and molecular modelling. In: Lambert BW (ed) Third SCI-RSC medicinal chemistry symposium, Cambridge, Sept 15–18. Royal Society of chemistry, London, pp 271–292

Boger J (1987) Clinical goal in sight for small molecule renin inhibitors. Trends Pharm Sci 8:370–372
Boger J, Lohr N, Ulm EH, Poe M, Blaine EM, Fanelli GM, Lin T-Y, et al. (1983) Novel renin inhibitors containing the amino acid statine. Nature 303:81–84
Boger J, Payne LS, Perlow DS, Lohr NS, Poe M, Blaine EH, Ulm EH, et al. (1985a) Renin inhibitors. Synthesis of subnanomolar, competitive, transition-state analogue inhibitors containing a novel analogue of statine. J Med Chem 28:1779–1790
Boger J, Bennett CD, Payne LS, Ulm EH, Blaine EH, Homnick CF, Schorn TW, et al. (1985b) Design of proteolytically-stable, peptidal renin inhibitors and determination of their fate in vivo. Regul Pept 11:8–13
Bolis G, Fung AKL, Greer J, Kleinert HD, Marcotte PA, Perun TJ, Plattner JJ, Stein HH (1987) Renin inhibitors. Dipeptide analogues of angiotensinogen incorporating transition-state, nonpeptidic replacements at the scissile bond. J Med Chem 30: 1729–1737
Bott R, Subramanian E, Davies DR (1982) Three-dimensional structure of the complex of the Rhizopus chinensis carboxyl proteinase and pepstatin at 2.5 Å resolution. Biochemistry 21:6956–6962
Breipohl G, Geiger R, Henke S, Kleemann H-W, Knolle J, Ruppert D, Schölkens BA, et al. (1987) Studies on renin inhibitors. Top Med Chem 4:101–127
Brunner HR, Nussberger J, Waeber B (1988) ACE inhibition and renin inhibition. Symposium: Renin inhibitors-present and future, Osaka, May 28
Bühlmayer P, Caselli A, Fuhrer W, Göschke R, Rasetti V, Rüeger H, Stanton JL, et al. (1988) Synthesis and biological activity of some transition-state inhibitors of human renin. J Med Chem 31:1839–1846
Burton J, Cody RJ Jr, Herd A, Haber E (1980) Specific inhibition of renin by an angiotensinogen analog: studies in sodium depletion and renin-dependent hypertension. Proc Natl Acad Sci USA 77:5476–5479
Burton J, Slater EE, Corvol P, Ménard J, Hartley LH (1982a) Use of anti-human renin antisera to inhibit renin in primates. Clin Exp Hypertens [A], 4:322–324
Burton J, Cody R Jr, Poulsen K, Hartley LH, Slater EE, Haber E (1982b) The design of specific inhibitors of renin which are active in vivo. In: Yashida Y, Hagihara Y, Ebashi S (eds) Advances in pharmacology and therapeutics, vol 2. Pergamon, London, pp 231–241
Burton J, Hyun H, TenBrink RE (1983) The design of substrate analog renin inhibitors. In: Hruby VB, Rich DH (eds) Peptides: structure and function. Pierce, Rockford, IL, pp 559–567
Campbell DJ (1985) The site of angiotensin production. J Hypertens 3:199–207
Campbell DJ (1987) Circulating and tissue angiotensin systems. J Clin Invest 79:1–6
Carlson W, Handschumacher M, Haber E (1984) Studies of the three-dimensional structure of human renin and its inhibitors. J Hypertens [Suppl 3] 2:S281–S284
Carlson W, Karplus M, Haber E (1985) Construction of a model for the three-dimensional structure of human renal renin. Hypertension 7:199–207
Carlson WD, Handschumacher M, Summers M, et al. (1987) Models for the three-dimensional structure of renin inhibitors bound in the active site of human renin: an analysis of the properties that produce tight binding. J Cardiovasc Pharmacol [Suppl 7] 10:S91–S93
Cody RJ, Burton J, Evin G, Poulsen K, Herd JA, Haber E (1980) A substrate analog inhibitor of renin that is effective in vivo. Biochem Biophys Res Commun 97: 230–235
Corvol P, Ménard J (1986) From the renin gene to renin inhibitors. Ann Endocrinol (Paris) 47:156–166
Corvol P, Michel JB, Evin G, et al. (1983) Inhibition of the renin system at the level of the renin-substrate reaction. Ann Endocrinol (Paris) 44:339–342
Cumin F, Evin G, Fehrentz J-A, Seyer R, Castro B, Ménard J, Corvol P (1985) Inhibition of human renin by synthetic peptides derived from its prosegment. J Biol Chem 260:9154–9157
Cumin F, Nisato D, Gagnol J-P, Corvol P (1987a) A potent radiolabeled human renin

inhibitor, ^{3}H-SR42128:Enzymatic, kinetic, and binding studies to renin and other aspartic proteases. Biochemistry 26:7615–7621

Cumin F, Nisato D, Gagnol J-P, Corvol P (1987b) Binding of a tritiated pepstatin analog to human renin. J Cardiovasc Pharmacol [Suppl 7] 10:S102–S104

Dann JG, Stammer DK, Harris CJ, Arrowsmith RJ, Davies DE, Hardy GW, Morton JA (1986) Human renin: A new class of inhibitors. Biochem Biophys Res Commun 134:71–77

De Clavière M, Fourment P, Richaud JP, Vukovic J, Gagnol J-P, Mague G (1985a) Haemodynamic effects of the renin inhibitor SR 42128 in conscious baboons. J Hypertens [Suppl 3] 3:S271–S273

De Clavière M, Cazaubon C, Lacoure C, Nisato D, Gagnol JP, Evin G, Corvol P (1985b) In vitro and in vivo inhibition of human and primate renin by a new potent renin inhibitor: SR 42128. J Cardiovasc Pharmacol [Suppl 4] 7:S58–S61

DeForrest JM, Waldron TL, Oehl RS, Scalese RJ, Free CA, Weller HN, Ryono DE (1988) Pharmacology of novel imidazole alcohol inhibitors of primate renin. Symposium: Renin Inhibitors—Present and Future, May 28, Osaka

Dellaria JF, Maki RG, Bopp BA, Cohen J, Kleinert HD, Luly JR, Mevits I, et al. (1987) Optimization and in vivo evaluation of a series of small, potent, and specific renin inhibitors containing a novel Leu-Val replacement. J Med Chem 30:2137–2144

Diaz, J (1987) Pepstatin analogs:promising antihypertensive compounds. Drugs Fut 12:1133–1144

Dzau VJ (1985) In vivo inhibition of renin by antirenin antibodies: Potential experimental and clinical applications. J Cardiovasc Pharmacol [Suppl 4] 7:S53–S57

Dzau VJ (1986) Significance of the vascular renin-angiotensin system. Hypertension 8:553–559

Dzau VJ, Kopelman RI, Barger AC, Haber E (1980) Renin-specific antibody for study of cardiovascular homeostasis. Science 207:1091–1093

Dzau VJ, Brenner A, Wolfsohn S, Haber E (1982) Characterization of antibodies to canine renal renin. Studies of interspecies homology of renin using antibodies as probe. Hypertension 4:341–343

Dzau VJ, Devine D, Mudgett-Hunter M, Kopelman RI, Barger AC, Haber E (1983) Antibodies as specific renin inhibitors: Studies with polyclonal and monoclonal antibodies and Fab fragments. Clin Exp Hypertens [A] 5:1207–1220

Dzau VJ, Kopelman RI, Barger AC, Haber E (1984) A comparison of renin specific IgG and Fab in studies of blood pressure regulation. Am J Physiol 246:H404–H409

Eid M, Evin G, Castro B, Ménard J, Corvol P (1981) New renin inhibitors homologous with pepstatin. Biochem J 197:465–471

Epps DE, Mao B, Staples DJ, Sawyer TK (1988) Structure-conformation relationships of synthetic peptide inhibitors of human renin studied by resonance energy transfer and molecular modeling. Int J Pept Protein Res 31:22–34

Evans BE, Rittle KE, Bock MG, Bennett CD, DiPardo RM, Boger J, Poe M, et al. (1985) A uniquely potent renin inhibitor and its unanticipated plasma binding component. J Med Chem 28:1755–1756

Fearon K, Spaltenstein A, Hopkins PB, Gelb MH (1987) Fluoroketones containing peptides as inhibitors of human renin. J Med Chem 30:1617–1622

Fehrentz JA, Heitz A, Castro B (1986) Synthesis of aldehydic peptides inhibiting renin. Int J Pept Protein Res 26(3):236–241

Fix JA, Engle K, Dorter PA, Leppert PS, Selk SJ, Gardner CR, Alexander J (1986) Acylcarnitins: drug absorbtion-enhancing agents in the gastrointestinal tract. Am J Physiol 251:G332–G340

Foundling SI, Cooper J, Watson FE, Cleasby A, Pearl LH, Sibanda BL, Hemmings AM, et al. (1987a) Crystallographic studies of reduced bond inhibitors complexed with an aspartic proteinase. J Cardiovasc Pharmacol [Suppl 7] 10:S59–S68

Foundling SI, Cooper J, Watson FE, Cleasby A, Peral LH, Sibanda BL, Hemmings A, et al. (1987b) High resolution X-ray analyses of renin inhibitor-aspartic proteinase complexes. Nature 327:349–352

Free CA, Ryono DE, Samaniego SG, Neubeck R, Petrillo EW Jr (1985) Potent and selective renin inhibitors based upon substrate analogs containing an aminoalcohol

function. Fed Proc 44 (5964):1431
Galen FX, Devaux C, Atlas S, Guyenne T, Ménard J, Corvol P, Simon D, et al. (1984) New monoclonal antibodies directed against human renin. J Clin Invest 74:732–735
Ganten D, Unger T, Lang RE (1984) Pharmacological interferences with the renin-angiotensin system. Arzneimittelforschung 34(10B):1391–1398
Gardes J, Evin G, Castro B, Corvol P, Ménard J (1980) Synthesis and renin inhibitory properties of a new soluble pepstatin derivative. J Cardiovasc Pharmacol 2:687–698
Greenlee WJ (1988) Renin inhibitors. Pharm Res 4:364–373
Guégan R, Diaz J, Cazamba C, Beaumont M, Carlet C, Clément J, Demorne H, et al. (1986) Pepstatin analogues as novel renin inhibitors. J Med Chem 29:1152–1159
Haber E, Burtonz (1979) Inhibitors of renin and their utility in physiological studies. Fed Proc 338:2768–2773
Haber E (1980) The fifth Volhard lecture. Specific inhibitors of renin. Clin Sci 59:7s–19s
Haber E (1983a) Peptide inhibitors of renin in cardiovascular studies. Fed Proc 42:3155–3161
Haber E (1983b) Inhibitors of renin: Present and future. Clin Exp Hypertens 5:1193–1205
Haber E (1984a) Renin inhibitors. N Engl J Med 311:1631–1633
Haber E (1984b) Potential tools for determing the role of renin in human essential hypertension. J Hypertens [Suppl 1] 2:95–103
Haber E (1984c) The first Sir George Pickering memorial lecture. Which inhibitors will give us true insight into what renin really does? J Hypertens 2:223–230
Haber E (1985a) Defining the physiologic and pathophysiologic roles of renin: the role of specific inhibitors. Am J Kidney Dis 5:A14–A22
Haber E (1985b) Will renin inhibitors influence decision-making in antihypertensive therapy? J Hypertens [Suppl 2] 3:S71–S80
Haber E (1986) Renin inhibitors. Hypertension 8:1093–1095
Haber E, Zusman R, Burton J, Dzau VJ, Barger AC (1983) Is renin a factor in the etiology of essential hypertension? Hypertension 5:V8–V15
Haber E, Hui KY, Carlson WD, Bernatowicz MS (1987) Renin inhibitors: a search for principles of design. J Cardiovasc Pharmacol [Suppl 7] 10:S54–S58
Hallett A, Jones DM, Atrash B, Szelke M, Leckie BJ, Beattie S, Dunn BM, et al. (1985) Inhibition of aspartic proteinases by transition state substrate analogs. In: Kostka V (ed) Aspartic proteinases and their inhibitors. Springer, Berlin Heidelberg New York, pp 467–478
Hanson GJ, Baran JS, Lindberg T, Walsh GM, Papaioannou SE, Babler M, Bittner SE, et al. (1985) Dipeptide glycols: A new class of renin inhibitors. Biochem Biophys Res Commun 132:155–161
Hanson GJ, Baran JS, Lowrie HS, Sarussi SJ, Yang PC, Babler M, Bittner SE, et al. (1987) Enhanced potency dipeptide glycol renin inhibitors: studies in vitro and in the conscious rhesus. Biochem Biophys Res Commun 146:959–963
Hiwada K, Kokubu T, Murakami E, Muneta S, Morisawa Y, Yabe Y, Koike H, Iijima Y (1988) A highly potent and long-acting oral inhibitor of human renin. Hypertension 11:708–712
Hofbauer KG, Wood JM (1984) Inhibition of renin: recent developments. Contrib Nephrol 43:144–152
Hofbauer KG, Wood JM (1985) Inhibition of renin, recent immunological and pharmacological advances. Trends Pharm Sci 6:173–177
Hofbauer KG, Führer W, Heusser C, Wood JM (1985) Comparison of different drug interference with the renin-angiotensin system. J Cardiovasc Pharmacol [Suppl 4] 7:S62–S68
Hui KY, Carlson WD, Bernatowicz MS, Haber E (1987) Analysis of structure-activity relationships in renin substrate analogue inhibitory peptides. J Med Chem 30: 1287–1298
Iizuka K, Kamiya T, Kubota T, Akahane K, Umeyama H, Kiso Y (1988a) New human renin inhibitors containing an unnatural amino acid, norstatine. J Med Chem 31:701–704
Iizuka K, Kamijo T, Kubota T, Akahane K, Harada H, Shimaoka I, Umeyama H, Kiso

Y (1988b) New potent renin inhibitors. In: Shiba T, Sakakibara S (eds) Peptide chemistry 1987. Protein Research Foundation, Osaka, pp 649–652
James MNG, Sielecki AR (1983) Stereochemical analysis of peptide bond hydrolysis catalyzed by the aspartic proteinase penicillopepsin. Biochemistry 24:3701–3713
James MNG, Sielecki AN, Fujinaga M, Muir AK, Murphy MEP, Carilli CT, Shine J (1988) The molecular structure of recombinant human renin. 18th Linderstrøm-Lang Conference on Aspartic Proteinases, July 4–8, Elsinore
Johnson RL (1984) Inhibition of renin by substrate analogue inhibitors containing the olefinic amino acid 5(S)-amino-7-methyl-3(E)-octenoic Acid. J Med Chem 27:1351–1354
Kati WM, Pals DT, Thaisrivongs S (1987) Kinetics of the inhibition of human renin by an inhibitor containing a hydroxyethylene dipeptide isostere. Biochemistry 16:7621–7626
Kay J (1985) Structure and activity of aspartic proteinases. Aspartic proteinases and their inhibitors. Biochem Soc Trans 13:1027–1029
Kempf DJ de Lara E, Stein RH, Cohen J, Plattner JJ (1987) Renin inhibitors based on novel dipeptide analogues. Incorporation of the dehydrohydroxyethylene isostere at the scissile bond. J Med Chem 30:1978–1983
Kleinert HD, Luly JR, Marcotte PA, Perun TJ, Plattner JJ, Stein H (1988a) Renin inhibitors: Improvements in the stability and biological activity of small peptides containing novel Leu-Val replacements. FEBS Lett 230:38–42
Kleinert HD, Martin D, Chekal MA, Kadam J, Luly JR, Plattner JJ, Perun TJ, Luther RR (1988b) Effects of the renin inhibitor A-64662 in monkeys and rats with varying baseline plasma renin activity. Hypertension 11:613–619
Kokubu T, Hiwada K (1987) Human renin inhibitors. Drugs Today 23:101–108
Kokubu T, Hiwada K, Ito T, Ueda E, Yamamura Y, Mitoguchi T, Shigezane K (1973) Peptide inhibitors of renin-angiotensin reaction system. Biochem Pharmacol 22:3217–3223
Kokubu T, Hiwada K, Sato Y, Iwata T, Imamura Y, Matsueda R, Yabe Y, et al. (1984) Highly potent and specific inhibitors of human renin. Biochem Biophys Res Commun 118:929–933
Kokubu T, Hiwada K, Murakami E, Imamura Y, Matsueda R, Yabe Y, Koike H, Iijima Y (1985) Highly potent and specific inhibitors of human renin. Hypertension [Suppl 1] 7:8–11
Kokubu T, Hiwada K, Nague A, Murakami E, Morisawa Y, Yabe Y, Koike H, Iijima Y (1986) Statine-containing dipeptide and tripeptide inhibitors of human renin. Hypertension [Suppl 2] 8:II1–II5
Kokubu T, Hiwada K, Murakami E, et al. (1987) In vitro inhibition of human renin by statine-containing tripeptide renin inhibitor (ES–1005). J Cardiovasc Pharmacol [Suppl 7] 10:S88–R90
Kokubu T, Hiwada K, Murakami E, Muneta S, Morisawa Y, Yabe Y, Koike H, Iijima Y (1988) A highly potent and long-acting inhibitor of human renin-derivative of thiazolylalanine cyclostatine. Clin Exp Hypertens [A] 10:512
Leckie BJ, Szelke M, Hallett A, Hughes M, Lever AF, McIntyre G, Merthen JJ, Tree M (1983) Peptide inhibitors of renin. Clin Exp Hypertens [A] 5:1221–1236
Leckie BJ, Szelke M, Atrash B, Beattie SR, Hallett A, Jones DM, McIntyre GD, et al. (1985) Human renin inhibitors. Biochem Soc Trans 13:1029–1032
Lee VHL (1986) Enzymic barriers to peptide and protein absorption and the use of penetration enhancers to modify absorption. NATO ASI Ser [A] 125:87–104
Liepina I, Nikiforovich GV, Paira ACM (1984) Conformational aspects of angiotensinogen analogues with renin inhibitory activity. Biochem Biophys Res Commun 122:700–705
Luly JR, Plattner JJ, Stein H, Yi N, Soderquist J, Marcotte PA, Kleinert HD, Perun TJ (1987) Modified peptides which display potent and specific inhibition of human renin. Biochem Biophys Res Commun 143:44–51
Luly JR, Bolis G, BaMaung N, Soderquist J, Dellaria JF, Stein H, Cohen J, et al. (1988) New inhibitors of human renin that contain novel Leu-Val replacements. Examination of the P1 site. J Med Chem 31:532–539

Marciniszyn J, Hartsuck JA, Tang J (1976) Mode of inhibition of acid proteases by pepstatin. J Biol Chem 251:7088–7094
Michel J-B, Wood J, Hofbauer K, Corvol P, Ménard J (1984) Blood pressure effects of renin inhibition by human renin antiserum in normotensive marmosets. Am J Physiol 246:F309–F316
Morris BJ (1988) Renin gene and protein structure; sites for renin blockade. Symposium: Renin Inhibitors-Present and Future, May 28, Osaka
Neisius D, Wood JM (1987) Antihypertensive effect of a renin inhibitor in marmosets with a segmental renal infarction. J Hypertens 5:721–725
Nisato D, Lacacer C, Roccon A, Gayvaud R, Cazaubon C, Carlet C, Plouzauc C, et al. (1987a) Discovery and pharmacological characterization of highly potent, picomolar-range, renin inhibitors. J Hypertens [Suppl 5] 5:S23–S25
Nisato D, Wagnon J, Callet G, Mettefeu D, Assens J-L, Plouzauc C, Tonnere B, et al. (1987b) Renin inhibitors. Free-Wilson and correlation analysis of the inhibitory potency of a series of pepstatin analogues on plasma renin. J Med Chem 30:2287–2291
Oldham AA, Arnstein MJA, Major JS, Crough DP (1984) In vivo comparison of the renin inhibitor H 77 with the angiotensin-converting enzyme inhibitor captopril. J Cardiovasc Pharmacol 6:672–677
Omura S, Imamura N, Kawakita K, Yamazaki Y, Masuma R, Takahashi Y, Tamaha H, et al. (1986) Ahpatinins, new acid protease inhibitors containing 4-amino-3-hydroxy-5-phenylpentanoic acid. J Antibiot (Tokyo) 39:1079–1085
Ondetti MB, Cushman DW (1982) Enzymes of the renin-angiotensin system and their inhibitors. Annu Rev Biochem 51:283–308
Pals DT, de Graaf GL, Kati WM, Lawson JA (1985) Cardiovascular effects of a renin inhibitor in relation to posture in nonhuman primates. Clin Exp Hypertens [A] 7:105–121
Pals DT, Thaisrivongs S, Lawson JA, Kati WM, Turner SR, de Graaf GL, Harris DW, Johnson GA (1986) An orally active inhibitor of renin. Hypertension 8:1105–1112
Papaioannou S, Hanson D Jr, Babler M, Yang P-C, Bittner S, Miller A, Clare M (1985a) New class of inhibitors specific for human renin. Clin Exp Hypertens [A] 7:1243–1257
Papaioannou S, Hanson D Jr, Babler M, Yang P-C, Bittner S, Clare M (1985b) New inhibitors specific for human renin. Fed Proc 44 (6487):1520
Pearl L, Blundell T (1984) The active site of aspartic proteinases. FEBS Lett 174:96–101
Plattner JJ, Creer J, Flung AKL, Stein H, Kleinert MD, Skan HL, Smital JR, Perun TJ (1986) Peptide analogues of angiotensinogen. Effect of peptide chain length on renin inhibition. Biochem Biophys Res Commun 139:982–990
Poulsen K, Burton J, Haber E (1973) Competitive inhibitors of renin. Biochemistry 12:3877–3882
Rich DH (1986) Inhibitors of aspartic proteinases. In: Barrett AJ, Salvesen G (eds) Proteinase inhibitors. Elsevier, Amsterdam, pp 129–217
Rosenberg S, Plattner JJ, Wood KJ, Skin HK, Marcotte PM, Cohen J, Perun TJ (1987) Novel renin inhibitors containing analogues of statine retro-inverted at the C-termini: specificity at the P_2 histidine site. J Med Chem 30:1224–1228
Roy P, Delepierre M, Wagnon J, Nisato D, Roques BP (1987) Conformational analysis of pepstatin and related renin inhibitors by 400 MHz ^{1}H N.M.R. spectroscopy. Int J Pept Protein Res 30:44–53
Samani NJ, Swales JD, Brammar WJ (1988) Expression of the renin gene in extrarenal tissues of the rat. Biochem J 253:907–910
Sawyer TK, Pals DT, Mao B, Maggiora LL, Staples DJ, de Vaux AE, Schostarez H, et al. (1988a) Structure-conformation-activity relationships of renin inhibitory peptides having P_1-P_1'XAAψ(CH_2NH)YAA substitutions: molecular modeling and crystallography studies. Tetrahedron 44:661–673
Sawyer TK, Pals DT, Mao B, Staples DJ, deVaux AE, Maggiora LL, Affholter JA, et al. (1988b) Design, structure-activity, and molecular modeling studies of potent renin inhibitory peptides having N-terminal N(In)-For-Trp (Ftr):angiotensinogen congeners modified by P_1-P_1'Phe-Phe, Sta, Leuψ(CH(OH)CH_2)Val or Leuψ(CH_2NH) Val substitutions. J Med Chem 31:18–30

Schölkens BA, Jung W (1974) Renin inhibition by pepstatin in experimental hypertension. Arch Int Pharmacodyn Ther 208:24–34
Serre M, Galindo G, Marion A, et al. (1987) Hemodynamic response to SR 42128A in normal and sodium-depleted baboons. J Cardiovasc Pharmacol [Suppl 7] 10:S99–S101
Sham HL, Rempel C, Plattner JJ, Stein H, Cohen J, Perun TJ (1986) Renin inhibitors: Tripeptides incorporating 2-substituted statine analogs which display potent and specific inhibition of human renin (Abstr 8). 191th American Chemical Society Meeting, New York
Sham HL, Stein H, Rempel CA, Cohen J, Plattner JJ (1987) Highly potent and specific inhibitors of human renin. FEBS Lett 220:299–301
Sham HL, Bolis G, Stein HH, Fesik SW, Marcotte PA, Plattner JJ, Rempel CA, Greer J (1988) Renin inhibitors. Design and synthesis of a new class of conformationally restricted analogues of angiotensinogen. J Med Chem 31:284–295
Skeggs LT, Lentz KE, Kahn JR, Hochstrasser H (1968) Kinetics of the reaction of renin with nine synthetic peptide substrates. J Exp Med 128:13–34
Smith CW, Saneii TK, Pals DT, Scahill TA, Kamdar BV, Lawson JA (1988) Synthesis and renin inhibitory activity of angiotensinogen analogues having dehydrostatine, Leuψ[CH_2S]Val or Leuψ[CH_2SO]Val at the P_1-P_1' cleavge site. J Med Chem 31: 1377–1382
Smith SG, Seymour AA, Mazack EK, Boger J, Blaine EH (1987) Comparison of a new renin inhibitor and enalaprilat in renal hypertensive dogs. Hypertension 9:150–156
Szelke M, Leckie BJ, Hallett A, Jones DM, Sueiras-Diaz J, Atrash B, Lever AF (1982) Potent new inhibitors of renin. Nature 299:555–557
Szelke M, Jones DM, Atrash B, Hallett A, Leckie BJ (1983) Novel transition state analog inhibitors of renin. In: Hruby VJ, Rich DH (eds) Peptides: structure and function. Pierce, Rockford, IL, pp 579–582
Szelke M, Tree M, Leckie BJ, Jones MD, Atrash B, Beattie S, Donovan B, et al. (1985) A transition-state analogue inhibitor of human renin (H 261): test in vitro and a comparison with Captopril in the anaesthetized baboon. J Hypertens 3:13–18
Takaori K, Donowitz M, Burton J (1984) Intact jejunal absorption of a synthetic nonapeptide renin inhibitor. Fed Proc 43 (943):446
Takaori K, Hartley LH, Burton J (1987) Hypotensive effects of the renin inhibitor (RI-78) and the converting enzyme inhibitor (teprotide) in conscious monkeys. Clin Exp Hypertens [A] 9:387–390
TenBrink RE, Pals DT, Harris DW, Johnson GA (1988) Renin inhibitors containing Psi(CH2O)pseudopeptide inserts. J Med Chem 31:671–677
Thaisrivongs S, Pals DT, Kati WM, Turner SR, Thomasco LM (1985) Difluorostatine- and difluorostatone-containing peptides as potent and specific renin inhibitors. J Med Chem 28:1553–1555
Thaisrivongs S, Pals DT, Harris DW, Kati WM, Turner SR (1986a) Design and synthesis of a potent and specific renin inhibitor with a prolonged duration of action in vivo. J Med Chem 29:2088–2093
Thaisrivongs S, Pals DT, Kati WM, Turner SR, Thomasco LM, Watt W (1986b) Design and synthesis of potent and specific renin inhibitors containing difluorostatine, difluorostatone, and related analogues. J Med Chem 29:2080–2087
Thaisrivongs S, Schostarez HJ, Pals DT, Turner SR (1987a) α,α-difluoro-β-aminodeoxystatine-containing renin inhibitory peptides. J Med Chem 30:1837–1842
Thaisrivongs S, Pals DT, Kroll DT, Turner SR, Han F-S (1987b) Renin inhibitors. Design of angiotensinogen transition-state analogues containing novel (2R, 3R, 4R, 5S)-5-amino-3,4-dihydroxy-2-isopropyl-7-methyloctanoic acid. J Med Chem 30:976–982
Thaisrivongs S, Pals DT, Lawson JA, Turner SR, Harris DW (1987c)α-Methylproline-containing renin inhibitory peptides: in vivo evaluation in an anesthetized, ganglion-blocked, hog renin infused rat model. J Med Chem 30:536–541
Thaisrivongs S, Pals DT, Turner SR, Krol LT (1988) Conformationally constrained renin inhibitory peptides: γ-lactam-bridged isosteres as conformational restriction. J Med Chem 31:1369–1376
Tree M, Atrash B, Donovan B, Gamble J, Hallett A, Hughes M, Jones DM, et al. (1983)

New inhibitors of human renin tested in vitro and in vivo in the anaesthetized baboon. J Hypertens 1:399–403
Tree M, Szelke M, Leckie B, Atrash B, Donovan B, Hallett A, Jones DM, et al. (1985) Renin inhibitors: their use in understanding the role of angiotensin II as a pressor hormone. J Cardiovasc Pharmacol [Suppl 4] 7:S49–S52
Umezawa H, Aoyagi T, Morishima M, Matsuzaki M, Hamada M, Takeuchi T (1970) Pepstatin, a new pepsin inhibitor produced by actinomycetes. J Antibiot (Tokyo) 23:259–262
Waeber B, Nussberger J, Brunner HR (1986) What have we learned about inhibitors of renin angiotensin system? Ann Endocrinol (Paris) 47:167–177
Webb DJ, Cumming AMM, Leckie BJ, Level AF, Morton JJ, Robertson JIS, Szelke M, Donovan B (1983) Reduction of blood pressure in man with H-142, a potent new renin inhibitor. Lancet 2:1486–1487
Webb DJ, Manhem PJO, Ball SG, Inglis GI, Leckie BJ, Lever AF, Morton LJ, et al. (1985) A study of the renin inhibitor H142 in man. J Hypertens 3:653–658
Webb DJ, Manhem PJO, Ball SG, Inglis GI, Leckie BJ, Lever AF, Morton LJ, et al. (1987) Clinical and biochemical effects of the renin inhibitor H142 in humans. J Cardiovasc Pharmacol [Suppl 7] 10:S69–S74
Wolfenden R (1976) Transition state analog inhibitors and enzyme catalysis. Annu Rev Biophys Bioeng 5:271–306
Wood JM, Gulati N, Forgiarini P, Führer W, Hofbauer KG (1985) Effects of a specific and long-acting renin inhibitor in the marmoset. Hypertension 7:797–803
Wood JM, Heusser C, Gulati N, Forgiarini P, Hofbauer KG (1986) Monoclonal antibodies against human renin. Blood pressure effects in the marmoset. Hypertension 8:600–605
Wood JM, Baum H-P, Jobber RA, Neisius D (1987a) Sustained reduction in blood pressure during chronic administration of a renin inhibitor to normotensive marmosets. J Cardiovasc Pharmacol [Suppl 7] 10:S96–S98
Wood JM, Jobber RA, Baum H-P, Hofbauer KG (1987b) Comparison of chronic inhibition of renin and converting enzyme in the marmoset. Clin. Exp Hypertens [A] 9:337–343
Wood JM, Stanton JL, Hofbauer KG (1987c) Inhibitors of renin as potential therapeutic agents. J Enzyme Inhib 1:169–185
Wood JM, Whitfield SL, Baum H-P, Jobber RA (1988) Effects of chronic administration of a renin inhibitor on renin-like activity in marmoset tissues (Abstr 1313). 12th Scientific Meeting of the International Society of Hypertension, May 22–26, Kyoto

CHAPTER 12

Prostaglandins

G. SCHRÖDER, R. GRYGLEWSKI, J. MEHTA, and G. STOCK

CONTENTS

1 Introduction

Arachidonic acid (AA) is converted by different mammalian enzymes to a variety of prostaglandins, thromboxanes, prostacyclin, and leukotrienes. Products of the AA metabolic pathway contribute to the regulation of circulatory (cardiovascular) homeostasis as well as to the pathogenesis of several conditions, such as thrombotic disorders, Bartter's syndrome, asthma, and inflammation. This review will focus on the impact of AA products on mechanisms of blood pressure regulation, such as renal function and vascular tone. The contribution of AA products to the pathogenesis of primary hypertension will be discussed.

2 Nomenclature of Arachidonic Acid Metabolites

The existence of biologically active prostaglandins was first described by VON EULER (1934, 1935) and GOLDBLATT (1935) in the early 1930s. In human prostatic tissue, in human semen, in sheep semen and vesicular glands they found a smooth muscle stimulating factor which lowered blood pressure.

As prostatic tissue was believed to be the main source of this compound VON EULER (1935) proposed the name prostaglandin.

The work of BERGSTRÖM et al. (1962a,b, 1963a,b), SAMUELSSON (1963, 1964a,b) and others in the 1960s led to the identification of the chemical structure of primary prostaglandins. These are 20-carbon unsaturated carboxylic acids containing a cyclopentane ring and two aliphatic side chains (Fig. 1). The substituents on the cyclopentane ring distinguish the main classes as denoted by the final capital letter; figures indicate the number of double bonds per molecule (e.g., prostaglandin E_2 has two double bonds in the side chains and PGE_1 has one).

In addition to the primary prostaglandins the endoperoxides PGG_2 and PGH_2, the bicyclic prostacyclin (PGI), and thromboxanes (TXA and TXB), have been described as products of the AA metabolic pathway (NUGTEREN and HAZELHOF 1973; HAMBERG and SAMUELSSON 1973, 1974; JOHNSON et al. 1976; HAMBERG et al. 1975).

In 1974, SAMUELSSON and colleagues discovered another pathway for AA metabolism. Products of this pathway were named leukotrienes because they were initially found in leukocytes (SAMUELSSON 1983). Leukotrienes do not possess a ring structure; they contain a conjugated triene system and can be divided into groups (A-F) according to their major structural differences (see Fig. 1).

A third pathway, first described in 1981 by OLIW and colleagues, leads to epoxides and 19- and 20-HETEs (hydroxyeicosatetraenoic acids, see Fig. 1).

3 Eicosanoid Synthesis and Metabolism

Eicosanoids are not stored intracellularly, rather they are generated rapidly from free fatty acids after an appropriate stimulus, which can be hormonal, neuronal, immunological, and/or chemical. After biosynthesis they exert their effects and are quickly metabolised. For these reasons eicosanoids have been termed local or tissue hormones or autacoids. Their physiological role seems to be that of a local modulator.

Eicosanoid synthesis begins with the liberation of 20-carbon polyunsaturated fatty acids derived from phospholipids stored in membrane tissue. The fatty acid precursors of the three main series of AA are dihomo-γ-linolenic acid (precursor of the 1 series), eicosapentanoic acid (precursor of the 3 series), and eicosatetraenoic acid or arachidonic acid, which is the precursor for the 2 series. The physiological relevance of the 1 series is largely unknown; products of the 3 series are known for their potential antithrombotic effects.

This review will mainly focus on arachidonic acid, as the main and most important precursor of prostaglandins and leukotrienes (Fig. 2). The key enzyme which liberates AA is phospholipase A_2, which can be pharmacologically blocked by glucocorticoids (GRYGLEWSKI et al. 1975). In addition to

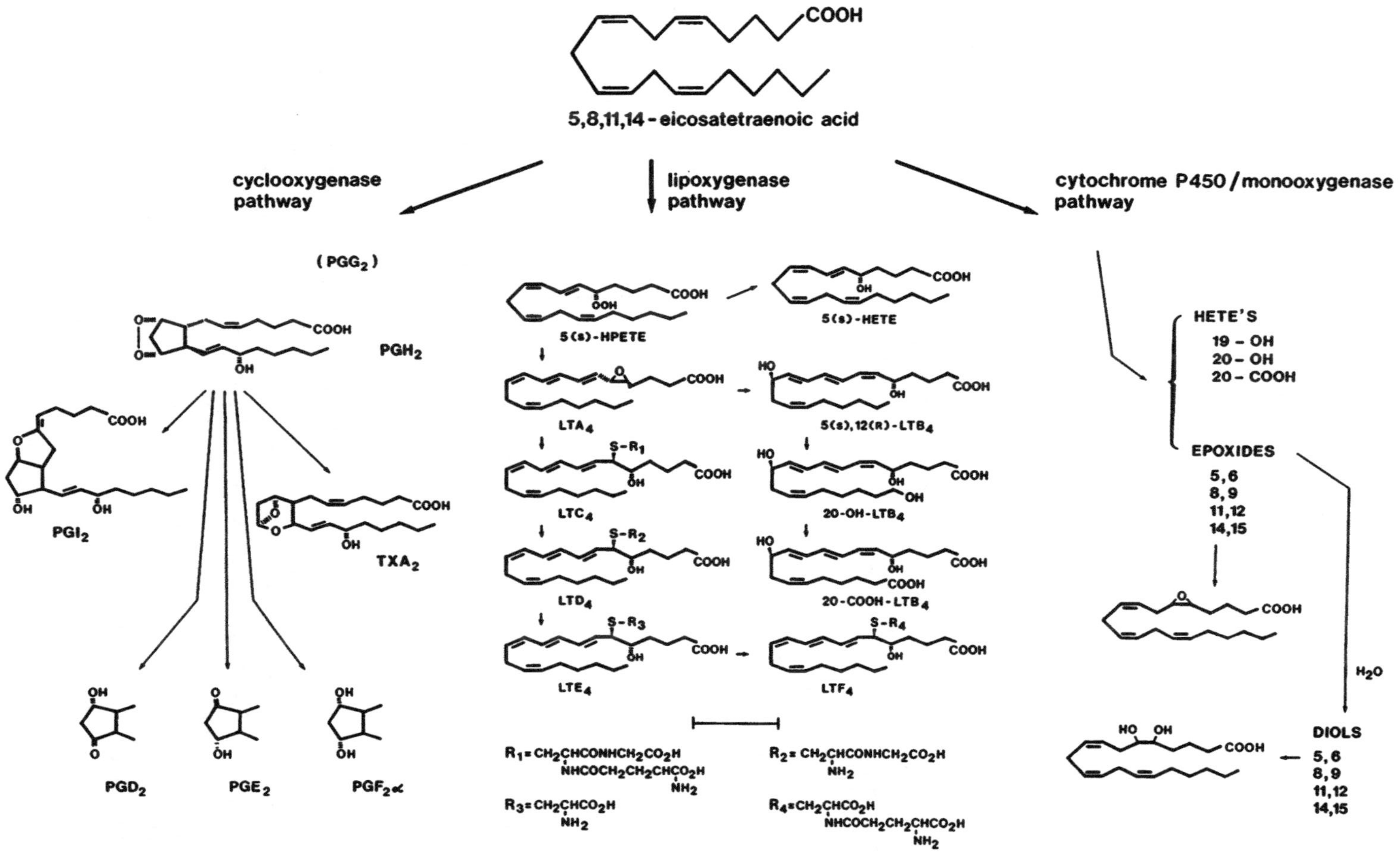

Fig. 1. Eicosanoid nomenclature: principle products of the cyclo-oxygenase, lipoxygenase, and cytochrome P-450 monooxygenase pathways. *PG*, prostaglandin; *HETE*, hydroxyeicosa tetraenoic acid; *HPETE*, hydroperoxyeicosatetraenoic acid; *LT*, leukotriene; *TX*, thromboxane

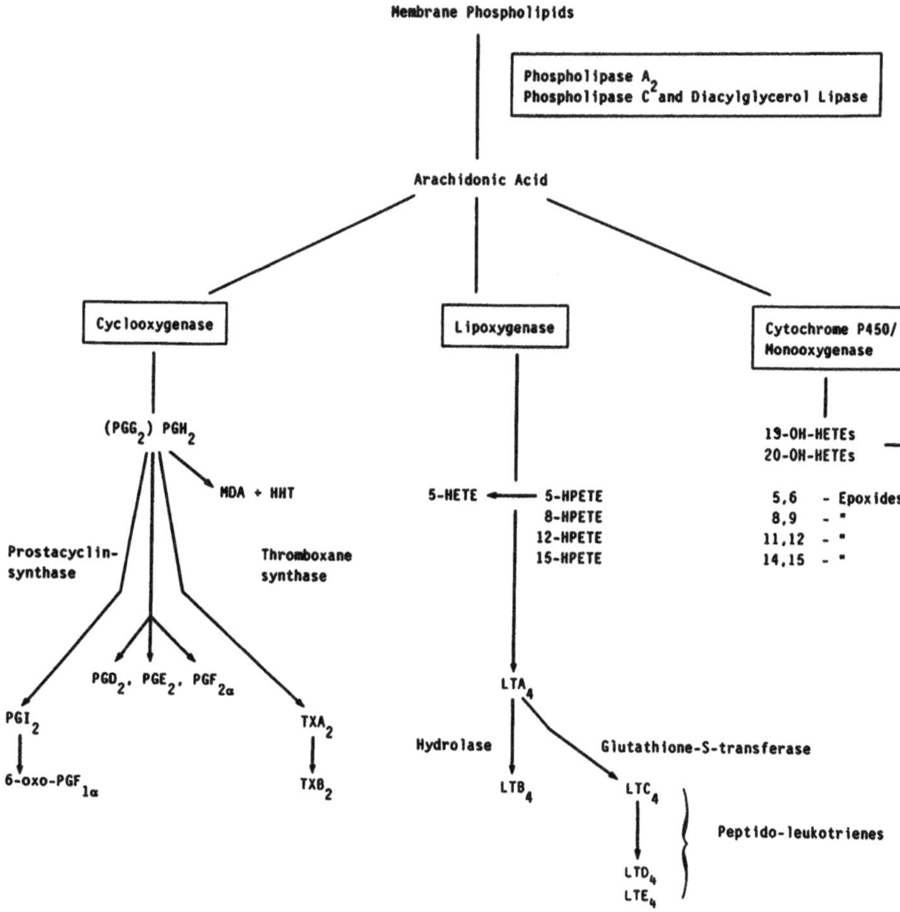

Fig. 2. Pathways of arachidonic acid metabolism. Three major pathways of eicosanoid formation are shown: cyclooxygenase, lipoxygenase, and cytochrome P450/monooxygenases. *PG*, prostaglandin; *TX*, thromboxane; *MDA*, malondialdehyde; *HHT*, hydroxyacid; *LT*, leukotriene; *HETEs*, hydroxyeicosatetraenoic acids; *HPETEs*, hydroperoxyeicosatetraenoic acids

phospholipase A_2, phospholipase C in collaboration with diacylglycerol lipase liberates AA. Metabolism of AA involves two main pathways, the cyclooxygenase and the lipoxygenase; both enzymatic pathways can be inhibited pharmacologically. Cyclooxygenase is blocked by nonsteroidal antiinflammatory agents e.g., aspirin, indomethacin, ibuprofen, phenylbutazone, and sulindac. Frequently described lipoxygenase inhibitors include BW 755C, nafrazatom, AA 861, and piroprost (HAMBERG 1976; HIGGS et al. 1979; RANDALL et al. 1980; MARDIN and BUSSE 1983; YOSHIMOTO et al. 1982; BACH et al. 1982) (Fig. 3).

Cyclooxygenase catalyses the formation of the unstable endoperoxides PGG_2 and PGH_2 from which primary prostaglandins, PGI_2, TXA_2, a C_{17}-hydroxy fatty acid (HHT), and malondialdehyde (MDA) are formed enzymatically or non-

Cyclooxygenase inhibitors:

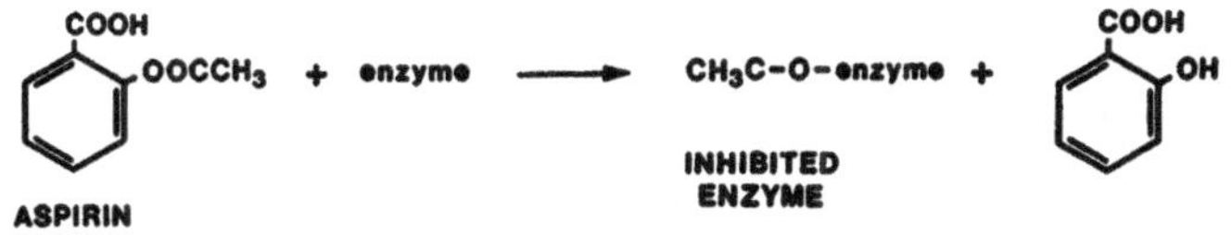

ASPIRIN

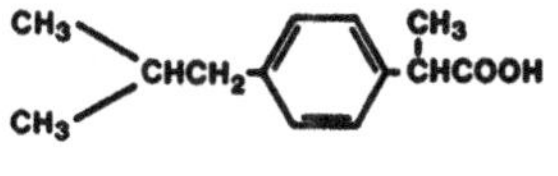

IBUPROFEN

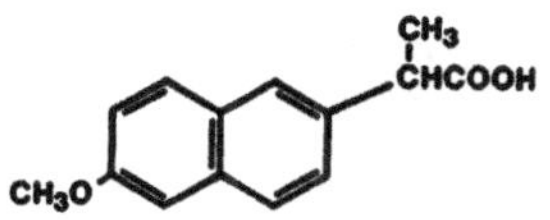

NAPROXEN

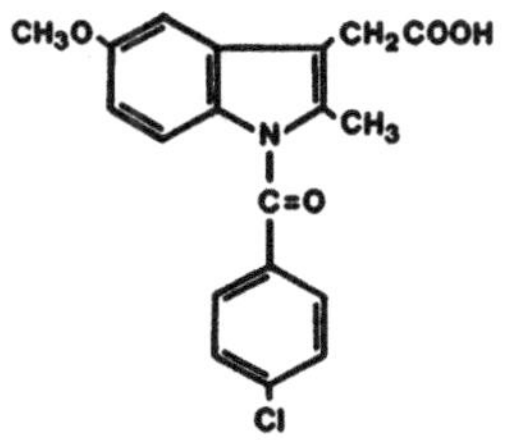

INDOMETHACIN

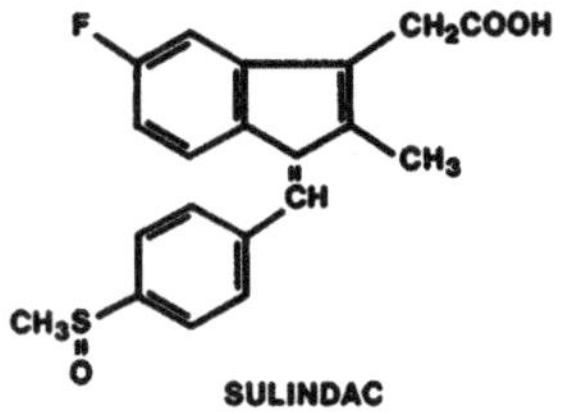

SULINDAC

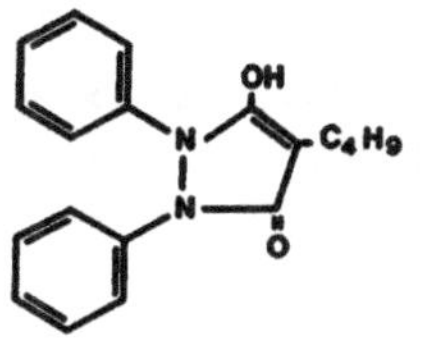

PHENYLBUTAZONE

Five-lipoxygenase inhibitors:

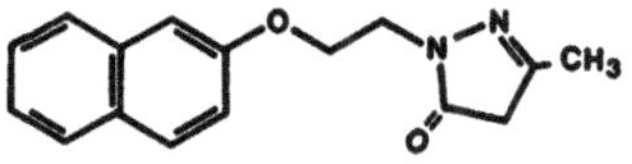

NAFAZATROM

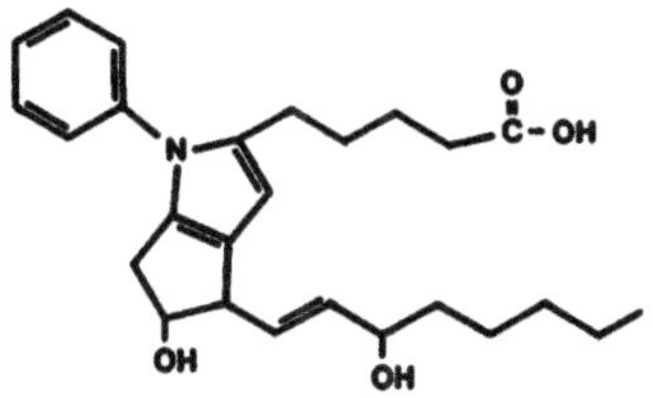

PIROPROST

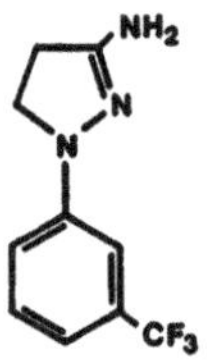

BW 755C

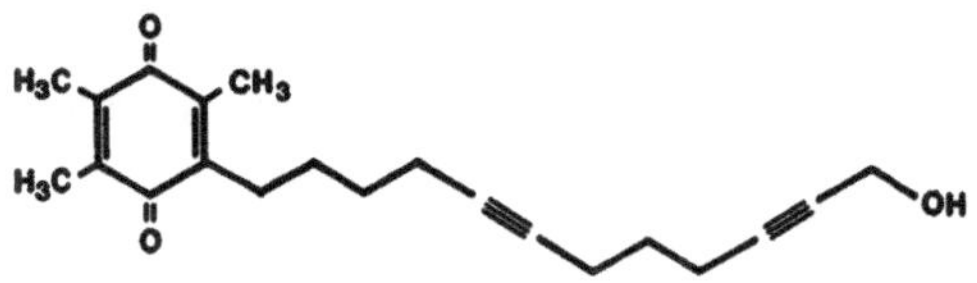

AA 861

Fig. 3. Structures of some compounds which inhibit cyclooxygenase or 5-lipoxygenase. The compounds are either relatively specific inhibitors of cyclooxygenase or 5-lipoxygenase or dual inhibitors of both enzymes enzymatically (see Fig. 2). The metabolites formed vary from cell to cell: blood platelets convert AA to TXA_2 whereas vascular endothelium mainly produces PGI_2.

The biological half-lives of PGI_2 and TXA_2 are very short (approx. 5 min and 3 s, respectively); normally they are hydrolysed to 6-keto-$PGF_{1\alpha}$ and TXB_2, respectively.

The lipoxygenase enzymes convert the fatty acid into hydroperoxyderivatives (hydroperoxyeicosatetraenoic acids, HPETEs), which are reduced to the corresponding hydroxyacids (HETEs) by glutathione peroxidase. Activity of 5- and 12-lipoxygenases has been described in biological tissues. The 5-hydroperoxy derivative, 5-HPETE is the most interesting, because it can be converted to the biologically active compounds known as leukotrienes (NUGTEREN 1975; BORGEAT et al. 1976). 5-HPETE is dehydrated to leukotriene A_4 (LTA_4), which is then hydrolysed to leukotriene B_4 (LTB_4) (BORGEAT and SAMUELSSON 1979a,b) by LTA_4 hydrolase. LTA_4 can be nonenzymatically transformed to 5,12- and 5,6-dihydroxyacids (BORGEAT and SAMUELSSON 1979a; see Fig. 2).

Under the influence of glutathione S-transferase, LTA_4 can react with glutathione. The reaction product is leukotriene C_4 (LTC_4), which then can be metabolized to leukotriene D_4 (LTD_4) and leukotriene E_4 (LTE_4) (MORRIS et al. 1980a,b). LTC_4, LTD_4, and LTE_4 are so-called peptidolipid leukotrienes, also known as "slow reacting substance of anaphylaxis" (SRS-A; BROCKLEHURST 1962; see Fig. 2).

As with prostaglandins, the different leukotrienes are formed in specific cell types. Human eosinophils and neutrophils synthesize LTC_4 and LTB_4, respectively, whereas monocytes and macrophages are able to produce LTB_4 and the peptidolipid leukotrienes (WELLER et al. 1983; SAMUELSSON 1983; see Fig. 2).

4 Arachidonic Acid Products and the Control of Blood Pressure

Blood pressure is determined by cardiac output and peripheral resistance. Because normally approximately 20% of cardiac output passes through the kidneys, renal vascular resistance is a major factor determining total peripheral resistance. Indeed, a reduction in renal blood flow, related to renal vasoconstriction, is among the early abnormalities in essential hypertension. In addition to renal hemodynamics the endocrinological and excretory functions of the kidney play important roles in blood pressure regulation. AA metabolites may be involved in blood pressure controlling mechanisms that regulate:

a) renal circulation and renal function;
b) endocrinological systems, such as the kallikrein-kinin system which opposes the pressor effects of the renin-angiotensin system;
c) the release of vasodilatory AA metabolites from the vascular wall, which alter smooth muscle response to pressor stimuli and may exert some vasoprotective effect by affecting endothelial cell function.

The following sections will deal with these three aspects.

4.1 Eicosanoids and the Kidney

4.1.1 Arachidonic Acid Metabolism in the Kidney

There are three enzymatic pathways involved in the renal synthesis of AA metabolites which include cyclooxygenase (DUNN and HOOD 1977; MCGIFF 1981), lipoxygenase (JIM et al. 1982; SRAER et al. 1983), and cytochrome P-450 monooxygenase (MORRISON and PASCOE 1981; OLIW et al. 1981). Cyclooxygenase converts AA into PG G_2 and PGH_2, which are enzymatically converted to PGE_2, $PGF_{2\alpha}$, PGD_2, PGI_2, and thromboxane A_2 (TXA_2). The renal medulla has a tenfold greater capacity to produce prostaglandins than the renal cortex (LARSSON and ÄNGGARD 1973; SHENG et al. 1983).

Lipoxygenase enzyme converts AA into HPETEs, which are then reduced to the corresponding to HETEs. Lipoxygenase activity is also greater in the renal medulla. Cytochrome P-450 monoxygenase has been described in the rabbit renal cortex, and activation of this enzyme leads to the generation of trihydroxyeicosatetraenoic acids formed via Ω- and (Ω-1)-hydroxylation of the di-HETEs (OLIW et al. 1981).

4.1.2 Renal Circulation

Infusion of AA into the renal arteries of rabbits and dogs causes a biphasic flow response (early vasoconstriction followed by vasodilatation) and a redistibution of blood flow towards the inner cortex; this effect can be blocked with cyclooxygenase inhibitors, thereby showing that these responses are a result of its conversion to vasoactive prostaglandins (DI BONA 1986).

Administration of certain endproducts of AA metabolism causes renal vasodilation and redistribution of blood flow ($PGI_2 > PGE_2 > PGD_2$). Intrarenal administration of $PFG_{2\alpha}$ and TXA_2 analogues causes the opposite effect, i.e., renal vasoconstriction, but no redistribution of cortical blood flow (DI BONA 1986; MAKHOUL and GEWERTZ 1986).

The effect of exogenous prostaglandins, however, may not reflect their physiological actions. Further evidence of a role for endogenously synthesised prostaglandins in the regulation of renal blood flow (RBF) has been provided by experiments using cyclooxygenase inhibitors. However, these studies are controversial: in some experiments these drugs caused an increase in RBF while in others they did not.

These results led many authors to conclude that in the stressed animal (e.g., anesthesia, hypovolemia, or major surgery) with states in which the activities of the renin-angiotensin system and the sympathoadrenal systems are increased, prostaglandins are necessary to counteract the ensuing vasoconstriction (GROENE and DUNN 1985; TERRAGNO et al. 1977; MAKHOUL and GEWERTZ 1986).

The role of lipoxygenase products in the regulation of renal blood flow is less clear. Peptido- LTC_4 administration to rats and pigs reduces RBF (DATA et al. 1978). LTC_4- and LTD_4-induced renal vasoconstriction can be blocked by LT-receptor antagonists.

Peptido-LTs have been shown to stimulate prostaglandin and TXA_2 synthesis and release in many organs (FEUERSTEIN et al. 1981; CRAMER et al. 1983;

WARGOVICH et al. 1985; SIMONSON and DUNN 1986); however, cyclooxygenase inhibition does not modify LT-induced vasoconstriction (WARGOVICH et al. 1985; SIMONSON and DUNN 1986). Recent studies show that LTC_4 and LTD_4 contract rat glomerular mesangial cells (SIMONSON and DUNN 1986). Whether renal tissues per se generate LTs is not yet settled.

Other lipoxygenase products generated in the kidney, such as HETEs, may be important in autoregulation of RBF as they are known inhibitors of PGI_2 synthetase (TURK et al. 1980; HAM et al. 1979). 15-HPETE may regulate medullary blood flow by inhibiting synthesis of vasodilator PGI_2 (MORRISON et al. 1982). It is noteworthy that HETEs and LTs are formed in the activated monocytes and polymorphonuclear leukocytes in large amounts, and immune injury to the glomerulus results in infiltration of these cell types. Leukocytes are necessary in lowering the ultrafiltration coefficient in glomerular injury (TUCKER et al. 1985), and this effect may be mediated via release of the lipoxygenase and cyclooxygenase products of AA metabolism.

The NADPH-dependent cytochrome P-450 monooxygenase present in the renal cortex also metabolizes AA (OLIW et al. 1981). Although the precise effects of this pathway of AA metabolism on renal hemodynamics are not clear, some studies suggest that inhibition of P-450 enzymes as well as lipoxygenase blocks the initial renal arterial constriction seen following AA infusion into the anaesthetized dog, suggesting that this part of the AA response may relate to conversion of AA to hydroxylated eicosanoids (FEIGEN 1984).

4.1.3 Eicosanoids and the Renin-Angiotensin System

The mechanisms known to control renin secretion are:

a) the intrarenal baroreceptor in the afferent arteriole;
b) the macula densa mechanism in the juxtaglomerulosa cells;
c) the intrarenal β-receptor.

Arachidonic acid, prostaglandin endoperoxides (WEBER et al. 1976), PGA_1, PGA_2 (ATALLAH and LEE 1982; HORNYCH 1978), PGE_1 (WERNING et al. 1971), PGE_2, PGD_2, prostacyclin (ABE 1981; BOLGER et al. 1978; PACE-ASCIAK 1980; SCHÖLKENS 1978; SEYMOUR et al. 1979), and, finally, 6-keto-PGE_1, (JACKSON et al. 1981; MCGIFF et al. 1982) all have been claimed to release renin from the kidney in either in vivo or in vitro experiments.

Although the glomeruli of the renal cortex are capable of synthesising a number of cyclooxygenase products (KONIECZKOWSKI et al. 1983; REMUZZI et al. 1978), some of which influence renin release by indirect mechanisms such as changes in blood flow, natriuresis, hemodynamic, and osmotic pressure changes, most researchers would agree that PGI_2 and PGE_2 directly stimulate renin release (BEIERWALTES et al. 1982). In fact, the most potent renin secretagogue is 6-keto-PGE_1, a stable, biologically active product of the biotransformation of PGI_2 (JACKSON et al. 1981; MCGIFF et al. 1982). Some researchers assume that the renin-stimulating effect of PGI_2 is not secondary to its metabolism to 6-keto-PGE_1 (SCHWERTSCHLAG et al. 1982) as has been proposed by MCGIFF and his colleagues (JACKSON et al. 1981; McGIFF et al. 1982). An interesting concept has been put forward that PGI_2 (or 6-keto-PGE_1) not only stimulates renin release but is also responsible for the proteolytic conversion of inactive renin to its active form through PGI_2-induced mobilization of the renal kallikrein system (OHDE et al. 1982).

Cyclooxygenase inhibitors such as indomethacin decrease basal plasma renin levels and inhibit the renin release induced by orthostasis, renal artery clamping, dietary hyponatremia, and furosemide (ATALLAH and LEE 1982; CHAN and CERVONI 1985; GERBER et al. 1979; JACKSON et al. 1982; PATAK et al. 1975; WEBER 1978; YLITALO et al. 1978). In patients with essential hypertension, indomethacin or captopril, an angiotensin-converting enzyme inhibitor, decrease angiotensin II plasma levels. However, indomethacin induces a significant rise in blood pressure whereas captopril is strongly hypotensive (ABE et al. 1980).

To determine via which mechanisms prostaglandins interact with the renin system, a series of studies was performed to isolate the various mechanisms of renin release. These studies indicated that the renal baroreceptor and the macula densa mechanism involve prostaglandin synthesis to release renin (DATA et al. 1978).

Since the isoprenaline-induced increase in plasma renin activity is not blocked by indomethacin and indomethacin lowers plasma renin activity in the presence of β-adrenergic receptor antagonists (OATES et al. 1979), renin release following β-receptor stimulation is independent of the prostaglandin system.

$PGF_{2\alpha}$ has been reported to decrease renin release in a dose-dependent manner (WEBER et al. 1976). A role of TXA_2 in renin release has not yet been elucidated. However, it may well be that an increased local generation of TXA_2, e.g., in a hydronephrotic kidney (ALBRIGHTSON et al. 1987) or in the kidneys of elderly patients (BAUD et al. 1983), exacerbates the reduction in renal perfusion by causing vasospasm and platelet aggregation, thereby increasing production of renin by the ischemic kidney (FITZGERALD and FITZGERALD 1984). In humans the urinary excretion of TXB_2 (2,3-dinor-TXB_2 has not been investigated) is not responsive to vasoactive hormones that increase urinary excretion of PGE_2 (ZIPSER and SMORLESI 1984).

A role of lipoxygenase products in renin release is not yet clear. Cultured phagocytosing rat glomerular mesangial cells generate superoxide anions, hydrogen peroxide, and lipid peroxides including 12-HPETE, 15-HPETE, and the corresponding monohydroxyacids (BAUD et al. 1983). In human, rat, and murine glomeruli, 12-HETE and 15-HETE are the major products of lipoxygenation of arachidonic acid (BAUD et al. 1983; HASSID et al. 1982; SRAER et al. 1983; WONG et al. 1987). The biosynthesis of LTs occurs only during the interaction of glomeruli and neutrophils of genetically hypertensive rats (WONG et al. 1987).

LTC_4, LTD_4, as well as LTB_4 have no effect on the PGI_2-induced release of renin from slices of rat kidney (ANTONIPILLAI et al. 1987). In this preparation 12-HPETE, 15-HPETE, and the corresponding monohydroxyacids are potent inhibitors of renin release (ANTONIPILLAI et al. 1987).

Cells of the renomedullary thick ascending limb of the loop of Henle contain a cytochrome P-450-dependent enzyme which transforms arachidonic acid to a series of epoxyeicosatrienoic acids (EETs), e.g., 5,6-EET. These epoxides are Na^+/K^+-ATPase inhibitors and vasorelaxants, and their generation is augmented in arterial hypertension (CHIBA et al. 1984). Perhaps this cytochrome P-450-dependent pathway of arachidonic acid metabolism acts as a common mechanism responsible for natriuresis evoked by endogenous "natriuretic factors" and by drugs. However, a direct effect (if any) of these monooxygenase products on renin release has not yet been investigated, and it is unlikely to occur because of the site of their generation.

Platelet-activating factor (PAF-acether) stimulates calcium-dependent activity of both phospholipase A_2 and a phosphatidylinositol-specific phospholipase C in renal epithelial cells, and, thus, PAF-acether enhances the biosynthetic capacity of prostanoids in the kidney (KAWAGUCHI and YASUDA 1986). In the perfused rat kidney these cyclooxygenase products act as vasoconstrictors which counteract the powerful direct vasodilatory effect of PAF-acether on the renal vasculature. PAF-acether, by an unknown mechanism, inhibits selectively the vasoconstrictor action of angiotensin II and stimulates renin release from the kidney, perhaps as a consequence of the PAF-acether-induced drop in renal perfusion pressure (SCHWERTSCHLAG et al. 1987).

It might seem a paradox that the product of enzymatic activity of renin (angiotensin I) and the product of its further enzymatic conversion (angiotensin II) are both potent stimulators of the release of PGI_2 or PGE_2 from the kidney (AIKEN and VANE 1973; GRYGLEWSKI et al. 1980; NEEDLEMAN et al. 1973), from the lung (GRYGLEWSKI et al. 1980), from strips of renal and femoral arteries (SATOH et al. 1984), from perfused mesenteric artery (DESJARDINS-GIASSON et al. 1982; GRODZINSKA and GRYGLEWSKI 1980), and from the cerebral circulation, but not from the hindquarters of dogs, cats, and rats (AIKEN and VANE 1973; GRYGLEWSKI et al. 1980). The PGI_2-releasing effect of angiotensin I is abolished by captopril (GRYGLEWSKI 1979). There must exist an unknown biological "servomechanism" which down-regulates the functioning of this apparent vicious cycle: PGI_2—renin—angiotensin I—angiotensin II—PGI_2. This unknown regulatory mechanism might be out of order in patients with Bartter's syndrome, in whom overproduction of prostanoids coexists with high plasma renin and aldosterone levels, hypokalemia, hypotension, and a suppressed pressor responsiveness to exogenous angiotensin II (WEBER 1978). On the other hand, vasodilatory prostanoids which attenuate the vasoconstrictor-antidiuretic action of angiotensin II must play an important role in protecting the kidney and possibly other organs against ischemic damage by endogenous vasoconstrictors (MCGIFF et al. 1970; MCGIFF and QUILLEY 1982).

Among the biologically active peptides (ZUSMAN and KEISER 1977), not only angiotensin II (AIKEN and VANE 1973) and vasopressin (WALKER et al. 1978) but also bradykinin (MCGIFF and NASJETTI 1976) are the potent stimulators of PGI_2 and PGE_2 release from the kidney, most likely through activation of acylhydrolases which liberate arachidonic acid from phospholipids (COOPER et al. 1985; SCHWARTZMAN et al. 1981). There exists a major difference between mechanisms of angiotensin II-induced and bradykinin-induced renal output of PGI_2. The first depends on intracellular calcium and calmodulin and the second one operates on a calcium/calmodulin-independent principle (COOPER et al. 1985). The PGI_2-releasing activity of angiotensin I is blocked by captopril, an inhibitor of angiotensin-converting enzyme and of kininase II (GRYGLEWSKI et al. 1980; MULLANE et al. 1980). Captopril has been shown to increase urinary excretion of PGE_2 (ABE et al. 1981; HORNYCH 1980), renal secretion of PGI_2 (MULLANE et al. 1980), and the release of PGI_2 into the blood of anesthetized cats, although in patients with essential hypertension captopril did not increase the urinary excretion of either 6-keto-$PGF_{1\alpha}$ or TXB_2 (VLASSES et al. 1983). Apart from this last finding the other data are in line with a concept of a unique bidirectional coupling of the kallikrein-kinin and prostanoid systems within the renal parenchyma (MCGIFF and NASJLETTI 1976; MCGIFF and QUILLEY 1982). The interaction between angiotensin II and prostanoids might be of importance for maintaining the tone of the renal vasculature (BJORO 1985), for platelet aggregation (SHEBUSKI and AIKEN 1980), central regulation of blood pressure (SCHÖLKENS et al. 1979), and modification by prostanoids of angiotensin II receptors in renal tubule cells (SIMPSON and GOODFRIEND 1984). Moreover, in stress situations the renin-angiotensin system supercedes the kallikrein-kinin system in determining the level of activity of renal prostaglandins (TERRAGNO et al. 1977).

4.1.4 Eicosanoids and the Kallikrein-Kinin System

MCGIFF and coworkers (1975; MCGIFF and NASJLETTI 1976) have discovered that the intrarenal activity of prostaglandins is regulated primarily by the kallikrein-kinin system, at least in the basal state. Renal prostanoids enhance the vasodilator-diuretic action of kinins (MCGIFF et al. 1975). When kinins are infused into the renal artery, the prostanoids level increases both in urine (FRÖLICH et al. 1975) and in venous blood (MCGIFF et al. 1970). Positive correlations have been found between PGE_2 and renin activity in renal venous blood as well as PGE_2 and kallikrein levels in urine (NASJLETTI et al. 1978). Changes in renal generation of PGI_2 are better reflected by an altered efflux of either 6-keto-$PGF_{1\alpha}$ or metabolites of PGI_2 into renal venous blood rather than by excretion of 6-keto-$PGF_{1\alpha}$ in urine (WONG et al. 1978). Unlike PGI_2, primary prostaglandins are effectively taken up by the lung. Their 13,14-dihydro-15-keto metabolites have relatively long biological half-lives, and changes in plasma levels of these metabolites may be indicative of alterations in the biosynthesis of prostaglandins.

The interstitial medullar cells, glomeruli, renal blood vessels, tubular and the collecting duct lining cells have a large capacity to generate prostanoids (KONIECZKOWSKI et al. 1983; SMITH and WILKIN 1977). However, the conditions in the distal nephron and the collecting duct are those most favorable for the kinin-prostaglandin interaction. PGE_2 released by kinins in the distal nephron contributes to the regulation of medullary blood flow, affects salt transport, and amplifies the effects of kinins on renal function (MCGIFF and QUILLEY 1982). Kinins release prostanoids through a calcium/calmodulin independent mechanism (COOPER et al. 1985) via the activation of renal phospholipases (SCHWARTZMAN et al. 1981). In addition, kinins have been claimed to activate renal and vascular 9-ketoreductase, an enzyme which not only converts PGE_2 to $PGF_{2\alpha}$

but also transforms PGI_2 to 6-keto-PGE_1 (HAM et al. 1979). This last prostaglandin is a potent renin releaser (TURK et al. 1980; HAM et al. 1979), and, thus, a complex network of renal interactions between kinins, angiotensin II, and prostanoids is likely to operate (ABE et al. 1980; Fig. 4).

4.1.5 Renal Excretory Function

The effect of prostaglandins on sodium and water excretion have been studied intensively. Many contradictory and confusing results have been obtained, but from some in vitro studies there is good evidence for a direct inhibitory effect of prostaglandins on NaCl transport distal to the proximal tubule (STOKES 1982).

PGE_2 seems to inhibit NaCl reabsorption in the medullary thick ascending limb of the loop of Henle and in the cortical and medullary collecting tubule. Urea absorption in the collecting tubule is decreased by PGE_2 (ROMAN and LECHENE 1981). In the isolated collecting tubule, PGE_2 can reduce the osmotic water permeability induced by vasopressin (LEVY 1977; SOLEZ et al. 1974). LTB_4 seems to amplify PGE_2-induced renal effects.

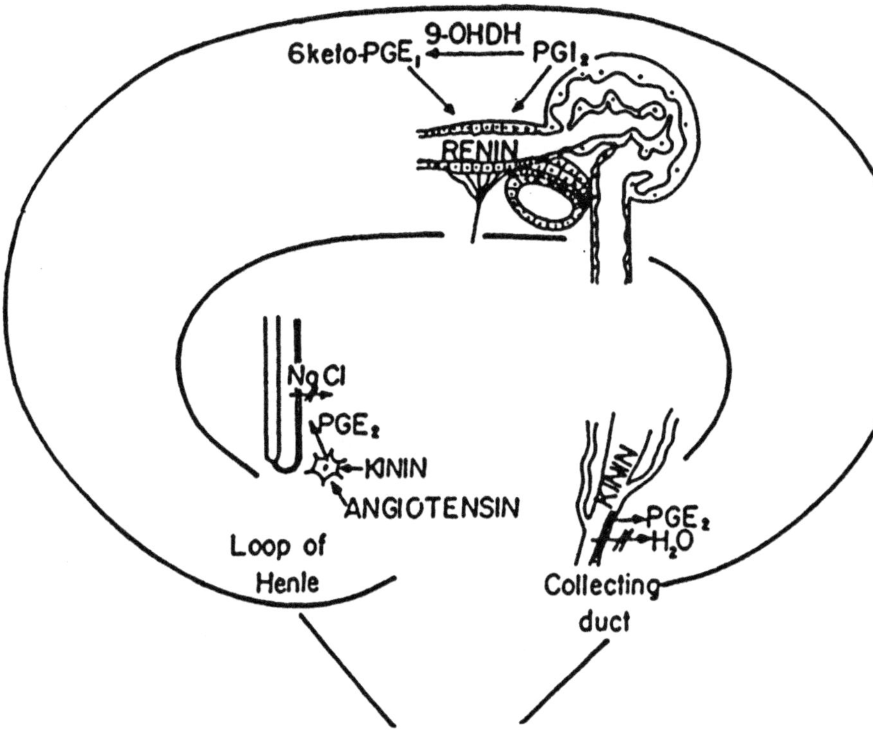

Fig. 4. Intrarenal prostaglandin (*PG*) actions and interactions with the kallikrein-kinin system and the renin-angiotensin system. Three major targets for renal PG activity are illustrated: the medulla and the loop of Henle on the *left side*, the juxtaglomerulosa apparatus in the *center*, and the distal nephron and the collecting duct on the *right side* (*9-OHDH*, 9-OH-prostaglandin dehydrogenase (from McGIFF 1981)

4.2 Eicosanoids and the Vascular Wall

4.2.1 Generation of Eicosanoids by the Vessel Wall

4.2.1.1 In Vitro Data

PGI_2 is the main product of AA cyclooxygenation, generated via PGH_2 by aortic microsomes (BUNTING et al. 1976; GRYGLEWSKI et al. 1975) and released from native and cultured aortic endothelial cells (GRYGLEWSKI et al. 1986a). The PGI_2-generating capacity diminishes across the arterial wall from intima to adventitia. There are profound differences in the amount of PGI_2 generated by various vascular beds in various mammalian species. Primary prostaglandins including PGE_2 (GRYGLEWSKI et al. 1986a; PIPILI and POYSER 1982) and PGD_2 (GERRITSEN 1983) as well as TXA_2 (BRUNKWALL et al. 1987; NERI et al. 1983) might also be released from blood vessels. Interestingly, the products of AA lipoxygenation, e.g., 15-HETE (LARRUE et al. 1985), LTB_4, and peptide LTs (PIPER and GALTON 1984), are also claimed to be produced by arteries. Vascular smooth muscle cells metabolize 12-HETE from platelets to 8-hydroxyhexadecatrienoic acid, whose biological activity is as yet unknown (HADJIAGAPIOU et al. 1987). Finally, a cytosolic lipoxygenase in endothelial cells converts linoleic acid to 13-hydroxyoctadienoic acid (13-HODE), which, in contrast to its AA-derived relatives (e.g., 15-HETE), has platelet-suppressant and chemorepellent properties.

In vitro studies performed in the arteries of animals fed atherogenic or vitamin E-deficient (CHAN and LEITH 1981) diets have shown that the PGI_2 synthetic capacity is decreased and plasma lipid peroxides increased (OKUMA et al. 1980).

In arteries of rats with spontaneous or experimentally induced hypertension, the generation of PGI_2 is enhanced (KONIECZKOWSKI et al. 1983; MOTOMIYA and YAMAZAKI 1981; PACE-ASCIAK et al. 1978; PIPILI and POYSER 1982; UEHARA et al. 1987), probably as a reflection of intravascular stress. This is brought about by the increased activity of both arterial phospholipase C and PGI_2 synthetase (UEHARA et al. 1987). A proposed explanation for the increased capacity to generate PGI_2 is to regard it as a compensatory arterial mechanism to blunt the elevated blood pressure in hypertensive animals (MOTOMIYA and YAMAZAKI 1981). These findings have been challenged by the results of SOMA and colleagues (1985) who reported a reduced production of PGI_2 in the perfused mesenteric vascular bed of spontaneously hypertensive rats.

4.2.1.2 In Vivo Data

The data obtained from in vitro experiments on PGI_2 synthesis rate in vessels especially from hypertensive animals are difficult to reconcile with data obtained from in vivo experiments.

FALARDEAU et al. (1985), by measuring urinary levels of 2,3-dinor-6-keto-$PGF_{1\alpha}$ in spontaneously hypertensive and Wistar-Kyoto normotensive rats, have shown that hypertensive rats do not produce more PGI_2 in vivo than normotensive rats. Using a similar approach in patients with low- and high-renin essential hypertension, FRÖHLICH et al. (1985) reached a similar conclusion. Although patients with high-renin hypertension excrete significantly more PGI_2 metabolite than do patients with low-renin hypertension, the urinary excretion of the PGI_2 metabolite in none of the hypertensive group was significantly different from that in normotensive subjects. A discrepancy between in vivo and in vitro data may reflect the fact that the urinary excretion of 2,3-dinor-6-keto-$PGF_{1\alpha}$ represents total turnover of body PGI_2 (including lungs, veins, leukocytes, macrophages, etc.) whereas we are really interested in the arterial generation of PGI_2.

4.2.2 Endothelial Cells in Hypertension

In recent years the role of the endothelial cell layer in blood vessels has been elucidated. It is regarded as a cell layer functioning both as a barrier involved in fluid and substrate exchange as well as having high synthetic activity for regulatory compounds such as PGI_2, EDRF (Endothelium derived relexing factor), tissue plasminogen activator, and most likely also for compounds with trophic functions such as EDGF (Endothelium derived growth factor).

There have been studies implicating the endothelial cell in pathophysiology. Especially in hypertension, enhanced permeability of arterial endothelium has been shown (PEACH and LOEB 1987).

During the acute phase of hypertension, hyperplasia of the endothelial cells occurs, whereas during sustained hypertension, hypertrophy of the cells with a tight homocellular junction is observed. Endothelium may also contribute to the increased smooth muscle mass or cell number. As will be shown later, there is evidence of altered prostaglandin synthesis and metabolism in endothelial cells derived from hypertensive animals. In addition, endothelial uptake or metabolism of noradrenaline and serotonin is increased during hypertension.

Functional studies have shown that the aortic contractile response to aggregating platelets is markedly enhanced in hypertensive rats. Response to endothelium-dependent vasodilators (acetylcholine, ionophore A23187, ADP) is impaired in both acute and in chronic hypertension, suggesting functional impairment in the endothelium (LÜSCHER and VANHOUTTE 1986; MILLER et al. 1987).

There is also evidence that not only impaired vasodilatation but also the release of constrictor substances contributes to the development and maintenance of hypertension. Upon stimulation with acetylcholine there is release of a constricting factor which is blocked by inhibition of cyclooxygenase. There is evidence that this factor is TXA_2 (Table 1). It is as yet unknown to what extent the recently discovered peptidergic endothelial derived constricting factor (YANNAGISAWA et al. 1988) is involved in this mechanism.

4.2.3 Cell-Cell Interactions in Relation to the Pathogenesis of Hypertension

In the intact animal blood flow to various organs is distributed according to a integrated activation of neurohumoral and local metabolic mechanisms. These include the production of local metabolites derived from the endothelial cell and smooth muscle cell but also from platelets and leucocytes. This synergism of

Table 1. Evidence for abnormalities in prostaglandin (PG) synthesis/release in essential hypertension

1. Decreased urinary excretion of PGE_2 and 6-keto-$PGF_{1\alpha}$
2. Increased urinary excretion of TXB_2
3. Increased plasma PGE_2
4. Increased renal systemic vascular resistance after nonsteroidal antiinflammatory drugs (NSAIDs)
5. Increase in blood pressure in hypertensive patients and normal subjects after NSAIDs
6. Attenuation of response to antihypertensive agents (diuretics, β-blockers, and converting enzyme inhibitors) after NSAIDs
7. Reduction in blood pressure by polyunsaturated fatty acids

local regulators—probably as yet underestimated—in their role for pathophysiological events in the circulation, especially the microcirculation will be addressed in the following section.

Degradation of EDRF and PGI_2 released from endothelial cells presumably involves neutrophil-derived oxygen free radicals (for EDRF) and HETEs (Turk et al. 1980; Ham et al. 1979; Gryglewski et al. 1986a,b). Endothelium becomes dysfunctional following temporary renal occulsion most likely related to the entry of neurophils (Mehta et al. 1988). Loss of synthesis of endothelium-derived vasodilators along with an increased vascular content of noradrenaline and serotonin may render the renal bed less sensitive to naturally occurring EDRF-dependent as well as EDRF-independent vasodilators. On the other hand, the vascular bed may exhibit enhanced sensitivity to peptido-LTs, serotonin, and other vasoconstrictors.

Activation of the lipoxygenase pathway with release of HETEs, particularly 12-HPETE from the renal medulla (Oliw and Oates 1981), is a potent stimulus for neutrophil chemotaxis and generation of LTs and 5-HETE (MacLouf et al. 1982). Peptido-LTs may then cause reduction in blood flow, and 5-HETE formation may accelerate the degradation of PGI_2. Selective TXA_2 inhibitors shunt accumulated cyclic endoperoxides to PGI_2 formation in neutrophils (Mehta et al. 1983) with subsequent reduction in neutrophil oxidative burst, chemotaxis, and LTB_4 formation. These observations may relate in part to the beneficial effect of TXA_2 synthetase inhibitors in animal models of hypertension.

Leukocytes also activate platelets, and this activation is mediated via peptido-LTs and release of oxygen free radicals. LTs ($LTE_4 > LTD_4 > LTC_4$) enhance the proaggregatory effects of subthreshold concentrations of adrenaline on platelets and cause release of TXA_2 with complete platelet aggregation (Mehta et al. 1986). This phenomenon can be prevented by selective TXA_2-synthetase or receptor blockers, but not by LT-receptor antagonists. In the arterial bed, peptido-LTs and TXA_2 analogues synergistically reduce blood flow (Nichols et al. 1988). This effect can also be blocked by TXA_2-synthetase inhibitors.

Recent studies from our laboratory indicate that peptido-LTs in very small concentrations significantly enhance the contractile effect of adrenaline and noradrenaline, but not of KCl or serotonin, on isolated rat aortic rings (Fig. 5; Lawson et al. 1986). Similar potentiation between peptido-LTs and α-agonists

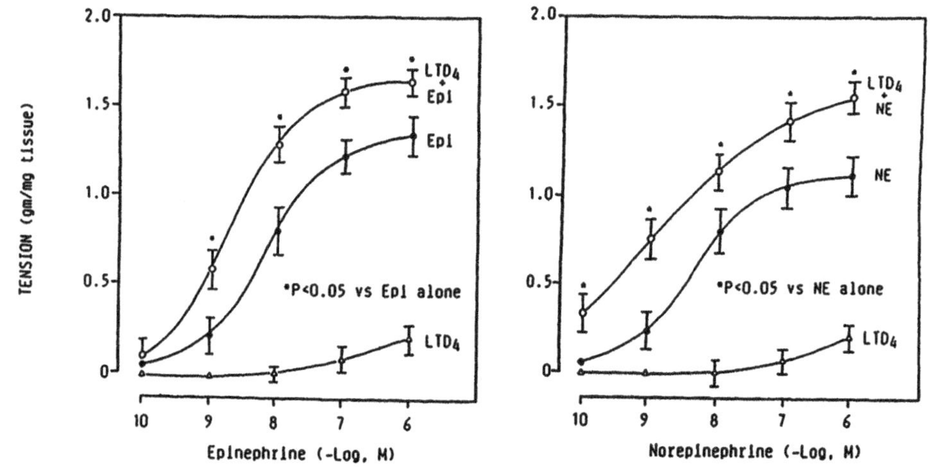

Fig. 5. Potentation of the contractile effects of adrenaline and noradrenaline by pretreatment of rat aortic rings by leukotriene (LTD_4) ($10^{-7} M$). Note that LTD_4 itself had very mild contractile effects on rat aorta. (From MEHTA et al. 1987)

or TXA_2 may occur in renal vessels, resulting in perpetuation and progression of hypertension.

The effects to LTs on the aorta appear to be endothelium-dependent. In the presence of endothelium, peptido-LTs can cause relaxation of precontracted aortic rings, presumably via release of EDRF. In contrast, in the absence of endothelium, LTs cause additional contraction of precontracted aortic rings (MEHTA et al. 1987).

It is believed that forthcoming research on the regulation of vascular tone will present clear evidence that vascular tone and vascular function, especially of small vessels, is determined more by an integration of various cellular interactions ("micromilieu") than by the impact of one or two major factors, such as sympathetic tone, alone. In this context the metabolites of the arachidonic acid pathways may have an important impact. Especially in the initiation phase of vascular disorders such as ischemic events but also hypertension, disturbances of the cell-cell interaction, imbalances of the "micromilieu" might be of significance. They may lead to regional, localised vascular dysfunction, thereby inducing a series of compensatory tropic events. If uninterrupted, such a sequence of events will eventually lead to permanent maladaptation. Early arteriosclerotic alterations could be explained by interactions between endothelial cells, platelets, leukocytes, and smooth muscle cells as proposed by R. Ross in his theory on the genesis of arteriosclerosis (ROSS and GLOMSET 1976). Such a mechanism would of course also be operative in aggravating atherosclerotic alterations. It has to be tested whether this hypothesis holds true in clinical practice and whether this sequence of events can be effectively interrupted by interfering with AA metabolism or by substituting e.g., prostacyclin or stable analogues thereof.

5 Effects of Antihypertensive Drug Therapy on Arachidonic Acid Metabolism

Several recent studies indicate a reduction in blood pressure following dietary supplementation with Ω-3 polyunsaturated fatty acids (eicosapentanoic acid), which modulate prostaglandin synthesis in favor of vasodilator PGs. In addition, such diets also reduce formation of LTs of the 4-series and de novo formation of relatively inactive LTs of the 5-series in conjunction with reduction in serum lipid concentrations. These trials suggest that modulation of AA metabolism at several steps may have a salutary effect by influencing the function of several cell types involved in hypertension and probably also in arteriosclerosis.

The antihypertensive potency of β-blockers, e.g., propanolol, has been shown to be attenuated by indomethacin. Mepindolol, a β-blocker with intrinsic sympathomimetic activity, stimulates the synthesis of PGI_2 in guinea pig hearts, and probably more importantly the inactivation of released PGI_2 was retarded after mepindolol (Kahlen and Schrör 1982).

Application of ACE inhibitors leads to an increase in the levels of kinins which again stimulate phospholipase A_2 activity and thereby lead to an increase of prostaglandin synthesis. In fact, several authors have shown an increase in prostaglandins in kidney and plasma during the course of therapy with ACE inhibitors. The finding that concomitant treatment with indomethacin diminished the effect of ACE inhibitors on blood pressure in hypertensive patients clearly supports this concept.

6 Conclusions

Prostanoids (i.e., products of cyclooxygenation of arachidonic acid) have a longer record of experimental and clinical studies concerning their role in arterial hypertension than the lipoxygenase and monooxygenase products (i.e., hydroxyeicosatetraenoic and epoxyeicosatrienoic acids, 13-hydroxyoctadecadienoic acid, leukotrienes, and lipoxins). Vascular endothelium generates vasodepressor prostanoids such as prostacyclin and PGE_2. The biosynthesis of prostacyclin is inhibited by lipid peroxides, hydrogen peroxide, and hydroxyl radicals. It seems that, in several types of arterial hypertension, a compensatory mechanism augments the generation of vasodepressor prostanoids, although obviously not to such an extent as to overcome the prevailing vasopressor mechanisms. Prostacyclin and EDRF decrease vascular resistance through two different biochemical mechanisms, i.e., the stimulation of receptors associated with membrane-bound adenylate cyclase and activation of the heme center in cytosolic soluble guanylate cyclase, respectively. Renal function is intimately modulated by eicosanoids, including the regulation of blood flow, natriuresis, activity of Na^+/K^+-ATPase, renin and kallikrein release, especially under the stress of ischemia or hypertension. The complex network of interrelationships between the opposing actions of PGE_2, prostacyclin, 6-keto-PGE_1, and 5,6-epoxyeicosatrienoic acid on the one hand and thromboxane A_2, leukotrienes, and lipoxins on the other will require more study, as will the role of eicosanoids in the functioning of the renin-angiotensin-aldosterone and kallikrein-kinin systems. A consensus is expected to be reached on the significance of a deficiency in renal vasodepressor prostanoids in primary hypertension with low and high plasma renin activity. Nonetheless, even given the present stage of knowledge, it seems reasonable to assume that synthetic analogues of prostacyclin and PGEs, the clinical usefulness of which has been justified by their effect on peripheral vascular resistance, will also serve as a valuable supplement in kidneys of patients with arterial hypertension. Although there is evidence that the antihypertensive drugs currently used in clinical practice also have important effects of AA metabolism which could explain—to a certain degree—their clinical efficacy, there is no conclusive evidence as yet that derivatives of AA metabolites (or stable analogues) would be clinically relevant antihypertensive drugs per se.

However, given that the role of eicosanoids is best defined in cell-cell interactions, in maintaining the integrity of a vascular micromilieu (vide supra), it is conceivable that eicosanoid agonists or antagonists have a considerable impact on the functional and morphological maladaptation seen in the early and late phases of the hypertension disease process. Arteriosclerotic lesions, renal dysfunction, and local circulatory disorders, which occur as primary or secondary events in the course of hypertension, could be regarded as primary targets for drugs mimicking (e.g., PGI_2, PGE, PGD analogues) or antagonizing (e.g., TXA_2, LT antagonists) eicosanoid functions. Hence it is conceivable to assume that drugs of this kind could gain clinical importance as adjuncts to standard antihypertensive drug therapy.

Summary

Arachidonic acid (AA)-metabolites of three different pathways (cyclooxygenase, lipoxygenase, and P_{450}monooxygenase) are supposed to be involved in blood pressure controlling mechanisms. Renal hemodynamics as one major determinant of blood pressure are regulated by PGI_2 and primary prostaglandins when the activity of the renin-angiotensin system and the sympathoadrenal system is increased.

In addition to renal hemodynamics, endocrinological systems of the kidney such as the renin-angiotensin system and the opposing kallikrein-kinin system are under the control of AA metabolites. PGI_2, 6-keto-PGE_1 (a stable, biologically active product of the biotransformation of PGI_2), and PGE_2 directly stimulate renin release. A series of studies indicate that the renal baroreceptor and the macula densa mechanism involve PG synthesis to release renin whereas renin release following β-receptor stimulation is independent of the PG system.

In addition to the regulation of renal hemodynamics and endocrinological functions of the kidney, there is good evidence for a direct inhibitory effect of PGE_2 on renal excretory functions in the loop of Henle and the collecting tubule.

Products of AA cyclooxygenation and lipoxygenation have been found in vascular cells. Release of vasodilatory AA metabolites from the vascular wall is increased under hypertensive conditions, probably in order to alter smooth muscle response to pressor stimuli. TXA_2 and products of the lipoxygenase pathway exert some vasocontricting activity and enhance the contractile response to pressor stimuli.

The potency of some antihypertensive agents (e.g. β-blockers, angiotensin converting enzyme inhibitors) is diminished by indomethacin, a cyclooxygenase inhibitor.

References

Abe K (1981) The kinins and prostaglandins in hypertension. Clin Endocrinol Metab 3:577

Abe K, Ito T, Sato M, Haruyama T, Sato K, Omata K, Hiwatari M, Sakurai Y, Imai Y, Yoshinaga K (1980) Role of prostaglandins in the antihypertensive mechanism of captopril in low renin hypertension. Clin Sci Mol Med 59:141S–144S

Abe K, Sato M, Imai Y, Haruyama T, Sato K, Hiwatari M, Kasai Y, Yoshinaga K (1981) Renal kallikrein-kinin: its relation to renal prostanglandins and renin-angiotensin-aldosterone in man. Kidney Int 19:869–880

Aiken JW, Vane JR (1973) Intrarenal prostaglandin release attenuates the renal vasoconstrictor activity of angiotensin. J Pharmacol Exp Ther 184:678–687

Albrightson CR, Evers AS, Griffin AC, Needleman P (1987) Effect of endogenously produced leukotrienes and thromboxane on renal vascular resistance in rabbit hydronephrosis. Circ Res 61:514–522

Antonipillai I, Robin EC, Nadler JL, Horton R (1987) Dual regulatory role of prostaglandins and lipoxygenase products on renin secretion. In: Samuelsson B, Paoletti R, Ramwell PW (eds) Advances in prostaglandin, thromboxane, and leukotriene research, vol 17B. Raven, New York, p 733

Atallah AA, Lee JB (1982) Prostaglandins, renal function and blood pressure regulation. In: Lee JB (ed) Prostaglandins. Elsevier, New York, p 251

Bach MK, Brashler JR, Smith HW, Fitzpatrick FA, Sun FF, McGuire JC (1982) 6,9-deepoxy-6,9-(phenylimino)-^{6,8}-prostaglandin I_1, (U-60,257), a new inhibitor of leukotriene C and D synthesis: in vitro studies. Prostaglandins 23:759–771

Baud L, Hagege J, Sraer J, Rondeau E, Perez J, Ardaillou R (1983) Reactive oxygen production by cultured rat glomerular mesangial cells during phagocytosis is associated with stimulation of lipoxygenase activity. J Exp Med 158:1836–1852

Beierwaltes WH, Schryver S, Sanders E, Strand J, Romero JC (1982) Renin release selectively stimulated by prostaglandin I_2 in isolated rat glomeruli. Am J Physiol 243:F276–F283

Bergström S, Dressler F, Krabisch L, Ryhage R, Sjövall J (1962a) The isolation and structure of a smooth muscle stimulating factor in normal sheeps and pig lungs. Ark Kemi 20:63–66

Bergrström S, Ryhage R, Samuelsson B, Sjövall J (1962b) The structure of prostaglandin E, F_1 and F_2. Acta Chem Scand 16 (2):501–528

Bergström S, Danielsson H, Samuelsson B (1963 a) The enzymatic formation of prostaglandin E_2 from arachidonic acid: prostaglandins and related factors, 32. Biochim Biophys Acta 90:207–210

Bergström S, Ryhage R, Samuelsson B, Sjövall J (1963 b) Prostaglandins and related factors: the structures of prostaglandin E_1, F_1a and F_1. J Biol Chem 238:3555–3564

Bjoro K Jr (1985) Effects of angiotensin I and II and their interactions with some prostanoids in perfused human umbilical arteries. Prostaglandins 30:989–998

Bolger PM, Eisner GM, Ramwell PW, Slotkoff LM, Corey EJ (1978) Renal actions of prostacyclin. Nature 271:467–469

Borgeat P, Samuelsson B (1979a) Arachidonic acid metabolism in polymorphonuclear leukocytes: unstable intermediate in formation of dihydroxy acids. Proc Natl Acad Sci USA 76:3213–3217

Borgeat P, Samuelsson B (1979b) Transformation of arachidonic acid by rabbit polymorphonuclear leukoctyes: formation of a novel dihydroxyeicosatetraenoic acid. J Biol Chem 254:2643–2646

Borgeat P, Hamberg M, Samuelsson B (1976) Transformation of arachidonic acid and homo-linolenic acid by rabbit polymorphonuclear leukocytes: monohydroxy acids from novel lipoxygenases. J Biol Chem 251:7816–7820

Brocklehurst WE (1962) Slow-reacting substance and related compounds. Prog Allergy 6:539–558

Brunkwall J, Bergqvist, Sjernquist U (1987) Prostacyclin and thromboxane release from the vessel wall—comparison between an incubation and a perfusion model. Prostaglandins 34:467–476

Bunting S, Gryglewski R, Moncada S, Vane JR (1976) Arterial walls generate from prostaglandin endoperoxides a substance (Prostaglandin X) which relaxes strips of mesenteric and coeliac arteries and inhibits platelet aggregation. Prostaglandins 12: 897–913

Chan PS, Cervoni P (1985) Hypertension. In: Cohen MM (ed) Biological protection with prostaglandins. CRC, Boca Raton

Chan AC, Leith MK (1981) Decreased prostacyclin synthesis in vitamin E-deficient rabbit aorta. Am J Clin Nutr 34:2341–2347

Chiba S, Abe K, Kudo K, Omata K, Yasujima M, Sato K, Seino M, Imai Y, Sato M, Yoshinaga K (1984) Sex and age-related differences in the urinary excretion of TXB_2 in normal human subjects: a possible pathophysiological role of TXA_2 in the aged kidney. Prostaglandins Leukotrienes Med 16:347–358

Cooper CL, Shaffer JE, Malik KU (1985) Mechanism of action of angiotensin II and bradykinin in prostaglandin synthesis and vascular tone in the isolated rat kidney. Circ Res 56:97–108

Cramer EB, Pologe L, Pawloski NA, Cohn ZA, Scott WA (1983) Leukotriene C_4 promotes prostacyclin synthesis by human endothelial cells. Proc Natl Acad Sci USA 80:4109–4113

Data JL, Gerber JG, Crump WJ, Frölich JC, Hollifield JW, Nies AS (1978) The prostaglandin system: a role in canine baroreceptor control of renin release. Circ Res 42:454–458

Desjardins-Giasson S, Gutkowska J, Garcia R, Genest J (1982) Effect of angiotensin II and norepinephrine on release of prostaglandins E_2 and I_2 by the perfused rat mesenteric artery. Prostaglandins 24:105–114

Di Bona G (1986) Prostaglandins and non-steroidal anti-inflammatoty drugs. Am J Med 80:12–21

Dunn MJ, Hood VL (1977) Prostaglandins and the kidney. Am J Physiol 233:F169–F184

Falardeau P, Robillard M, Martineau A (1985) Urinary levels of 2,3-dinor-6-oxo-PGF_1 alpha: a reliable index of the production of PGI2 in the spontaneously hypertensive rat. Prostaglandins 29:621–628

Feigen LP (1984) Influence of renal lipoxygenase activity on the renal vascular response to arachidonic acid. J Pharmacol Exp Ther 228:140–146

Feuerstein N, Foegh M, Ramwell PW (1981) Leukotrienes C_4 and D_4 induce prostaglandin and thromboxane release from rat peritoneal macrophages. Br J Pharmacol 72:389–391

Fitzgerald GA, Fitzgerald DJ (1984) Biosynthesis of thromboxane A_2 in renovascular hypertension. JAMA 251:3121–3122

Frölich JC, Wilson TW, Sweetman BJ, Smigel M, Nies AS, Carr K, Watson JT, Oates JA (1975) Urinary prostaglandins—identification and origin. J Clin Invest 55:763–770

Frölich JC, Filep J, Yoshizawa M, Förstermann U, Fejes-Toth G (1985) Role of eicosanoids in regulation of blood pressure. In: Hayaishi O, Yamamoto S (eds) Advances in prostaglandin, thromboxane, and leukotriene research, vol 15. Raven New York, pp 455–460

Gerber JG, Keller RS, Nies JA (1979) Prostaglandins and renin release. Circ Res 44: 796–809

Gerritsen ME (1983) PGD_2 formation in the vasculature: characteristics of rat tail vein prostaglandin endoperoxide—Disomerase. Prostaglandins 25:105–120
Goldblatt MW (1935) Properties of human seminal plasma. J Physiol (Lond) 84:208–218
Grodzinska L, Gryglewski RJ (1980) Angiotensin-induced release of prostacyclin from perfused organs. Pharmacol Res Commun 12:339–347
Groene HJ, Dunn MJ (1985) The role of prostaglandins in arterial hypertension: a critical review. Adv Nephrol 14:241–272
Gryglewski RJ (1979) Prostacyclin as a circulatory hormone. Biochem Pharmacol 28: 3161–3166
Gryglewski RJ, Panczenko B, Korbut R, Grodzinska L, Ocetkiewicz A (1975) Corticosteroids inhibit prostaglandin release from perfused mesenteric blood vessels of rabbit and from perfused lungs of sensitized guinea pig. Prostaglandins 10:343–355
Gryglewski RJ, Splawinski J, Korbut R (1980) Endogenous mechanisms that regulate prostacyclin release. In: Samuelsson B, Ramwell PW, Paoletti R (eds) Advances in prostaglandin and thromboxane research, vol 7. Raven, New York, pp 777–787
Gryglewski RJ, Moncada S, Palmer RMJ (1986 a) Bioassay of prostacyclin and endothelium derived relaxing factor (EDRF) from porcine aortic endothelial cells. Br J Pharmacol 87:685–694
Gryglewski RJ, Palmer RMJ, Moncada S (1986 b) Superoxide anion is involved in the breakdown of endothelium-derived vascular relaxing factor. Nature 320:454–460
Hadjiagapiou C, Sprecher H, Kaduce TL, Figard PH, Spector AA (1987) Formation of 8-hydroxyhexadecatrienoic acid by vascular smooth muscle cells. Prostaglandins 34: 579–589
Ham EA, Egan RW, Soderman DD, Gale PA, Kuehl FA (1979) Peroxidase-dependent deactivation of prostacyclin synthetase. J Biol Chem 254:2191–2194
Hamberg M (1976) On the formation of thromboxane B_2 and 12L-hydroxy-5,8,10,14-Eicosatetraenoic acid (12 ho-20:4) in tissues from the guinea pig. Biochim Biophys Acta 431:651–654
Hamberg M, Samuelsson B (1973) Detection and isolation of an endoperoxide intermediate in prostaglandin biosynthesis. Proc Natl Acad Sci USA 70:899–903
Hamberg M, Samuelsson B (1974) Prostaglandin peroxides VII. Novel transformations of arachidonic acid in guinea pig lung. Biochem Biophys Res Comun 61:942–949
Hamberg M, Svensson J, Samuelsson B (1975) Prostaglandin endoperoxides: Novel transformations of arachidonic acid in human platelets. Proc Natl Acad Sci USA 71:3400–3404
Hassid AH, Sun F, Dunn MS (1982) Lipoxygenase activity in rat kidney glomeruli, glomerular epithelial cells and cortical tubules. J Biol Chem 257:1024S–1029S
Higg GA, Flower RJ, Vane JR (1979) A new approach to anti-inflammatory drugs. Biochem Pharmacol 28:1959–1961
Hornych A (1978) Prostaglandins and high blood pressure. Contrib Nephrol 12:54–68
Hornych A (1980) Role of prostaglandins in control of blood pressure. In: Ramwell P (ed) Prostaglandin synthetase inhibitors: new clinical applications. Liss, New York, p 291
Jackson EK, Herzer WA, Zimmerman JB, Branch RA, Oates JA, Gerkens JF (1981) 6-Keto-prostaglandin E_1 is more potent than prostaglandin I_2 as a renal vasodilator and renin secretagogue. J Pharmacol Exp Ther 216:24–27
Jackson EK, Branch RA, Oates JA (1982) Participation of prostaglandins in control of renin release. In: Oates JA (ed) Prostaglandins and the cardiovascular system. Raven, New York, p 255
Jim K, Hassid A, Sun F, Dunn MJ (1982) Lipoxygenase activity in rat kidney glomeruli, glomerular epithelial cells and cortical tubules. J Biol Chem 257:10294–10299
Johnson KL, Morton DR, Kumer JH, Gorman RR, McGuire JC, Sun FF, Whitacker N, Bunting S, Salomon J, Moncada S, Vane JR (1976) The chemical structure of prostaglandin X (prostacyclin). Prostaglandins 12:915–928
Kahlen I, Schrör K (1982) Mepindolol protection of prostacyclin formation. Subsequent increase in arachidonic acid-induced prostacyclin release in isolated guinea pig heart. Eur J Pharmacol 82:81–84
Kawaguchi H, Yasuda H (1986) Effect of platelet activating factor on arachidonic acid

metabolism in renal epithelial cells. Biochim Biophys Acta 875:525–534
Konieczkowski M, Dunn MJ, Stork JE, Hassid A (1983) Glomerular synthesis of prostaglandins and thromboxane in spontaneously hypertensive rats. Hypertension 5: 446–452
Larrue J, Razaka G, Daret D, Henri J, Rigaud M, Bricaud H (1985) Lipoxygenase derived products in cultured human aortic smooth muscle cells. In: Neri Serneri GG, McGiff JC, Paoletti R, Born GVR (eds) Advances in prostaglandin, thromboxane, and leukotriene research, vol 13. Raven, New York, pp 55–58
Larsson C, Änggard E (1973) Increased juxtamedullary blood flow on stimulation of intrarenal prostaglandine biosynthesis. Eur J Pharmacol 25:326–334
Lawson D, Smith C, Katovich M et al. (1986) Cumulative contractile effects of leukotriene D_4 and epinephrin on isolated rat aortic rings. Circulation 74:11–15
Levy JV (1977) Changes in systolic arterial blood pressure in normal and spontaneously hypertensive rats produced by acute administration of inhibitors of prostaglandin biosynthesis. Prostaglandins 13:153
Lüscher TF, Vanhoutte PM (1986) Endothelium-dependent responses to platelets and serotonin in spontaneously hypertensive rats. Hypertension 8 [Suppl II]:55–60
MacLouf J, Fruteau DeLaclos B, Borgeat P (1982) Stimulation of leukotriene biosynthesis in human blood leukocytes by platelet-derived 12-hydroperoxy-icosatetraenoic acid. Proc Natl Acad Sci USA 79:6042–6046
Makhoul RG, Gewertz BL (1986) Renal prostaglandins. J Surg Res 40:181–192
Mardin M, Busse W-D (1983) Effect of Nafazatrom on the lipoxygenase pathways in PMN leukocytes and RBL-1 cells. In: Piper PJ (ed) Leukotrienes and other lipoxygenase products. Research Studies, Chichester, pp 263–274
McGiff JC (1981) Prostaglandins, prostacyclin, and thromboxanes. Annu Rev Pharmacol Toxicol 21:479–509
McGiff JC, Nasjletti A (1976) Kinins, renal function and blood pressure regulation. Fed Proc 35:172–174
McGiff JC, Quilley J (1982) Prostaglandins act as modulators and mediators of the vascular and renal actions of kinins. In: McConn R (ed) Role of chemical mediators in the pathophysiology of acute illness and injury. Raven, New York, p 37
McGiff JC, Crowshaw K, Terragno NA, Lonigro AJ (1970) Renal prostaglandins: possible regulators of the renal actions of pressor hormones. Nature 225:1255–1257
McGiff JC, Iskowitz HD, Terragno NA (1975) The actions of bradykinin and eledoisin in the canine isolated kidney: relationship to prostaglandins. Clin Sci Mol Med 49: 125–131
McGiff JC, Spokas EG, Wong PY-K (1982) Stimulation of renin release by 6-oxoprostaglandin E_1 and prostacyclin. Br J Pharmacol 75:137–144
Mehta J, Mehta P, Lawson D, Ostrowski N, Brigman L (1983) Influence of selective thromboxane synthetase blocker CGS-13080 on thromboxane and prostacyclin biosynthesis in whole blood: evidence for synthesis of prostacyclin by leukocytes from platelet-derived endoperoxides. J Lab Clin Med 106:246
Mehta P, Mehta J, Lawson D et al. (1986) Leukotrienes potentiate the effects of epinephrine and thrombin on human platelet aggregation. Thromb Res 41:731–738
Mehta J, Lawson D, Mehta P et al. (1987) Leukotriene-induced relaxation of precontracted rat aortic rings: dependence on endothelial integrity. Clin Res 5:573A
Mehta J, Nichols WW, Mehta P (1988) Neutrophils as potential participants in acute myocardial ischemia: relevance to reperfusion. J Am Coll Cardiol 11:1309–1316
Miller MJS, Pinto A, Mullane KM (1987) Impaired endothelium-dependent relaxations in rabbits subjected to aortic coarctation hypertension. Hypertension 10:164–170
Morris HR, Taylor GW, Piper PJ, Tippins JR (1980a) Structure of slow-reacting substance of anaphylaxis from guinea-pig lung. Nature 285:104–106
Morris HR, Taylor GW, Piper PJ, Samhoun MN, Tippins JR (1980b) Slow reacting substances (SRSs): the structure identification of SRSs from rat basophil leukaemia (RBL-I) cells. Prostaglandins 19:185–201
Morrison AR, Pascoe N (1981) Metabolism of arachidonate through NADPH-dependent oxygenase of renal cortex. Proc Natl Acad Sci USA 78:7375–7378
Morrison AR, Winokur TS, Brown WA (1982) Inhibition of soyabean lipoxygenase by

mannitol. Biochem Biophys Res Commun 108:1757–1762
Motomiya T, Yamazaki H (1981) Vascular smooth muscle reactivity to rabbit aorta contracting substance (RCS) and production of prostacyclin-like substance in normotensive and hypertensive rats. Jpn Circ J 45:680–686
Mullane KM, Moncada S, Vane JR (1980) Prostacyclin release induced by bradykinin may contribute to the antihypertensive action of angiotensin-converting enzyme inhibitors. In: Samuelsson B, Ramwell PW, Paoletti R (eds) Advances in prostaglandin and thromboxane research, vol 7. Raven, New York, p 1159
Nasjletti A, McGiff JC, Colina-Chourio J (1978) Interrelations of the renal kallikrein-kinin system and renal prostaglandins in the conscious rat. Circ Res 43:799–807
Needleman P, Kauffman AH, Douglas JR Jr, Johnson EM Jr, Marshall GR (1973) Specific stimulation and inhibition of renal prostaglandin release by angiotensin analogs. Am J Physiol 224:1415–1419
Neri Serneri GG, Abbate R, Gensini GF, Panetta A, Casolo GC, Carini M (1983) TXA_2 production by human arteries and veins. Prostaglandins 25:753–766
Nichols WW, Mehta J, Thompson L Donnelly WH (1988) Synergistic effects of LTC_4 and TXA_2 on coronary flow and myocardial function. Am J Physiol 255:H153–H159
Nugteren DH (1975) Arachidonate lipoxygenase in blood platelets. Biochim Biophys Acta 380:299–307
Nugteren DH, Hazelhof E (1973) Isolation and properties of intermediates in prostaglandin biosynthesis. Biochim Biophys Acta 326:448–461
Oates JA, Whorton AR, Gerkens JF, Branch RA, Hollifield JW, Frölich JC (1979) The participation of prostaglandins in the control of renin release. Fed Proc 38:72–74
Ohde H, Ogihara T, Nakamaru M, Higaki J, Gotoh S, Masuo K, Ohtsuka A, Saeki S, Kumahara Y (1982) Effect of prostacyclin infusion on active and inactive renin release in the isolated perfused kidney. Life Sci 31:3031–3035
Okuma M, Takayama H, Uchino H (1980) Generation of prostacyclin-like substance and lipid peroxidation in vitamin E-deficient rats. Prostaglandins 19:527–536
Oliw EH, Oates JA (1981) Rabbit renal cortical microsomes metabolize arachidonic acid to trihydroxyeicosatrienoic acids. Prostaglandins 22:863–871
Oliw EH, Lawson JA, Brash AR, Oates JA (1981) Arachidonic acid metabolism in rabbit renal cortex. J Biol Chem 256:9924–9931
Pace-Asciak CR (1980) Prostacyclin and hypertension. Mater Med Pol 3:181
Pace-Asciak CR, Carrara MC, Rangaraj G, Nicolaou KC (1978) Enhanced formation of PGI_2, a potent hypotensive substance, by aortic rings and homogenates of the spontaneously hypertensive rats. Prostaglandins 15:1005–1012
Patak RV, Mookerjee KB, Bentzel CJ, Hysert PE, Babej M, Lee JB (1975) Antagonism of the effects of furosemide by indomethacin in normal and hypertensive man. Prostaglandins 10:649–659
Peach MJ, Loeb AL (1987) Changes in vascular endothelium and its function in systemic arterial hypertension. Am J Cardiol 14:1101–1151
Piper PJ, Galton SA (1984) Generation of leukotriene B_4 and leukotriene E_4 from porcine pulmonary artery. Prostaglandins 28:905–914
Pipili E, Poyser NL (1982) Release of prostaglandins I_2 and E_2 from the perfused mesenteric arterial bed of normotensive and hypertensive rats. Effects of sympathetic nerve stimulation and norepinephrine administration. Prostaglandins 23:543–549
Randall RW, Eakins KE, Higgs GA, Salmon JA, Tateson JE (1980) Inhibition of arachidonic acid cyclo-oxygenase and lipoxygenase activities of leukocytes by indomethacin and compound BW 755C. Agents Actions 10:553–555
Remuzzi G, Cavenaghi AE, Mecca G, Donati MB, DeGaetano G (1978) Human renal cortex generates prostacyclin-like activity. Thromb Res 12:363–366
Roman RJ, Lechene C (1981) Prostaglandin E_2 and F_2 reduces urea reabsorbtion from the rat collecting duct. Am J Physiol 241:F53
Ross R, Glomset JA (1976) The pathogenesis of atherosclerosis. N Engl J Med 295: 369–377, 420–425
Samuelsson B (1963) Prostaglandins and related factors 17: the structure of prostaglandin E_3. J Am Chem Soc 85:1878–1879
Samuelsson B (1964 a) Identification of a smooth muscle stimulating factor in bovine

brain: prostaglandins and related factors, 25. Biochim Biophys Acta 84:218–219
Samuelsson B (1964 b) Identification of prostaglandin F_3a in bovine lung: prostaglandins and related factors, 26. Biochim Biophys Acta 84:707–713
Samuelsson B (1983) Leukotrienes: mediators of immediate hypersensitivity reactions and inflammation. Science 220:568–575
Satoh H, Hosono M, Satoh S (1984) Distinctive effect of angiotensin II on prostaglandin production in dog renal and femoral arteries. Prostaglandins 27:807–820
Schölkens BA (1978) Antihypertensive effect of prostacyclin (PGI_2) in experimental hypertension and its influence on plasma renin activity in rats. Prostaglandins Med 1:359
Schölkens B, Steinbach R, Ganten D (1979) Blood pressure effects of endogenous brain angiotensin in rats are increased by inhibition of prostaglandin biosynthesis. Clin Sci 57:271s–274s
Schwartzman M, Liberman E, Raz A (1981) Bradykinin and angiotensin II activation of arachidonic acid deacylation and prostaglandin E_2 formation in rabbit kidney. J Biol Chem 256:2329–2333
Schwertschlag U, Stahl T, Hackenthal E (1982) A comparison of the effects of prostacyclin and 6-keto-prostaglandin E_1 on renin release in the isolated rat and rabbit kidney. Prostaglandins 23:129–138
Schwertschlag U, Scherf H, Gerber JG, Mathias M, Nies AS (1987) L-platelet activating factor induces changes on renal vascular resistance, vascular reactivity and renin release in the isolated perfused rat kidney. Circ Res 60:534–539
Seymour AA, Davis JO, Freeman RH, DeForrest JM, Williams GM (1979) Renin release filtering and non-filtering kidneys stimulated by PGI_2 and PGD_2. Am J Physiol 237:F285–290
Shebuski RJ, Aiken JW (1980) Angiotensin II-induced renal prostacyclin release suppresses platelet aggregation in the anesthetized dogs. In: Samuelsson B, Ramwell PW, Paoletti R (eds) Advances in prostaglandin and thormboxane research, vol 7. Raven, New York, p 1149
Sheng WY, Lysz TA, Wyche A, Needleman P (1983) Kinetic comparison and regulation of the cascade of microsomal enzymes involved in renal arachidonate and endoperoxide metabolism. J Biol Chem 258:2188–2192
Simonson MS, Dunn MJ (1986) Leukotriene C_4 and D_4 contract rat glomerular mesangial cells. Kidney Int 30:524–531
Simpson RU, Goodfriend TL (1984) Angiotensin and prostaglandin interactions in cultured kidney tubules. J Lab Clin Med 103:255–271
Smith WL, Wilkin GP (1977) Immunochemistry of prostaglandin endoperoxide-forming cyclooxygenases: the detection of the cyclooxygenases in rat, rabbit and guinea-pig kidneys by immunofluorescence. Prostaglandins 13:873–892
Solez K, Fox JA, Miller M et al. (1974) Effects of indomethacin on renal inner medullary plasma flow. Prostaglandins 7:91
Soma M, Manku MS, Jenkins DK, Horrobin DF (1985) Prostaglandins and thromboxane outflow from the perfused mesenteric vascular bed in spontaneously hypertensive rats. Prostaglandins 29:323–333
Sraer J, Rigaud M, Bens M, Rabinovitch H, Ardaillou R (1983) Metabolism of arachidonic acid via the lipoxygenase pathway in human and murine glomerguli. J Biol Chem 258:4325–4330
Stokes JG (1982) Tubular actions of arachidonic acid metabolites. Effects on NaCl and water transport. In: Dunn MJ, Patrono C, Cinotti GA (eds) Prostaglandins and the kidney. Plenum, New York, pp 133–149
Terragno NA, Terragno DA, McGiff JC (1977) Contribution of prostaglandins to the renal circulation in conscious, anaesthetized and laparotomized dogs. Circ Res 40: 590–595
Tucker BJ, Gushwa LC, Wilson CB, Blantz RC (1985) Effect of leukocyte depletion on glomerular dynamics during acute glomerular immune injury. Kidney Int 28:28–35
Turk J, Wyche A, Needleman P (1980) Inactivation of vascular prostacyclin synthetase by platelet lipoxygenase products. Biochem Biophys Res Commun 95:1628–1634
Uehara Y, Ishimitsu T, Ishii M, Sugimoto T (1987) Prostacyclin synthetase and phos-

pholipases in the vascular wall of experimental hypertensive rats. Prostaglandins 34:423–432

Vlasses PH, Ferguson RK, Smith JB, Rotmensch HH, Swanson BN (1983) Urinary excretion of prostacyclin and thromboxane A_2 metabolites after angiotensin converting enzyme inhibition in hypertensive patients. Prostaglandins Leukotrienes Med 11:143–150

von Euler US (1934) Zur Kenntnis der pharmakologischen Wirkungen von Nativsekreten und Extraktenmännlicher accessorischer Geschlechtsdrüsen. Naunyn-Schmiedeberg's Arch Exp Pathol Pharmacol 175:78–84

von Euler US (1935) kurzwissenschaftliche Mitteilungen über die spezifische blutdruck—senkende Substanz des menschlichen Prostata—und Samenblasensekrets. Klin Wochenschr 14:1182–1184

Walker LA, Whorton AR, Smigel M, France R, Frölich JC (1978) Antidiuretic hormone increases renal prostaglandin synthesis in vivo. Am J Physiol 235:F180–F185

Wargovich T, Mehta J, Nichols WW, Pepine CJ, Conti CR (1985) Reduction in blood flow in normal and narrowed coronary arteries of dogs by leukotriene C_4. Am J Coll Cardiol 6:1047–1051

Weber PC (1978) Renal prostaglandins in the control of renin. Contrib Nephrol 12: 92–103

Weber PC, Larsson C, Anggard E, Hamberg M, Corey EJ, Nicolaou KC, Samuelsson B (1976) Stimulation of renin release from rabbit renal cortex by arachidonic acid and prostaglandin endoperoxides. Circ Res 39 (6):868–874

Weller PF, Lee CW, Foster DW, Corey EJ, Austen KF, Lewis RA (1983) Generation and metabolism of 5-lipoxygenase pathway leukotrienes by human eosinophils: predominant production of leukotriene C_4. Proc Natl Acad Sci USA 80:7626–7630

Werning C, Vetter W, Weidmann P, Schweikert HU, Stiel D, Siegenthaler W (1971) Effect of prostaglandin E_1 on renin in the dog. Am J Physiol 220:852–856

Wong PY-K, McGiff JC, Cagen L, Malik KU, Sun FF (1978) Metabolism of prostacyclin in the rabbit kidney. J Biol Chem 254:12–14

Wong PY-K, Spur B, Hejny P, Chao PH-W, Lam BK (1987) Biosynthesis and metabolism of leukotrienes in response to glomeruli and neutrophil interaction of genetically hypertensive rats. In: Samuelsson B, Paoletti R, Ramwell PW (eds) Advances in prostaglandin, thromboxane, and leukotriene research, vol 17B. Raven, New York, p 736

Yannagisawa M, Kurihara H, Kimura S, Tomobe Y, Kobayashi M, Mitsui Y, Yazaki Y, Goto K, Masaki T (1988) A novel potent vasoconstrictor peptide produced by vascular endothelial cells. Nature 332:411–415

Ylitalo P, Pitkäjärvi T, Metsä-Ketelä T, Vapaatalo H (1978) The effect of inhibition of prostaglandin synthesis on plasma renin activity and blood pressure in essential hypertension. Prostaglandins Med 1:479–488

Yoshimoto T, Yokoyama C, Ochi K, Yamamoto S, Maki Y, Ashida Y, Terao S, Shiraishi M (1982) 2,3,5-trimethyl-6-(12-hydroxy-5,10-dodecadiynyl)-1,4-benzoquinone (AA861), a selective inhibitor of the 5-lipoxygenase reaction and the biosynthesis of slow-reacting substance of anaphylaxis. Biochim Biophys Acta 713:470–473

Zipser RD, Smorlesi C (1984) Regulation of urinary thromboxane B_2 in man: influence of urinary flow rate and tubular transport. Prostaglandins 27:257–271

Zusman RM, Keiser HR (1977) Prostaglandin E_2 biosynthesis by rabbit renomedullary interstitial cells in tissue culture: mechanism of stimulation by angiotensin II, bradykinin and arginine vasopressin. J Biol Chem 252:2069–2071

CHAPTER 13

Interferences with 5-Hydroxytryptamine

P.R. SAXENA and W. WOUTERS

CONTENTS

1 Introduction

5-Hydroxytryptamine (5-HT, serotonin) is present both in the periphery and in the CNS, where it functions as a neurotransmitter. In the periphery 5-HT is mainly synthesized in the enterochromaffin cells from whence it is released into the portal circulation to be taken up by blood platelets. The physiological role of 5-HT in cardiovascular regulation is still unclear, but the amine has powerful pharmacological effects on the heart (see SAXENA 1986) and blood vessels. Its vascular effects depend upon several factors (species, vascular bed, dose, etc.), and it can elicit either vasodilatation or vasoconstriction directly, which can be modified indirectly, via neural mechanisms. Recent investigations suggest that the cardiovascular and, indeed, other effects of 5-HT are mediated by at least three types of receptors for 5-HT. In this chapter we deal first with the subdivision, nomenclature, and function of 5-HT receptors and subsequently with the antihypertensive effects of agents acting via interferences with the 5-HT system.

2 5-Hydroxytryptamine Receptors

2.1 Historical "D" and "M" Receptors

More than 30 years ago GADDUM and PICARELLI (1957) showed that 5-HT-induced contractions of the guinea pig isolated ileum are only partially antagonized by phenoxybenzamine (Dibenzyline) or morphine but are completely blocked by their combination. Furthermore, atropine, methadone, and cocaine do not modify the response to 5-HT in morphine-treated ileum but almost completely block it in phenoxybenzamine-treated ileum; the reverse is true for 5-benzyloxygramine, lysergide, and dihydroergotamine. GADDUM and PICARELLI (1957) concluded that 5-HT stimulates two different types of receptors named "D" (dibenzyline, 5-benzyloxygramine, lysergide, or dihydroergotamine sensitive) and "M" (morphine, methadone, atropine, or cocaine sensitive), which are located on the intestinal smooth muscle and intramural neurons, respectively. Later, several other drugs — 2-bromolysergide, cyproheptadine, methysergide, methiothepin, metergoline, and mianserin — became known as selective D 5-HT receptor antagonists. Nevertheless, from time to time, it was pointed out that some pharmacological effects of 5-HT, for example, common carotid artery vasoconstriction in the dog (SAXENA et al. 1971), did not entirely fit into the "D" and "M" 5-HT receptor classification.

2.2 Binding Sites

The next advance was in 1979 when in rat brain membranes PEROUTKA and SNYDER demonstrated two different binding sites, 5-HT_1 and 5-HT_2, having high affinities for, respectively, [^{3}H]5-HT and [^{3}H]spiperone. These and other authors also showed that 5-carboxamidotryptamine (5-CT) possesses a high and selective affinity for the 5-HT_1 binding site while ketanserin, cyproheptadine, mianserin, and cinanserin are selective for the 5-HT_2 binding site; lysergide, 2-bromolysergide, methiothepin, and metergoline have affinities for both binding sites (PEROUTKA and SNYDER 1979; LEYSEN 1981; ENGEL et al. 1983). Subsequent studies showed that the 5-HT_1 binding site is heterogeneous (PEDIGO et al. 1981), and so far four subtypes (5-HT_{1A}, 5-HT_{1B}, 5-HT_{1C}, and 5-HT_{1D}) have been recognized (see HOYER et al. 1985; PEROUTKA 1986; HEURING and PEROUTKA 1987; WAEBER et al. 1988) (Table 1). More recently, the 5-HT_3 binding site has been located (KILPATRICK et al. 1987; HOYER and NEIJT 1988).

Table 1. Arrangement of some drugs in order of affinities (pK_1) at $5\text{-}HT_1$ binding site subtypes

$5\text{-}HT_{1A}$	$5\text{-}HT_{1B}$	$5\text{-}HT_{1C}$	$5\text{-}HT_{1D}$
Putative agonists			
9.7 5-CT	8.4 RU 24969	7.5 5-HT	8.8 5-CT
8.8 Flesinoxan	8.3 5-CT	6.5 Indorenate	7.9 5-HT
8.7 8-OH DPAT	7.6 5-HT	6.4 RU 24969	7.4 RU 24969
8.5 5-HT	6.7 BEA 1654	6.2 5-CT	6.0 8-OH-DPAT
8.3 RU 24969	5.4 Indorenate	5.3 Flesinoxan	
7.8 Indorenate	5.0 Flesinoxan	5.3 BEA 1654	
7.6 BEA 1654	4.5 Urapidil	5.1 8-OH-DPAT	
7.0 Urapidil	4.2 8-OH-DPAT		
Putative antagonists			
8.4 Spiroxatrine	9.5 (±)Cyanopindolol	9.3 Metergoline	8.7 Metergoline
8.2 Metergoline	7.6 Metergoline	8.8 Mesulergine	8.4 Methiothepin
8.1 (±)Cyanopindolol	7.3 Methiothepin	8.0 Mianserin	6.4 Mianserin
7.6 Methysergide	7.3 (−)Propranolol	7.6 Methiothepin	6.3 Methiothepin
7.4 8-MeO-CLEPAT	7.1 (−)Pindolol	7.2 Methysergide	6.1 (±)Cyanopindolol
7.6 (−) Pindolol	6.3 Methysergide	6.4 Ketanserin	5.8 Mesulergine
7.2 Spiperone	5.8 8-MeO-CLEPAT	6.4 (−)Propranolol	5.2 (−)Propranolol
7.1 Methiothepin	5.7 Ketanserin	5.9 Spiperone	4.8 Ketanserin
6.7 (−)Propranolol	5.7 Mianserin	5.1 (±)Cyanopindolol	4.8 (−)Pindolol
6.2 Mesulergine	5.3 Spiperone	4.3 (−)Pindolol	4.7 Spiperone
6.0 Ketanserin	5.0 Spiroxatrine		
5.9 Mianserin	4.9 Mesulergine		

Data for $5\text{-}HT_{1A}$, $5\text{-}HT_{1B}$, and $5\text{-}HT_{1C}$, except for methysergide (PEROUTKA 1986), flesinoxan, urapidil, 8-MeO-CLEPAT, BEA 1654 (TULP, personal communication) and spiroxatrine (NELSON and TAYLOR 1986), are from HOYER et al. (1985), and data for $5\text{-}HT_{1D}$ are from WAEBER et al. (1988). $5\text{-}HT_{1A}$ pig cortex; $5\text{-}HT_{1B}$, rat cortex; $5\text{-}HT_{1C}$, pig choroid plexus; $5\text{-}HT_{1D}$, pig caudate.
5-CT, 5-carboxamidotryptamine; 8-OH DPAT, 8-hydroxy-2-(di-*N*,*N*- *n*-propylamino) tetralin; RU 24969, 5-methoxy-3-(1,2,3,6-tetrahydro-4-pyridinyl-1H-indole; BEA 1654, *N*-(3-acetylaminophenyl) piperazine; 8-MeO-CLEPAT, 8-methoxy-2-(*N*-2-chloroethyl-*N*-*n*-propyl)-aminotetraline.

2.3 Present Classification of Receptors

Since the above classifications — D and M receptors (GADDUM and PICARELLI 1957) or 5-HT_1 and 5-HT_2 receptors (PEROUTKA and SNYDER 1979) — did not adequately cover the pharmacological effects of 5-HT, an international working group was set up to try to classify 5-HT receptors in a more meaningful way incorporating recent knowledge. Based on certain criteria (Table 2), three distinct receptor types mediating functional response to 5-HT were recognized, and the working group proposed that they be called 5-HT_1-like, 5-HT_2, and 5-HT_3 receptors (BRADLEY et al. 1986; SAXENA et al. 1986). It has to be emphasized that only 5-HT_2 and 5-HT_3 receptors have so far been well-characterized using selective antagonists. Since no selective antagonists are available for the 5-HT_1-like receptors, this group cannot yet be fully characterized, hence the suffix "like". The 5-HT_1-like receptor appear to be heterogeneous in nature (BRADLEY et al. 1986; HUMPHREY and RICHARDSON 1989; Table 3), but the exact association with the 5-HT_1 binding site subtypes is still unclear since sufficiently selective drugs (except for the 5-HT_{1A} site; see Table 1) are not yet available.

3 Effects of 5-Hydroxytryptamine and Related Drugs on Arterial Blood Pressure

3.1 Nature of the Blood Pressure Effect

In a number of species 5-HT elicits a triphasic response on arterial blood pressure, consisting of an initial, transient, depressor phase, a middle hypertensive phase, and a late, long-lasting, hypotensive phase (PAGE and MCCUBBIN 1953; PAGE 1957). The initial transient depressor phase is due to the Von Bezold-Jarisch reflex mediated by 5-HT_3 receptors (FOZARD 1984; KALKMAN et al. 1984; SAXENA and LAWANG 1985; SAXENA et al. 1985). The hypertensive phase is due either to a direct action of 5-HT on blood vessels as in the rat (LEYSEN et al. 1984; KALKMAN et al. 1984; SAXENA and LAWANG 1985) or to a release of adrenomedullary catecholamines as in the dog (FENIUK et al. 1981); however, in both cases 5-HT_2 receptors are involved. The long-lasting depressor phase is mediated by 5-HT_1-like receptors (KALKMAN et al. 1984; SAXENA and LAWANG 1985; CONNOR et al. 1986) and may involve different mechanisms (SAXENA et al. 1987) that will be discussed below. At this juncture, however, three points may be made. Firstly, contrary to the connotation conveyed by the word "serotonin", 5-HT is much more potent in eliciting vasodepressor responses than in evoking either the Von Bezold-Jarisch reflex or pressor responses (Fig. 1; BLAUW et al. 1987, 1988). Secondly, evidence is accumulating to suggest that the distribution of 5-HT receptors differs along the arterial tree: 5-HT_2 receptors mediating vasoconstriction are probably greater in number in large conduit arteries, whereas 5-HT_1-like receptors mediating vasodilatation predominate in the resistance vessels (arterioles) (SAXENA and VERDOUW 1982; HOLLENBERG 1987). Thirdly, it should be realized that 5-HT influences blood flow distribution in a complex way. By using the radioactive microsphere technique, it has been

Table 2. Classification and characterization of functional 5-HT receptors

Receptor type	Criteria for identification			Relationship to classic receptors	Relationship to binding sites
	Antagonism by	Resistance to antagonism by	Selectively mimicked by		
5-HT_1-like	Methiothepin[a] or methysergide[b,c]	Ketanserin or cyproheptadine, MDL 72222 or ICS 205–930	5-CT	D	5-HT_1[a]
5-HT_2	Ketanserin, cyproheptadine, or methysergide	MDL 72222, ICS 205–930 BRL 24924, or GR 38032F	$\alpha\text{-CH}_3\text{-5-HT}$	D	5-HT_2
5-HT_3	MDL 72222, ICS 205-930, BRL 43694, or GR 38032F	Methiothepin, ketanserin, cyproheptadine, or methysergide	$2\text{-CH}_3\text{-5-HT}$	M	5-HT_3

[a] Relationship with subtypes is as yet uncertain.
[b] Nonselective antagonist (also blocks 5-HT_2 receptors).
[c] Partial agonist at some 5-HT_1-like receptors. Based on SAXENA et al. (1986). BRL 43694, endo-*N*-(9-methyl-9-azabicyclo [3,3,1]non-3-yl)-1-methyl-indazole-3-carboxamide; GR 38032F, 1,2,3,9-tetrahydro-9-methyl-3-methyl-3[(2-methyl-1H-imidazol-1-yl)methyl]-4H-carbazol-4-one.

Table 3. Heterogeneity of 5-HT_1-like receptors[a]

Subtype	Responses	Agonists	Antagonists
5-HT_{1A}	Decrease in acetylcholine release in the guinea pig ileum, centrally induced hypotension in several species.	5-CT, 8-OH-DPAT, RU 24969	Methiothepin, cyanopindolol, methysergide
5-HT_{1B}	Autoreceptor in the rat brain, mouse urinary bladder contraction	5-CT, RU 24969	Methiothepin, cyanopindolol, methysergide
Unnamed[b]	Vascular and nonvascular smooth muscle relaxation, tachycardia in the cat	5-CT	Methiothepin, methysergide
Unnamed[b]	Contraction of dog saphenous vein, and cephalic arteries and arteriovenous anastomoses in several species	5-CT, GR43175[c]	Methiothepin, methysergide[d]

[a] Due to lack of selective drugs, no functional response can be convincingly associated with the 5-HT_{1C} or 5-HT_{1D} binding sites.
[b] Relationship with binding site subtypes is uncertain.
[c] Binding data have not yet been reported.
[d] Seems to be a partial agonist.
GR43175, 3-[2-dimethylamino]ethyl-*N*-methyl-1*H*-indole-5-methane sulphonamide.

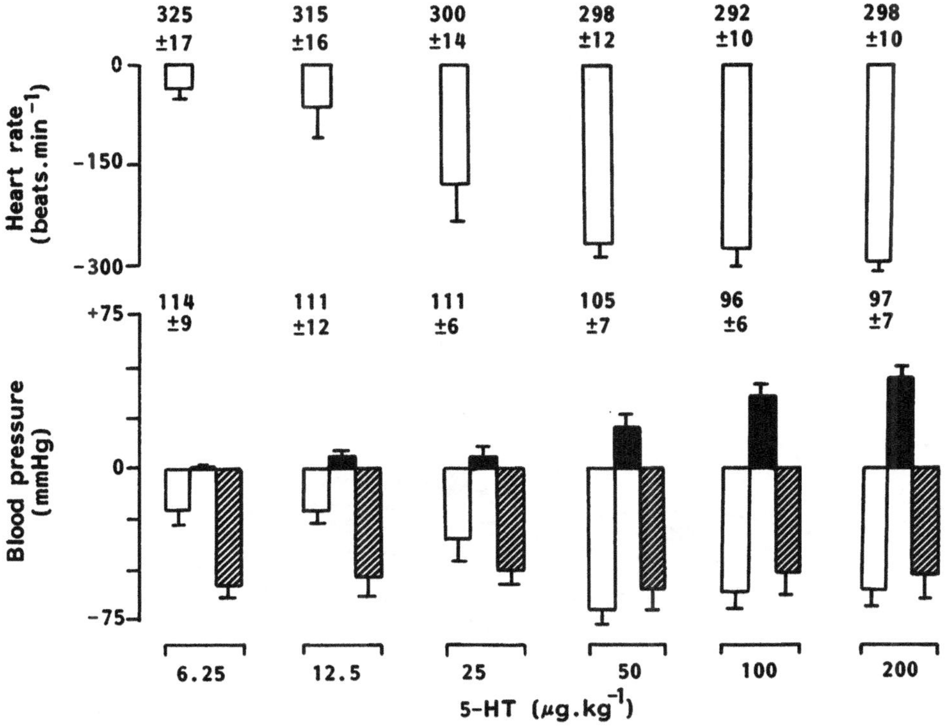

Fig. 1. The effects of 5-HT on heart rate and mean arterial blood pressure in rats. The three *columns* in the blood pressure panel represent the initial hypotensive, associated with bradycardia (*open*), middle pressor (*solid*), and late (*hatched*) hypotensive phases. The *number above each column* represent mean (± SE) values of heart rate and blood pressure at the time a certain dose of 5-HT was given. (From SAXENA and LAWANG 1985)

demonstrated that 5-HT and some selective agonists at 5-HT_1-like receptors (5-CT and BEA 1654) redistribute blood to the nutrient compartment (arteriolar dilatation) from the nonnutrient compartment (constriction of arteriovenous anastomoses), especially in the skin and ears (SAXENA and VERDOUW 1982, 1984, 1985; VERDOUW et al. 1985).

3.2 Long-Lasting Depressor Effect

The depressor response to 5-HT is observed in several animal species like the rat (KALKMAN et al. 1983a; SAXENA and LAWANG 1985; DALTON 1986; MARTIN et al. 1987), rabbit (BOLT and SAXENA 1985; WRIGHT and ANGUS 1987), cat (CONNOR et al. 1986), and pig (SAXENA and VERDOUW 1984). Since the hypotensive activity in a small series of tryptamine analogues correlates with their affinities to the 5-HT_1 binding site, KALKMAN et al. (1983a) suggested the involvement of 5-HT_1-like receptors in the hypotensive action. The high potency of the 5-HT_1 receptor agonist 5-CT in the rat (SAXENA and LAWANG 1985; DOCHERTY 1986; MARTIN et al. 1987), cat (CONNOR et al. 1986), rabbit (WRIGHT and ANGUS 1987), and pig

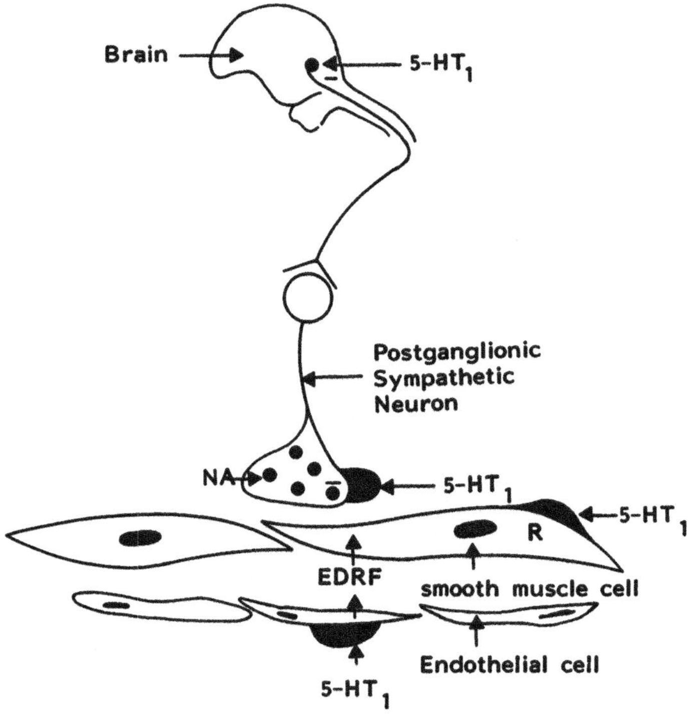

Fig. 2. Schematic representation of a sympathetic neuron innervating blood vessels. *NA*, noradrenaline; *EDRF*, endothelium-derived relaxant factor; *R*, relaxation; *minus sign* inhibition; *5-HT₁*, 5-HT₁-like receptor. Note that 5-HT₁-like receptors mediating vascular relaxation and hypotension are located at four different sites

(SAXENA and VERDOUW 1985), and the antagonism of the hypotensive response by methiothepin and methysergide confirms mediation via 5-HT_1-like receptors. These 5-HT_1-like receptors are located at different parts of the cardiovascular regulatory sites (Fig. 2), and, depending upon their location, the activation of these receptors leads to a decrease in blood pressure by at least four different mechanisms: (a) within the CNS via a decrease in sympathetic outflow; (b) presynaptically via reduced transmitter release from postganglionic sympathetic nerves; (c) at the endothelium via a release of endothelium-derived relaxant factor (EDRF) which may be identical to nitric oxide (PALMER et al. 1987); and (d) on smooth muscle cells to elicit a "direct" vasodilatation. In subsequent paragraphs these four mechanisms are elucidated further.

3.2.1 Hypotensive and Antihypertensive Effects of 5-HT_1-like Receptor Agonists via the CNS

In 1959 BHARGAVA and TANGRI, demonstrating the hypotensive action of intracerebroventricularly administered 5-HT in the dog, suggested that 5-HT may be involved in the CNS in the regulation of cardiovascular activity. Indeed, similarities between the central serotonergic neurons and the pathways involved in cardiovascular regulation seem to bear out the above suggestion (CHALMERS 1975; KUHN et al. 1980; WOLF et al. 1985). However, this role is still only incompletely understood and appears to be rather complex (KUHN et al. 1980). The increase in 5-HT concentrations in the CNS by 5-hydroxytryptophan and depletion of central 5-HT stores by *p*-chloro-phenylalanine or by chemical destruction of 5-HT pathways often yield opposite effects on blood pressure and heart rate in different species and experimental models. Also, injections of 5-HT into the CNS result mainly in pressor responses in the rat but in depressor responses in the cat or dog (KUHN et al. 1980). More recent studies indicate that, both in the cat and rat, centrally-administered 5-HT can evoke pressor, depressor, or biphasic blood pressure responses, largely depending on the exact site of application, the doses employed, and whether conscious or anesthetized, normotensive or hypertensive animals are used (SUKAMOTO et al. 1984; KRSTIC 1985; DALTON 1986; COOTE et al. 1987). With the demonstration of three distinct types of 5-HT receptors (5-HT_1-like, 5-HT_2, and 5-HT_3) and the heterogeneous nature of the 5-HT_1 binding site in the CNS, it is quite possible that pressor and depressor effects of 5-HT are associated with different 5-HT receptors. Therefore, a part of the existing confusion may be resolved by the use of selective compounds. Indeed, such attempts have been made with new compounds (Fig. 3) which show a high affinity and selectivity for the 5-HT_{1A} binding site and, in addition, either elicit (or block) hypotensive and antihypertensive actions. In particular, 8-hydroxy-2-(di-*N*,*N*-*n*-propylamino) tetralin (8-OH-DPAT) and flesinoxan have been studied more extensively (GRADIN et al. 1985; MARTIN and LIS 1985; FOZARD et al. 1987; WOUTERS et al. 1988a, b). 8-OH-DPAT lowers blood pressure in normotensive and spontaneously hypertensive rats and in normotensive cats (GRADIN et al. 1985; MARTIN and LIS 1985; RAMAGE and FOZARD 1987; DOODS et al. 1985), and flesinoxan lowers blood pressure in spontaneously hypertensive rats, renal hypertensive rabbits, and normotensive cats, dogs, and baboons. The decrease in blood pressure is accompanied by a moderate (flesinoxan) or strong (8-OH-DPAT) bradycardia in conscious rats and by a strong bradycardia in anesthetized cats at higher doses (WOUTERS et al. 1988a, b; WOUTERS, unpublished results).

The involvement of the CNS in the cardiovascular response to putative 5-HT_{1A} receptor agonists is supported by several observations. Administration directly into the CNS via either the vertebral arteries or the atlanto-occipital membrane considerably increases the potency of 8-OH-DPAT and flesinoxan compared with their i.v. administration in cats (DOODS et al. 1987; WOUTERS et al. 1988a, b). Though in rats central administration of 8-OH-DPAT is no more efficacious than its i.v. administration (GRADIN et al. 1985; MARTIN and LIS 1985), the cardiovascular responses to 8-OH-DPAT can be effectively blocked by central administration of the putative 5-HT_{1A} receptor antagonist, 8-methoxy-2-(*N*-2-chloroethyl-*N*-*n*-propyl) aminotetraline (8-MeO-CLEPAT; FOZARD et al. 1987). Prominent hypotensive effects of these compounds, which could be attributed to stimulation of putative peripheral 5-HT_{1A} receptors, have not been observed. 8-OH-DPAT does not lower blood pressure in pithed rats with artificially raised blood pressure nor does it affect the cardiovascular responses

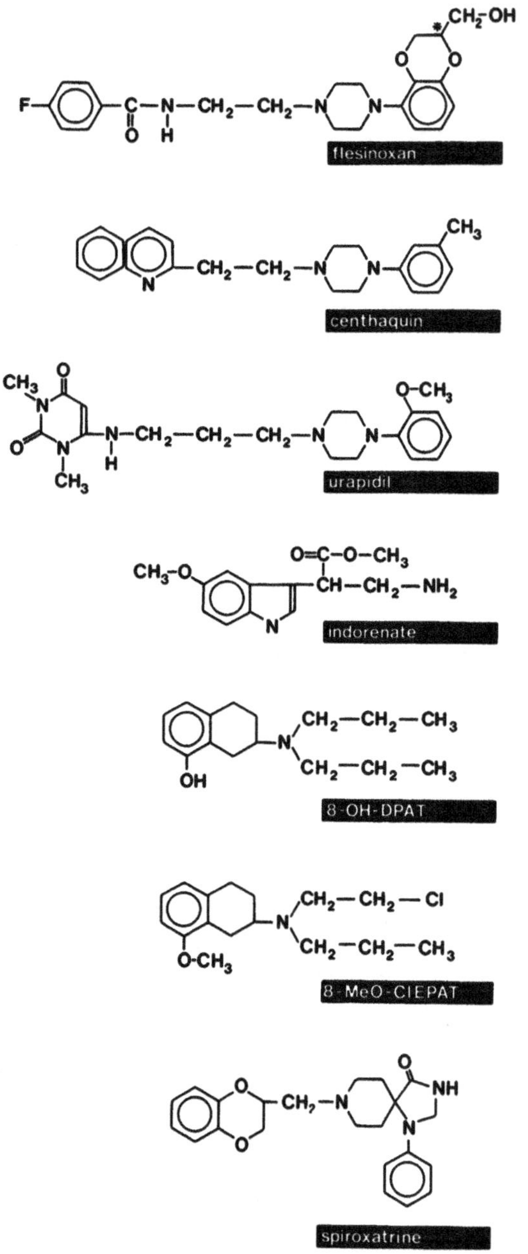

Fig. 3. Structural formulae of some drugs which have high and selective affinity for the 5-HT_{1A} binding sites. The *asterisk* in the formula of flesinoxan indicates an asymmetrical C-atom. Flesinoxan represents the (+)−enantiomere

to spinal stimulation or to phenylephrine in rats (GRADIN et al. 1985; FOZARD et al. 1987). Similarly, flesinoxan does not affect nictitating membrane contractions evoked by pre- or postganglionic stimulation of the cervical sympathetic nerve or the hypertensive response to phenylephrine in the cat (WOUTERS et al. 1988a, b). Thus, ganglion blockage, presynaptic inhibition, or α_1-adrenoceptor antagonism do not contribute to the cardiovascular effects of these compounds. Furthermore, conclusive evidence in favor of a central antihypertensive mechanism is provided by experiments in which the effects of drugs acting at 5-HT_1-like receptors have been studied on the sympathetic nerve activity. Both 8-OH-DPAT and flesinoxan reduce central sympathetic outflow (RAMAGE and FOZARD 1987; MCCALL et al. 1987; RAMAGE et al. 1988) and, interestingly, when activity of the renal, splanchnic, and cardiac nerves are recorded simultaneously, it appears that the renal nerve activity is affected most and the cardiac nerve activity, least by these drugs (Fig. 4; RAMAGE AND WILKINSON 1988; RAMAGE, personal communication). In contrast to 8-OH-DPAT and flesinoxan, the well-known, centrally acting, antihypertensive drug clonidine decreases activity in the cardiac nerve more than in the renal nerve (RAMAGE and WILKINSON 1988). Since the bradycardia induced by 8-OH-DPAT and flesinoxan is abolished by vagotomy or atropine, it seems that the CNS action of these drugs increases vagal tone (GRADIN et al. 1985; RAMAGE and FOZARD 1987; RAMAGE et al. 1988). Hypotension, along with bradycardia and a decrease in the renal nerve activity, has also recently been shown to occur with the administration of 5-HT into the fourth ventricle of the cat (COOTE et al. 1987) as has the centrally induced increases in the vagal tone in the rat (DALTON 1986).

In an extensive pharmacological analysis of the cardiovascular effects of 8-OH-DPAT in rats, FOZARD et al. (1987) made a number of important observations. The cardiovascular effects of 8-OH-DPAT are not antagonized by ketanserin or 1αH, 3α, 5αH-tropan-3yl-3,5-dichlorobenzoate (MDL 72222), thus excluding the involvement of 5-HT_2 or 5-HT_3 receptors. Clear antagonism is observed with the mixed 5-HT_1-like and 5-HT_2 receptor antagonists metergoline and methiothepin and the putative 5-HT_{1A} receptor antagonist 8-MeO-CLEPAT, indicating the involvement of 5-HT_{1A} receptors in the CNS. Similar results have been obtained with flesinoxan (Fig. 5; DRETELER et al., unpublished data). The β-adrenoceptor antagonists (±)pindolol and (±)cyanopindolol which have appreciable affinities for the 5-HT_{1A} binding site (see Table 1) clearly prevent the effects of 8-OH-DPAT and flesinoxan on blood pressure and heart rate. However, these compounds also antagonize the hypotension and bradycardia induced by clonidine (FOZARD et al. 1987; WOUTERS et al. 1988b). Antagonism of the responses to 8-OH-DPAT is also observed with the putative 5-HT_{1A} receptor antagonist spiroxatrine in the rat (DABIRÉ et al. 1987) and with methiothepin and (−)pindolol in the cat (DOODS et al. 1987). Lastly, there is a high degree of correlation between the hypotensive activities in cats and the affinities for the 5-HT_{1A} binding sites in a large series of analogues of flesinoxan (WOUTERS et al., unpublished data).

As the relationship between the CNS regulation of blood pressure and 5-HT becomes better defined, some already existing compounds with a central

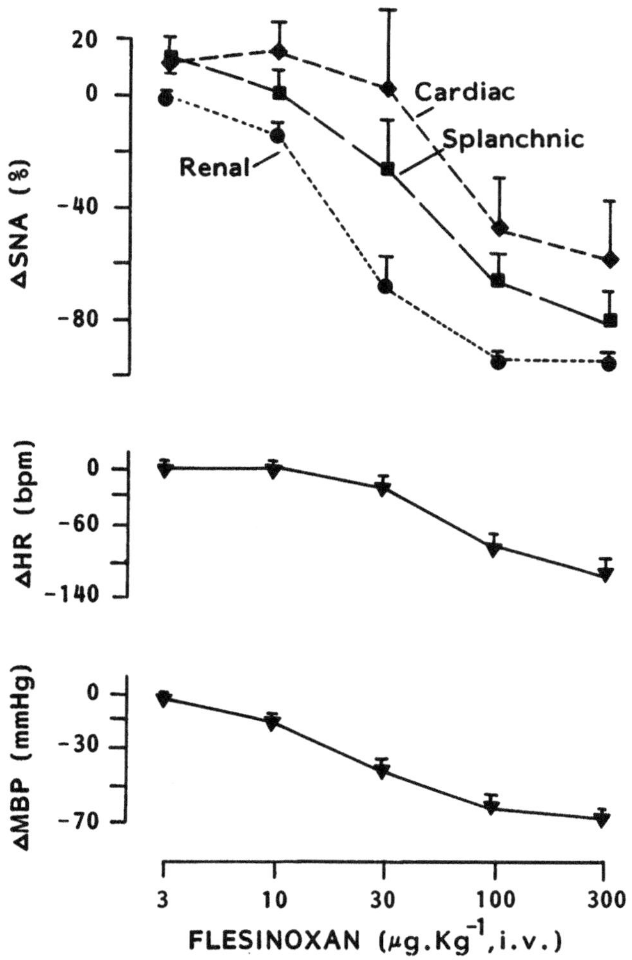

Fig. 4. Changes by flesinoxan in the activities of *cardiac, splanchnic,* and *renal* sympathetic nerves (*SNA*), heart rate (*HR*), and mean arterial blood pressure (*MBP*) in cats anesthetized with α-chloralose. Note the difference in the sensitivity to the inhibitory action of flesinoxan on the nerve activities recorded simultaneously. (Data courtesy of Dr. A.G. RAMAGE)

antihypertensive action, such as the tryptamine analogue indorenate (HONG et al. 1983) and the phenylpiperazine derivative centhaquin (SRIMAL et al. 1984) (Fig. 3), might well act via putative CNS 5-HT_{1A} receptors. Interestingly, the well-known, α_1-antagonistic antihypertensive, urapidil (Fig. 3), has an equal affinity to the 5-HT_{1A} binding site (GILLIS et al. 1987; GROSS et al. 1987), and a central hypotensive component is evident (VAN ZWIETEN et al. 1987a).

3.2.2 Activation of Presynaptic 5-Hydroxytryptamine Receptors on Sympathetic Nerves Causing Reduced Noradrenaline Release

The existence of 5-HT receptors on the presynaptic elements of postganglionic sympathetic nerves has been demonstrated in the organs of different species,

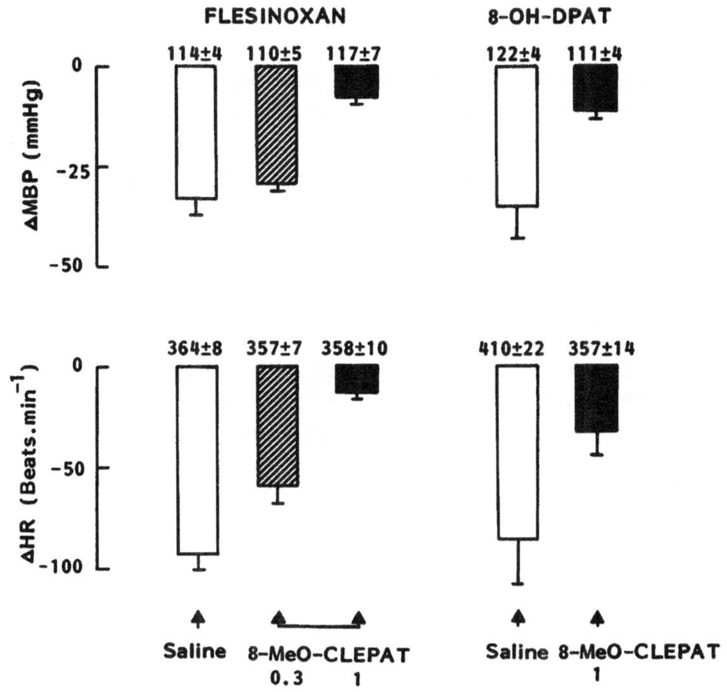

Fig. 5. Antagonism by 8-MeO-CLEPAT of the hypotensive and bradycardiac effects induced by flesinoxan (100 $\mu g.kg^{-1}$, i.v.) or 8-OH-DPAT (32 $\mu g.kg^{-1}$, i.v.) in pentobarbital-anesthetized rats. Saline and 8-MeO-CLEPAT (0.3 or 1.0 $mg.kg^{-1}$, i.v.) were administered 60 min before flesinoxan or 8-OH-DPAT. *Numbers above the different columns* represent values of mean blood pressure (*MBP*) or heart rate (*HR*) just before the administration of flesinoxan or 8-OH-DPAT. (Data courtesy of Dr. G.H. DRETELER)

like the canine and human saphenous vein (McGRATH 1977; FENIUK et al. 1979; GÖTHERT et al. 1986), rat kidney (CHARLTON et al. 1986), and rat vena cava (MOLDERINGS et al. 1987). Activation of these receptors by 5-HT (10^{-9} – $10^{-6}M$) causes a reduction of noradrenaline release in response to transmural stimulation by up to about 40%. Consequently, the end-organ response is diminished by 5-HT as shown, for example, in vitro by a reduction of the relaxation of canine coronary arteries induced by transmural electrical stimulation (COHEN 1985) and in vivo by a suppression of tachycardia in electrically stimulated pithed rats (GÖTHERT et al. 1986). The reduction in the release of the sympathetic transmitter by 5-HT and/or 5-CT is not antagonized by the 5-HT_2-selective antagonists ketanserin and 4-isopropyl-7-methyl-9-(2-hydroxy-l-methylpropoxycarbonyl)4,6,6a,7,8,9,10,10a-octahydroindolol[4,3-*fg*]quinoline maleate (LY 53857) (COHEN 1985; CHARLTON et al. 1986; GÖTHERT et al. 1986) or by metoclopramide (CHARLTON et al. 1986), which has 5-HT_3 receptor antagonistic property; therefore, mediation by 5-HT_2 or 5-HT_3 receptors can be excluded. The involvement of 5-HT_1-like receptors is favored by the high agonist potency of 5-CT (CHARLTON et al. 1986; MOLDERINGS et al. 1987) and by the fact that methiothepin, metergoline, and methysergide antagonize the effect of 5-HT

(COHEN 1985; LORENZ and VANHOUTTE 1985; CHARLTON et al. 1986; GOTHERT et al. 1986).

A further classification related to 5-HT_1 binding subsites (see Table 1) is still controversial. CHARLTON et al. 1986) using the isolated perfused rat kidney concluded that the prejunctional 5-HT receptor is distinct from the designated 5-HT_{1A}, 5-HT_{1B}, or 5-HT_{1C} subtypes. In their preparation 8-OH-DPAT and 5-methoxy-3-(1,2,3,6-tetrahydro-4-pyridinyl)-1H-indole (RU 24969) are inactive or only moderately potent as agonists, and the β-adrenoceptor antagonists, (−)propranolol, (±)pindolol, and (±)cyanopindolol, which have affinities for 5-HT_{1A} and 5-HT_{1B} binding sites, are inactive in antagonizing 5-HT-induced prejunctional effects. However, using rat vena cava, MOLDERINGS et al. (1987) found rather opposite results, i.e., a very high potency for RU 24969 and antagonism by propranolol. Whether these differences reflect differences in the receptor subtype or are due to changes in experimental conditions is not clear.

3.2.3 Relaxation of Blood Vessels due to Release of Endothelium-Derived Relaxant Factor by 5-Hydroxytryptamine-related Drugs

It has been amply shown that 5-HT-induced relaxations are markedly attenuated and 5-HT-induced contractions are exaggerated in isolated coronary and other vessels of the pig, dog, chick, and rabbit when endothelium is absent as compared with when it is present (COCKS and ANGUS 1983; R.A. COHEN et al. 1983; GRIFFITH et al. 1984; IMAIZUMI et al. 1984; LEFF et al. 1987; MARTIN et al. 1987; HOUSTON and VANHOUTTE 1988). The endothelium-dependent relaxation induced by 5-HT is not sensitive to ketanserin or MDL 72222 but is antagonized by methiothepin, methysergide, or metergoline (COCKS and ANGUS 1983; R.A. COHEN et al. 1983; MARTIN et al. 1987; HOUSTON and VANHOUTTE 1988), thus excluding the involvement of 5-HT_2 or 5-HT_3 receptors and indicating mediation by 5-HT_1-like receptors. These 5-HT_1-like receptors on the endothelium show no affinity for the 5-HT_{1A}-selective ligand 8-OH-DPAT or the 5-HT_{1A} and 5-HT_{1B} ligand cyanopindolol (HOUSTON and VANHOUTTE 1988) and also differ from some other 5-HT_1-like receptors (see BRADLEY et al. 1986) as cyproheptadine behaves as an antagonist (IMAIZUMI et al. 1984; LEFF et al. 1987), and 5-CT is a less potent agonist than 5-HT or α-methyl 5-HT (LEFF et al. 1987; MARTIN et al. 1987).

In vivo, 5-HT-induced endothelium-dependent vasodilatation has thus far been studied to a limited extent, and the evidence for a role of 5-HT is rather indirect. LAMPING et al. (1985) showed that removal of endothelium from the left anterior descending artery in anesthetized dogs strongly potentiates the constrictor responses to 5-HT but not to angiotensin II or phenylephrine.

3.2.4 Activation of 5-Hydroxytryptamine Receptors on Vascular Smooth Muscle Cells Resulting in Vasodilatation

The issue whether vasodilatation induced by 5-HT is mediated by 5-HT receptors on the endothelium (releasing EDRF) and/or on vascular smooth muscle cells has been recently studied in the rabbit jugular vein (MARTIN et al. 1987) and the canine coronary artery (HOUSTON and VANHOUTTE 1988). In both tissues, as compared with the preparations with intact endothelium higher concentrations of 5-HT are required for vasorelaxation after denudation of endothelium. Notwithstanding, 5-HT-induced relaxation in the endothelium-denuded preparations also qualifies as a 5-HT_1-like receptor-mediated response since methysergide and methiothepin, but not ketanserin and MDL 72222, are effective as antagonists (MARTIN et al. 1987; HOUSTON and VANHOUTTE 1988). However, the affinities and efficacies of a series of tryptamine agonists differ substantially for the 5-HT_1-like receptors on the endothelium and smooth muscle. Furthermore, unlike at the endothelial receptors, both *N,N*-dimethyl tryptamine and spiperone are competitive antagonists at the smooth muscle receptors.

It is not yet known to what extent vasodilatation induced by 5-HT in vivo is due to endothelial and/or vascular smooth muscle cell 5-HT_1-like receptors. In pentobarbital-anesthetized rats, however, the potency sequence of these tryptamines in inducing depressor responses shows close agreement with the affinity sequence at the smooth muscle 5-HT_1-like receptors (LEFF et al. 1987). The same appears to be the case with respect to arteriolar dilatation in the cat and pig (SAXENA et al. 1985; SAXENA and VERDOUW 1985; CONNOR et al. 1986). Further, 5-CT-induced depressor responses in the rat as well as 5-HT-induced relaxations of the rat jugular vein after endothelium removal are susceptible to antagonism by spiperone, whereas the endothelium-mediated relaxations of the rat jugular vein are not. These data support the veiw that 5-HT-induced vasodilatation in vivo is mediated by 5-HT_1-like receptors on vascular smooth muscle cells.

3.3 Clinical Effects of 5-Hydroxytryptamine Receptor Agonists

Little is known about the clinical efficacy of selective 5-HT receptor agonists in the treatment of human hypertension. Urapidil has been marketed in some countries, and initial clinical experience suggests that the drug is effective. However, it is not known to what extent 5-HT_{1A} receptor agonism contributes to the well-known α_1-adrenolytic effect of the drug in lowering blood pressure. Another 5-HT_{1A} receptor agonist that is undergoing clinical trial is flesinoxan. In a small, placebo-controlled, double-blind trial in hypertensive subjects, daily oral doses of 0.6–1.6 mg of flesinoxan lowered blood pressure and heart rate; the effects peaked (decreases of 18/11 mmHg and 13 beats. min^{-1} with 1.6-mg dose) after 1–2 h and lasted for about 6 h. The side effects noticed were dizziness, nausea, vomiting, and paleness (DE VOOGD 1988).

4 Antihypertensive Effects of 5-Hydroxytryptamine Receptor Antagonists

Amongst the antagonists of 5-HT only ketanserin has an undisputed antihypertensive effect in both animals and man. The mechanism of the antihypertensive effect of ketanserin still generates debate (see BOLT and SAXENA 1985; VAN-

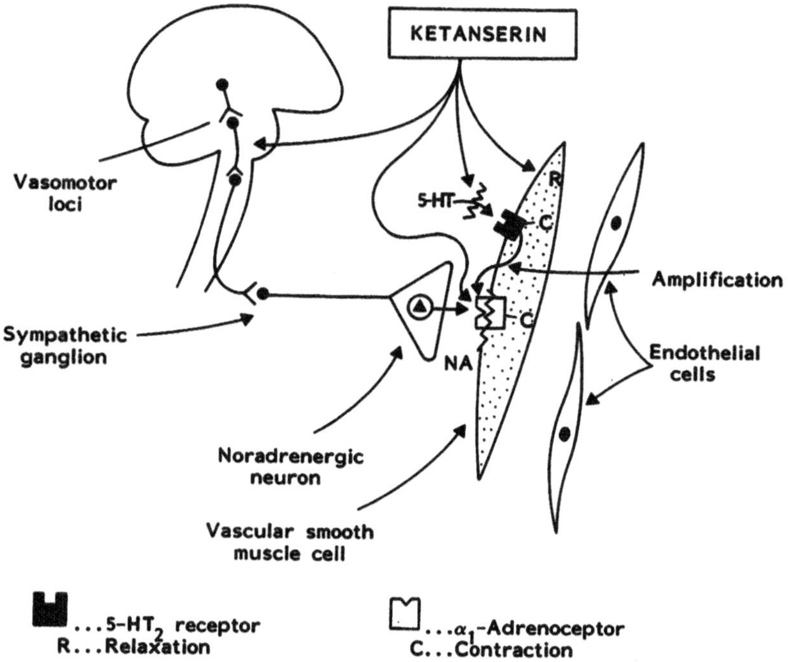

Fig. 6. The possible sites and mechanisms of antihypertensive action exerted by ketanserin. *NA*, noradrenaline

HOUTTE et al. 1986, 1988) and probably involves several factors (Fig. 6; SAXENA et al. 1987) contributing to different degrees as discussed below.

4.1 Blockade of 5-HT$_2$ Receptor-Mediated Vasoconstriction

Since both in animals and humans ketanserin possesses a high antagonistic activity against 5-HT-induced vasoconstriction (mediated by 5-HT$_2$ receptors) and unmasks the vasodilator effects of 5-HT (see, VAN NUETEN et al. 1981, 1987; BOLT and SAXENA 1985; VERDOUW et al. 1984; BLAUW et al. 1987, 1988; VANHOUTTE et al. 1988), many investigators immediately concluded that the antihypertensive effect of ketanserin is mainly related to 5-HT$_2$ receptor blockade (VAN NUETEN et al. 1981; WENTING et al. 1982; VANHOUTTE et al. 1983; JANSSEN 1985). The above conclusion is seemingly not valid for several reasons. Firstly, though some abnormalities in the metabolism of 5-HT may exist during hypertension (SYMOENS and VANHOUTTE 1985), 5-HT is present in very low concentrations in the plasma, and there is no convincing evidence to suggest a major role of 5-HT in the development or maintenance of hypertension. Secondly, though not often realized, the vasodilator effect of 5-HT on resistance vessels is much more marked than its vasconstrictor response (See Sect. 3.1). Thirdly, there is a poor correlation between 5-HT$_2$ receptor antagonism and the antihypertensive potential of a number of drugs (M.L. COHEN et al. 1983; KALKMAN et al. 1983b), and several highly selective 5-HT_2 antagonists—LY 53857 (M.L. COHEN et al. 1983), ritanserin (HOSIE et al. 1987; VAN ZWIETEN et al. 1987b; BLAUW et al. 1988), 2-(2-dimethylamino-2-methylpropylthio)-3-phenylquindine hydrochloride (ICI 170809; BLACKBURN et al. 1988)—do not seem to be effective as antihypertensive agents.

4.2 α_1-Adrenoceptor Blockade

It is now well-established that ketanserin has an appreciable α_1-adrenoceptor blocking activity. In experimental animals this effect is observed at doses which, though higher than needed for 5-HT_2 receptor antagonism, show antihypertensive activity (FOZARD 1982; KALKMAN et al. 1982; WRIGHT and ANGUS 1983; MARWOOD and STOKES 1984; BOLT and SAXENA 1985), and there is a remarkable similarity in the regional hemodynamic profiles of ketanserin and prazosin in hypertensive rabbits (BOLT and SAXENA 1985). In normal volunteers and hypertensive subjects also, distinct (though perhaps weaker than prazosin) α_1-adrenoceptor antagonism has been demonstrated with ketanserin after acute or chronic administration in several investigations (REIMANN and FROHLICH 1983; BALL et al. 1983; FAGARD et al. 1984; CASIGLIA et al. 1986; BERDEAUX et al. 1987; BLAUW et al. 1987, 1988). It should, however, be noted that acute administration of ketanserin can lower blood pressure for a short time in hypertensive subjects without concomitant α_1-adrenoceptor blockade (WENTING et al. 1982, 1984) or in normotensive subjects with autonomic insufficiency (WENTING et al. 1984).

Recently, two more compounds—irindalone (DRAGSTED and BOECK 1988) and 4-{3-[3-(4-(4-fluorobezoyl)-1-piperidinyl)-propoky]-4-methoryphenyl}-1-pyrolidone (ZK 33.839; SCHRÖDER et al. 1988)—have been described which, like ketanserin, possess 5-HT_2 receptor and α_1-adrenoceptor blocking actions. Both these compounds decrease arterial blood pressure in hypertensive animals.

4.3 Inhibition of Central Vasomotor Loci

Contrary to initial suggestions, ketanserin does seem to enter into the CNS as it causes sedation and electroencephalographic changes in humans (HERRMANN and BAUMGARTNER 1986; REIMANN et al. 1986). It also interferes with central cardiovascular control mechanisms. Thus, ketanserin-induced hypotension (a) is accompanied by a decrease in sympathetic nerve discharges after i.v. administration to baroreceptor denervated (MCCALL and SCHUETTE 1984) or innervated (RAMAGE 1985) cats and spontaneously hypertensive rats (HEDNER et al. 1986); (b) can be obtained in cats upon intracarotid (COPELAND and BENTLEY 1985) or intravertebral (VAN ZWIETEN et al. 1987b) infusions; (c) is associated with suppression of centrally integrated pressor responses (carotid occlusion and nicotine) in doses after low i.v. doses that do not affect peripheral sympathetic transmission (PHILLIPS et al. 1985); (d) is exerted without clear changes in baroreceptor sensitivity (VANHOUTTE et al. 1986); and (e) is not accompanied by sustained reflex increases in heart rate (FOZARD 1982; KALKMAN et al. 1982; WENTING et al. 1982; WRIGHT and ANGUS 1983; BOLT and SAXENA 1985; WOITTIEZ et al. 1986; HEDNER et al. 1987) and plasma renin or catecholamine levels (WOITTIEZ et al. 1986; HENDER et al. 1987) in both hypertensive animals and humans.

The receptors mediating the central antihypertensive action are not clearly delineated. The mixed 5-HT_1 and 5-HT_2 receptor antagonist methysergide, which may function as a partial agonist at some 5-HT_1-like receptors (BRADLEY et al. 1986; SAXENA 1974), reduces blood pressure, heart rate, pressor responses to bilateral carotid occlusion, and sympathetic nerve activity (SAXENA 1974; ANTONACCIO and TAYLOR 1977; RAMAGE 1985), but the other highly selective 5-HT_2 receptor antagonists, LY 53857 (RAMAGE 1985) and ritanserin (HOSIE et al. 1987; VAN ZWIETEN et al. 1987b; BLAUW et al. 1988), do not exhibit hypotensive activity. Although like ketanserin, the α_1-adrenoceptor antagonist prazosin shows central hypotensive activity (MCCALL and SCHUETTE 1984), the involvement of central α-adrenoceptors is not borne out by corynanthine and rauwolscine (VAN ZWIETEN et al. 1987b). Further investigation is needed to establish the role of 5-HT_2 and/or α_1-adrenoceptors in the antihypertensive activity of ketanserin as well as in the central regulation of cardiovascular activity.

4.4 Combined Blockade of α_1-Adrenoceptors and 5-HT_2 Receptor-Mediated Amplification of Noradrenaline Response

Since at levels giving similar antihypertensive effects ketanserin may be weaker than prazosin as an α_1-adrenoceptor antagonist and since ritanserin and LY 53857 are devoid of antihypertensive properties (see Sect. 4.2), VAN NUETEN et al. (1986) suggest that a combination of 5-HT_2 receptor (responsible for the potentiation of noradrenaline-induced vasoconstriction) and α_1-adrenoceptor blockade is needed for the antihypertensive action of ketanserin. Some evidence for this is provided by the observation that ritanserin, which has no effect against phenylephrine-induced vasoconstriction, potentiates the hypotensive action of prazosin or phentolamine (VAN DER STARRE 1988; VAN NUETEN et al. 1988).

4.5 "Direct" Vasodilatation

In renal hypertensive rabbits, ketanserin produces a biphasic hypotensive effect, consisting of a short-lasting but pronounced phase and a longer-lasting but more moderate phase (BOLT and SAXENA 1985). Since the initial hypotensive effect persists after blockade of autonomic ganglia by hexamethonium, ketanserin also has a "direct" vasodilator activity (BOLT and SAXENA 1985) that may play a limited role in the antihypertensive action of the drug in some circumstances.

4.6 Clinical Effects of 5-Hydroxytryptamine Receptor Antagonists

Among the 5-HT receptor antagonists only ketanserin, which blocks 5-HT_2 receptors but also has other properties (see above), has been shown to lower arterial blood pressure in hypertensive patients (see review by VANHOUTTE et al. 1988). Acute administration of ketanserin (10 mg, i.v.) lowers both systolic and diastolic pressures with only small increases in heart rate and cardiac output, showing that the drug mainly decreases total peripheral resistance. It does not consistently lower pressure in patients with uncontrolled hypertension and, therefore, is not suitable for use in hypertensive emergencies, except perhaps for hypertensive episodes during or after coronary artery bypass surgery or in carcinoid syndrome. Long-term use of ketanserin in several placebo-controlled trials has established the antihypertensive effect of the drug. The magnitude of the depressor effect of ketanserin is comparable to that of β-adrenoceptor antagonists or diuretics which with it shows an additive (not synergistic) effect. Several studies have indicated that the antihypertensive effect of ketanserin is more marked in patients over 60 years of age (VANHOUTTE et al. 1988). It should, however, be pointed out that ketanserin may not be unique in this respect because, with increasing age and arterial calcification, the wall to luman ratio is altered, and many drugs acting via arterial vasodilatation can show an age-related hyperresponsiveness.

The side effects of ketanserin (drowsiness, sleepiness, lack of concentration, and lightheadedness) are usually mild and disappear after a few days. In early studies using high doses (60 mg or more) side effects, mainly drowsiness, fatigue, dizziness, and headache, were often noted. In addition, ketanserin seems to prolong the Q-Tc interval particularly in patients who have low blood potassium levels or are also receiving antiarrhythmics (VANHOUTTE et al. 1988).

The exact place of ketanserin in the therapy of hypertension is not yet clear. More extensive use of the drug, as is expected after its marketing in several countries, will determine its value in comparison with other drugs in the treatment of hypertension.

5 Conclusions

The receptors for 5-HT can now be subdivided into three distinct groups named 5-HT_1-like (agonist: 5-CT; antagonists: methysergide and methiothepin), 5-HT_2 (antagonists: ketanserin and cyproheptadine besides methysergide and methiothepin), and 5-HT_3 [agonist: 2-methyl-5-HT; antagonists: MDL 72222 and (3α-tropanyl)-1H-indole-3-carboxylic acid ester (ICS 205-930)]. These receptors mediate the pharmacological effects of 5-HT, including those in the cardiovascular system, but the physiological role of the amine in the regulation of cardiovascular activity is still unclear.

Upon injection into the CNS 5-HT elicits either a pressor or a depressor response that seems to depend upon the dose, the site of administration, and the receptor type involved. Recent findings suggest that the depressor effect may be mediated by central 5-HT_1-like receptors. Peripherally, 5-HT elicits vasodilatation (both directly and indirectly via presynaptic sympathoinhibition and the release of EDRF) or vasoconstriction with associated amplification of noradrenaline response mediated by, respectively, 5-HT_1-like and 5-HT_2 receptors.

The above account suggests that antihypertensive drug therapy can be achieved via 5-HT in mainly three ways. Firstly, activation of central 5-HT_1-like receptors by compounds which exhibit a high affinity for the 5-HT_{1A} binding site lowers blood pressure in both hypertensive and normotensive animals. Such compounds are undergoing clinical investigation. Secondly, selective agonists at peripheral 5-HT_1-like receptors can lead to vasodilatation and reduced blood pressure mainly by a direct action on blood vessels as well as indirectly by interfering with the release of noradrenaline from the postganglionic sympathetic nerve fibers. Such drugs are yet to be tried in humans. The third approach may be via 5-HT_2 receptor blockade. However, of the various antagonists of 5-HT_2 receptors, arterial blood pressure is lowered by ketanserin which has other properties such as the α_1-adrenoceptor antagonism and central sympathoinhibition. Therefore, it is doubtful that 5-HT_2 receptor antagonism plays a primary role in the antihypertensive action of ketanserin. Early clinical experiences with ketanserin seems to suggest that its antihypertensive effect is equivalent to that of β-adrenoceptor antagonists or thiazide diuretics and is apparently more marked in elderly patients. Clinical data with ketanserin is so far limited and, therefore, its right place in the antihypertensive regimen is yet to be determined.

Acknowledgements. We are grateful to Dr. A.G. Ramage and Dr. G.H. Dreteler for the use of their unpublished data and to the *Journal of Cardiovascular Pharmacology* and the *Journal of Drug Research* for the use of figures.

Summary

5-Hydroxytryptamine (5-HT) has complex effects on arterial blood pressure. Central injection of 5-HT induces either a pressor or a depressor response depending upon dose, site of administration and receptor type involved. The depressor effect seems to be mediated by central 5-HT_1-like receptors (putative 5-HT_{1A} subtype). Peripherally, 5-HT elicits vasodilatation (both by a direct action on the vascular smooth muscle and indirectly via presynaptic sympathoinhibition and the release of relaxant factor(s) from the endothelium) or vasoconstriction with associated amplification of noradrenaline response mediated by, respectively, 5-HT_1-like and 5-HT_2 receptors. Therefore, antihypertensive action via 5-HT mechanisms can be achieved mainly with compounds that are (a) agaonists at the central 5-HT_{1A} receptors, (b) agonists at the peripheral 5-HT_1-like receptors on blood vessels and/or postganglionic sympathetic neurons, or (c) antagonists at the vascular 5-HT_2 receptors. However, of the various 5-HT_2 receptor antagonists, only ketanserin lowers artieral blood pressure, and it has other properties such as the α_1-adrenoceptor antagonism and central sympathoinhibition.

References

Antonaccio MJ, Taylor DJ (1977) Reduction in blood pressure, sympathetic nerve discharge and centrally evoked pressor responses by methysergide in anaesthetized cats. Eur J Pharmacol 42:331–338

Ball SG, Zabludowski JR, Robertson JIS (1983) Mechanism of antihypertensive action of ketanserin in man. Br Med J 287:1065

Berdeaux A, Edouard A, Samii K, Giudicelli JF (1987) Ketanserin and the arterial baroreceptor reflex in normotensive subjects. Eur J Clin Pharmacol 32:27–33

Bhargava KP, Tangri KK (1959) The central vasomotor effects of 5-hydroxytryptamine. Br J Pharmacol 14:411–414

Blackburn TP, Haworth SJ, Jessup CL, Morton PB, Williams C (1988) ICI 170809, a selective 5-hydroxytryptamine antagonist, inhibits human aggregation in vitro and ex vivo (Abstr P37). International Congress on Cardiovascular Pharmacology of 5-HT, Oct 4–7, Amsterdam

Blauw GJ, van Brummelen P, Chang PC, van Zwieten PA (1987) Vascular effects of serotonin and ketanserin in man. J Hypertens [Suppl 5] 5:S201–S203

Blauw GJ, van Brummelen P, Chang PC, van Zwieten PA (1988) Regional vascular effects of serotonin and ketanserin in young, healthy subjects. Hypertension 11: 256–263

Bolt GR, Saxena PR (1985) Cardiovascular profile and hypotensive mechanism of ketanserin in the rabbit. Hypertension 7:499–506

Bradley PB, Engel G, Feniuk W, Fozard JR, Humphrey PPA, Middlemiss DN, Mylecharane JE, Richardson B, Saxem PR (1986) Proposals for the classification and nomenclature of functional receptors for 5-hydroxytryptamine. Neuropharmacology 25:563–575

Casiglia E, Gava R, Semplicini A, Nicolin P, Pessina AC (1986) The mechanism of the antihypertensive effects of ketanserin: a comparison with metoprolol. Br J Clin Pharmacol 22:751–752

Chalmers JP (1975) Brain amines and models of experimental hypertension. Circ Res 36:469–480

Charlton KG, Bond RA, Clarke DE (1986) An inhibitory prejunctional 5-HT_1-like receptor in the isolated perfused rat kidney. Naunyn Schmied ebergs Arch Pharmacol 332:8–15

Cocks TM, Angus JA (1983) Endothelium-dependent relaxation of coronary arteries by noradrenaline and serotonin. Nature 305:627–630

Cohen ML, Fuller RW, Kurz KD (1983) LY 53857, a selective new potent serotonergic (5-HT_2) receptor antagonist, does not lower blood pressure in the spontaneously hypertensive rat. J Pharmacol Exp Ther 227:327–332

Cohen RA (1985) Serotonergic prejunctional inhibition of canine coronary adrenergic nerves. J Pharmacol Exp Ther 235:76–80

Cohen RA, Shepherd JT, Vanhoutte PM (1983) 5-Hydroxytryptamine can mediate endothelium-dependent relaxation of coronary arteries. Am J Physiol 245: H1077–H1080

Connor HE, Feniuk W, Humphrey PPA, Perren MJ (1986) 5-Carboxamidotryptamine is a selective agonist at 5-hydroxytryptamine receptors mediating vasodilation and tachycardia in anaesthetized cats. Br J Pharmacol 87:417–426

Coote JH, Dalton DW, Feniuk W, Humphrey PPA (1987) The central site of the sympatho-inhibitory action of 5-hydroxytryptamine in the cat. Neuropharmacology 26:147–154

Copeland IW, Bentley GA (1985) A possible central action of prazosin and ketanserin to cause hypotension. J Cardiovasc Pharmacol 7:822–825

Dabiré H, Cherqui C, Fournier B, Schmitt H (1987) Comparison of effects of some 5-HT_1 agonists on blood pressure and heart rate of normotensive anesthetized rats. Eur J Pharmacol 140:259–266

Dalton DW (1986) The cardiovascular effects of centrally administered 5-hydroxytryptamine in the conscious normotensive and hypertensive rat. J Auton Pharmacol 6:67–75

De Voogd JM (1988) Early clinical experience with flesinoxan, a new selective 5-HT_{1A} agonist (Abstr P42). International Congress on Cardiovascular Pharmacology of 5-HT, Oct 4–7, Amsterdam
Docherty JR (1986) 5-Hydroxytryptamine receptors involved in vasodilation in the pithed rat. Br J Pharmacol 89:753P
Doods HN, Kalkman HO, de Jonge A, Thoolen JMC, Wilffert B, Timmermans PBMWM, van Zwieten PA (1985) Differential selectivities of RU 24969 and 8-OH-DPAT for the purported 5-HT_{1A} and 5-HT_{1B} binding sites. Correlation between 5-HT_{1A} affinity and hypertensive activity. Eur J Pharmacol 112:363–370
Doods HN, Kalkman HO, Mathy MJ (1987) Central hypertensive activity in the cat of compounds with high affinity for 5-HT_{1A}-receptors. Naunyn Schmied ebergs Arch Pharmacol 335:R90
Dragsted N, Boeck V (1988) Cardiovascular effects of irindalone, a novel 5-HT_2 antagonist with antihypertensive activity (Abstr P43). International Congress on Cardiovascular Pharmacology of 5-HT, Oct 4–7, Amsterdam
Engel G, Göthert M, Müller-Schweinitzer E, Schlicker E, Sistonen L, Stadler PA (1983) Evidence for common pharmacological properties of [^{3}H]5-hydroxytryptamine binding sites, presynaptic 5-hydroxytryptamine autoreceptors in CNS and inhibitory presynaptic 5-hydroxytryptamine receptors on sympathetic nerves. Naunyn Schmied ebergs Arch Pharmacol 324:116–124
Fagard R, Fioli R, Lijnen P, Staessen J, Moeman E, de Schaepdryver A, Amery A (1984) Haemodynamic and humoral responses to chronic ketanserin treatment in essential hypertension. Br Heart J 51:149–156
Feniuk W, Humphrey PPA, Watts AD (1979) Presynaptic inhibitory action of 5-hydroxytryptamine in dog isolated saphenous vein. Br J Pharmacol 67:247–254
Feniuk W, Humphrey PPA, Watts AD (1981) Analysis of the mechanism of 5-hydroxytryptamine-induced vasopressor responses in ganglion-blocked anaesthetized dogs. J Pharm Pharmacol 33:155–160
Fozard JR (1982) Mechanism of the hypotensive effect of ketanserin. J Cardiovasc Pharmacol 4:829–838
Fozard JR (1984) MDL 72222: a potent and highly selective antagonist at neuronal 5-HT receptors. Naunyn Schmied ebergs Arch Pharmacol 326:36–44
Fozard JR, Mir AK, Middlemiss DN (1987) The cardiovascular response to 8-hydroxy-2-(Di-N-propylamino)-tetralin (8-OH-DPAT) in the rat: site of action and pharmacological analysis. J Cardiovasc Pharmacol 9:328–347
Gaddum JH, Picarelli ZP (1957) Two kinds of tryptamine receptors. Br J Pharmacol 12:323–328
Gillis RA, Hill K, Kirbt JS, Martino-Barrows A, Gatti PJ, Quest JA, Norman WP, Kellar KJ (1987) Possible sites and mechanisms where by urapidil and its analogue B695–40 exert CNS mediated hypotensive effects. In Rand MJ, Raper C (eds) Pharmacology. Elsevier, Amsterdam, pp 31–36
Göthert M, Schlicker E, Kollecker P (1986) Receptor mediated effects of serotonin and 5-methoxytryptamine on noradrenaline release in the rat vena cavia and in the heart of the pithed rat. Naunyn Schmied ebergs Arch Pharmacol 336:124–130
Gradin K, Pettersson A, Hedner T, Persson B (1985) Acute administration of 8-hydroxy-2-(Di-N-propylamino) tetralin (8-OH-DPAT), a selective 5-HT-receptor agonist, causes a biphasic blood pressure response and a bradycardia in the normotensive Sprague-Dawley rat and in the spontaneously hypertensive rat. J Neural Transm 62:305–319
Griffith TM, Henderson AH, Hughes ED, Lewis MJ (1984) Isolated perfused rabbit coronary artery and aortic strip preparations: The role of endothelium-derived relaxant factor. J Physiol (Lond) 351:12–24
Gross G, Hanft G, Kolassa N (1987) Derivatives of urapidil with hypotensive properties high affinity for 5-HT_{1A} receptors. Br J Pharmacol 92:753P
Hedner T, Pettersson A, Gradin K, Persson B (1986) Peripheral serotonergic mechanisms in cardiovascular regulation in the spontaneously hypertensive rat. J Hypertens [Suppl 3] 4:S223–S225
Hedner T, Andersson OK, Pettersson A, Persson B (1987) Cardiovascular effects of

ketanserin during cold pressure and during isometric and dynamic exercise in hypertensive patients. J Cardiovasc Pharmacol [Suppl 3] 10:S73–S77

Herrmann WM, Baumgartner P (1986) Combined pharmaco-EEG and pharmacopsychological study to estimate CNS effects of ketanserin in hypertensive patients. Neuropsychobiology 16:47–56

Heuring RE, Peroutka SJ (1987) Characterization of a novel ^{3}H-5-hydroxytryptamine binding site subtypes in bovine brain membranes. J Neurosci 7:894–903

Hollenberg NK (1987) Collateral arterial tree and responses to serotonin. J Cardiovasc Pharmacol [Suppl 3] 10:S35–S38

Hong E, Rion R, Vidrio M (1983) Stimulation of central serotonin receptors as a novel mechanism of antihypertensive activity. In: Bevan JA, Fujiwara M, Maxwell RA, Mohri K, Shibata S, Toda N (eds) Vascular neuroeffector mechanisms. Raven, New York, pp 273–277

Hosie J, Stott DJ, Robertson JIS, Ball SG (1987) Does acute serotenergic type-2 antagonism reduce blood pressure? Comparative effects of single doses of ritanserin and ketanserin in essential hypertension. J Cardiovasc Pharmacol [Suppl 3] 10:S86–S88

Houston DS, Vanhoutte PM (1988) Comparison of serotonergic receptor subtypes on the smooth muscle and endothelium of the canine coronary artery. J Pharmacol Exp Ther 244:1–10

Hoyer D, Neijt HC (1988) Identification of serotonin 5-HT_3 recognition sites in membranes of N1E-115 neuroblastoma cells by radioligand binding. Mol Pharmacol 33:303–309

Hoyer D, Engel G, Kalkman HO (1985) Molecular pharmacology of 5-HT_1 and 5-HT_2 recognition sites in rat and pig brain membranes: radioligand binding studies with [^{3}H]5-HT, [^{3}H]8-OH-DPAT, (−)[125I]iodocyano-pindolol, [^{3}H]mesulergine and [^{3}H]ketanserin. Eur J Pharmacol 118:13–23

Humphrey PPA, Richardson BP (1989) 5-HT receptor classification: a current view based on a workshop debate. In: Mylecharane EJ, Angus A, de la Lande I, Humphrey PPA (eds) Serotonin. Macmillan, Basingstoke (in press)

Imaizumi Y, Baba M, Imaizumi Y, Watanabe M (1984) Involvement of endothelium in the relaxation of isolated chick jugular vein by 5-hydroxytryptamine. Eur J Pharmacol 97:335–336

Janssen PAJ (1985) Pharmacology of potent and selective S_2-serotonergic antagonists. J Cardiovasc Pharmacol [Suppl 7] 7:S2–S11

Kalkman HO, Timmermans PBMWM, van Zwieten PA (1982) Characterization of the antihypertensive properties of ketanserin (R41468) in rats. J Pharmacol Exp Ther 222:227–231

Kalkman HO, Boddeke HWGM, Doods HN, Timmermans PBMWM, van Zwieten PA (1983a) Hypertensive activity of serotonin receptor agonists in rats is elated to their affinity for 5-HT_1 receptors. Eur J Pharmacol 91:155–156

Kalkman HO, Harms YM, van Gelderen EM, Batink HD, Timmermans PBMWM, van Zwieten PA (1983b) Hypotensive activity of serotonin antagonists; correlation with α_1-adrenoceptor and serotonin receptor blockade. Life Sci 32:1499–1505

Kalkman HO, Engel G, Hoyer D (1984) Three distinct types of serotonergic receptors mediate the triphasic blood pressure response to serotonin in rats. J Hypertens [Suppl 2] 6:S421–S428

Kilpatrick GJ, Jones BJ, Tyers MB (1987) Identification and distribution of 5-HT_3 receptors in rat brain using radioligand binding. Nature 330:746–748

Krstic MK (1985) Central serotonergic and tryptaminergic regulation of the cardiovascular system. Period Biol 87:131–140

Kuhn DM, Wolf WA, Lovenberg W (1980) Review of the role of the central serotonergic neuronal system in blood pressure regulation. Hypertension 2:243–255

Lamping KG, Marcus ML, Dole WP (1985) Removal of endothelium potentiates canine large coronary artery constrictor responses to 5-hydroxytryptamine in vivo. Circ Res 57:46–54

Leff P, Martin GR, Morse JM (1987) Differential classification of vascular smooth muscle and endothelial cell 5-HT receptors by use of tryptamine analogues. Br J Pharmacol 91:321–331

Leysen JE (1981) Serotonergic receptors in brain tissue: properties and identification of various ^{3}H-ligand binding sites in vitro. J Physiol (Paris) 77:351–362
Leysen JE, de Chaffoy de Courcelles D, de Clerck F, Niemegeers CJE, van Nueten JM (1984) Serotonin-S_2 receptor binding sites and functional correlates. Neuropharmacology 23:1493–1501
Lorenz RR, Vanhoutte PM (1985) Prejunctional adrenergic inhibition by aggregating platelets in canine blood vessels. Am J Physiol 249:H685–H689
Martin GE, Lis EV (1985) Hypertensive action of 8-hydroxy-2-(Di-N-propylamino) tetralin (8-OH-DPAT) in spontaneously hypertensive rats. Arch Int Pharmacodyn 273:251–261
Martin GR, Leff P, Cambridge D, Barrett VJ (1987) Comparative analysis of two types of 5-hydroxytryptamine receptor mediating vasorelaxation: differential classification using tryptamines. Naunyn Schmiedebergs Arch Pharmacol 336:365–373
Marwood JF, Stokes GS (1984) Studies on the mechanism of action of the hypotensive effect of ketanserin. Clin Exp Pharmacol Physiol 11:125–132
McCall RB, Schuette MR (1984) Evidence for an alpha-1 receptor-mediated central sympathoinhibitory action of ketanserin. J Pharmacol Exp Ther 228:704–710
McCall RB, Patel BN, Harris LT (1987) Effects of serotonin$_1$ and serotonin$_2$ receptor agonists and antagonists on blood pressure, heart rate and sympathetic nerve activity. J Pharmacol Exp Ther 242:1152–1159
McGrath MA (1977) 5-Hydroxytryptamine and neurotransmitter release in canine blood vessels. Inhibition by low and augmentation by high concentrations. Circ Res 41:428–435
Molderings GJ, Fink K, Schlicker E, Göthert M (1987) Inhibition of noradrenaline release via presynaptic 5-HT_{1B} receptors of the rat vena cava. Naunyn Schmiedebergs Arch Pharmacol 336:245–280
Nelson DL, Taylor ET (1986) Spiroxatrine: A selective serotonin$_{1A}$ receptor antagonist. Eur J Pharmacol 124:207–208
Page IH (1957) Cardiovascular actions of serotonin (5-hydroxytryptamine). In: Lewis GP (ed) 5-Hydroxytryptamine. Pergamon, London, pp 93–108
Page IH, McCubbin JW (1953) Modification of vascular responses to serotonin. Am J Physiol 174:436–440
Palmer RMJ, Ferrige AG, Moncada S (1987) Nitric oxide release accounts for the biological activity of endothelium-derived relaxing factor. Nature 327:524–526
Pedigo NW, Yamamura HI, Nelson DL (1981) Discrimination of multiple [^{3}H]5-hydroxytryptamine binding sites by the neuroleptic spiperone in rat brain. J Neurochem 36:220–226
Peroutka SJ (1986) Pharmacological identification of 5-HT_{1A}, 5-HT_{1B} and 5-HT_{1C} binding sites in rat frontal cortex. J Neurochem 47:529–540
Peroutka SJ, Snyder SH (1979) Multiple serotonin receptors differential binding of [^{3}H]-5-hydroxytryptamine, [^{3}H]-lysergic acid diethylamide and [^{3}H]-spiroperidol. Mol Pharmacol 16:687–699
Phillips CA, Mylecharane EJ, Markus JK, Shaw J (1985) Hypotensive actions of ketanserin in dogs: involvement of a centrally mediated inhibition of sympathetic vascular tone. Eur J Pharmacol 111:319–327
Ramage AG (1985) The effects of ketanserin, methysergide and LY 53857 on sympathetic nerve activity. Eur J Pharmacol 113:295–303
Ramage AG, Fozard JR (1987) Evidence that the putative 5-HT_{1A} receptor agonists, 8-OH-DPAT and ipsapirone, have a central hypertensive action that differs from that of clonidine in anaesthetized cats. Eur J Pharmacol 38:179–191
Ramage AG, Wilkinson SJ (1988) Evidence for differentiation sympathoinhibitory action of 8-OH-DPAT and clonidine in anaesthetized cats. Br J Pharmacol 93:121P
Ramage AG, Wouters W, Bevan P (1988) Evidence that the novel antihypertensive agent flesinoxan causes differential sympathoinhibition and also increases vagal tone by a central action. Eur J Pharmacol 151:373–379
Reimann IW, Frohlich JC (1983) Mechanism of antihypertensive action of ketanserin in man. Br Med J 287:381–383
Reimann IW, Ziegler G, Ludwig L, Frohlich JC (1986) Central and autonomic nervous

system side effects of ketanserin. Arzneimittel forschung 36(2):1681–1684
Saxena PR (1974) Selective vasoconstriction in the carotid vascular bed by methysergide: possible relevance to its antimigraine effect. Eur J Pharmacol 27:99–105
Saxena PR (1986) Nature of the 5-hydroxytryptamine receptors in mammalian heart. Prog Pharmacol 6:173–185
Saxena PR, Lawang A (1985) A comparison of cardiovascular and smooth muscle effects of 5-hydroxytryptamine and 5-carboxamidotryptamine, a selective agonist of 5-HT_1-like receptors. Arch Int Pharmacodyn Ther 227:235–252
Saxena PR, Verdouw PD (1982) Redistribution by 5-hydroxytryptamine of carotid arterial blood at the expense of arteriovenous blood flow. J Physiol (Lond) 332: 501–520
Saxena PR, Verdouw PD (1984) Effects of methysergide and 5-hydroxytryptamine on carotid blood flow distribution in pigs: further evidence of the presence of atypical 5-HT receptors. Br J Pharmacol 82:817–826
Saxena PR, Verdouw PD (1985) 5-Carboxamide tryptamine, a compound with high affinity for 5-hydroxytryptamine binding sites, dilates arterioles and constricts arteriovenous anastomoses. Br J Pharmacol 84:533–544
Saxena PR, van Houwelingen P, Bonta IL (1971) The effect of mianserin hydrochloride on the vascular responses to 5-hydroxytryptamine and related substances. Eur J Pharmacol 13:295–305
Saxena PR, Mylecharane EJ, Heiligers J (1985) Analysis of the heart rate effects of 5-hydroxytryptamine in the cat; mediation by 5-HT_1-like receptors. Naunyn Schmiedebergs Arch Pharmacol 330:121–129
Saxena PR, Richardson B, Mylecharane EJ, Middlemiss DN, Humphrey PPA, Fozard JR, Feniuk W, et al. (1986) Functional receptors for 5-hydroxytryptamine. Trends Pharmacol Sci 7(7):Centrefold
Saxena PR, Bolt GR, Dhasmana KM (1987) Serotonin agonists and antagonists in experimental hypertension. J Cardiovasc Pharmacol [Suppl 3] 10:S12–S18
Schröder G, Beckmann R, Müller B, Schulz BG, Stock G (1988) Pharmacological profile of ZK 33.839, a new $5\text{-HT}_2/\alpha_1$-antagonist (Abstr P38). International Congress on Cardiovascular Pharmacology of 5-HT, Oct 4–7, Amsterdam
Srimal RC, Gulati AK, Dhawan BN (1984) Centhaquin, a new centrally acting hypotensive agent (Abstr). 9th IUPHAR Congress, London
Sukamoto TT, Yamamoto S, Watanabe S, Ueki S (1984) Cardiovascular responses to centrally administered serotonin in conscious normotensive and spontaneously hypertensive rats. Eur J Pharmacol 100:173–179
Symoens J, Vanhoutte PM (1985) The role of serotonin in blood pressure regulation. In: Smith JAR, Watkins J (eds) Care of the postoperative patient. Butterworth, London, pp 141–164
Van der Starre PJA (1988) Ketanserin and hypertension in cardiac surgery. Thesis, State University of Limburg, Maastricht
Vanhoutte PM, van Nueten JM, Symoens J, Janssen PAJ (1983) Antihypertensive properties of ketanserin (R7 41 468). Fed Proc 42:182–185
Vanhoutte PM, Ball SG, Berdeaux A, Cohen ML, Hedner T, McCall R, Ramage AG, et al. (1986) Mechanism of action of ketanserin in hypertension. Trends Pharmacol Sci 7:58–59
Vanhoutte PM, Amery A, Birkenhäger W, Breckenridge A, Bühler F, Distler A, Dormandy J. et al. (1988) Serotonergic mechanisms in hypertension: Focus on the effects of ketanserin. Hypertension 11:111–133
Van Nueten JM, Janssen PAJ, van Beek J, Xhonneux R, Verbeuren TJ, Vanhoutte PM (1981) Vascular effects of ketanserin (R 41 468), a novel antagonist of 5-HT_2 serotonergic receptors. J Pharmacol Exp Ther 218:217–230
Van Nueten JM, Schuurkes JAJ, de Ridder WJE, Kuyps JJMD, Janssens WJ (1986) Comparative pharmacological profile of ritanserin and ketanserin. Drug Dev Res 8:187–195
Van Nueten JM, Janssen PAJ, Symoens J, Janssens WJ, Heykants J, de Clerck F, Leysen J, et al. (1987) Ketanserin. In: Scriabine A (ed) New cardiovascular drugs 1987. Raven, New York, pp 1–56

Van Nueten JM, Xhonneux R, Janssens WJ, Schuurkes JAJ, Janssen PAJ (1988) Interaction between S_2-serotonergic and $alpha_1$-adrenergic receptors and control of blood pressure. In: Vanhoutte PM (ed) Vasodilatation. Raven, New York, pp 267–272

Van Zwieten PA, Mathy MJ, Doods HN (1987a) Demonstration of the central hypotensive activity of α_1-adrenoceptor antagonists. Focus on urapidil. In: Rand MJ, Raper C (eds) Pharmacology. Elsevier, Amsterdam, pp 47–51

Van Zwieten PA, Mathy MJ, Boddeke HWGM, Doods HN (1987b) Central hypotensive activity of ketanserin in cats. J Cardiovasc Pharmacol [Suppl 3] 10:S54–S58

Verdouw PD, Jennewein HM, Heiligers J, Duncker DJ, Saxena PR (1984) Redistribution of carotid artery blood flow by 5-HT: effects of the 5-HT_2 receptor antagonist ketanserin and WAL 1307. Eur J Pharmacol 102:499–509

Verdouw PD, Jennewein HM, Mierau J, Saxena PR (1985) N-(3-acetylaminophenyl) piperazine hydrochloride (BEA 1654), a putative 5-HT_1 agonist, causes constriction of arteriovenous anastomoses and dilatation of arterioles. Eur J Pharmacol 107: 337–346

Waeber C, Schoeffter P, Palacios JM, Hoyer D (1988) Molecular pharmacology of 5-HT_{1D} recognition site: radioligand binding studies in human, pig and calf brain membranes. Naunyn Schmiedebergs Arch Pharmacol, 337:595–601

Wenting GJ, Man in't Veld AJ, Woittiez AJJ, Boomsma F, Schalekamp MADH (1982) Haemodynamic effects of ketanserin, a selective 5-hydroxytryptamine (serotonin) receptor antagonist, in essential hypertension. Clin Sci 63:435S–438S

Wenting GJ, Woittiez AJJ, Man in't Veld AJ, Schalekamp MADH (1984) 5-HT, alpha-adrenoceptors, and blood pressure; effects of ketanserin in essential hypertension and autonomic insufficiency. Hypertension 6:100–109

Woittiez AJJ, Wenting GJ, van der Meiracker AH, Ritsma van Eck HJ, Man in't Veld AJ, Zantvoort FA, Schalekamp MADH (1986) Chronic effect of ketanserin in mild to moderate essential hypertension. Hypertension 8:167–173

Wolf WA, Kuhn DM, Lovenberg W (1985) Serotonin and central regulation of arterial blood pressure. In: Vanhoutte PM (ed) Serotonin and the cardiovascular system. Raven, New York, pp 63–73

Wouters W, Hartog J, Bevan P (1988a) Flesinoxan. Cardiovasc Drug Rev 6:71–83

Wouters W, Tulp MTM, Bevan P (1988b) Flesinoxan lower blood pressure and heart rate in rats via 5-HT_{1A} receptors. Eur J Pharmacol 149:213–223

Wright CE, Angus JA (1983) Haemodynamic response to ketanserin in rabbits with page hypertension: Comparison with prazosin. J Hypertens 1:183–190

Wright CE, Angus JA (1987) Diverse vascular responses to serotonin in the conscious rabbit. Effects of serotonin antagonists on renal artery spasm. J Cardiovasc Pharmacol 10:415–423

CHAPTER 14

Interferences with Dopamine

B.-G. SCHULZ, R. CASTO, A. JÖDICKE, and G. STOCK

CONTENTS

1 Introduction

Dopamine (DA), a precursor in catecholamine synthesis, was first described as a catecholaminergic transmitter in the brain in its own right only in 1958 (CARLSSON 1959; CARLSSON et al. 1960). Since then data from preclinical and clinical research have provided evidence that DA has important CNS functions with relevance for a variety of neurologic, psychiatric, and endocrine disorders. In contrast to the noradrenergic fiber system in the brain, the projection pattern of DA fibers seems to be more restricted, more specific, and less arborized along their pathway and less widespread in the terminal projection area. It is only quite recently that DA has received attention as a transmitter within the cardiovascular regulatory system, originating from the early work of GOLDBERG (1972) and GOLDBERG et al. (1978). they could demonstrate that DA dilates renal arteriolar vessels by a specific mechanism. Clinically, the intravenous administration of DA in the treatment of shock has become widely used.

A role for DA in the central cardiovascular regulation was only postulated after the findings of BJÖRKLUND et al. (1970) that dopamine existed in sympathetic ganglia and BELL and LANG (1973), who suggested that dopamine is a physiological neurotransmitter also in the peripheral nervous system. Together with accumulating functional data these discoveries led to GOLDBERG's proposal (1984) that there is an intrinsic role for DA in the etiology of hypertension.

This development explains why only then different approaches—as yet not fully successful—were under taken to search for specific ligands for the DA subtypes, aimed at treatment for cardiovascular diseases, e.g., heart failure, renal failure and specifically hypertension.

In the following sections an overview is given on peripheral and central actions of DA and related compounds in the cardiovascular system, its regulation, and the clinical implications of the use of dopaminergic agents.

2 Synthesis of Dopamine

The precursor for endogenous DA synthesis is phenylalanine as shown in the following scheme. In neurons or tissues lacking the enzyme DA hydroxylase, synthesis stops at the level of DA. Where the enzyme is present, DA is converted to noradrenaline (Fig. 1).

3 Cardiovascular Actions of Dopamine

Cardiovascular actions of exogenous DA have been known since 1910 when BARGER and DALE observed its pressor potency in the spinal cat (cf. GOLDBERG 1972). Depressor effects were first demonstrated after pretreatment with ergotoxine in the spinal cat and yohimbine in the anesthetized dog (HAMET 1931; TAINTER 1930). In 1942 HOLTZ and CREDNER demonstrated that in guinea pigs and rabbits DA differed in its action from norepinephrine, lowering blood pressure at low doses. From many studies it became clear that the pressor effect of DA can be blocked by α-adrenergic blocking agents in humans, dogs, cats, and rats (cf. GOLDBERG 1972). The depressor effect cannot be blocked by atropine or β-blockers. In the heart DA has positive inotropic and chronotropic effects which can be antagonized to a great extent by β-blockers (cf. GOLDBERG 1972). In the cat there is recent evidence that stimulation of cardiac DA receptors has inotropic effects also when β-receptors are fully blocked by β-receptor antagonists (unpublished results).

4 Dopamine Receptors and Ligands

Since 1972 the evolution of knowledge of central and peripheral DA receptors has been discussed in several reviews (GOLDBERG et al. 1978; SCHMIDT et al. 1981; BRODDE 1982; KEBABIAN 1984). Due to the development of a variety of more or less specific tools, different DA receptors were described in the CNS (designated as D_1 and D_2) and in the periphery (Da_1 and Da_2) (Fig. 2).

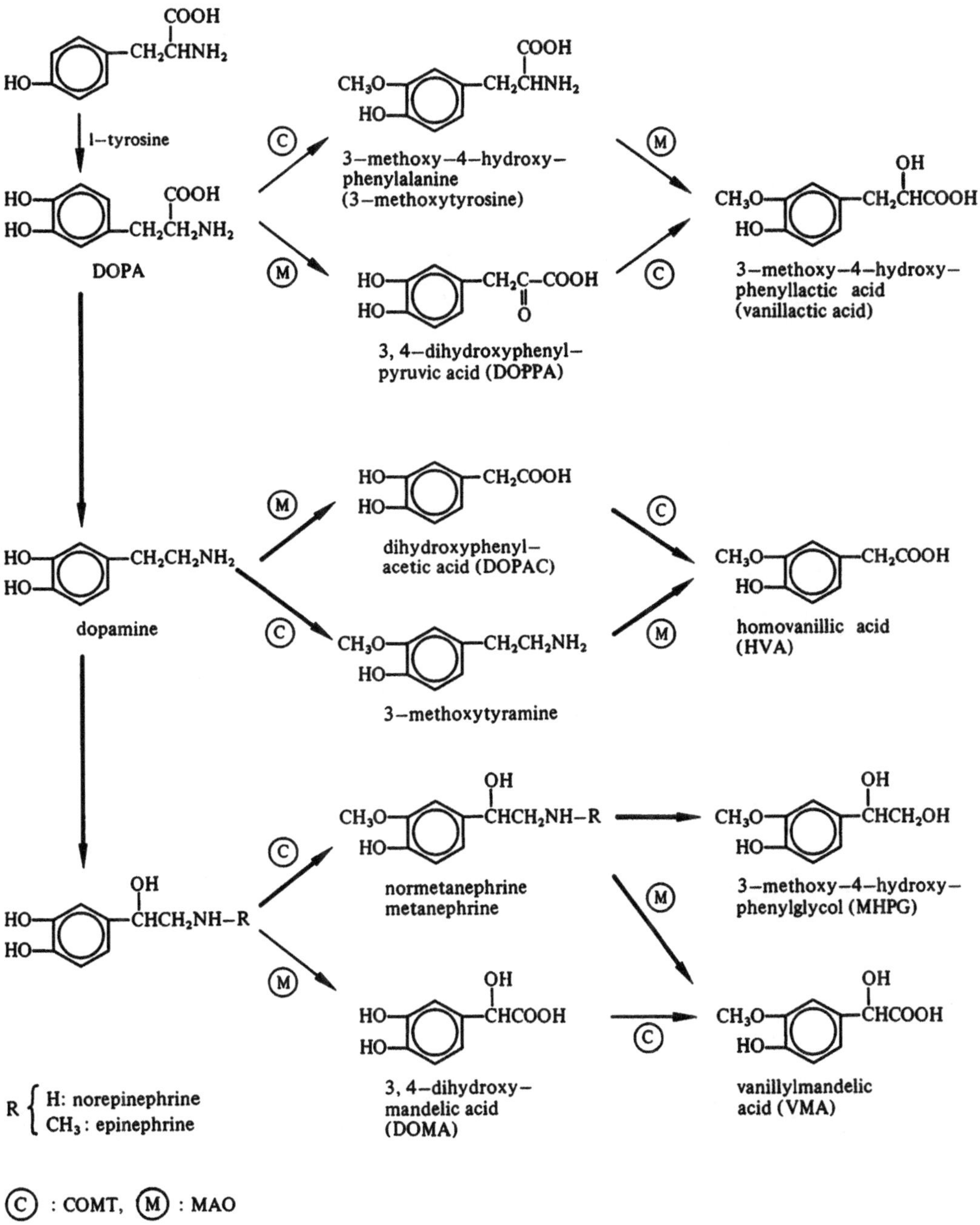

Fig. 1. Synthesis and metabolism of dopamine

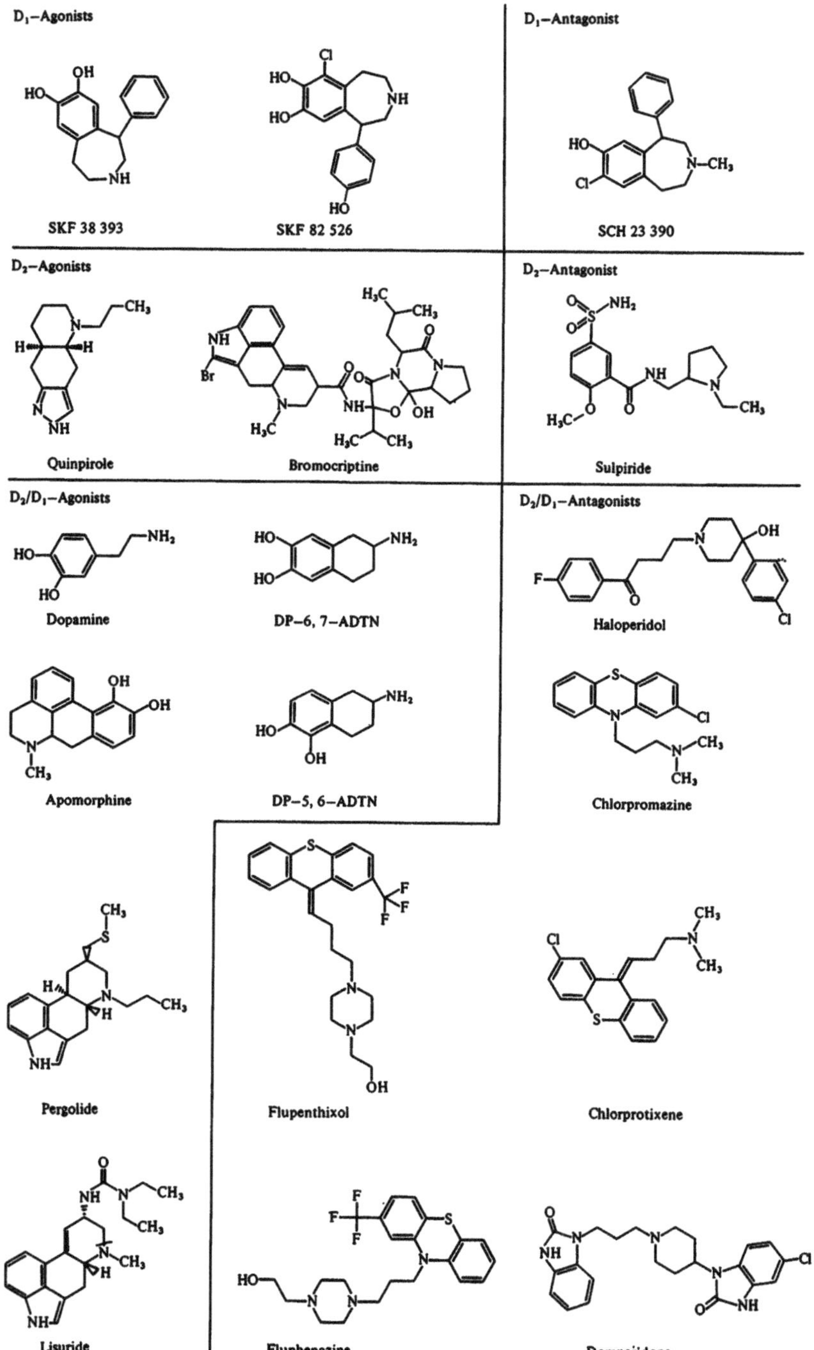

Fig. 2. Structural formulas of agonists and antagonists at the dopamine receptors. SKF 82 526, fenoldopam

From studies in brain homogenates, KEBABIAN and CALNE in 1979 separated two classes of DA receptors in the CNS. The D_1 receptor is linked to a DA-specific adenylate cyclase and mainly found in the striatum, whereas the D_2 receptor is not or even negatively linked to adenylate cyclase as found on mammotrophs (KEBABIAN 1984; STOFF and KEBABIAN 1984). Since then several groups of investigators using radioligand assays have suggested the existence of as many as four different types of DA receptors (SEEMAN 1980; CREESE and LEFF 1982; CREESE et al. 1984; SOKOLOFF et al. 1980). The D_1 receptor displays high affinities for thioxanthenes and phenothiazines and low affinities for butyrophenones and benzamides (KEBABIAN and CALNE 1979; HYTTEL 1981; CROSS and OWEN 1980). The D_2 receptor has a high affinity for all neuroleptics, especially for butyrophenones such as haloperidol or spiroperidol (STOOF and KEBABIAN 1981; ONALI et al. 1984; KEBABIAN 1984).

GOLDBERG and KOHLI (1979) functionally investigated peripheral DA receptors in the femoral and renal vascular bed of the dog using different agonists and antagonists. They propose a Da_1 receptor linked to adenylate cyclase on vascular smooth muscle in the renal and mesenteric bed and a Da_2 receptor located on sympathetic nerve endings. These receptors differ from the central receptors on the basis of different potencies of agonists and antagonists. Nevertheless, central and peripheral receptors have many similarities (HILDITCH and DREW 1987). Therefore, the differences in nomenclature (D_1 versus Da_1 and D_2 versus Da_2) will probably fade in the future. Using the hamster β_2-adrenergic receptor gene as a hybridization probe Bunzow et al. (1988) have recently isolated related genes including a cDNA encoding the rat D_2 dopamine receptor. This receptor has been characterized on the basis of three criteria: the deduced amino-acid sequence which reveals that it is a member of the family of G-protein-coupled receptors; the tissue distribution of the mRNA which parallels that of the D_2 dopamine receptor; and the pharmacological profile of mouse fibroblast cells transfected with the cDNA. A detailed analysis with different agonists and antagonists of vascular and neuronal peripheral DA receptors in different tissues and species was recently elaborated by HILDITCH and DREW (1987) (Table 1).

Several ergot derivatives used in the treatment of Parkinsonism or hyperprolactinoma act on D_2/Da_2 receptors but not on D_1/Da_1 receptors. The specificity of these compounds is, however, not fully proven; they often also act on α-adrenergic and/or serotonergic receptors (CLARK 1979).

Intense synthetical efforts reveal that the structural requirements for Da_1 agonists are much stricter than for Da_2. Therefore, only very few compounds meet the criteria of a specific Da_1 receptor agonist, fenoldopam (SK&F 82526) being the most selective up to now (HAHN et al. 1982; ACKERMAN et al. 1983). More recent studies, however, have shown that fenoldopam also blocks α_1-receptors very weakly and blocks α_2-receptors with moderate potency (FOLEY and SARAU 1984; OHLSTEIN et al. 1985). According to NAKAMURA et al. (1986) the EC_{50} of fenoldopam as a Da_1 agonist is only two to three fold lower than its α_2-adrenolytic activity as determined by the pA_2 value. Also in vivo in the pithed rabbit, fenoldopam increases noradrenaline spillover, indicative of α_2-receptor

Table 1. Functional comparison of dopamine receptor ligands (from HILDITCH and DREW 1987)

	Postsynaptic (vascular) Da_1 receptor	Presynaptic (neuronal) Da_2 receptor
Receptor distribution in the peripheral cardiovascular system	Coronary, mesenteric, renal artery, renal tubules	Sympathetic nerve terminals, sympathetic ganglia
Animal model	Mesenteric vascular bed (dog)	Heart (cat)
Effects measured	Relaxation of vascular smooth muscle	Modulation of norepinephrine release
Relative potencies of receptor agonists	SK&F 82526 [a]>dopamine =DP-5,6-ADTN≥DP-6,7-ADTN >DPDA>>DEDA	DP-5,6-ADTN>DP-6,7-ADTN >6,7-ADTN>dopamine≥DPDA >DEDA>>SK&F 82526
Relative potencies of receptor antagonists	SCH 23390>*cis*-α-flupenthixol >fluphenanzine>sulpiride >>domperidone=haloperidol	Domperidone=fluphenazine =haloperidol≥cis-α-flupenthixol=sulpiride >SCH 23390
Ergot derivatives (mixed receptor profile)	inactive	active

[a] In other vascular preparations, e.g., rabbit splenic artery, SK&F 82526 was less potent than dopamine.

DEDA, *N,N*-diethyldopamine; DPDA, *N,N*-di-*n*-propyldopamine; 5,6-ADTN, 6-amino-5,6,7,8-tetrahydro-1,2-napthalendiol; DP-5,6-ADTN, *N,N*-di-*n*-propyldopamine-6-amino-5,6,7,8-tetrahydro-1,2-napthalendiol; DP-6,7-ADTN, *N,N*-di-*n*-propyldopamine-6-amino-5,6,7,8-tetrahydro-2,3-napthalendiol; SK&F 82526, 6-chloro-2,3,4,5-tetrahydro-1(4-hydroxypheny)-1-*H*-3-benzazepine-7,8-diol; SCH 23390, (R)−(+)8-chloro-2,3,4,5-tetrahydro-3-methyl-5-phenyl-1*H*-benzazepine-7-01; 6,7-ADTN, 6-amino-5,6,7,8-tetrahydro-2,3-naphthalenediol.

antagonism (SZABO et al. 1986). A recently developed tool used to characterize Da_1 receptors is the benzodiazepine derivative SCH 2330, which binds to Da_1 receptors in subnanomolar concetrations and to Da_2 receptors only in micromolar concentrations (KEBABIAN 1986). This compound also binds very weakly to α_2-receptors (CROSS et al. 1983) and potently blocks 5-HT_2 receptors (HICKS et al. 1984; OHLSTEIN et al. 1985).

5 Distribution and Physiology of Peripheral Dopamine Receptors

5.1 Postsynaptic Da_1 Receptors

The Da_1 receptor is thought to be located postsynaptically (GOLDBERG and Kohli 1979; LOKHANDWALA and BARRET 1982). In the cardiovascular system it is mainly found in the efferent arterioles of the glomeruli of the kidney and in the mesenteric, coeliac, and cardiac vascular beds (GOLDBERG and KOHLI 1979, 1983; LEE 1982; LOKHANDWALA and BARRET 1982; LOKHANDWALA et al. 1987).

More recent investigations suggest that the distribution of vascular Da_1 receptors is more generalized than initially thought (LOKHANDWALA and BARRET 1982). For example, HUGHES et al. (1986) reported an increase in forearm blood flow in humans, which could be blocked by *R*-sulpiride. In the canine hindlimb BELL et al. (1975) and LISTINSKY et al. (1980) found Da_1 receptor-mediated vasodilation, whereas GREGA et al. (1984) using fenoldopam were unable to show this in the canine forelimb. It remains an open question whether these are contradictory results or reflect forelimb-hindlimb differences.

Stimulation of vessel Da_1 receptors leads to an increase in cAMP (AMENTA et al. 1984; MISSALE et al. 1985, 1986; DREW et al. 1987; ALKADHI et al. 1986; SABOUNI et al. 1987) and vasodilation and in the kidney elicits natriuresis via a mechanism directly linked to the Da_1 receptor (MURTHY et al. 1976; GOLDBERG 1978; GOLDBERG and KOHLI 1979).

5.2 Presynaptic Da_2 Receptors

The Da_2 receptor is generally thought to be located presynaptically on sympathetic nerve terminals and in sympathetic ganglia (BOGAERT et al. 1977; WILLEMS et al. 1979; for review, see WILLEMS et al. 1985). LANGER (1973) and ENERO and LANGER (1975) were the first to describe a peripheral presynaptic DA receptor in the nictitating membrane of the cat in an in vitro study. This type of receptor was also found on the cardioaccelerator nerve in the rabbit heart (for review, see WILLEMS et al. 1985, pp 170–171).

Stimulation of the presynaptic Da_2 receptor inhibits the release of noradrenaline from sympathetic nerve terminals, thereby antagonizing the tonic influence of the sympathetic system on vessels and heart (LANGER 1981; CAVERO et al. 1982b; LOKHANDWALA and BASSET 1982).

Dilation of innervated blood vessels or inhibition of nerve stimulation-induced vasoconstriction could be achieved with different dopaminergic compounds in different vessels, e.g., renal, mesenteric, and femoral arteries of dog, rabbit, cat, and rat (WILLEMS et al. 1985).

In vitro a widely used model to study the Da_2 receptor is the electrically stimulated rabbit ear artery in which DA and related agonists clearly inhibit the release of noradrenaline (MCCULLOCH et al. 1973; HOPE et al. 1976, 1979; ZIEGLER et al. 1979). Application of a selective DA_2 receptor antagonist like domperidone blocks this effect.

In rats and guinea pigs the presynaptic effect of DA is attributed to its affinity to α_2-receptors (HICKS and CANNON 1979; CAVERO et al. 1981; WILFFERT et al. 1984).

The physiological role of the presynaptic DA receptors is still in debate. Experiments with the canine hindlimb gave the first clear hints that inhibition of transmitter release from sympathetic nerve endings via a presynaptic DA receptor might indeed have a significant effect on vascular resistance (LAUBIE et al. 1977; BUYLAERT et al. 1978). The short-lasting vasodilation caused by injection of apomorphine into the femoral artery could not be antagonized by α-adrenoceptor blocking agents or atropine but was antagonized by haloperidol in doses that did not influence the response to isoprenaline, acetylcholine, histamine, or nitroglycerin. That this vasodilatation was due to interference with the sympathetic vasconstrictor tone was shown by the fact that it disappeared after transection of the lumbar sympathetic chain or the femoral nerve and after administration of the ganglionic blocker hexamethonium. Moreover, after sympathetic denervation the vasodilation induced by apomorphine was restored when vascular tone was raised by electrical stimulation of the sympathetic nerve but not when tone was increased by noradrenaline infusion. In the dog renal vasculature a presynaptic inhibitory effect has been described for DA which was antagonized by pimozide. In humans a presynaptic effect was observed in the omental vein (STJÄRNE and BRUNDIN 1975).

In addition to the neuronal localization of Da_2 receptors, a postsynaptic localization in the periphery was recently also suggested, activation of which causes inhibition of adenylate cyclase in rabbit cerebral vessels (AMENTA et al. 1984) as well as renal and mesenteric artery and adrenal cortex (MISSALE et al. 1985, 1986). These findings speak in favor of vascular Da_2 receptor activation, which may lower cAMP in certain vascular beds. This can be compared with the pituitary, where D_2 receptors inhibit adenylate cyclase whereas in other cerebral tissues they do not (STOOF and KEBABIAN 1984).

6 Dopamine and Kidney

The kidney is thought to play a central role in the etiology of essential hypertension. Therefore, the finding of MCDONALD et al. (1963) that DA i.v. in humans reduces renal vascular resistance and causes an increase in renal plasma flow and natriuresis stimulated interest in DA as a natural natriuretic factor. In dogs MCNAY et al. (1965) found that low doses of DA (0.76–7 mg/kg) cause renal vasodilation. Vasoconstriction occurs after doses between 96 and 192 mg/kg, which could be prevented by phenoxybenzamine. DA-induced renal vasodilation could not be blocked by adrenergic antagonists but was blocked by haloperoidl, *R*-sulpiride, metoclopramide, or SCH 23390 (GOLDBERG 1972; GOLDBERG et al. 1978, 1986). all these compounds are more or less specific dopaminergic antagonists.

In all species studied the kidney is the organ most abundantly supplied with Da_2 receptor—containing adrenergic nerves, besides being rich in postsynaptic Da_1 receptors. In the kidney both Da_1 and Da_2 receptors are present in the vascular bed, Da_2 receptors located mainly in the glomeruli (BRODDE 1980; FELDER et al. 1984a; GOLDBERG and KOHLI 1979; SCHMIDT et al. 1981), though the effects of DA on renal blood flow and glomerular filtration rate are mostly attributed to Da_1 receptors. However, bromocriptine, a Da_2 agaonist, also increases renal blood flow in the isolated perfused rat kidney (SCHMIDT et al. 1981). To investigate specific DA effects, often α- and β-adrenergic blockade is used. Using phenoxybenzamine as an α-blocker, Da_2 receptors are also alkylated (CREESE et al. 1981). Under such conditions treatment with Da_2 antagonists cannot attenuate the vasodilatation induced by DA. Therefore, it is concluded that only a Da_1 receptor is involved, because the expression of Da_2 receptor—mediated inhibition of noradrenaline release is prevented, and the contribution of Da_2 receptors on renal hemodynamics cannot be evaluated (SCHMIDT et al. 1987). In the isolated perfused rat kidney [^{3}H] noradrenaline release is inhibited by the Da_2 receptor agonist quinpirole, which could be blocked by *R*/*S*-sulpiride but not by SCH 23390 (LOKHANDWALA and STEENBERG 1984a). In male Sprague-Dawley rats with an intact adrenergic system, micropuncture studies show a prompt and significant increase of single nephron GFR after injection of quinpirole (SERI and APERIA 1988).

The question of whether natriuresis results from a direct action of DA on renal tubules or secondary to renal vascular changes is still unresolved. Several investigators report that intrarenal infusion of DA can also cause natriuresis independent of changes in renal blood flow and GFR, pointing to a tubular effect (DAVIS et al. 1968; PELAYO et al. 1983). In rat and rabbit Da_1 receptors in the proximal convoluted tubule and the pars recta have been demonstrated. These receptors are positively linked to adenylate cyclase and could be stimulated by fenoldopam and blocked by SCH 23390 (FELDER et al. 1984b). NAKAJIMA et al. (1977) also report stimulation of adenylate cyclase in the rat kidney. In rabbit proximal tubule DA decreases fluid and sodium reabsorption, which could be prevented by haloperidol (10^{-8} *M*) or metoclopramide (10^{-7} *M*) (BELLO-REUSS et al. 1982). The concentrations of DA in these experiments were in the micromolar range (FELDER et al. 1984b; BELLO-REUSS et al. 1982), and BELL et al. (1978a) reported that the naturally occurring DA concentrations in the renal cortex are about 10^{-6} *M*.

An interesting hypothesis was recently proposed by APERIA et al. (1987), that locally synthesized DA inhibits Na K-ATPase activity in isolated proximal tubules of the rat. This cannot be prevented by metoclopramide. It is speculated that this reflects an intracellular effect of DA not involving the surface receptor (BERTORELLO and APERIA 1987).

Furthermore, natriuresis by DA can be caused indirectly by inhibition of aldosterone secretion (see also sect. 7).

Several lines of evidence show that besides its pharmacological effects DA plays a physiological role in the kidney, i.e., it is a natural natriuretic factor (LEE 1982). This raises the question whether DA is present in the kidney at concentrations sufficient to elicit different actions and what its source is.

ANTON and SAYRE (1964) report for the first time that in human urine 5–20 times more unconjugated DA is excreted than noradrenaline. These amounts must be either produced or released by the kidney, because the plasma concentrations of DA are extremely low, and therefore urinary levels cannot be explained by glomerular filtration (KUCHEL et al. 1978). Three theories address the source of DA:

(a) The kidney deconjugates dopaminsulfate or -glucuronate, which are found in the plasma in considerable amounts (UNGER et al. 1980; BUU et al. 1981).
(b) DA is released by dopaminergic nerves innervating glomeruli, arterioles, and tubules (BELL et al. 1978a; DINERSTEIN et al. 1979; FELDER et al. 1984).
(c) DA is synthesized by proximal tubules from L-dopa by the enzyme dopa decarboxylase and secreted into the tubular lumen dependent on sodium status. This latter mechanism is responsible for at least one-half of the DA in urine, and approximately all urinary DA stems from nonneuronal sources (CHAN 1976; ULLRICH et al. 1974; BALL et al. 1982; BROWN and ALLISON 1981; BAINES et al. 1985; STEPHENSON et al. 1982).

Assuming that DA plays a physiological role in the cardiovascular system, the question arises whether deficits in the dopaminergic system are involved in the genesis of hypertension. In humans and animals expansion of the extracellular fluid by infusion, water immersion, or sodium loading leads to an increase in plasma and urinary levels of DA and natriuresis (ALEXANDER et al. 1974; CAREY et al. 1981; SAITO et al. 1986; SOWERS et al. 1985; BALL et al. 1978; MACCLANAHAN et al. 1985).

Low sodium intake reverses this (BAINES 1982). Inhibition of DA synthesis by carbidopa or DA blockers like metoclopramide, *cis*-flupenthixol, or SCH 23390 blocks natriuresis (BALL et al. 1978; FREDERICKSON et al. 1985; IMONDI et al. 1979; KRISHNA et al. 1985; PELAYO et al. 1983; SOWERS et al. 1982a,b; CORUZZI 1987; CHAPMAN et al. 1980; BENNET et al. 1982).

The concept of DA as a physiological natriuretic factor is reinforced by reports of abnormally low plasma DA to noradrenaline ratios in a subgroup of patients with essential hypertension and by the fact that some essential hypertensive patients—especially those with a low renin status—do not respond to salt loads with either natriuresis or DA excretion (FRANCO-MORSELLI et al. 1977; ERHARDT and SCHWARTZ 1978; MESSERLI et al. 1981; SHIKUMA et al. 1986; KRSTULOVIC et al. 1981; HARVEY et al. 1984; PERKINS et al. 1980; CRITCHLEY and LEE 1986; GOLDBERG 1984). This is the group of the so-called salt-sensitive hypertensive patients.

In SH rats compared with normotensive WKY control rats an increased DA content in the adrenal glands as well as in the kidney and enhanced urinary excretion of DA are observed (YOSHIMURA et al. 1987; RACZ et al. 1985; MAEMURA et al. 1982). On the contrary LUTOLD et al. (1979) reported a decreased DA metabolism in sympathetic celiac ganglia of young SHR. In humans a relatively high output of urinary DA with lower sodium excretion is found in normotensive subjects with a positive family history of hypertension, which may be indicative of a compensatory attempt (SAITO et al. 1986).

7 Dopaminergic Control of Aldosterone Secretion

Since EDWARDS et al. in 1975 observed that the DA agonist bromocriptine partially blocks the furosemide-induced increase in aldosterone secretion, an inhibitory action of DA on aldosterone has been suspected (SOWERS 1984; CAMPBELL et al. 1981a,b; GANGULY 1984). The DA antagonist metoclopramide increases aldosterone secretion in humans and animals (NORBIATO et al. 1977; CAREY et al. 1979). DA infusion markedly attenuates the aldosterone response to metoclopramide (CAREY et al. 1979). It does not reduce basal aldosterone levels, which leads to the hypothesis that aldosterone is under maximal dopaminergic inhibition (CAREY et al. 1980). Functionally, a connection between sodium status and the DA-aldosterone relation is hypothesized. DRAKE and CAREY (1984) reported a direct effect of DA on aldosterone secretion in normal sodium-restricted subjects. Angiotensin II-induced aldosterone secretion is also inhibited by DA, dependent on salt intake (AGUILERA and CATT 1984; MCKENNA et al. 1979). In humans on low sodium intake, infusion of DA changes the angiotensin-aldosterone response curve, making it similar to that obtained during high sodium intake. In the presence of high sodium intake angiotensin II does not stimulate aldosterone secretion. Addition of metoclopramide restores the effects of angiotensin II (AGUILERA and CATT 1984; GORDON et al. 1983). The interpretation of the above data is complicated by the limited specificity of some of the drugs used in the experiments and the differential effects of DA_1 and DA_2 agonists on renin secretion thereby interfering with aldosterone regulation.

The site of action of DA on aldosterone is not yet clear. In vitro studies demonstrate DA receptors in human, rat, and calf in the aldosterone-producing zona glomerulosa of the adrenal cortex (DUNN and BOSMANN 1981; BEVILACQUA et al. 1982). These receptors belong to the Da_2 subtype (BEVILACQUA et al. 1982) Furthermore, the adrenal cortex generates large amounts of DA not derived from the adrenal medulla. An indirect effect of DA on aldosterone secretion has also been suggested. INGLIS et al. (1987) propose that DA inhibits aldosterone secretion by increasing the clearence of angiotensin II.

HUANG et al. (1987) by intracerebroventricular application of DA provided evidence for a central mechanism. In these experiments DA in doses that are ineffective when given intravenously depresses aldosterone levels. The precise physiological role of DA in the regulation of aldosterone secretion and its potential pathophysiological role, especially in hypertension, are not yet defined.

8 Atrial Natriuretic Factor and Dopamine

Recent investigations indicate that the natriuretic effect of atrial natriuretic factor (ANF) depends on DA. In DA-depleted rats the effect of ANF is significantly reduced (Felder and Carey 1987). After reserpinization of rats the effect of ANF is inhibited and can be restored by DA infusion. ANF-induced natriuresis is inhibited by the Da_1 receptor antagonist SCH 23390 and *R*- but not *S*-sulpiride. Marin-Grez et al. (1985) could block the ANF response by haloperidol and chlorpromazine. Petterson et al. (1986) found an attenuation of the ANF response by the Da_2/α_2 agonist BHT 920. So the issue is not yet settled, and the DA receptor subtype involved is unclear.

9 Summary of Actions of Dopamine

The following summarizes receptor binding data and results from physiological and pharmacological experiments indicating that DA interacts with Da_1 and Da_2 receptors in the peripheral autonomic nervous system and the cardiovascular system:

Da_1: Vasodilatation (primarily in renal, mesenteric, cerebral, and coronary vascular bed) in dog, rabbit, cat, humans.
Increase in renal plasma flow, GFR, sodium excretion, diuresis (probably also Da_2) in kidney of dog, cat, humans.
Increase of cellular cAMP in brain and peripheral tissue from rat, cow, dog, guinea pig, and rabbit.
Increase of renin secretion.

Da_2: Inhibition of neurotransmitter release in sympathetic nerve terminals in cat, dog, humans.
Inhibition of ganglionic transmission in autonomic ganglia (probably also Da_1).
Inhibition of aldosterone secretion.
Inhibition of renin release.

Furthermore, DA itself in higher doses interacts with β_1- and β_2-receptors as well as α_1- and α_2-receptors with the following effects on the cardiovascular system:

β_1: Increase in cardiac contractility, heart rate, AV conduction
β_2: Vasodilatation primarily in the skeletal muscle
α_1: Vasoconstriction
α_2: Vasoconstriction and inhibition of transmitter release

10 Sources of Dopamine

Despite the indisputable pharmacological effects of DA, it is still a highly debatable question whether peripheral DA, besides being a precursor of norepinephrine in sympathetic nerves, plays a physiological role via specific peripheral dopaminergic neurons. A prerequisite of this is proof of dopaminergic nerves in which DA is synthesized, is stored, is released by nerve activity, acts on a specific postsynaptic receptor, is degraded, or is reuptaken. The presence alone of DA even in high concentrations in different tissues is not a sufficient precondition (BELL 1982). For example, in splanchnic and genitofemoral nerves and urinary bladder the amount of DA is up to 30% that of noradrenaline. High DA to noradrenaline ratios are also reported in the renal cortex of dog and cat.

11 Small Intensively Fluorescent Cells

In 1963 ERÄNKO and HARKONNEN found small intensively fluorescent (SIF) cells in rat superior cervical ganglia. By histofluorescence and microspectrofluorometry BJÖRKLUND et al. in 1970 demonstrated that the neurotransmitter of these SIF cells is DA. Physiologically, the dopaminergic SIF cells modulate ganglionic transmission (LIBET 1977; LIBET and TOSAKIA 1970; LIBET and OWMAN 1974). It was also shown that exogenous DA inhibits ganglionic transmission (BOGAERT et al. 1977; QUENZER et al. 1979). However, this may be due to α- or β-receptor stimulation (DE GROAT and VOLLE 1966). These SIF cells are found especially in paravertebral ganglia innervating the kidney and mesenteric arteries.

Initially, the DA receptor on the cell body of postganglionic sympathetic neurons was believed to belong to the Da_2 receptor subtype (CAVERO et al. 1982b). The DA receptor subtype was especially studied by SABOUNI et al. (1987) in the dog stellate and the rat superior cervical ganglion using the specific Da_1 receptor agonist fenoldopam, the Da_2 receptor agonist quinpirole, and DA itself. Ganglionic transmission was blocked by fenoldopam as well as by quinpirole and dopamine. This effect is due to stimulation of two different receptors. The effect of fenoldopam was blocked by *R*-sulpiride but not by the highly selective Da_1 antagonist SCH 23390. The DA_2 antagonist *S*-sulpiride was ineffective against fenoldopam but effective against the DA_2 agonist quinpirole. DA was not antagonized by SCH 23390. Therefore, the ganglionic receptors appear not to belong to the classic Da_1 or Da_2 subtype. This is also found in the dog hindlimb (LOKHANDWALA et al. 1987).

12 Other Dopaminergic Nerves

In addition to SIF cells biochemical, pharmocological, and histological methods have identified dopaminergic nerves in different species. In the dog BELL et al. (1978a,b) identified dopaminergic axons supplying the kidney and arteriovenous anastomoses of the hindpaw. The presence of dopaminergic axons in the kidney was confirmed by DINERSTEIN et al. (1979, 1983). Renal nerves contain dopa decarboxylase but lack DA β-hydroxylase, i.e., they can synthesize DA but are unable to convert it to noradrenaline (MULLER and BELL 1986).

The terminals of renal nerves contain far higher concentrations of dopa decarboxylase than expected for noradrenergic neurons (HARRIS et al. 1986). Both cell bodies and nerve terminals are more efficient to process exogenous L-dopa than noradrenergic nerves (BELL and MCLACHLAN 1982). In the dog the possible origin of dopaminergic outflow to kidney and hindpaw are the spinal segments T11 to T12 and L6 to S2 (ROLEWICZ and ZIMMERMAN 1972; BELL and LANG 1979). In humans LACKOVIC et al. (1981; LACKOVIC and Neff 1980) found that in spinal nerve roots and the vagus nerve the concentration of DA was higher than that of noradrenaline, and in the splanchnic and genitofemoral nerves, DA levels represented more than 20% of those of noradrenaline. The amount of hydroxymandelic acid was usually higher than the amount of DA, indicating that a large portion of DA is catabolized and not converted to noradrenaline.

Besides these specific dopaminergic nerves which show high species dependency, DA could also play a physiological role when coreleased with noradrenaline, stimulating either postsynaptic Da_1 or presynaptic Da_2 receptors. DA in catecholaminergic neurons is regarded to be localized only in the cell body, where it is converted to noradrenaline. By ultracentrifugation it is shown that 30%–50% of DA is localized in axon terminals in large synaptic vesicles whereas noradrenaline is released from small and large vesicles (THURESON-KLEIN et al. 1979; NEUMANN et al. 1984; MÜLLER and BELL 1986; BELL 1987; SOAREZ-DA SILVA and AZEVEDO 1987; FILLENZ and HOWE 1975). DA storage in large vesicles is compatible with the hypothesis that it is released as a normal component of evoked transmitter release from noradrenergic neurons. WILLEMS et al. (1985) speculated that the ratio of DA to noradrenaline released is dependent on sympathetic nerve activity. In situations of prolonged nerve activity coreleased DA represents a mechanism to decrease the noradrenaline release via a presynaptic Da_2 receptor (HEAD and BERKOWITZ 1979; HOPE et al. 1979; WILLEMS et al. 1985). Exercise or upright tilting results in generalized sympathetic activation, elevating concentrations of noradrenaline in the blood with minimal effects on DA levels (FRANCO-MORSELLI et al. 1977; ERHARDT and SCHWARTZ 1978; MEFFORD et al. 1981; PEQUIGNOT et al. 1985). Hemorrhage, for example, in adrenalectomized animals elevates DA and noradrenaline levels in the blood to a similar extent (ANDERSSON et al. 1982; FREDHOLM et al. 1979; KVETNANSKY et al. 1979), whereas hypoxia increases DA with little effect on the other catecholamines (PEQUIGNOT et al. 1985).

Peripheral DA actions upon injections of DA or DA analogues have been shown unequivocally despite the fact that there are as yet no conclusive data explaining the source of endogenous DA to act on the peripheral receptors. As outlined above there are as yet only speculations as to what extent a "resting tone" of a peripheral dopaminergic system contributes to cardiovascular regulation.

Within the CNS morphological, biochemical, and functional data are now available which clearly indicate that DA not only plays a major role in the integration of motor and psychomotor behavior but also of mood. Since these complex behavioral patterns always include autonomic, especially cardiovascular components (STOCK 1982; SCHULZ et al. 1986), it is conceivable to assume that neurally released DA has an impact on these as well. In fact, recent evidence clearly indicates that DA has a very specific action on central nervous cardiovascular regulation.

13 Central Dopamine Pathways and Cell Groups

Central actions of DA were first suggested by CARLSSON in 1958 long before knowledge of DA-containing neuropathways. Recent advances in immunohistochemical and histofluorescent tracing techniques are providing evidence of a diverse network of DA-containing cells in the CNS innervating structures with known function in basic cardiovascular regulation as well as higher centers involved in psychomotor behavior.

13.1 Distribution of Dopaminergic Neurons

DA-synthesizing neurons are distributed in the mesencephalon, diencephalon, and telencephalon. Within the mesencephalon, dopaminergic cells form three distinct cell groups: A8, A9, and A10 (cf. FELTEN et al. 1974; MOORE and BLOOM 1978). Groups A8 and A9 appear to be bilateral, whereas A10 lies in the midline within the ventral tegmental area. A9 constitutes the substantia nigra and gives rise to the nigrostriatal pathway (UNGERSTEDT 1971), forming an extremely dense terminal network in the caudate and putamen where it appears to be involved in complex motor behavior and appropriate reaction to sensory information. With potential cardiovascular importance, the A10 group gives rise to a mesolimbic DA system whose projections include the lateral septal nuclei and the basal and central amygdala. The dorsal raphe nucleus demonstrates DA histofluorescence (HÖKFELT et al. 1976; LINDVALL and BJÖRKLUND 1974) and immunocytochemical staining for DA (OCHI and SHIMIZU 1978; MAICHON et al. 1984), but the projection of these cell bodies is presently not known.

Within the diencephalon, four distinct dopaminergic cell groups, A11–A14, give rise to five efferent projections, four of which have terminal fields within known cardiovascular regulatory sites. The A11 and A13 groups form a complex but diffuse bundle which projects to the adjacent dorsal and rostral portions of the hypothalamus (BJÖRKLUND et al. 1975). This projection has been referred to as the incerto-hypothalamic tract (for review, see NIEUWENHUYS 1985). A caudally oriented projection has also been demonstrated originating from these two groups, which has among its terminal fields the locus coeruleus, dorsal vagal nucleus, and nucleus tractus solitarii. Axons of the A12 group pass through the infundibulum and terminate mainly in the external layer of the median eminence. There is evidence that these fibers transport DA to the anterior pituitary to inhibit the release of prolactin (MACLEOD and LEHMEYER 1974; BEN-JONATHAN et al. 1977).

At least two descending dopaminergic pathways project directly to areas of the brain stem and spinal cord primarily involved in regulation of sympathetic

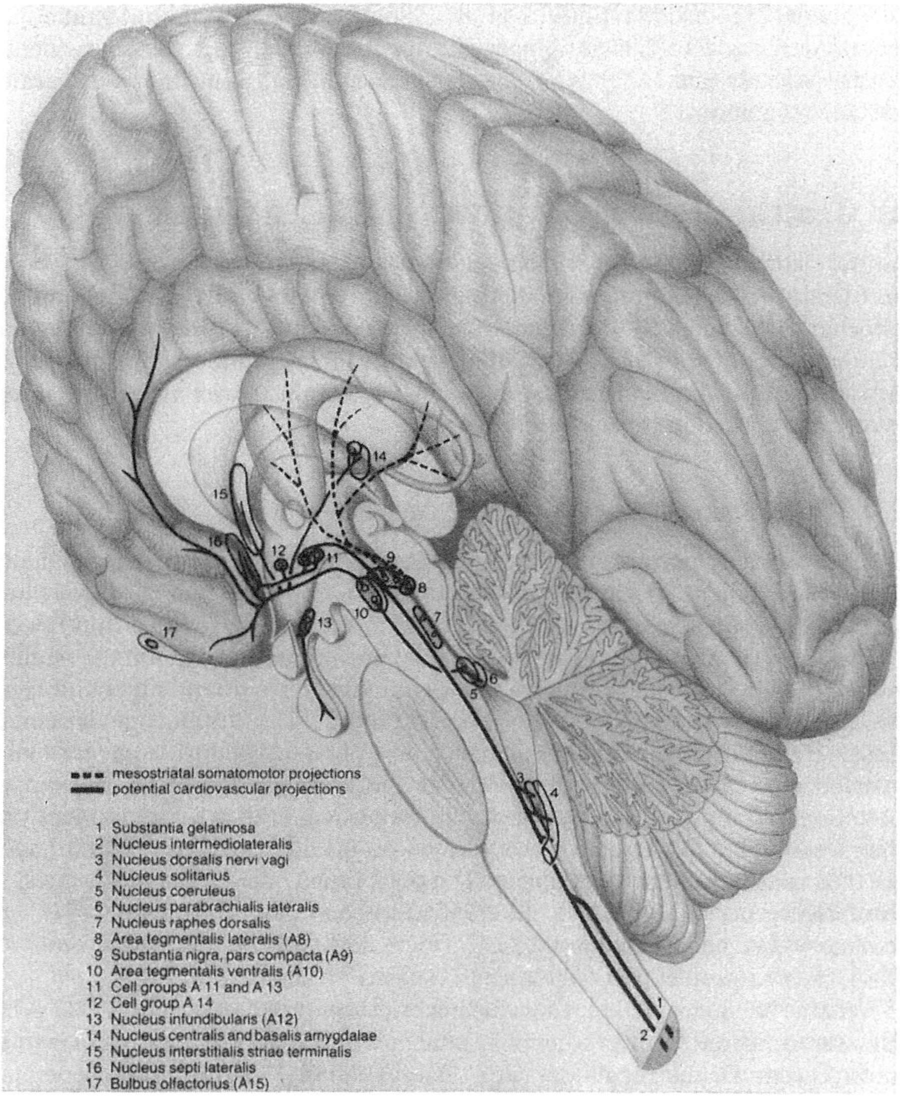

Fig. 3. Central dopaminergic neurons and projections

and parasympathetic tone (Fig. 3). Recently a pathway has been shown originating within the dorsal hypothalamus and projecting to the spinal cord (BLESSING and CHALMERS 1979). The exact course of these fibers is not known, but their terminal fields include the dorsal horn, dorsolateral funiculus, and the intermedio-lateral cell column of the spinal cord, the origin of preganglionic sympathetic neurons (BJÖRKLUND and SKAGERBERG 1979; HÖKFELT et al. 1979; SKAGERBERG et al. 1982; LINDVALL and BJÖRKLUND 1983). According to SWANSON et al. (1981), tyrosine hydroxylase-positive neurons may be found in the parvocellular portion of the paraventricular nucleus, which project to the dorsal vagal complex and thoracic spinal cord. Finally, LINDVALL et al. (1984) provide evidence that the A11–A14 cell groups also project to the supraoptic and dorsomedial nuclei of the hypothalamus, which participate in the regulation of oxytocin and vasopressin release from the pituitary.

13.2 Dopamine Receptor Distribution in the Central Nervous System

Two categories of functionally independent DA receptors, D_1 and D_2, can be identified in the CNS by pharmacological and biochemical criteria (cf. STOOF and KEBABIAN 1984). The D_1 subtype appears positively coupled to adenylate cyclase while the D_2 is not coupled (or negatively coupled to this enzyme). The D_2 receptor is located both pre- and postsynaptically.

There is evidence that each DA receptor exists either in high or low affinity state. Guanosine triphosphate modulates the interconversion from high to low affinity, while divalent cations like Mg^{2+} favor the high affinity state.

With specific tritiated agonists and antagonists SCATTON and DUBOIS (1985) demonstrated in the rat the highest concentration of D_1 receptors in the caudate putamen. Intermediate receptor density was found in the septum, substantia nigra, amygdaloid complex, and portions of the cortex. In the rat the density of D_2 receptors generally parallels that of DA innervation and D_1 receptor distribution in the areas mentioned above (BOUTHENET et al. 1987). D_2 receptors are also found in the dorsal vagal nucleus and the nucleus of the solitary tract which are apparently innervated by descending DA projections from the hypothalamus (BJÖRKLUND et al. 1975; SWANSON et al. 1981).

Many major DA cell groups also contain D_2 receptors. Their density is greatly reduced after injections of the neurotoxin 6-hydroxydopamine, suggesting a localization of D_2 autoreceptors on dendrites or perikarya of DA neurons in this area. The studies have also shown that there are areas in which receptors but no known projections occur, or projections but no known receptors exist. Probably, histochemical methods have not the sensitivity to detect minor DA innervation, particularly in areas in which DA fibers and terminals are combined with heavy noradrenergic projections. It is also possible that some neurons express DA receptors which respond to DA released by noradrenergic or even noncatecholaminergic neurons.

Of particular importance for this discussion is the observation that the distribution of D_1 and D_2 receptors in the brain stem is not superimposable, as only D_2 receptors have been described within the brain stem or spinal cord (SCATTON and DUBOIS 1985; BOUTHENET et al. 1987).

14 Central Cardiovascular Actions of Dopamine

The first evidence of an influence or a contribution of central DA systems on cardiovascular activity can be credited to DUTTA et al. (1974) who showed that intracerebroventricular administration of DA in the cat decreased blood pressure and heart rate. OSBORNE (1976) later reported that DA neurons in the midbrain could alter superficial and cutaneous vein capacitance. Since the initial report of DUTTA et al. (1974) several seemingly contradictory reports regarding the central role of DA systems in cardiovascular regulation have appeared in the literature, as both pressor and depressor actions have been reported (see Table 2). The probable explanation for this contradiction is twofold. The first is that dopamine and many dopaminergic agonists share α-adrenergic (and β-adrenergic) as well as dopaminergic activity. In contrast to the peripheral circulation in which these effects are opposite (vasoconstriction versus vasodilation) and can be easily separated, central α-adrenergic systems are thought to be generally depressor. Secondly, the adrenergic-dopaminergic balance of a particular dopaminergic compound in both the center and the periphery can be easily altered by experimental conditions, such as the type and level of anesthesia. This is illustrated by examination of the reports of cardiovascular effects of central DA in the years subsequent to the original work of DUTTA et al. (1974) and summarized in Table 2. In the rat, DA is reported to decrease blood pressure when given to thiobutabarbital Inactin (HUTCHINSON et al. 1983) or thiopental (PAZOS et al. 1982) anesthetized or conscious rats (KONDO et al. 1981). Alternatively, DA is reported to increase arterial pressure and heart rate in the conscious dog (LANG and WOODMAN 1979) and cat (DAY and ROACH 1976) and again to decrease blood pressure and heart rate in the anesthetized cat (DUTTA et al. 1975). Attempts to block the central effects of DA by adrenergic, ganglionic, and dopaminergic antagonists are equally confusing. The depressor effects of DA are reportedly blocked by ganglionic or dopaminergic antagonists (KONDO et al. 1981) as well as by phentolamine but not by haloperidol (PAZOS et al. 1982). Depressor effects in the cat can be blocked by either haloperidol or cholinergic antagonism (DUTTA et al. 1974, 1975). In addition, studies in conscious cats and dogs are often complicated by DA activation of the chemoreceptor trigger zone and the production of emesis with stress-induced pressor and tachycardic episodes (BOGAERT et al. 1978; LANG and WOODMAN 1979).

The use of more specific DA receptor agonists has greatly reduced this confusion. Results of studies with apomorphine, a highly selective DA receptor agonist, clearly demonstrate the central cardiovascular effects of DA receptor activation in the dog, cat, and rat. Apomorphine produces central depressor responses and bradycardia in conscious (PETITJEAN et al. 1984) and anesthetized (FINCH and HERSOM 1976) rats, anesthetized dogs (MONTASTRUC and GUIOL 1984), and anesthetized cats (DUTTA et al. 1974, 1975).

While the somatomotor effects of DA are predominantly localized within the neostriatum, the cardiovascular site of action within the CNS is less well understood. In the original studies of DUTTA et al. (1975), direct microinjection of apomorphine indicated that the dorsal vagal nucleus and hypothalamus could mediate the central cardiovascular effects of DA agonists, which matches with the distribution of dopaminergic terminals. To localize better the site and mechanism of action, compounds were delivered either intracerebroventricularly (i.c.v.), or intracisternally (i.c.) in a small volume (10 μl saline) bolus. Application of apomorphine i.c. (1–10 μg/kg) produces a slow-onset, long-duration depressor response with the maximum decrease observed after between 1 and 2 min followed by a return to baseline within 10 min. Also present is a significant decrease in heart rate which is temporally delayed relative to the depressor response. Maximum bradycardia occurs after between 5 and 10 min, and in some animals the heart rate is significantly depressed at 30 min (CASTO et al. 1988; JÖDICKE et al. 1988).

Application of apomorphine i.c.v. within the dose range studied (1–10 μg/kg) produces no significant cardiovascular response. Increasing the dose to 25 and 75 μg/kg elicits a response qualitatively similar to that witnessed with 5 and 10 μg/kg, i.c. By relative potency, administration of apomorphine i.c. produces the greatest decrease in blood pressure and heart rate. This supports studies by DAY and ROACH (1976) in which i.c. administration of DA in the conscious cat produced depression of arterial pressure and heart rate while i.c.v. application produced a transient increase then prolonged decrease in both cardiovascular parameters. These results may be interpreted as indicating that the actual site of action is closer to the fourth cerebral ventricle than the lateral ventricle.

Similarly, GEORGIEV et al. (1978) studied reflex hypertension produced by sciatic nerve stimulation in anesthetized cats following injection of apomorphine into the lateral, third, and fourth ventricles. Only the fourth ventricular site of injection effectively inhibited reflexogenic hypertension. ZANDBERG et al. (1979) later reported a specific depressor effect when DA was injected into the nucleus of the solitary tract. This nucleus receives terminal fields of descending dopaminergic projections from midbrain nuclei and represents a major site of cardiovascular regulation as the first synapse of baroreceptor reflex afferents (SELLER and ILLERT 1969). Thus, a fourth ventricular site of action appears most likely for the central depressor response and bradycardia induced by central administration of DA agonists. Since the blood-brain barrier is permeable for many compounds at this site, a central action of drugs administered peripherally could also happen.

Recent reports suggest that a spinal site may also be important in the central cardiovascular effect of apomorphine (PETITJEAN et al. 1984). Both a brain stem and spinal site of action would agree with the known distribution of D_2 receptors in central cardiovascular areas.

Although the exact site of action within the hindbrain remains unknown, receptor distribution and direct microinjection studies suggest brain stem nuclei such as the dorsal vagal nucleus or nucleus of the solitary tract as the most likely focus (ZANDBERG et al. 1979). It thus appears plausible that the diencephalic (A11, A13, A14) and mesencephalic (A10) origin of descending DA-containing fibers which project to the dorsal vagal complex and the spinal cord are primarily depressor and bradycardic in nature.

The nature of the receptor subtype was investigated using i.c. administrations of the D_2 receptor agonist pergolide and the D_1 receptor agonist fenoldopam (JÖDICKE et al. 1988). Pergolide i.c. produces depression of blood pressure and heart rate similar to apomorphine which is in agreement with studies in the dog by LOKHANDWALA et al. (1984) and i.c.v. studies in the rat (JADHAV et al. 1983). Fenoldopam in this setting is virtually without effect when administered

Table 2. Cardiovascular actions of some centrally administered dopaminergic compounds in various experimental animals

Primary receptor activity	Agonist	Change in						
		Route	Species	Blood pressure	Heart rate	Anesthetic state	Dose	Reference
α, β	Dopamine	icv	dog	no change[a]	no change[a]	pentobarbital	0.2–1 mg	McCUBBIN et al. (1960)
D_1, D_2			dog	increase[b]	increase[b]	conscious	100–500 μg	LANG and WOODMAN (1979)
			cat	decrease	decrease	α-chloralose	25–100 μg/kg	DUTTA et al. (1974)
			cat	decrease	decrease	conscious	1.7×10^{-3}	HEISE (1976)
			cat	inc/dec[c]	inc/dec[c]	conscious	30–45 μg	DAY and ROACH (1976)
			rat	decrease	decrease	dial-urethane	1–10 μg	BAUM and SHROPSHIRE (1973)
			rat	decrease	decrease	thiopental	30–300 μg/kg	PAZOS et al. (1982)
			rat	decrease		Inactin	400 μg/kg	HUTCHINSON et al. (1983)
			rat	decrease		conscious	50–200 μg/kg	KONDO et al. (1981)
		ic	cat	decrease	decrease	conscious	30–45 μg/kg	DAY and ROACH (1976)

D_1	Fenoldopam	ic	dog	no change	no change	pentobarbital	10–40 µg/kg	Lokhandwala et al. (1985)
D_2	Apomorphine	icv	cat	decrease	decrease	α-chloralose	25–100 µg	Dutta et al. (1974)
			rat	decrease	decrease	urethane	1–100 µg	Finch and Hersom (1976)
			rat	decrease	decrease	α-chloralose	25–75 µg/kg	Casto et al. (1988)
		ic	dog	increase		pentobarbital	1.25 µg/kg	Bogaert et al. (1978)
			dog	decrease	increase	α-chloralose	200 µg/kg	Montastruc and Guiol (1984)
			rat	decrease	decrease	α-chloralose	1–10 µg/kg	Casto et al. (1988)
		it	rat	decrease	decrease	conscious	35–80 µg	Petitjean et al. (1984)
D_2	Pergolide	icv	rat	decrease		pentobarbital	12–50 µg/kg	Jadhav et al. (1983)
		ic	dog	decrease	decrease	pentobarbital	12.5 µg/kg	Lokhandwala et al. (1984)

ic, intracisternal; icv, intracerebroventricular; it, intrathecal
[a] Blood pressure and heart rate decrease observed with monoamine oxidase inhibition.
[b] Increase accompanied with retching/vomiting.
[c] Short increase followed by prolonged decrease.

centrally, further suggesting that the centrally mediated response to apomorphine results from activity at D_2 receptors.

15 Role of Central Dopamine Systems in Hypertension

DA may play a role in the centrally mediated maintenance of arterial pressure. A contribution of a central dopaminergic dysfunction in the etiology of essential hypertension is a matter of debate.

Recent studies have revealed that central dopaminergic activity is related not only to the control of basal secretion of pituitary hormones such as prolactin and growth hormone (MACLEOD and LEHMEYER 1974; MACLEOD 1976) but also to peripheral sympathetic activity (BAUM and SHROPSHIRE 1973; DAY and ROACH 1976; FINCH and HERSOM 1976; KAYE et al. 1976; WATANABE et al. 1974). STUMPE et al. (1977) found that in essential hypertensive patients the secretion of prolactin, which is under permanent dopaminergic inhibition, is increased. Bromocriptine, a dopaminergic agonist, reduces blood pressure in such patients. This led to the assumption that a defiency in central dopaminergic activity contributes to hypertension. The findings of MCMURTRY et al. (1979), KOLLOCH et al. (1980, 1981), and SARUTA et al. (1983) support this hypothesis. Also in SHR prolactin is reported to be elevated. FUXE et al. (1979) describe lower DA levels in the hypothalamus of young and adult SHRSP. KONDO et al. (1981) and NAGAHAMA et al. (1984) found that the depressor activity of bromocriptine in SHR is attenuated by metoclopramide, which passes the blood-brain barrier, whereas domperidone, a purely peripheral DA antagonist, has no effect. DA i.c.v. causes a greater drop in blood pressure in SHR than in normotensive WKY.

KAWABE et al. (1983) reported that SHR have significantly higher sensitivity to the central depressor actions of DA than DOCA-salt hypertensive or normotensive rats. HUTCHINSON et al. (1983) reported a central dopaminergic insufficiency in SHR by studying the response of normotensive and hypertensive animals to L-dopa, the precursor to DA. BHARGAVE (1983) showed a DA receptor supersensitivity in SHR. CHIU et al. (1984) also reported supersensitivity of DA receptors in the mesolimbic and striatum of SHR and suggested a functional attenuation in central dopaminergic transmission in this hypertensive model.

Other groups did not find elevated prolactin levels in hypertensive patients (MEIER et al. 1980; MODLINGER and GRETKIN 1978; LENGYEL et al. 1982). In the study of STERN et al. (1983) prolactin was insignificantly higher in hypertensive patients, but they had a much greater response to metoclopramide than the normotensive control group, which indicates that dopaminergic activity is reduced. This is supported by the work of OS et al. (1987). SOWERS et al. (1982b) state that it is probably not the basal secretion of prolactin that is altered but its response to stress factors.

In an editorial comment SLATER (1983) states that, considering together the divergent results, only a subgroup of hypertensive patients show a decreased dopaminergic activity. Patients with elevated prolactin levels should give a good response to a centrally acting, dopaminergic, antihypertensive agent.

Since DA decreases blood pressure by activation of D_2 receptors in the CNS and by interaction with presynaptic D_2 receptors on peripheral sympathetic neurons, both central and peripheral nervous components of an antihypertensive effect of DA or an analogue can become important. The relative contribution of central versus peripheral DA systems in hypertension may be assessed by comparing the antihypertensive efficacy of peripherally versus centrally acting DA agonists.

16 Clinical use of Dopamine and Related Compounds in the Treatment of Cardiovascular Diseases

DA is a substrate for the enzymes monoamine oxidase and catechol-*o*-methyl transferase and is therefore not effective when orally administered. In addition, peripherally administered dopamine usually has no central effects because it does not readily cross the blood-brain barrier. The native compound has nevertheless been utilized acutely to take advantage of its peripheral multiple receptor activity. In the peripheral circulation, DA increases systolic pressure and heart rate due β_1-agonistic activity. There is little effect on total peripheral resistance at low or therapeutic doses due to a balance between α-mediated vasoconstriction and DA receptor-mediated vasodilation. Due to the presence of specific DA receptors, a reduction in arterial resistance occurs in the mesenteric and renal beds with only minor changes in other vascular beds. The result is an increase in GFR, renal blood flow, and sodium excretion. DA is therefore especially useful in the management of circulatory shock, where a generalized increase in sympathetic activity might compromise renal function (WEINER 1980). DA has also been of value in treating chronic refractory congestive heart failure (GOLDBERG 1984).

The usefulness of specific dopaminergic compounds for the treatment of hypertension is not yet established, although beneficial effects can be expected and were observed in limited clinical studies. Owing to the different target sites divergent cardiovascular profiles will result if either Da_1 and Da_2 receptors are stimulated.

Despite extensive chemical efforts only fenoldopam, a benzodiazepine derivative, has been shown to activate vascular Da_1 receptors, having a limited oral availability (HAHN et al. 1981; ACKERMAN et al. 1982, 1983).

After oral application in normotensive and SH rats, dogs, and monkeys, fenoldopam lowers blood pressure accompanied by slight tachycardia (HIEBLE et al. 1987; McCOY et al. 1986; CAVERO and HICKS 1985). Blood pressure effects can be blocked by specific Da_1 receptor antagonists. The most characteristic hemodynamic effect in these animals is an increase in renal blood flow (HAHN et al. 1981; ACKERMAN et al. 1983; BATH et al. 1986).

Fenoldopam has been clinically studied as an antihypertensive drug in patients with essential hypertension. A single oral dose reduces both supine and standing blood pressure for 1–4 h (Carey et al. 1984; Harvey et al. 1986; Ventura et al. 1984). In normotensive subjects little effect on blood pressure was seen although renal blood flow increased in both groups (Carey et al. 1984). Blood pressure reduction is accompanied by tachycardia and an increase in renin secretion (Carey et al. 1984; Harvey et al. 1986; Dupont et al. 1986), plasma aldosterone (Harvey et al. 1986), and plasma norepinephrine (Glück et al. 1987) levels. These effects are thought to be counterregulatory, limiting the blood pressure-lowering effect of fenoldopam, which would also relate to future Da_1 agonists.

In a 4-week study a single oral dose of fenoldopam retained its efficacy on blood pressure, with signs of tachyphylaxis concerning heart rate, plasma renin, and plasma aldosterone effects (Harvey et al. 1986). In an 8-week study fenoldopam administered twice daily caused only a small, statistically insignificant, blood pressure reduction after each dose (Caruana et al. 1987). In hypertensive patients a marked variability in responsiveness to fenoldopam is seen, which is attributed to the fact that the compound undergoes extensive first pass metabolism (Ziemniak et al. 1981).

In conclusion fenoldopam is an hypotensive agent and renal vasodilator with a short duration of action.

Da_2 receptor agonists will be most effective in hypertensive patients with high sympathetic tone due to their mode of action. For Da_2 agonists the structural requirements are much less restrictive, so several compounds with oral availability can be found, mainly ergot alkaloids and their derivatives. These compounds usually also act on other receptors, e.g., α, 5-HT, or histamine receptors, either as agonists or antagonists (Clark 1979; Goldberg and Murphy 1987).

In patients treated for Parkinson's disease these drugs also have been found to decrease blood pressure (Klawans and Weiner 1981; Johns et al. 1984). A common side effect is nausea and vomiting, which is attributed to central D_2 receptor stimulation.

Bromocriptine, a Da_2 receptor agonist, was studied for its antihypertensive effect. It inhibits the release of norepinephrine evoked by sympathetic stimulation in the pithed rat, dog, the isolated perfused cat spleen, and central ear artery of the rabbit (Lokhandwala et al. 1979; Ziegler et al. 1979; Clark 1987). The cardiovascular effects in normotensive and hypertensive animals and the inhibition of norepinephrine release are selectively antagonized by Da_2 receptor antagonists (Ziegler et al. 1979; Ensinger et al. 1985; Clark 1981). In hypertensive patients bromocriptine administered orally twice daily lowers blood pressure significantly in both the supine and upright postures. This effect was maintained for 4 weeks (Stumpe et al. 1977). The authors report that bromocriptine was more effective in patients with high renin and prolactin levels. The antihypertensive effect of bromocriptine and the reduction of plasma norepinephrine levels at rest and during exercise were also shown in other studies (Ziegler et al. 1979; Johns et al. 1984; Mercuro et al. 1985). These effects are blocked by domperidone (Gessa et al. 1986).

This limited survey on studies with Da_1 and Da_2 prototypes indicates that dopaminergic compounds will be effective in the treatment of essential hypertension. The major limitation of peripherally acting Da_1 agonists in the treatment of hypertension is reflex activation of the sympathetic nervous system. Yet this compromise can be prevented by the simultaneous withdrawal of sympathetic tone by activation of central and peripheral D_2 receptors. The combination of direct peripheral vasodilation, increased renal perfusion, and reduced sympathetic tone provides a new approach to the treatment of hypertension. Thus, the development of orally active dopamine agonists holds promise as an effective antihypertensive treatment for a variety of forms of hypertension.

Summary

An overview is given on the peripheral and central actions of dopamine and related compounds in the cardiovascular system, their regulation, and the clinical implications of the use of dopaminergic agents. In the periphery dopamine acts on two different receptors. The Da_1 receptor is located primarily on renal, mesenteric, cerebral, and coronary vessels, causing vasodilatation, and in the kidney also natriuresis. The Da_2 receptor is found in sympathetic ganglia and on sympathetic nerve terminals, inhibiting the release of noradrenaline, thereby reducing sympathetic tone. As sources of dopamine in the periphery, dopaminergic neurons, colocalization with noradrenaline in sympathetic nerve terminals, and production by extraneuronal tissue are discussed. In the central nervous system dopaminergic neurons are widely distributed, influencing cardiovascular regulatory sites, especially in the brain stem. Central dopamine produces depressor and bradycardiac effects in different species. A defiency in central dopaminergic activity is suspected to contribute to hypertension. According to the central and peripheral functions of dopamine in the cardiovascular system, the treatment of hypertensive patients with dopamine analogues seems a promising new therapy.

References

Ackerman DM, Weinstock J, Wiebelhaus VD, Berkowitz BA (1982) Renal vasodilators and hypertension. Drug Dev Res 2:283–297

Ackerman DM, Blumberg AL, McCafferty JP, Sherman S, Weinstock J, Kaiser C, Berkowitz BA (1983) Potential usefulness of renal vasodilators in hypertension and renal disease. Fed Proc 42:186–190

Adam WR (1980) Aldosterone and dopamine receptors in the kidney a site for pharmacologic manipulation of renal function. Kidney Int 19:623–635

Aguilera G, Catt KJ (1984) Dopaminergic modulation of aldosterone secretion in the rat. Endocrinology 114:176–181

Alexander RW, Gill TR, Yamabe H, Lovenberg W, Keiser HR (1974) Effect of dietary sodium and acute saline infusion on the interrelationship between dopamine excretion and adrenergic activity in man. J Clin Invest 54:194–200

Alkadhi KA, Sabouni MH, Ansari AF, Lokhandwala MF (1986) Activation of Da-receptors by dopamine or fenoldopam increases cyclic AMP levels in the renal artery but not the superior cervical ganglion of the rat. J Pharmacol Exp Ther 238:547–553

Amenta F, Convallotti C, de Rossi M, Thione MF (1984) Dopamine sensitive c-AMP generating system in rat extra cerebral arteries. Eur J Pharmacol 97: 105–116
Andersson FO, Farnebo LO, Fredholm B, Hamberger B, Holst J, Jarhult J (1982) Metabolic and hormonal adjustements during hemorrhage in cats after interference with the sympatho-adrenal system. Acta Physiol Scand 114:111–119
Anton AH, Sayre DF (1964) The distribution of dopamine and dopa in various animals and a method for their determination in diverse biological material. J Pharmacol Exp Ther 145:326–336
Aperia A, Bertorello A, Seri I (1987) Dopamine causes inhibition of Na-KATPase from rat proximal tubule segments. Am J Physiol 252:F39–F45
Ball SG, Lee MR (1977) The effects of carbidopa administration on urinary sodium excretion in man: is dopamine an intrarenal natriuretic hormone? Br J Clin Pharmacol 4:115–119
Baines AD (1982) Effect of salt intake and renal denervation on catecholamine catabolism and excretion. Kidney Int 21:316–322
Baines AD, Drangova R, Hatcher C (1985) Dopamine production by isolated glomeruli and tubules from rat kidneys. Can J Physiol Pharmacol 63:155–161
Ball SG, Oats NS, Lee MR (1978) Urinary dopamine in man and rat: Effects of inorganic salts on dopamine excretion. Clin Sci Mol Med 55:167–173
Ball SG, Gunn IG, Douglas IHS (1982) Renal handling of dopa, dopamine, norepinephrine and epinephrine in the dog. Am J Physiol 242:F56–F62
Barger G, Dale HH (1910) Chemical structure and sympathomimetic action of amines. J Physiol (Lond) 41:18–59
Bath S, Churchill M, Churchill P, McDonald T (1986) Renal effects of SK&F 82526 in anesthetized rats. Life Sci 38:1565–1571
Baum T, Shropshire AT (1973) Reduction of sympathetic outflow by central administration of L-dopa, dopamine and norepinephrine. Neuropharmacology 12:49–56
Bell C (1982) Dopamine as a postganglionic autonomic neurotransmitter. Neuroscience 7:1–8
Bell C (1987) Dopamine: Precursor or neurotransmitter in sympathetically innervated tissues? Blood Vessels 24:234–239
Bell C, Lang WJ (1973) Neural dopaminergic vasodilator control in the kidney. Nature New Biol 246:27–29
Bell C, Lang WJ (1979) Evidence for dopaminergic vasodilator innervation of the canine paw pad. Br J Pharmacol 67:337–343
Bell C, McLachlan EM (1982) Dopaminergic neurones in sympathetic ganglia of the dog. Proc R Soc Lond [Biol] 215:175–190
Bell C, Muller B (1982) Absence of dopamine-β-hydroxlase in some catecholamine-containing sympathetic ganglion cells of the dog: Evidence for dopaminergic autonomic neurons. Neurosci Lett 31:31–35
Bell C, Conway EL, Lang WJ, Padanyi R (1975) Vascular dopamine receptors in the canine hindlimb. Br J Pharmacol 55:167–172
Bell C, Lang WJ, Laska F (1978a) Dopamine-containing vasomotor nerves in the dog kidney. J. Neurochem 31:77–83
Bell C, Lang WJ, Laska F (1978b) Dopamine-containing axons supplying the arterio-venous anastomoses of the canine paw pad. J Neurochem 31:1329–1333
Bello-Reuss E, Higashi Y, Kaneda Y (1982) Dopamine decreases fluid reabsorption in straight portions of rabbit proximal tubule. Am J Physiol 242:F634–F640
Ben-Jonathan N, Oliver C, Weiner HJ, Mical RS, Porter JC (1977) Dopamine in hypophysial portal plasma of the rat during the estrous cycle and throughout pregnancy. Endocrinology 100:452–458
Bennet ED, Tighe D, Wegg W (1982) Abolition by dopamine blockade of the natriuretic response produced by lower-body positive pressure. Clin Sci 63:361–366
Bertorello A, Aperia A (1987) Effect of L-dopa, dopamine, dihydroxyphenylacetic acid and homovanillic acid on Na-K-ATPase activity in rat proximal tubule segments. Acta Physiol Scand 130:571–574
Bevilacqua M, Vago T, Scorza D, Norbiato G (1982) Characterization of dopamine receptors of ^{3}H-ADTN binding in calf adrenal zona glomerulosa. Biochem Biophys

Res Commun 108:1661–1669
Bhargava HN (1983) Effect of cyclo (leu-gly) on the supersensitivity of dopamine receptors in spontaneously hypertensive rats. Life Sci 32:2131–2137
Björklund A, Skagerberg G (1979) Evidence for a major spinal cord projection from the diencephalic A11 dopamine cell group in the rat using transmitter-specific fluorescent retrograde tracing. Brain Res 177:170–175
Björklund A, Cegrell L, Falck B, Ritzin M, Rosengren E (1970) Dopamine-containing cells in sympathetic ganglia. Acta Physiol Scand 78: 334–338
Björklund A, Lindvall O, Nobin A (1975) Evidence of an incerto-hypothalamic dopamine neurone system in the rat. Brain Res 89: 29–42
Blessing WW, Chalmers JP (1979) Direct projections of catecholamine (presumably dopamine)- containing neurons from hypothalamus to spinal cord. Neurosci Lett 11:35–40
Bogaert MG, de Schaepdryer AF, Willems JL (1977) Dopamine induced neurogenic vasodilatation in the intact hindleg of the dog. Br J Pharmacol 59:283–292
Bogaert MG, Buylaert WA, Willems JL (1978) Hypotension produced by intravenous apomorphine in the anesthetized dog is not centrally mediated. Br J Pharmacol 63:481–484
Bouthenet ML, Matres MP, Sales N, Schwartz JC (1987) A detailed mapping of dopamine D-$_2$ receptors in rat central nervous system by autoradiography with ^{125}J jodosulpiride. Neuroscience 20:117–155
Brodde OE (1980) Demonstration of vascular dopamine receptors in membranes from rabbit renal artery using ^{3}H-Spiroperidol binding. Experientia 37:1099–1101
Brodde OE (1982) Vascular dopamine receptors: Demonstration and characterization by in vitro studies. Life Sci 31:289–306
Brown MJ, Allison DJ (1981) Renal conversion of plasma DOPA to urine dopamine. Br J Clin Pharmacol 12:251–253
Bunzow JR, Vain Tol HHU, Grandy DK, Albert P, Salon J, Christie M, Machida CA, Neve KA, Civelli O (1988) Cloning and expression of a rat D_2 dopamine receptor cDNA. Nature 336:783–787
Buu NT, Nair G, Kuchel O, Genest J (1981) The extra-adrenal synthesis of epinephrine in cats: Possible involvement of dopamine sulfate. J Lab Clin Med 98:527–535
Buylaert WA, Willems JL, Bogaert MG (1977) Vasodilatation produced by apomorphine in the hindleg of the dog. J Pharmacol Exp Ther 201:738–746
Buylaert WA, Willems JL, Bogaert MG (1978) The receptor mediating the apomorphine vasodilatation in the hindleg of the dog. J Pharm Pharmacol 30:113–115
Calne DB (1977) Developments in the pharmacology and therapeutics of parkinsonism. Ann Neurol 1:111–119
Campbell DJ, Mendelsohn FAO, Adam W, Funder JW (1981a) Metoclopramide does not elevate aldosterone in the rat. Endocrinology 109:1484–1491
Campbell DJ, Mendelsohn FAO, Adam W, Funder JW (1981b) is aldosterone secretion under dopaminergic control? Circ Res 49:1217–1227
Carey RM, Thorner MO, Ortt EM (1979) Effects of metoclopramide and bromocriptine on the renin-angiotensin-aldosterone system in man. J Clin Invest 58:71–76
Carey RM, Thorner MO, Ortt EM (1980) Dopaminergic inhibition of metoclopraminde induced aldosterone secretion in man. J Clin Invest 66:10–18
Carey RM, van Loon GR, Baines AD, Ortt EM (1981) Decreased plasma and urinary dopamine during dietary sodium depletion in man. J Clin Endocrinol Metab 52: 903–909
Carey RM, Stote RM, Dubb JW, Townsend LH, Rose CE, Kaiser DL (1984) Selective peripheral dopamine-1 receptor stimulation with fenoldopam in human essential hypertension. J Clin Invest 74:2198–2207
Carlsson A (1959) The occurrence, distribution and physiological role of catecholamines in the nervous system. Pharmacol Rev 11:490–495
Carlsson A, Lindquist A, Magnusson T (1960) On the biochemistry and possible functions of dopamine and noradrenaline in brain. In: Vane JR, Wolstenholme GEW, O'Connor M (eds) Adrenergic mechanisms. Churchill, London, pp 432–439
Caruana MP, Heber M, Brigden G, Raftery EB (1987) Effects of fenoldopam, a specific

dopamine receptor agonist, on blood pressure and left ventricular function in systemic hypertension. Br J Clin Pharmacol 24:721–727
Casto R, Jödicke A, Stock G (1988) Central cardiovascular effects of dopamine receptor activation. FASEB J 2:A500
Cavero I, Hicks PE (1985) Studies on the transient hypotensive effect of fenoldopam, a Da_1 dopamine receptor agonist in rats. Br J Pharmacol 86:436P
Cavero I, Lefevre Borg F, Gomeni R (1981) Heart rate lowering effects of *N, N*-di-*n*-propyl-dopamine in rats: evidence for stimulation of peripheral dopamine receptors leading to inhibition of sympathetic vascular tone. J Pharmacol Exp Ther 218: 515–524
Cavero I, Massingham R, Lefevre-Borg (1982a) Peripheral dopamine receptors, potential targets for a new class of antihypertensive agents. I. Subclassification and functional description. Life Sci 31:939–948
Cavero I, Massingham R, Lefevre-Borg (1982b) Peripheral dopamine receptors, potential targets for a new class of antihypertensive agents. II. Sites and mechanisms of action of dopamine receptor agonists. Life Sci 31:1059–1069
Chan YC (1976) Cellular mechanisms of renal tubular transport of L-dopa and its derivatives in the rat: microperfusion studies. J Pharmacol Exp Ther 199:17–24
Chapman BJ, Horn NM, Munday KA, Robertson MJ (1980) The actions of dopamine and of sulpiride on regional blood flows in the rat kidney. J Physiol (Lond) 298: 437–452
Chiu P, Rajakumar G, Chiu S, Kwan CY, Mishra RK (1984) Differential changes in central serotonin and dopamine receptors in spontaneous hypertensive rats. Prog Neuropsychopharmacol Biol Psychiatry 8:665–668
Clark BJ (1979) Cardiovascular effects of ergot alkaloids. J Pharmacol (Paris) 10:439–453
Clark BJ (1981) Dopamine receptors and the cardiovascular system. Postgrad Med J 57:45–54
Clark BJ (1987) Is stimulation of prejunctional dopamine receptors an antihypertensive principle? Clin Exper Theor Pract A9:1045–1068
Clark BJ, Bucher T, Waite R (1985) Analysis of the cardiovascular effects of codergocrine (hydergine). J Pharmacol [Suppl 3] 16:115–127
Coruzzi P (1987) Dopa blockade abolishes the exaggerated natriuresis of essential hypertension. J Hypertens 5:587–591
Creese I, Leff SE (1982) Dopamine receptors: a classification. J Clin Psychopharmacol 2:329–335
Creese I, Sibley DR, Leff SE, Hamblin M (1981) Dopamine receptors: subtypes, localization and regulation. Fed Proc 40:147–152
Creese I, Sibley DR, Leff SE (1984) Agonist interaction with dopamine receptors: focus on radioligand-binding studies. Fed Proc 43:2779–2784
Critchley JAJH, Lee MR (1986) Salt sensitive hypertension in West Africans: an uncoupling of the renal sodium dopamine relation. Lancet 8504:460
Cross AJ, Owen F (1980) Characteristics of 3H-cis-flupenthixol binding to calf brain membranes. Eur J Pharmacol 65:341–347
Cross A, Marshal RD, Johnson JA, Owen F (1983) Preferential inhibition of ligand binding to calf striatal dopamine D_1 receptors by SCH 23390. Neuropharmacology 22:1327–1329
Davis BB, Walter MJ, Murdaugh HV (1968) The mechanism of the increase in sodium excretion following dopamine infusion. Proc Soc Exp Biol Med 129:210–213
Day MD, Roach AG (1976) Cardiovascular effects of dopamine after central administration into conscious cats. Br J Pharmacol 58:505–515
De Groat WC, Volle RL (1966) The actions of the catecholamines on transmission in the superior cervical ganglion of the cat. J Pharmacol Exp Ther 154:1–13
Dinerstein RJ, Vannice J, Henderson RC, Roth LJ, Goldberg LI, Hoffmann PC (1979) Histofluorescence techniques provide evidence for dopamine-containing neuronal elements in canine kidney. Science 205:497–499
Dinerstein RJ, Jones RT, Goldberg LI (1983) Evidence for dopamine-containing renal nerves. Fed Proc 42:3005–3008

Drake CR, Carey RM (1984) Dopamine modulates sodium-dependent aldosterone responses to angiotensin II in man. Hypertension [Suppl 1] 6:119–123
Drew GM, Hilditch A, Clark KL (1987) IBMX and forskolin potentiate the effect of dopamine in the rabbit isolated splenic artery. Clin Exp Hypertens [A]9:1085
Dunn MG, Bosmann GH (1981) Peripheral dopamine receptor identification: properties of a specific dopamine receptor in the rat adrenal zona glomerulosa. Biochem Biophys Res Commun 99:1081–1087
Dupont AG, Vanderniepen P, Volckaert A, Smits J, van Steirteghem AC, Sic RO (1986) Effect of fenoldopam on the aldosterone response to metoclopramide in man. Clin Endocrinol (Oxf) 24:203–208
Dutta SN, Guha D, Pradhan SN (1974) Mechanism of centrally induced hypotensive effect of apomorphine. Pharmacologist 16:509
Dutta SN, Guha D, Pradhan SN (1975) Cardiovascular effects of central microinjections of apomorphine in cats. Arch Int Pharmacodyn Ther 215:259–265
Ehringer H, Hornykiewicz O (1960) Verteilung von Noradrenalin und Dopamin (3-Hydroxytryptamin) im Gehirn des Menschen und ihr Verhalten bei Erkrankungen des extrapyramidalen Systems. Klin Wochenschr 38:1236–1239
Edwards CRW, Miall PA, Hauber JP, Thorner MO, Al Dujaili EAS, Besser GM (1975) Inhibition of the plasma aldosterone response to furosemide by bromocriptine. Lancet 2:903–904
Enero MA, Langer SZ (1975) Inhibition of dopamine of ^{3}H-noradrenaline release elicited by nerve stimulation in the isolated cat's nictitating membrane. Naunyn Schmiedebergs Arch Pharmacol 289:179–203
Ensinger H, Majewski H, Hedler L, Starke K (1985) Neuronal and postjunctional components in the blood pressure effects of dopamine and bromocriptine in rabbits. J Pharmacol Exp Ther 234:681–690
Eranko O, Harkonen M (1963) Histochemical demonstration of fluorogenic amines in the cytoplasm of sympathetic ganglion cells of the rat. Acta Physiol Scand 58:285–286
Erhardt J, Schwartz J (1978) A gas chromatography-mass spectrometry assay of human plasma catecholamines. Clin Chim Acta 88:71–79
Felder RA, Carey RM (1987) Dopamine in cardiovascular function. In: Buckley JP, Ferrario CM (eds) Brain peptides and catecholamines. Raven, New York, pp 79–91
Felder RA, Blecher M, Eisner GM, Jose PA (1984a) Cortical tubular and glomerular dopamine receptors in the rat kidney. Am J Physiol 246:F557–F568
Felder RA, Blecher M, Calcagno PL, Jose PA (1984b) Dopamine receptors in the proximal tubule of the rabbit. Am J Physiol 247:F499–F505
Felten DL, Laties AM, Carpenter MB (1974) Monoamine-containing cell bodies in the squirrel monkey brain. Am J Anat 139:153–166
Fillenz M, Howe PRC (1975) Depletion of noradrenaline stores in sympathetic nerve terminals. J Neurochem 24:683–688
Finch I, Hersom A (1976) Studies on the centrally mediated cardiovascular effects of apomorphine in the anesthetized rat. Br J Pharmacol 56:336P
Foley JJ, Sarau HM (1984) Adrenergic binding studies of SK&F 82526 and its enantiomers. Fed Proc 43:555
Fox M, Thier S, Rosenberg L, Segal S (1964) Ionic requirements for amino acid transport in the rat kidney cortex slice. I. Influence of extracellular ions. Biochem Biophys Acta 79:167–176
Franco-Morselli R, Elghozi JL, Joly E, di Guiglio S, Meyer P (1977) Increased plasma adrenaline concentrations in benign essential hypertension. Br Med J 2:1251–1254
Frederickson ED, Bradley T, Goldberg LI (1985) Blockade of renal effects of dopamine in the dog by the DA_1 antagonist SCH 23390. Am J Physiol 249:F236–F240
Fredholm BB, Farnebo LO, Hamberger B (1979) Plasma catecholamines, cyclic AMP and metabolic substrates in hemorrhagic shock of the rat. The effect of adrenal demedullation and 6-OH dopamine tratment. Acta Physiol Scand 105:481–495
Fuxe K, Ganten D, Jonsson G, Agnati LF, Andersson K, Hökfelt T, Bome P, et al. (1979) Catecholamine turnover changes in hypothalamus and medulla oblongata of spontaneously hypertensive rats. Neurosci Lett 15:283–288
Ganguly A (1984) Dopaminergic regulation of aldosterone secretion: how credible? Clin

Sci 66:631–637
Georgiev VP, Doda M, Gyorgy L (1978) Influence of intraventricularly applied apomorphine on somatovegetative reflexes in cats. Arch Int Pharmacodyn Ther 231:131–138
Gessa GL, Mercuro G, Rossetti ZL (1986) Peripheral dopamine receptors controlling norepinephrine release in man. In: Biggio G, Spano PF, Toffano G, Gessa GL (eds) Modulation of central and peripheral transmitter function. Liviana, Podova, pp 203–217 (Fidia research series)
Glück Z, Lossen L, Weidmann P, Gnädinger MP, Peheim E (1987) Cardiovascular and renal profile of acute peripheral dopamine$_1$-receptor agonism with fenoldopam. Hypertension 10:43–54
Goldberg LI (1972) Cardiovascular and renal actions of dopamine: Potential clinical applications. Pharmacol Rev 24:1–29
Goldberg LI (1984) Dopamine receptors and hypertension. Physiological and pharmacological implications. Am J Med 77:37–44
Goldberg LI, Kohli JD (1979) Peripheral pre- and postsynaptic dopamine receptors: are they different from dopamine receptors in the central nervous system? Commun Psychpharmacol 3:447–456
Goldberg LI, Kohli JD (1983) Peripheral dopamine receptors: a classification based on potency series and specific antagonists. Trends Pharmacol Sci 4:64–66
Goldberg LI, Murphy MB (1987) Potential use of Da$_1$ and Da$_2$ receptor agonists in the treatment of hypertension. Clin Exp Hypertens [A]9:1023–1035
Goldberg LI, Volkmann PH, Kohli JD (1978) A comparison of the vascular dopamine receptor with other dopamine receptors. Annu Rev Pharmacol Toxicol 18:57–79
Goldberg LI, Glock D, Kohli JD, Barnett A (1984) Separation of peripheral dopamine receptors by a selective Da$_1$ antagonist, SCH 23390. Hypertension [Suppl 1] 6:25–30
Goldberg LI, Kohli JD, Glock D (1986) Conclusive evidence for two subtypes of peripheral dopamine receptors. In: Woodruff GN, Poat JA, Roberts JP (eds) Dopaminergic systems and their regulation. Macmillan, London, pp 195–212
Gordon MB, Moore TJ, Dluhy RS, Willians GH (1983) Dopaminergic modulation of aldosterone responsiveness to angiotensin II with changes in sodium intake. J Clin Endocrinol Metab 56:340–345
Grega GJ, Barret RJ, Adamski SW, Lokhandwala MF (1984) Effects of dopamine and SK&F 82526, a selective DA$_1$-receptor agonist, on vascular resistances in the canine forelimb. J Pharmacol Exp Ther 22:756–762
Hahn RA, Wardell JR, Sarau HM, Ritley PT (1982) Characterization of the peripheral and central effects of SK&F 82526, a novel dopamine receptor agonist. J Pharmacol Exp Ther 223:305–313
Hamet R (1931) Contribution à l'étude de la dihydroxyphenylethylamine. Arch Int Pharmacodyn Ther 40:427–443
Harris T, Muller BD, Cotton RGH, Voltatorni B, Bell C (1986) Dopaminergic and noradrenergic nerves of the dog have different DOPA decarboxylase activities. Neurosci Lett 65:155–160
Harvey JN, Casson IF, Claydon AD, Cope GF, Perkins CM, Lee MR (1984) A paradoxical fall in urinary dopamine when patients with essential hypertension are given dietary salt. Clin Sci 67:83–88
Harvey JN, Worth DP, Brown J, Lee MR (1986) Studies with fenoldopam, a dopamine receptor Da$_1$ agonist in essential hypertension. Br J Clin Pharmacol 21:53–61
Head RJ, Berkovitz BA (1979) Concentration and function of dopamine in normal and diseased blood vessels. In: Imbs JL, Schwartz J (eds) Peripheral dopamine receptors. Pergamon, Oxford, pp 173–181
Heise A (1976) Hypotensive actions by central α-adrenergic ad dopaminergic receptor stimulation. In: Scriabine A, Sweet CS (eds) New antihypertensive drugs. Spectrum, New York, pp 135–145 (Monographs of the Physiological Society of Philadelphia, vol 2)
Hicks PE, Cannon JG (1979) N,N dialkyl derivatives of 2-amino-5,6, dihydroxy-1,2,3,4 tetrahydronaphtalene as selective agonists at presynaptic α-adrenoceptors in the rat. J Pharm Pharmacol 31:494–496
Hicks PE, Shoemaker H, Langer SZ (1984) 5-HT-receptor antagonistic properties of

SCH 23390 in vascular smooth muscle and brain. Eur J Pharmacol 105:339–342
Hieble JP, Owen DAA, Harvey CA, Blumberg AL, Valocik RE, DeMarinio RM (1987) Hemodynamic effects of selective dopamine receptor agonists in the rat and dog. Clin Exp Hypertens [A]9:889–912
Hilditch A, Drew GM (1987) Subclassification of peripheral dopamine receptors. Clin Exp Ther Pract A9:853–872
Hökfelt T, Johansson O, Fuxe K, Goldstein M, Park D (1976) Immunohistochemical studies on the localization and distribution of monoamine neuron systems in the rat brain. Med Biol 54:427–453
Hökfelt T, Phillipson O, Goldstein M (1979) Evidence for a dopaminergic pathway in the rat descending from the A11 cell group to the spinal cord. Acta Physiol Scand 107:393–395
Holtz P, Credner K (1942) Die enzymatische Entstehung von Oxytyramin im Organismus und die physiologische Bedeutung der Dopadecarboxylase. Arch Pharmakol Exp Pathol 200:356–388
Hope W, Law M, McCulloch MW, Rand MJ, Story DF (1976) Effects of some catecholamines on noradrenergic transmission in the rabbit ear artery. Clin Exp Pharmacol Physiol 3:15–28
Hope W, Majewski H, McCulloch MW, Rand MJ, Story DF (1979) Modulation of sympathetic transmission by neuronally released dopamine. Br J Pharmacol 67:185–192
Huang BS, Malvin RL, Lee J, Grehin RJ (1987) Central dopaminergic regulation of aldosterone secretion in sheep. Hypertension 10:157–163
Hughes A, Thom S, Martin G, Redman D, Hasan S, Sever P (1986) The action of a dopamine (DA_1) receptor agonist, fenoldopam in human vasculature in vivo and in vitro. Br J Clin Pharmacol 22:535–540
Hutchinson JS, DiNicolantonio R, Veroni M, Cleverdon M (1983) Evidence for a functional central dopaminergic insufficency in the spontaneously hypertensive rat. Clin Exp Pharmacol Physiol 10:311–314
Hyttel J (1981) Similarities between the binding of 3H-pifluxitol and 3H-flupentixol to rat striatal dopamine receptors in vitro. Life Sci 28:563–569
Imondi AR, Hageman LM, Belair EG (1979) Inhibition of saline induced diuresis in the rat by sulpiride. Experientia 35:251–252
Inglis GC, Kenyon SJ, Hannah IAM, Connell IMC, Ball SG (1987) Does dopamine regulate aldosterone secretion in the rat? Clin Sci 73:93–97
Jadhav AL, Willette RN, Sapru HN, Lokhandwala MF (1983) Involvement of central dopamine receptors in the hopotensive action of pergolide. Naunyn Schmiedebergs Arch Pharmacol 324:281–286
Jödicke A, Casto R, Hilbig J, Kersten G, Stock G (1988) Dopamine receptor activation modulates central cardiovascular regulation. Pflügers Arch 412:R59
Johns DW, Ayers CR, Carey RM (1984) The dopamine agonist bromocriptine induces hypotension by venous and arteriolar dilation. J Cardiovasc Pharmacol 6:582–587
Kawabe H, Kondo K, Saruta T (1983) Effect of the intracerebroventricular injection of dopamine on blood pressure in the spontaneously hypertensive rat. Clin Exp Hypertens 5:1703–1716
Kaye SB, Shaw KM Ross EJ (1976) Bromocriptine and hypertension. Lancet 7970: 1176–1177
Kebabian JW (1984) Pharmacological and biochemical characterization of two categories of dopamine receptors. In: Poste G, Crooke ST (eds) Dopamine receptor agonists. Plenum, New York, pp 3–22
Kebabian JW, Calne DB (1979) Multiple receptors for dopamine. Nature 277:93–96
Kebabian JW, Agni T, van Oene JC, Shigematsu K, Saavedra JM (1986) The D_1 dopamine receptor: new perspectives. Trends Pharmacol Sci 7:96–99
Klawans HL, Weiner WJ (1981) Parkinsonism. In: Klawans HL, Weiner WJ, Nausieda PA, Guetz (Gleds) Textbook of clinical neuropharmacology. Raven, New York, pp 1–35
Kohli JD, Glock D, Goldberg LI (1988) Relative DA_1-Dopamine receptor agonist and α-adrenoceptor antagonist activity of Fenoldopam in the anesthetized dog. J Cardiovasc Pharmacol 11:123–126

Kolloch RE, Kobayashi K, DeQuattro V (1980) Dopaminergic control of sympathetic tone and blood pressure: evidence in primary hypertension. Hypertension 2:390–394
Kolloch RE, Stumpe KO, Ismer U, Kletzy O, DeQuattro V (1981) Central dopaminergic mechanisms in young patients with essential hypertension. Clin Sci 61:231s–234s
Kondo K, Suzuki H, Handa M, Nagahama S, Saruta T (1981) Effects of intracerebroventricular administration of dopamine and metoclopramide on blood pressure in rats. Arch Int Pharmacodyn Ther 250:273–278
Krishna GG, Danovitch GM, Beck FW, Sowers JR (1985) Dopminergic mediation of the natriuretic response to volume expansion. J Lab Clin Med 105:214–218
Krstulovic AM, Dziedzic SW, Bertani-Dziedzic L, di Rico DE (1981) Plasma catecholamines in hypertension and pheochromocytoma determined using ion-pair reversed phase chromatography with amperometric detection. Investigation of the separation mechanisms and clinical methodology. J Chromatogr 217:523–537
Kuchel O, Buu NT, Unger T, Genest J (1978) Free and conjugated catecholamines in human hypertension. Clin Sci Mol Med 55:77s–80s
Kvetnansky R, Weise VK, Thoa NB, Kopin IJ (1979) Effects of chronic guanethidine treatment and adrenal medullectomy on plasma levels of catecholamines and corticosterone in forcibly immobilized rats. J Pharmacol Exp Ther 209:287–291
Lackovic Z, Neff NH (1980) Evidence for the existence of peripheral dopaminergic neurons. Brain Res 193:289–292
Lackovic Z, Kleinman J, Karoum F, Neff NH (1981) Dopamine and its metabolites in human peripheral nerves: is there a widely distributed system of peripheral dopaminergic nerves? Life Sci 29:912–922
Lang WJ, Woodman OL (1979) Cardiovascular responses produced by the injection of dopamine into the cerebral ventricles of the unanesthetized dog. Br J Pharmacol 66:235–240
Langer SZ (1973) The regulation of transmitter release elicited by nerve stimulation through a presynaptic feed-back mechanism. In: Usdin E, Synder JH (eds) Frontiers in catecholamine research. Pergamon New York pp 543–549
Langer SZ (1981) Presynaptic regulation of the release of catecholamines. Pharmacol Rev 32:337–362
Laubie M, Schmitt H, Falq E (1977) Dopamine receptors in the femoral vascular bed of the dog as mediators of a vasodilator and sympatho inhibitory effect. Eur J Pharmacol 42:307–310
Lee MR (1982) Dopamine and the kidney. Clin Sci 62:439–448
Lengyel AMJ, Vieira JGH, Chacra AR, Abucham-Filho JZ, Lima MPC, Ribeiro AB, Ramos OL (1982) Dynamic evaluation of prolactin secretion in essential hypertension: evidence against hypothalamic-pituitary dopaminergic dysfunction. J Clin Endocrinol Metab 54:849–853
Libet B (1977) The role SIF-cells play in ganglionic transmission. Adv Biochem Psychopharmacol 16:541–546
Libet B, Owman C (1974) Concomitant changes in formaldehyde-induced fluorescence of dopamine interneurons and in slow inhibitory postsynaptic potentials of the rabbit superior cervical ganglion, induced by stimulation of the preganglionic nerve or by a muscarinic agent. J Physiol (Lond) 237:635–662
Libet B, Tosaka T (1970) Dopamine as a synaptic transmitter and modulator in sympathetic ganglia: a different mode of synaptic action. Proc Nat Acad Sci USA 67: 667–673
Lindvall O, Björklund A (1974) The organization of the ascending catecholamine neuron systems in the at brain as revealed by glyoxlic acid fluorescence method. Acta Physiol Scand [Suppl] 412:1–48
Lindvall O, Björklund A (1983) Dopamine- and norepinehrine-containing neuron systems: Their anatomy in the rat brain. In: Emson PC (ed) Clinical neuroanatomy. Raven, New York, pp 229–255
Lindvall O, Björklund A, Skagerberg G (1984) Selective histochemical demonstration of dopamine terminal systems in rat di- and telencephalon: New evidence for dopaminergic innervation of hypothalamic neurosecretory nuclei. Brain Res 306:19–30
Listinsky JJ, Kohli JD, Goldberg LI (1980) Consistent unmasking of dopamine-induced

dilation of the canine femoral vascular bed. J Pharmacol Exp Ther 215:662–667
Lokhandwala MF (1987a) Preclinical and clinical studies on the cardiovascular and renal effects of fenoldopam: A Da_1-receptor agonist. Drug Dev Res 10:123–134
Lokhandwala MF (1987b) Dopamine receptor agonists and cardiovascular neuroeffector function. In: Buckley JP, Ferrario CM (eds) Brain peptides and catecholamines in cardiovascular regulation. Raven, New York, pp 65–77
Lokhandwala MF, Barret RJ (1982) Cardiovascular dopamine receptors: physiological, pharmacological and therapeutic implications. J Auton Pharmacol 3:189–215
Lokhandwala MF, Steenberg ML (1984) Selective activation by LY141865 and apomorphine of presynaptic dopamine receptors in the rat kidney and influence of stimulation parameters in the action of dopamine. J Pharmacol Exp Ther 228:161–167
Lokhandwala MF, Steenberg ML (1984a) Evaluation of the effect of SK&F 82526 and LY 171555 on presynaptic (DA_2) and postsynaptic dopamine receptors in rat kidney. J Auton Pharmacol 4:273–277
Lokhandwala MF, Tadepalli AS, Jandhyala BS (1979) Cardiovascular actions of bromocriptine: Evidence for a neurogenic mechanism. J Pharmacol Exp Ther 211:620–625
Lokhandwala MF, Kivlighn SD, Jandhyala BS (1984) Characterization of the neurogenic vasodilation elicited by central dopamine receptor stimulation with pergolide. J Pharmacol Exp Ther 228:696–703
Lokhandwala MF, Watkins HO, Sabouni MH, Alkadhi KA (1985) Pharmacological analysis of the actions of SKF 82526 on cardiovascular dopamine receptors. J Pharmacol Exp Ther 234:337–344
Lokhandwala MF, Watkins HO, Dlewati A (1987) Different dopamine receptor subtypes mediate the neurogenic vasodilatation produced by fenoldopam and SKF 85174 in the dog hindlimb. Eur J Pharmacol 143:383–390
Lutold BE, Karoum F, Neff NH (1979) Activationof rat sympathetic ganglia SIF cell dopamine metabolism by muscarinic agonists. Eur J Pharmacol 54:21–26
MacLeod RM (1976) Regulation of prolactin secretion. In: Martini L, Ganong WA (eds) Frontiers in neuroendocrinology. Raven, New York, pp 169–194
MacLeod RM, Lehmeyer JE (1974) Studies on the mechanism of the dopamine-mediated inhibition of prolactin secretion. Endocrinology 94:1077–1085
Maemura S, Niva M, Ozaki M (1982) Characteristic alterations in adrenal catecholamine content in SHR, SHRSP and WKY during development of hypertension and stroke. Jpn Heart J 23:593–603
Maichon S, Bérod A, Leger L, Chat M, Hartman B, Pujol JF (1984) Identification of catecholamine cell bodies in the pons and pons-mesencephalon junction of the cat brain, using tyrosine hydroxylase and dopamine-β-hydroxylase immunohistochemistry. Brain Res 305:369–374
Marin-Grez M, Briggs JP, Schubert G, Schnermann J (1985) Dopamine receptor antagonists inhibit the natriuretic response to atrial natriuretic factor (ANF). Life Sci 16:2171–2176
Matthews MR (1980) Ultrastructural studies relevant to the possible functions of small granule-containing cells in the rat superior cervical ganglion. Adv Biochem Psychopharmacol 25:77–86
McCoy CE, Douglas FL, Goldberg LI (1986) Selective antagonism of the hypotensive effects of dopamine agonists in spontaneously hypertensive rats. Hypertension 8:298–302
McClanahan M, Sowers JR, Beck FWJ, Mohanty PK, McKenzie T (1985) Dopaminergic regulation of natriuretic response to acute volume expansion in dogs. Clin Sci 68: 263–269
McCubbin JW, Kaneko Y, Page IH (1960) Ability of serotonin and norepinephrine to mimic the central effects of reserpine on vasomotor activity. Circ Res 8:849–858
McCulloch AW, Rand MJ, Story DF (1973) Evidence for a dopaminergic mechanism for modulation of adrenergic transmission in the rabbit ear artery. Br J Pharmacol 49:141P
McDonald RH, Goldberg LI, McNay JC, Tuttle EP (1963) Augmentation of sodium excretion and blood flow by dopamine in man. Clin Res 11:248
McDonald RH, Goldberg LI, McNay JC, Tuttle EP (1964) Effects of dopamine in man:

Augmentation of sodium excretion glomerular filtration rate and renal plasma flow. J Clin Invest 43:1116–1124
McKenna TJ, Island DP, Nickolson WP, Liddle GW (1979) Dopamine inhibits angiotensin-stimulated aldosterone biosynthesis in bovine adrenal cells. J Clin Invest 64:287–291
McMurtry JP, Kazama N, Wexler BC (1979) Effects of bromocriptine on hormone and blood pressure levels in the spontaneously hypertensive rat. Proc Soc Exp Biol Med 161:186–188
McNay JL, McDonald RH, Goldberg LI (1965) Direct vasodilation produced by dopamine in the dog. Circ Res 16:510–517
Mefford IN, Ward MM, Miles L, Taylor B, Chesney MA, Keegan DL, Barchas JD (1981) Determination of plasma catecholamines and free 3,4-dihydroxyphenylacetic acid in continuously collected human plasma by high performance liquid chromatography with electrochemical detection. Life Sci 28:477–483
Meier A, Weidman P, Hennes V, Ziegler WH (1980) Plasma prolactin in normal and hypertensive subjects: relationship with age, posture, blood pressure, catecholamines and renin. J Clin Endocrinol Metab 50:304–308
Mercuro G, Rossetti ZL, Tocco L, Rivano CA, Cherchi A, Gessa GL (1985) Bromocriptine reduces plasma noradrenaline and 3,4-dihydropphenylacetic acid in normal and hypertensive subjects. Eur J Clin Pharmacol 27:671–675
Messerli FH, Frohlich ED, Suarez DH, Reisin E, Dreslinski GR, Dunn FG, Cole FE (1981) Borderline hypertension: relationship between age, hemodynamics and circulating catecholamines. Circulation 64:760–764
Missale C, Memo M, Liberini P, Carruba MD, Spano P (1985) Evidence for the presence of D_1 and D_2 receptors in the rat adrenal cortex. Eur J Pharmacol 109:315–316
Missale C, Castelletti L, Liberini P, Memo M, Carruba MO, Spano PF (1986) Evidence for the presence of postsynaptic D_1 and D_2 receptors in the cardiovascular system. Soc Neurosci 12:385
Modlinger RA, Gretkin H (1978) Plasma prolactin in essential and renovascular hypertension. J Lab Clin Med 91:693–697
Mok JSL, Sim MK (1987) The actions of dopamine on the blood pressure and heart rate of conscious hypertensive rats: evidence for reduced dopaminergic activity in rats of the Japanese strains. Clin Exp Hypertens [A]9:1615–1635
Montastruc JL, Guiol C (1984) Experimental study of the hypotensive effect of apomorphine. Arch Mal Coeur 77:1176–1180
Moore RY, Bloom FE (1978) Central catecholamine neuron systems: Anatomy and physiology of the dopamine systems. Annu Rev Neurosci 1:129–169
Muller BD, Bell D (1986) Vesicular storage of dopamine and noradrenaline in terminal sympathetic nerves of dog spleen and kidney. J Neurochem 47:1370–1375
Murthy VV, Gilbert JC, Goldberg LI, Kuo JF (1976) Dopamine-sensitive adenylate cyclase in canine renal artery. J Pharm Pharmacol 28:567–571
Nagahama S, Chen Y, Oparil S (1984) Mechanism of the depressor effect of bromocriptine in the spontaneously hypertensive rat. J Pharmacol Exp Ther 220:370–375
Nakajima T, Naitoh F, Kurowa I (1977) Dopamine sensitive adenylate cyclase in the rat kidney particulate preparation. Eur J Pharmacol 41:163–169
Nakamura S, Kohli JD, Rajfer SI (1986) α-Adrenoceptor blocking activity of fenoldopam (SK&F 82526), a selective DA_1 agonist. J Pharm Pharmacol 38:113–117
Neumann B, Wiedermann CJ, Fischer Colbrie R, Schober M, Sperk G, Winkler H (1984) Biochemical and functional properties of large and small dense-core vesicles in sympathetic nerves of rat and ox vas deferens. Neuroscience 13:921–931
Nieuwenhuys RN (1985) Chemoarchitecture of the brain. Springer, Berlin Heidelberg New York, pp 14–19
Norbiato GM, Bevilacqua M, Reggi U, Micossi P, Moroni C (1977) Metoclopramide increases plasma aldosterone concentration in man. J Clin Endocrinol Metab 45: 1313–1321
Ochi J, Shimizu K (1978) Occurrence of dopamine-containing neurons in the midbrain raphe nuclei of the rat. Neurosci Lett 8:317–320
Ohlstein EH, Berkovitz BA (1985) SCH 23390 and SK&F 83566 are antagonists at

vascular dopamine and serotonin receptors. Eur J Pharmacol 108:205–208
Ohlstein EH, Zabko-Potapovich B, Berkovitz BA (1985) The Da_1 receptor agonist fenoldopam (SK&F 82526) is also an alpha$_2$-adrenoceptor antagonist. Eur J Pharmacol 118:321–329
Onali P, Olianas MC, Gessa GL (1984) Selective blockade of dopamine D_1 receptors by SCH 23390 discloses striatal dopamine D_2 receptors mediating the inhibition of adenylate cyclase in rats. Eur J Pharmacol 99:127–128
Os I, Kjeldsen SE, Westheim A, Aakesson I, Norman N, Enger E, Hjermann I, Eide I (1987) Decreased central dopaminergic activity in essential hypertension. J Hypertens 5:191–197
Osborne MW (1976) On the genesis of essential hypertension—the possible role of central nervous dopaminergic neurons. In: Scriabine A, Swett CS (eds) New antihypertensive drugs. Spectrum, New York, pp 105–134 (Monographs of the Physiological Society of Philadelphia, vol 2)
Pazos A, Mediavilla A, Florez J (1982) Cardiovascular effects of intracerebroventricular injection of dopamine after selective MAO inhibition in rats. Neuropharmacology 21:317–322
Pelayo JC, Fildes RD, Eisner GM, Jose PA (1983) The effects of dopamine blockade on renal sodium excretion. Am J Physiol 245:F247–F263
Pequignot JM, Favier R, Desplanches D, Peyrin L, Flandrois R (1985) Free dopamine in dog plasma: lack of relationship with sympathoadrenal activity. J Appl Physiol 58:763–769
Perkins CM, Casson IF, Cope GF, Lee MR (1980) Failure of salt to mobilize renal dopamine in essential hypertension. Lancet 2:1370
Petitjean P, Mouchet P, Pellissier G, Manier M, Feuerstein C, Demenge P (1984) Cardiovascular effects in the rat of intrathecal injections of apomorphine at the thoracic spinal cord level. Eur J Pharmacol 105:355–359
Petterson A, Hedner J, Hedner T (1986) The diuretic effect of atrial natriuretic peptide (ANP) is dependent on dpomainergic activation. Acta Physiol Scand 126:619–621
Quenzer L, Yahn D, Alkadhi K, Volle RL (1979) Transmission blockade and stimulation of adenylate cyclase by catecholamines. J Pharmacol Exp Ther 208:31–36
Racz K, Kuchel O, Buu NT, Tenneson S (1985) Peripheral dopamine synthesis and metabolism in spontaneously hypertensive rat. Circ Res 57:889–897
Rolewicz TF, Zimmerman BG (1972) Peripheral distribution of cutaneous sympathetic vasodilator system. Am J Physiol 223:939–943
Sabouni MH, Alkadhi KH, Lokhandwala MF (1987) Biochemical and pharamacological characterization of ganglionic dopamine receptors. Clin Exp Hypertens [A]9:873–887
Saito I, Takeshita E, Saruta T, Nagano S, Sekihara T (1984) Plasma prolactin, renin and catecholamines in young normotensive and borderline hypertensive subjects. J Hypertens 2:61–64
Saito I, Takeshita E, Saruta T, Nagano S (1986) Urinary dopamine excretion in normotensive subjects with or without family history of hypertension. J Hypertens 4: 57–60
Saruta T, Kawabe H, Fujimaki M, Nagahama S, Saito I, Kondo K (1983) Prolactin, renin and catecholamines in essential hypertension. Clin Exp Hypertension 5:531–541
Scatton B, Dubois A (1985) Autoradiographic localization of D_1 dopamine receptors in the rat brain with ^{3}H-SKF 38393. Eur J Pharmacol 111:145–146
Scatton B, Simon H, Le Moal M, Bischoff S (1980) Origin of dopaminergic innervation of the rat hippocampal formation. Neurosci Lett 18:125–131
Schmidt M, Imbs JL (1980) Pharmacological characterization of renal vascular dopamine receptors. J Cardiovasc Pharmacol 2:595–605
Schmidt M, Schmidt JL, Schwartz J (1981) The vascular dopamine receptor: A review. J Pharmacol 12:355–382
Schmidt M, Krieger JP, Giesen-Crouse EM, Imbs JL (1987) Vascular effects of selective dopamine agonists and antagonists in the rat kidney. Arch Int Pharmacodyn Ther 286:195–205

Schulz G, Lambertz M, Stock G, Langhorst P (1986) Neuronal activity in the amygdala related to somatomotor and vegetative components of behaviour in cats. JANS [Suppl]:639–648

Seeman P (1980) Brain dopamine receptors. Pharmacol Rev 32:229–313

Seller H, Illert M (1969) The localization of the first synapse in the carotid sinus baroreceptor reflex pathway and its alteration of afferent input. Pflügers Arch 306:1–19

Seri I, Aperia A (1988) Contribution of dopamine receptors to dopamine induced increase in glomerular filtration rate. Am J Physiol 254:F196–F201

Shikuma R, Yoshimura M, Kambara S, Yamazaki H, Takashina R, Takahashi H, Takeda K, Ijichi H (1986) Dopaminergic modulation of salt sensitivity in patients with essential hypertension. Life Sci 38:915–922

Skagerberg G, Björklund A, Lindvall O, Schmidt RH (1982) Origin and termination of the diencephalospinal dopamine system in the rat. Brain Res Bull 9:237–244

Slater IH (1983) Editorial comment prolactin, dopaminergic mechanisms and hypertension. Clin Exp Hypertens [A]5:559–561

Soarez-da Silva P, Azevedo I (1987) Differential effects of 6-hydroxydopamine on the two types of nerve vesicles and dopamine and noradrenaline content in mesenteric arterial vessels. J Auton Pharmacol 8:1–10

Sokoloff P, Matres MP, Schwartz SC (1980) Three classes of dopamine receptors (D-$_2$, D-$_3$, D-$_4$) identified by binding studies with ^{3}H-apomorphine and ^{3}H-domperidone. Naunyn Schmiedebergs Arch Pharmacol 35:89–102

Sowers JR (1984) Dopaminergic regulation of renin and aldosterone secretion. A review. J Hypertens [Suppl] 2:67–73

Sowers JR, Crane PD, Beck FWJ, McClanahan M, King ME, Mohonty PK (1985) Relationship between urinary dopamine production and natriuresis after acute intravascular volume expansion with sodium chloride in dogs. Endocrinology 115: 2085–2090

Sowers JR, Gollub MS, Berger ME, Whitfield LA (1982a) Dopaminergic modulation of pressor and hormonal responses in essential hypertension. Hypertension 4:424–430

Sowers JR, Nyby M, Jasberg K (1982b) Dopaminergic control of prolactin and blood pressure: altered control in essential hypertension. Hypertension 4:431–438

Stephenson RK, Sole MJ, Baines AD (1982) Neural and extraneural catecholamine production by rat kidneys. Am J Physiol 242:F261–F266

Stern N, Eshkol A, Lunenfeld B, Rosenthal T (1983) Prolactin secretion in essential hypertension. Clin Exp Hypertens [A]5:543–558

Stjärne L, Brundin J (1975) Affinity of noradrenaline and dopamine for neural α-receptors mediating negative feedback control of noradrenaline secretion in human vasoconstrictor nerves. Acta Physiol Scand 95:89–94

Stock G (1982) Neurobiology of REM sleep. A possible role for dopamine. In: Ganten D, Pfaff D (eds) Sleep, clinical and experimental aspects Springer, Berlin Heidelberg New York, pp 1–36 (Current topics in neuroendocrinology)

Stoof JC, Kebabian JW (1981) Opposing roles for D_1 and D_2 dopamine receptors in efflux of cyclic AMP from rat neostriatum. Nature 294:366–368

Stoof JC, Kebabian JW (1984) Two dopamine receptors: Biochemistry, physiology and pharmacology. Life Sci 35:2281–2296

Stumpe KO, Higuchi M, Kolloch R, Krück F, Vetter H (1977) Hyperprolactinaemia and antihypertensive effect of bromocriptine in essential hypertension. Lancet 2 (8031): 211–214

Swanson LW, Sawchenko PE, Bérod A, Hartman BK, Helle KB, Vanorden DE (1981) An immunohistochemical study of the organization of catecholaminergic cells and terminal fields in the paraventricular and supraoptic nuclei of the hypothalamus. J Comp Neurol 196:271–285

Szabo B, Hedler L, Starke K (1986) Dopamine$_1$ receptor agonist and α-$_2$-adrenoceptor antagonist effects of fenoldopam in rabbits. J Pharmacol Exp Ther 239:881–886

Tainter ML (1930) Comparative action of sympathomimetic compounds: The influence of cocaine and certain related compounds upon the action of a group of sympathomimetic amines. Q J Pharmacol 3:584–589

Thureson-Klein A, Klein RL, Johansson O (1979) Catecholamine-rich cells and varicosities in bovine splenic nerve, vesicle contents and evidence for exocytosis. J

Neurobiol 10:309–324
Ullrich KJ, Rumrich G, Klöss S (1974) Sodium dependency of the amino acid transport in the proximal convolution of the rat kidney. Pflügers Arch Gesamte Physiol 351: 49–60
Unger T, Buu NT, Kuchel O, Schurch W (1980) Conjugated dopamine: peripheral origin, distribution and response to acute stress in the dog. Can J Physiol Pharmacol 58:22–27
Ungerstedt U (1971) Stereotaxic mapping of the monoamine pathways in the rat brain. Acta Physiol Scand [Suppl]367:1–49
Ventura HO, Messerli FH, Fröhlich ED, Kobin I, Oigman W, Dunn FG, Carey RM (1984) Immediate hemodynamic effects of a dopamine receptor agonist (Fenoldopam) in patients with essential hypertension. Circulation 69:1142–1145
Watanabe AM, Judy WV, Cardon PV (1974) Effect of L-dopa on blood pressure and sympathetic nerve activity after decarboyxlase inhibitor in cats. J Pharmacol Exp Ther 188:107–113
Weiner N (1980) The role of cyclic nucleotides in the regulation of neurotransmitter release from adrenergic neurons by neuromodulators. Essays Neurochem Neuropharmacol 4:69–124
Weiner N (1985) Norepinephrine, epinephrine and the sympathomimetic amines. In: Gilman AG, Goodman LS, Rall TW, Murad F (eds) The pharmacological basis of therapeutics. Macmillan, New York pp 145–180
Wilffert B, Smit G, de Jonge A, Thoolen MJ, Timmermans PB, van Zwieten PA (1984) Inhibitory dopamine receptors on sympathetic neurons innervating the cardiovascular system in the pithed rat. Characterization and role in relation to presynaptic α_2-adrenoceptors. Naunyn Schmiedebergs Arch Pharmacol 326:91–98
Willems JL, Buylaert WA, Bogaert MG (1979) Evidence that dopamine receptors mediate the neurogenic vasodilatation by dopaminergic agents. In: Imbs JL, Schwartz J (eds) Peripheral dopaminergic receptors. Pergamon, Oxford, pp 299–307
Willems JL, Buylaert WA, Lefebvre RA, Bogaert MG (1985) Neuronal dopamine receptors on autonomic ganglia and sympathetic nerves and dopamine receptors in the gastrointestinal system. Pharmacol Rev 37:165–216
Williams TH, Chiba T, Black AC, Bhalla RC, Jew J (1976) Species variation in SIF cells of superior cervical ganglia: Are there two functional types? In: Eranko O (ed) SIF cells: Structure and function of the small intensely fluoresecent sympathetic cells. Department of Health, Education and Welfare, Washington, pp 143–162 (DHEW publication no (NIH) 76–942)
Wilson TA, Kaiser DZ, Carey RM (1983) Dopaminergic inhibition of aldosterone secretion in man is independent of the autonomic nervous system. J Clin Endocrinol Metab 57:200–203
Yoshimura M, Kambara S, Okabashi H, Takehashi H, Jichi H (1987) Effect of decreased dopamine synthesis on the development of hypertension induced by salt loading in spontaneously hypertensive rats. Clin Exp Hypertens [A]9:1141–1157
Zandberg P, de Jong W, de Wied D (1979) Effect of catecholamine-receptor stimulating agents on blood pressure after local application in the nucleus tractus solitarii of the medulla oblongata. Eur J Pharmacol 55:43–56
Ziegler MG, Lake CR, Williams AC, Teychenne PF, Shoulson I, Steinsland O (1979) Bromocriptine inhibits norepinephrine release. Clin Pharmacol Ther 25:137–142
Ziemñiak J, Allison N, Boppana VK, Dubb J, Stote R (1981) The effect of acetoaminophen on the disposition of fenoldopam: a competition for sulfatation. Clin Pharmacol Ther 41:275

CHAPTER 15

Peptides in Hypertension

R.E. LANG

CONTENTS

1 Introduction

It is now well-established that blood pressure control is exerted by the concerted action of hormonal, renal, vascular, and neural mechanisms and that a variety of substances differing in chemical nature are involved in the mediation of these effects. Peptides have been among the first implicated in considerations concerned with the pathogenesis of hypertension.

Research on vasoactive peptides started more than 30 years ago, when angiotensin and vasopressin became available in pure form. The successful development and application of compounds which potently interfere with the synthesis and action of angiotensin II revealed, in confirmation of earlier suggestions, that this peptide plays a pivotal role in blood pressure regulation, under both physiological and pathophysiological conditions, and opened up new avenues for drug therapy. During the 1970s it was recognized that the function of the nervous system does not solely rely on the action of classical transmitters such as catecholamines but also requires the presence of a variety of neuropeptides (HÖKFELT et al. 1980). In fact, angiotensin II was one of the first vasoactive peptides to be discovered in the brain as a neuropeptide (GANTEN et al. 1971, 1983, 1984). Some of them have been shown to affect vascular tone and cardiac performance, which launched a huge surge in research activities aimed at elucidating the possible role of neuropeptides in hypertension. Another burst in peptide research was kindled very recently when it was found that the heart is the site of synthesis of hormones capable of lowering blood pressure and of inducing diuresis following systemic administration (DE BOLD et al. 1981). The most recent spectacular discovery in the long history of vasoactive peptides is the isolation and characterization of a peptide called endothelin, which is produced by vascular endothelial cells and which is considered the most potent vasoconstrictor yet found (YANAGISAWA et al. 1988).

The importance of most of the vasoactive peptides described thus far with respect to hypertension cannot be viewed with sufficient perspective to permit more than an initial understanding. This is mainly due to the lack of sufficiently potent and specific antagonists suited to block the action of endogenous peptides. One of the rare exceptions is angiotensin, which is being dealt with in a separate chapter of this book. The peptides selected for a more detailed presentation in the following sections are those which appear to be of particular importance with respect to their possible role in blood pressure regulation and the development or maintenance of hypertension and which might gain importance either as targets or tools in the treatment of cardiovascular disease.

The first section of the chapter is concerned with vasoactive peptides of neuronal origin with special emphasis on neuropeptide Y and calcitonin gene related peptide. The second part is devoted to atrial natriuretic peptide and summarizes our knowledge about the chemistry and action of this hormone which recently attracted much interest as a putative antihypertensive agent due to its broad spectrum of effects on blood pressure regulating mechanisms. The third part deals with endothelin, a constrictor peptide synthetized in endothelial cells.

2 Neuropeptides

During the past years more than 30 novel biologically active peptides have been discovered. A few are produced in endocrine glands and circulate as hormones in the blood. Some are contained in the enterochromaffin cells of the gut and may be involved in the regulation of intestinal functions. The vast majority, however, have been detected in the central and peripheral nervous system, where they are synthesized in distinct neurons and stored in neurovesicles. These neuropeptides have been shown to be released in response to appropriate stimuli such as electrical or chemical depolarization and to produce certain biological effects which are mediated by specific receptors. This led to the assumption that they represent a new category of neurotransmitters forming a third component of the autonomic nervous system which, in analogy to the cholinergic and adrenergic one, was termed the peptidergic system of nerves (Hökfelt et al. 1980; Snyder 1980).

It has now become clear that many, if not all, of these peptides co-exist with classical transmitters or other neuropeptides in individual neurons, which suggests that they may not exclusively have neurotransmitter functions but may also interfere with classical neurotransmitters, i.e., they may act as neuromodulators (Kaczmarek and Levitan 1987; Siggins and Gruol 1986). The designation neuromodulator is being applied to substances which, as opposed to neurotransmitters, show no direct effects on their own but are capable of modulating the response of a cell to a neurotransmitter or to electrical stimulation or of interfering with the release of neurotransmitters. Modulation by neuropeptides of the action of neurotransmitters is particularly observed in the situation of co-localization within the same nerve fibers. Neuromodulation can take place both pre- and postjunctionally. For instance, in neurons in the tegmental area of the brain that contain both cholecystokinine and dopamine, cholecystokinin not only attenuates the potassium-evoked dopamine release but also increases the number of dopamine binding sites and blocks the dopamine action in activating adenylate cyclase (Agnati et al. 1983; Studler et al. 1986). A particular form of neuromodulation may be the regulation of the expression of a neurotransmitter receptor gene by a neuropeptide. One of the most exciting examples for this kind of interaction is calcitonin gene related peptide (CGRP), which has been found to increase severalfold the mRNA concentration of the acetylcholine receptor at the motor endplate of skeletal muscle (Fontaine et al. 1987).

Potential physiological roles in the control of cardiovascular functions for neuropeptides are suggested by their distribution in the brain and peripheral nerves. For example, neurons containing enkephalins, substance P (SP), CGRP, vasoactive intestinal peptide, or neuropeptide Y (NPY) have been demonstrated to innervate cardiovascular centers in the medulla oblongata or in the hypothalamus (Hökfelt et al. 1984). As for the periphery, most of these peptides are also present in nerve fibers and terminals within the wall of systemic blood vessels. Beyond that they have been localized in cardiac structures such as the sinoatrial node, specialized conducting tissue, atrial and ventricular myocardium, and the wall of coronary vessels (Reinecke 1987). Experimental studies support this view of the importance of neuropeptides in blood pressure control and regulation of cardiac performance. Neuropeptides have been demonstrated to alter blood pressure and heart rate following central administration, to exert inotropic and chronotropic effects when given systemically or to isolated hearts and to affect vascular tone profoundly both in vivo and in vitro. Some neuropeptides appear to be true neurotransmitters, i.e., they show postjunctional effects upon their release such as vasoactive intestinal peptide, which produces marked vasodilatation in the salivary gland both when administered exogenously and following liberation by nerve stimulation (Lundberg and Hökfelt 1983). Others, such as enkephalins, have been reported to exert their action mainly by neuromodulation (Ensinger et al. 1984; Illes et al. 1985).

Table 1. Vasoactive peptides and their blood pressure effects upon systemic administration. +, pressor; −, depressor

Angiotensin II	+
Atrial natriuretic peptide	−
Bradykinin	−
Endothelin	+/−
Calcitonin gene related peptide	−
Neuropeptide Y	+
Neurotensin	+/− (depends on species)
Opioid peptides	−
Somatostatin	+
Substance P	−
Vasoactive intestinal peptide	−
Vasopressin	+

A list of neuropeptides reported to interfere with the cardiovascular system is given in Table 1. The peptides indicated do not provide a complete enumeration of vasoactive neuropeptides. Their selection is based on the observation that they affect blood pressure following acute administration. The action of neuropeptides over a longer time period may, however, also have considerable impact on blood pressure. It has long been recognized that the vascular system responds to changes in blood pressure with remarkable structural adaptations (FOLKOW et al. 1982). Little is known about the mechanisms involved. There are many examples for mitogenic and trophic effects of peptide hormones and neuropeptides in various systems (HANLEY 1985; SCHELLING et al. 1979). It is therefore intriguing to speculate that neuropeptides may affect blood pressure not only by their acute effects on vascular tone but, beyond that, might be involved in the control of proliferation and hypertrophy of vascular smooth muscle cells. This "trophic" hypothesis appears very attractive in the face of the slow and gradual development of hypertension and certainly deserves a detailed exploration in the future.

With respect to the limited space available, it appears more practical to concentrate in this chapter on only a few examples of neuropeptides thought to play a role in cardiovascular regulation and to present these in greater detail, rather than to give an exhaustive description of all peptides so far implicated in blood pressure control. Two peptides, NPY and CGRP, have been chosen, which are particularly conspicuous with respect to their effects on blood pressure. CGRP exists together with SP in sensory nerve fibers. Both substances are known to lower blood pressure very potently; in contrast to SP, however, CGRP does not induce extravasation. NPY, which is co-stored with noradrenaline in sympathetic nerve fibers, is one of the most effective pressor substances when administered systemically. Both peptides have been shown to exert their cardiovascular actions not only in experimental animals but also in humans. NPY might well be involved in the pathogenesis or maintenance of hypertension. The development of specific antagonists appears, therefore, at least from the experimental point of view, an interesting task. Analogues of CGRP could be useful as a new class of vasodilators given their selectivity for vascular receptors.

2.1 Calcitonin Gene Related Peptide

2.1.1 Chemistry

The calcitonins are single chain peptides of 32 amino acids with an N-terminal disulfide bridge linking positions 1 and 7 and with an amide group on the C-terminal proline residue. The amino acid sequences of the calcitonin molecule from a variety of species such as humans, cows, pigs, sheep, rats, and salmon, reveal close homologies for only 9 of the 32 amino acid residues. All of them share the C-terminal proline amide and have close homologies in the N-terminal seven-membered ring but show marked heterogeneity in the central three-fourths of the molecule. Despite the close homology in the N-terminal part of the molecule the entire 32-amino acid sequence of calcitonin is required for biological activity (FOSTER et al. 1972).

Messenger RNA encoding calcitonin is present in large amounts in the normal thyroid gland, medullary thyroid carcinoma, and lung cancer cells. The observation that a serially transplanted rat medullary carcinoma of the thyroid largely lost its ability to synthesize calcitonin and instead started to produce a new and larger cytoplasmic RNA encoding a different peptide led to the discovery of the calcitonin gene related peptide (CGRP; AMARA et al. 1982). Using the nucleotide sequence CGRP as a probe, its mRNA was detected in neural tissues of the rat. Complementary sequences to the mRNA encoding calcitonin and CGRP were used to identify the calcitonin/CGRP gene in the rat genomic library. The calcitonin gene was unexpectedly found to encode two different mRNA with identical 5′sequences but with distinct 3′sequences (ROSENFELD et al. 1983). In the C-cells of the thyroid the first three of the six exons contained in the chain are spliced to the fourth calcitonin-coding exon to generate the mature calcitonin mRNA. In the nervous system, pituitary, and, to a lesser extent, thyroid C-cell the first three exons are spliced to the fifth and sixth exons. The fourth calcitonin-coding exon is excised and not expressed. The tissue specificity of this so-called alternative splicing determines the pattern of expression of calcitonin and CGRP in their respective tissues of origin (Fig. 1).

CGRP is a unique 37-amino acid peptide which, like calcitonin, contains an intrachain disulfide bridge and is amidated at the C-terminus (Fig. 2). The close homology of the peptide to calcitonin and in particular salmon calcitonin has invited speculation as to the potential origin of the calcitonin and CGRP exons from a common primordial gene.

2.1.2 Anatomical Distribution

CGRP is predominantly synthesized in the nervous system as revealed by the presence of mRNA encoding the peptide. Antisera raised against synthetic rat CGRP have been used to demonstrate immunoreactive material in both the central and peripheral nervous system (FRANCO-CERECEDA et al. 1987c; LUNDBERG et al. 1985a; SKOFITSCH and JACOBOWITZ 1985; UDDMAN et al. 1986; JU et al. 1987). In brain CGRP-positive nerve cell bodies are present in the preoptic area and hypothalamus, ventromedial thalamus, medial amygdala, hippocampus,

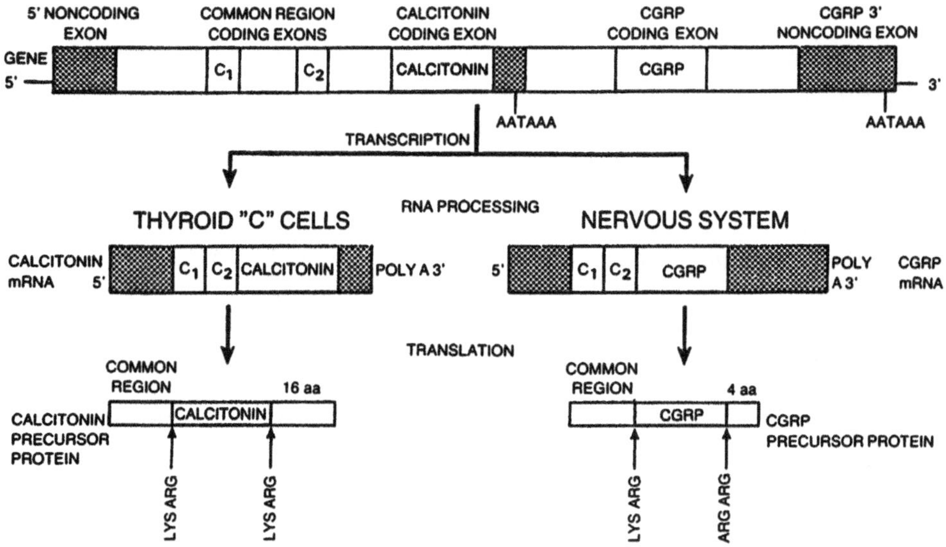

Fig. 1. The calcitonin gene encodes two biologically active peptides, calcitonin and calcitonin gene related peptide. The gene transcript is spliced in a way that results either in the synthesis of calcitonin(thyroid gland) or calcitonin gene related peptide (nervous tissue)

superior colliculus, lateral lemniscus, dentate gyrus, Purkinje's cells of the cerebellum, and in sensory and motor nuclei of cranial nerves. Fibers are particularly abundant in the inferior colliculus, cranial nerve nuclei, and spetum. The presence of CGRP in many peripheral tissues may reflect the presence of the peptide in the distal terminals of sensory nerves. Thus, CGRP is found in the epidermis with the highest levels in the nose and lowest in skin from the back. Many sensory cells in the jugular, thoracic spinal, and nodose ganglia are CGRP-positive and stain with antibodies directed against SP, suggesting colocalization of these peptides. This is further supported by studies demonstrating the presence of CGRP together with SP-like immunoreactivity in peripheral nerve fibers which are predominantly associated with blood vessels (FRANCO-CERECEDA et al. 1987c; LUNDBERG et al. 1985a; UDDMAN et al. 1986). In the heart CGRP- and SP-containing nerve fibers are found around coronary vessels, close to myocardial cells, as well as under and within the peri- and endocardia (GERSTHEIMER and METZ 1986; MULDERRY et al. 1985). These fibers are also associated

Calcitonin Gene Related Peptide
(CGRP, Human)
Ala-Cys-Asp-Thr-Ala-Thr-Cys-Val-Thr-His-
Arg-Leu-Ala-Gly-Leu-Leu-Ser-Arg-Ser-Gly-
Gly-Val-Val-Lys-Asn-Asn-Phe-Val-Pro-Thr-
Asn-Val-Gly-Ser-Lys-Ala-Phe-NH_2

Fig. 2. Amino acid sequence of human calcitonin gene related peptide(CGRP)

with the sinoatrial node and the cardiac valves. In the ventricles, CGRP- and SP-immunoreactive (IR) nerves are also mainly associated with blood vessels and endo- and pericardia. In addition, varicose CGRP- and SP-IR nerve terminals can be observed around local parasympathetic ganglion cells associated with the atria of the heart as well as close to some sympathetic ganglion cells in the stellate ganglia. Generally, arteries receive a richer supply of CGRP- and SP-IR nerve fibers than veins. The carotid arteries and the thoracic aorta show a dense network, whereas the supply diminishes as the aorta descends to the abdomen (MULDERRY et al. 1985). Brachial and femoral arteries contain few CGRP fibers. In the gastrointestinal tract muscular arteries such as the superior and inferior mesenteric arteries and the gastroepiploic artery as well as the small arteries and arterioles in the gut wall are richly innervated. Small arteries in the parenchyma of the liver, spleen, kidney, and pancreas receive very few CGRP fibers. A very scarce supply of CGRP fibers also accompanies the small blood vessels in skeletal muscle.

The location of CGRP together with SP in sensory nerve fibers is suggested by studies using capsaicin. Capsaicin is a neurotoxic agent known to cause selective degeneration of a certain population of primary sensory neurons of the C-fiber type and the type B cells of sensory ganglia. Systemic treatment of rats or guinea pigs with capsaicin has been demonstrated to extinguish most of the CGRP- and SP-IR present in nerve fibers of the heart and lung, in the wall of the large arteries, and in spinal root ganglia (LUNDBERG et al. 1985a; FRANCO-CERECEDA et al. 1987c).

2.1.3 Functions

CGRP is not likely to participate in calcium and phosphorus homeostasis, since in contrast to calcitonin intravenous administration of the peptide does not affect plasma calcium and phosphorus concentrations (LENZ et al. 1985). Both peptides, however, decrease gastric secretion and food intake in rats following intracerebral or intravenous administration (LENZ et al. 1985).

Intravenous administration of CGRP has been reported to result in peripheral vasodilatation and hypotension in animals and humans, whereas central administration in experimental animals appears to activate sympathetic outflow with a pressor response and an increase in plasma noradrenaline levels (LAPPE et al. 1987; FRANCO-CERECEDA et al. 1987b; STRUTHERS et al. 1985; FISHER et al. 1983; BRAIN et al. 1985). In spontaneously hypertensive rats (SHR) bolus injection of CGRP 0.1–5 μg/kg has been shown to produce a dose-dependent fall in mean arterial pressure with a maximal change of nearly 50 mmHg (LAPPE et al. 1987). This was accompanied by a large increase in heart rate and significant reductions in the renal, mesenteric, and hindquarter vascular resistances. The vasodilator actions of CGRP failed to demonstrate any regional selectivity in these studies, which is in contrast to other peptides such as SP or atrial natriuretic peptide (ANP), which dilate preferentially the hindquarter vascular bed and the renal vasculature, respectively (LAPPE et al. 1987). The hypotension observed following sytemic administration of CGRP probably reflects its direct action at the vasculature rather than a centrally or reflexly mediated response, since this depressor effect can also be demonstrated in pithed rats, which are completely devoid of centrally mediated circulatory reflexes (HAASS and SKOFITSCH 1985). This is further supported by the direct microscopic observation that CGRP causes dilatation of the major resistance vessels, the arterioles, and by the strong relaxant effect of the peptide on the vascular tone of isolated blood vessels in vitro (BRAIN et al. 1985; UDDMAN et al. 1986; THOM et al. 1987). Topical application of CGRP at concentrations in the femtomolar to picomolar range have been reported to induce a long-lasting increase in skin blood flow in rabbits and humans and to dilate the arterioles in the hamster cheek pouch (BRAIN et al. 1985). Rat aortic strips precontracted with noradrenaline were shown to relax in response to CGRP at concentrations as little as 2.5×10^{-11} *M*. Similar effects were observed in brain vessels, femoral, mesenteric, and gastroepiploic arteries (UDDMAN et al. 1986).

CGRP is also a powerful dilator of coronary arteries (THOM et al. 1987). This has been demonstrated both in vitro and in vivo (McEWAN et al. 1986). When injected intracoronarily in humans, a dose-dependent increase in coronary diameter is observed. Ergonovine-induced coronary arterial spasm was not prevented by prior infusion of the peptide, suggesting that CGRP is not involved in the pathogenesis of variant angina.

In addition to its vascular effects CGRP has positive inotropic and chronotropic properties (FRANCO-CERECEDA and LUNDBERG 1985, 1987). The chronotropic effect of the peptide is more pronounced than the inotropic response and is observed at a threshold concentration of 10^{-9} *M* whereas the inotropic response starts at 10^{-8} *M* CGRP in isolated guinea pig atria (FRANCO-CERECEDA and LUNDBERG 1985). The effects are slow in onset and long-lasting, as suggested by studies in the isolated perfused heart. The response to the continuous presence of CGRP ceases with time due to the development of tachyphylaxis (FRANCO-CERECEDA and LUNDBERG 1985).

2.1.4 Mechanism of Action

The CGRP-evoked vasodilatation is not mediated by adrenergic, cholinergic, or histaminergic mechanisms since it is not modified by β-adrenoceptor blockers, cholinergic blockers, or histamine H_1- and H_2-receptor blockers (BRAIN et al. 1985). In experiments on rat aorta, it has been noted that inhibitors of prostaglandin synthesis attenuate the relaxation induced by CGRP (BRAIN et al. 1985). Thus, prostaglandin generation may be responsible for a part of the responses to the peptide, at least in some areas of the vascular bed. A major role in the mediation of CGRP-induced vasodilation appears to be played the endothelium. When rat aortic strips preconstricted by noradrenaline are exposed to CGRP a dose-dependent relaxation is obtained, which is completely absent after the endothelial cells have been removed (BRAIN et al. 1985). Similar observations have been made in human radial, coronary, gastric, and cerebral arteries, in which the relaxation in response to CGRP is abolished after luminal rubbing (THOM et al. 1987). This might indicate involvement of the endothelium-derived relaxant factor (EDRF) in the mediation of the vascular effects of CGRP. The mechanism underlying the actions of this factor has been shown to be cGMP-linked (RAPAPORT et al. 1983). If the response to CGRP involved EDRF, a rise in guanylate cyclase activity might be expected. Indeed, methylene blue and hemoglobin, both of which are held to be inhibitors of soluble guanylate cyclase, have been reported to reverse the vascular response to CGRP (THOM et al. 1987). A conceptual difficulty in accepting the role of EDRF in the response to CGRP arises with the consideration of its storage in perivascular nerves, which may be considerably far away from the endothelium. However, the peptide has been demonstrated in the circulation (ZAIDI et al. 1985). It appears, therefore, not unlikely that CGRP might reach the endothelium from the blood to exert its effects.

In certain vessels, such as cerebral vessels from cat, CGRP has been demonstrated to stimulate adenylate cyclase activity (EDVINSSON et al. 1985). Moreover, an increase in cAMP content in response to CGRP has been observed in cultured vascular smooth muscle cells (KUBOTA et al. 1985). Whether the changes in cAMP contribute to the vasorelaxant effect of CGRP is presently not known.

There is some evidence that the reported stimulation of adenylate cyclase by CGRP plays an important role in the mediation of the effects of this peptide on the heart. Half-maximal stimulation of adenylate cyclase activity in rat atria has been observed with 3 n*M* CGRP which corresponds very closely to the concentration of the peptide required to displace 50% of the binding of [^{125}I]CGRP to heart membranes (SIGRIST et al. 1986). These values are about one order of magnitude lower than the concentration at which half-maximal stimulation in heart rate and contraction amplitude are observed. The reason for this discrepancy is not clear but may indicate that mediators other than cAMP are involved in the cardiac response to CGRP.

Very recently, it was proposed that SP, which is co-released with CGRP from sensory nerve fibers and is known to activate most cells, is involved in the control of the vascular effects of CGRP in cutaneous tissue (BRAIN et al. 1988). It was demonstrated that injection of CGRP together with SP into human skin results in a shortening of the long-lasting vasodiiatation observed in response to CGRP alone and that this effect is due to inactivation of CGRP through the action of tryptic enzymes released from mast cells by SP. This is the first example that peptide transmitters contained in the same nerve fibers can interact by affecting the metabolism of each other. It sheds a light also for the first time on the role of mast cells in the mediation of the vascular action of neuropeptides.

2.2 Neuropeptide Y

Neuropeptide Y (NPY) is a 36-amino acid peptide isolated from the porcine brain by a novel method for detecting peptides possessing a C-terminal α-amide (TATEMOTO 1982). The peptide is characterized by an N-terminal and C-terminal tyrosine (Y), according to the single letter amino acid abbreviation, and is a member of a larger peptide family which includes the pancreatic polypeptide (PP) and peptide YY (PYY), a hormone from the lower intestine with which it

NPY (Neuropeptide Y) (Human)
Tyr-Pro-Ser-Lys-Pro-Asp-Asn-Pro-Gly-Glu-
Asp-Ala-Pro-Ala-Glu-Asp-Met-Ala-Arg-Tyr-
Tyr-Ser-Ala-Leu-Arg-His-Tyr-Ile-Asn-Leu-
Ile-Thr-Arg-Gln-Arg-Tyr-NH_2

Fig. 3. Amino acid sequence of human neuropeptide Y(NPY)

shares considerable sequence homologies (LEITER et al. 1984; TATEMOTO 1982). It has 19 of the total of 36 amino acids in common with avian pancreatic polypeptide (APP) and with PYY (Fig. 3). All of these peptides probably possess similar tertiary structures (GLOVER et al. 1985). X-ray crystallographic studies have shown APP to contain an extended polyproline-like helix (residues 1–8), an α-helix (residues 14–31) that runs roughly antiparallel to this first region, and a C-terminal segment (residues 32–36) which possesses considerable conformation flexibility (ALLEN et al. 1987a; BLUNDELL et al. 1981). This flexible C-terminal segment shows very little sequence variation across all PP-related peptides, which might indicate that it plays an important role in the affinity of PP molecules for their binding sites.

As with other neuropeptides, NPY is produced as a larger molecule which is processed enzymatically to the biologically active 36-amino acid peptide. This processing is thought to take place in analogy with other peptides during transport within the neurosecretory vesicles to the nerve endings. The amino acid sequence for human prepro-NPY as deduced from a clone harboring the NPY cDNA has recently been reported (MINTH et al. 1986). A clone was obtained from total RNA isolated from a human pheochromocytoma, a tumor of adrenal medullary origin which overproduces NPY. Prepro-NPY comprises 98 amino acids. Cleavage by a signal peptidase produces pro-NPY (69 residues), from which the mature active NPY peptide and a 30-amino acid terminal peptide are generated by proteolysis within the region Gly^{66}-Lys^{67}-Arg^{68}, followed by an enzymatically catalyzed amidation in which the Tyr at the C-terminal end of NPY is converted to Tyr-NH_2.

2.2.1 Anatomical Distribution

NPY is widely distributed within neurons of the central and peripheral nervous systems and occurs in mammalian brain in higher concentrations than hitherto described for any other peptide (ALLEN et al. 1983; ADRIAN et al. 1983a). In the brain, areas with the highest concentrations include the paraventricular and arcuate nuclei of the hypothalamus. High levels of NPY immunoreactivity are also found within the periventricular, dorsomedial, anterior, suprachiasmatic, and medial preoptic hypothalamus, septum, and medial amygdala. This distribution corresponds well with the distribution of NPY-immunoreactive terminals as reported by immunocytochemical experiments (EVERITT et al. 1983; LUNDBERG et al. 1984b; DE QUIDT and EMSON 1986). The paraventricular, periventricular, and arcuate nuclei and the preoptic portion of the bed nucleus of the stria terminalis contain an especially dense plexus of NPY-immunoreactive terminals.

A large number of cell bodies, positive for NPY, occur within the ventromedial aspect of the arcuate nucleus. In the mesencephalon many cell bodies are located within the dorsal part of the locus coeruleus, and most of these cells contain noradrenaline (EVERITT et al. 1983). In the medulla oblongata NPY-like immunoreactivity is observed in virtually all adrenaline neurons in the medial part of the nucleus tractus solitarii, which is considered the first relay station in the baroreflex arch. There are in addition several NPY-immunoreactive cell bodies scattered throughout the dorsal vagal complex. These areas contain a dense network of NPY-positive nerve terminals. High concentrations of NPY have been identified throughout the cardiovascular system. The peptide has been localized by immunocytochemistry to the dense plexus of nerve fibers found around the adventitia of blood vessels (EMSON and DE QUIDT 1984) and within the muscle layers of the media. Few NPY-containing nerve fibers are found in the aortic arch and the thoracic and anterior portion of the abdominal aorta, whereas an abundant network of NPY-positive nerve fibers is observed in the wall of the posterior portion of the abdominal aorta, bifurcation of the aorta, left and right common iliac artery, superior and inferior mesenteric arteries, and renal arteries (LUNDBERG et al. 1982; ALLEN et al. 1985). The number of NPY-containing nerve fibers in the heart is similar or even more abundant than in other parts of the cardiovascular system (GU et al. 1984; STERNINI and BRECHA 1985). Radioimmunoassay of extracts shows that the heart contains collossal concentrations of NPY, which as deduced by chromatographic analysis using HPLC, is identical with the NPY originally extracted from the brain by TATEMOTO and MUTT (POLAK and BLOOM 1984). NPY-positive nerves have been identified in all areas of the heart, perivascular plexus, and intramuscular fascicles, as well as in the conduction system. Varicose nerve fibers containing NPY are also found in close relation to cardiac muscle. Clusters of nerve cell bodies, which show a positive reaction with antibodies directed against NPY have been reported to occur in close proximity to the sinus node and AV node (GU et al. 1984; HASSALL and BURNSTOCK 1986). NPY has also been demonstrated to be present in the adrenal medulla of several species including humans (VARNDELL et al. 1984). According to immunohistochemical studies the peptide appears to be produced in chromaffin cells of the adrenaline type, where it was found together with the adrenaline-synthesizing enzyme phenylethanolamine N-methyltransferase and enkephalin. High levels of NPY have been found in plasma and tumors from pheochromocytoma patients (ALLEN et al. 1987b).

Of major interest has been the observation of NPY coexistence with catecholamines in both central and peripheral neurons (HÖKFELT et al. 1983; LUNDBERG et al. 1982). Investigation of the sympathetic nervous system using NPY-directed antisera has revealed numerous NPY-positive neurons in superior cervical, stellate, and coeliac ganglia (LUNDBERG et al. 1982). Removal of the appropriate ganglion results in a parallel depletion of both NPY and catecholamine-containing terminals from the innervated tissue. Treatment with the catecholamine neurotoxin 6-hydroxydopamine, or with reserpine which depletes catecholamine stores, has also been shown to deplete NPY-containing sympathetic fibers of their peptide immunoreactivity (LUNDBERG et al. 1985b). Additional evidence for the existence of NPY in sympathetic neurons and nerve endings comes from immunohistochemical studies in which analysis of adjacent sections or elution-restained sections of blood vessels from various vascular beds revealed that the same processes contain both NPY and tyrosine-hydroxylase-like immunoreactivity (STERNINI and BRECHA 1985). Furthermore, it has been demonstrated that the peptide is released together with noradrenaline from sympathetic nerve endings. The concentrations of both NPY and noradrenaline in the perfusion medium from isolated perfused hearts increase in a concentration-dependent manner in response to stimulation with nicotine (RICHARDT et al. 1988). Similarly, NPY and noradrenaline are concomitantly released upon stimulation of the sympathetic nerves of the guinea pig vas deferens (KASAKOV et al. 1988). In the blood-perfused pig spleen, splenic nerve stimulation induces a severalfold increase in NPY-like immunoreactivity in the blood which accompanies that of noradrenaline (LUNDBERG et al. 1986). Interestingly, intermittant bursts at high frequency are more active than continuous stimulation at a low frequency in eliciting NPY release, which led to the speculation that NPY comes into play as an additional sympathetic transmitter under emergency conditions. Costorage of NPY with noradrenaline is also supported by the observation that in humans plasma levels of NPY and noradrenaline increase in parallel in stressful situations such as thoracotomy, which is known to activate the sympathetic nervous system (LUNDBERG et al. 1985c). The NPY detected in plasma under these conditions may have its main origin from sympathetic nerves and not from the adrenal gland, since plasma adrenaline levels do not correlate with those of NPY.

2.2.2 Functions

Systemic administration of NPY has been shown to induce a long-lasting increase in arterial blood pressure which is obviously due to the vasoconstrictor effect of the peptide, since total peripheral resistance is elevated while cardiac index and stroke volume are reduced (ZUKOWSKA-GROJEC et al. 1987; LUNDBERG and TATEMOTO 1982). The threshold for the blood pressure response is 10^{-9} M, which is of the same order of potency as angiotensin II and less than for noradrenaline. It is unlikely that the NPY levels circulating in plasma, which are in the picomolar range, are sufficient to cause a general vasoconstriction (LUNDBERG et al. 1985c). In patients with pheochromocytoma, however, who display greatly elevated NPY levels, the peptide may well contribute to the hypertension characteristic for this disease (ADRIAN et al. 1983b). The pressor effect of NPY following i.v. injection is resistant to adrenoceptor blocking agents, indicating that the peptide exerts its blood pressure effect by acting directly on the blood vessels (LUNDBERG and TATEMOTO 1982). A number of reports have demonstrated a relatively small, if any, contractile effect of NPY on the relatively large conduit blood vessels such as the femoral artery (EKBLAD et al. 1984; EDVINSSON et al. 1984; PERNOW et al. 1986). The pressure action of the peptide appears rather to be mediated by the small arteries and arterioles. This is suggested by intravital microscopic studies using skeletal muscle blood vessels, in which NPY at a concentration of 10^{-7} *M* contracted arterioles to a similar extent as noradrenaline 10^{-6} *M* (PERNOW et al. 1987a). A higher vasoconstrictor potency of NPY as compared with noradrenaline has also been observed in segments of small human skeletal muscle arteries, where similar maximal contractile effects were obtained at 20 times lower concentrations for NPY than for noradrenaline (PERNOW et al. 1987b). The effect of NPY on the small arteries of skeletal muscle is of particular interest with respect to blood pressure regulation, since skeletal muscle tissue is considered to contribute greatly to total peripheral resistance, especially at the arteriolar level.

In some arteries and under certain conditions, NPY may potentiate the vasoconstrictor effects of noradrenaline. This has been demonstrated using the isolated rat femoral artery (EDVINSSON et al. 1987). The contractile response to electrical stimulation, which is sensitive to phentolamine and guanethidine, is considerably enhanced in the presence of low concentrations of NPY, which per se are without effect. Similar observations have been made in the isolated portal vein of rat or in human submandibular arteries, where NPY in low concentrations (10^{-9} *M*) was found to potentiate the contractile effects of noradrenaline or transmural nerve stimulation, while constrictor activation of the peptide per se was noticed at higher concentrations (DAHLÖF et al. 1985b; LUNDBERG et al. 1985c). A potentiating effect of NPY on the response to adrenergic agents has also been observed in vivo. In the pithed rat low doses of NPY, which by themselves are without effect, were reported to enhance the pressor response to phenylephrine (DAHLÖF et al. 1985a). The potentiation of the contractile response by NPY is not limited to noradrenaline but can also be seen with histamine (EDVINSSON et al. 1984). It is, on the other hand, not obtained following vasoconstriction with 5-HT, prostaglandin $F_{2\alpha}$, or high potassium. The mechanism underlying the potentiating effect of NPY is presently not understood.

There is good evidence that NPY in addition to its postsynaptic effects acts also at a presynaptic level and is involved in the control of noradrenaline release. Thus, NPY has been found to inhibit transmural nerve stimulation-evoked contraction of mouse and rat vas deferens, rat uterus, and rat and guinea pig heart, as well as mesenteric arteries (ALLEN et al. 1982; LUNDBERG and STJÄRNE 1984; STJERNQUIST et al. 1983; WESTFALL et al. 1987; LUNDBERG et al. 1984a). The effect has been shown to be due to a presynaptic inhibitory action of the peptide on the release of noradrenaline (LUNDBERG et al. 1984a; WESTFALL et al. 1987; DAHLÖF et al. 1985b). In the isolated perfused mesenteric arterial bed of the rat inhibition of the electrically stimulated release of noradrenaline was observed over a concentration range of NPY of 10^{-10}–10^{-7} *M*. Lower concentrations (10^{-10} and 10^{-9} *M*) decreased the effect of nerve stimulation on perfusion pressure, whereas higher concentrations (10^{-7} *M*) produced a marked potentiation (WESTFALL et al. 1987). The NPY-induced inhibition of preganglionic nerve stimulation-evoked release of noradrenaline has recently been confirmed by experiments in vivo (DAHLÖF et al. 1988). Systemic infusion of NPY in pithed rats markedly reduced the increase in plasma noradrenaline levels evoked by preganglionic nerve stimulation but enhanced at the same time the blood pressure response. These observations support the suggestion that

NPY may have a transmitter conserving role under certain conditions of stimulation (STJÄRNE et al. 1986). Transmitter stores could be conserved by the presynaptic inhibitory action of NPY without compromising the magnitude of the postjunctional response which would be enhanced by the peptide.

NPY may affect the heart in at least three ways: by acting as a vasoconstrictor at the coronary arteries, by inhibiting noradrenaline release from sympathetic nerve endings, and by attenuation of vagal activity. The peptide has been shown to produce a prompt reduction in perfusate flow in isolated hearts prepared according to the Langendorff technique (ALLEN et al. 1983). The reported concurrent inhibition of the cardiac contractility is most likely secondary to the resulting hypoxia, since NPY has no effect on inotropic or chronotropic parameters of isolated atria or electrically driven papillary muscle (ALLEN et al. 1986; WAHLESTEDT et al. 1987). NPY also has potent effects on the vascular tone of human coronary arteries in vitro and in vivo. The peptide has been demonstrated to induce long-lasting contractions of human epicardial coronaries at a threshold concentration of 5×10^{-9} M (FRANCO-CERECEDA and LUNDBERG 1987). According to clinical studies NPY may be more effective at the more distal part of the coronary system. The arteriographic appearance following infusion of NPY into coronary arteries of patients with angina suggested preferential constriction of small vessels rather than constriction of epicardial coronary arteries (CLARKE et al. 1987). From these studies it appears not unlikely that NPY is involved in the pathogenesis of coronary spasm.

In addition to its inhibitory presynaptic effects on noradrenaline release NPY has been implicated in the mediation of the noradrenergic inhibition of the vagal action on the heart which occurs after intense sympathetic stimulation (POTTER 1987). NPY has been shown to attenuate cardiac slowing induced by stimulation of vagal nerve terminals in isolated atria as well as in dogs, an effect which is not exerted postsynaptically at the cardiac pacemaker cells but presynaptically, since slowing of the heart in response to addition of cholinomimetic agents is not affected by the peptide.

The distribution of NPY in the brain suggests that the peptide might play a role in the central regulation of the cardiovascular system. Administration of NPY into the cisterna magna has been reported to cause hypotension (FUXE et al. 1983). When administered intracerebroventricularly at low concentrations, a dose-dependent increase in blood pressure and heart rate is observed, whereas higher doses induce a fall in blood pressure (CARTER et al. 1985). The pressor effect appears to be mediated by the activation of the sympathetic nervous system and does not depend on the action of circulating vasopressin (VALLEJO and LIGHTMAN 1986).

2.2.3 Neuropeptide Y Receptors and Structure-Activity Relationship

Binding sites for NPY have been characterized in the brain of rat and humans (WESTLIND-DANIELSSON et al. 1987; CHANG et al. 1985; UNDÉN and BARTFAI 1984; LEYS et al. 1987; SARIA et al. 1984). In all tissues studied so far a single class of high affinity binding sites was found with dissociation constant values in the

10^{-10} *M* range. Biochemical data on the structure and size of the putative NPY receptor have as yet not been presented. A number of studies using peptide fragments or natural or synthetic analogues of NPY have been performed to determine which part of the peptide is needed for the production of the biological effects and for the interaction with the receptor. All studies came to the conclusion that the C-terminal part of NPY is essential for binding and mediates the vasoconstrictor effects and the prejunctional inhibition of NPY release (WAHLESTEDT and HAKANSON 1986; RIOUX et al. 1986; LUNDBERG et al. 1988). The C-terminal amide appears to be crucial since desamido NPY has been reported to be inactive in a number of test systems commonly employed to determine the biological activity of NPY (WAHLESTEDT and HAKANSON 1986). Shortening of the molecule by removal of Tyr 1 through Glu 15 or Tyr 1 through Ala 18 causes marked losses of the vasoconstrictor potency without detectable reduction of the intrinsic activity (RIOUX et al. 1986; LUNDBERG et al. 1988). The shortest C-terminal fragment reported to be capable of displacing [^{125}I]NPY from its binding to chicken brain membranes was NPY 30–36 (PERLMAN et al. 1987). The affinity is drastically reduced by substitution of the Arg residues in positions 35 and 33 by ornithine or by lysine. This suggests that the guanidinium side chain of Arg plays an important part in the binding of the peptide. Deletion of the N-terminal amino acid Tyr 1 reduces the NPY potency as a coronary constrictor by about one order of magnitude (RIOUX et al. 1986). The biological activity of the peptide depends therefore not solely on the C-terminal part. This is of considerable interest in view of the proposed tertiary structure of NPY (ALLEN et al. 1987a). Due to the hairpin shape of the molecule, the N- and C-terminal parts are in close vicinity to each other and may thus both participate in binding.

2.2.4 Mechanism of Action

The mechanism underlying the vasoconstrictor effects of NPY is presently ill understood. As outlined above, the direct effects of NPY on blood vessels are resistant to adrenoceptor blockade (PERNOW et al. 1987a; LUNDBERG et al. 1982). The potentiation of the noradrenaline-induced vasoconstriction by NPY appears not to be due to an interference of the peptide with adrenoceptors, since neither number nor affinity of α_1- or α_2-adrenoceptors are altered in the rat femoral artery in response to NPY (PERNOW et al. 1986). There is good evidence that extracellular calcium is involved in the vascular effects of NPY. Calcium channel blockers such as verapamil or nifedipine have been reported to abolish NPY-induced contraction of cerebral coronary or skeletal muscle arteries and to prevent the increase in perfusion pressure obtained following infusion of the peptide into the isolated heart or spleen (EMSON and DE QUIDT 1984; PERNOW et al. 1986, 1987b; LUNDBERG et al. 1985b, 1988; RIOUX et al. 1986). This is in contrast to the prejunctional effects on NPY, which have been reported to be resistant to calcium channel blockers (PERNOW et al. 1987b). It is presently not clear how calcium metabolism in vascular tissues is affected by NPY. A number of studies, in which the possibility of NPY stimulating phosphoinositide hydrolysis was investigated, failed to detect any effect of the peptide on this system. The tissues tested were vascular smooth muscle cells, vas deferens, and spleen (REYNOLDS and SHINJI 1988; HÄGGBLAD and FREDHOLM 1987; LUNDBERG et al. 1988). On the other hand, inhibition of stimulated cAMP accumulation by NPY, which appears to be due to a direct effect of the peptide on adenylate cyclase activity, has consistently been found in these tissues (WESTLIND-DANIELSSON et al. 1987). The effect is totally abolished following treatment with pertussis toxin to inactivate inhibitory G-proteins. Pertussis toxin treatment has also been reported to attenuate the increase in renal vascular resistance following administration of NPY into the isolated perfused rat kidney (HACKENTHAL et al. 1987). Since it is hard to imagine that NPY exerts its vascular effects solely by inhibition of adenylate cyclase, it appears not unjustified to speculate that there is another pertussis toxin-sensitive transmembrane signalling mechanism which mediates its actions on vascular tone. In the light of the recent finding that in the adrenal gland coupling of ANG II to Ca^{2+} channels involves a pertussis toxin-sensitive G-protein, it appears likely that a similar mechanism underlies the vascular effects of NPY (HESCHELER et al. 1988).

3 Atrial Natriuretic Peptide

A central theme of research in cardiovascular physiology has been the attempt to understand how the heart interacts with the peripheral circulation. Historically, the heart was considered a pump that responded to changes in blood volume and circulatory pressure by adjusting the kinetics of stretch and contraction. The observation that atrial myocytes contain granules that vary in concentration depending on the water and electrolyte balance led to the discovery that the heart is the site of production and storage of a peptide which initiates a prompt diuresis, natriuresis, and fall in blood pressure upon intravenous administration (DE BOLD et al. 1981). It has been suggested that this atrial natriuretic peptide (ANP) may gain some importance in the treatment of hypertension as it possesses a uniquely desirable combination of antihypertensive properties: it is both a vasorelaxant and a diuretic. As opposed to drugs sharing these effects it blocks the activation of salt- and water-conserving hormone systems and prevents at the same time potassium loss. Beyond that, it functionally resembles converting enzyme blockers due to its inhibitory action on renin and aldosterone.

3.1 Chemistry

The family of natriuretic and diuretic peptides was originally isolated from mammalian atrial tissue (FLYNN et al. 1983; KANGAWA et al. 1984). These peptides, which share a common amino acid core, were found to be fragments of differing length hydrolyzed from a common precursor molecule of 126 amino acids which is the predominant storage form of the atrial natriuretic peptide in the heart (Fig. 4) (LEWICKI et al. 1986; MAKI et al. 1984; NEMER et al. 1984;

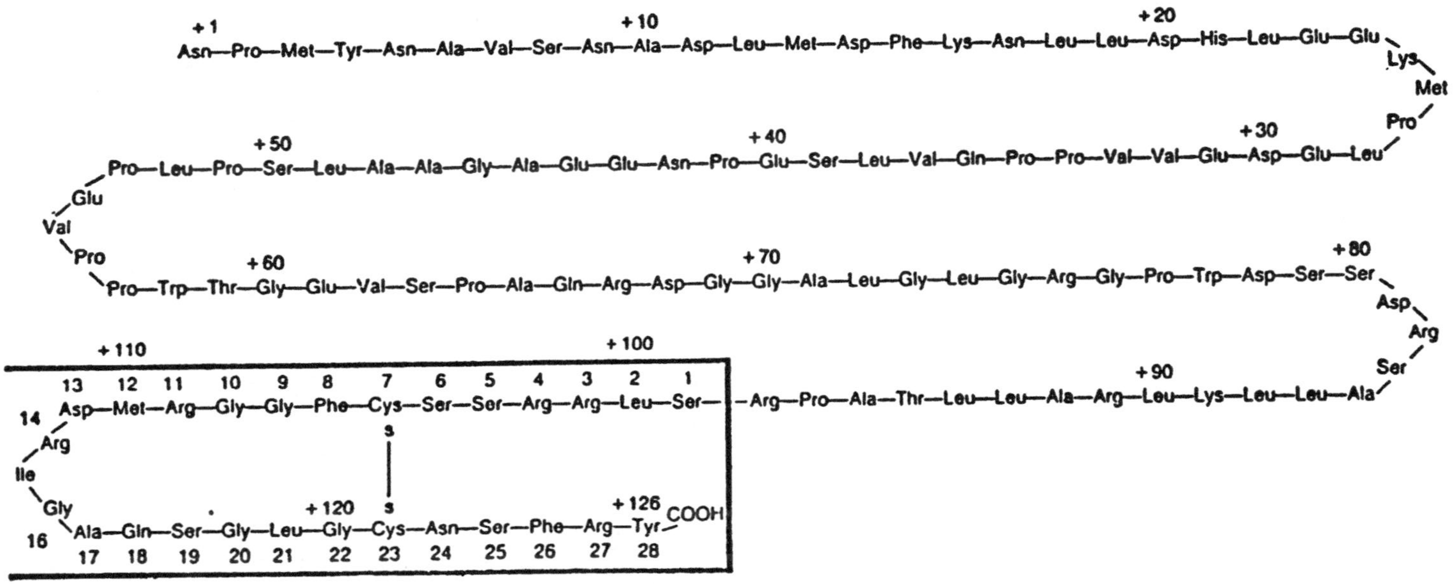

Fig. 4. Structure of human proatrial natriuretic peptide (ANP). The sequence 99-126 corresponds to the biologically active peptide, ANP 99-126, previously termed alpha-ANP

OIKAWA et al. 1984; SEIDMAN et al. 1984; YAMANAKA et al. 1984). The precursor is found in large amounts in both the left and right atrium but has also been detected, albeit in smaller concentrations, in ventricular tissue. It appears that immediately before, during, or after release from the myocytes the prohormone is cleaved by a specific processing enzyme to yield the biologically active C-terminal, pro-ANF 99–126, and the N-terminal portion. Different investigators reported isolation of natriuretic peptides from the heart which meant that a variety of names were used for similar peptides, leading to confusion and complicating scientific communication (MAACK 1985).

A nomenclature committee, established jointly by the International Society of Hypertension, the American Heart Association, and the World Health Organization, has recently proposed a standard approach to the naming and reporting of these compounds: they recommended that the term "atrial natriuretic peptide (or factor)" be adopted and that the prefix "h" for human or "r" for rat be used for species designation. They further proposed that the specific amino acid composition of each peptide be designated with reference to the common precursor molecule with peptide sequence 1–126 numbering from the N-terminus and excluding the signal peptide (Joint Nomenclature and Standardization Committee 1987).

The major circulating form of the peptide in human blood accordingly is correctly designated hANP99–126 and in rat blood, rANP99–126 (SCHWARTZ et al. 1985; THIBAULT et al. 1985).

3.2 Regulation of Synthesis and Release

Synthesis and release of ANF are induced by perturbations associated with a rise in atrial pressure. Thus, high plasma levels have been measured in animals and in humans during volume expansion, salt loading, exercise, head down tilt, and water immersion (ANDERSON et al. 1986; ESKAY et al. 1986; LANG et al. 1985; LAROSE et al. 1985; SAGNELLA et al. 1985; YAMAJI et al. 1985). ANP seems to be released from the heart by the direct effect of increased atrial stress on the myocytes rather than by a neuroreflex mediated through stimulation of left atrial receptors. This is suggested by experiments in dogs which demonstrate that atrial stretch in response to mitral obstruction induces ANP release even after cervical vagotomy and adrenergic blockade (LEDSOME et al. 1985). Furthermore, it can also be released in response to atrial distension from isolated perfused hearts (DIETZ 1984; LANG et al. 1985). The successful cloning of pro-ANP cDNA has permitted studies of the regulation of ANP gene expression in the heart and the search for possible extra-atrial sites of synthesis. Both synthesis and release extra-atrial sites of synthesis. Both synthesis and release of ANP in the heart are regulated by sodium balance (NAKAYAMA et al. 1984). This is suggested by experiments demonstrating a marked reduction of atrial prepro-ANP mRNA levels following water deprivation and an increase following dietary salt loading. Administration of glucocorticoids has been shown to stimulate ANP mRNA levels in vivo in the rat atria as well as in vitro in cultured cardiocytes (DAY et al. 1986). Mammalian ventricular myocytes, originally felt to lack ANP-synthesizing capability, have recently been shown to contain small amounts of ANP mRNA. The levels of ventricular ANP mRNA are about 1/100 of those found in the atria. Cardiac ventricular wall stretch may be a stimulus for ANP mRNA transcription since left ventricular mRNA levels have been reported to increase up to tenfold in response to chronic volume overload produced by an arterial arteriovenous fistula (LATTION et al. 1986). It remains to be elucidated how the translation product is processed and whether it contributes to the levels of circulating ANP.

The technique of ANP mRNA determination by in situ or in vitro hybridization with specific cDNAs has been employed to study extracardiac sites of ANP production. Prepro-ANP mRNA has been identified in the lungs, pituitary hypothalamus, and adrenal gland (GARDNER et al. 1986).

3.3 Biological Effects

Continuous infusion of ANF into healthy subjects at doses which raise plasma ANF levels to the upper range observed in pathophysiological states has been shown to cause an acute fall in blood pressure and to increase glomerular filtration rate, filtration fraction, urinary sodium excretion, and free water clearance (RICHARDS et al. 1985a; WEIDMANN et al. 1986b). Plasma renin and aldosterone levels are suppressed. When administered at rates that elevate plasma ANF concentrations only to the upper part of the physiological range, blood pressure and heart rate remain unchanged in normal subjects (ANDERSON et al. 1987). In contrast, both urinary sodium excretion and urine flow increase, whereas plasma renin activity is suppressed. These observations are evidence for the physiological role of ANF as a factor in salt-water homeostasis.

The mechanisms involved in the mediation of the renal effects of ANP have been the subject of some controversy. The distribution of ANP binding sites in the kidney indicates that the glomeruli are the primary site of action of ANP in the kidney cortex, but it may also act in the medulla (BIANCHI et al. 1985). In binding studies on isolated kidney cells, the highest concentration of ANP receptor sites was found on the glomeruli, followed by the collecting ducts, and thick ascending limbs of Henle's loops (DE LEAN et al. 1985). In the glomeruli the receptors were confined to the mesangial cells. Proximal tubules are completely devoid of receptors. This receptor distribution along the nephron correlates well with the pattern of ANP-induced cGMP production in the various nephron segments and the localization of labeled ANP by autoradiographic studies. These studies also suggest a high density of binding sites in the renal vasculature such as the vasa recta (BIANCHI et al. 1985). The observations would favour, in part, the view that the natriuretic effect of ANP is due to its renal hemodynamic and vascular actions and in particular to an increase in the glomerular filtration rate and medullary washout (MAACK 1985). Indeed, significant increments in the glomerular filtration rate and filtration fraction, irrespective of renal blood flow, have been found following administration of relatively high doses of ANP to rats, dogs, or humans (BURNETT et al. 1984; HUANG et al. 1985; MAACK et al. 1984; RICHARDS et al. 1985a; WEIDMANN et al. 1986b). The mechanism for the increased glomerular filtration rate is not known exactly. Constriction of efferent and dilatation of afferent glomerular arterioles leading to an elevation in hydraulic pressure in the glomerular capillaries has been postulated (Maack 1985). An increase in glomerular capillary permeability in response to ANP could be another explanation (Maack 1985). There is good evidence that the increase in glomerular filtration rate cannot fully account for the enhanced natriuresis and diuresis observed upon administration of ANP. It was found both in vivo and in vitro that low-dose infusions of ANP increased sodium excretion, although changes in the glomerular filtration rate were not detectable (Briggs et al. 1982; Murray et al. 1985; Sonnenberg et al. 1982; Yukimura et al. 1984).

Natriuretic and diuretic effects not dependent on the glomerular filtration rate might be mediated by a redistribution of renal blood flow or a direct effect of ANP on sodium reabsorption. A shift of blood flow toward the superficial and midcortical regions of the kidney in conscious dogs has been demonstrated in response to a synthetic ANP (Maack et al. 1985). The ANP-induced natriuresis may therefore be achieved in part by shunting blood flow away from the salt-retaining nephrons. The increase in medullary or papillary blood flow observed during infusion of atrial extracts could also contribute to natriuresis by washing out the medullary osmotic gradient, with a resultant fall in distal tubular reabsorption. The observation of reduced urine osmolality without a change in free water clearance during ANP-induced natriuresis would support such an idea (Sonnenberg et al. 1982). Evidence has been presented that ANF might, in addition, specifically inhibit sodium reabsorption from the medullary collecting duct. This has been shown in rats by measuring the sodium concentration in samples of duct fluid collected by retrograde catheterization via the exposed papillar tip (Sonnenberg et al. 1986). Further support for this view comes from a recent study in isolated, inner medullary, collecting duct cells (Zeidel et al. 1986). In this system, ANP reduced the sodium-potassium-ATPase-mediated oxygen consumption. Since the activity of this enzyme depends on the concentration of intracellular sodium, and because ANP did not affect oxygen consumption when sodium was artificially introduced into the cells, it was concluded that this effect was due to the direct blockade of normal sodium reabsorption into the duct cells. The mode of action of ANP may, therefore, in some way resemble that of amiloride.

3.4 Effect on Renin and Aldosterone Secretion

Renin release has been demonstrated to be blocked by ANP when the basal secretion rate of renin is high. Thus, a fall in renin secretion and plasma renin activity was observed in anesthetized dogs and in unconscious dogs' inferior vena cava ligation or in two-kidney, one-clip Goldblatt hypertensive or slat-depleted, one-kidney one-clip Goldblatt hypertensive rats (Freeman et al. 1985; Volpe et al. 1985). There are some controversies concerning the possible mechanism by which ANP could inhibit renin secretion. Since renin-producing juxtaglomerular cells in afferent glomerular arterioles respond to changes in arteriolar wall stretch by altering the rate of renin secretion, ANP could block renin release by causing renal vasodilatation. An increase in sodium load to the macula densa, generated by the ANP-induced increase in glomerular filtration rate which exerts a negative feedback signal to the juxtaglomerular cells, might be another mechanism reducing renal secretion. Studies in dogs with a single, denervated, nonfiltering kidney argue against the latter mechanism (OPGENORTH et al. 1986; VILLARREAL et al. 1986). Finally, ANP could act directly on juxtaglomerular cells to suppress renin secretion. This is supported by studies in cultured renal cortical cells, in which renin activity has been reported to drop after addition of ANP (KURTZ et al. 1986).

Inhibition of aldosterone production by ANP is suggested by experiments in isolated rat or bovine glomerulosa cells, demonstrating that since synthetic ANP attenuates basal aldosterone secretion as well as the release induced by angiotensin II, ACTH, prostaglandin E_2, forskolin, and potassium (ATARASHI et al. 1985; CHARTIER et al. 1984; DE LEAN et al. 1984; GOODFRIEND et al. 1984; KUDO and BAIRD 1984). Lowering of plasma aldosterone levels of response to ANP infusion has been documented in dogs, rats, and humans (CHARTIER et al. 1984; VOLPE et al. 1985; WEIDMANN et al. 1986c). Aldosterone inhibition has been observed even in the presence of increased or normal plasma renin levels, supporting the idea of a direct action of ANP on the glomerulosa cells. ANP is thought to exert its action at a step prior to the formation of progesterone and 25-hydroxycholesterol, since synthesis of aldosterone from these compounds is not reduced by the peptide (GOODFRIEND et al. 1984).

3.5 Blood Pressure Effects

Synthetic ANP has been shown to relax aortic rings contracted by noradrenaline, methoxamine, histamine, serotonin, or angiotensin II (WINQUIST et al. 1984a). Aortic contractions elicited by high concentrations of potassium are less affected by ANP than those induced by low potassium concentrations, suggesting that events which result in profound membrane depolarization functionally antagonize the relaxing effects of the hormone (GARCIA et al. 1984). This is supported by the observation that ANP potently relaxes the tonic myogenic tone of, for instance, the rabbit facial vein but is much less active against the phasic myogenic tone of the rat portal vein induced by cell membrane depolarizations (WINQUIST et al. 1984a). Agonist-contracted central arteries such as the aorta, carotid, mesenteric, or renal arteries are much less effectively relaxed by ANP than more distal arteries including the iliac, saphenous, femoral, ear, or basilar arteries (FAISON et al. 1985). This heterogeneity in the response of blood vessels from different vascular beds is not dependent on the contractile agent used and is not observed when sodium nitroprusside is employed as the vasodilator (COHEN and SCHENCK 1984). ANP exerts a pronounced relaxant effect on rat renal arcuate arteries contracted with potassium, noradrenaline, or 5-hydroxytryptamine (AALKJAER et al. 1985). Small resistant vessels from rat cerebral or mesenteric arteries, however, were shown not to alter their contractile response to vasoconstrictors in the presence of ANP (OSOL et al. 1986). This is consistent with the finding that intravenous administration of ANP to rats preferentially reduced vascular resistance in the kidney but not in other organs, except when very high concentrations of ANP were infused (WAKITANI et al. 1985).

The C-terminal segment of the ANP molecule appears to be of particular importance for the vasorelaxant activity of the peptide (GARCIA et al. 1985b; KATSUBE et al. 1985). Cleaving of Tyr^{126} from ANP101–126 has been shown to decrease significantly the inhibitory potency of the peptide on the noradrenaline-induced contraction of rabbit aorta in vitro, whereas no difference in the vasodilator effect on the dog kidney was found. Removal of Arg^{125}-Tyr^{125} or Phe^{124}-Arg^{125}-Tyr^{126} results in a further reduction of vasorelaxant potency in rabbit aortic strips and also decreases the effects on renal blood flow (WAKITANI et al. 1985). Deletion of all C-terminal residues after Cys^{121} renders the molecule almost inactive. The N-terminal region of ANP appears to be less critical for the bioactivity. In the dog there is little difference in renal vasodilatation whether elicited by administration of ANP99–126, ANP101–126, or ANP103–126 (KATSUBE et al. 1985). Relaxation of the rabbit aorta is still observed with the N-terminally truncated ANP105–126 (GARCIA et al. 1985b). The intramolecular cysteine bridge in the ANP molecule may be of importance for the stabilization and the bioactive conformation of the peptide but is not an absolute requirement for biological activity. This is suggested by a recent study demonstrating that a linear fragment of ANP, unable to form the cysteine bridge (ANP106–125) still possesses some smooth muscle relaxant activity (SCHILLER et al. 1985).

With respect to the effects of ANP on isolated blood vessels, direct vasodilatation would be expected to be the most likely mechanism accounting for the hypertensive response. However, most authors have failed to demonstrate a decrease in peripheral resistance (BREUHAUS et al. 1985; LAPPE et al. 1985a; MARSH et al. 1985; SASAKI et al. 1985). In fact, the renal, mesenteric, and hindquarter blood flow in rats has been shown to decrease in parallel with arterial blood pressure during the infusion of ANP (LAPPE et al. 1985a). At the same time, total peripheral resistance was significantly elevated, whereas central venous pressure, cardiac output, and stroke volume were reduced. Infusion of ANP (0.3 μg/kg·min) into dogs also resulted in a drop of cardiac output and stroke volume associated with a slight but not significant rise in peripheral resistance (KLEINERT et al. 1986). A similar pattern with the same dose of ANP was observed in sheep (BREUHAUS et al. 1985). Cardiac output, stroke volume, atrial pressure, and blood pressure were found to be reduced while peripheral resistance as well as heart rate increased. Chemical sympathectomy or ganglionic blockade prevented the increase in heart rate and peripheral resistance but did not effect the other parameters (BREUHAUS et al. 1985; LAPPE et al. 1985b). This suggests that the unexpected rise of peripheral resistance was due to a reflex activation of the sympathetic nervous system elicited by the fall in blood pressure. The fall in blood pressure has, in turn, to be ascribed to the decreased cardiac output (BREUHAUS et al. 1985; KLEINERT et al. 1986; LAPPE et al. 1985a). In this context a direct negative effect of ANP on the heart is not very likely to play a role, since in vivo right atrial pressure is lowered rather than increased, as one would expect in the case of a negative inotropic effect of the hormone (BREUHAUS et al. 1985). Moreover, ANP has been reported not to affect the force of contraction or heart rate when administered to isolated spontaneously beating heart atria or electrically driven papillary muscle (Hiwatari et al. 1986). The fall in cardiac output is thought to be due to ANP-induced relaxation of venous smooth muscles, leading to an augmentation of venous capacitance and a reduction of venous return, as reflected by the decrease in central venous pressure (Breuhaus et al. 1985). Acutely, rapid contraction of blood volume may play an additional role. It has been observed that the hematocrit quickly goes up during infusion of ANP, which is also observed in anephric rats in which infusion of 1 μg/mg·min of ANP for 25 min reduces plasma volume by 14% (Almeida et al. 1986; Maack 1985; Weidmann et al. 1986b). This suggests that short-term administration of ANP decreases blood volume not only by inducing diuresis but also by causing intravascular fluid to shift into the interstitium.

Although studies in normotensive animals do not suggest that ANP induces a reduction in peripheral resistance, which might explain the blood pressure lowering effect, there is some evidence from recent investigations that in vasoconstricted hypertensive animal models or in patients with peripheral vasoconstriction such as in severe cardiac failure, the peptide induces arterial relaxation (Cody et al. 1986; Gellai et al. 1986; Volpe et al. 1986).

ANP effects blood pressure when administered at high doses but not at doses which increase ANP plasma levels within the physiological range (Anderson et al. 1987; Cody et al. 1986; Richards et al. 1985a; Weidmann et al. 1986b). An ANP effect on blood pressure in humans was first demonstrated in a study of normal volunteers who were given an intravenous bolus of 100 μg human ANP99–126 (Richards et al. 1985a). Immediately after ANP administration, there was a sudden drop in blood pressure and a reflex increase in heart rate. At the same time, facial flushing was observed, which was attributed to dilatation of subcutaneous vessels. The hypertensive effect was long lasting, probably reflecting a combined action of vasodilatation and volume contraction. The physiological implications of this study are not clear, since the plasma ANP levels during administration of the peptide were not determined. In another study, ANP102–126 was infused intravenously into salt-loaded normal volunteers at a rate of either 0.5 or 5 μg/min for 4 h (Bussien et al. 1986). No change in blood pressure or heart rate was observed with the lower dose. However, the higher dose markedly reduced systolic and diastolic blood pressure after a latency period of 2–3 h. Heart rate exhibited a slight increase. The fall in blood pressure in response to the systemic administration of ANP may, at least partly, be related to the direct vasorelaxant effect of the peptide. Forearm blood flow increases markedly after intra-arterial infusion of ANP99–126 (Müller et al. 1986). Moreover, skin blood flow has been found to increase dose-dependently in response to an intravenous infusion of 1–40 μg/min ANP102–126 (Bussien et al. 1986). These observations are consistent with the contention that the decrease in blood pressure following ANP administration at lower doses relies on the vasodilatory effect of the peptide. Suppression of the renin-angiotensin system by ANP may also contribute to the blood pressure lowering effect of this hormone (Biollaz et al. 1986; Weidmann et al. 1986c).

3.6 Atrial Natriuretic Peptide Receptor and Mechanism of Action

The vasorelaxation of blood vessel segments with ANP is obtained regardless of whether the endothelium is intact or destroyed (WINQUIST et al. 1984b). Thus, ANP seems to exert its vasorelaxant effects in an endothelium-independent way. This is surprising, since not only vascular smooth muscle cells but also endothelial cells show specific binding sites for radiolabeled ANP. The number of ANP receptors is higher in smooth muscle cells; the endothelial cells, however, show a much greater affinity for the hormone (LEITMAN and MURAD 1986; SCHENK et al. 1985a). The physiological role of ANP receptors on endothelial cells is not known. The possibility that ANP may modify the effects of endothelium-dependent vasodilators or vasoconstrictors (e.g., endothelin) at this site is still a matter of speculation.

Receptor binding studies using vascular smooth muscle cells demonstrated a good correlation between the receptor affinities of ANP fragements and their respective vasorelaxant potencies (HIRATA et al. 1985). The binding of ANP molecules is greatly reduced upon removal of residues from the C-terminal party but only slightly affected by N-terminal site deletions. Furthermore, a hydrophobic amino acid residue within the ring structure appears to play an important role in receptor binding, since sulfoxidation of the methionine residue in position 12 results in a marked loss of affinity (HIRATA et al. 1985; GARCIA et al. 1985b).

The distribution of ANP binding sites in the body has been assessed by receptor binding studies and in situ autoradiography. ANP binding sites have been localized in the kidney, blood vessels, adrenal gland, small intestine, colon, and certain brain areas (BIANCHI et al. 1985; DE LEAN et al. 1985; NAPIER et al. 1984; SCHIFFRIN et al. 1985). A high density of receptors in the kidney was found in glomeruli and a smaller concentration in the vasa recta bundles in the inner part of the outer medulla. In the adrenal gland, a high density of binding sites has been reported in the zona glomerulosa, which is consistent with the inhibitory effects of ANP on aldosterone synthesis and secretion. As mentioned above, specific binding sites for ANP have also been demonstrated in vascular smooth muscle cells and in endothelial cells. The affinity of the vascular receptor (k_D approximately 0.05–2 nmol/l) has been reported to correspond well with the inhibitory concentration of ANP required for relaxation of blood vessels (NAPIER et al. 1984). Both functional and pharmacological studies indicate that there exist at least two distinct ANP receptors. Whereas an important receptor-mediated effect of ANP is the stimulation of particulate guanylate cyclase activity, several truncated analogues of ANP which neither stimulate guanylate cyclase nor antagonize the ANP-mediated stimulation of guanylate cyclase have been reported nevertheless to bind with high affinity to the major class of receptors observed in vascular smooth muscle cells (LEITMAN et al. 1988). Confirmation that there are multiple populations of ANP receptors, part of which do not couple to guanylate cyclase, comes from cross-linking studies in various cell lines and tissues including the kidney, in which two types of ANP binding sites were identified, one a molecular size of 130000 daltons and the other of 66000 daltons (LEITMAN et al. 1988). Under reducing conditions more than 90% of the high molecular weight material is converted to a 66000 dalton protein. This finding gave rise to speculation that there are two subclasses of 130000 dalton receptors represented by two different proteins. Only the nonreducible form with high molecular weight shows guanylate cyclase activity. The overwhelming majority of renal and ANP receptors corresponds to the low molcular weight form and may be biologically silent, since they do not couple to cGMPase and do not mediate any of the known effects (MAACK et al. 1987). The latter type of receptor appears to be subject preferentially to down-regulation and internalization in the presence of high concentrations of ANP and has therefore been termed clearance or c-receptor. It was proposed that these clearance binding sites act as a hormonal buffer system to modulate plasma levels of ANP (MAACK et al. 1987). The c-receptor protein has recently been isolated from vascular smooth muscle cells. Corresponding cDNA clones were isolated using a partial amino acid sequence, and the entire amino acid sequence of the c-receptor was established. It appears to consist of 496 amino acids with a single potential transmembrane domain predicting a 37-amino acid cytoplasmic domain and a large, acidic extracellular domain, which is rich in cysteine and is assumed to contain attached carbohydrates. The identity of the cloned material with an ANP receptor was confirmed by expression in *Xenopus* oocytes which resulted in high affinity, membrane-associated binding sites for ANP (FULLER et al. 1988).

The receptor which is coupled to guanylate cyclase contains a binding subunit which is about 130K under reducing conditions. This polypeptide exhibits both high affinity ANP binding as well as intrinsic guanylate cyclase activity, which led to the suggestion that ANP binding and guanylate cyclase activity reside in the same macromolecular complex (SCHENK et al. 1985b). cGMP accumulation is clearly associated with vascular smooth muscle relaxation (HAMET et al. 1984; WALDMAN et al. 1984). The intracellular increase in cGMP-dependent protein kinase activity in vascular smooth muscle cells results in an altered phosphorylation of numerous smooth muscle proteins finally leading to myosin light chain dephosphorylation. cGMP-dependent protein kinase activation is thought to increase the activity of a membrane calcium ATPase, thus decreasing cytosolic concentrations of calcium. This would result in a decreased activity of myosin light chain kinase, a calcium calmodulin-dependent enzyme, which would finally account for decreased phosphorylation of myosin light chain.

3.7 Atrial Natriuretic Peptide and Hypertension

In view of the well-known link between sodium homeostasis and blood pressure regulation, it has been speculated that ANP might be involved in the development and maintenance of hypertension either due to inadequate secretion or to a failure of endorgan response to the hormone. Current data, however, provide little evidence supporting this idea. Hypertension has been found to be associated with high ANP plasma levels both in animals and in humans (GUTKOWSKA et al. 1986; HAASS et al. 1986; IMADA et al. 1985; MORII et al. 1986; SAGNELLA et al. 1986; Snajder and Rapp 1986; Sugarawa et al. 1986). Two animal models of genetic hypertension, namely, the spontaneoulsy hypertensive rats (SHR) and the stroke-prone substrain (SHRSP), have been reported to increase plasma ANP concentrations with the development of hypertension (Haass et al. 1986; Morii et al. 1986). At the age of 15–16 weeks, when mean arterial blood pressure in SHR has reached a plateau of about 180 mmHg, plasma ANP was found to be about fourfold higher than in 3-week-old SHR. These observations are very similar to the findings in another animal model of hypertension, the Dahl salt-sensitive rat. The rise in blood pressure in response to high salt intake in these animals is also accompanied by an increase in plasma ANP. Increased plasma ANP levels are also observed in human hypertension (Sagnella et al. 1986; Sugawara et al. 1986). The levels show a good correlation with systolic as well as with diastolic blood pressure in patients with low plasma renin activity; compared with patients with high renin values, plasma ANP concentrations appear to be elevated. The increased release of ANP in hypertensive sufferers probably reflects an attempt by the heart to reduce its working load. Only part of the ANP found in the plasma of hypertensives may originate from the heart atria. In severe hypertension the left ventricular tissue may also contribute to circulating ANP levels, since it has been demonstrated both in experimental and clinical studies that ventricular hypertrophy is associated with ANP gene induction (Lattion et al. 1986; Saito et al. 1987).

Infusion of ANP has been reported to reduce blood pressure both in hypertensive animals and in patients with hypertension (Gellai et al. 1986; Lappe et al. 1985b; Richards et al. 1985b; Volpe et al. 1986; Weidmann et al. 1986a). When administered intravenously as a continuous infusion of 1 μg/kg·min for 30 min, a large fall in mean arterial blood pressure was observed in conscious SHR. The concomitant increase in peripheral vascular resistance could be abolished by chemical sympathectomy or surgical ablation of the vagus, suggesting that the increase in peripheral vascular resistance was caused by reflex stimulation of the sympathetic tone due to the reduced cardiac output and not by a direct vasoconstrictor action of ANP (Lappe et al. 1985b).

The study further indicated that the hypotensive effect of ANP does not depend on a direct interaction of the hormone with the nervous system. Experiments in hypertensive animals suggest that very low doses of ANP are sufficient to decrease blood pressure provided the peptide is administered chronically. In SHR, blood pressure is reduced to almost normal levels after chronic infusion of as little as 100 μg/h of rat ANP101–126 for 7 days (Garcia et al. 1985a). When administered to normotensive rats the same dose over the same time period did not significantly change blood pressure. Natriuresis and diuresis were not significantly affected by this treatment in either normotensive or hypertensive rats. Similarly, prolonged infusion of low doses of ANP which per se did not change basal blood pressure, urine volume, or sodium excretion has been shown to prevent the expected increase in arterial blood pressure following a continuous infusion of norepinephrine (Yasujima et al. 1985). Neither body weight nor urine volume were altered during the experimental period in this study. It was therefore concluded that ANP exerts its hypertensive effects by direct interaction with norepinephrine at the blood vessels. This would agree with the observation that as opposed to normal animals ANP decreases peripheral vascular resistance in certain models of hypertension. In two-kidney, one-clip, renin-dependent, Goldblatt hypertension, infusion of ANP caused a marked reduction in peripheral resistane (VOLPE et al. 1986). In SHR an increased sensitivity to the antihypertensive action of ANP has been found as compared with normotensive Wistar-Kyoto rats (GELLAI et al. 1986).

The effect of ANP on blood pressure has also been investigated in human hypertension. When administered as a bolus of 100 μg ANP99–126 only a very brief hypotensive response was reported in hypertensive subjects, which is in contrast to a sustained, albeit small, decrease in blood pressure in normotensive volunteers (RICHARDS et al. 1985b). This is an unexpected finding, since blood pressure lowering maneuvers usually produce greater effects when basal blood pressure is increased. Interestingly, the diuretic response in hypertensive patients was more pronounced than in normotensive ones.

In another study infusion of ANP over 45 min to patients with primary hypertension induced a slightly more pronounced increase in systolic and diastolic blood pressure in a hypertensive as compared with a normotensive control group. Plasma renin activity and angiotensin II concentrations tended to increase during the infusion in hypertensive patients but were not altered in normotensiveones. Similarly, the increase in plasma norepinephrine was greater in hypertensive compared with normal subjects. Both observations may be explained by a secondary activation due to the differences in the blood pressure response (WEIDMANN et al. 1986a).

ANP may act at multiple sites to reduce blood pressure in hypertension. The peptide may exert its action by both acute and more chronic effects. The acute effects include a reduction in cardiac output and vasorelaxation. Besides an increase in venous capacitance, a reduction of blood volume may be responsible for the fall in cardiac output. The reduction in blood volume appears to be secondary to an ANP-induced shift of fluid to the extravascular compartment. This is indicated by the rapidly developing rise in hematocrit, which can be observed in intact as well as in nephrectomized animals and therefore cannot be due to diuresis alone. The increase in peripheral resistance in response to ANP, which has been observed in many studies, particularly in those in which high doses of the peptide have been administered, most likely reflects an activation of the sympathetic nervous system through the reduction in cardiac output. Lowering of peripheral resistance in response to ANP has been observed in experimental forms of hypertension associated with an increased vascular tone such as in Goldblatt hypertension. The long-term pressure effects of ANP in hypertension may be based on both its renal action as well as its effects on other hormonal systems. The enhanced natriuresis may cause a reduction of blood pressure by the contraction of extracellular blood volume and reduced cardiac output. The associated loss of sodium could, in addition, lower the sensitivity of vascular smooth muscle cells to the action of vasoconstrictor agents. Sodium depletion and volume contraction normally activate the renin-angiotensin-aldosterone system and stimulate vasopressin release. Both systems, which represent functional antagonists of ANP, are blocked by the hormone. This should result in an unopposed diuretic and natriuretic effect of the hormone.

4 Endothelin

Recent studies suggest that besides humoral, neural, and myogenic factors the endothelium may be an important modulator of vascular tone. The realization that endothelium is involved in vasoregulation first came with the discovery of prostacyclin, which is, among others, produced by endothelial cells and is a vasodilator in many vascular beds (Moncada et al. 1976). Subsequently, Furchgott and Zawadzki (1980) demonstrated in their elegant experiments that acetylcholine-induced relaxation of arterial smooth muscle required the presence of endothelial cells. This stimulated intense interest in the role of endothelium in modulating vascular responsiveness. A host of other agents were found in the following years acting on specific endothelial receptors to cause release of a factor which provokes relaxation of the associated smooth muscles (Cocks and Angus 1983; De Mey et al. 1982). The factor was termed endothelium-derived relaxant factor (EDRF), and recent observations suggest that nitric oxide is equivalent to it (Palmer et al. 1987). In addition, the endothelium also appears to be involved with the vasoconstrictor action of some stimuli such as hypoxia, anoxia, arachidonic acid, or thrombin (De Mey and Vanhoutte 1983; Holden and McCall 1984; Rubany and Vanhoutte 1985). This implies that endothelial cells may also release substances that increase vascular smooth muscle tone. In fact, Hickey et al. (1985) were able to demonstrate that bovine aortic endothelial cells in culture release a constrictor of coronary arteries. The constrictor activity increased progressively in the culture medium over 2–12 h of incubation and was heat stable, not extractable by organic solvents, and totally destroyed by trypsin and neutral protease. These properties and the results of gel filtration experiments suggest that the endothelium-derived constricting factor (EDCF) is a peptide with a molecular weight of about 3000 daltons (Gillespie et al. 1986; O'Brien et al. 1987). In vascular ring preparations, constriction, which was typically preceded by a small, transient dilatation, developed gradually, achieving a maximum in tension only after 15–45 min. Constriction was little affected by washing and was reversed partly by verapamil and acetylcholine, and completely by nitroprusside and isoproterenol (O'Brien et al. 1987). Thrombin stimulated the release of the constrictor activity from cultured endothelial cells into the culture medium, whereas anoxia or hypoxia were without effect (O'Brien et al. 1987).

In 1988 Yanagisawa and coworkers succeeded in isolating from the supernatant of porcine aortic endothelial cells in culture a constrictor peptide which was probably identical with the vasoconstrictor substance previously described by Hickey et al. and Gillespie and coworkers (Yanagisawa et al. 1988a). The peptide, now termed endothelin, consists of 21 amino acid residues, causes an endothelium-independent, slow-onset contraction when added to coronary artery strips, and induces a long-lasting increase in arterial blood pressure upon

1 3
ET 1 Cys—Ser—Cys—Ser—Ser—Leu—Met—Asp—Lys—Glu—
11 15
—Cys—Val—Tyr—Phe—Cys—His—Leu—Asp—Ile—Ile—Trp
ET 2 Cys—Ser—Cys—Ser—Ser—*Trp*—*Leu*—Asp—Lys—Glu—
—Cys—Val—Tyr—Phe—Cys—His—Leu—Asp—Ile—Ile—Trp
ET 3 Cys—*Thr*—Cys—*Phe*—*Thr*—*Tyr*—*Lys*—Asp—Lys—Glu—
—Cys—Val—Tyr—*Tyr*—Cys—His—Leu—Asp—Ile—Ile—Trp

Fig. 5. Amino acid sequences of endothelin 1, endothelin 2, and endothelin 3 (ET 1, ET 2, ET 3). The human genome contains three different genes encoding three different endothelins. ET 1 was originally isolated from media of cultured porcine endothelial cells. ET 3 was originally considered specific for the rat

intravenous administration to anesthetized, chemically denervated rats (Fig. 5) (YANAGISAWA et al. 1988a). The data suggested that endothelin is one of the most potent vasoconstrictors so far known. This makes the substance particularly attractive for studies concerned with the regulation of blood pressure and the pathophysiology of hypertension. The present state of research in this field, about half a year after the discovery of endothelin, is summarized in the following sections.

4.1 Structure

According to its production by porcine endothelial cells in culture, porcine endothelin is a 21-amino acid peptide with free N- and C-termini. It has a relative molecular mass of 2492 and has four cysteine residues forming two sets of intrachain disulfide bonds (YANAGISAWA et al. 1988a). There is a cluster of charged residues within the first ring (residues 8–10) and a hydrophobic C-terminal tail (residues 16–21). The peptide appears to be synthesized and processed similarly to other peptide hormones. Endothelial cells contain mRNA encoding the preproform of endothelin, and the deduced amino acid sequence for preproendothelin reveals an eukaryotic translation initiation site followed by a characteristic secretory signal sequence (YANAGISAWA et al. 1988a). As expected, paired basic amino-acid residues (Lys51-Arg52) precede the endothelin sequence, suggesting processing by typical endopeptidases at this site. Interestingly, however, no dibasic pair of amino acids is found at the end of the endothelin sequence, which indicates that the mature peptide is generated by unusual proteolytic processing between Trp 73-Val 74 through an endopeptidase with specificity similar to chymotrypsin (YANAGISAWA et al. 1988a).

Human endothelin is identical with porcine endothelin (ITOH et al. 1988). This was found by comparison of porcine endothelin cDNA with the nucleotide sequence of a cDNA clone isolated from a human placenta cDNA library. Cloning and sequencing of the rat endothelin gene revealed that rat endothelin is similar to, but distinct from porcine and human endothelin (YANAGISAWA et al. 1988b). The positions of the four cysteine residues as well as the last six amino acids at the C-terminal part are perfectly conserved. Major differences are found only in the apolar region of the ring.

Sequence evaluation has shown that endothelins are similar to certain scorpion toxins, which bind to tetrodotoxin-sensitive sodium channels, and are also closely related to certain newly isolated toxins from the burrowing asp, *Atractaspis engaddensis*, which are called sarafotoxins (Takagi et al. 1988; Lee et al. 1988). Animals bitten by this asp die of myocardial infarction due to the potent coronary constrictor effect of sarafotoxins.

4.2 Cardiovascular Effects

Intravenous bolus injection of porcine/human or rat endothelin (1 nmol/kg) causes a slowly developing and sustained rise in arterial pressure in anesthetized, chemically denervated, or awake rats (Yanagisawa et al. 1988a,b). In contrast to other vasoconstrictors such as angiotensin, the increase in blood pressure in response to endothelin is preceded by a transient antihypertensive response, which is dose-dependent and lasts less than a minute (Yanagisawa et al. 1988b; Wright and Fozard 1988). The fall in blood pressure has been shown to be associated with increases in hindquarter and carotid vascular conductances but marked decreases in conductance in the renal and mesenteric vascular beds (Wright and Fozard 1988). The subsequent gradual rise in systemic pressure coincided with an intense vasoconstriction in all four vascular beds. The pressor effect of endothelin in autonomically uncompromised rats is accompanied by a marked suppression in heart rate, wheres reflex tachycardia is observed during the initial drop in blood pressure (Yanagisawa et al. 1988). In contrast to other vasoconstrictors, the pressor response to endothelin in rats is slow in onset, that is, it takes several minutes after bolus injection before the peak increase in blood pressure is reached. Conversely, it takes 1 h or longer until pressure has returned to baseline levels (Wright and Fozard 1988; Yanagisawa et al. 1988a,b). Similar observations were recently made in dogs (Goetz et al. 1988). Intravenous administration of the porcine/human peptide at rates of 10 and 30 ng/kg·min for 60 min increased dose-dependently arterial pressure, left and right atrial pressures, and total peripheral resistance. Heart rate and cardiac output were reduced. On a molar basis, endothelin appeared to be slightly less potent than vasopressin as a pressor agent in this study. A decline in circulating norepinephrine was observed at endothelin 10 ng/kg·min, probably indicating a decrease in sympathetic neural discharge mediated by a reflex from the arterial baroreceptors. At higher infusion rates both norepinephrine and epinephrine plasma levels increased, either by a direct effect of the peptide on the chromaffin cells of the adrenal medulla or due to acidosis resulting from the endothelin-induced reduction in blood flow (Goetz et al. 1988). The higher infusion rate caused an increase in plasma vasopressin, renin, aldosterone, and ANP. Elevated vasopressin plasma levels were only measured in those animals showing brief episodes of vomiting during peptide administration. Since vomiting is a well-known stimulus for vasopressin secretion, the endothelin effect on vasopressin was most likely mediated by this mechanism (Goetz et al. 1988). The observed increase in renin secretion following endothelin may be attributed to vasoconstriction of renal vessels proximal to the juxtaglomerular cells. Another possibility is a reduction in the amount of sodium reaching the macula densa. Stimulation of renin release by a direct action at the juxtaglomerular apparatus appears not very likely, considering the recent finding that endothelin attenuates renin release from dispersed rat juxtaglomerular cells (TAKAGI et al. 1988). The rise in ANP was probably due to the increase in atrial pressure observed during endothelin infusion (GOETZ et al. 1988). Whether the plasma concentrations of endothelin achieved in these experiments were sufficient to stimulate directly ANP release from the heart (see below) is uncertain.

As already suggested by the pressor effects of the peptide, endothelin is a powerful vasoconstrictor. This has been demonstrated in preparations of isolated blood vessels from various vascular beds (YANAGISAWA et al. 1988a; DE NUCCI et al. 1988). Venous strips appear to be more sensitive to endothelin than arterial strips. The rabbit jugular and mesenteric veins were reported to contract in response to as little as 0.5–2.5 pmol of the peptide (DE NUCCI et al. 1988). Similar to the blood pressure response the endothelin-induced contraction of arterial vessels is slow in onset and long-lasting (YANAGISAWA et al. 1988a,b). The maximum increase in tension of the rat aortic strips following administration of rat endothelin was found to be higher than that obtained with high concentrations of potassium chloride. The estimated EC_{50} values in this preparation were $5-6 \times 10^{-8}$ M for rat endothelin and 3×10^{-9} M for porcine/human endothelin (YANAGISAWA et al. 1988b). This compares very well with the response of ring segments of rat renal arteries and porcine coronary arteries, which were reported to contract at concentrations as low as 10^{-10} M with an EC_{50} for porcine/human endothelin of 2×10^{-9} M (TOMOBE et al. 1988; YANAGISAWA et al. 1988a).

Endothelin has at least three distinct effects on the heart. It is a potent coronary constrictor, increases cardiac contractility, and stimulates the release of ANP (YANAGISAWA et al. 1988a,b; HU et al. 1988a,b; ISHIKAWA et al. 1988; FUKUDA et al. 1988). As demonstrated in isolated hearts perfused at a constant rate, bolus injections of endothelin produce a marked, gradually developing rise in perfusion pressure, which in the case of porcine/human endothelin lasts for more than 1 h (YANAGISAWA et al. 1988a). We and others have found that the peptide increases the contraction amplitude of isolated, electrically driven left atria or spontaneously beating right atria from various species including humans (Fig. 1, HU et al. 1988a; ISHIKAWA et al. 1988). As observed in blood vessels, the tension that develops rises gradually over a period of 3–4 min after administration of the peptide to the organ bath until a stable plateau is reached. The threshold concentration required for obtaining a reproducible effect in rat atria is, according to our experiments, in the 10^{-9} M range (HU et al. 1988a). A maximal response, which is about 170% of the control, can be observed at concentrations between 10^{-8} and 10^{-7} M. Autonomic nerves appear not to be involved in the mediation of this effect, since it is not significantly affected by addition of adrenergic or cholinergic blockers. Heart rate is little affected in isolated, spontaneously beating left atria. The inotropic effect is long-lasting and persists even after repeated washing. As revealed by electrophysiological studies in guinea pig atria, endothelin increases the amplitude and duration of the plateau phase of the action potential (ISHIKAWA et al. 1988). Neither time to peak force nor relaxation are altered in the presence of the peptide (ISHIKAWA et al. 1988).

Endothelin is, at least in our hands, the only naturally occurring substance capable of increasing ANP release by a direct site of action at the heart (HU et al. 1988b). When added to isolated rat atria, it induces a gradual rise in ANP concentration in the bath medium, reaching a plateau after 5–10 min. At 10^{-7} *M* endothelin the levels increase to about 300% of control. The secretory response to endothelin is not significantly altered by the administration of α-, β-, and cholinergic blockers, which indicates that transmitter release from endogenous nerve endings is not involved in the mediation of this effect. Recent studies in cultured atrial cells support the view that endothelin acts directly at the heart muscle cells to induce ANP release (FUKUDA et al. 1988).

4.3 Mechanism of Action

In their first report, YANAGISAWA and coworkers proposed that endothelin induces vasoconstriction by acting directly on plasma membrane calcium channels (YANAGISAWA et al. 1988a). This speculation was based on the observation that endothelin shares some structural homologies with certain peptide toxins such as conotoxins or nuerotoxins from scorpion venoms which are known to bind to ion channels in the plasma membranes. Furthermore, these authors had found that the endothelin-induced contraction of vascular smooth muscle depends on extracellular calcium ions and can be inhibited by calcium channel blockers such as nicardipine. More recent studies, however, do not support the idea of endothelin being an endogenous calcium channel agonist (AUGUET et al. 1988; VAN RENTERGHEM et al. 1988; SUGIURA et al. 1989). When added to rabbit aortic vascular strips, partial constriction was observed in the absence of extracellular calcium, indicating that endothelin acts at least not exclusively by opening calcium channels (SUGIURA et al. 1989). In rat aortic smooth muscle cells in primary culture, endothelin has been shown to induce a rapid and sustained increase in cytosolic free calcium (HIRATA et al. 1988; KAI et al. 1989). The first component of this response, the rapid increase in calcium, was also observed in medium from which calcium was omitted. The sustained elevation, however, could be blocked by addition of calcium entry blockers (KAI et al. 1989).

Endothelin may therefore increase the intracellular free calcium concentration not only by an extracellular calcium-dependent mechanism but also by releasing calcium from intracellular stores. Such an action would be compatible with the activation of the phosphoinositol system by endothelin. In fact, quite a number of studies have now demonstrated that in cultured vascular smooth muscle cells endothelin provokes marked breakdown of phosphatidylinositol, producing inositol mono-, bis-, and triphosphates (VAN RENTERGHEM et al. 1988; RESINK et al. 1988; MARSDEN et al. 1989; SUGIURA et al. 1989). In accordance with the vasoconstrictor response to endothelin the increase in phosphatidylinositol metabolites is slow, reaching a maximum after several minutes as opposed to other vasoconstrictors such as angiotensin II (SUGIURA et al. 1989). Endothelin also promotes the production of diacylglycerol as demonstrated by experiments in smooth muscle cells prelabeled with [^{3}H]arachidonic acid (RESINK et al. 1988). Diacylglycerol is known to activate in the presence of calcium protein kinase C, which in turn has been proposed to be involved in the regulation of the sustained phase of agonist-induced vasoconstriction. Indirect evidence for a role of protein kinase C in the mediation of the vasoconstrictor effect of endothelin has been provided by experiments in which addition of the protein kinase C antagonist H7 induced relaxation of blood vessels preconstricted with the peptide (SUGIURA et al. 1989).

Endothelin may, however, operate not only through the activation of phospholipase C, resulting in an enhanced phosphoinositol turnover, but also by stimulating phospholipase A_2, the key enzyme in the sequence of events leading to the synthesis of biologically active metabolites of arachidonic acid (DE NUCCI et al. 1988; RESINK et al. 1989). This is suggested by the observation that indomethacin potentiates the pressor response to endothelin in pithed rats and, furthermore, by the fact that the peptide is a potent stimulator of prostacyclin and thromboxane A_2 release from the guinea pig lung (DE NUCCI et al. 1988). Moreover, endothelin has been reported to induce extracellular release of arachidonic acid products from rat and bovine aortic smooth muscle cells (RESINK et al. 1989). This effect is blocked by the phospholipase A_2 inhibitor quinacrine, whereas phospholipase C inhibitors are ineffective. Release of arachidonic acid metabolites might in part explain the transient fall in blood pressure observed after intravenous administration of endothelin (DE NUCCI et al. 1988; WRIGHT and FOZARD 1988). Another factor possibly involved in this effect is EDRF. DE NUCCI and coworkers (1988) observed dose-dependent vasodilatations when perfusing the rat mesentery with low concentrations (1–3 pmol) of endothelin. This effect was suppressed by oxyhemoglobin, which is known to inactivate EDRF, and largely reduced after removal of the endothelial cells in which EDRF is produced.

Specific binding sites for porcine/human endothelin have been demonstrated in cultured rat aortic smooth muscle cells (HIRATA et al. 1988). Scatchard analysis suggested a single class of high affinity binding sites; the maximal binding capacity was estimated at 11 000–13 000 sites per cell with a K_d of $2-4 \times 10^{-10}$ *M*. Bound [^{125}I]-endothelin showed little dissociation even after repeated washing. This may partly account for the long-lasting vasoconstrictor effect of the peptide, which is characteristically difficult to wash off.

4.4 Future Prospects

The discovery of endothelin, one of the most potent vasoconstrictor peptides, provides a new outlook on the mechanism of controlling vascular tone, peripheral resistance, and thereby blood pressure. Much of the current wave of data in this field has focussed on its purification, elucidation of the structure, and initial descriptions of the biological effectiveness of exogenously administered endothelin. Its participation in physiological and pathophysiological processes, however, still remains to be defined. The answer to this question will necessitate, first of all, the establishment of sensitive assays for the detection of endothelin. This would enable the evaluation of physiological stimuli for their ability to manipulate endothelin release. Since endothelial cells show only very few secretory granules, it appears most likely that this peptide is produced and immediately released without any storage. This would imply that the amount of endothelin leaving the cell is mainly determined by the rate of its synthesis. The only agents so far reported to stimulate preproendothelin synthesis at the level of mRNA transcription are thrombin, adrenaline, and the calcium ionophore A23 187 (YANAGISAWA et al. 1988a). Whether other stimuli previously described to induce endothelium-dependent vasoconstriction, such as hypoxia or sudden stretch, have similar effects awaits to be investigated. As hypoxic contractions are very rapid and readily reversible upon return to control oxygen tension, whereas contractions to endothelin are long-lasting and most difficult to wash out, it is not very likely that endothelin plays a part in the vascular response to hypoxia. Early studies in cultured endothelial cells, in which the vasoconstrictor activity in the media was determined by bioassay, also do not support a role of hypoxia in the control of endothelin production (O'BRIEN et al. 1987). The reported stimulation of endothelin gene expression by thrombin as well as the observation that thrombin increases the concentration of a vasoconstrictor activity in the supernatant of cultured endothelial cells would be consistent with the role of endothelin in blood pressure homeostasis. The rate of release of the vasoconstrictor activity in culture is low, both under basal conditions and following administration of thrombin (HICKEY et al. 1985; GILLESPIE et al. 1986). If this substance is identical with endothelin and if its release from cultured cells corresponds to in vivo conditions, one should anticipate that endothelin is not involved in the rapid control of vascular tone, but rather has a function in long-term regulation. This possibility is further strengthened by the characteristic time course of vasoconstriction in response to the peptide. In view of the extremely potent, long-lasting vasoconstrictor activity, it is intriguing to speculate that endothelin plays not only an important part in long-term blood pressure control but is also involved in the pathogenesis or maintenance of high blood pressure.

There is little hope that serum assays will help to uncover disturbances in the production of endothelin. Its presumably slow rate of release and rapid removal from circulation by the lungs (more than 50% in a single passage) suggest very low plasma levels of the peptide which probably do not reflect the events at the abluminal site of the endothelial cells (DE NUCCI et al. 1988). Approaches to answer the question of whether endothelin is a factor in the pathogenesis of hypertension should include studies concerned with the analysis of the endothelin gene, the enzymatic processing of the propeptide, and the characterization of respective receptors. Another obvious strategy would be the development of analogues which block the action of the peptide, thereby uncovering the contribution of endogenous endothelin to the regulation of vascular tone.

References

Aalkjaer C, Mulvany MJ, Nyborg NCB (1985) Atrial natriuretic factor causes specific relaxation of rat renal arcuate arteries. Br J Pharmacol 86:447–453

Adrian TE, Allen JM, Bloom SR, Ghatei MA, Rosser MN, Roberts GW, Crow TJ, Tatemoto K, Polak JM (1983a) Neuropeptide distribution in human brain. Nature 306:584–586

Adrian TE, Terenghi G, Brown MJ, Allen JM, Bacarese-Hamilton AJ, Polak JM, Bloom SR (1983b) Neuropeptide Y in pheochromocytomas and ganglioneuroblastomas. Lancet ii:540–543

Agnati LF, Fuxe K, Benfenati F, Celani MF, Battistini N et al. (1983) Differential modulation by CCK-8 and CCK-4 of [3H]spiperone binding sites linked to dopamine and 5-hydroxytryptamine receptors in the brain of the rat. Neurosci Lett 35:179–183

Allen JM, Adrian TE, Tatemoto K, Polak JM, Hughes J, Bloom SR (1982) Two novel related peptides, neuropeptide Y (NPY) and peptide YY (PYY) inhibit the contraction of the electrically stimulated mouse vas deferens. Neuropeptides 3:71–77

Allen JM, Bircham PMM, Edwards AV, Tatemoto K, Bloom SR (1983) Neuropeptide Y (NPY) reduces myocardial perfusion and inhibits the force of contraction of the isolated perfused rabbit heart. Regul Pept 6:247–253

Allen JM, Polak JM, Rodrigo J, Darcy K, Bloom SR (1985) Localisation of neuropeptide Y in nerves of the rat cardiovascular system and the effect of 6-hydroxydopamine. Cardiovasc Res 19:570–577

Allen JM, Gjorstrup P, Bjorkman JA, Ek L, Abrahamsson T, Bloom SR (1986) Studies on cardiac distribution and function of neuropeptide Y. Acta Physiol Scand 126: 405–411

Allen JM, Novotny J, Martin J, Heinrich G (1987a) Molecular structure of mammalian neuropeptide Y: analysis by molecular cloning and computer-aided comparison with crystal structure of avian homologue. Proc Natl Acad Sci USA 84:2532–2536

Allen JM, Yeats JC, Causon R, Brown MJ, Bloom SR (1987b) Neuropeptide Y and its flanking peptide in human endocrine tumors plasma. J Clin Endocrinol Metab 64:1199–1204

Allen YS, Adrian TE, Allen JM, Tatemoto K, Crow TJ, Bloom SR, Polak JM (1983) Neuropeptide Y distribution in rat brain. Science 221:877–879

Almeida FA, Suzuki M, Maack T (1986) Atrial natriuretic factor increases hematocrit and decreases plasma volume in nephrectomized rats. Life Sci 39:1193–1199

Amara SG, Jonas V, Rosenfeld MG, Ong ES, Evans RM (1982) Alternative RNA processing in calcitonin gene expression generates mRNA's encoding different polypeptide products. Nature 298:240–243

Anderson JV, Donckier J, McKenna WJ, Bloom SR (1986) The plasma release of atrial natriuretic peptide in man. Clin Sci 71:151–155

Anderson JV, Donckier J, Payne NN, Beacham J, Slater JDH, Bloom SR (1987) Atrial natriuretic peptide: evidence of action as a natriuretic hormone at physiological plasma concentrations in man. Clin Sci 72:305–312

Atarashi K, Mulrow PJ, Franco-Saenz R (1985) Effect of atrial peptides on aldosterone production. J Clin Invest 76:1807–1811

Auguet M, Delaflotte S, Chabrier P-E, Pirotzky E, Clostre F, Braquet P (1988) Endothelin and Ca^{++} agonist Bay K 8644: different vasoconstrictive properties. Biochem Biophys Res Commun 156:186–192

Bianchi C, Gutkowska J, Thibault G, Garcia R, Genest J, Cantin M (1985) Radioautographic localization of ^{125}I-atrial natriuretic factor (ANF) in rat tissues. Histochemistry 82:441–452

Biollaz J, Nussberger J, Porchet M, Brunner-Ferber F, Otterbein E, Gomez H, Waeber B, Brunner HR (1986) Four-hour infusions of synthetic atrial natriuretic peptide in normal volunteers. Hypertension 8:II96–II105

Blundell TL, Pitts JE, Tickle IJ, Wood SP, Wu CW (1981) X-ray analysis of avian pancreatic polypeptide: small globular protein hormone. Proc Natl Acad Sci USA 78:4175–4179

Brain SD, Williams TJ, Tippins JR, Morris HR, MacIntyre I (1985) Calcitonin gene-related peptide is a potent vasodilator. Nature 313:54–56
Brain SD, Williams TJ (1988) Substance P regulates the vasodilutor activity of calcitonin gene-related peptide. Nature 335:73–75
Breuhaus BA, Saneii HH, Brandt MA, Chimoskey JE (1985) Atriopeptin II lowers cardiac output in conscious sheep. Am J Physiol 249:R776–R780
Briggs JP, Steipe B, Schubert G, Schnermann J (1982) Micropuncture studies of the renal effects of atrial natriuretic substance. Pflügers Arch 395:271–276
Burnett JC Jr, Granger JP, Opgenorth TS (1984) Effects of synthetic atrial natriuretic factor on renal function and renin release. Am J Physiol 247:F863–F866
Bussien JP, Biollaz J, Waeber B, Nussberger J, Turini GA, Brunner HR, Brunner-Ferber F, Gomez HJ, Otterbein ES (1986) Dose-dependent effect of atrial natriuretic peptide on blood pressure, heart rate, and skin blood flow of normal volunteers. J Cardiovasc Pharmacol 8:216–220
Carter DA, Vallejo M, Lightman SL (1985) Cardiovascular effects of neuropeptide Y in the nucleus tractus solitarius of rats: relationship with noradrenaline and vasopressin. Peptides 6:421–425
Chang RSL, Lotti VL, Chen T, Cerino DJ, Kling PJ (1985) Neuropeptide Y (NPY) binding sites in rat brain labelled with ^{125}J-Bolton-Hunter NPY: comparative potencies of various polypeptides on brain NPY binding and biological responses in the rat vas deferens. Life Sci 37:2111–2122
Chartier L, Schiffrin E, Thibault G, Garcia R (1984) Atrial natriuretic factor inhibits the stimulation of aldosterone secretion by angiotensin II, ACTH and potassium in vitro and angiotensin II-induced steroidogenesis in vivo. Endocrinology 115:2026–2028
Clarke JG, Kerwin R, Larkin S, Lee Y, Yacoub M, Davies GJ, Hackett D, Dawbarn D, Bloom SR, Maseri A (1987) Coronary artery infusion of neuropeptide Y in patients with angina pectoris. Lancet:1057–1059
Cocks TM, Angus JA (1983) Endothelium-dependent relaxation of coronary arteries by noradrenaline and serotonin. Nature 305:627–630
Cody RJ, Atlas SA, Laragh JH et al. (1986) Atrial natriuretic factor in normal subjects and heart failure patients. J Clin Invest 78:1362–1374
Cohen ML, Schenck KW (1984) Atriopeptin II: differential sensitivity of arteries and veins from the rat. Eur J Pharmacol 108:103–104
Dahlöf C, Dahlöf P, Lundberg JM (1985a) Neuropeptide Y (NPY): Enhancement of blood pressure increase upon α-adrenoceptor activation and direct pressor effects in pithed rats. Eur J Pharmacol 109:289–292
Dahlöf C, Dahlöf P, Tatemoto K, Lundberg JM (1985b) Neuropeptide Y (NPY) reduces field stimulation evoked release of noradrenaline and enhances force of contraction in the rat portal vein. Naunyn Schmiedeberg's Arch Pharmacol 328:327–330
Dahlöf P, Persson K, Lundberg JM, Dahlöf C (1988) Neuropeptide Y (NPY) induced inhibition of preganglionic nerve stimulation evoked release of adrenalin and noradrenaline in the pithed rat. Acta Physiol Scand 132:51–57
Day ML, Schwartz D, Rodi C, Rankin A, Needleman P, Wiegand R (1986) Enhanced atriopeptin mRNA and immunoreactivity in atria and ventricles treated with dexamethasone. Fed Proc 45:601–607
De Bold AJ, Borenstein HB, Veress AT, Sonnenberg H (1981) A rapid and potent natriuretic response to intravenous injection of atrial myocardial extract in rats. Life Sci 28:89–94
De Lean A, Racz K, Gutkowska J, Nguyen TT, Cantin M, Genest J (1984) Specific receptor-mediated inhibition by synthetic atrial natriuretic factor of hormone-stimulated steroidogenesis in cultured bovine adrenal cells. Endocrinology 115:1636–1638
De Lean A, Vinay P, Cantin M (1985) Distribution of atrial natriuretic factor receptors in dog kidney fractions. FEBS Lett 193:239
De Mey JG, Vanhoutte PM (1983) Anoxia and endothelium-dependent reactivity of the canine femoral artery. J Physiol (Lond) 335:65–74
De Mey JG, Claeys M, Vanhoutte PM (1982) Endothelium-dependent inhibitory effects of acetylcholine, adenosine triphosphate, thrombin and arachidonic acid in the canine femoral artery. J Pharmacol Exp Ther 222:166–173

De Nucci G, Thomas R, D'Orleans-Juste P, Antunes E, Walder C, Warner TD, Vane JR (1988) Pressor effects of circulating endothelin are limited by its removal in the pulmonary circulation and by the release of prostacyclin and endothelium-derived relaxing factor. Proc Natl Acad Sci USA 85:9797–9800

De Quidt ME, Emson PC (1986) Distribution of neuropeptide Y-like immunoreactivity in the rat central nervous system—II. Immunohistochemical analysis. Neuroscience 18:545–618

Dietz JR (1984) Release of natriuretic factor from heart-lung preparation by atrial distension. Am J Physiol 247:R1093–R1096

Edvinsson L, Ekblad E, Hakanson R, Wahlestedt C (1984) Neuropeptide Y potentiates the effect of various vasoconstrictor agents on rabbit blood vessels. Br J Pharmacol 83:519–525

Edvinsson L, Fredholm B, Hamel E, Janssen I, Verechia C (1985) Perivascular peptides relax cerebral arteries concomittant with stimulation of cyclic adenosine monophosphate accumulation or release of an endothelium-derived relaxing factor in the cat. Neurosci Lett 58:213–217

Edvinsson L, Hakanson R, Wahlestedt C, Uddman R (1987) Effects of neuropeptide Y on the cardiovascular system. Trends Pharmacol Sci 8:231–235

Ekblad E, Edvinsson L, Wahlestedt C, Uddman R, Hakanson R, Sundler F (1984) Neuropeptide Y co-exists and co-operates with noradrenaline in perivascular nerve fibers. Regul Pept 8:225–235

Emson PC, de Quidt ME (1984) NPY—a new member of the pancreatic polypeptide family. Trends Neurol Sci 7:1–4

Ensinger H, Hedler L, Schurr C, Starke K (1984) Ethyletocyclazocine decreases noradrenaline release and blood pressure in the rabbit at a peripheral opioid receptor. Naunyn-Schmiedeberg's Arch Pharmacol 328:20–23

Eskay R, Zukowska-Grojec Z, Haass M, Dave JR, Zamir N (1986) Circulating atrial natriuretic peptides in conscious rats: regulation of release by multiple factors. Science 232:636–639

Everitt BJ, Hökfelt T, Terenius L, Tatemoto K, Mutt V, Goldstein M (1983) Differential coexistence of neuropeptide Y (NPY)-like immunoreactivity with catecholamines in the central nervous system of the rat. Neuroscience 11:443–462

Faison EP, Siegl PKS, Morgan G, Winquist RJ (1985) Regional vasorelaxant selectivity of atrial natriuretic factor in isolated rabbit vessels. Life Sci 37:1073–1079

Fisher LA, Kikkawa DO, Rivier JE, Amara R, Rosenfeld MG, Vale WW, Brown MR (1983) Stimulation of noradrenergic sympathetic outflow by calcitonin gene-related peptide. Nature 305:534–536

Flynn TG, de Bold ML, de Bold AJ (1983) The amino acid sequence of an atrial peptide with potent diuretic and natriuretic properties. Biochem Biophys Res Commun 117:859–865

Folkow B, Hallback M, Lundgren R, Sivertsson R, Weiss L (1982) Importance of adaptive changes in vascular design for establishment of primary hypertension studied in man and in spontaneously hypertensive rats. Circ Res 32,33:I2–I16

Fontaine B, Klarsfeld A, Changeux J-P (1987) Calcitonin gene related peptide and muscle activity regulate acetylcholine receptor α-subunit mRNA levels by distinct intracellular pathways. J Cell Biol 105:1337–1342

Foster GV, Byfield PGH, Gudmunsson TV (1972) Calcitonin. Clin Endocrinol Metab 1:93–101

Franco-Cereceda A, Lundberg JM (1985) Calcitonin gene-related peptide (CGRP) and capsaicin-induced stimulation of heart contractile rate and force. Naunyn-Schmiedeberg's Arch Pharmacol 331:146–151

Franco-Cereceda A, Lundberg JM (1987) Potent effects of neuropeptide Y and calcitonin gene-related peptide on human coronary vascular tone in vitro. Acta Physiol Scand 131:159–160

Franco-Cereceda A, Bengtsson L, Lundberg JM (1987a) Inotropic effects of calcitonin gene-related peptide, vasoactive intestinal polypetide and somatostatin on the human right atrium in vitro. Eur J Pharmacol 134:69–76

Franco-Cereceda A, Gennarini C, Nami R, Agnusdei D, Pernow J, Lundberg JM,

Fischer JA (1987b) Cardiovascular effects of calcitonin gene-related peptides I and II in man. Circ Res 60:393–397
Franco-Cereceda A, Henke H, Lundberg JM, Petermann JB, Hökfelt T, Fischer JA (1987c) Calcitonin gene-related peptide (CGRP) in capsaicin-sensitive substance P-immunoreactive sensory neurons in animals and man: distribution and release by capsaicin. Peptides 8:399–410
Freeman RH, Davis JO, Vari RC (1985) Renal response to atrial natriuretic factor in conscious dogs with caval constriction. Am J Physiol 248:R495–R500
Fukuda Y, Hirata Y, Yoshimi H, Kojima T, Kobayashi Y, Yanagisawa M, Masaki T (1988) Endothelin is a potent secretagogue for arterial natriuretic peptide in cultured rat atrial myocytes. Biochem Biophys Res Commun 155:167–172
Fuller F, Porter JG, Arfsten AE, Miller J, Schilling JW, Scarborough RM, Lewicki JA, Schenk DB (1988) Atrial natriuretic peptide clearance receptor: complete sequence and functional expression of cDNA clones. J Biol Chem 263:9395–9401
Furchgott RF, Zawadzki JV (1980) The obligatory role of endothelial cells in the relaxation of arterial smooth muscle by acetylcholine. Nature 288:373–376
Fuxe K, Agnati LF, Härfstrand A, Zini I, Tatemoto K, Pich EM, Hökfelt T (1983) Central administration of neuropeptide Y induces hypotension, bradypnoe and EEG synchronization in the rat. Acta Physiol Scand 118:189–192
Ganten D, Minnich JL, Granger P, Hayduk K, Brecht HM, Barbeau A, Boucher R, Genest J (1971) Angiotensin-forming enzyme in brain tissue. Science 173:64–65
Ganten D, Hermann K, Bayer C, Unger T, Lang RE (1983) Angiotensin Synthesis in the brain and increased turnover in hypertensive rats. Science 221:869–871
Ganten D, Lang RE, Lehmann E, Unger T (1984) Commentary; Brain angiotensin: on the way to becoming a well-studied neuropeptide system. Biochem Pharmacol 33 (22):3523–3528
Garcia R, Thibault G, Cantin M, Genest J (1984) Effect of a purified atrial natriuretic factor on rat and rabbit vascular strips and vascular beds. Am J Physiol 247:R34–R39
Garcia R, Thibault G, Gutkowska J, Horky K, Hamet P, Cantin M, Genest J (1985a) Chronic infusion of low doses of atrial natriuretic factor (ANF arg 101-tyr 126) reduces blood pressure in conscious SHR without apparent changes in sodium excretion. Proc Soc Exp Biol Med 179:396–401
Garcia R, Thibault G, Seidah NG, Lazure C, Cantin M, Genest J, Chretien M (1985b) Structure-activity relationships of atrial natriuretic factor (ANF) II. Effect of chain-length modifications on vascular reactivity. Biochem Biophys Res Commun 126: 178–184
Gardner DG, Deschepper CF, Ganong WF, Hane S, Fiddes J, Baxter JD, Lewicki J (1986) Extra-atrial expression of the gene for atrial natriuretic factor. Proc Natl Acad Sci USA 83:6697–6701
Gellai M, DeWolf RE, Kiner LB, Beeuwkes R III (1986) The effect of atrial natriuretic factor on blood pressure, heart rate, and renal functions in conscious, spontaneously hypertensive rats. Circ Res 59:56–62
Gerstheimer FP, Metz J (1986) Distribution of calcitonin gene related peptide-like immunoreactivity in the guinea pig heart. Anat Embryol (Berl) 175:255–260
Gillespie MN, Owasoyo JO, McMurtry IF, O'Brien RF (1986) Sustained coronary vasoconstriction provoked by a peptidergic substance released from endothelial cells in culture. J Pharmacol Exp Ther 236:339–343
Glover ID, Bartlow DI, Pitts JE, Wood SP, Tickle IJ, Blundell TL, Tatemoto K, Kimmel JR, Wollmer A, Strassburger W, Zhang Y (1985) Conformational studies on the pancreatic polypeptide hormone family. Eur J Biochem 142:379–385
Goetz KL, Wang BC, Madwed JB, Zhu JL, Leadley RJ Jr (1988) Cardiovascular, renal, and endocrine responses to intravenous endothelin in conscious dogs. Am J Physiol 255:R1064–R1068
Goodfriend TL, Elliott M, Atlas SA (1984) Actions of synthetic atrial natriuretic factor on bovine adrenal glomerulosa. Life Sci 35:1675–1682
Gu J, Polak JM, Allen JM, Huang WM, Sheppard MN, Tatemoto K, Bloom SR (1984) High concentrations of a novel peptide, neuropeptide Y, in the innervation of mouse and rat heart. J Histochem Cytochem 32:467–472

Gutkowska J, Kuchel O, Racz K, Buu NT, Cantin M, Genest J (1986) Increased plasma immunoreactive atrial natriuretic factor concentrations in salt sensitive Dahl rats. Biochem Biophys Res Commun 136:411–416

Haass M, Skofitsch G (1985) Cardiovascular effects of calcitonin gene-related peptide in the pithed rat: comparison with substance P. Life Sci 37:2085–2090

Haass M, Zamir N, Zukowska-Grojec Z (1986) Plasma levels of atrial natriuretic peptides in conscious adult spontaneously hypertensive rats. Clin Exp Hypertens [A] 8:277–287

Hackenthal E, Aktories K, Jakobs KH, Lang RE (1987) Neuropeptide Y inhibits renin release by a pertussis toxin-sensitive mechanism. Am J Physiol 252:F543–F550

Häggblad J, Fredholm BB (1987) Adenosine and neuropeptide Y enhance α_1-adrenoceptor-induced accumulation of inositol phosphate and attenuate forskolin-induced accumulation of cyclic AMP in rat vas deferens. Neurosci Lett 82:211–216

Hamet P, Tremblay J, Pang SC, Garcia R, Thibault G, Gutkowska J, Cantin M, Genest J (1984) Effect of native and synthetic atrial natriuretic factor on cyclic GMP. Biochem Biophys Res Commun 123:515–527

Hanley MR (1985) Neuropeptides as mitogens. Nature 315:14–15

Hassall CJS, Burnstock G (1986) Intrinsic neurons and associated cells of the guinea-pig heart in culture. Brain Res 364:102–113

Hescheler J, Rosenthal W, Hinsch K-D, Wulfern M, Trautwein W, Schultz G (1988) Angiotensin II-induced stimulation of voltage-dependent Ca^{2+} currents in an adrenal cortical cell line. EMBO J 7:619–624

Hickey KA, Rubany G, Paul RJ, Highsmith RF (1985) Characterization of a coronary vasoconstrictor produced by cultured endothelial cells. Am J Physiol 248:C550–C556

Hirata Y, Tomita M, Takada S, Yoshimi H (1985) Vascular receptor binding activities and cyclic GMP responses by synthetic human and rat atrial natriuretic peptides (ANF) and receptor down-regulation by ANP. Biochem Biophys Res Commun 128:538–546

Hirata Y, Yoshimi H, Takata S, Watanabe TX, Kumagai S, Nakajima K, Sakakibara S (1988) Cellular mechanism of action by a novel vasoconstrictor endothelin in cultured rat vascular smooth muscle cells. Biochem Biophys Res Commun 154:868–875

Hiwatari M, Satoh K, Angus JA, Johnston CI (1986) No effect of atrial natriuretic factor on cardiac rate, force and transmitter release. Clin Exp Pharmacol Physiol 13: 163–168

Hökfelt T, Johansson O, Ljungdahl A, Lundberg JM, Schultzberg M (1980) Peptidergic neurones. Nature 284:515–521

Hökfelt T, Lundberg JM, Lagercrantz H, Tatemoto K, Mutt V, Lundberg JM, Terenius L, Everitt BJ, Fuxe K, Agnati LF, Goldstein M (1983) Occurrence of neuropeptide Y (NPY)-like immunoreactivity in catecholamine neurons in the human medulla oblongata. Neurosci Lett 36:217–222

Hökfelt T, Johansson O, Goldstein M (1984) Chemical anatomy of the brain. Science 225:1326–1334

Holden WE, McCall E (1984) Hypoxia-induced contractions of porcine pulmonary artery strips depend on intact endothelium. Exp Lung Res 7:101–112

Hu JR, Berninger UG, Lang RE (1988a) Endothelin stimulates atrial natriuretic peptide (ANP) release from rat atria. Eur J Pharmacol 158:177–178

Hu JR, von Harsdorf R, Lang RE (1988b) Endothelin has potent inotropic effects in rat atria. Eur J Pharmacol 158:275–278

Huang CL, Lewicki J, Johnson LK, Cogan MG (1985) Renal mechanism of action of rat atrial natriuretic factor. J Clin Invest 75:769–773

Illes P, Pfeiffer N, Kügelgen IV, Starke K (1985) Presynaptic opioid receptor subtypes in the rabbit ear artery. J Pharmacol Exp Ther 232:526–533

Imada T, Takayanagi R, Inagami T (1985) Changes in the content of atrial natriuretic factor with the progression of hypertension in spontaneously hypertensive rats. Biochem Biophys Res Commun 133:759–765

Ishikawa T, Yanagisawa M, Kimura S, Goto K, Masaki T (1988) Positive inotropic action of novel vasoconstrictor peptide endothelin on guinea pig atria. Am J Physiol 255: H970–H973

Itoh Y, Yanagisawa M, Ohkubo S, Kimura C, Kosaka T, Inoue A, Ishida N, Mitsui Y, Onda H, Fujimo M, Masaki T (1988) Cloning and sequence analysis of cDNA encoding the precursor of a human endothelium-derived vasoconstrictor peptide, endothelin: identity of human and porcine endothelin. FEBS Lett 231:440–444
Joint Nomenclature and Standardization Committee of the International Society of Hypertension American Heart Association and the World Health Organization (1987) J Hypertens 5
Ju G, Hökfelt T, Brodin E, Fahrenkrug J, Fischer JA, Frey P, Elde RP, Brown JC (1987) Primary sensory neuron of the rat showing calcitonin gene-related peptide immunoreactivity and their relation to substance P-, somatostatin-, galanin-, vasoactive intestinal polypeptide- and cholecystokinin-immunoreactive ganglion cells. Cell Tissue Res 247:417–431
Kaczmarek LK, Levitan IB (1987) What is neuromodulation? In: Kacmarek LK, Levitan IB (eds) Neuromodulation. Oxford University Press, New York, p 3
Kai H, Kanaide H, Nakamura M (1989) Endothelin-sensitive intracellular Ca^{2+} store overlaps with caffeine-sensitive one in rat aortic smooth muscle cells in primary culture. Biochem Biophys Res Commun 158:235–243
Kangawa K, Fukuda A, Kubota I, Hayashi Y, Matsue H (1984) Identification in rat atrial tissue of multiple forms of natriuretic polypeptides of about 3000 daltons. Biochem Biophys Res Commun 121:585–591
Kasakov L, Ellis J, Kirkpatrick K, Milner P, Burnstock G (1988) Direct evidence for concomitant release of noradrenaline, adenosine 5′-triphosphate and neuropeptide Y from sympathetic nerve supplying the guinea-pig vas deferens. J Auton Nerv Syst 22:75–82
Katsube N, Wakitani K, Fok FK, Tjoeng FS, Zupec ME, Eubanks SR, Adams SP, Needleman P (1985) Differential structure-activity relationships of atrial peptides as natriuretics and renal vasodilators in the dog. Biochem Biophys Res Commun 128:325–330
Kleinert HD, Volpe M, Odell G, Marion D, Atlas SA, Camargo MJ, Laragh JH, Maack T (1986) Cardiovascular effects of atrial natriuretic factor in anesthetized and conscious dogs. Hypertension 8:312–316
Kubota M, Mosely JM, Butera L, Dusting GJ, MacDonald PS, Martin TJ (1985) Calcitonin gene-related peptide stimulates cyclic AMP formation in rat aortic muscle cells. Biochem Biophys Res Commun 132:88–94
Kudo T, Baird A (1984) Inhibition of aldosterone production in the adrenal glomerulosa by atrial natriuretic factor. Nature 312:756–757
Kurtz A, Bruna RD, Pfeilschifter J, Tangner R, Bauer C (1986) Atrial natriuretic peptide inhibits renin release from juxtaglomerular cells by a cGMP-mediated process. Proc Natl Acad Sci USA 83:4769–4773
Lang RE, Thölken H, Ganten D, Luft FC, Ruskoaho H, Unger T (1985) Atrial natriuretic factor—a circulating hormone stimulated by volume loading. Nature 314: 264–266
Lappe RW, Smits JFM, Todt JA, Debets JJM, Wendt RL (1985a) Failure of atriopeptin II cause arterial vasodilation in the conscious rat. Circ Res 56:606–612
Lappe RW, Todt JA, Wendt RL (1985b) Mechanisms of action of vasoconstrictor responses to atriopeptin II in conscious SHR. Am J Physiol 249:R781–R786
Lappe RW, Todt JA, Wendt RL (1987) Regional vasodilator actions of calcitonin gene-related peptide in conscious SHR. Peptidess 8:747–749
Larose P, Meloche S, de Suich P, De Lean A, Ong H (1985) Radio-immunoassay of atrial natriuretic factor: human plasma levels. Biochem Biophys Res Commun 130:553–558
Lattion AL, Michel JB, Arnauld E, Corrol P, Soubrier F (1986) Myocardial recruitment during ANF mRNA increase in response to volume overload in the rat. Am J Physiol 251:H890–H896
Ledsome JR, Wilson N, Courneya CA, Rankin AJ (1985) Release of atrial natriuretic peptide by atrial distension. Can J Physiol Pharmacol 63:739–742
Lee CY, Takasaki C, Yanagisawa M, Kimura S, Goto K, Masaki T (1988) Similarity of endothelin to snake venom toxin. Nature 335:303
Leiter AB, Keutmann HT, Goodman RH (1984) Structure of a precursor to human

pancreatic polypeptide. J Biol Chem 259:14702–14705
Leitman DC, Murad F (1986) Comparison of binding and cyclic GMP accumulation by atrial natriuretic peptides in endothelial cells. Biochem Biophys Res Commun 885: 74–79
Leitman DC, Andresen JW, Catalano RM, Waldman SA, Tuan JJ, Murad F (1988) Atrial natriuretic peptide binding, crosslinking, and stimulation of cyclic GMP accumulation and particulate guanylate cyclase activity in cultured cells. J Biol Chem 263:3720–3728
Lenz HJ, Rivier JE, Brown MR (1985) Biological actions of human and rat calcitonin gene-related peptide. Regul Pept 12:81–89
Lewicki JA, Greenberg B, Yamanaka M, Vlasuk G, Brewer M, Gardner D, Baxter J, Johnson LK, Fiddess JC (1986) Cloning, sequence analysis, and processing of the rat and human atrial natriuretic peptide precursors. Fed Proc 45:2086–2090
Leys K, Schachter M, Sever P (1987) Autoradiographic localisation of NPY receptors in rabbit kidney: comparison with rat, guinea-pig and human. Eur J Pharmacol 134: 233–237
Lundberg JM, Hökfelt T (1983) Coexistence of peptides and classical transmitters. Trendo Neurol Sci 6:325–333
Lundberg JM, Stjärne L (1984) Neuropeptide Y (NPY) depresses the secretion of ^{3}H-noradrenaline and the contractile response evoked by field stimulation, in the rat vas deferens. Acta Physiol Scand 120:477–479
Lundberg JM, Tatemoto K (1982) Pancreatic polypeptide family (APP, BPP, NPY and PYY) in relation to α-adrenoceptor-resistant sympathetic vasoconstriction. Acta Physiol Scand 116:393–402
Lundberg JM, Terenius L, Hökfelt T, Martling C-R, Tatemoto K, Mutt V, Polak JM, Bloom SR (1982) Neuropeptide Y (NPY)-like immunoreactivity in peripheral noradrenergic neurons and effects of NPY on sympathetic function. Acta Physiol Scand 116:477–480
Lundberg JM, Hua XY, Franco-Cereceda A (1984a) Effects of neuropeptide Y (NPY) on mechanical activity and neurotransmission in the heart, vas deferens and urinary bladder of the guinea-pig. Acta Physiol Scand 121:325–332
Lundberg JM, Terenius L, Hökfelt T, Tatemoto K (1984b) Comparative immunohistochemical and biochemical analysis of pancreatic polypetide-like peptides with special reference to presence of neuropeptide Y in central and peripheral neurons. J Neurosci 4:2376–2386
Lundberg JM, Franco-Cereceda A, Hua X, Hökfelt T, Fischer JA (1985a) Co-existence of substance P and calcitonin gene-related peptide immunoreactivities in sensory nerves in relation to cardiovascular bornchoconstrictor effects of capsaicin. Eur J Pharmacol 108:315–322
Lundberg JM, Saria A, Franco-Cereceda A, Hökfelt T, Terenius L, Goldtein M (1985b) Differential effects of reserpine and 6-hydroxydopamine on neuropeptide Y (NPY) and noradrenaline in peripheral neurons. Naunyn-Schmiedeberg's Arch Pharmacol 328:386–401
Lundberg JM, Torssell L, Sollevi A, Theodorsson-Norheim E, Pernow J, Änggard A, Hamberger B (1985c) Neuropeptide Y and sympathetic vascular control in man. Regul Pept 13:41–52
Lundberg JM, Rudehill JM, Sollevi A, Theodorsson-Norheim E, Hamberger B (1986) Frequency- and reserpine-dependent chemical coding of sympathetic transmission: differential release of noradrenaline and neuropeptide Y from pig spleen. Neurosci Lett 36:96–100
Lundberg JM, Hemsen A, Larsson O, Rudehill A, Saria A, Fredholm BB (1988) Neuropeptide Y receptor in pig spleen: binding characteristics, reduction of cyclic AMP formation and calcium antagonist inhibition of vasoconstriction. Eur J Pharmacol 145:21–29
Maack T (1985) Atrial natriuretic factor: structure and functional properties. Kidney Int 27:607–615
Maack T, Marion DN, Camargo MJF, Kleinert HD, Laragh JH, Vaughan ED Jr, Atlas SA (1984) Effect of auriculin (atrial natriuretic factor) on blood pressure, renal

function and the renin-aldosterone system in dogs. Am J Med 77:1069–1075
Maack T, Suzuki M, Almeida FA et al. (1987) Physiological role of silent receptors of atrial natriuretic factor. Science 238:675–677
Maki M, Takayanagi R, Misono KS, Pandey KN, Tibbetts C, Inagami T (1984) Structure of rat atrial natriuretic factor precursor deduced from cDNA sequences. Nature 309:722–724
Marsden PA, Danthuluri NR, Brenner BM, Ballermann BJ, Brock TA (1989) Endothelin action on vascular smooth muscle involves inositol triphosphate and calcium mobilization. Biochem Biophys Res Commun 158:86–93
Marsh EA, Seymour AA, Haley AB, Whinney MA, Napier MA, Nutt RF, Blaine EH (1985) Renal blood pressure responses to synthetical atrial natriuretic factor in spontaneously hypertensive rats. Hypertension 7:386–391
McEwan J, Larkin S, Davies G, Chierchia S, Brown M, Stevenson J, MacIntyre I, Maseri A (1986) Calcitonin gene-related peptide: a potent dilator of human epicardial coronary arteries. Circulation 74:1243–1247
Minth CD, Andrews PC, Dixon JE (1986) Characterization, sequence, and expression of the cloned human neuropeptide Y gene. J Biol Chem 261:11974–11979
Moncada S, Glryglewski R, Bunting S, Vane JR (1976) An enzyme isolated from arteries transforms prostaglandin endoperoxidase to an unstable substance that inhibits platelet aggregation. Nature 263:663–665
Morii N, Nakao K, Kihara M, Sugawara A, Skamoto M, Yamori Y, Imura H (1986) Decreased content in left atrium and increased plasma concentration of atrial natriuretic polypeptide in spontaneously hypertensive rats (SHR) and SHR stroke-prone. Biochem Biophys Res Commun 135:74–81
Mulderry PK, Ghatei MA, Rodrigo J, Allen JM, Rosenfeld MG, Polak JM, Bloom SR (1985) Calcitonin gene-related peptide in cardiovascular tissue of the rat. Neuroscience 14:947–954
Müller FB, Erne P, Raine AEG, Bolli P, Linder L, Resink TJ, Cottier C, Bühler FR (1986) Atrial antipressor natriuretic peptide: release mechanisms and vascular action in man. J Hypertens 4:S109–S114
Murray RD, Itoh S, Inagami T, Misono K, Seto S, Scicli AG, Carretero OA (1985) Effects of synthetic atrial natriuretic factor in the isolated perfused rat kidney. Am J Physiol 249:F603–F609
Nakayama K, Ohkubo H, Hirose T, Inayama S, Nakanishi S (1984) mRNA sequence for human cardiodilatin-atrial natriuretic factor precursor and regulation of precursor mRNA in rat atria. Nature 23:699–701
Napier MA, Vandlen RL, Albers-Schöberg G, Nutt RF, Brady S, Lyle T, Winquist R, Faison EP, Heinel LA, Blaine EH (1984) Specific membrane receptors for atrial natriuretic factor in renal and vascular tissues. Proc Natl Acad Sci USA 81:5946–5950
Nemer M, Chamberland M, Sirois D, Argentin S, Drouin J, Dixon RAF, Zivin RA, Condra JH (1984) Gene structure of the human cardiac hormone precursor, pronatriodilatin. Nature 312:654–656
O'Brien RF, Robbins RJ, McMurty IF (1987) Endothelial cells in culture produce a vasoconstrictor substance. J Cell Physiol 132:263–270
Oikawa S, Imai M, Veno A, Tanaka S, Nogushi T, Nkazato H, Kangawa K, Fukuda A, Matsuo H (1984) Cloning and sequence analysis of cDNA encoding a precursor for human atrial natriuretic polypeptide. Nature 309:724–726
Opgenorth TJ, Burnett JC Jr, Granger JP, Scriven TA (1986) Effects of atrial natriuretic peptide on renin secretion in nonfiltering kidney. Am J Physiol 250:F798–F801
Osol G, Halpern W, Tesfamarian B, Nakayama K, Weinberg D (1986) Synthetic atrial natriuretic factor does not dilate resistance-sized arteries. Hypertension 8:606–610
Palmer RMJ, Ferrige AG, Moncada S (1987) Nitric oxide release accounts for the biological activity of endothelium-derived relaxing factor. Nature 327:524–526
Perlman MO, Perlman JM, Adamo ML, Hazelwood RL, Dyckes DF (1987) Binding of C-terminal segments of neuropeptide Y to chicken brain. Int J Pept Protein Res 30:153–162
Pernow J, Saria A, Lundberg JM (1986) Mechanisms underlying pre- and postjunctional effects of neuropeptide Y in sympathetic vascular control. Acta Physiol Scand 126:

239–249

Pernow J, Öhlen A, Hökfelt T, Nilsson O, Lundberg JM (1987a) Neuropeptide Y: presence in perivascular noradrenergic neurons and vasoconstrictor effects on skeletal muscle blood vessels in experimental animals and man. Regul Pept 19: 313–324

Pernow J, Svenberg T, Lundberg JM (1987b) Actions of calcium antagonists on pre- and postjunctional effects of neuropeptide Y on human peripheral blood vessels in vitro. Eur J Pharmacol 136:207–218

Polak JM, Bloom SR (1984) Regulatory peptides the distribution of two newly discovered peptides: PHI and NPY Peptides: 5 (Suppl) 79–89

Potter E (1987) Presynaptic inhibition of cardiac vagal postganglionic nerves by neuropeptide Y. Neurosci Lett 83:101–106

Rapaport RM, Dmeznim MB, Murad F (1983) Endothelium-dependent relaxation in rat aorta may be mediated through cyclic GMP-dependent protein phosphorylation. Nature 306:174–176

Reinecke M (1987) Untersuchungen zur peptidergen Innervation des Herzens. Verh Anat Ges 81:115–127

Resink TJ, Scott-Burden T, Bühler FR (1988) Endothelin stimulates phospholipase C in cultured vascular smooth muscle cells. Biochem Biophys Res Commun 157:1360–1368

Resink TJ, Scott-Burden T, Bühler FR (1989) Activation of phospholipase A_2 by endothelin in cultured vascular smooth muscle cells. Biochem Biophys Res Commun 158:279–286

Reynolds EE, Shinji Y (1988) Neuropeptide Y receptor-effector coupling mechanisms in cultured vascular smooth muscle cells. Biochem Biophys Res Commun 151:919–925

Richards AM, Nicholls MG, Ikram H, Webster MW, Yandle TG, Espiner EA (1985a) Renal, hemodynamic and hormonal effects of human α atrial natriuretic peptide in healthy volunteeers. Lancet 1:545–548

Richards AM, Nicholls MG, Espiner EA, Ikram H, Yandle TG, Joyce SL, Cullens MM (1985b) Effects of α-human atrial natriuretic peptide in essential hypertension. Hypertension 7:812–817

Richardt G, Haass M, Neeb S, Hock M, Lang RE, Schömig A (1988) Nicotine-induced release of noradrenaline and neuropeptide Y in guinea-pig heart. Klin Wochenschr 66:21–27

Rioux F, Bachelard H, Martel J-C, St-Pierre S (1986) The vasoconstrictor effect of neuropeptide Y and related peptides in the guinea-pig isolated heart. Peptides 7: 27–31

Rosenfeld MG, Mermod JJ, Amava SG, Swanon LW, Sawchenko PE, Rivier J, Vale WW, Evans RM (1983) Production of a novel neuropeptide encoded by the calcitonin gene via tissue-specific RNA processing. Nature 304:240

Rubany GM, Vanhoutte PM (1985) Hypoxia releases a vasoconstrictor substance from the canine vascular endothelium. J Physiol (Lond) 34:45–56

Sagnella GA, Markandu NM, Shore AC, MacGregor GA (1985) Effects of changes in dietary sodium intake and saline infusion on immunoreactive atrial natriuretic peptide in human plasma. Lancet ii:1208–1211

Sagnella GA, Markandu NM, Shore AC, MacGregor GA (1986) Raised circulating levels of atrial natriuretic peptides in essential hypertension. Lancet i:179

Saito Y, Nakao K, Arai H et al. (1987) Atrial natriuretic polypetide (ANP) in human ventricle increased gene expression of ANP in dilated cardiomyopathy. Biochem Biophys Res Commun 148:211–217

Saria A, Theodorsson-Norheim E, Lundberg JM (1984) Evidence for specific neuropeptide Y-binding sites in rat brain synaptosomes. Eur J Pharmacol 107:105–107

Sasaki A, Kida O, Kangawa K, Matsuo H, Tanaka K (1985) Hemodynamic effects of α-human atrial natriuretic polypeptide (α-hANP) in rats. Eur J Pharmacol 109: 405–407

Schelling P, Ganten D, Speck G, Fischer H (1979) Effects of angiotensin II and antagonist saralasin on cell growth and renin in 3T3 and SV3T3 cells. J Cell Physiol 98 (3):503–513

Schenk DB, Johnson LK, Schwartz K, Sista H, Scarborough RM, Lewicki JA (1985a) Distinct atrial natriuretic factor receptor sites on cultured bovine aortic smooth muscle and endothelial cells. Biochem Biophys Res Commun 127:433–442

Schenk DB, Phelps MN, Porter JG, Scarborough RM, McEnroe GA, Lewicki JA (1985b) Identification of the receptor for atrial natriuretic factor on cultured vascular cells. J Biol Chem 260:14887–14890

Schiffrin EL, Chartier L, Thibault G, St Louis J, Cantin M, Genest J (1985) Vascular and adrenal receptors for atrial natriuretic factor in the rat. Circ Res 56:801–807

Schiller PW, Maziak L, Nguyen TMD, Godin J, Garcia R, De Leadn A, Cantin M (1985) Synthesis and biological activity of a linear fragment of the atrial natriuretic factor (ANF). Biochem Biophys Res Commun 131:1056–1062

Schwartz D, Geller DM, Manning PT, Siegel NR, Fok KF, Smith CE, Needleman P (1985) Ser-leu-arg-arg-atriopeptin III: the major circulating form of atrial peptide. Science 229:397–400

Seidman CE, Duby AD, Choi E, Graham RM, Haber E, Homcy C, Smith JA, Seidman JG (1984) The structure of rat preproatrial natriuretic factor as defined by a complementary DNA clone. Science 225:324–326

Siggins GR, Gruol DL (1986) Mechanisms of transmitter action in the vertebrate central nervous system. In: Mountcastle VB, Bloom FE, Geiger SR (eds) The nervous system. Intrinsic regulatory systems of the brain. Am Physiol Soc, Bethesda, p 1 (Handbook of physiology, vol 4)

Sigrist S, Franco-Cereceda A, Muff R, Henke H, Lundberg JM, Fischer JA (1986) Specific receptor and cardiovascular effects of calcitonin gene-related peptide. Endocrinology 119:381–389

Skofitsch G, Jacobowitz DM (1985) Quantitative distribution of calcitonin gene-related peptide in the rat central nervous system. Peptides 6:1069–1073

Snajder RM, Rapp JP (1986) Elevated atrial natriuretic polypeptide in plasma of hypertensive Dahl salt-sensitive rats. Biochem Biophys Res Commun 137:876–883

Snyder SH (1980) Brain peptides as neurotransmitters. Science 209:976–981

Sonnenberg H, Cupples WA, de Bold AJ, Veress AT (1982) Intrarenal localization of the natriuretic effect of cardiac atrial extract. Can J Physiol Pharmacol 60:1149–1152

Sonnenberg H, Honrath U, Chuong CK, Wilson DR (1986) Atrial natriuretic factor inhibits sodium transport in medullary collecting duct. Am J Physiol 250:F936–F966

Sternini C, Brecha N (1985) Distribution and colocalization of neuropeptide Y- and tyrosine hydroxylase-like immunoreactivity in the guinea-pig heart. Cell Tissue Res 241:93–102

Stjärne L, Lundberg JM, Astrand P (1986) Neuropeptide Y—a cotransmitter with noradrenaline and adenosine 5′-triphosphate in the sympathetic nerves of mouse vas deferens? A biochemical, physiological and electropharmacological study. Neuroscience 18:151–166

Stjernquist M, Emson P, Owman C, Sjöberg N-O, Sundler F, Tatemoto K (1983) neropeptide Y in the female reproductive tract of the rat. Distribution of nerve fibers and motor effects Neurosci Lett 39:279–284

Struthers AD, Brown MJ, Beacham JL, Morris HR, MacIntyre I, Stevenson JC (1985) The acute effect of human calcitonin generelated peptide in man. J Endocrinol 104:129–136

Studler JM, Reibaud M, Herve D, Blanc G, Glowinski J, Tassin JP (1986) Opposite effects of sulfated cholecystokinin in DA-sensitive adenylate cyclase in two areas of the rat nucleus accumbens. Eur J Pharmacol 126:125–128

Sugawara A, Nakao K, Sakamoto M, Morii N, Yamada T, Itoh H, Shiono S, Imura H (1986) Plasma concentration of atrial natriuretic polypeptide in essential hypertension. Lancet ii:1426

Sugiura M, Inagami T, Hare GMT, Johns JA (1989) Endothelin action: inhibition by a protein kinase C inhibitor and involvement of phosphoinositols. Biochem Biophys Res Commun 158:170–176

Takagi M, Matsuoka H, Atarashi K, Yagi S (1988) Endothelin: a new inhibitor of renin release. Biochem Biophys Res Commun 157:1164–1168

Tatemoto K (1982) Neuropeptide Y: complete amino acid sequence of the brain peptide.

Proc Natl Acad Sci USA 79:5485–5491
Thibault G, Lazure C, Schiffrin EL, Gutkowska J, Chartier L, Garcia R, Seidah NG, Chretien M, Genest J, Cantin M (1985) Identification of a biologically active circulating form of rat atrial natriuretic factor. Biochem Biophys Res Commun 130: 981–986
Thom SM, Hughes AD, Goldberg P, Martin G, Schachter M, Sever PS (1987) The actions of calcitonin gene-related peptide and vasoactive intestinal peptide as vasodilators in man in vivo and in vitro. Br J Clin Pharmacol 24:139–144
Tomobe Y, Miyauchi T, Saito A, Yanagisawa M, Kimura S, Goto K, Masaki T (1988) Effects of endothelin on the renal artery from spontaneously hypertensive and Wistar Kyoto rats. Eur J Pharmacol 152:373–374
Uddman R, Edvinsson L, Ekblad E, Hakanson R, Sundler F (1986) Calcitonin gene-related peptide (CGRP): perivascular distribution and vasodilator effects. Regul Pept 15:1–23
Undén A, Bartfai T (1984) Regulation of neuropeptide Y (NPY) binding by guanine nucleotides in the rat cerebral cortex. FEBS Lett 177:125–128
Vallejo M, Lightman SL (1986) Pressor effect of centrally administered neuropeptide Y in rats: role of sympathetic nervous system and vasopressin. Life Sci 38:1859–1866
Van Renterghem C, Vigne P, Brahanin J, Schmid-Alliana A, Frelin C, Lazdunski M (1988) Molecular mechanism of action of the novel vasoconstrictor peptide endothelin Biochem Biophys Res Commun 157:977–985
Varndell NM, Polak JM, Allen JM, Terenghi G, Bloom SR (1984) Neuropeptide tyrosine (NPY) immunoreactivity in norepinephrine-containing cells and nerves of the mammalian adrenal gland. Endocrinology 114:1460–1462
Villarreal D, Freeman RH, Davis JO, Verburg KM, Vari RC (1986) Renal mechanisms for suppression of renin secretion by atrial natriuretic factor. Hypertension 8: II28–II35
Volpe M, Odell G, Kleinert HD, Camargo MJF, Laragh JH, Maack T, Vaughan ED Jr, Atlas SA (1985) Effects of atrial natriuretic factor on blood pressure, renin and aldosterone in renovascular hypertensive rats. Hypertension 7:I43–I48
Volpe M, Sosa RE, Müller FB, Camargo MJF, Glorioso N, Laragh JH, Maack T, Atlas SA (1986) Differing hemodynamic response to atrial natriuretic factor in two models of hypertension. Am J Physiol 250:H871–H878
Wahlestedt C, Hakanson R (1986) Effects of neuropeptide Y (NPY) at the sympathetic neuroeffector junction. Can pre- and postjunctional receptors be distinguished? Med Biol 64:85–88
Wahlestedt C, Wohlfart B, Hakanson R (1987) Effects of neuropeptide Y (NPY) on isolated guinea-pig heart. Acta Physiol Scand 129:459–463
Wakitani K, Osshima T, Loewy AD, Holmberg SW, Cole BR, Adams SP, Fok KF, Currie MG, Needleman P (1985) Comparative vascular pharmacology of the atriopeptins. Circ Res 56:621–627
Waldman SA, Rapaport RM, Murad R (1984) Atrial natriuretic factor selectively activates particulate guanylate cyclase and elevates cyclic GMP in rat tissue. J Biol Chem 259:14332–14334
Weidmann P, Gnädinger MP, Ziswiler HR, Shaw S, Bachmann C, Rascher W, Uehlinger DE, Hasler L, Reubi FC (1986a) Cardiovascular, endocrine and renal effects of atrial natriuretic peptide in essential hypertension. J Hypertens 4:S71–S83
Weidmann P, Hasler L, Gnädinger MP, Lang RE, Uehlinger DE, Shaw S, Rascher W, Reubi FC (1986b) Blood levels and renal effects of atrial natriuretic peptide in normal man. J Clin Invest 77:734–742
Weidmann P, Hellmüller B, Uehlinger DE, Lang RE, Gnädinger MP, Hasler L, Shaw S, Bachmann C (1986c) Plasma levels and cardiovascular, endocrine, and excretory effects of atrial natriuretic peptide during different sodium intakes in man. J Clin Endocrinol Metab 62:1027–1036
Westfall TC, Carpentier S, Chen X, Beinfeld MC, Naes L, Meldrum MJ (1987) Prejunctional and postjunctional effects of neuropeptide Y at the noradrenergic neuroeffector junction of the perfused mesenteric arterial bed of the rat. J Cardiovasc Pharmacol 10:716–722

Westlind-Danielsson A, Undén A, Abens J, Andell S, Bartfai T (1987) Neuropeptide Y receptors and the inhibition of adenylate cyclase in the human frontal and temporal cortex. Neurosci Lett 74:237–242
Winquist RJ, Faison EP, Nutt RF (1984a) Vasodilator profile of synthetic atrial natriuretic factor. Eur J Pharmacol 102:169–173
Winquist RJ, Faison EP, Waldman SA, Schwartz K, Murad F, Rapaport RM (1984b) Atrial natriuretic factor elicits an endothelium-independent relaxation and activates particulate guanylate cyclase in vascular smooth muscle. Proc Natl Acad Sci USA 81:7661–7664
Wright CE, Fozard JR (1988) Regional vasodilation is a prominent feature of the haemodynamic response to endothelin in anaesthetized, spontaneously hypertensive rats. Eur J Pharmacol 155:201–203
Yamaji T, Ishibashi M, Takaku F (1985) Atrial natriuretic factor in human blood. J Clin Invest 76:1705–1709
Yamanaka M, Greenberg B, Johnson L, Seilhamer J, Brewer M, Friedemann T, Miller J, Atlas S, Laragh J, Lewicki J, Fiddes J (1984) Cloning and sequence analysis of cDNA for the rat atrial natriuretic factor precursor. Nature 309:719–722
Yanagisawa M, Kurihara H, Kimura S, Tomobe Y, Kobayajhi M, Mitsci Y, Yazaki Y, Soto K, Masaki T (1988a) A movel potent vasoconstrictor peptide produced by vascular endothelial cells. Nature 332:411–415
Yanagisawa M, Inoue A, Ishikawa T, Kasuya Y, Kimura S, Kumagaye S-I, Nakjima K, Watanabe TX, Sakakibara S, Goto K, Masaki T (1988b) Primary structure, synthesis, and biological activity of rat endothelin, an endothelium-derived vasoconstrictor peptide. Proc Natl Acad Sci USA 85:6964–6967
Yasujima M, Abe K, Konzuki M, Tanno M, Kasai Y, Sato M, Omata K, Kudo K, Tsunoda K, Takeuchi K, Yoshinaga K, Inagami T (1985) Atrial natriuretic factor inhibits the hypertension induced by chronic infusion of norepinephrine in conscious rats. Circ Res 57:470–474
Yukimura TK, Ito K, Takenaga T, Yamamoto K, Kangawa K, Matsuo H (1984) Renal effects of synthetic human atrial natriuretic polyepitde in anesthetized dogs. Eur J Pharmacol 103:363–366
Zaidi M, Bevis PJ, Girgis SF, Lynch C, Stevenson JC, MacIntyre I (1985) Circulating CGRP comes from the perivascular nerves. Eur J Pharmacol 11:283–284
Zeidel ML, Seifter JL, Lear S, Brenner BM, Silva P (1986) Atrial peptides inhibit oxygen consumption in kidney medullary collecting duct cells. Am J Physiol 251:F379–F383
Zukowska-Grojec Z, Marks ES, Haass M (1987) Neuropeptide Y is a potent vasoconstrictor and a cardiodepressant in rat. Am J Physiol 253:H1234–H1239

CHAPTER 16

Antihypertensive Agents Which Open Smooth Muscle K Channels

A.H. WESTON

CONTENTS

1 Principle of K-Channel Opening as an Inhibitory Mechanism in Vascular Smooth Muscle

The resting membrane potential of most excitable cells lies between −50 and −80mV. This potential is the result of a complex balance between the different permeabilities which the plasma membrane exhibits towards diffusible ions, the intracellular synthesis of non-diffusible ions giving rise to the Gibbs-Donnan effect and the presence of membrane pumps (especially the Na^+/K^+ pump) which transport pairs of ions unequally. In vascular smooth muscle, probably no ionic species is at equilibrium at the typical resting membrane potential of about − 60mV. For potassium (K^+) ions to be at equilibrium ($[K^+{}_i] \simeq 150$ m*M*; $[K^+{}_o] \simeq 6$ m*M*), the membrane potential of the smooth muscle cell must lie close to −90mV at the so-called potassium equilibrium potential (E_K).

The opening of potassium channels by neurotransmitters and hormones constitutes an important physiological inhibitory mechanism (Fig. 1). One of the best-known examples of this is seen in the amphibian and mammalian heart in which acetylcholine liberated from parasympathetic neurons opens K channels following interaction with muscarinic receptors. The resulting decrease in the

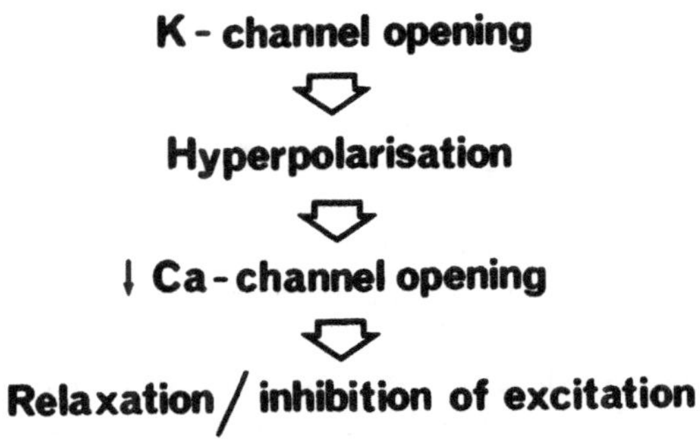

Fig. 1. Basic principle believed to underlie the smooth muscle relaxant and antihypertensive action of smooth muscle K channel opening molecules

slope of pacemaker potentials in nodal tissues and action potential shortening in atrial cells are responsible for the characteristic decrease in cardiac rate and force of contraction mediated by vagal nerve stimulation (NOBLE 1984).

In this example and in others involving K-channel opening, membrane resistance decreases, and efflux of K occurs. The membrane potential moves towards E_K and away from the threshold potential at which ion channels associated with membrane depolarisation (e.g. Na^+ or Ca^{2+}) are able to open. Any tendency towards depolarisation may be countered by further efflux of K^+, giving rise to a form of chemical voltage clamping.

In mammalian smooth muscle, such an effect is associated with α-adrenoceptor-mediated relaxation of the gastrointestinal tract, which is associated with the opening of an apamin-sensitive K-channel (BÜLBRING and TOMITA 1987). In the vascular system, the endothelium-derived hyperpolarising factor (EDHF) dilates blood vessels by a mechanism which also involves the opening of smooth muscle K-channels (TAYLOR and WESTON 1988). However, in both these instances physiological mechanisms, e.g. transmitter uptake, ensure that the inhibition is relatively short lived. In contrast, the synthetic agents cromakalim and pinacidil produce a long-lasting relaxant effect which seems well-correlated with their ability to open K channels (HAMILTON and WESTON 1989). The resulting hyperpolarisation moves the membrane potential away from the potential at which depolarisation-dependent Ca channels open and furthermore tends to negate the effects of excitatory, depolarising pressor agents by chemical voltage clamping as already discussed. Hyperpolarisation may also enhance relaxation by stimulating Ca loss via the voltage-dependent Na^+/Ca^{2+} exchange mechanism (KACZOROWSKI et al. 1988). Inhibition of Ca storage and release from intracellular Ca stores may also occur (BRAY, personal communication).

2 Pinacidil

2.1 Chemistry and History of Development

The development of pinacidil is described by AHNFELT-RØNNE (1988a, b). In 1972 a chemical research team led by H J Petersen synthesised a series of hypotensive alkylpyridylthioureas, one of the most potent of which was designated P950 [*N*-(3-pyridyl)-*N*′-(1,1-dimethylpropyl)thiourea; Fig. 2]. Toxicological problems in experimental animals resulted in the synthesis of a compound designated P1075 in which the sulphur atom in P950 was replaced with an NCN moiety. From P1075, a series of pyridylcyanoguanidines was developed. Good hypotensive activity in rat was achieved with 3-substituted pyridine derivatives in which a branched alkyl residue was attached to the guanidyl nitrogen atom (Fig. 2, P1060 ; PETERSEN et al. 1978). Derivatives based on 4-substituted pyridines were generally less active than 3-substituted molecules. However, P1134, one of the 4-substituted pyridines, was selected for final development as an antihypertensive agent and was given the generic name pinacidil (Fig. 2).

Pinacidil [(±)*N*″-cyano-*N*-4-pyridyl-*N*′-1,2,2-trimethylpropylguanidine monohydrate] is sparingly soluble in water but is soluble in dilute acid and in ethanol. It exists in two enantiomeric forms with a chiral carbon atom in the pinacolyl (1,2,2-trimethylpropyl) moiety (Fig. 2). Biological activity resides in the (−)enantiomer (PETERSEN, personal communication; Sect. 2.3.1.4 and

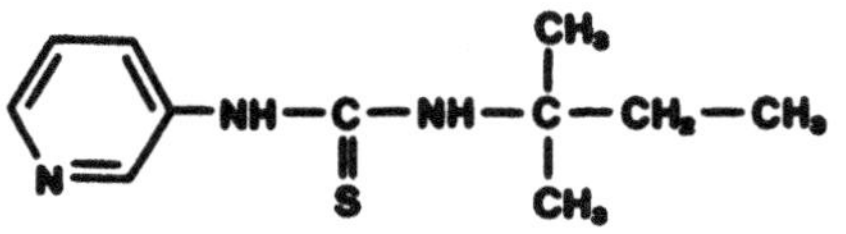

P950

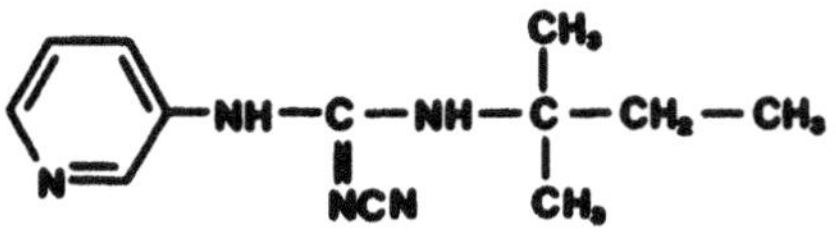

P1075

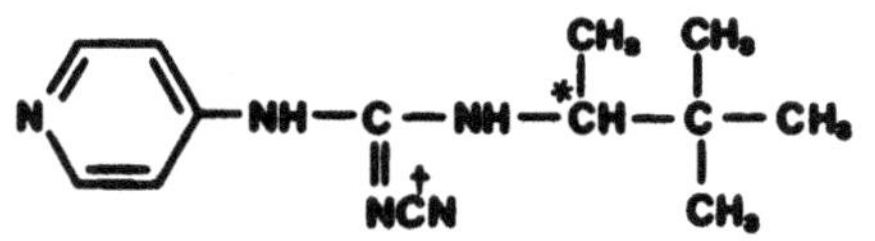

(±)-Pinacidil

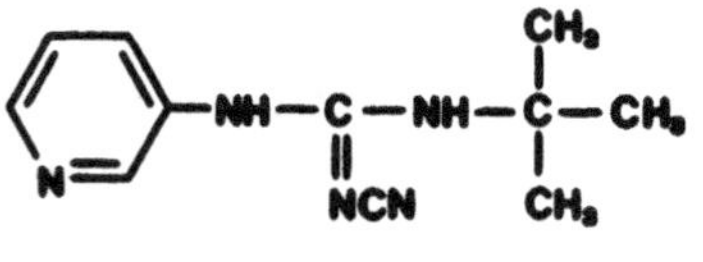

P1060

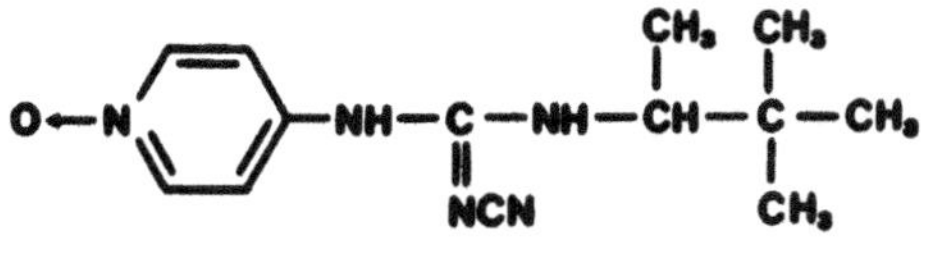

P1368

Fig. 2. Chemical structure of the alkylpyridylthiourea (*P950*) and two alkylpyridylguanidines (*P1060* and *P1075*) from which (±) *pinacidil* was selected for clinical development. The position of the chiral carbon atom in pinacidil is indicated by an *asterisk*, and † denotes the position of the ^{14}C used in the pharmacokinetic studies of EILERTSEN et al. (1982a, b). The major metabolite of pinacidil is pinacidil-*N*-oxide (*P1368*). For further details, see PETERSEN et al. (1978)

2.3.2.4). The assay of pinacidil in biological fluids and extracts is described by EILERTSEN et al. (1982a,b).

2.2 Pharmacokinetics, Tissue Distribution and Metabolism

The pharmacokinetics and metabolism of (±)pinacidil have been studied using (±) [^{14}C] pinacidil in rats and dogs and (±)pinacidil in humans (EILERTSEN et al. 1982a, b). No similar data on the enantiomeric components of pinacidil are available.

2.2.1 Pharmacokinetics and Tissue Distribution

After oral administration to rats, pinacidil is rapidly absorbed, and peak plasma concentrations are achieved 0.5–1 h after dosing. After either oral or intravenous administration, the plasma half-life is 1.1–1.2 h (EILERTSEN et al. 1982a). In the dog, limited studies ($n = 2$) have also shown rapid absorption after oral administration. Peak concentrations are achieved 0.5–1.5 h after dosing, with a plasma half-life ranging from 1.8 to 2.3 h. Similar plasma half-life values are seen after intravenous administration (EILERTSEN et al. 1982a).

In fasting human volunteers, peak plasma concentrations are detected 0.5–1.2 h after dosing, with plasma half-life values in the range 1.6–2 h. In postprandial volunteers, absorption is delayed, and the plasma half-life is increased to 2.2 h. Binding studies indicate that there is substantial plasma protein binding in the rat (60%) and dog (66%), with the majority associated with the albumin fraction (EILERTSEN et al. 1982a).

In both the rat and dog, the volume of distribution of pinacidil is relatively high, indicating substantial tissue binding. Whole animal autoradiographic studies followed by tissue analysis show that the order of binding in the rat following oral administration is liver>small intestine>kidney>stomach>spleen >heart>muscle. Very similar results are obtained following intravenous administration (EILERTSEN et al. 1982b).

2.2.2 Metabolism

Studies in the rat, dog and humans show that the *N*-oxide derivative of pinacidil (P1368, Fig. 2) is the major metabolite detectable in plasma. Three other metabolites have been detected but not identified. Little unchanged pinacidil is found in urine and faeces (EILERTSEN et al. 1982b).

The *N*-oxide metabolite is probably formed in the liver and excreted largely in the urine with little delay (EILERTSEN et al. 1982b). It exerts both blood pressure-lowering activity in vivo (GODTFREDSEN, personal communication) and smooth muscle relaxant actions in vitro (COHEN and COLBERT 1986; WESTON et al. 1988b). Although this agent is less potent that pinacidil itself, it may accumulate during chronic pinacidil treatment in humans and contribute to the antihypertensive and/or toxic effects of the parent compound (MCBURNEY et al. 1988).

2.3 Pharmacodynamics

2.3.1 Effects on the Cardiovascular System In Vivo

2.3.1.1 Effects on Basal Blood Pressure and Heart Rate

In a variety of animal models (±)pinacidil produces a dose-dependent fall in blood pressure accompanied by reflex tachycardia.

In conscious rats, a single oral dose of 2.5 mg/kg produces a lowering of blood pressure which is maximal 2 h after dosing and which remains significantly reduced for several hours. These hypotensive effects are greater in SHR than in normotensive rats and are accompanied by a reflex tachycardia. Pinacidil also produces a lowering of blood pressure in renal and neurogenically hypertensive rats (ARRIGONI-MARTELLI et al. 1980).

An acute dose-response study in SHR showed that oral administration of pinacidil (0.3–3 mg/kg) produces a dose-related fall in blood pressure. Furthermore, there is no difference between the hypotensive effects of pinacidil on the 3rd and 5th days of treatment, indicating the absence of tachyphylaxis (ARRIGONI-MARTELLI et al. 1980; COHEN and KURZ 1988).

In conscious, normotensive dogs, oral administration of pinacidil (0.1–0.5 mg/kg) produces a dose-related depressor effect and reflex tachycardia, with a duration of action from 2–5 h over this dose range (ARRIGONI-MARTELLI and FINUCAINE 1985). In conscious, renal hypertensive dogs, pinacidil (0.25–2 mg/kg) also produces a dose-related fall in blood pressure with no evidence of tachyphylaxis (ARRIGONI-MARTELLI et al. 1980). Intra-arterial injection of pinacidil in both normotensive and SHR produces maximum blood pressure lowering within 0.5 min at a dose of 0.3 mg/kg, an effect which is greatest in SHR (THOOLEN et al. 1983; ARRIGONI-MARTELLI and FINUCAINE 1985). In anaesthetised cats, pinacidil has no apparent effect on baroreceptor sensitivity to pressor challenge (CLAPHAM and COOPER 1988).

2.3.1.2 Effects on Regional Blood Flow

Changes in blood flow to a variety of mammalian vascular beds have been studied by several groups of workers. The changes observed depend on the dose of pinacidil employed and are species-specific for a given vascular bed.

In dogs, subhypotensive doses of pinacidil produce an increase in carotid, coronary, femoral and renal blood flow (BANG-OLSEN and ARRIGONI-MARTELLI 1983; ARRIGONI-MARTELLI and FINUCAINE 1985). At concentrations which produce a moderate fall in blood pressure, pinacidil produces an increase in renal blood flow and function with little effect on femoral perfusion (ARRIGONI-MARTELLI et al. 1980; BANG-OLSEN and ARRIGONI-MARTELLI 1983). At higher concentrations, renal and femoral blood flow is little affected (BANG-OLSEN and ARRIGONI-MARTELLI 1983). In rats, DIEPERINK et al. (1983) found that pinacidil produces no change in renal blood flow. Similarly in cats, no change in renal vascular resistance is seen on oral or intravenous infusion of pinacidil at a dose which produces a significant decrease in mesenteric vascular resistance (CLAPHAM 1988; LONGMAN et al. 1988).

In chronically hypoxic rat skeletal muscle, pinacidil (0.3–3 mg/kg intraduodenally) produces an increase in skeletal muscle blood cell flux and pO_2 (ANGERSBACH and NICHOLSON 1988).

2.3.1.3 Effect on Agonist-Induced Pressor Responses

In pithed rats, THOOLEN et al. (1983) showed that the pressor responses produced by cirazoline, an α_1-adrenoceptor-selective agonist, and by B-HT 920, an α_2-adrenoceptor-selective agonist, are reduced by pretreatment with pinacidil. The pressor responses to 8-lysine vasopressin are also inhibited by pinacidil. In anaesthetised rats, COOK et al. (1988a) found that intravenous administration of pinacidil (0.3–1 mg/kg) is relatively ineffective at inhibiting pressor responses to angiotensin II, in contrast to the inhibition produced by the calcium entry blocking agent, isradipine.

2.3.1.4 Stereospecificity of Cardiovascular Actions

The hypotensive effects of oral administration of the separated enantiomers of pinacidil (see Fig. 2) have been studied in SHR (ARRIGONI-MARTELLI et al. 1980). Both forms are capable of lowering blood pressure, and their relative potencies can be assessed on the basis of the dose required to produce a blood pressure fall of 30 mmHg. From this (−)pinacidil is approximately four times more potent than (+)pinacidil, assuming identical pharmacokinetics and distribution (which was not confirmed). Although the (+)enantiomer was contaminated with the more active (−)enantiomer (< 1% contamination: AHNFELT-RØNNE, personal communication), it is unlikely that this low level can account for the hypotensive activity of (+)pinacidil.

2.3.2 Effects on Isolated Vascular Tissues

2.3.2.1 Effects on Spontaneous Mechanical Activity

Pinacidil inhibits the spontaneous mechanical activity characteristic of mammalian portal vein, an effect which has been examined in the rat (BRAY et al. 1987a; SOUTHERTON et al. 1988), guinea pig (COOK et al. 1988a) and rabbit (LONGMAN et al. 1988). In the rat, pinacidil (0.1–1 μM) produces a reduction in the amplitude and duration of each phasic tension wave. Only at the upper end of this concentration range is the frequency of tension waves reduced and finally abolished (BRAY et al. 1987a). In the guinea pig, pinacidil (0.1–1 μM) decreases both the amplitude and frequency of the waves until they are abolished (COOK et al. 1988a).

2.3.2.2 Effects on Agonist-Induced Contractions

In rat aorta and portal vein, pretreatment with pinacidil (0.3–100 μM) produces a reduction in maximum responses to noradrenaline with some rightward shift in the noradrenaline dose-response curve (BRAY et al. 1987a). A similar inhibitory effect is produced by pinacidil (0.3–30 μM) against angiotensin II-induced contractions in rabbit aorta (COOK et al. 1988a). In canine cephalic vein, pinacidil (0.01–10 μ*M*) produces a concentration-dependent relaxation of an established phenylephrine-induced contraction (STEINBERG et al. 1988).

Pretreatment of rat aorta and portal vein with pinacidil (0.3–100 μ*M*) produces a reduction in responses to KCl (5–80 m*M*) with some rightward shift of the dose-response curve and evidence of a selective inhibition at the lower end of the KCl concentration range (BRAY et al. 1987a). A similar effect is observed in rabbit aorta (COOK et al. 1988a). In rat aorta, pinacidil (0.1–10 μ*M*) is able to relax completely an established contraction to 20 m*M* KCl. In contrast, over this concentration range little inhibition of responses to 80 m*M* KCl is observed (SOUTHERTON et al. 1988; WESTON et al. 1988a, b).

2.3.2.3 Stereospecificity of In Vitro Effects

The inhibitory effects of the isolated (+) and (−)enantiomers of pinacidil have been examined on spontaneous mechanical changes in rat portal vein and against established contractions to 20 m*M* KCl in rat aorta (BRAY et al. 1987b; SOUTHERTON et al. 1988). In both tissues (−)pinacidil is approximately 20 times more potent than (+)pinacidil.

2.3.2.4 Effects on Membrane Potential

In rat portal vein, pinacidil (0.3–10 μ*M*) abolishes spontaneous electrical multispike complexes and produces a concentration-dependent membrane hyperpolarisation (SOUTHERTON et al. 1988) (Fig. 3). At the lower end of this concentration range (0.3 μ*M*), only the duration of multispike electrical complexes is reduced, with no effect on the frequency of these discharges within a complex, or on the rate of spike rise or fall. In the concentration range 3–10 μ*M*, exposure to pinacidil abolishes the spikes and produces a concentration-dependent hyperpolarisation which raises the membrane potential to the region of the theoretical E_K (SOUTHERTON et al. 1988). On exposure of rat aorta to pinacidil (3–10 μ*M*) a concentration-dependent hyperpolarisation is produced which raises the membrane potential by a maximum of approximately 25 mV (SOUTHERTON et al. 1988). A concentration-dependent hyperpolarisation by pinacidil (0.3–10 μ*M*) has also been reported by VIDEBAEK et al. (1988a, b) in rat mesenteric artery.

2.3.2.5 Effects on ^{86}Rb and ^{42}K Efflux

In rat portal vein and aorta pinacidil (0.3–10 μ*M*) produces a concentration-dependent increase in ^{86}Rb efflux (BRAY et al. 1987a; SOUTHERTON et al. 1987b, 1988). When the effects of the analogues P1060 and P1368 (Fig. 2) on ^{86}Rb exchange in rat portal vein are compared with those of pinacidil, the potency series for this effect is P1060 $\geqslant$ pinacidil $>$ P1368 (WESTON et al. 1988b). In rat portal vein the stimulatory effect of pinacidil on ^{42}K efflux is slightly greater than that seen when ^{86}Rb is used (SOUTHERTON et al. 1988). In rat mesenteric artery, pinacidil produces a concentration-dependent increase in ^{42}K exchange, with relatively little effect on ^{86}Rb efflux (VIDEBAEK et al. 1988a, b).

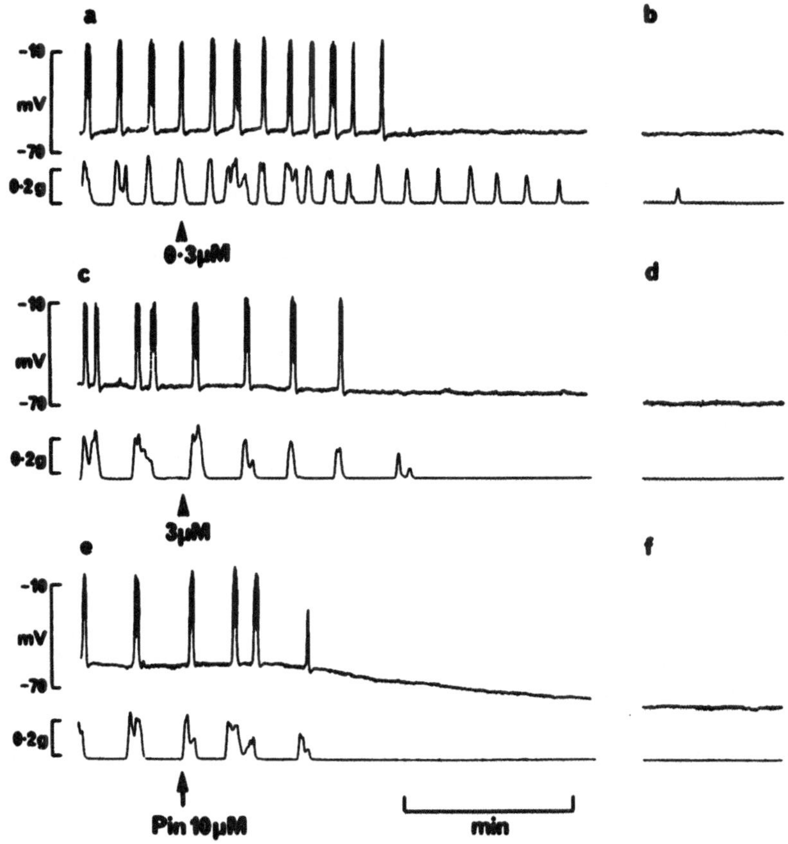

Fig. 3a–f. Effect of pinacidil on electrical (*upper traces*) and mechanical (*lower traces*) activity in rat portal vein. The records are part of a continuous recording with washout of pinacidil (*Pin*) between panels **b** and **c**, **d** and **e**. The records in **b**, **d** and **f** were obtained 4.5 min, 5 min and 7 min after exposure to pinacidil in **a**, **c** and **e**, respectively. From SOUTHERTON et al. (1988), with permission

2.3.3 Effects on Non-Vascular Tissue

2.3.3.1 Cardiac Muscle

In spontaneously beating guinea pig atria, pinacidil (100 μ*M*) produces a reduction in both rate and force of contraction. Pinacidil-*N*-oxide is without effect (COHEN and COLBERT 1986). A detailed study of the effects of pinacidil and its analogues in dog and cat cardiac muscle has been made by SMALLWOOD and STEINBERG (1988) and by STEINBERG et al. (1988). In canine Purkinje fibres and ventricular muscle, pinacidil (1–100 μ*M*) reduces the action potential duration with no inhibitory effect on action potential maximum upstroke velocity or conduction time at concentrations which produce action potential shortening. Pinacidil also decreases Ba^{2+}-induced automaticity in Purkinje fibres. In electrically stimulated cat papillary muscle, pinacidil (1–30 μ*M*) produces a concentration-dependent reduction in twitch tension (STEINBERG et al. 1988).

2.3.3.2 Trachea

The effects of pinacidil on guinea pig trachea have been studied by COHEN and COLBERT (1986) and BRAY et al. (1987a). Pinacidil (1–100 μ*M*) relaxes the spontaneous tone characteristic of guinea pig trachea (COHEN and COLBERT, 1986; BRAY et al. 1987a); pinacidil-*N*-oxide is 50 times less potent than pinacidil itself (COHEN and COLBERT 1986). Pinacidil (10–100 μ*M*) is also capable of relaxing segments of trachea pre-contracted with KCl 20 m*M* (BRAY et al. 1987a), histamine and carbachol (COHEN and COLBERT 1986).

2.3.3.3 Bladder

In both normal and hypertrophied bladder detrusor muscle from the rat, pinacidil (1–10 μ*M*) inhibits spontaneous contractions and contractile responses to KCl (≤40 m*M*), effects which are greater in hypertrophied than normal muscle samples (ANDERSSON et al. 1988). Pinacidil also shifts the carbachol spasmogenic dose-response curve to the right and antagonises the effects of electrical field stimulation in both normal and hypertrophied muscle. In the mechanoinhibitory concentration range, pinacidil (1–30 μ*M*) increases the rate of ^{86}Rb efflux from samples of both normal and hypertrophied muscle (ANDERSSON et al. 1988). Similar inhibitory effects of pinacidil on mechanical activity and the ability of pinacidil to stimulate ^{86}Rb efflux are seen in segments of normal human bladder (FOVAEUS et al. 1989).

2.3.3.4 Gastrointestinal Tract

In guinea pig ileum, pinacidil (0.1–100 μ*M*) inhibits contractions resulting from electrical field stimulation and those produced by carbachol or histamine. Pinacidil-*N*-oxide produces similar inhibition of electrical stimulation and of carbachol spasms but is 50–125 times less potent than pinacidil (COHEN and COLBERT 1986). Pinacidil (0.1–100 μ*M*) also relaxes basal tone in rat fundus strips and produces non-competitive inhibition of contractile responses to 5-HT. Pinacidil-*N*-oxide is less potent than pinacidil (COHEN and COLBERT 1986). In guinea pig taenia caeci, pinacidil (0.1–10 μ*M*) produces a concentration-dependent relaxation of spontaneous tone, an effect which is not antagonised by the presence of apamin (BRAY et al. 1987a).

2.3.3.5 Reproductive Tract

Pinacidil (>10 μ*M*) inhibits spontaneous mechanical activity in the rat uterus and produces a slight inhibition of responses to oxytocin. Similar effects are produced by pinacidil-*N*-oxide. Both compounds also inhibit contractile responses to electrical field stimulation of rat vas deferens, with pinacidil approximately 60 times more potent than pinacidil-*N*-oxide (COHEN and COLBERT 1986).

2.4 Mechanism of Action

2.4.1 Evidence for the Role of K Channels

Data derived from several different types of in vitro experiment suggest that the smooth muscle relaxant effects of pinacidil result from the opening of plasmalemmal K channels. The ensuing hyperpolarisation lowers intracellular calcium levels as described in Sect. 1.

Using microelectrodes, pinacidil-induced hyperpolarisation has been measured in a variety of rat blood vessels (SOUTHERTON et al. 1988; VIDEBAEK et al. 1988a, b). The magnitude of the recorded change is itself suggestive of the opening of K channels as the membrane potential increases to approach the theoretical E_K. In cardiac muscle, the shortening of action potentials described by STEINBERG et al. (1988) is also consistent with the opening of membrane K channels. In a study of several pinacidil analogues, there is an excellent correlation between action potential shortening in canine Purkinje fibres and relaxation of canine cephalic veins (STEINBERG et al. 1988; Sect. 2.3.3.1).

Ion flux studies have confirmed the K channel opening action of pinacidil. At concentrations which produce mechanical inhibition of smooth muscle, a marked increase in ^{86}Rb exchange (BRAY et al. 1987a; COOK et al. 1988a; SOUTHERTON et al. 1988; WESTON et al. 1988a) or ^{42}K exchange (SOUTHERTON et al. 1988; VIDEBAEK et al. 1988a, b) is produced by pinacidil (0.3–10 μM). In a study of pinacidil analogues, there was a correlation between mechano-inhibitory effects and the increase in ^{86}Rb exchange (WESTON et al. 1988b).

A characteristic feature of the inhibitory profile of pinacidil is its ability to relax contractions produced by low KCl concentrations ($\leq$20 mM) but to have relatively little inhibitory effect on responses to higher KCl concentrations ($\geq$80 mM) (BRAY et al. 1987a; SOUTHERTON et al. 1988). Addition of KCl to the physiological salt solution alters E_K to a less negative value, the magnitude of which can be estimated using the Nernst equation. If the resulting E_K is more negative than the potential at which L-type Ca channels open (probably between −40 and −50 mV; BOLTON et al. 1984), a K channel opening drug will ensure that membrane permeability to K^+ becomes dominant over other ion permeabilities. The membrane potential will thus tend to move towards the E_K predicted by the Nernst equation. Thus, relaxation of a contraction produced by 20 mM KCl ($E_K \triangleq -50$ mV) should occur, but the contraction produced by 80 mM KCl ($E_K \triangleq -20$ mV) should be unaffected. The observed differential ability of pinacidil to relax high/low KCl-induced contractions (BRAY et al. 1987a; COOK et al. 1988a; SOUTHERTON et al. 1988) is thus consistent with a K channel opening action.

2.4.2 Causal Relationship Between K Channel Opening In Vitro and Hypotensive Effects In Vivo

In vitro, the electrical changes produced by pinacidil, which are characteristic of K-channel opening, are observed in the concentration range 0.3–10 μM (SOUTHERTON et al. 1988; VIDEBAEK et al. 1988a, b). This range is similar to the plasma concentrations of pinacidil (0.2–1 μ*M*) associated with hypotensive effects in the rat, dog and humans (EILERTSEN et al. 1982a, b; ZACHARIAH et al. 1986; CALLAGHAN et al. 1988).

There is a good correlation between the in vivo and in vitro potency ratios of a series of pinacidil analogues. The studies of WESTON et al. (1988b) show that the potency of a series of pinacidil analogues to relax vascular smooth muscle and to increase ^{86}Rb efflux from such tissues is the same as that for their hypotensive effects (PETERSEN et al. 1978). In addition, STEINBERG et al. (1988) showed a good correlation between the inhibitory potency of a large series of pinacidil analogues in cardiac and vascular muscle with that observed in vivo (PETERSEN et al. 1978). In vivo, the (−)enantiomer of pinacidil is more potent than the (+)enantiomer (ARRIGONI-MARTELLI et al. 1980), a result also obtained in vitro (SOUTHERTON et al. 1988) (Sects. 2.3.1.4 and 2.3.2.3).

All attempts to show that pinacidil has an alternative mechanism of action to that of K-channel opening have been unsuccessful. Early studies demonstrated that the effects of pinacidil are unchanged by antagonists at cholinergic, histaminergic, α- and β-adrenergic sites (PETERSEN et al. 1978). No binding to α-adrenoceptors was detected (THOOLEN et al. 1983). Later studies have shown that pinacidil does not increase tissue levels of cAMP or cGMP (KAUFFMAN et al. 1986; SOUTHERTON et al. 1988; YANAGISAWA et al. 1988), and no calcium antagonist activity has been detected (KAERGAARD-NIELSEN and ARRIGONI-MARTELLI 1981; MIKKELSEN and PEDERSEN 1982). Removal of the vascular endothelium does not affect responses to pinacidil (TODA et al. 1985; KAUFFMAN et al. 1986).

These factors combine to suggest strongly that K channel opening is the mechanism which underlies the in vivo and in vitro effects of pinacidil.

2.4.3 Type of K Channel Modulated by Pinacidil

The mechanoinhibitory effects of pinacidil in rat portal vein are antagonised by tetraethylammonium (TEA) or by procaine. In contrast, 3,4-diaminopyridine (DAP) (up to 1 m*M*) is without effect (SOUTHERTON et al. 1988). Neither TEA nor procaine is a very selective blocker of any particular K channel, and both agents are capable of blocking a Ca^{2+}-dependent and a voltage-dependent K channel (BENHAM et al. 1985; BOLTON et al. 1985). In contrast, DAP is somewhat selective for Ca-independent K channels (BOWMAN and SAVAGE 1981; BOWMAN 1982; COOK and HAYLETT 1985), and thus the lack of effect of DAP suggests that pinacidil may interact with a Ca-dependent K channel.

Evidence in favour of this has recently been obtained by HERMSMEYER (1988). In isolated cells from rat azygous vein, pinacidil increases the K current in the whole cell patch configuration. In isolated inside-out patches, pinacidil increases the number of openings of a K channel with characteristics similar to the 200pS Ca-dependent K channel.

Data which suggest that the K channel with which pinacidil interacts is impermeable to ^{86}Rb, at least in rat mesenteric artery, have also been obtained by VIDEBAEK et al. (1988a, b). However, it is a common finding that vascular K channels are impermeable to ^{86}Rb relative to ^{42}K or ^{43}K (SMITH et al. 1986). In other rat blood vessels, the pinacidil-induced increase in ^{86}Rb efflux is also smaller than that seen with ^{42}K (SOUTHERTON et al. 1988) but within the normal limits described by SMITH et al. (1986).

2.5 Clinical Studies

2.5.1 Effects in Hypertensive Patients

Early clinical observations on the effects of oral pinacidil in essential hypertension (CARLSEN et al. 1981; KARDEL et al. 1981) were made using relatively simple formulations of pinacidil in tablet form. However, the short half-life of the agent prompted the development of slow-release formulations (EILERTSEN et al. 1982a, b; CARLSEN et al. 1983). All subsequent human studies have been carried out using retarded release formulations.

In an early study in hypertensive patients, CARLSEN et al. (1981) showed that a single oral dose of pinacidil (25 mg) produces a marked decrease in blood pressure with an increase in heart rate. Total peripheral resistance and forearm resistance are decreased. KARDEL et al. (1981) showed that a fall in blood pressure could be achieved with single doses of pinacidil (10–25 mg) in both supine and erect patients. More recently, ZACHARIAH et al. (1986) found that dosing with pinacidil (12.5–75 mg twice daily) significantly lowers daytime blood pressure with little effect on nightime pressure. NICHOLLS et al. (1984) investigated the acute effects of intravenous administration of pinacidil (0.2 mg/kg iv.). A rapid reduction in mean arterial pressure together with an increase in heart rate was observed. In a follow-up study to their early work, CARLSEN et al. (1985) found that the effects of pinacidil on heart rate could be reduced by iv. administration of metoprolol. The combined results of these studies show that in the dose range 12.5–75 mg twice daily pinacidil is an effective antihypertensive agent with the profile of a peripheral vasodilator. These conclusions have been supported by the results of recent multicentre trials (CALLAGHAN et al. 1988; GOLDBERG 1988; GOLDBERG and OFFEN 1988; JÜRGENSEN 1988; STEENSGARD-HANSEN and CARLSEN 1988; STERNDORRF and JOHANSEN 1988).

Weight gain is a common adverse effect of pinacidil treatment (Sect. 2.5.2), and several investigators have found evidence of activation of the renin-angiotensin system in patients receiving pinacidil. MUIESAN et al. (1983) observed an increase in both plasma catecholamines and renin activity, findings which were also reported by BYYNY et al. (1987) and IZZO et al. (1987). However, ABRAHAM et al. (1987) failed to confirm these observations and reported a slight reduction in plasma aldosterone levels, together with changes consistent with an increase in renal blood flow. The origin of the weight gain in pinacidil patients does not seem to be simply related to a reduction of renal blood flow and secondary activation of the renin-angiotensin system. It is possible that pinacidil can directly hyperpolarise the cells of the juxtaglomerular apparatus with a consequent increase in renin release (HACKENTHAL and TAUGNER 1986).

When used as monotherapy, pinacidil produces a reduction in total serum cholesterol and triglycerides (GOLDBERG and ROCKHOLD 1986). This effect is reduced on combined administration with a thiazide (CALLAGHAN et al. 1988).

2.5.2 Adverse Reactions

When used as monotherapy, adverse reactions in decreasing order of severity and typical of a peripheral vasodilator are headache, oedema, palpitation, dizziness and rhinitis (GOLDBERG 1988). The incidence of these effects is greatly reduced by co-administration of a thiazide diuretic. Other adverse effects include hypertrichosis (2% in males, 13% in females) and flattening or inversion in the ECG T wave (GOLDBERG 1988). The mechanism underlying hypertrichosis is unknown. However, since it is shared by both minoxidil and diazoxide (see Sect. 5), it may be related to selective dilation of blood vessels supplying hair follicles. The T wave changes may be associated with the effects of pinacidil on cardiac muscle in vitro (Sect. 2.3.3.1); no adverse clinical consequences of this ECG change are apparent (GOLDBERG 1988).

3 Cromakalim

3.1 Chemistry and History of Development

The original synthesis of a series of benzopyran derivatives with the ability to lower blood pressure in rats is described by EVANS et al. (1983). Introduction of a carbonyl group into the pyrrolidine ring of (±) BRL20673, the lead compound from this work yielded BRL34915: (±)-6-cyano-3,4-dihydro-2,2-dimethyl-*trans*-4-(2-oxopyrrolidin-1-yl)-2*H*-1-benzopyran-3-ol (ASHWOOD et al. 1984, 1986; Fig. 4).

The molecular structure of BRL34915 contains two chiral carbon atoms at positions 3 and 4, and the two enantiomeric forms of the molecule have been separated (ASHWOOD et al. 1986). The biological activity of BRL34915 resides largely in the (−)3S, 4R enantiomer (ASHWOOD et al. 1986; BUCKINGHAM et al. 1986a, BRAY et al. 1987b; ARCH et al. 1988a; HOF et al. 1988). This active form has been designated BRL38227 and the (+)3R,4S enantiomer, BRL38226 (GILL et al. 1988a, b), while the racemic BRL34915 has been given the generic name cromakalim.

The racemic *cis*-diastereoisomer of cromakalim, (±)-6-cyano-3,4-dihydro-2,2-dimethyl-*cis*-4-(2-oxopyrrolidyn-1-yl)-2*H*-1-benzopyran-3-ol has also been synthesised and found to be approximately tenfold less active than cromakalim as an antihypertensive agent in rats (ASHWOOD et al. 1986). The biological activity of the individual *cis*-enantiomers has not yet been reported.

No detailed comment has been made on the general features of the structure-activity relationships within the series of substituted benzopyrans apart from the data given in EVANS et al. (1983) and in ASHWOOD et al. (1986). However, the presence of the carbonyl group in the pyrrolidine ring is a critical feature, while the size and type of substituent at position 4 have marked effects on anti-

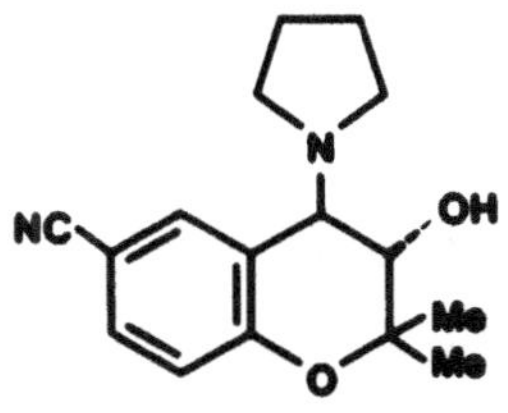

(±)-BRL 20673

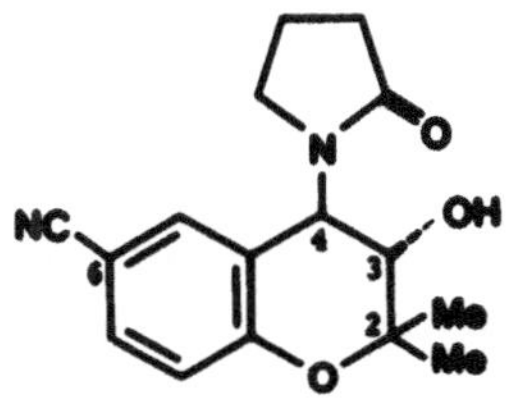

(±)-BRL 34915
Cromakalim

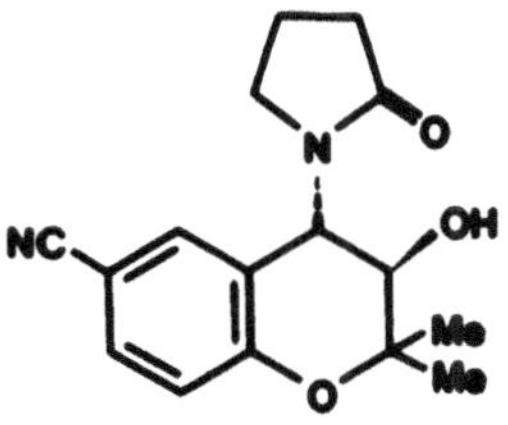

BRL 38226
(+)-3R,4S

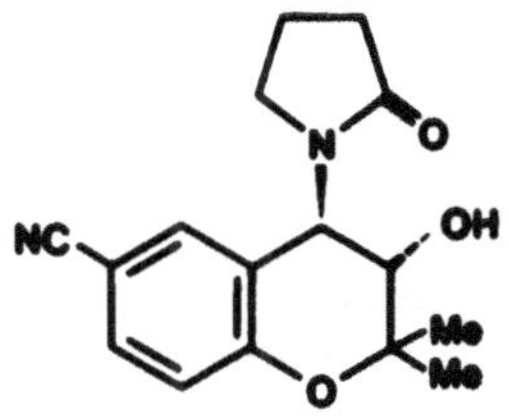

BRL 38227
(−)-3S,4R

Fig. 4. Development of cromakalim. Insertion of a carbonyl group into the racemate (±) *BRL20673* yields *BRL34915*, a racemic mixture of the *trans* enantiomers *BRL38226* and *BRL38227*. The biological activity of BRL34915, now known as *cromakalim*, resides in the 3S, 4R enantiomer BRL38227

hypertensive activity (Ashwood et al. 1986). Additional requirements are the presence and precise location of electron-withdrawing groups in the benzene component of the benzopyran ring (Ashwood et al. 1986; see also Lang and Wenk 1988) and the gem dimethyl group at position 2.

Cromakalim is sparingly soluble in water but is soluble in ethanol and in water:ethanol or water:polyethyleneglycol 400 mixtures. For in vitro studies, the agent is usually dissolved in a 70% v/v ethanol:water mixture with subsequent dilutions in saline or physiological salt solution.

3.2 Pharmacokinetics, Distribution and Metabolism

No published data are available on the pharmacokinetics, tissue distribution or metabolism of cromakalim in animals.

In humans, single oral administration of cromakalim (0.5–2 mg) produces mean maximum plasma concentrations in the range 4.4–17.3 ng/ml (DAVIES et al. 1988). Bioavailability is unaffected by the prandial state. DAVIES et al. (1988) also compared the pharmacokinetics of single dose and repeated daily dosing of 1 mg cromakalim in healthy male subjects. No differences were detected, yielding mean values for maximum plasma concentration and half-life of 9.3 ng/ml and 22.5 h, respectively.

In subsequent studies, GILL et al. (1988a, b) showed differences between the pharmacokinetics of the (+) and (−)enantiomeric components of cromakalim detected after oral administration (0.5–2 mg) to male volunteers. The mean maximum plasma concentrations of the (−)enantiomer (BRL38227) are greater than those of the (+)enantiomer (BRL38226) at all dose levels. In contrast the half-life of BRL38227 is less than that of BRL38226. The basis of these differences has not been investigated.

No published information is available on the tissue distribution or metabolism of cromakalim in humans.

3.3 Pharmacodynamics

3.3.1 Effects on the Cardiovascular System In Vivo

3.3.1.1 Effects on Basal Blood Pressure and Heart Rate

In the conscious normal or renal hypertensive cat, cromakalim (0.007–0.1 mg/kg, p.o. or 0.002 mg/kg per min, i.v.) produces a dose-dependent fall in blood pressure accompanied by reflex tachycardia, effects which last for several hours (BUCKINGHAM et al. 1986b; CLAPHAM and BUCKINGHAM 1988; LONGMAN et al. 1988). In the anaesthetised cat, CLAPHAM and COOPER (1988) found that cromakalim sensitised baroreceptors to pressor challenge.

Similar hypotensive effects were seen in conscious or anaesthetised rats (BUCKINGHAM et al. 1986b; BUCKINGHAM 1988; COOK and HOF 1988), in renal hypertensive dogs (BUCKINGHAM et al. 1986b) and in anaesthetised rabbits (COOK and HOF 1988; HOF et al. 1988). The increase in heart rate seen in animals is antagonised by β-adrenoceptor blockade (BUCKINGHAM et al. 1986b; COOK and HOF 1988), indicating the reflex nature of the response. Repeated oral administration of cromakalim to dogs produces no evidence of tachyphylaxis to the hypotensive effect (BUCKINGHAM et al. 1986b).

3.3.1.2 Effects on Regional Blood Flow

Using electromagnetic flow probes, BUCKINGHAM et al. (1988b) detected a moderate cromakalim-induced increase in renal blood flow in the anaesthetised cat with smaller increments in carotid, femoral and mesenteric perfusion. The effect on renal blood flow was confirmed by CLAPHAM and BUCKINGHAM (1988) and by LONGMAN et al. (1988) in the conscious cat. In the anaesthetised rabbit, cromakalim (0.003–0.03 mg/kg, intraduodenally) dilates gastric blood vessels and increases blood flow (as measured using radioactive microspheres) to the heart and small intestine. Cerebral perfusion is also increased while skeletal muscle and renal blood flow are essentially unchanged (COOK and HOF 1988; HOF et al. 1988). In the anaesthetised dog, cromakalim increases renal blood flow (DUMEZ et al. 1988). In the conscious SHR, cromakalim reduces the systemic blood pressure, an effect associated with an antidiuresis and excretion of hypertonic urine (DUMEZ et al. 1988).

In the rat, cromakalim (0.03–0.3 mg/kg, intraduodenally) causes some increase in skeletal muscle blood cell flux and pO_2 in normal muscle but produces a marked increase in these parameters in chronically hypoxic muscle. This increase occurs despite a fall in systemic blood pressure (ANGERSBACH and NICHOLSON 1985, 1988).

3.3.1.3 Effects on Agonist-Induced Pressor Responses

In anaesthetised, ganglion-blocked SHR, cromakalim (0.1–0.3 mg/kg, i.v.) antagonises pressor responses to intravenous infusion of noradrenaline or phenylephrine. No significant inhibition of responses to methoxamine, angiotensin II, or vasopressin was detected. In pithed SHR cromakalim (0.3 mg/kg, i.v.) inhibits pressor responses produced by electrical stimulation of the spinal cord (BUCKINGHAM 1988).

3.3.1.4 Stereospecificity of In Vivo Effects

In conscious SHR, BRL38227 is at least 100 times more potent than BRL38226 at lowering blood pressure (ASHWOOD et al. 1986; BUCKINGHAM et al. 1986a; see also Sect. 3.1 and 3.3.2.3). In anaesthetised rabbits, BRL38227 is 100–200 times more potent than BRL38226 as a hypotensive agent (HOF et al. 1988).

3.3.2 Effects on Vascular Tissues In Vitro

3.3.2.1 Effects on Spontaneous Mechanical Activity

The ability to inhibit the spontaneous mechanical activity of mammalian portal veins is one of the characteristics of cromakalim (0.1–1 μM). This inhibitory action has been reported in the rat (HAMILTON et al. 1986; HOF et al. 1988), guinea pig (QUAST 1987; COOK et al. 1988a) and rabbit (LONGMAN et al. 1988). In the rat, HAMILTON et al. (1986) observed that the amplitude of contractions is progressively reduced by cromakalim with little effect on the frequency of tension waves. In contrast, HOF et al. (1988) reported that tension amplitude is essentially unchanged by cromakalim while contraction frequency is reduced. In the guinea pig both contraction amplitude and frequency are diminished (COOK et al. 1988a). In rabbit basilar and pig coronary arteries, cromakalim (0.1–10 μM) relaxes tissue spontaneous tone (CAIN and NICHOLSON 1988).

3.3.2.2 Effects on Agonist-Induced Contractions

Pretreatment with cromakalim (0.1–10 μ*M*) reduces maximum responses to noradrenaline in rat aorta and portal vein with some rightward shift in the agonist dose-response curves (HAMILTON et al. 1986; WEIR and WESTON 1986b). Similar inhibitory effects are seen in rabbit mesenteric artery (CLAPHAM and WILSON 1987) and against angiotensin II (rabbit aorta; COOK et al. 1988a; HOF et al. 1988) and 5-HT (rabbit basilar and mesenteric arteries, pig coronary artery; CAIN and NICHOLSON 1988). Pretreatment with cromakalim has no effect on the initial contractile response of rabbit aorta to noradrenaline. However, cromakalim (0.3–10 μ*M*) relaxes an established noradrenaline contraction in this tissue (BRAY et al. 1988).

Pretreatment with cromakalim produces selective inhibition of responses to low concentrations of KCl (≤30 m*M*) in a variety of tissues, whereas contractions generated by higher concentrations of KCl (≥80 m*M*) are little affected (HAMILTON et al. 1986; WEIR and WESTON 1986b; CLAPHAM and WILSON 1987; CAIN and NICHOLSON 1988; COOK et al. 1988a, c).

3.3.2.3 Stereospecificity of In Vitro Effects

The inhibitory effects of the separated enantiomeric components of cromakalim have been examined in rat and rabbit isolated blood vessels. In rat portal vein, BRL38227 was 50–200 times more potent than BRL38226 as an inhibitor of spontaneous mechanical activity and as a stimulator of ^{86}Rb efflux (BUCKINGHAM et al. 1986b; BRAY et al. 1987b; HOF et al. 1988). Similar potency differences are seen when the inhibitory effects of the enantiomers on KCl-induced contractions are compared in segments of rat and rabbit aorta (BRAY et al. 1987b; HOF et al. 1988) or on angiotensin II-induced contractions in rabbit aorta (HOF et al. 1988).

3.3.2.4 Effects on Membrane Potential

In rat portal vein, low concentrations of cromakalim (0.3–1 μ*M*) reduce the duration of electrical multispike complexes with no effect on the frequency of spikes within a complex (HAMILTON et al. 1986; WESTON, unpublished data). At higher concentrations, multispike complexes are abolished and a concentration-dependent hyperpolarisation is detected (HAMILTON et al. 1986). In the concentration range 0.4–10 μ*M*, cromakalim produces hyperpolarisation in rat and rabbit aorta and in rabbit mesenteric and pulmonary arteries (KREYE et al. 1987a, b; SOUTHERTON et al. 1987a, MCHARG et al. 1988; NAKAO et al. 1988; TAYLOR et al. 1988b).

3.3.2.5 Effects on ^{86}Rb and ^{42}K Efflux

In rat portal vein cromakalim (10 μ*M*) produces an increase in ^{86}Rb efflux (HAMILTON et al. 1986), an effect which in later studies was shown to be dependent on the concentration of cromakalim (0.3–10 μ*M*) (Fig. 5; SOUTHERTON, unpublished data). The ability of cromakalim to increase ^{86}Rb exchange in rat

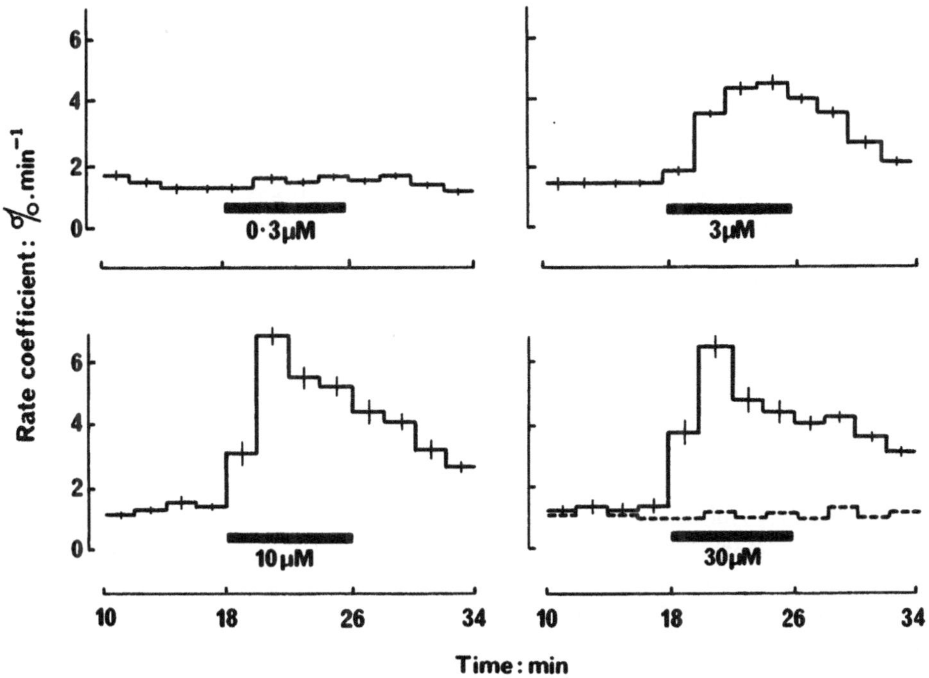

Fig. 5. Effect of cromakalim (0.3–10 µ*M*) on the loss of ^{86}Rb from rat aorta. Tissues were exposed to cromakalim between the 18th and 26th min of the efflux period (*solid bar*). From Southerton, unpublished observations

portal vein is due to the (−)enantiomeric component, BRL38227 (Hof et al. 1988). Similar changes in ^{86}Rb efflux have been detected in rat aorta (Weir and Weston 1986b), in guinea pig portal vein (Quast 1987) and in the aorta, pulmonary, ear and mesenteric arteries of the rabbit (Coldwell and Howlett 1987; Kreye et al. 1987a, b; McHarg et al. 1988). In a comparative study the increase in ^{42}K efflux produced by cromakalim is greater than the comparable rise in ^{86}Rb exchange, suggesting that the K channels involved are more permeable to ^{42}K than to ^{86}Rb (Quast 1988).

3.3.3 Effects on Non-Vascular Tissue

3.3.3.1 Cardiac Muscle

In segments of guinea pig papillary muscle, cromakalim (1–100 µ*M*) shortens the duration of cardiac action potentials (Cain and Metzler 1985). These findings were confirmed by Grosset and Hicks (1986) and by Scholtysik (1987). Analysis of the changes produced by cromakalim (1–100 µ*M*) in guinea pig isolated cardiac myocytes was described by Osterrieder (1988). Cromakalim shortens the duration of electrically induced action potentials and slightly increases the resting membrane potential. Under voltage clamp conditions, this effect of cromakalim is associated with removal of the inward rectifying properties of the K outward current at potentials positive to approximately −50 mV (OSTERRIEDER 1988).

3.3.3.2 Trachea

The ability of cromakalim (1−10 μ*M*) to relax spontaneous tone in guinea pig isolated trachea was first described by ALLEN et al. (1986). Similar observations were made subsequently by BUCKLE et al. (1987), ARCH et al. (1988a, b) and TAYLOR et al. (1988a). Although cromakalim is able to inhibit contractions produced by histamine, 5-HT, leukotriene D_4 and prostaglandin E_2 in the guinea pig, it is relatively ineffective against contractions produced by acetylcholine (ALLEN et al. 1986; ARCH et al. 1988a, b; TAYLOR et al. 1988a). In the innervated isolated guinea pig trachea, cromakalim may inhibit acetylcholine release from intramural cholinergic neurons (HALL and MACLAGAN 1988). In anaesthetised guinea pigs, cromakalim (3−10 mg/kg, intraduodenally) inhibits 5-HT-induced bronchospasm, while in conscious animals, protection against the effects of a histamine aerosol is observed (ARCH et al. 1988a). In conscious, antigen-sensitised animals, cromakalim (2.5 mg/kg, p.o.) reduces the bronchial effects of antigen challenge (ARCH et al. 1988a). In contrast to the guinea pig, cromakalim is an effective inhibitor of carbachol-induced spasm in segments of human bronchiole (TAYLOR et al. 1988a).

3.3.3.3 Bladder

Cromakalim (0.1−10 μ*M*) abolishes spontaneous contractions of detrusor muscle from pigs and guinea pigs, and from pigs and humans with detrusor instability. In contrast, contractions in response to stimulation of intrinsic nerves or exposure to carbachol are little affected (FOSTER and BRADING 1987). In guinea pig bladder cromakalim (0.5−10 μ*M*) abolishes spontaneous spike discharges, hyperpolarises the membrane and increases membrane conductance (FUJII 1987).

3.3.3.4 Gastrointestinal Tract

In guinea pig taenia caeci, cromakalim (0.1−10 μ*M*) relaxes the spontaneous tone of the preparation (WEIR and WESTON 1986a).

3.3.3.5 Reproductive Tract

In the term-pregnant rat, cromakalim (1−10 μ*M*) abolishes spontaneous mechanical activity. Contractions produced by low concentrations of KCl (⩽20 m*M*) are inhibited, while responses to high (⩾80 μ*M*) concentrations are little affected. Some inhibition of the increase in tension produced by oxytocin is also seen (HOLLINGSWORTH et al. 1987, 1988). In the anaesthetised rat, cromakalim rapidly inhibits uterine contractions with a selective action on contraction frequency. On repeated exposure to cromakalim, evidence of tolerance to these in vivo inhibitory effects is obtained (DOWNING et al. 1989).

3.3.3.6 Central Nervous System

Little information is available on the possible CNS effects of cromakalim. However, TRICKLEBANK et al. (1988) have shown that administration of cromakalim (0.01–1 μg, i.c.v.) reduces the behavioural responses to subsequent exposure to pilocarpine (5 mg/kg, i.p.). In guinea pig hippocampal slices, cromakalim (30–300 μ*M*) reduces the EPSP and population spike components of evoked potentials and reduces the bursting rate of pacemaker neurons (ALZHEIMER and TEN BRUGGENCATE 1988).

3.4 Mechanism of Action

3.4.1 Evidence for the Role of K Channels

Information derived from a combination of microelectrode, ion flux and organ bath techniques strongly indicates that the smooth muscle relaxant effects of cromakalim are the indirect consequence of the opening of K channels (Sect. 1, Fig. 1).

Electrophysiological measurements indicate that cromakalim produces a cessation of continuing electrical discharges and/or membrane hyperpolarisation in a wide variety of smooth muscles (HAMILTON et al. 1986; HOLLINGSWORTH et al. 1987; MCHARG et al. 1988, 1989; NAKAO et al. 1988). The changes in membrane potential are usually maintained in the presence of cromakalim, and in some tissues the hyperpolarisation approaches the theoretical E_K. At concentrations which produce cessation of spontaneous electrical discharges, a small increase in ^{42}K or ^{86}Rb efflux can sometimes be detected (MCHARG et al. 1988, 1989; SOUTHERTON, unpublished data; Fig. 5). At concentrations of cromakalim which generate hyperpolarisation, all tissues studied except rat uterus show a marked increase in ^{42}K or ^{86}Rb exchange (HAMILTON et al. 1986; HOLLINGSWORTH et al. 1987; QUAST 1987; HOF et al. 1988; MCHARG et al. 1988, 1989; TAYLOR et al. 1988b). In organ bath experiments, the ability of cromakalim to relax contractions produced by low concentrations of KCl (≤20 m*M*) but to have little inhibitory action on responses to high concentrations (≥80 m*M*) is consistent with the ability to open K channels (see Sect. 2.4.1).

In cardiac muscle, concentrations of cromakalim generally 30–100 times greater than those required to produce smooth muscle relaxation shorten the duration of evoked action potentials (CAIN and METZLER 1985; GROSSET and HICKS 1986; SCHOLTYSIK 1987; OSTERRIEDER 1988). Such an effect is also consistent with the ability to open K channels (see Sect. 16 3.4.3). In both cardiac and smooth muscle, cromakalim has no effect on cAMP and cGMP concentrations (COLDWELL and HOWLETT 1987; GILLESPIE and SHENG 1988; NEWGREEN et al. 1988a, b; TAYLOR et al. 1988b; YANAGISAWA et al. 1988).

In rabbit aorta, tonic responses to noradrenaline are inhibited by cromakalim, a property not shared with calcium antagonists. However, this inhibition is not seen under depolarising conditions, suggesting that K channel opening is also involved in this aspect of cromakalim-induced inhibition (BRAY et al. 1988; COOK et al. 1988c).

3.4.2 Causal Relationship Between K Channel Opening In Vitro and Hypotensive Effects In Vivo

No data are available on the relative potencies for in vitro K channel opening and in vivo hypotensive activity in a series of cromakalim analogues. However, the (−)enantiomer (BRL38227) is both a potent stimulator of ^{86}Rb exchange in vitro and a potent hypotensive agent (HOF et al. 1988). Contrary to an early report than the K channel blocking agent glibenclamide was unable to antagonise the hypotensive action of cromakalim (WILSON et al. 1988a), further investigations have shown that intravenous administration of glibenclamide can antagonise the depressor action of cromakalim (CAVERO et al. 1988; HAMILTON, personal communication).

In a comprehensive study, COLDWELL and HOWLETT (1987) showed that cromakalim does not interact with known binding sites in a variety of tissues and has no effect on phosphodiesterase activity.

3.4.3 Type of K Channel Modulated by Cromakalim

K channel blocking agents have been extensively used in an attempt to confirm the mechanism of K-channel opening and to clarify the type of channel involved in the action of cromakalim. The neuropeptide apamin (HABERMANN 1984) has no effect on responses to cromakalim, either in vitro (WEIR and WESTON 1986a) or in vivo (COOK and HOF 1988). Procaine is an effective antagonist of the actions of cromakalim, whereas the ability of TEA or 4-aminopyridine to modify the inhibition of cromakalim varies from tissue to tissue (ALLEN et al. 1986; BEECH and BOLTON 1987; FUJII 1987; SOUTHERTON and WESTON 1987; HOLLINGSWORTH et al. 1988; WILSON et al. 1988b). Some actions of cromakalim are also inhibited by a component contained in *Leiurus quinquestriatus* venom (QUAST and COOK 1988).

In cells isolated from rabbit portal vein, BEECH and BOLTON (1987) found that cromakalim produces an increase in outward K current. Using TEA and 4-aminopyridine they concluded that this current is essentially voltage and Ca independent. Other studies in whole tissues or isolated cells have indicated that the cromakalim-induced outward K current is Ca dependent and may be carried through a large conductance K channel. (KUSANO et al. 1987; GELBAND et al. 1988; NAKAO et al. 1988; TALVENHEIMO et al. 1988; TRIESCHMAN et al. 1988). The site of action of cromakalim in stimulating K currents is unknown. Pertussis toxin has no effect on cromakalim-induced changes in rat heart and blood vessels (QUAST et al. 1988). Protein kinase C is not involved in the actions of cromakalim in rabbit mesenteric artery (COLDWELL 1988).

In isolated cardiac myocytes, cromakalim stimulates a time-dependent K current which is relatively voltage insensitive (ESCANDE et al. 1988b). This effect is antagonised by glibenclamide, a potent, selective blocker of ATP-dependent K channels in pancreatic β-cells (FOSSET et al. 1988). In isolated membrane patches, cromakalim activates ATP-dependent K channels (ESCANDE et al. 1988b). These data together with the ability of glibenclamide to inhibit the relaxant effects of cromakalim in smooth and cardiac muscle (MESTRE et al.

1988; QUAST and COOK 1988; WILSON et al. 1988b; NEWGREEN et al. 1989) and its hypotensive effects in vivo (CAVERO et al. 1988) suggest that cromakalim may interact with a smooth muscle K channel not unlike the ATP-dependent K channel found in cardiac muscle (NOMA 1987).

Cromakalim may interact with ATP-dependent K channels in pancreatic β-cells (COOK et al. 1988b), although the evidence for this is weak (ASHFORD et al. 1989; WILSON et al. 1988a).

3.4.4 Comparative Studies Between Pinacidil, Cromakalim, Nicorandil and Calcium Antagonists

Many studies have been reported in which the effects of cromakalim have been compared with those of pinacidil, nicorandil and various calcium antagonists (BUCKINGHAM et al. 1986b; HAMILTON et al. 1986; WEIR and WESTON 1986a, b; CLAPHAM and WILSON 1987; COLDWELL and HOWLETT 1987; ANGERSBACH and NICHOLSON 1988; ARCH et al. 1988a, b; CLAPHAM 1988; CLAPHAM and COOPER 1988; COOK et al. 1988a, c; GOTANDA et al. 1988; LONGMAN et al. 1988; WILSON et al. 1988b). In vitro, the anti-vasoconstrictor effects of pinacidil, cromakalim and nicorandil display a profile different from that of the calcium antagonists. Within the substances showing K channel opening properties, the potency series is cromakalim > pinacidil > nicorandil. In vivo, no general systematic differences between the K channel openers and calcium antagonists have emerged. However, within a given species, marked differences exist between individual K channel openers and between these agents and calcium antagonists. In lowering blood pressure, the general potency series is cromakalim > pinacidil > nicorandil.

3.5 Clinical Studies

Reports of the effects of cromakalim in humans are limited to those derived from single-dose studies or from relatively short duration trials. These have allowed a preliminary profile of the effects of the drug in humans to be established and have indicated the dose ranges for use in longer trials.

3.5.1 Volunteer Studies

In a study using six male volunteers, NGUYEN et al. (1987) showed that a single oral dose (1–2 mg) of cromakalim has little effect on resting systolic or diastolic blood pressure. However, the pressor effects of noradrenaline or angiotensin II administered intravenously are reduced by cromakalim treatment. Fox et al. (1987) administered cromakalim (0.5–2 mg) as single oral doses to eight male volunteers. A significant reduction in supine and standing blood pressure is seen after 2 mg cromakalim, together with an increase in heart rate. Fox et al. (1987) also showed that cromakalim increases forearm blood flow with no effect on venous capacitance. GLUCK et al. (1987) have studied the effects of a single oral dose of 1 mg cromakalim in six volunteers and in hypertensive patients; results were pooled. The diastolic blood pressure decreased, while plasma noradrenaline levels together with renal plasma flow and GFR increased. Some changes in K excretion were detected, and it was concluded that cromakalim produces systemic and renal vasodilation with a decrease in aldosterone production.

The effects of cromakalim on the respiratory tract have been examined by BAIRD et al. (1988) in seven volunteers. After oral administration of cromakalim (2 mg), the bronchoconstrictor effects of a histamine inhalation are reduced. These effects are accompanied by a small reduction in diastolic blood pressure and an increase in heart rate similar to that seen in the same patients after administration of salbutamol.

3.5.2 Effects in Hypertensive Patients

In a single-dose, multicentre study involving 40 patients with essential hypertension (VANDENBURG et al. 1986), cromakalim (0.5–1.5 mg) decreased supine mean arterial pressure. Erect blood pressure was lowered in the dose range 1–1.5 mg, but postural hypotension was not reported. Some tachycardia was also detected. In a related study (VANDENBURG et al. 1987b) the duration of antihypertensive action of cromakalim following a single oral dose (1–1.5 mg) was 6–10 h. In a 6-week study, daily administration of 0.75 mg cromakalim decreased systolic and diastolic blood pressure in seated patients within 14 days. Reflex tachycardia was observed, but oedema and electrolyte changes were absent (ECKL and GREB 1987). During a 1-week, dose-ranging investigation (VANDENBURG et al. 1987a,b) cromakalim (0.5–1.5 mg) produced a dose-related decrease in supine mean arterial pressure. Postural hypotension was not detected. In apparently the same patient group, minor ECG changes were seen in cromakalim-treated patients (PILGRIM et al. 1987). In a 3-day study LEBEL et al. (1988) showed that cromakalim lowers mean supine blood pressure without producing postural hypotension or alteration of renal haemodynamics.

3.5.3 Adverse Effects

A dose-related headache in some patients is an adverse reaction common to both the volunteer and hypertensive patient studies (see VANDENBURG et al. 1987a).

4 RP 49356

4.1 Chemistry and History of Development

RP 49356 [(±)*N*-methyl-2-(3-pyridinyl)-tetrahydrothiopyran-2-carbothioamide-1-oxide] (Fig. 6) was developed from a series of compounds with anti-ulcer activity (ALOUP et al. 1987). RP 49356 is one of a series of substituted thiopyrans with blood pressure-lowering properties currently under development. The molecule contains a single chiral carbon atom at position 2 of the thiopyran ring (Fig. 6). Biological activity resides in the (−)enantiomer (WITHNALL, personal communication), the absolute stereochemistry of which has not been disclosed.

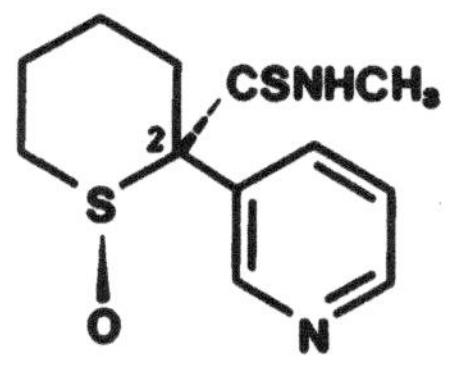

(±)-RP 49356

Fig. 6. Chemical structure of RP 49356. The biological activity of this molecule resides in the (−)enantiomer

4.2 Pharmacological Profile

The effects of RP 49356 in vivo and in vitro have been briefly described by ESCANDE et al. (1988a) and by MONDOT et al. (1988). The general profile of this agent is similar to those of pinacidil and cromakalim. RP 49356 (0.1–1 mg/kg, p.o.) lowers blood pressure in a variety of hypertensive rat models and in anaesthetised dogs and cats. These effects are associated with a reflex tachycardia sensitive to β-adrenoceptor blockade. In rat aortic rings, it selectively relaxes contractions produced by low concentrations of KCl (≤20 m*M*) but has no effect on responses to 80 m*M* KCl. These vasorelaxant effects are accompanied by an increase in ^{86}Rb efflux (LONGMORE and WESTON, unpublished data). In guinea pig papillary muscle, it (300 μ*M*) shortens the duration of evoked action potentials. Its in vitro effects can be antagonised by glibenclamide (MONDOT et al. 1988). In isolated cardiac myocytes RP 49356 activates an ATP-dependent K channel (ESCANDE et al. 1988a).

4.3 Clinical Studies

RP 49356 is in the early stages of clinical development as a potential antihypertensive agent. No information on its status is available.

5 Diazoxide and Minoxidil Sulphate

The development and current status of diazoxide and of minoxidil are described elsewhere in this volume (Chap. 9). Until recently, the mode of action of these agents was unknown. However, recent experiments with diazoxide (BRAY et al. 1988; COOK et al. 1986) and with the active sulphate metabolite of minoxidil (JOHNSON et al. 1982; McCALL et al. 1983) have shown that both agents possess K channel opening properties in smooth muscle (BRAY et al. 1988; MEISHERI et al. 1988; WILDE and LEE, 1988; NEWGREEN et al. 1989). It is not yet known whether this property can fully account for the blood pressure-lowering action of these agents.

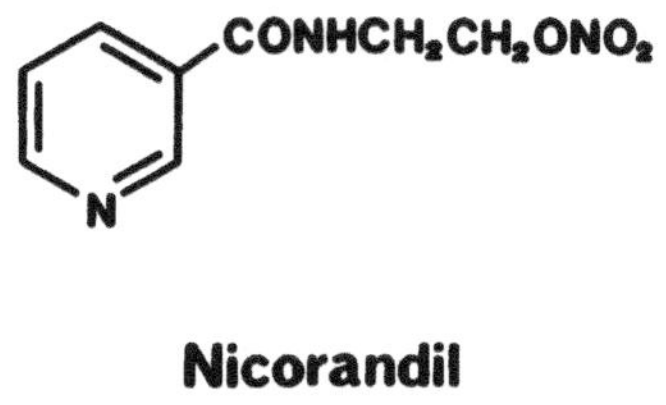

Fig. 7. Chemical structure of nicorandil

6 Nicorandil

Nicorandil (2-nicotinamidoethyl nitrate, Fig. 7) was developed in Japan, and its coronary vasodilator properties were first described by UCHIDA et al. (1978). Nicorandil exhibits both K channel opening and guanylate cyclase-activating properties. It is currently under development as an anti-anginal agent (for review, see HAMILTON and WESTON 1988).

Acknowledgements. I am very grateful to Dr J.M. Evans (Beecham) and to Dr T.C. Hamilton (Beecham) for their helpful advice and comments.

Summary

Cromakalim (BRL34915) and pinacidil (P1134) are recently developed vasodilator drugs which belong to a newly recognised class of agent—the smooth muscle K channel openers. The mechanism of the antihypertensive action of these substances was first recognised in vitro from a combination of ion flux and microelectrode studies and is primarily exerted by the opening of K channels in vascular smooth muscle. The resulting membrane hyperpolarisation indirectly reduces the intracellular Ca^{2+} concentration and functionally antagonises the effects of a variety of circulating pressor agents. The in vitro actions of cromakalim and pinacidil on smooth muscle can be antagonised by K channel blockers such as tetraethylammonium, procaine, 4-aminopyridine and glibenclamide and may thus be mediated via a K channel similar to the ATP-dependent K channel in cardiac muscle. The clinical use of cromakalim and pinacidil in hypertension is under development, and their application in peripheral vascular diseases is also indicated. The relaxant action of these agents is not restricted to vascular smooth muscle, and possibilities for their use in the treatment of bronchial asthma and in the irritable bladder syndrome are also emerging. New developments in this field include RP 49356 and the recognition that minoxidil sulphate and diazoxide also exhibit K channel opening actions.

References

Abraham PA, Halstenson CE, Matzke GR, Kean WR (1987) Comparison of antihypertensive, renal hemodynamic and humoral effects of pinacidil and hydralazine monotherapy. J Clin Hypertens 3:439–451

Ahnfelt-Rønne I (1988a) Pinacidil: history, basic pharmacology and therapeutic implications. J Cardiovasc Pharmacol 12 (Suppl 2):51–54

Ahnfelt-Rønne I (1988b) Pinacidil preclinical investigations. Drugs 36 (Suppl 7):4–9

Allen SL, Boyle JP, Cortijo J, Foster RW, Morgan GP, Small RC (1986) Electrical and mechanical effects of BRL 34915 in guinea-pig isolated trachealis. Br J Pharmacol 89:395–405

Aloup JC, Bouchaudon J, Farge D, James C, Deregnaucourt J, Houis MH (1987) Synthesis and antisecretory and antiulcer activities of derivatives and analogues of 2-(2-pyridyl) tetrahydrothiophene-2-carbothioamide. J Med Chem 30:24–29

Alzheimer C, ten Bruggencate G (1988) Actions of BRL34915 (cromakalim) upon convulsive discharges in guinea-pig hippocampal slices. Naunyn Schmiedebergs Arch Pharmacol 337:429–434

Andersson KE, Andersson P-O, Fovaeus M, Hedlund H, Malmgren A, Sjögren C (1988) Effects of pinacidil on bladder muscle. Drugs 36 (Suppl 7):55–63

Angersbach D, Nicholson CD (1985) The effect of the novel antihypertensive agent BRL34915 on the nutritional blood flow of rat chronically ischaemic skeletal muscle. Naunyn Schmiedebergs Arch Pharmacol 329:241R

Angersbach D, Nicholson CD (1988) Enhancement of muscle blood cell flux and pO_2 by cromakalim (BRL34915) and other compounds enhancing membrane K^+ conductance, but not by Ca^{2+} antagonists or hydralazine in an animal model of occlusive arterial disease. Naunyn Schmiedebergs Arch Pharmacol 337:341–346

Arch JRS, Buckle DR, Bumstead J, Clarke GD, Taylor JF, Taylor SG (1988a) Evaluation of the potassium channel activator cromakalim (BRL34915) as a bronchodilator in the guinea-pig: comparison with nifedipine. Br J Pharmacol 95:763–770

Arch JRS, Buckle DR, Bumstead J, Taylor JF (1988b) Comparison of the effects of cromakalim (BRL34915) and pinacidil in guinea-pig models of bronchoconstriction. Br J Pharmacol Proc 95 (Suppl):794

Arrigoni-Martelli E, Finucaine J (1985) Pinacidil. In: Scriabine A (ed) New cardiovascular drugs. Raven, New York, pp 133–151

Arrigoni-Martelli E, Kaergaard-Nielsen C, Bang Olsen U, Petersen HJ (1980) N″-cyano-N-4-pyridyl(-N′-1,2,2,-trimethylpropylguanidine monohydrate (P1134): new potent vasodilator. Experientia 36:445–447

Ashford MLJ, Hales CN, Kozlowski RZ (1989) Diazoxide but not BRL34915 activates ATP-sensitive potassium channels in a rat insulinoma cell line. J Physiol 409:53p

Ashwood VA, Cassidy F, Evans JM, Faruk EA, Hamilton TC (1984) *Trans*-4-cyclicamido-3,4-dihydro-2H-benzopyran-3-ols as antihypertensive agents. In: Dahlbom R, Nilsson JLG (eds) Proceedings of VIIIth international medicinal chemistry symposium (Uppsala), vol 7. Swedish Pharmaceutical, Stockholm, pp 316–317

Ashwood VA, Buckingham RE, Cassidy F, Evans JM, Faruk EA, Hamilon TC, Nash JD, Stemp G, Willcocks K (1986) Synthesis and antihypertensive activity of 4-(cyclic amido)-2H-1-benzopyrans. J Med Chem 29:2194–2201

Baird A, Hamilton TC, Richards DH, Tasker T, Williams AJ (1988) Inhibition of histamine induced bronchoconstriction in normal healthy volunteers by a potassium channel activator, cromakalim, BRL34915. Br J Clin Pharmacol 25:114P

Bang Olsen U, Arrigoni-Martelli E (1983) Vascular effects in dogs of pinacidil (P1134), a novel vasoactive antihypertensive agent. Eur J Pharmacol 88:389–392

Beech DJ, Bolton TB (1987) Effects of BRL 34915 on membrane currents recorded from single smooth muscle cells from rabbit portal vein. Br J Pharmacol 92:550P

Benham CD, Bolton TB, Lang RJ, Takewaki T (1985) The mechanism of action of Ba and TEA on single Ca activated K-channels in arterial and intestinal smooth muscle cell membranes. Pflügers Arch 403:120–127

Bolton TB, Lang RJ, Takewaki T (1984) Mechanisms of action of noradrenaline and

carbachol on smooth muscle of guinea-pig anterior mesenteric artery. J Physiol 351: 549–572
Bolton TB, Lang RJ, Takewaki T (1985) Patch and whole cell voltage clamp of single mammalian visceral and vascular smooth muscle cells. Experientia 4:887–894
Bowman WC (1982) Aminopyridines and similarly acting drugs. Effects on nerves muscles and synapses. In: Lechat P, Thesleff S, Bowman WC (eds) Advances in the biosciences, vol 35. Pergamon, New York, pp 335–341
Bowman WC, Savage AO (1981) Pharmacological actions of aminopyridines and related compounds. Pure App Pharmacol Sci 2:317–371
Bray KM, Brown BS, Duty S, Kay PB, Longmore J, McHarg AD, Newgreen DT, Southerton JS, Waterfall JF, Weston AH (1988) Studies on the mode of action of minoxidil sulphate and diazoxide: a comparison with cromakalim. Br J Pharmacol Proc (Suppl) 95:733P
Bray KM, Newgreen DT, Small RC, Southerton JS, Taylor SG, Weir SW, Weston AH (1987a) Evidence that the mechanism of the inhibitory action of pinacidil differs from that of glyceryl trinitrate. Br J Pharmacol 91:421–429
Bray KM, Newgreen DT, Weston AH (1987b) Some effects of the enantiomers of the potassium channel openers BRL 34915 and pinacidil on rat blood vessels. Br J Pharmacol Proc (Suppl) 91:357P
Bray KM, Weston AH, McHarg AD, Newgreen DT, Southerton JS, Duty S (1988) Further studies on the actions of the K-channel openers, cromakalim (BRL34915) and pinacidil, in rabbit aorta. Pflügers Arch 411:R202
Buckingham RE, Clapham JC, Coldwell MC, Hamilton TC, Howlett DR (1986a) Stereospecific mechanism of action of the antihypertensive agent BRL 34915. Br J Pharmacol 87:78P
Buckingham RE, Clapham JC, Hamilton TC, Longman SD, Norton J, Poyser RE (1986b) BRL 34915, a novel antihypertensive agent: comparison of effects on blood pressure and other haemodynamic parameters with those of nifedipine in animal models. J Cardiovasc Pharmacol 8:798–804
Buckingham RE (1988) Studies on the anti-vasoconstrictor activity of BRL34915 in spontaneously hypertensive rats; a comparison with nifedipine. Br J Pharmacol 93:541–552
Buckle DR, Bumstead J, Clarke GD, Taylor JF, Taylor SG (1987) Reversal of agonist-induced bronchoconstriction in the guinea pig by the potassium channel activator BRL34915. Br J Pharmacol 92:744P
Bülbring E, Tomita T (1987) Catecholamine action on smooth muscle. Pharmacol Rev 39:49–96
Byyny RL, Niers AS, Loverde ME, Mitchell, WB (1987) A double blind randomised controlled trial comparing pinacidil to hydralazine in essential hypertension. Clin Pharmacol Ther 42:50–57
Cain CR, Metzler V (1985) Electrophysiological effects of the antihypertensive BRL 34915 on guinea-pig papillary muscle. Naunyn Schmiedebergs Arch Pharmacol 329:R53
Cain C, Nicholson CD (1988) A comparison of the effects of BRL34915 on basilar, coronary and mesenteric arteries. Br J Pharmacol Proc (Suppl) 93:208P
Callaghan JT, Goldberg MR, Brunelle R (1988) Double-blind comparator trails with pinacidil, a potassium channel opener. Drugs 36 (Suppl 7):77–82
Carlsen JE, Kardel T, Hilden T, Tango M, Trap-Jensen J (1981) Immediate central and peripheral haemodynamic effects of a new vasodilating agent pinacidil (P1134) in hypertensive man. Clin Physiol 1:375–384
Carlsen JE, Kardel T, Jensen HE, Tango M, Trap-Jensen J (1983) Pinacidil a new vasodilator: pharmacokinetics of a new retarded release tablet in essential hypertension. Eur J Pharmacol 25:557–561
Carlsen JE, Kardel T, Lund JO, McNair A, Trap-Jensen J (1985) Acute haemodynamic effects of pinacidil and hydralazine in essential hypertension. Clin Pharmacol Ther 37:253–259
Cavero I, Mondot S, Mestre M, Escande D (1988) Haemodynamic and pharmacological mechanisms of the hypotensive effects of cromakalim in rats: blockade by gliben-

clamide. Br J Pharmacol Proc (Suppl) 95:643P
Clapham JC (1988) Renal haemodynamic effects of cromakalim, nifedipine and pinacidil in the conscious cat. Br J Pharmacol Proc 95(Suppl):793P
Clapham JC, Buckingham RE (1988) The haemodynamic profile of cromakalim in the cat. J Cardiovasc Pharmacol 12:555–567
Clapham JC, Cooper SM (1988) Effect of cromakalim (BRL34915) and pinacidil on baroreceptor sensitivity in the anaesthetised cat. Br J Pharmacol Proc (Suppl) 93:200P
Clapham JC, Wilson C (1987) Antispasmogenic and spasmolytic effects of BRL34915: a comparison with nifedipine and nicorandil. J Auton Pharmacol 7:233–242
Cohen ML, Colbert WE (1986) Comparison of the effects of pinacidil and its metabolite, pinacidil-N-oxide in isolated smooth and cardiac muscle. Drug Dev Res 7:111–124
Cohen ML, Kurz KD (1988) Pinacidil-induced vascular relaxation: comparison to other vasodilators and to classical mechanisms of vasodilation. J Cardiovasc Pharmacol 12 (Suppl 2):55–59
Coldwell MC (1988) Interaction between cromakalim (BRL34915) and protein kinase C activation in rabbit mesenteric artery. Br J Pharmacol Proc (Suppl) 93:207P
Coldwell MC, Howlett DR (1987) Specificity of action of the novel antihypertensive agent, BRL34915, as a potassium channel activator. Comparison with nicorandil. Biochem Pharmacol 36:3663–3669
Cook NS, Haylett DG (1985) Effects of apamin, quinine and neuromuscular blocking agents on calcium activated potassium channels in guinea pig hepatocytes. J Physiol 358:373–394
Cook NS, Hof RP (1988) Cardiovascular effects of apamin and BRL34915 in rats and rabbits. Br J Pharmacol 93:121–131
Cook NS, Quast U, Hof RP, Baumlin Y, Pally C (1988a) Similarities in the mechanism of action of two new vasodilator drugs: pinacidil and BRL34915. J Cardiovasc Pharmacol 11:90–99
Cook NS, Quast U, Weir SW (1988b) In vitro and in vivo comparison of two K^+ channel openers, diazoxide and BRL34915. Pflügers Arch 411:R46
Cook NS, Weir SW, Danzeisen MC (1988c) Anti-vasoconstrictor effects of the K^+ channel opener cromakalim on the rabbit aorta – comparison with the calcium antagonist isradipine. Br J Pharmacol 95:741–752
Davies BE, Dierdorf D, Eckl KM, Greb WH, Mellows G, Thomsen T (1988) The pharmacokinetics of cromakalim, BRL34915, a new antihypertensive agent, in healthy male subjects. Br J Clin Pharmacol 25:136P–137P
Dieperink H, Kemp E, Jorgensen KA, Starklint H (1983) Pinacidil: effects on function and perfusion of normal kidneys and renal xerografts. J Hypertens 1:357–360
Downing SJ, Hollingsworth M, Miller M (1989) Tolerance to cromakalim in the rat uterus in vivo. Br J Pharmacol 96:732–738
Dumez D, Zazzi-Sudriez E, Pautrel C, Armstrong JM, Hicks PE (1988) Comparison of the cardiovascular and renal effects of BRL34915 with those of nitrendipine in dogs and SHR. Br J Pharmacol Proc (Suppl) 93:201P
Eckl KM, Greb WH (1987) Potassium channel activation in the vascular smooth muscle cell membrane – a new mechanism of action in antihypertensive treatment – early clinical results with BRL34915. Clin Exp Ther 49:160
Eilertsen E, Hart JW, Magnussen MP, Sorensen H, Arrigoni-Martelli E (1982a) Pharmacokinetics and distribution of the new antihypertensive agent pinacidil in rat, dog and man. Xenobiotica 12:177–185
Eilertsen E, Magnussen MP, Petersen HJ, Rastrup-Andersen N, Sorensen H, Arrigoni-Martelli E (1982b) Metabolism of the new antihypertensive agent pinacidil in rat, dog and man. Xenobiotica 12:187–196
Escande D, Thuringer D, Laville M, Courteix J, Cavero I (1988a) RP 49356 is a potent opener of ATP-modulated potassium channels in cardiac myocytes. Br J Pharmacol Proc (Suppl) 95:814P
Escande D, Thuringer D, Leguern S, Cavero I (1988b) The potassium channel opener cromakalim (BRL34915) activates ATP-dependent K^+-channels in isolated cardiac myocytes. Biochem Biophys Res Commun 154:620–625
Evans JM, Fake CS, Hamilton TC, Poyser RH, Watts EA (1983) Synthesis and anti-

hypertensive activity of substituted trans-4-amino-3,4-dihydro-2,2-dimethyl-2H-1-benzopyran-3-ols. J Med Chem 26:1582–1589
Fosset M, DeWeille JR, Green RD, Schmid-Antomarchi H, Lazdunski M (1988) Antidiabetic sulphonylureas control action potential properties in heart cells via high affinity receptors that are linked to ATP-dependent K^+-channels. J Biol Chem 236:7933–7936
Foster CD, Brading AF (1987) The effect of potassium channel antagonists on the BRL34915 activated potassium channel in guinea pig bladder. Br J Pharmacol 92:751P
Fovaeus M, Andersson K-E, Hedlund H (1989) The action of pinacidil in the human bladder. J Urol 141:637–640
Fox JS, Whitehead E, Shanks RG (1987) Cardiovascular effects of the novel antihypertensive agent BRL34915 in normal volunteers. Br J Clin Pharmacol 23:600P
Fujii K (1987) An electrophysiological investigation of the mechanism of action of BRL34915 on the guinea pig bladder. Br J Pharmacol 92:705P
Gelband CH, Lodge NJ, Talvenheimo JA, Van Breeman C (1988) BRL34915 increases Popen of the large conductance Ca^{2+} activated K^+ channel isolated from rabbit aota in planar lipid bilayers. Biophys J 53:149a
Gill TS, Davies BE, Allen GD, Greb WH (1988a) Stereospecific pharmacokinetics of cromakalim enantiomers in healthy male subjects. Br J Clin Pharmacol 25:669P
Gill TS, Davies BE, Tasker TCG, Whitehead EM, Fox J, Shanks RG (1988b) Stereospecific pharmacokinetics of cromakalim enantiomers at various oral dose levels in healthy male subjects. Br J Clin Pharmacol Proc 26 (Suppl):658P
Gillespie JS, Sheng H (1988) The lack of involvement of cyclic nucleotides in the smooth muscle relaxant action of BRL34915. Br J Pharmacol 94:1189–1197
Glück Z, Windemann P, Gnädinger MP, Weidmann P (1987) Cardiovascular, endocrine and renal actions of acute potassium channel activation by BRL34915 in man. Cardiovasc Drugs Ther 1 (3):241
Goldberg MR (1988) Clinical pharmacology of pinacidil, a prototype for drugs which affect potassium channels. J Cardiovasc Pharmacol 12 (Suppl 2):541–549
Goldberg MR, Offen WW (1988) Pinacidil with and without hydrochlorothiazide: dose-response relationships from results of a 4 × 3 factorial design study. Drugs 36 (Suppl 7):83–92
Goldberg MR, Rockhold RW (1986) Beneficial effects of pinacidil on plasma lipids. J Hypertens 4 (Suppl 5):S575
Gotanda K, Satoh K, Taira N (1988) Is the cardiovascular profile of BRL34915 characteristic of potassium channel activators? J Cardiovasc Pharmacol 12:239–246
Grossett A, Hicks PE (1986) Evidence for blood vessel selectivity of BRL34915. Br J Pharmacol 89:500P
Habermann E (1984) Apamin. Pharmacol Ther 25:255–270
Hackenthal E, Taugner R (1986) Hormonal signals and intracellular messengers for renin secretion. Mol Cell Endocrinol 47:1–12
Hall AK, Maclagan J (1988) Effect of cromakalim on cholinergic neurotransmission in the guinea-pig trachea. Br J Pharmacol Proc 95 (Suppl):792P
Hamilton TC, Weir SW, Weston AH (1986) Comparison of the effects of BRL 34915 and verapamil on electrical and mechanical activity in rat portal vein. Br J Pharmacol 88:103–111
Hamilton TC, Weston AH (1989) Cromakalim, nicorandil and pinacidil: novel drugs which open potassium channels in smooth muscle. Gen Pharmacol 20:1–9
Hermsmeyer K (1988) Ion channel effects of pinacidil in vascular muscle. Drugs 36 (Suppl 7):29–32
Hof RP, Quast U, Cook NS, Blarer S (1988) Mechanism of action of and systemic and regional hemodynamics of the potassium channel activator BRL34915 and its enantiomers. Circ Res 62:679–686
Hollingsworth M, Amédée T, Edwards D, Mironneau J, Savineau JP, Small RC, Weston AH (1987) The relaxant action of BRL34915 in rat uterus. Br J Pharmacol 91: 803–813
Hollingsworth M, Edwards D, Rankin JR, Weston AH (1988) BRL34915 and relaxation

of rat uterus – role of K^+ channels. Br J Pharmacol Proc (Suppl) 93:199P
Izzo JL, Licht MR, Smith RJ, Larrabee PS, Radke KJ, Kallay MC (1987) Chronic effects of direct vasodilation (pinacidil), alpha adrenergic blockade (prazosin) and angiotensin-converting enzyme inhibition in systemic hypertension. Am J Cardiol 60:303–308
Johnson GA, Barsuhn KJ, McCall JM (1982) Sulfation of minoxidil by liver sulphontransferase. Biochem Pharmacol 31:2949–2954
Jürgensen HJ (1988) Comparative effects of pinacidil and nifedipine in the treatment of arterial hypertension. Drugs 36 (Suppl 7):67–69
Kaczorowski GJ, Slaughter RS, Garcia ML, King VF (1988) The role of the sodium-calcium exchange in excitable cells. Trans Biochem Soc 16:529–532
Kaergaard Nielsen C, Arrigoni-Martelli E (1981) Effect of a new vasodilator pinacidil (P1134) on potassium, noradrenaline and serotonin induced contractions in rabbit vascular tissues. Acta Pharmacol Toxicol 49:427–431
Kardel T, Hilden T, Carlsen JE, Trap-Jensen J (1981) N″-cyano-N-4-pyridyl-N′-1,2,2-trimethyl propylguanidine, a new vasodilating agent: acute effect on blood pressure and pharmacokinetics in hypertensive patients. J Cardiovasc Pharmacol 3:1002–1007
Kauffman RF, Schenk KW, Conery BG, Cohen ML (1986) Effects of pinacidil on serotonin-induced contractions and cyclic nucleotide levels in isolated rat aortae: comparison with nitroglycerin, minoxidil and hydralazine. J Cardiovasc Pharmacol 8:1195–1200
Kreye VAW, Gerstheimer F, Weston AH (1987a) Effects of the antihypertensive BRL34915 on membrane potential and ^{86}Rb efflux in rabbit tonic vascular smooth muscle. Pflugers Arch 408:R79
Kreye VAW, Gerstheimer F, Weston AH (1987b) Effects of BRL34915 on resting membrane potential and ^{86}Rb efflux in rabbit tonic vascular smooth muscle. Naunyn Schmiedebergs Arch Pharmacol 335:R64
Kusano K, Barros F, Katz G, Garcia M, Kaczorowski G, Reuben JP (1987) Modulation of K channel activity in aortic smooth muscle by BRL 34915 and a scorpion toxin. Biophys J 51:55a
Lang RW, Wenk PF (1988) Synthesis of selectively trifluoromethylated pyridine derivatives as potential antihypertensives. Helv Chim Acta 71:596–601
Lebel M, Grose JH, Lacourciere Y (1988) Effects of the novel antihypertensive agent BRL34915 on endocrine sodium regulation in essential hypertension. Am J Hypertens 1:32 (abstract 1211)
Longman SD, Clapham JS, Wilson C, Hamilton TC (1988) Cromakalim a potassium channel activator: a comparison of its cardiovascular haemodynamic profile and tissue specificity with those of pinacidil and nicorandil. J Cardiovasc Pharmacol 12: 535–542
McBurney A, Henry JA, Ward JW (1988) Accumulation of pinacidil N-oxide during chronic treatment with pinacidil. Eur J Clin Pharmacol 35:93–95
McCall JM, Aiken JW, Chidester CG, DuCharme DW, Wendling MG (1983) Pyrimidine and triazine 3-oxide sulfates: a new family of vasodilators. J Med Chem 26:1791–1793
McHarg AD, Southerton JS, Weston AH (1988) An investigation into the inhibitory action of cromakalim in rabbit isolated mesenteric artery. Br J Pharmacol 95:642P
McHarg AD, Southerton JS, Weir SW, Weston AH (1989) A comparison of the effects of cromakalim, noradrenaline and isoprenaline in guinea pig isolated taenia caeci. Br J Pharmacol Proc 96 (Suppl):27P
Meisheri KD, Cipkus LA, Taylor CJ (1988) Mechanism of action of minoxidil sulphate-induced vasodilation: a role for increased K^+ permeability. J Pharmacol Exp Ther 245:751–760
Mestre M, Escande D, Cavero I (1988) Glibenclamide blocks the transmembrane action potential shortening evoked by cromakalim in guinea-pig papillary muscle. Br J Pharmacol Proc (Suppl) 95:571P
Mikkelsen E, Pedersen OL (1982) Comparison of the effects of a new vasodilator pinacidil and nifedipine on isolated blood vessels. Act Pharmacol Toxicol 51:407–412
Mondot S, Mestre M, Caillard CG, Cavero I (1988) RP49356: a vasorelaxant agent with potassium channel activating properties. Br J Pharmacol Proc 95 (Suppl):813P

Muiesan G, Fariello R, Muiesan ML (1983) Effects of pinacidil on blood pressure, plasma catecholamines and plasma renin activity in essential hypertensive patients. Clin Pharmacol Ther 33:229

Nakao K, Okabe K, Kitamura A, Kuriyama H, Weston AH (1988) Characteristics of cromakalim-induced relaxations in smooth muscle cells of guinea-pig mesenteric artery and vein. Br J Pharmacol 95:795–804

Newgreen DT, Bray KM, Southerton JS, Weston AH (1988a) The action of glyceryl trinitrate and sodium nitroprusside on rat aorta: a comparison with nicorandil and BRL34915. Br J Pharmacol Proc (Suppl) 93:17P

Newgreen DT, Bray KM, Southerton JS, Weston AH (1988b) The relationship between K-channel opening and cGMP concentration in rat aorta. Pflügers Arch 411:R198

Newgreen DT, Longmore J, Weston AH (1989) The effect of glibenclamide on the action of cromakalim, diazoxide and minoxidil on rat aorta. Br J Pharmacol Proc 96 (Suppl):776P

Nguyen PV, Davis A, Tasker TCG, Leenen FHH (1987) Effects of BRL34915 on pressor and chronotropic responses to IV norepinephrine, angiotensin II and isoproterenol in normal men. Cardiovasc Drugs Ther 1 (3):270

Nicholls DP, O'Keefe DB, Marton P, Murtagh JG, Scott ME, Shanks RG (1984) Cardiovascular effects of pinacidil in man. Ir J Med Sci 153:80–81

Noble D (1984) The surprising heart: a review of recent progress in cardiac electrophysiology. J Physiol 353:1–50

Noma A (1987) Chemical-receptor-dependent potassium channels in cardiac muscles. In: Noble D, Powell T (eds) Electrophysiology of single cardiac muscle cells. Academic Press, New York, pp 223–246

Osterrieder W (1988) Modification of K^+ conductance of heart cell membrane by BRL34915. Naunyn Schmiedebergs Arch Pharmacol 337:93–97

Petersen HJ, Kaergaard-Nielsen C, Arrigoni-Martelli, E (1988) Synthesis and hypotensive activity of N-alkyl-N^{11}-N^{1}-pyridylguanidines. J Med Chem 21:773–781

Pilgrim AJ, Vandenburg MJ, Arr-Woodward M, Marks C, Tasker TC (1987) Potassium channel activators: antihypertensive activity and effects on resting surface ECG: a study with BRL34915. Cardiovasc Drugs Ther 1 (3):276

Quast U (1987) Effect of the K^+efflux stimulating vasodilator BRL34915 on $^{86}Rb^+$ efflux and spontaneous activity in guinea-pig portal vein. Br J Pharmacol 91:569–578

Quast U (1988) Comparison of $^{86}Rb^+$ and $^{42}K^+$ effluxes stimulated by the K^+ channel opener BRL34915 in vascular smooth muscle. Br J Pharmacol Proc (Suppl) 93:19P

Quast U, Cook NS (1988) *Leiurus quinquestriatus* venom inhibits BRL34915-induced $^{86}Rb^+$ efflux from the rat portal vein. Life Sci 42:805–810

Quast U, Scholtysik G, Weir SW, Cook NS (1988) Pertussis toxin treatment does not inhibit the effects of the potassium channel opener BRL34915 on rat isolated vascular and cardiac tissues. Naunyn-Schmiedebergs Arch Pharmacol 337:98–104

Scholtysik G (1987) Evidence for inhibition by ICS-250 and stimulation by BRL34915 of K^+ conductance in cardiac muscle. Naunyn Schmiedebergs Arch Pharmacol 335: 692–696

Smallwood JK, Steinberg MI (1988) Cardiac electrophysiological effects of pinacidil and related pyridylcyanoguanidines: relationship to antihypertensive activity. J Cardiovasc Pharmacol 12:102–109

Smith JM, Sanchez AA, Jones AW (1986) Comparison of rubidium-86 and potassium-42 fluxes in rat aorta. Blood vessels 23:297–309

Southerton JS, Taylor SG, Weston AH (1987a) Comparison of the effects of BRL34915 and of acetylcholine-liberated EDRF on rat isolated aorta. J Physiol 382:50P

Southerton JS, Taylor SG, Weir SW, Weston AH (1987b) An investigation into the mechanism of action of pinacidil in rat blood vessels. Br J Pharmacol 90:126P

Southerton JS, Weston AH (1987) Some effects of Ca^{2+} and K^+-channel-blocking agents on responses to BRL 34915 and pinacidil in the isolated rat portal vein. J Physiol 391:77P

Southerton JS, Weston AH, Bray KM, Newgreen DT, Taylor SG (1988) The potassium channel opening action of pinacidil; studies using biochemical, ion flux and electrophysiological techniques. Naunyn Schmiedebergs Arch Pharmacol 338:310–318

Steensgaard-Hansen F, Carlsen JE (1988) Effects of long-term treatment with pinacidil and nifedipine on left ventricular anatomy and function in patients with mild-moderate systemic hypertension. Drugs 36 (Suppl 7):70–76
Steinberg MI, Ertel P, Smallwood JK, Wyss V, Zimmerman K (1988) The relation between vascular relaxant and cardiac electrophysiological effects of pinacidil. J Cardiovasc Pharmacol 12 (Suppl 2):530–540
Sterndorff B, Johansen P (1988) Comparative trial of pinacidil versus prazosin in mild to moderate arterial hypertension. Drugs 36 (Suppl 7):64–66
Talvenheimo JA, Lam G, Gelband C (1988) Charybdotoxin inhibits the 250 pS Ca^{2+}-activated K^+ channel in aorta and contracts aorta smooth muscle. Biophys J 53:258a
Taylor SG, Bumstead J, Morris JEJ, Shaw DJ, Taylor JF (1988a) Cromakalim inhibits cholinergic-mediated responses in human isolated bronchioles but not in guinea-pig airways. Br J Pharmacol Proc 95 (Suppl):795P
Taylor SG, Southerton JS, Weston AH, Baker JRJ (1988b) Endothelium dependent effects of acetylcholine in rat aorta. A comparison with sodium nitroprusside and cromakalim. Br J Pharmacol 94:853–863
Taylor SG, Weston AH (1988) Endothelium-derived hyperpolarising factor: a new endogenous inhibitor from the vascular endothelium. Trends Pharmacol Sci 9:272–274
Thoolen MJMC, Van Meel MCA, Wilffert B, Timmermans PBMWM, Van Zwieten PA (1983) Haemodynamic characterization of pinacidil in rats. Comparison with hydralazine. Pharmacology 27:245–254
Toda N, Nakajima S, Miyazaki M, Ueda M (1985) Vasodilatation induced by pinacidil in dogs. Comparison with hydrolazine and nifedipine. J Cardiovasc Pharmacol 7: 1118–1126
Tricklebank MD, Flockhart G, Freedman SB (1988) The potassium channel activator, BRL34915, antagonises a behavioural response to the muscarinic receptor agonist, pilocarpine. Eur J Pharmacol 151:349–350
Trieschmann U, Pichlmaier M, Klöckner U, Isenberg G (1988) Vasorelaxation due to K-agonists. Single channel recordings from isolated human vascular myocytes. Pflügers Arch 411:R199
Uchida Y, Yoshimoto N, Murao A (1978) Effect of 2-nicotinamidoethyl nitrate (SG75) on coronary circulation. Jpn Heart J 19:112–124
Vandenburg MJ, Arr-Woodward M, Hossain M, Stewart-Long P, Tasker TCG (1986) Potassium channel activators lower blood pressure: an initial study of BRL34915 in hypertensive patients. J Hypertens 4 (Suppl 6):S166–S167
Vandenburg MJ, Arr-Woodward M, Stewart-Long P, Tasker T, Pilgrim AJ, Dews IM, Fairhurst G (1987a) Potassium channel activators: antihypertensive activity and adverse effect profile of BRL34915. J Hypertens 5 (Suppl 5):S193–S195
Vandenburg MJ, Kakad J, Wiseman WT, Stephens D, Stewart-Long PM, Tasker T (1987b) BRL34915 a novel potassium channel activator: duration of antihypertensive action. Cardiovasc Drugs Ther 1 (3):299
Videbaek LM, Aalkjaer C, Mulvany MJ (1988a) Pinacidil opens K^+-selective channels causing hyperpolarization and relaxation of noradrenaline contractions in rat mesenteric resistance vessels. Br J Pharmacol 95:103–108
Videbaek LM, Aalkjaer C, Mulvany MJ (1988b) Vasodilation with pinacidil: mode of action in rat resistance vessels. Drugs 36 (Suppl 7):33–40
Weir SW, Weston AH (1986a) Effect of apamin on responses to BRL 34915, nicorandil and other relaxants in the guinea-pig taenia caeci. Br J Pharmacol 88:113–120
Weir SW, Weston AH (1986b) The effects of BRL34915 and nicorandil on electrical and mechanical activity and on ^{86}Rb efflux in rat blood vessels. Br J Pharmacol 88:121–128
Weir SW, Weston AH (1988) Effects of apamin on the inhibitory actions of sodium nitroprusside and sodium azide on the guinea-pig taenia caeci. Br J Pharmacol Proc (Suppl) 93:18P
Weston AH, Bray KM, Duty S, McHarg AD, Newgreen DT, Southerton JS (1988a) In vitro studies on the mode of action of pinacidil. Drugs 36 (Suppl 7):10–28
Weston AH, Southerton JS, Bray KM, Newgreen DT, Taylor SG (1988b) The mode of action of pinacidil and its analogs P1060 and P1368: results of studies in rat blood

vessels. J Cardiovasc Pharmacol 12 (Suppl 2) S10–S16
Wilde DW, Lee KS (1988) Inward and outward ionic currents of isolated dog coronary smooth muscle cells and effects of ACh and minoxidil sulfate. Biophys J 53:262a
Wilson C (1988) Comparative effects of cromakalim on contractions to noradrenaline and caffeine in rabbit isolated renal artery. Br J Pharmacol Proc (Suppl) 95:570P
Wilson C, Buckingham RE, Mootoo S, Parrott LS, Hamilton TC, Pratt SC, Cawthorne MA (1988a) In vivo and in vitro studies of cromakalim (BRL34915) and glibenclamide in the rat. Br J Pharmacol Proc (Suppl) 93:126P
Wilson C, Coldwell MC, Howlett DR, Cooper SM, Hamilton TC (1988b) Comparative effects of K^+ channel blockade on the vasorelaxant activity of cromakalim, pinacidil and nicorandil. Eur J Pharmacol 152:331–339
Yanagisawa T, Hashimoto H, Taira N (1988) The negative inotropic effect of nicorandil is independent of cyclic GMP changes: a comparison with pinacidil and BRL34915 in canine atrial muscle. Br J Pharmacol 95:393–398
Zachariah PK, Sheps SG, Schirger A, Fisher LD, Shub C, Collins JB, Spiekerman RE (1986) Antihypertensive efficacy of pinacidil – automatic ambulatory blood pressure monitoring. Eur J Clin Pharmacol 31:133–141

CHAPTER 17

Principles in the Combination of Antihypertensive Drugs

K.H. Rahn

CONTENTS

1 Use of Sygnergism of Antihypertensive Drugs

During chronic treatment of hypertension, two or more antihypertensive drugs are often combined. The rationale for this procedure is based on the fact that many hypotensive agents have been shown to possess a synergistic effect on elevated blood pressure. Furthermore, there is no blood pressure lowering drug which is able to normalize the elevated blood pressure in all hypertensive patients.

Data from numerous studies demonstrate that diuretics, β-receptor blocking agents, calcium antagonists, and angiotensin-converting enzyme (ACE) inhibitors are able to decrease elevated blood pressure to levels below 150/100 mmHg only in about one-half or two-thirds of subjects with mild to moderate primary hypertension. In a comparative study 81 patients with mild to moderate hypertension (with diastolic blood pressures in the range of 90–114 mmHg) were treated with propranolol in daily doses of 120–480 mmHg for a total of 18 months (Veterans Administration Cooperative Study Group on Antihypertensive Agents 1977). In 52% of the patients, the β-receptor blocking drug decreased the diastolic blood pressure to levels below 90 mmHg. Similary, atenolol in daily doses from 50–100 mg decreased the diastolic blood pressure to less than 95 mmHg in 57% of hypertensive patients treated for 12 weeks (Nifedipine-Atenolol Study Review Committee 1988). In the same study, the target level of diastolic blood pressure was obtained in 64% of the patients treated with the calcium antagonist nifedipine in doses of 20–40 mg daily. In a placebo-controlled study, the diuretic hydrochlorothiazide in a dose of 25 mg daily decreased diastolic blood pressure to less than 91 mmHg in 56% of 59 patients with mild to moderate hypertension (Veterans Administrations Cooperative Study Group on Antihypertensive Agents 1982).

Several studies have been performed to test the efficacy of ACE inhibitors in patients with hypertension. The Veterans Administration Cooperative Study Group on Antihypertensive Agents (1982) demonstrated that in 59%–70% of 399 hypertensive subjects captopril in doses of 12.5–50 mg three times daily caused diastolic blood pressure to decrease below 91 mmHg. Similarly, in about 60% of the patients with mild to severe primary hypertension enalapril was sufficiently effective when given as monotherapy in daily doses of 10–40 mg (Gavras et al. 1981; Sassano et al. 1984). Pool et al. (1987) reported that in 55% of patients with mild to moderate primary hypertension the target diastolic blood pressure — i.e., less than 90 mmHg — was obtained with lisinopril doses of 20–80 mg per day.

The combination of two of the above-mentioned antihypertensive agents (Table 1) increases considerably the percentage of hypertensive patients in whom the therapeutic goal is reached. Thus, in 81% of hypertensive patients treated with the combination of propranolol and hydrochlorothiazide blood pressure was decreased sufficiently, whereas the therapeutic goal during monotherapy with the β-blocker was reached in only 52% (Veterans Administration Cooperative Study Group on Antihypertensive Agents 1977). Similarly, the combination of hydrochlorothiazide with propranolol or metoprolol was considerably more effective in lowering blood pressure than monotherapy with the diuretic or with one of the β-blockers alone (Weber and Drayer 1984).

There are controversial results concerning the synergistic effects of diuretics and calcium blockers in the treatment of hypertension (Weinberger 1988). Poulter et al. (1986) observed a further decrease of blood pressure when mefruside was added to nifedipine in hypertensive patients. Similar results were obtained by Schoenberger et al. (1984) for nitrendipine added to hydrochlorothiazide. Furthermore, data by Hallin et al. (1983) suggest an additive effect of nifedipine and bendroflumethiazide. In contrast, Massie et al. (1987) found that in hypertensive patients whose blood pressure was inadequately controlled by diltiazem, addition of hydrochlorothiazide had only a small antihypertensive effect which was not statistically significant. Interestingly enough, in this study addition of hydrochlorothiazide also did not lead to a significant reduction of blood pressure in hypertensive patients inadequately controlled by propranolol. One may, therefore, assume that the discrepancies between the studies by Poulter et al. (1986) and Schoenberger et al. (1984) on one side and by Massie et al. (1987) on the other are due to different patient populations. In a double-

Table 1. Useful combinations of two antihypertensive drugs

β-Blocker and diuretic
ACE inhibitor and diuretic
Calcium antagonist and diuretic
β-Blocker and calcium antagonist
ACE inhibitor and calcium antagonist

ACE, angiotensin-converting enzyme.

blind study CAPPUCCIO et al. (1987) found that the addition of bendrofluazide had little additive effect on blood pressure in hypertensive patients already on treatment with atenolol and nifedipine. However, in this study, therapy with atenolol and nifedipine had resulted in almost normal blood pressure levels. One could imagine that the blood pressure lowering effect of bendrofluazide would have been more pronounced in hypertensive patients with higher blood pressure levels prior to the addition of the diuretic. Taken together, there is evidence from controlled studies that calcium antagonists and diuretics act in a synergistic way on elevated blood pressure.

There are numerous studies demonstrating that addition of a diuretic to treatment with an ACE inhibitor causes a further reduction of blood pressure in hypertensive patients. This is true for captopril (FERGUSON et al. 1980b; Veterans Administration Cooperative Study Group on Antihypertensive Agents 1982; MACGREGOR et al. 1982), enalapril (VIDT 1984), and lisinopril (POOL et al. 1987).

In the study by MACGREGOR et al. (1982), addition of the β-blocker propranolol to treatment with captopril caused no further decrease of blood pressure in patients with primary hypertension. However, in this study therapy with the ACE inhibitor had already resulted in almost normal blood pressure levels. FERGUSON et al. (1980a) found that propranolol added to treatment with captopril and a diuretic caused a further decrease of blood pressure which was not statistically significant in the small group of eight hypertensive patients studied.

There is no doubt that ACE inhibitors and calcium antagonists have a synergistic effect on elevated blood pressure. This has particularly been demonstrated for captopril and nifedipine in patients with severe or resistant hypertension (GUAZZI et al. 1984; WHITE et al. 1986). There are now numerous clinical observations demonstrating that the combination of an ACE inhibitor, a diuretic, and a calcium antagonist is effective in lowering blood pressure in most patients with otherwise drug-resistant hypertension.

It has been demonstrated that calcium antagonists and β-blockers have a synergistic effect on elevated blood pressure (AOKI et al. 1978; FRANZ and WIEWEL 1984). β-Blockers and verapamil both have a negative dromotropic and negative inotropic effect when given in antihypertensive doses. This may result in bradycardia and hypotension when verapamil and a β-blocker are combined (WAYNE et al. 1982). In view of the possibility of this adverse interaction, this combination should be avoided in the treatment of hypertensive patients. The same is true for diltiazem combined with a β-blocker.

Besides these combinations of two antihypertensive drugs, there are several other possible combinations such as reserpine and a diuretic, methyldopa and a diuretic, and clonidine and a diuretic. However, there is no logic in concurrently administering drugs with a similar mechanism of action such as methyldopa and clonidine or two differing types of β-blockers. One cannot expect a greater blood pressure lowering effect and fewer side effects with such a combination than with an optimal dose of a single agent.

Table 2. Useful combinations of three antihypertensive drugs

β-Blocker, diuretic, and vasodilator (hydralazine, calcium antagonist, ACE inhibitor, post-synaptic α_1-blocker)
β-Blocker, diuretic, and methyldopa
ACE inhibitor, diuretic, and calcium antagonist

ACE, angiotensin-converting enzyme.

If the use of two antihypertensive drugs together has proven to be insufficiently effective in lowering blood pressure, triple drug therapy should be considered (Table 2). A combination of three blood pressure lowering agents should always include a diuretic. The reason for this recommendation is that many patients requiring more than two drugs for the control of their elevated blood pressure have at least partially volume-dependent hypertension. Furthermore, diuretics have been shown to have a synergistic effect with practically all other antihypertensive drugs. Finally, as will be discussed later, many antihypertensive agents cause salt and water retention which antagonizes their antihypertensive action. There are several drugs which have been shown to cause a further decrease of blood pressure in hypertensive patients who are treated with the combination of a β-blocker and a diuretic; such drugs are hydralazine (Veterans Administration Cooperative Study Group on Antihypertensive Agents 1977; McAREAVEY et al. 1984), methyldopa, prazosin, and minoxidil (McAREAVEY et al. 1984), as well as nifedipine (MURPHY et al. 1983). As has been discussed earlier, there are also data suggesting that β-blockers have an additional blood pressure lowering effect when added to the combination of an ACE inhibitor and a diuretic (FERGUSON et al. 1980a). In otherwise drug-resistant hypertensive patients, the combination of an ACE inhibitor, a diuretic, and a calcium antagonist, preferably of the dihydropyridine type, or minoxidil should be considered (RAINE and LEDINGHAM 1982; WHITE et al. 1986).

2 Influence on Compensatory Mechanisms Working Against Blood Pressure Reduction by Drugs

Several antihypertensive agents cause salt and water retention during chronic treatment (FINNERTY et al. 1970). This is particularly true for strongly acting vasodilating agents such as minoxidil (GILMORE et al. 1970). Due to the salt and water retention, the antihypertensive action of blood pressure lowering drugs may decrease with time or even completely disappear. On the other hand, it is understandable that antihypertensive agents causing salt and water retention are rendered more effective when a diuretic is added. This additive effect is well documented for reserpine, methyldopa, guanethidine, vasodilators, clonidine (CONWAY 1977) and prazosin (BROGDEN et al. 1977). These agents, therefore, should always be used in combination with a diuretic. Besides diuretic drugs, the only antihypertensive agents not causing salt and water retention and thereby not increasing plasma volume are β-blockers (TARAZI et al. 1971), calcium antagonists (GUAZZI et al. 1980), and ACE inhibitors (TODD and HEEL 1986). Therefore, diuretics, β-blockers, calcium antagonists, and ACE inhibitors are the only antihypertensive agents to be used chronically in monotherapy.

There are several antihypertensive drugs which cause reflex activation of the sympathetic nervous system. By doing so, they increase heart rate and cardiac output. The reflex elevation of cardiac output antagonizes the blood pressure lowering effect of the antihypertensive agent. This is particularly true for arteriolar vasodilating drugs, such as hydralazine and minoxidil (GILMORE et al. 1970). The blood pressure lowering effect of these vasodilators can be enhanced by combining them with an agent inhibiting sympathetic function. These considerations are the basis of combinations consisting of an arteriolar vasodilator with drugs like β-blocker reserpine, clonidine, and methyldopa. Particularly useful is the combination of a vasodilating agent and a β-blocker (GILMORE et al. 1970; Veterans Administration Cooperative Study Group on Antihypertensive Agents 1977). The specific antagonism of the reflex increase of heart rate by β-blockers can easily be demonstrated.

Diuretic agents cause reflex activation of the sympathetic nervous system, too (FUJITA et al. 1980). In hypertensive patients, this can be demonstrated by measurement of plasma noradrenaline levels (VAN HOOFF et al. 1983; RAHN 1985). Antagonism of the effects of reflex sympathetic activation may contribute to the synergism of diuretics and drugs inhibiting sympathetic function, such as methyldopa (DRAYER et al. 1982), or of diuretics and β-blockers (WEBER and DRAYER 1984).

During treatment with diuretics, plasma renin activity and plasma angiotensin II levels increase (CONWAY 1977). Plasma renin activity starts rising within 30 min after i.v. application of furosemide (VAN HOOFF et al. 1983). The elevation of plasma renin activity persists during long-term treatment with diuretics (CONWAY 1977; WEBER and DRAYER 1984). One may assume that the diuretic-induced rise of plasma angiotensin II concentration counteracts the decrease of blood pressure caused by these drugs. It has been shown that drugs interfering with the sympathetic nervous system antagonize the effect of diuretics on plasma renin activity and thereby plasma angiotensin II levels. This is particularly true for β-blockers (WEBER and DRAYER 1984) and may contribute to the synergistic effect of diuretics and drugs interfering with the sympathetic nervous function. ACE inhibitors decrease angiotensin II concentrations (ROBERTSON et al. 1987), and this action probably contributes to their marked antihypertensive effect in combination with diuretics.

3 Decrease of Incidence of Side Effects

The various groups of antihypertensive agents differ in their pattern of side effects. Because of the synergistic effect on blood pressure, smaller doses of the individual drug can be used during combination therapy than during monotherapy of hypertension. The severity and the frequency of side effects of many antihypertensive agents are dose-dependent. By using smaller doses in the combination therapy, the severity and the frequency of side effects may be diminished.

This has clearly been shown for reserpine, a drug which, at high doses, exhibits major side effects (Participating Veterans Administration Medical Centers 1982). In a multicenter, controlled study with 329 patients with mild to moderate hypertension, the effect of a combination therapy consisting of chlorthalidone 50 mg/day and reserpine in daily doses of 0.05, 0.125, or 0.25 mg was studied. With the highest dose of reserpine 6.8% of the patients complained of lethargy and of sexual dysfunction. The frequency of these complaints was considerably less, that is 2.6%, in the hypertensive patients receiving 0.05 mg reserpine daily. In the same study, the effect of chlorthalidone on serum potassium levels was measured. Serum potassium concentrations of less than 3 mmol/l were found in 11% of hypertensive patients receiving 50 mg chlorthalidone daily for a total of 4 weeks. In contrast, only 4% of the patients receiving 25 mg/day chlorthalidone developed hypokalemia, with serum potassium levels of less than 3 mmol/l.

One of the major potential adverse actions of hydralazine is the lupus erythematosus-like syndrome. The frequency of this side effect progressively increases with doses of hydralazine exceeding 200 mg daily (Perry 1973). On the other hand, a lupus erythematosus-like syndrome is rarely observed in patients receiving less than 200 mg hydralazine per day.

Shortly after its introduction into hypertension therapy, the ACE inhibitor captopril was given in rather high oral doses of up to 1 g daily. With these doses, proteinuria developed not infrequently (Heel et al. 1980). For several years since then, captopril has usually been given in doses as low as 6.25 mg and not exceeding 150 mg/day. With this dosage, proteinuria is extremely rare (Chalmers et al. 1987).

In conclusion, combination of antihypertensive drugs often allows the use of relatively low doses of the individual agent, resulting in a decrease of the severity and the frequency of side effects. In addition, blood pressure lowering drugs can sometimes be combined in such a way that one agent antagonizes the side effects of another one. This is definitively true for the combination of thiazide diuretics with potassium-sparing diuretics. In a study by Holzgreve (1980) treatment of hypertensive patients with hydrochlorothiazide in doses of up to 100 mg daily resulted in hypokalemia with serum potassium levels of less than 3.6 mmol/l in 22% of the patients. Addition of potassium-sparing diuretics or of oral potassium considerably diminished the frequency of hypokalemia to a level of 7%.

Besides hypokalemia, thiazide diuretics may cause a rise of serum uric acid concentrations. ACE inhibitors in general have only a minor effect on serum potassium and on serum uric acid levels. However, they markedly attenuate the hypokalemia and the hyperuricemia induced by thiazide diuretics (Todd and Heel 1986).

4 Summary and Conclusions

Numerous antihypertensive agents act in a synergistic way on elevated blood pressure when they are combined with each other. Part of this synergism is due to an additive blood pressure lowering effect. Another part is due to the antagonism by one antihypertensive drug of compensatory mechanisms working against blood pressure reduction by another antihypertensive agent.

Combination therapy makes it possible to use relatively small doses of antihypertensive drugs in patients with hypertension. Thus, the frequency and severity of side effects of individual antihypertensive agents may be decreased. Furthermore, the side effects of some blood pressure lowering drugs may be antagonized by combination with other antihypertensive agents.

In view of the above-mentioned considerations, it may now be recommended to start with one single drug and observe the patient for a sufficient time, but to limit the doses of antihypertensive agents given in the form of a monotherapy in order to avoid a disproportionate increase of side effects. According to these recommendations, for monotherapy with a β-blocker daily doses of 100–200 mg atenolol or the equieffective blood pressure lowering doses of other β-receptor blocking agents should not be exceeded. The respective figures for diuretics are about 50 mg hydrochlorothiazide daily, for ACE inhibitors about 75 mg captopril daily, for calcium antagonists about 240 mg verapamil daily. Specific recommendations for drug combinations, interactions and contraindications are discussed in the respective chapters of this book.

References

Aoki K, Kondo S, Mochizaki A, Yoshida T, Kato S, Kato K, Takikawa K (1978) Antihypertensive effect of cardiovascular Ca 2+ antagonists in hypertensive patients in the absence and presence of beta-adrenergic blockade. Am Heart J 96:218–226

Brogden RN, Heel RC, Speight TM, Avery GS (1977) Prazosin: a review of its pharmacological properties and therapeutic efficacy. Drugs 14:163–185

Cappuccio FP, Markandu ND, Tucker FA, Shore AC, Mac Gregor GA (1987) A double-blind study of the blood pressure lowering effect of a thiazide diuretic in hypertensive patients already on nifedipine and a beta-blocker. Hypertension 5:733–738

Chalmers D, Dombey SL, Lawson DH (1987) Post marketing surveillance of captopril (for hypertension): a preliminary report. Br J Clin Pharmacol 24:343–349

Conway J (1977) Antihypertensive effect of diuretics. In: Gross F (ed) Antihypertensive agents. Springer, Berlin Heidelberg NewYork, pp 477–494 (Handbuch der experimentellen Pharmakologie, vol XXXIX)

Drayer JIM, Weber MA, Lipson JL, Megaffin BB (1982) Differential effects of diuresis and beta-adrenoreceptor blockade during angiotensin converting enzyme inhibition in patients with severe hypertension. J Clin Pharmacol 22:179–186

Ferguson RK, Vlasses PH, Koplin JR, Shirivian A, Burke JF, Alexander JC (1980a) Captopril in severe treatment-resistant hypertension. Am Heart J 99:579–585

Ferguson RK, Vlasses PH, Swanson BN (1980b) Effects of captopril diuretic and their combination in low-renin essential hypertension. Life Sci 27:2519–2522

Finnerty FA Jr, Davidov M, Mroczek WJ, Gavrilovick L (1970) Influence of extracellular fluid volume on response to antihypertensive drugs. Circ Res 26 [Suppl I]: 71–80

Franz IW, Wiewel D (1984) Antihypertensive effects on blood pressure at rest and during exercise of calcium antagonists, β-receptor blockers, and their combination in hypertensive patients. J Cardiovasc Pharmacol 6:S1037–1042
Fujita T, Henry WL, Bartter FC, Lake CR, Delea CS (1980) Factors influencing blood pressure in salt sensitive patients with hypertension. Am J Med 69:334–344
Gavras H, Biollaz J, Waeber B, Brunner HR, Gavras I, Davies RO (1981) Antihypertensive effect of the new oral angiotensin converting enzyme inhibitor 'MK-421'. Lancet ii:543–547
Gilmore E, Weil J, Chidsey C (1970) Treatment of essential hypertension with a new vasodilator in combination with beta-adrenergic blockade. N Engl J Med 282:521–527
Guazzi MD, Fiorentini C, Olivari MT, Bartorelli A, Necchi G, Polese A (1980) Short and long-term efficacy of a calcium-antagonistic agent (nifedipine) combined with methyldopa in the treatment of severe hypertension. Circulation 61:913–918
Guazzi MD, Decesare N, Galli C, Salvioni A, Tramontana C, Tamborini G, Bartorelli A (1984) Calcium-channel blockade with nifedipine and angiotensin converting-enzyme inhibition with captopril in the therapy of patients with severe primary hypertension. Circulation 70:279–284
Hallin L, Andrén L, Hansson L (1983) Controlled trial of nifedipine and bedroflumethiazide in hypertension. J Cardiovasc Pharmacol 5:1083–1086
Heel RC, Brogden RN, Speight TM, Avery GS (1980) Captopril. Drugs 20:409–452
Holzgreve H (1980) Nebenwirkungen der Antihypertensiva. In: Heidland A, Wetzels E (ed) Pharmakotherapie bei Niereninsuffizienz. Springer, Berlin Heidelberg New-York, pp 86–93
Massie BM, MacCarthy EP, Ramanathan KB (1987) Diltiazem and propranolol in mild-to-moderate essential hypertension as monotherapy or with hydrochlorothiazide. Ann Intern Med 107:150–157
MacGregor GA, Markandu ND, Banks RA, Bayliss J, Roulston JE, Jones JC (1982) Captopril in essential hypertension: contrasting effects of adding hydrochlorothiazide or propranolol. Br Med J 284:693–696
McAreavey D, Ramsey L, Latham L, McLaren A, Lorimer A, Reid JL, Robertson J, Robertson M, Weir R (1984) 'Third drug' trial: comparative study of antihypertensive agents added to treatment when blood pressure remains uncontrolled by a beta blocker plus thiazide diuretic. Br Med J 288:106–111
Murphy MB, Scriver AJI, Dollery CT (1983) Efficacy of nifedipine as step 3 antihypertensive drug. Hypertension 5 [Suppl II]:118–121
Nifedipine-Atenolol-Study Review Committee (1988) Nifedipine and atenolol singly and combined for treatment of essential hypertension: comparative multicentre study in general practice in the United Kingdom. Br Med J 296:468–472
Participating Veterans Administration Medical Centers (1982) Low dose v standard dose of reserpine. JAMA 248:2471–2477
Perry HM Jr (1973) Late toxicity to hydralazine resembling systemic lupus erythematosus or rheumatoid arthritis. Am J Med 54:58–72
Pool JL, Gennari J, Goldstein R, Kochar MS, Lewin AJ, Maxwell MH, McChesney JA, Mehta J, Nash DT, Nelson EB, Rastogi S, Rofman B, Weinberger M (1987) Controlled multicenter study of the antihypertensive effects of lisinopril, hydrochlorothiazide, and lisinopril plus hydrochlorothiazide in the treatment of 394 patients with mild to moderate essential hypertension. J Cardiovasc Parmacol 9 [Suppl 3]:S 36–S 42
Poulter N, Thompson AV, Sever PS (1986) Do diuretics enhance the hypotensive effect of nifedepine? A double-blind trial in black hypertensive patients. J Hypertens 4:792–793
Rahn KH (1985) Einsatz von hochdosiertem Furosemid beim Hochdruck niereninsuffizienter Patienten. Nieren Hochdruckkr 6:261–263
Raine AEG, Ledingham JGG (1982) Clinical experience with captopril in the treatment of severe drug-resistant hypertension. Am J Cardiol 49:1475–1479
Robertson JIS, Tillman DM, Ball SG, Lever AF (1987) Angiotensin converting enzyme inhibition in hypertension. J Hypertens 5 [Suppl 3]:S 19–S 25

Sassano P, Chatellier G, Alhenc-Gelas F, Carvol P, Menard J (1984) Antihypertensive effect of enalapril as first-step treatment of mild and moderate uncomplicated essential hypertension. Am J Med 77:18–22

Schoenberger JA, Glasser SP, Ram CVS, MacMahon SG, Vanov SK, Leibowitz DA (1984) Comparison of nitrendipine combined with low-dose hydrochlorothiazide to hydrochlorothiazide alone in mild to moderate essential hypertension. J Cardiovasc Pharmacol 6 [Suppl 7]:S 1105–S 1108

Tarazi RC, Frohlich ED, Dustan HP (1971) Plasma volume changes with long-term beta-adrenergic blockade. Am Heart J 82:770–776

Todd PA, Heel RC (1986) Enalapril: a review of its pharmacodynamic and pharmacokinetic properties, and therapeutic use in hypertension and congestive heart failure. Drugs 31:198–248

Van Hooff MEJ, Does RJMM, Rahn KH, van Baak MA (1983) Time course of blood pressure changes after intravenous administration of propanolol or furosemide in hypertensive patients. J Cardiovasc Pharmacol 5:773–777

Veterans Administration Cooperative Study Group on Antihypertensive Agents (1977) Propranolol in the treatment of essential hypertension. JAMA 237:2303–2310

Veterans Administration Cooperative Study Group on Antihypertensive Agents (1982) Captopril: evaluation of low doses, twice-daily doses and the addition of diuretic for the treatment of mild to moderate hypertension. Clin Sci 63:443s–445s

Vidt DG (1984) A controlled multiclinic study to compare the antihypertensive effects of MK-421, hydrochlorothiazide and MK-421 combined with hydrochlorothiazide in patients with mild to moderate essential hypertension. J Hypertens 2 [Suppl 2]: 81–88

Wayne VS, Harper RW, Laufer E, Federman J, Anderson ST, Pitt A (1982) Adverse interaction between beta-adrenergic blocking drugs and verapamil-report of three cases. Aust N Z J Med 12:285–289

Weber MA, Drayer JIM (1984) Single-agent and combination therapy of essential hypertension. Am Heart J 108:311–316

Weinberger MH (1988) Additive effects of diuretics or sodium restriction with calcium channel blockers in the treatment of hypertension. J Cardiovas Pharmacol 12 [Suppl 4]:S 72–S 75

White WB, Viadero JJ, Lane TJ, Podesla S (1986) Effects of combination therapy with captopril and nifedipine in severe or resistant hypertension. Clin Pharmacol Ther 39:43–48

CHAPTER 18

Electrolyte Intake in the Treatment of Hypertension

F.C. LUFT

CONTENTS

1 Introduction

Hypertension is the most common chronic disease in acculturated societies and is a major contributor to the development of cardiovascular disease, stroke, and renal failure (KANNEL 1979). The pharmacological treatment of hypertension is effective in reducing the incidence of complications in hypertensive patients; however, the treatment must be life long, has side effects, and is often expensive. Nonpharmacological approaches, especially dietary modifications, have appeal, particularly given the possibility that such interventions may ameliorate or protect against the development of hypertension. The dietary content of four electrolytes, namely sodium, potassium, calcium, and magnesium, has received special attention. Epidemiological studies have investigated the role of the intake of each of these cations in the development of hypertension. Animal models have been used to document and elucidate the mechanisms by which these cations may influence blood pressure. Clinical trials have been conducted in normal and hypertensive individuals to examine the effect of modifying the dietary intake of each of these cations on blood pressure. Firm conclusions with respect to the safety and efficacy of these nonpharmacological approaches is of particular interest to those formulating health care policy. Further, clinicians applying these interventions must be confident that they are effective and safe. The purpose of this review is to examine the efficacy of each of these dietary interventions by presenting the currently available data. Prior to that presentation, a brief discussion of the rationale behind these approaches is appropriate.

2 Electrolyte Effects on Blood Pressure

2.1 Sodium

Epidemiological evidence has been presented to support the notion that by reducing dietary sodium intake, blood pressure may be lowered or the development of hypertension may be avoided. Hypertension is virtually nonexistent in many unacculturated societies, and blood pressure does not increase with age (FREIS 1976). Investigators who examined numerous societies of different ethnic and genetic backgrounds in various parts of the world concluded that the lack of hypertension was not attributable to malnutrition, thin body habitus, or to different amounts of stress. Instead, they explained the lack of hypertension by the extremely low dietary salt intake exhibited by these peoples (KAMINER and LUTZ 1960; PAGE et al. 1974; PRIOR et al. 1968). MADDOCKS (1967) compared different populations in New Guinea and found that while in the highlands there is no hypertension, and blood pressure does not increase with age, in coastal communities, in which people consume salted, canned foods, blood pressure increases with age, and hypertension is present. PAGE and co-workers (1974) reached similar conclusions on the basis of their studies of Solomon islanders. Studies in other primitive societies confirm a relation between blood pressure and sodium intake (LOWENSTEIN 1961; OLIVER et al. 1975; PAGE et al. 1974; PRIOR et al. 1968; SINNETT and WHYTE 1973). Subjects from primitive societies with low blood pressure have a very low sodium intake; however, they also ingest large amounts of potassium, are smaller and leaner, and are more physically active than their industrialized counterparts. Certain epidemiological studies have been criticized because the blood pressure measurements were not standardized, and sodium intake was estimated based on dietary recall or on spot urine collections without matching age, sex, and weight (GRIM et al. 1980; PICKERING 1980; SIMPSON et al. 1979; MCCARRON et al. 1984). Extrapolation from these data to the role of sodium intake in the pathogenesis of hypertension in industrialized societies remains speculative.

As opposed to cross-cultural studies, studies of the correlation between habitual sodium intake and blood pressure *within* industrialized populations have been almost uniformly negative. Dahl relied on dietary questionnaires to estimate sodium intake and reported that similar mean blood pressures are present in three groups whose intake of salt was characterized as low, average, or high (DAHL and LOVE 1954). MIALL in Scotland and the Framingham Study found no relationship between sodium intake as estimated by 24-h urinary sodium excretion and dietary history reported by test subjects (DAWBER et al. 1967; MIALL 1959). SCHLIERF et al. (1980) were unable to identify a correlation between 24-h sodium excretion and blood pressure in residents of Heidelberg, Federal Republic of Germany. Simpson's group in New Zealand was unable to demonstrate correlations of blood pressure with sodium excretion or urinary sodium-potassium or sodium-creatinine ratio (SIMPSON et al. 1978). Finally, several analyses of the huge National Health and Nutrition Examination Survey (NHANES I) data base found no direct correlations between salt intake and blood pressure (HARLAN et al. 1984). In one such analysis, an inverse correlation between salt intake and blood pressure was identified (McCARRON et al. 1984). The reason why no relationship was found between sodium intake and hypertension in industrialized societies may be because of the relatively high range of habitual sodium intake in these populations (100–250 mmol/day, in contrast to unacculturated societies with sodium intake of less than 50 mmol/day). It is also likely that sodium intake in industrialized societies is high enough to raise blood pressure only in genetically susceptible salt-sensitive individuals, who represent a minority of the population (LUFT and WEINBERGER 1982; FUJITA et al. 1980). For this reason, no correlation between blood pressure and sodium intake in the entire population would be expected. Since habitual salt intake is culturally determined, it may be anticipated that within a given population, salt intakes should be similar regardless of blood pressure.

Certain forms of experimental hypertension may be induced in animals by increasing salt intake (DAHL 1972; KOLETSKY 1959; LENEL et al. 1948; MENEELY and DAHL 1961; SAPERSTEIN et al. 1950) with or without the administration of mineralocorticoids or reduction of renal mass (CARRETERO and ROMERO 1977; KOLETSKY and GOODSITT 1960). It is easier to produce salt-induced hypertension in young rats than in adult rats. DAHL (1972, 1977) demonstrated variability in the response to salt loading in normal rats and by inbreeding was able to develop two strains, one of which was sensitive to the hypertensinogenic effects of salt, while the other was not. Cross-transplantation experiments have shown the importance of the kidney in this form of experimental hypertension (DAHL et al. 1974; BIANCHI et al. 1975). TOBIAN and colleagues (1979) showed that the kidneys of young, still normotensive, Dahl salt-sensitive rats excrete only half as much sodium as kidneys from resistant rats at equal levels of inflow pressure. Sensitive Dahl rats also fail to develop hypertension while receiving an 8% salt diet, if sodium retention is prevented by the administration of a thiazide diuretic (TOBIAN et al. 1979). The implications of these and other animal studies are uncertain. The relative amounts of salt required to induce hypertension in animals is far in excess of the usual content of human diets. The 8% salt diet fed to salt-sensitive Dahl rats is equivalent to a 40 g/day sodium diet given to humans. In the Kyoto SHR, which is another popular model of human hypertension, similar clear-out salt sensitivity has not been demonstrated. Moreover, in some rat models, blood pressure *increases* rather than decreases with reduced salt intake. SEYMOUR and colleagues (1980) produced hypertension in sodium-depleted, unilaterally nephrectomized rats. MUNOZ-RAMIREZ et al. (1980) found that salt restriction aggravated hypertension in rats with two-kidney Goldblatt hypertension. WEBB and associates (1987) found that dietary sodium deprivation could raise blood pressure in normal rats even without producing irreversible hyperaldosteronism.

Salt loading studies in humans have been short term. LUFT and colleagues (1979) gave human volunteers up to 1500 mmol sodium chloride per day and found an increase in blood pressure in some subjects but not in others. Black subjects were more salt sensitive than white subjects. Similar studies by others reported even more modest increases in blood pressure in response to salt loading (Roos et al. 1985).

Folkow (1978) described the structural adaptations of blood vessels to hypertension and the role of that adaptation to the maintenance of the elevation in blood pressure. Yet the favored pathogenetic model of hypertension resulting from salt intake is based on the cybernetic framework of Guyton and associates (1980). According to their explanation, in early hypertension cardiac output increases in response to renal sodium retention. Thereafter, due to general total body autoregulation, the peripheral resistance increases, blood pressure increases further, a diuresis ensues, and cardiac output decreases to normal, i.e., the state of affairs identified in established hypertension. However, Guyton's (1980) hypothesis is based largely on experimental animal studies in partially nephrectomized animals. Neither reduced renal mass models nor salt-dependent hypervolemic models such as DOCA-salt rats or primary aldosteronism or chronic renal failure in humans can readily be extrapolated to essential hypertension.

From the available evidence, the pathogenesis or perpetuation of essential hypertension cannot be attributed to sodium retention. Sodium intake cannot be adduced as a unifying hypothesis to account for the disorder. However, a subset of salt-sensitive individuals has been identified in several human studies (Skrabal et al. 1985; Weinberger et al. 1986). The responses to salt loading have been shown to be influenced by genetic variance. Further, a concordance in the blood pressure responses of children and their parents has been identified (Luft et al. 1987). Phenotypes of haptoglobin have been shown to be associated either with salt sensitivity or with salt resistance (Weinberger et al. 1987). It is probable that a subset of salt-sensitive individuals exists in whom salt intake is an important determinant in the development of hypertension.

Recently, attention has been drawn to the fact that only sodium accompanied by the anion chloride appears to influence blood pressure. A recent, carefully done, metabolic balance study (Kurtz et al. 1987) performed in a small number of salt-sensitive subjects with hypertension showed that only increased sodium chloride intake elevated blood pressure, while sodium citrate did not. The degree of sodium retained inside the body with both interventions does not differ. This study confirms the results of animal investigations and earlier human trials. The data are reviewed in more detail elsewhere (Luft and Ganten 1987; Weinberger 1987). This issue may be important in societies in which a substantial amount of the dietary sodium intake may be in the form of a nonchloride accompanying anion.

2.2 Potassium

Diets very low in sodium are invariably also very high in potassium. Thus, an alternative explanation for the low blood pressure found in some unacculturated societies is the contribution of large amounts of potassium rather than small amounts of sodium. Blood pressure is inversely correlated with urinary potassium excretion, and urinary sodium excretion correlates directly with the sodium/potassium ratio in epidemiologic studies in Japan, where high sodium diets and hypertension are widespread (YAMORI et al. 1981). Another Japanese study demonstrated a decreased incidence of hypertension in a population subgroup that consumed large amounts of apples compared with a neighboring community with similar sodium intakes but with low potassium intake (SASAKI 1962). Similar results have been reported in the United States of America and Sweden (LJUNGMAN et al. 1981; WALKER et al. 1979; WATSON et al. 1980). An inverse correlation between serum potassium and blood pressure was shown in Japan, and an inverse correlation between blood pressure and exchangeable and total body potassium in young hypertensive persons was reported in Scotland (LEVER et al. 1981; UESHIMA et al. 1981). However, other investigations have not shown any relationship between potassium intake and blood pressure (BERENSON et al. 1979).

A protective effect of increased potassium intake was shown in some models of experimental hypertension, particularly in Dahl salt-sensitive rats (BATTERBEE et al. 1979; DAHL et al. 1972). The Wistar-Kyoto strain of SHR has been reported to be protected from the pressor effect of a high dietary sodium intake by the concurrent administration of potassium (LOUIS et al. 1971). In rat models, the potassium loads were very large and the blood pressure responses, small and variable. Furthermore, in some animal experiments, reduced potassium intake lowered blood pressure, while potassium repletion increased it (FREED et al. 1951).

In human investigations, LUFT and associates (1979a) were able to attenuate the hypertensive effect of massive sodium loading by potassium supplementation. KHAW and THOM (1982) reported a modest but significant decrease in blood pressure in young healthy men during potassium supplementation of 64 mmol per day and unrestricted sodium intake. On the other hand, MILLER et al. (1987), who gave potassium as other than the chloride salt, found no effect on blood pressure of normal children and their normotensive parents.

Potassium intake may influence vascular disease independent of blood pressure. KHAW and BARRETT-CONNOR (1987) recently reported the results of an epidemiological investigation demonstrating a significant decrease in the incidence of stroke in Southern Californians who ate more potassium than those who did not. TOBIAN et al. (1989) also reported that a high intake to potassium appears to protect hypertensive rats from vascular disease, independent of any blood pressure-lowering effects.

The mechanisms whereby a high potassium intake may lower blood pressure include direct arteriolar dilatation, increased loss of water and sodium from the body, suppression of renin and angiotensin secretion (BAUER and GAUNTER 1979), decreased adrenergic tone (GOTO and TOBIAN et al. 1981), and stimulation of the sodium-potassium pump activity (HADDY 1975; for reviews, TREASURE and PLOTH 1983; LUFT and WEINBERGER 1987). A natriuretic effect of potassium chloride has been consistently demonstrated (ZOCALLI et al. 1985; OVERLACK et al. 1985) and may explain the fact that the magnitude of the decrease in blood pressure observed in patients receiving potassium supplements in different human studies seems to be related to the concomitant sodium intake. The higher the sodium intake, the better the blood pressure response (Berliner 1960; Berliner et al. 1950; Birkenhager et al. 1972).

2.3 Calcium

Contraction of smooth muscle and, therefore, peripheral vascular resistance depends on and is initiated by an increase in intracellular cytosolic calcium concentration. A keen interest in the role of calcium in the etiology, pathophysiology, and treatment of hypertension has developed. Epidemiologic studies examining the relationship between the intake of calcium-rich foods and blood pressure in various populations indicate that an inverse relationship exists between dietary calcium intake and blood pressure (McCarron et al. 1984; Ackley et al. 1983; Garcia-Palmieri et al. 1984; Harlan et al. 1985; Reed et al. 1985). Analysis of the data from the 1971–1974 NHANES I by McCarron and associates (1984) revealed an inverse relation between dietary intake of calcium and blood pressure. A similar relationship between potassium intake and blood pressure was also found. Harlan and coworkers (1984) interpreted these same data as showing a more tenuous relationship that does not hold for all subgroups of the population. Another analysis of the same data base by Gruchow and colleagues (1985) detected such a relationship in black populations only. As with other epidemiological studies directed at sodium and potassium, these investigations are open to certain criticisms. The methods of dietary recall vary in accuracy and reliability. Differences in other nutrients and ions that could affect blood pressure independently of calcium, such as potassium, could not always be eliminated in these population studies. Feinstein (1985) showed that the correlations between calcium intake and blood pressure are not strong and reach statistical significance in several of these studies only because the population sample sizes were very large. The Finns, who have a very high prevalence of hypertension, have a high calcium intake as well (Pietinen et al. 1984). Nevertheless, a growing number of epidemiological investigations have reached similar conclusions. Blood pressure and dietary calcium intake appear to be inversely correlated.

Serum calcium values have been evaluated in normal and hypertensive subjects. Several large studies including more than 10000 people demonstrated a significant increase in systolic and diastolic blood pressure with increasing levels of total serum calcium (Bulpitt et al. 1976; Kesteloot et al. 1984a; Robinson et al. 1982). Strazzulo and coworkers (1983) found no difference in total or ionized calcium concentrations between 55 patients with hypertension and a matched normotensive group. On the other hand, McCarron (1982) reported that hypertensive subjects have lower mean serum-ionized calcium levels than control subjects. Resnick and associates (1983) found low ionized calcium only in low-renin hypertensive patients. Folsom and associates (1986) reported a small decrease in ionized calcium values of hypertensive men but not women.

Intravenous calcium administration results in increased blood pressure and systemic vascular resistance in normotensive subjects are in patients with essential hypertension (BIANCHETTI et al. 1983; MARONE et al. 1980; PAK 1970; VLACHKIS et al. 1982; YAMAMOTO et al. 1982).

Calcium metabolism in experimental animal hypertension has been recently reviewed by YOUNG et al. (1988). In SHR, plasma ionized calcium values are decreased, parathyroid hormone values are generally found to be increased, urinary calcium excretion may be increased, calcium absorption from the intestine appears to be decreased, and bone mass is decreased compared with controls. In a number of dietary calcium-loading studies performed in SHR as well as in other rat models of hypertension, a decrease in blood pressure is observed compared with Wistar-Kyoto or appropriate control rats. MCCARRON et al. (1989) also observed that the blood pressure-lowering effects of calcium appear to be more prominent if the dietary salt intake is generous. On the other hand, LUFT et al. (1988) did not find that increased calcium intake lowers the blood pressure of SHRSP, although they did observe an attenuated release of catecholamines in response to stress in calcium-supplemented animals compared with controls. Increasing the dietary salt intake increased rather than decreased the blood pressure further in that study.

Cellular calcium metabolism is altered in hypertension at both the whole animal and cellular level. A unifying hypothesis to explain these apparent paradoxical observations, namely, increased cytosolic calcium as responsible for mediation of smooth muscle contraction and decreased dietary calcium intake or disordered calcium handling as contributing to hypertension, has not as yet been forthcoming. However, as YOUNG and colleagues (1988) point out, an underlying defect manifested in many cell lines may explain abnormal calcium handling not only at the cellular level but also at the organ and whole animal levels. That defect, be it related to cell membrane Ca-ATPase (ROULET et al. 1987), an intrinsic membrane-binding protein (Kowarski et al. 1986), a cell membrane Ca channel, or perhaps some other process, has not yet been identified.

2.4 Magnesium

Magnesium is the second most prevalent intracellular cation, and may play a role in the control of blood pressure as well as in the development of hypertension. SANGAL and BEEVERS (1982) found an inverse relationship between serum magnesium and blood pressure in Danish men and women aged 60 years and older. Similar relationships have been reported by others (ALBERT et al. 1958; PETERSEN et al. 1977). An inverse relationship between urinary magnesium excretion and diastolic blood pressure was reported in a subset of a population in Belgium (KESTELOOT 1984a). These data are not consistent with earlier reports suggesting that hypertension, in the absence of overt renal disease, is associated with increases in serum magnesium values (WALKER and WALKER 1936). No relationship between magnesium excretion and blood pressure was identified in a Korean population or in the NHANES I data (HARLAN et al. 1984; KESTELOOT

1984a). RESNICK and colleagues (1983) report an inverse correlation between plasma renin activity and serum magnesium values in patients with essential hypertension, suggesting that low-renin hypertensive patients have higher magnesium values than high-renin patients. ALTURA et al. (1984) observed a correlation between magnesium deficiency and hypertension in rats. Further, they were able to correlate microcirculatory changes with magnesium deficiency. The changes include reduced capillary, postcapillary, and venular blood flow, as well as decreases in lumen sizes. On the other hand, LUFT et al. (1988) found that in rats receiving a high calcium intake in the face of magnesium deficiency, blood pressure values were reduced compared with controls. EVANS et al. (1987) reported similar findings.

3 Blood Pressure Response to Changes in Dietary Electrolytes

3.1 Sodium

More than 50 studies have investigated the effect of altered sodium intake on blood pressure. MORGAN and NOWSON (1986) reviewed these investigations and found that decreases in blood pressure with salt restriction are related to the initial blood pressure values, i.e., the higher the blood pressure, the greater the reduction to be expected with salt restriction. They calculated a regression line which suggests that a decrease in blood pressure of about 10 mmHg per every 100 mmol reduction in dietary sodium intake per day could be expected on the basis of the data given in the studies. Others have also analyzed the results of studies examining the effects of reduced sodium intake on blood pressure (GROBBEE and HOFMAN 1986b); HOUSTON 1986; KAPLAN 1987; MAXWELL and WAKS 1987). GROBBEE and HOFMAN (1986b) subjected the data from 13 trials performed since 1970 to statistical analysis. The results from these trials appear as the first 13 examples in Table 1. They were randomized and controlled. Although the results of their analysis generally support the hypothesis that a reduction in sodium intake may lower blood pressure, GROBBEE and HOFMAN (1986b) found that only three of the studies show a significant fall in blood pressure with sodium restriction. The falls in systolic and diastolic blood pressure are directly correlated with the initial blood pressure and are also directly correlated withthe age of the subjects. Thus, the data from 13 randomized, controlled trials of the effects of reduced sodium intake on blood pressure suggest that the intervention results in small effects, generally restricted to systolic blood pressure. Three additional trials not included in Grobbee's review are included in Table 1. Of these, two show a significant decrease in blood pressure. Sodium restriction seems to provide only limited benefit for those who are most eligible for nonpharmacologic interventions, namely young patients with mild hypertension. Age-related effects were also observed by MILLER et al. (1987), who found that sodium restriction reduces the blood pressure of normotensive adults by 2 mmHg but has no effect on their identical twin children.

Investigations of sodium restriction in patients receiving antihypertensive drugs have also been carried out. In the course of a project to demonstrate the utility of dietary sodium restriction in hypertensive patients, WEINBERGER et al. (1988) found that only half of the subjects were able to reach goal compliance of 80 mmol/day urinary sodium excretion. The other half lowered their sodium intake from 170 to 110 mmol/day but were unable to reduce it further. One-half of the patients reaching goal compliance were able to reduce their medications; those patients not attaining goal compliance were not. This study illustrates several features of dietary sodium restriction. Compliance is difficult to attain, even if the subjects are motivated and the instruction in intensive. A reduction in intake to 80 mmol/day or below appears to be necessary to achieve the desired effect. In those subjects compliant to the regimen, sodium sensitivity appears to

Table 1. Effect of dietary sodium restriction on blood pressure in essential hypertension

Trial reference	No. of subjects	Duration of study (days)	UNaV (mEq/d) Baseline	Change	Blood pressure change (mmHg) Systolic	Diastolic	Significant *P* value
PARIJS et al. (1973)	22	28	191	−98	−7.6	+3.2	<0.05
MORGAN et al. (1978)	62	730	191	−38	−2.0	−7.0	<0.05
SKRABAL et al. (1981)	20	14	210	−170	−2.7	−3.0	NS
MACGREGOR et al. (1982)	19	28	162	−76	−10.0	−5.0	<0.05
BEARD et al. (1982)[a]	90	84	150	−113	−5.2	−3.4	NS
WATT et al. (1983)	18	28	143	−65	−0.5	−0.03	NS
SILMAN et al. (1983)	28	365	149	−21	−8.7	−6.3	NS
RICHARDS et al. (1984)	12	35	200	−100	−5.2	−1.8	NS
ERWTEMAN et al. (1984)	94	28	130	−58	−3.0	−2.5	NS
COOPER et al. (1984)	113	24	113	−70	−0.6	−1.4	NS
WATT et al. (1985)	31	28	128	−60	−0.5	+0.4	NS
GROBBEE et al. (1988)	35	28	131	−74	−1.4	+1.2	NS
GIBSON and CHAPMAN (1950)	40	42	129	−72	−0.8	−0.8	NS
MAGNANI (1976)	37	>365	—	—	−14	−14	<0.05
KAWASAKI et al. (1978)	19	—	109	—	−3	−3	NS
PARFREY et al. (1981)	41	5	244	−222	−14	−6	<0.05

NS, not significant. UNaV, urinary sodium excretion.
[a] Medications reduced.

be present in about 50%, similar to what one would estimate from previous reports on the prevalence of sodium sensitivity (WEINBERGER et al. 1986). The role of dietary sodium restriction as an adjunctive measure to pharmacological intervention is reviewed elsewhere (LUFT and WEINBERGER 1988). Sodium restriction may facilitate the management of numerous antihypertensive agents. Ca-channel blocking drugs appear to be an exception; they appear to be more effective if the subjects are ingesting a diet with a more generous (150 mmol/day) sodium content. Dietary sodium restriction trials in subjects previously identified as sodium sensitive have not yet been performed. The identification of a putative genetic marker (WEINBERGER et al. 1987) may facilitate such an endeavor. A final issue is whether or not dietary sodium restriction could possibly be harmful. Such a possibility appears unlikely in normal individuals, although it has not been entirely excluded (LUFT et al. 1988). A report by LONGWORTH et al. (1980) suggests that the blood pressure of some patients with essential hypertension may increase with dietary sodium restriction.

3.2 Potassium

For the most part, the more recent controlled trials of potassium supplementation in hypertensive patients involved small numbers of subjects and were of short duration (Table 2). A double-blind, randomized, crossover trial by MACGREGOR's group (1982) showed that the addition of 60 mmol/day potassium as the chloride salt causes a small but significant decrease in mean blood pressure in subjects with mild to moderate essential hypertension. However, the responses are heterogeneous, and some subjects do not respond at all. IIMURA and coworkers (1981) also performed a randomized, crossover trial and also observed a small but significant decrease in mean blood pressure. RICHARDS et al. (1984) increased potassium intake from 60 to 200 mmol/day for 4–6 weeks and found variable responses with no significant overall change. SVETKEY et al. (1987) found that potassium chloride lowers blood pressure in hypertensive subjects; however, the subjects randomized to the treatment group had significantly higher blood pressures than those randomized to the placebo group. SIANI et al. (1987) reported the most impressive results to date for potassium supplementation. They performed a 15-week, randomized, double-blind, placebo-controlled experiment with a supplement of 48 mmol/day in 37 patients. Impressive decreases in supine systolic (−14 mmHg), supine diastolic (−11 mmHg), standing systolic (−11 mmHg), and standing diastolic (−7 mmHg) reductions in blood pressure in treated patients were reported.

Adverse effects related to potassium supplementation were not identified in the studies reported in Table 2. However, the investigators excluded subjects with renal insufficiency for the trials. Clinicians must remain vigilantly aware of generalized distal renal tubular acidosis (Type IV) in patients with diminished renal function related to interstitial nephritis or diabetes mellitus, particularly if concomitant β-blocking drugs, converting enzyme inhibitors, potassium-retaining diuretics, nonsteroidal anti-inflammatory drugs, or digitalis preparations are given.

Table 2. Effect of dietary potassium supplementation on blood pressure in essential hypertension

Trial reference	No. of subjects	Duration of study (days)	UKV (mEq/d) Baseline	UKV (mEq/d) Change	Blood pressure change (mmHg) Systolic	Blood pressure change (mmHg) Diastolic	Significant *P* value
MACGREGOR et al. (1982)	23	28	62	+52	−7	−4	<0.05
IIMURA et al. (1981)	20	21	41	+82	−11	−11	NS
MORGAN et al. (1982)	8	14	46	+67	−10	−8	<0.05
RICHARDS et al. (1984)	12	28	60	+140	−2	−1	NS
SMITH et al. (1983)	10	12	65	+63	−8	−2	NS
OVERLACK et al. (1985)	16	56	66	+87	−17	−10	NS
SVETKY et al. (1987)	101	56	–	+120	−6.4	−4.1	<0.05
SIANI et al. (1987)	37	105	62	+48	−13	−9.6	<0.05
MILLER et al.[a] (1987)	64	28	58.6	+33	+0.4	+0.8	NS

NS, not significant. UKV, urinary potassium excretion.
[a] Supplement given as anonchloride salt.

3.3 Calcium

The results of calcium supplementation trials appear in Table 3. The calcium supplementation indicated in the table was in addition to that available in the diet of the study participants. Oral calcium loading in normotensive and hypertensive subjects has been reported to cause either a modest decrease or no change in blood pressure. BELIZAN and associates (1983a) studied 30 young, normotensive subjects who supplemented their diet with 25 mmol of calcium per day for 22 weeks and reported a 5%–9% decrease in supine diastolic pressure. The same group also reported a small blood pressure decrease in 36 pregnant women who were taking a supplement of 2 g calcium per day. JOHNSON and colleagues (1985) conducted a 4-year study in 81 normal and 34 hypertensive women, some of whom were taking a daily supplement of 1.5 g calcium and found no significant differences in blood pressure among the normotensive women between those taking the supplement and those who were not. In contrast, in the hypertensive group, the calcium-supplemented women had a 13 mmHg decrease in systolic pressure compared with a 7 mmHg decrease in the control hypertensive women over the course of the observations. LYLE et al. (1987) reported small but consistent (2–3 mmHg) decreases in systolic, diastolic, and mean arterial blood pressure in a group of 75 normal, younger men, treated either with a supplement of calcium (1.5 g/day) or placebo. GROBBEE and

Table 3. Effect of dietary calcium supplementation on blood pressure in essential hypertension

Trial reference	No. of subjects	Duration of study (days)	Ca (mg/day)	Blood pressure change (mmHg) Systolic	Diastolic	Significant *P* value
BELIZAN et al. (1983)	57	154	1000	−1.2	−5.6	<0.05
RESNICK and LARASH (1983)	10	5	2000	–	−7	<0.05 (low PRA)
JOHNSON et al. (1985)	95	56	1500	−10	0	<0.05
MCCARRON and Morris (1985)	80	56	1000	−6	−2	<0.05 (upright)
MEESE et al. (1986)	27	56	800	–	–	NS
GROBBEE and Hofman (1986[a])	90	84	1000	–	−2.4	<0.05
LUFT et al. (1986)	16	8	1000	−4	−2	<0.05 (systolic)
BLOOMFIELD et al. (1986)	32	28	1500	–	–	NS
LYLE et al. (1987)	75	84	1500	−3	−2	<0.05
STRAZULLO et al. (1986)	17	105	1000	−9	0	<0.05 (systolic)
BIERENBAUM et al. (1987)	200	180	1400 (milk)	−7	−6	<0.05
GILLILAND et al. (1987)	24	168	400	−6	−2	<0.05
THOMSEN et al. (1987)	28	365	2000	−0.6	+2	NS
VINSON et al. (1987)	15	42	1000	+1.1	−5	<0.05 (diastolic)
CAPPUCIO et al. (1987)	18	28	1600	+3.5	+1.1	NS

Absolute blood pressure values not available in some abstracts.
NS, not significant.
PRA, plasma renin activity.

HOFMAN (1986a) observed that mild hypertensives given 1 g per day experience a decrease in diastolic blood pressure at 6 and 12 weeks of 3.1 and 2.4 mmHg, respectively, compared with placebo. Subjects with higher parathyroid hormone values respond better than those with lower values. STRAZZULO et al. (1986) observed a decrease in systolic blood pressure in patients receiving calcium supplementation. LUFT et al. (1986) similarly noted a decrease in systolic blood pressure in older subjects receiving calcium (1 g/day) as opposed to those who were not given the supplement. MCCARRON's group (1985), in a double-blind study, reported no change in the standing blood pressure of 32 normal subjects after 8 weeks of supplementation but did observe a decrease of 3.8 mmHg and 2.3 mmHg systolic and diastolic supine blood pressure, respectively. Half of the hypertensive patients in that trial and 17% of the normotensive subjects

Table 4. Effect of dietary magnesium supplementation on blood pressure in essential hypertension

Trial reference	No. of subjects	Duration of study (days)	Mg (mmol/day) Baseline	Change	Blood pressure change (mmHg) Systolic	Diastolic	Significant *P* value
Dyckner and Wester (1983)	20	180	–	+15	−12	−8	<0.05
Cappuccio et al. (1985)	17	28	–	+15	−1	−0.5	NS
Henderson et al. (1986)	40	180	–	+9.4	−4	+1	NS

NS, not significant.

exhibited a decrease in blood pressure. The notion that subsets of hypertensive patients may respond is supported by the report of Resnick and Laragh (1983), who found that responders are those with low ionized calcium values. Cappuccio et al. (1987) performed a randomized, crossover, double-blind study in 18 unselected patients and found no effect with 1 month's treatment with calcium lactate gluconate, even though total serum calcium and urinary calcium excretion increased during calcium administration.

3.4 Magnesium

Magnesium has a well-recognized, blood pressure-lowering effect in patients with eclampsia and pre-eclampsia. The data from human intervention trials are scanty (Table 4). Dyckner and Wester (1983) conducted a study on 20 patients with hypertension or congestive heart failure who had had long-term treatment with diuretics. Magnesium supplementation resulted in a significant (21/8 mmHg) decrease in blood pressure. However, Cappuccio and coworkers (1985) found no change in blood pressure in a randomized, crossover study in 17 hypertensive subjects treated with 15 mmol per day of magnesium aspartate hydrochloride. Henderson et al. (1986) performed a randomized, controlled trial of magnesium supplementation in patients receiving diuretics. They were unable to confirm the work of Dyckner and Wester and found no significant difference between treated and placebo patients.

4 Conclusions and Summary

The evidence that too little or too much dietary sodium, potassium, calcium, or magnesium is responsible for the genesis of essential hypertension or that changes in the intake of these cations will consistently lower elevated blood pressure to lower value in patients with hypertension is incomplete. However, in certain patients or in subpopulations, alterations in cation metabolism may be important. Even though the *mean* change in blood pressure after altered cation intake in most of the studies is absent or modest, individual changes are often substantial.

Despite the general enthusiasm for the putative role of a high salt intake in the genesis of essential hypertension, firm conclusions that can be reached are few. In terms of therapy, it appears clear that a sizeable subgroup of patients with essential hypertension are salt sensitive. These patients appear to be older, may have higher blood pressures, and may more commonly be black than white. Prospective techniques to identify such patients are still not at hand, so a trial and error approach in likely patients appears warranted. It seems that sodium chloride intake must be reduced, since sodium accompanied by nonhalide anions has not been shown to influence blood pressure. The mechanisms of blood pressure reduction with sodium chloride restriction remain speculative.

The data for potassium chloride as a suitable intervention are not firm enough to allow guidelines for its general use. The overall safety of the intervention can be called into question in some patients with hypertension, particularly those with diabetes or those receiving drugs which impair the elimination of potassium or its deposition into cells. A palatable and inexpensive potassium supplement has not been developed. Data that nonchloride potassium supplements lower blood pressure are not available. It is possible that with increased potassium intake through natural means, the incidence of vascular complications could be reduced independent of effects on blood pressure.

The dietary calcium supplementation intervention is interesting and appears to be at low risk, although potential problems with renal calculi or increased intakes of saturated fats from dairy products have been mentioned as possible side effects from this particular intervention. It may also be suitable only for subgroups of patients with hypertension. Its general applicability and mechanism of action are not known.

There are no data to define the etiologic role of magnesium deficiency in human hypertension or to support the use of magnesium supplementation as antihypertensive therapy in patients with essential hypertension.

Interactions between these electrolytes may be important. For example, sodium and calcium compete for reabsorption in the proximal tubule, so that increasing the filtered load of either causes increased excretion of the other (Walser 1961). The effect of potassium intake on sodium excretion has already been mentioned. Dietary sources of calcium and magnesium are also rich in potassium (Engstrom and Tobelman 1983). Magnesium may function in part as a calcium antagonist (Levine and Coburn 1984). The interactions between calcium and magnesium are complex and imperfectly defined. A reduced sodium intake usually requires the removal of food sources rich in calcium in Western diets. With respect to any dietary intervention being a preventative in the development of hypertension, no prospective studies have been published thus far to support such a view.

Essential hypertension is a complicated disorder, which is heterogeneous and multifactorial. The National Institutes of Health recently appointed an advisory committee to review the evidence regarding nonpharmacological interventions (Final Report 1986). This committee of experts could only recommend weight control, alcohol restriction, and sodium restriction as adjuncts to therapy with antihypertensive drugs. The committee concluded that the data on potassium, calcium, and magnesium are insufficient for any current recommendations for hypertensive patients. Further, the data regarding the intake of any electrolyte and hypertension would appear not to warrant any health care policies for the general nonhypertensive population.

In summary, the treatment of hypertension by modification of dietary intake of sodium, potassium, calcium, and magnesium is suppoted in theory by several epidemiological, physiological, and experimental observations. However, data concerning the safety and efficacy of deliberate supplementation or limitation of these cations are incomplete, and few recommendations for treatment can be drawn from current information. Aside from restriction of dietary sodium chloride, by now a well-accepted component of therapy, panels of experts have been unable to reach a consensus regarding other electrolyte intake modifications as a treatment for hypertensive patients in general. Nevertheless, these forms of therapy can have important effects in certain individuals and subpopulations.

There is evidence that populations with a diet naturally high in potassium have a lower risk of vascular complications of hypertension. Potassium supplementation studies in rats with hypertension support these observations but the benefit of long-term supplementation in humans is still to be determined.

Dietary calcium supplementation has few associated risks and may be useful in subgroups of patients, but the advisability of this approach is not established. To date there is little to support the use of magnesium supplementation in hypertension treatment. Interactions between the electrolytes probably play a role in the modification of blood pressure, but these observations have not yet led to therapeutic recommendations. Similarly, current knowledge does not support the use of any particular alteration of electrolyte intake as a preventive measure for nonhypertensive people. The numerous investigations which have contributed to our imperfect understanding of the role of the principle cations in hypertension development and therapy have been reviewed in this chapter.

References

Ackley S, Barrett-Conner E, Suarez L (1983) Dairy products, calcium, and blood pressure. Am J Clin Nutr 38:457

Albert DG, Morita Y, Iseri LT (1958) Serum magnesium and plasma sodium levels in essential vascular hypertension. Circulation 17:761

Altura B, Atura B, Gebrewold A et al. (1984) Magnesium deficiency and hypertension: correlation between magnesium-deficient diets and microcirculatory changes in situ. Science 2232:1315–1317

Battarbee HD, Funch DP, Dailey JW (1979) The effect of dietary sodium and potassium upon blood pressure and catecholamine excretion in the rat. Proc Soc Exp Biol Med 171:32

Bauer JH, Gaunter W (1979) Effect of potassium chloride on plasma renin activity and plasma aldosterone during sodium restriction in normal man. Kidney Int 15:286

Beard TC, Cooke HM, Gray WR et al. (1982) Randomized controlled trial of a no-added-sodium diet for mild hypertension. Lancet 2:455

Belizan JM, Villar J, Pineda O et al. (1983a) Reduction of blood pressure with calcium supplementation in young adults. JAMA 249:1161

Belizan JM, Villar J, Salazar A et al. (1983b) Preliminary evidence of the effect of calcium supplementation on blood pressure in normal pregnant women. Am J Obstet Gynecol 146:175

Berenson GS, Voors AW, Dalferes ER et al. (1979) Creatinine clearance, electrolytes, and plasma renin activity related to the blood pressure of white and black children: the bogalusa heart study. J Lab Clin Med 93:535

Berliner RW (1960) Ion exchange mechanisms in the nephron. Circulation 21:892

Berliner RW, Kennedy TJ, Hilton JG (1950) Renal mechanisms for excretion of potassium. Am J Physiol 162:348

Bianchetti MG, Beretta-Piccoli C, Weidman P et al. (1983) Calcium and blood pressure regulation in normal and hypertensive subjects. Hypertension 5:57

Bianchi G, Baer PG, Fox U et al. (1975) Changes in renin, water balance, and sodium balance during development of high blood pressure in genetically hypertensive rats. Circ Res 36–37 (Suppl 1):153

Bierenbaum ML, Wolf E, Raff M, Maginnis WP (1987) The effect of dietary calcium supplementation on blood pressure and serum lipid levels, preliminary report. Nutr Rep Int 36:1147–1157

Birkenhager WH, Schalekamp MADH, Kraus KH et al. (1972) Consecutive hemodynamic pattern in essential hypertension. Lancet 1:560

Bloomfield RL, Young LD, Zurek G, Felts JH, Straw MK (1986) Effects of oral calcium carbonate on blood pressure in subjects with mildly elevated arterial pressure. J Hypertens 4(Suppl 5):351–354

Bulpitt CJ, Hodes C, Everitt MG (1976) The relationship between blood pressure and biochemical risk factors in a general population. Br J Prev Soc Med 30:158

Cappuccio FP, Markandu DN, Beynon GW et al. (1985) Lack of effect of oral magnesium on high blood pressure: a double-blind study. Br Med J 291:235

Cappuccio FP, Markandu ND, Singer DRJ, Smith SJ, Shore AC, MacGregor GA (1987) Does oral calcium supplementation lower high blood pressure? A double-blind study. J Hypertens 5:67–71

Carney S, Morgan T, Wilson M et al. (1975) Sodium restriction and thiazide diuretics in the treatment of hypertension. Med J Aust 1:803–897

Carretero OA, Romero JC (1977) Hypertension. McGraw-Hill, New York, p 497

Cooper R, Van Horn L, Liu K et al. (1984) A randomized trial on the effect of decreased dietary sodium intake on blood pressure in adolescents. J Hypertens 2:361–6

Dahl LK (1972) Salt and hypertension. Am J Clin Nutr 25:231

Dahl LK (1977) Hypertension. McGraw-Hill, New York, p 548

Dahl LK, Heine M, Thompson K (1974) Genetic influence of the kidney on blood pressure. Evidence from chronic renal homografts in rats with opposite predisposition to hypertension. Circ Res 34:94

Dahl LK, Leitt G, Heine M (1972) Influence of dietary potassium and sodium potassium molar ratios on the development of salt hypertension. J Exp Med 136:318

Dahl LK, Love RM (1954) Evidence of relationship between sodium (chloride) intake and human hypertension. Arch Intern Med 94:525

Dawber TR, Kanel WB, Kagan A et al. (1967) The epidemiology of hypertension. Grune and Stratton, New York, p 255

Dyckner T, Wester PO (1983) Effect of magnesium on blood pressure. Br Med J 286:1847

Engstrom AM, Tobelman RC (1983) Nutritional consequences of diet modification to reduce sodium intake. Ann Intern Med 98:870

Erwteman TM, Nagelkerke N, Lubsen J, Koster M, Dunning AJ (1984) Beta blockade, diuretics, and salt restriction for the management of mild hypertension: a randomized double blind trial. Br Med J 289:1525–8

Evans G, Weaver CM, Harrington DD, Babbs CF (1987) Dietary calcium and magnesium in the development of hypertension in the SHR. Fed Proc 45:709 (abstr 3220)

Feinstein AR (1985) Tempest in a P pot? Hypertension 7:313

Folkow B (1978) Cardiovascular structural adaptation: its role in the initiation and maintenance of primary hypertension. Clin Sci Mol Med 55 (Suppl 3):103–109
Folson AR, Smith CL, Prineas RJ et al. (1986) Serum calcium fractions in essential hypertensive and matched normotensive subjects. Hypertension 8:11
Freed SC, Friedman M (1951) Depressor effect of potassium restriction on blood pressure of the rat. Proc Soc Exp Biol Med 78:74
Freis ED (1976) Salt volume and the prevention of hypertension. Circulation 53:589
Fujita T, Henry WL, Bartter FC et al. (1980) Factors influencing blood pressure in salt-sensitive patients with hypertension. Am J Med 69:334
Garcia-Palmieri MR, Costos R Jr, Cruz-Videl M et al. (1984) Milk consumption, calcium intake, and decreased hypertension in Puerto Rico. Hypertension 67:322
Gibson CB, Chapman TB (1950) The diet and hypertension. Medicine 29:29–69
Gilliland M, Zawada ET, McClung D, TerWee J (1987) Preliminary report: natriuretic effect of calcium supplementation in hypertensive women over forty. J Am Coll Nutr 6:139–143
Goto A, Tobian L, Iwai J (1981) Potassium feeding reduces hyperactive central nervous system pressor responses in Dahl salt sensitive rats. Hypertension 3(Suppl I):I128
Grim CE, Luft FC, Miller JZ et al. (1980) Racial differences in blood pressure in Evans County, Georgia: relationship to sodium and potassium intake and plasma renin activity. J Chronic Dis 33:87
Grobbee DE, Hofman A (1986a) Effect of calcium supplementation on diastolic blood pressure in young people with mild hypertension. Lancet 2:703
Grobbee DE, Hofman A (1986b) Does sodium restriction lower blood pressure? Br Med J 293:27–29
Grobbee DE, Hofman A, Roelandt JTRC, Boomsma F, Schalekamp MADH, Valkenburg HA (1987) Sodium restriction and potassium supplementation in young people with mild hypertension. J Hypertens 5:115–120
Gruchow WH, Sobocinski KA, Barboriak JJ (1985) Alcohol, nutrient intake, and hypertension in US adults. JAMA 253:1567
Guyton AC (1980) Circulatory physiology III. Saunders, Philadelphia
Haddy FJ (1975) Minireview: potassium and blood vessels. Life Sci 16:1489
Harlan WR, Hull AL, Schmouder RL et al. (1984) Blood pressure and nutrition in adults: the national health and nutrition examination survey. Am J Epidemiol 120:17
Harlan WR, Landis JR, Schmouder RL et al. (1985) Relationship of blood lead and blood pressure in the adolescent and adult US population. JAMA 253:530
Henderson DG, Schierup J, Schoedt T (1986) Effect of magnesium supplementation on blood pressure and electrolyte concentrations in hypertensive patients receiving long term diuretic treatment. Br Med J 293:664–665
Houston MC (1986) Sodium and hypertension: a review. Arch Intern Med 146:179–185
Iimura O, Kijima T, Kikuchi K et al. (1981) Studies on the hypotensive effect of high potassium intake in patients with essential hypertension. Clin Sci 61:77s
Johnson NE, Smith EL, Freudenheim JL (1985) Effects on blood pressure of calcium supplementation of women. Am J Clin Nutr 42:12
Kaminer B, Lutz WPW (1960) Blood pressure in bushman of the Kalahari Desert. Circulation 22:289
Kannel WB (1979) On the cardiovascular hazards of hypertension. In: Onesti G, Klimt CR (eds) Hypertension: determinants, complications, and intervention. Grune and Stratton, New York, pp 143–149, pt 2, Chap 2
Kaplan NM (1987) Nonpharmacological therapy of hypertension. Med Clin North Am 71:921–933
Kawasaki T, Delea CS, Bartter FC et al. (1978) The effect of high-sodium and low-sodium intakes on blood pressure and other related variables in human subjects with idiopathic hypertension. Am J Med 64:193
Kesteloot H (1984a) Epidemiological studies on the relationship between sodium, potassium, calcium, and magnesium, and arterial blood pressure. J Cardiovasc Pharmacol 6:5192
Kesteloot H (1984b). Urinary cations and blood pressure population studies. Ann Clin Res 16 (Suppl 43):72

Kesteloot H, Geboers J, Math L et al. (1983) Epidemiological study of the relationship between calcium and blood pressure. Hypertension 5(Suppl II):II-52
Khaw KT, Barrett-Connor E (1987) Dietary potassium and stroke-associated mortality. N Engl J Med 316:235–240
Khaw KT, Thom S (1982) Randomized double-blind cross-over trial of potassium on blood pressure in normal subjects. Lancet 2:1127
Kirkendall WM, Conner WE, Abboud F et al. (1976) The effect of dietary sodium chloride on blood pressure, body fluids, electrolytes, renal function, and serum lipids of normotensive man. J Lab Clin Med 87:418
Koletsky S (1959) Hypertensive vascular disease produced by salt. Lab Invest 7:377
Koletsky S, Goodsitt AM (1960) Natural history and pathogenesis of renal ablation hypertension. Arch Pathol 69:654
Kowarski S, Cowen LA, Schachter D (1986) Decreased content of integral membrane calcium binding protein (IMCAL) in tissues of the spontaneously hypertensive rat. Proc Natl Acad Sci USA 83:1097–1100
Kurtz TW, Al-Bander HA, Morris RC Jr (1987) Salt-sensitive essential hypertension in man: is the sodium ion alone important? N Engl J Med 317:1043–1048
Lange J, Tobian L, Johnson MA et al. (1985) High K diets markedly reduce brain infarcts and death rate in SHRSP rats even when BP and body Na and K are precisely equal in the groups being compared. Proc Am Soc Nephrol 18:101A
Lenel R, Katz LN, Rodbard S (1948) Arterial hypertension in the chicken. Am J Physiol 152:557
Lever AF, Beretta-Piccoli C, Brown JJ et al. (1981) Sodium and potassium in essential hypertension. Br Med J 283:463
Levine BS, Coburn JW (1984) Magnesium, the mimic/antagonist of calcium. N Engl J Med 310:1253
Ljungman S, Aurell M, Hartford M et al. (1981) Sodium excretion and blood pressure. Hypertenson 3:318
Longworth DK, Drayer JIM, Weber MA et al. (1980) Divergent blood pressure responses during short-term sodium restriction in hypertension. Clin Pharmacol Ther 27:544
Louis WJ, Tabei R, Spector S (1971) The effects of sodium intake on inherited hypertension in the rat. Lancet 2:1283
Lowenstein FW (1961) Blood pressure in relation to age and sex in the tropics and subtropics. A review of the literature and an investigation in two tribes of Brazil Indians. Lancet 1:389
Luft FC, Aronoff GR, Sloan RS, Fineberg NS, Weinberger MH (1986) Short-term augmented calcium intake has no effect on sodium homeostasis. Clin Pharmacol Ther 39:414–419
Luft FC, Ganten D (1987) Salz ist nicht gleich Salz. Dtsch Med Wochenschr 112:1391–1394
Luft FC, Ganten U, Meyer D, Steinberg H, Gless KH, Unger TH, Ganten D (1988) Effect of high calcium diet on magnesium, catecholamines, and blood pressure of stroke-prone spontaneously hypertensive rats. Proc Soc Exp Biol Med 187:474–481
Luft FC, Miller JZ, Weinberger MH, Grim CE, Daugherty SA, Christian JC (1987) Influence of genetic variance on sodium sensitivity of blood pressure. Klin Wochenschr 65:101–109
Luft FC, Rankin LI, Bloch R et al. (1979a) Cardiovascular and humoral responses to extremes of sodium intake in normal black and white men. Circulation 60:697
Luft FC, Rankin LI, Henry DP (1979b) Plasma and urinary norepinephrine values at extremes of sodium intake in normal man. Hypertension 1:261
Luft FC, Weinberger MH (1982) Sodium intake and essential hypertension. Hypertension 4(Suppl III):III-14
Luft FC, Weinberger MH (1987) Potassium and blood pressure regulation. Am J Clin Nutr 45:1289–1294
Luft FC, Weinberger MH (1988) Effect of salt intake on the response to antihypertensive drugs. Hypertension 11:(Suppl. 4):I-229-I-232.
Lyle RM, Melby CL, Hyner GC, et al (1987) Blood pressure and metabolic effects of

calcium supplementation in normotensive white and black men. JAMA 257:1772
MacGregor GA, Markandu ND, Best FE et al. (1982) Double-blind randomized cross-over trial of moderate sodium restriction in essential hypertension. Lancet 1:351
MacGregor GA, Smith SJ, Markandu ND et al. (1982) Moderate potassium supplementation in essential hypertension. Lancet 2:567
Maddocks I (1967) Blood pressure in Melanesians. Med J Aust 1:1123
Magnani B, Ambrosioni E, Agosta R et al. (1976) Comparison of the effects of pharmacological therapy and a low sodium diet on mild hypertension. Clin Sci 51:625s–626s
Mark AL, Gordon FJ, Becker PA (1981) Mechanisms of the antihypertensive action of high dietary potassium (abstr). Clin Res 29:525A
Mark AL, Lawton WJ, Abboud FM et al. (1975) Effect of high and low sodium intake on arterial pressure and forearm vascular resistance in borderline hypertension. A preliminary report. Circ Res 36–37(Suppl 1):194
Marone C, Beretta-Piccoli C, Weidmann P (1980) Acute hypercalcemic hypertension in man: role of hemodynamics, catecholamines, and renin. Kidney Int 20:92
Maxwell MH, Waks AU (1987) Cations and hypertension: sodium, potassium, calcium, and magnesium. Med Clin North Am 71:859–875
McCarron DA (1982) Low serum concentrations of ionized calcium in patients with hypertension. N Engl J Med 307:226
McCarron DA (1989) Calcium metabolism and hypertension. Kidney Int 35:717–736
McCarron DA, Henry HJ, Morris CD (1982) Human nutrition and blood pressure regulation: an integrated approach. Hypertension 4(5 pt 2):III 2
McCarron DA, Lucas PA, Schneideman RS et al. (1985) Blood pressure development of the spontaneously hypertensive rat after concurrent manipulation of calcium and sodium: relation to intestinal fluxes. J Clin Invest 78:1147–1154
McCarron DA, Morris CD, Henry HJ et al. (1984) Blood pressure and nutrient intake in the United States. Science 224:1392
McCarron DA, Morris CD (1985) Blood pressure response to oral calcium in persons with mild to moderate hypertension: a randomized double-blind, placebo-controlled, crossover trial. Ann Intern Med 103:825
Messe RB, Gonzalez DG, Casparian JM, Ram CVS, Pak CYC, Kaplan NM (1986) Failure of calcium supplements to relieve hypertension. Clin Res 34:A218
Meneely GR, Dahl LK (1961) Electrolytes in hypertension. The effects of sodium chloride. Med Clin North Am 45:271
Miall WE (1959) Follow-up study of arterial pressure in the population of a Welsh mining valley. Br Med J 2:1201
Miller JZ, Weinberger MH (1986) Blood pressure response to sodium restriction and potassium supplementation in health normotensive children. Clin Exp Hypertens [A] 7:823–828
Miller JZ, Weinberger MH, Christian JC et al. (1987) Blood pressure response to potassium supplementation in normotensive adults and children. Hypertension 10: 437–442
Morgan TO (1982) The effect of potassium and bicarbonate ions on the rise in blood pressure caused by sodium chloride. Clin Sci 63:407s
Morgan T, Adam W, Gillies A, Wilson M, Morgan G, Carney S (1978) Hypertension treated by salt restriction. Lancet 1:227–30
Morgan T, Nowson C (1986) The role of sodium restriction in the management of hypertension. Can J Physiol Pharmacol 64:786–792
Munoz-Ramirez H, Chatelain RE, Bumpus FM, Khairallah PA (1980) Development of two-kidney Goldblatt hypertension in rats under dietary sodium restriction. Am J Physiol 238:H889–H894
Oliver WJ, Cohen EL, Neel JV (1975) Blood pressure, sodium intake and sodium related hormones in the Yanomamo Indians, a "no-salt" culture. Circulation 52:146
Overlack A, Stumpe KO, Moch B (1985) Hemodynamic, renal and hormonal responses to changes in dietary potassium in normotensive and hypertensive man: long-term antihypertensive effect of potassium supplementation in essential hypertension. Klin Wochenschr 63:3520360

Page LB, Danion A, Moellering RC Jr (1974) Antecedents of cardiovascular disease in six Soloman Islands societies. Circulation 49:1132
Pak CYC (1970) Osteoporosis. Current Therapy. Saunders, Philadelphia, p 337
Parfrey PS, Markandu ND, Roulston JE et al. (1981) Relationship between arterial pressure, dietary sodium intake, and renin system in essential hypertension. Br Med J 283:94
Parijs J, Joosens JV, Van Der Linden L et al. (1973) Moderate sodium restriction and diuretics in the treatment of essential hypertension. Am Heart J 85:22–33
Petersen B, Schroll M, Christiansen C et al. (1977) Serum and erythrocyte magnesium in normal elderly Danish people: relationships to blood pressure and serum lipids. Acta Med Scand 201:31
Pickering GW (1980) Salt intake and essential hypertension. Cardiovasc Rev Rep 1:13
Pietinen P, Dougherty R, Mutanen M (1984) Dietary intervention study among 30 free-living families in Finland. J Am Diet Assoc 84:313
Prior AM, Evans JG, Harvey HBP et al. (1968) Sodium intake and blood pressure in two Polynesian populations. N Engl J Med 279:515
Reed D, McGee D, Yano K et al. (1985) Diet, Blood pressure, and multicollinearity. Hypertension 7:405
Resnick LM, Laragh JH (1983) The hypotensive effect of short-term oral calcium loading in essential hypertension (abstr). Clin Res 31:334A
Resnick LM, Laragh JH, Sealey JE et al. (1983) Divalent cations in essential hypertension: relations between serum ionized calcium, magnesium, and plasma renin activity. N Engl J Med 309:888
Richards AM, Nicholls MG, Espiner EA et al. (1984) Blood pressure response to moderate sodium restriction and to potassium supplementation in mild essential hypertension. Lancet 1:757
Robinson D, Bailey AR, Williams PT (1982) Calcium and blood pressure. Lancet 2:1215
Roos JC, Koomans HA, Dorhout Mees EJ, Delawi IMK (1985) Renal sodium handling in normal humans subjected to low, normal, and extremely high sodium supplies. Am J Physiol 249:F941–F947
Roullet C, Drüeke T, McCarron D (1987) Calcium influx of SHR's isolated enterocytes: normalization by dietary calcium. Kidney Int 31:308
Sakahashi E, Saaski N, Takeda J et al. (1957) The geographic distribution of cerebral hemorrhage and hypertension in Japan. Hum Biol 29:139
Sangal AK, Beevers DG (1982) Serum calcium and blood pressure (letter). Lancet 2:493
Saperstein LA, Brandt WL, Drury DR (1950) Production of hypertension in the rat by substituting hypertonic sodium chloride for drinking water. Proc Soc Exp Biol Med 73:82
Sasaki N (1962) High blood pressure and the salt intake of the Japanese. Jpn Heart J 3:313
Schlierf G, Arab L, Schellenberg B, Oster P, Mordasini H, Schmidt-Gayk H, Vogel H (1980) Salt and hypertension: data from the Heidelberg study. Am J Clin Nutr 33:872–875
Sempos C, Cooper R, Kovar MG et al. (1986) Dietary calcium and blood pressure in national health and nutrition examination surveys I and II. Hypertension S:1067
Seymour AA, Davis JO, Freeman RH, De Forrest JM, Rowe BP, Stephens GA, Williams GM (1980) Hypertension produced by sodium depletion and unilateral nephrectomy; a new experimental model. Hypertension 2:125–129
Siani A, Strazzullo P, Russo L, Guglielmi S, Iacoviello L, Aldo Ferrara L, Mancini M (1987) controlled trial of long-term oral potassium supplements in patients with mild hypertension. Br Med J 294:1453–1456
Silman AJ, Locke C, Mitchell P et al. (1983) Evaluation of the effectiveness of a low sodium diet in the treatment of mild to moderate hypertension. Lancet 1:1179
Simpson FO (1979) Salt and hypertension: a skeptical review of the evidence. Clin Sci 57(Suppl 5):463
Simpson FO, Waal-Manning HJ, Bolli P et al. (1978) Relationship of blood pressure to sodium excretion in a population survey. Clin Sci Mol Med 55(Suppl 4):373
Sinnett PF, Whyte HM (1973) Epidemiological studies in a total highland population.

Tukisenta, New Guinea: cardiovascular disease and relevant clinical, electrocardiographic, radiological and biochemical findings. J Chronic Dis 26:265
Skrabal F, Aubock J, Hortnagel H (1981) Low sodium, high potassium diet for prevention of hypertension: probable mechanism of action. Lancet ii: 895–900
Skrabal F, Hamberger L, Gruber G, Meister B, Doll P, Cerny E (1985) Hereditäre Salzsensitivität als Ursache der essentiellen Hypertonie: Untersuchungen des Membrantrasportes und der intrazellulären Elektrolyte. Klin Wochenschr 63:891–896
Smith SJ, Markandu ND, Sagnella GA, et al (1983) Does potassium lower blood pressure by increasing sodium excretion? A metabolic study in patients with mild to moderate essential hypertension. J Hypertension 1(Suppl 2):27
Strazzullo P, Nunziata V, Cirillo M et al. (1983) Abnormalities of calcium metabolism in essential hypertension Clin Sci 65:137
Strazzullo P, Siani A, Guglielmi S et al. (1986) Controlled trial of long-term oral calcium supplementation in essential hypertension. Hypertension 8:1084–1088
Svetkey LP, Yarger WE, Feussner JR, DeLong E, Klotman PE (1987) Double-blind, placebo-controlled trial of potassium chloride in the treatment of mild hypertension. Hypertension 9:444–450
Thomsen K, Nilas L, Christiansen C (1987) Dietary calcium intake and blood pressure in normotensive subjects. Acta Med Scand 222:51–56
Tobian L (1989) High potassium diets during hypertension reduce arterial endothelial injury, stroke mortality rate, arterial hypertrophy, and renal lesions without lowering blood pressure. In: Retting R, Ganten D, Luft F (eds) *Salt and hypertension*. Springer, Berlin Heidelberg New York, pp 218–234
Tobian L, Lange J, Iwai J et al. (1979) Prevention with thiazide of NaCl induced hypertension in Dahl "S" rats: evidence for a Na retaining humoral in "S" rats. Hypertension 1:316
Treasure J, Ploth D (1983) Role of dietary potassium in the treatment of hypertension. Hypertension 5:864–872
Ueshima H, Tanigaki M, Iida M et al. (1981) Hypertension, salt and potassium. Lancet 1:504
Vinson JA, Mazur T, Bose P (1987) Comparison of different forms of calcium on blood pressure of normotensive young males. Nutr Rep Int 36:497–505
Vlachakis ND, Frederics R, Velasquez M et al. (1982) Sympathetic system function and vascular reactivity in hypercalcemic patients. Hypertension 4:452
Walker BS, Walker EW (1936) Normal magnesium metabolism and its significant disturbances. J Lab Clin Med 21:713
Walker WG, Whelton PK, Saito H et al. (1979) Relation between blood pressure and renin, renin substrate, angiotensin II, aldosterone and urinary sodium and potassium in 574 ambulatory subjects. Hypertension 1:287
Walser M (1961) Ion association. VII. Dependence of calciuresis on natriuresis during sulfate infusion. Am J Physiol 201:769
Watson RL, Langord HG, Abernethy J et al. (1980) Urinary electrolytes, body weight and blood pressure: pooled cross-sectional results among four groups of adolescent females. Hypertension 2(Suppl 1):93
Watt GCM, Edwards C, Hart JT et al. (1983) Dietary sodium restriction for mild hypertension in general practice. Br Med J 286:432
Watt GCM, Foy CJW, Hart JT et al. (1985) Dietary sodium and arterial blood pressure: evidence against genetic susceptibility. Br Med Jour 291:1525–1528
Webb DJ, Clark SA, Brown WB, Fraser R, Lever AF, Murray GD, Robertson JIS (1987) Dietary sodium deprivation raises blood pressure in the rat but does not produce irreversible hyperaldosteronism. J Hypertens 5:525–531
Weinberger MH (1987) sodium chloride and blood pressure. N Engl J Med 317:1084–1085
Weinberger MH, Cohen SJ, Miller JZ, Luft FC, Grim CE, Fineberg NS (1988) Dietary sodium restricition a adjunctive treatment of hypertension. JAMA 259:2561–2565
Weinberger MH, Miller JZ, Fineberg NS, Luft FC, Grim CE, Christian JC (1987) Association of haptoglobin with sodium sensitivity and resistance of blood pressure. Hypertension 10:443–446

Weinberger MH, Miller JZ, Luft FC, Grim CE, Fineberg NS (1986) Definitions and characteristics of sodium sensitivity and blood pressure resistance. Hypertension 8(II):127–134

Yamamoto I, Morimoto S, Uchida K et al. (1982) Reversible hypertension caused by calcium overloading in a patient with postoperative hypoparathyroidism. Endocrinol Jpn 29:725

Yamori Y, Kihara M, Nara Y et al. (1981) Hypertension and diet: multiple regression analysis in a Japanese farming community. Lancet 1:1204

Young EW, Bukoski RD, McCarron DA (1988) Calcium metabolism in experimental hypertension. Proc Soc Exp Biol Med 187:123–141

Zoccali C, Cumming AMM, Hutcheson MJ, Barnett P, Semple PF (1985) Effects of potassium on sodium balance, renin, noradrenaline and arterial pressure. J Hypertens 3:67–72

CHAPTER 19

Natural Agents and Extracts

H. Becker

CONTENTS

1 Introduction

Natural sources (microorganisms, plants, and animals) contain a large variety of pharmacologically active compounds which are used therapeutically as such. In many other cases natural compounds have been used as models for the synthesis of a whole series of drug families. To the first group belong, e.g., cardiac glycosides, cancerostatic indol alkaloids (vincristine and vinblastine), anthraquinones, and many antibiotics. To the second group belong the local anesthetics which have been derived from cocaine, the muscle relaxants derived from *Strychnos* and *Menispermaceous* alkaloids, spasmolytics derived from atropine, or analgesics derived from morphine.

As only a small part of the microorganisms, plants, and animals have been chemically and pharmacologically checked for active ingredients, it can be supposed that more ingredients active against a variety of diseases may be found. The search for those substances parallels the screening of synthetic products. The difficulty compared with synthetic products lies in the fact that raw extracts have to be used which contain a mixture of substances. Also, the concentration may be too low to be detected in a pharmacological test. The isolation of pure substances is very time consuming. Often, the amounts that can be isolated in a pure state are adequate for structure elucidation but not for pharmacological tests.

The *Rauwolfia* alkaloids, the *Veratrum* alkaloids, and the diterpenes (forskolin) from *Coleus* species are known plant ingredients with a marked hypertensive effect. Numerous other plants are used in the ethnic medicine of various geographic and cultural areas. These ethnically used vegetal antihypertonica must be scientifically checked for two reasons:

a) To develop new effective drugs. These new drugs may be active ingredients of plants themselves or synthetic derivatives of the active principles.

Especially for Third World countries the discovery of plants with active compounds could mean an economically important saving of foreign currency.

b) To prove the effectiveness or ineffectiveness of ethnically used plants. Thus, patients could be prevented from taking inactive medications.

The subject of this article has been reviewed repeatedly during the past 10 years (PETKOV 1979; FUNAYAMA and HIKINO 1981a; VILLAR et al. 1986). This present chapter updates the literature according to the chemistry of the active principle, if an active principle has been defined. Another group of compounds that have been claimed to be effective in treating hypertension but have not been chemically characterized will be discussed. In many countries, including Third World countries, an orientation towards traditional medicine is currently under way.

2 Alkaloids

2.1 Rauwolfia Alkaloids (Reserpine)

These alkaloids are treated in detail in Chap. 7 and will not be mentioned here.

2.2 Veratrum Alkaloids

Alkaloids have been extracted from a number of Liliaceae, e.g., *Veratrum*, *Schoenocaulon*, *Zygadenus*, and *Fritillaria*. Their chemistry has been reviewed by SCHLITTLER (1977), their pharmacological action, including hypotension, cardiotonic activity, respiratory depression, apnea, and emetic effect as well as their therapeutic use have been reviewed in detail by KRAYER and MEILMAN (1977).

The authors concluded that hypotensive *Veratrum* ester alkaloids continue to have their main therapeutic usefulness in the treatment of acute hypertensive states, such as eclampsia, malignant hypertension, hypertensive pulmonary edema, and hypertensive encephalopathy. *Veratrum* alkaloids are no longer used therapeutically.

2.3 Ergot Alkaloids

Ergot alkaloids in the form of co-dergocrinmesilat (a mixture of dihydroergocristine, dihydroergocryptine, dihydroergocornine) are in rare cases still used as antihypertensive agents (PALM et al. 1987). They cause a slight reduction of blood pressure within 2 weeks in elderly patients (>65 years). A recent patent describes the synthesis and hard gelatin capsule formulation of semisynthetic dihydroergoline derivatives (LAGUZZA 1986). Another patent deals with a controlled release formulation for oral administration of ergot alkaloid derivatives for the treatment of hypertension and migraine (ZUGER 1986).

2.4 Spermidine Alkaloids

2.4.1 Ephedradines

Ephedra plants have been clinically employed as an antisudorific (reducing increased perspiration) in China. Pharmacological investigation of their roots revealed hypotensive activity. As one of the hypotensive principles a series of spermidine alkaloids was isolated. Detailed studies have been conducted with ephedradine B (see *1*) (Hikino et al. 1983b). Administration of 0.1–3 mg/kg,

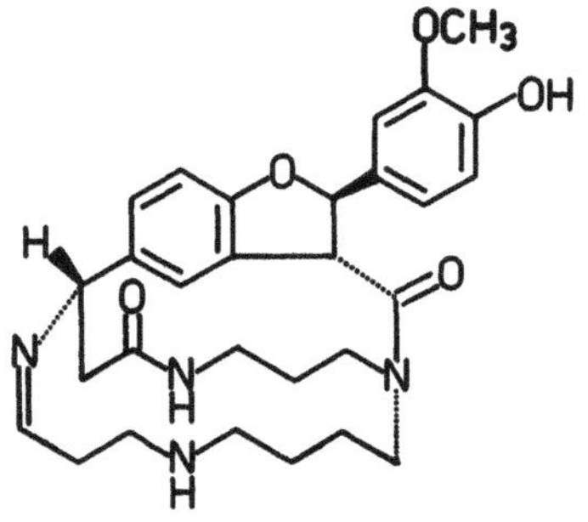

1

i.v., to Wistar rats and to SHR reduces blood pressure in a dose-dependent manner. In the hypogastric nerve vas deferens of the guinea pig, application of 3 $\times 10^{-7}-10^{-5}$ g/ml to the ganglion inhibits the contraction of the vas deferens induced by electrical preganglionic nerve stimulation and by acetylcholine ($10^{-4} - 10^{-3}$ g/ml) applied to the ganglion. It is thus concluded that the hypotensive activity of ephedradine B is exerted mainly by ganglion block. Ephedradines are not the only antihypertensive compounds from *Ephedra* roots. In addition, besides spermidine alkaloids, feruloylhistamine (see *2*) (Hikino et al. 1983a) and

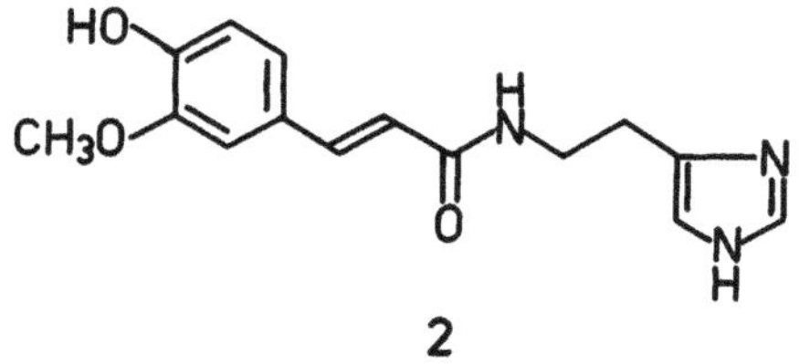

2

biflavonoids (see *3*) were found as antihypertensive compounds in Ephedra roots (Hikino et al. 1982). Administration of feruloylhistamine hydrochloride to rats at a dose of 5 mg/kg, i.v., causes significant hypotension. It is interesting to note that not only hypotensive compounds but also a hypertensive compound, maokonine, has been isolated from *Ephedra* roots. It shows structural and pharmacological similarities to ephedrine.

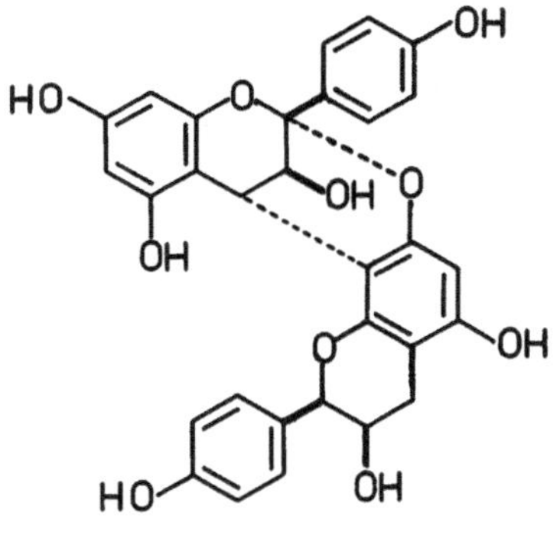

3

2.4.2 Kukoamine A

The oriental medicine "jikoppi", the root bark of *Lycium chinense* Miller (Solanaceae), has been shown to be clinically effective for hypertension and has been reported to exhibit hypotensive, hypoglycemic, antipyretic, and antistress ulcer activity in experimental animals (FUNAYAMA et al. 1980, and literature cited therein). FUNAYAMA et al. isolated the spermidine alkaloid, kukoamine A (see *4*), by monitoring various fractions for hypotensive activity. Kukoamine 4 induced apparent hypotension in rats (5 mg/kg, i.v.).

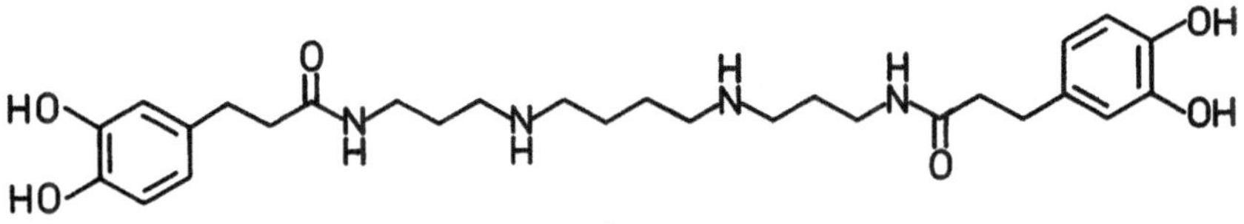

4

2.5 Isoquinoline and Tetrahydroisoquinoline Alkaloids

2.5.1 Neferine

Neferine (see *5*) a dimeric benzyltetrahydroisoquinoline alkaloid from the embryos of the Indian lotus, *Nelumbo nucifera* (Nympheaceae), exhibits antihypertensive activity in anesthetized SHR (NISHIBE et al. 1986).

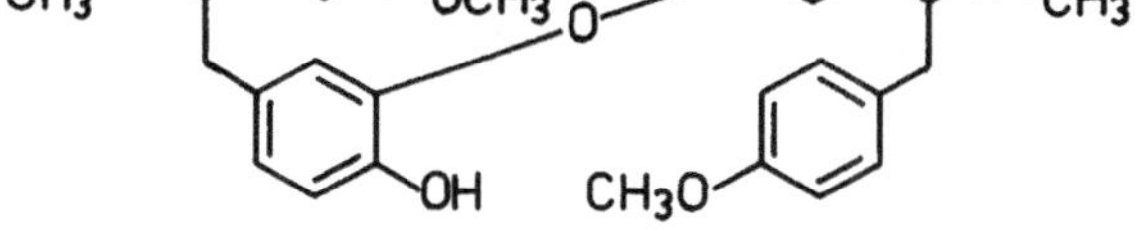

5

2.5.2 Thalystyline and Obamegine

Thalystyline (see *6*), a monoquarternary bisbenzylisoquinoline alkaloid, and obamegine (see *7*), a similar structure but lacking quarternary nitrogen, were both isolated from *Thalictrum* species (BANNING et al. 1982). They lower blood

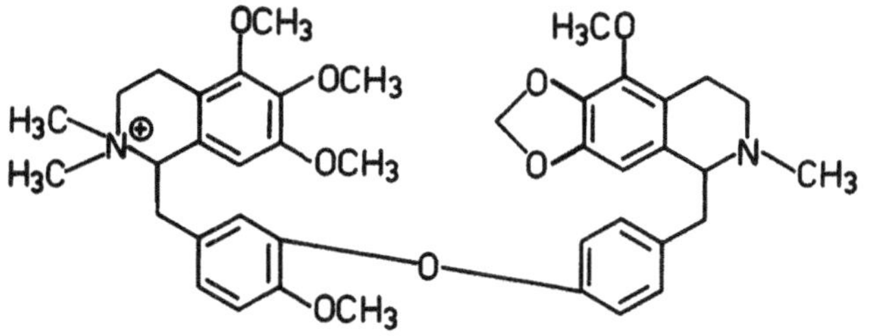

6

pressure in normotensive dogs. The effect is transient. Repeated injections of the alkaloids result in tachyphylaxis to blood pressure-lowering effects. Although alkaloids exhibit α-adrenergic blockade in the vascular preparation, the mechanism for the hypotensive effect remains to be established.

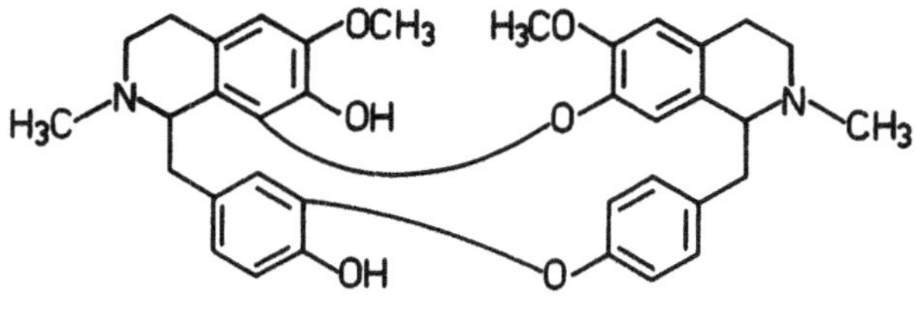

7

2.5.3 Majarol

Majarol (see *8*) prepared semisynthetically from the alkaloid majorine, isolated from *Berberis koreana*, shows atypical, transient hypotensive effects in rats and a subsequent prolonged decrease in arterial pressure accompanied by a decrease in heart rate (LEE et al. 1986).

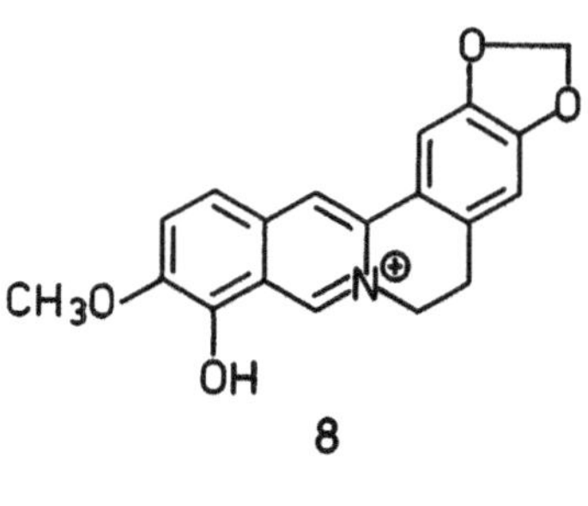

8

2.5.4 Hemanthamine

Hemanthamine (see *9*) decreases blood pressure in cats at a dose of 0.3–0.5 mg/kg. Hypotensive effects of vagal nerve stimulation and of acetylcholine injections are increased at doses of 0.5–2.0 mg/kg (ZAKIROV and KAMILOV 1967).

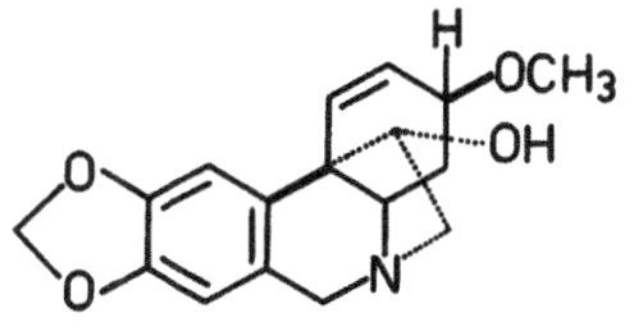

9

2.5.5 Magnoflorine

Magnoflorine (see *10*), a quarternary ammonium base, is isolated from the Chinese herb "tu qing mu xiang" (roots of *Aristolochia debilis*) as a hypotensive principle. In anesthetized cats intravenous injection of 2 mg/kg produces a prompt and significant fall in blood pressure lasting about 1–2 h. Oral administration (20 and 40 mg/kg) also results in hypotension. The alkaloid is equally effective when administered i.p. or i.v. in anaesthetized dogs. Its hypotensive action can be explained through its ganglionic blockade (CHANG et al. 1964).

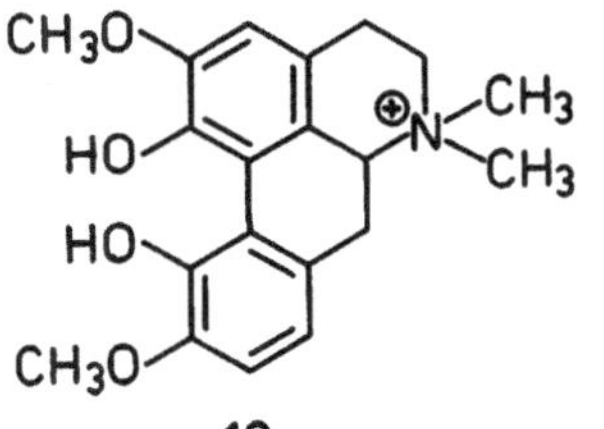

10

2.5.6 Morphine

Small doses of morphine injected i.v. into anaesthetized dogs cause a marked transient fall in blood pressure; repeated injections of morphine result in acute tolerance and a lesser fall in blood pressure (MURANO and TANAKA 1957).

2.6 β-Carboline-Derived Alkaloids

β-Carboline alkaloids possess a tricyclic ring system (see *11*); the 6-membered nitrogen-containing ring is often hydrogenated. The alkaloids are biogenetically derived from tryptamine. More than 1200 representatives of this group are known (LUCKNER 1984). Among those exerting a hypotensive action, *Rauwolfia* alkaloids (mentioned in Sect. 2.1) are the most prominent. Besides them, the following β-carboline-derived alkaloids were reported to be hypotensive.

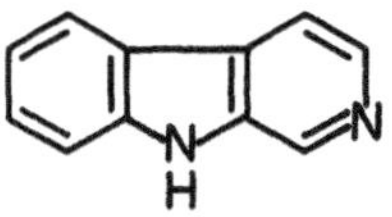

11

2.6.1 Tabernulosine

Tabernulosine (see *12*) isolated from *Tabernaemontana glandulosa*, Apocynaceae, shows significant antihypertensive activity which lasts several hours when given i.v. (18 mg/kg) to genetically hypertensive rats (ACHENBACH et al. 1982). An indole alkaloid isolated from the seeds of another *Taberaemontana* species (*T. dichotoma*) also shows hypotensive activity and also weak muscle relaxant activity. The same pharmacological properties were described for perivine, vobasine, coronaridine, and dichomine found in the leaves, fruit, and bark of *T. dichomata* (PERERA et al. 1985).

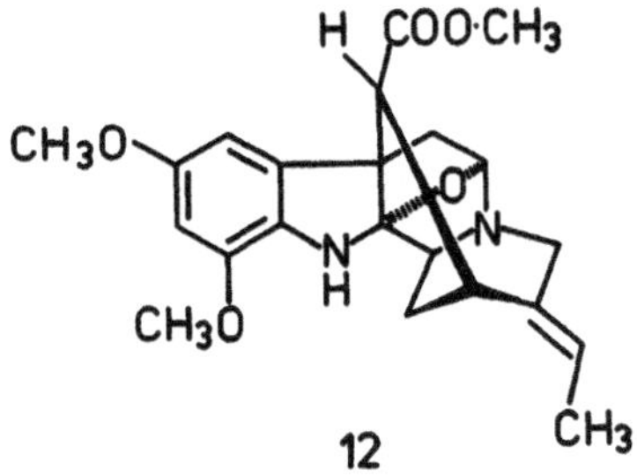

12

2.6.2 Nitramarine

Nitramarine (see *13*) an alkaloid of *Nitraria komorovii* possesses hypotensive and spasmolytic activities (TULYAGANOV et al. 1984).

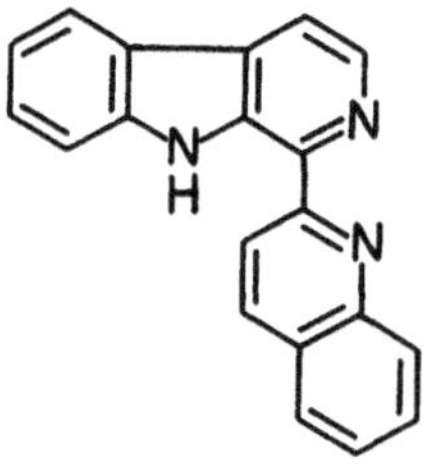

13

2.6.3 Vincamine

Vincamine (see *14*), an alkaloid isolated from the common periwinkle, *Vinca minor*, is used as a vasodilator. In cats and dogs i.v. administration of pure vincamine and isovincamine in doses of 2.5 mg/kg results in a fall of blood pressure and partial respiratory paralysis (KACZMAREK et al. 1962).

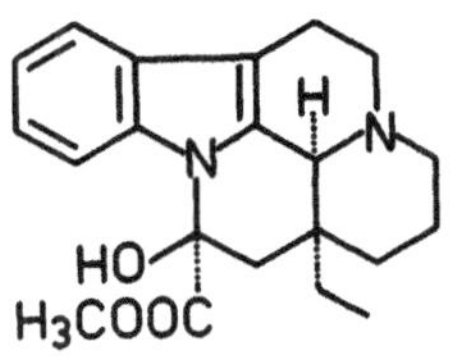

14

2.6.4 Trichotomine

A Japanese patent describes the isolation of trichotomine (see *15*), a dimeric β-carboline alkaloid, from two Verbenaceae plants, *Clerodendron trichotomum* and *Premna microphylla* (IWADARE et al. 1976) (see *15*). It shows hypotensive as well as sedative activities.

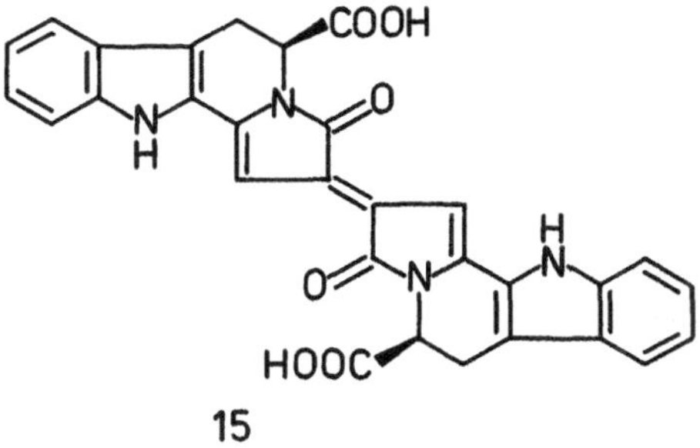

15

2.6.5 *β*-Carboline Derivative from Picrasma quassioides

1-(β-*carbolin-1-yl)-2-methoxy-4-(4,8-dimethoxy*-β-carbolin-1-yl)butan-1-one (see *16*) exhibits antihypertensive activity, as well as antiulcer, antithrombotic and antitumor activity (Kaken Pharmaceutical Co 1985). It is an inhibitor of phosphodiesterase. The extraction of 50 kg wood chips of *Picrasma quassioides* yields only 31 mg of this compound.

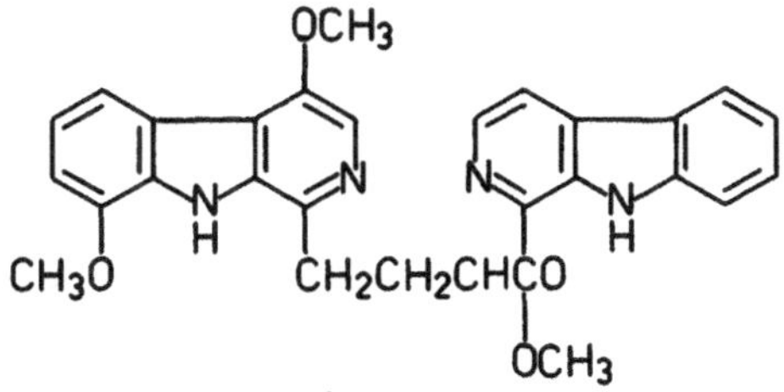

16

2.6.6 Cinchona Alkaloids

Two alkaloids isolated from *Cinchona ledgeriana*, cinchophylline and cinchophyllamine (see *17*), are hypotensive by virtue of their mild adrenolytic action (QUEVAUVILLER et al. 1969).

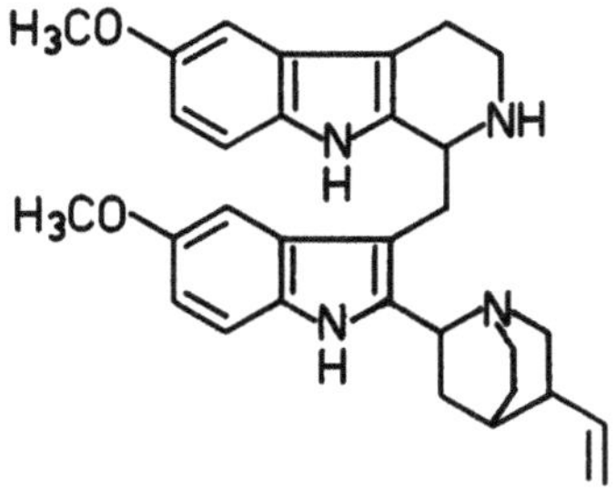

17

2.7 Quinolizidine and Pyrrolizidine Alkaloids

2.7.1 Calpurnine

Calpurnine (see *18*) was isolated from various plants belonging to the leguminoseae family. The antihypertensive properties are highest in narcotized dogs, monkeys, and rats (0.2 mg/kg, i.v.) but less in nonnarcotized animals. A dose of 0.5 mg/kg given to dogs i.p. reduces blood pressure. A relatively high toxicity (LD_{50}: i.v.: mouse and rat 3 mg/kg; orally: mouse 32 mg, rat: 132 mg; s.c.: rat 41 mg/kg) prevents therapeutic use of this quinolizidine alkaloid (see BAUMGARTH 1980, for references).

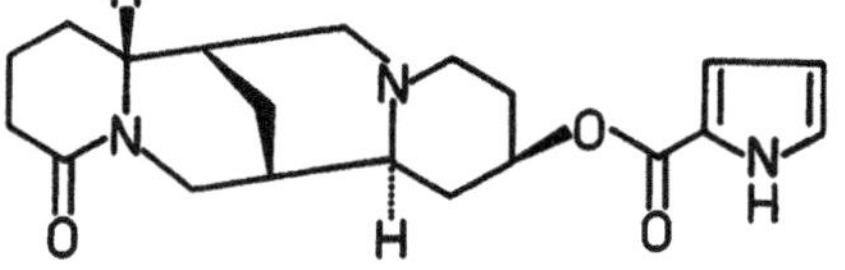

18

2.7.2 Heliosupine

Heliosupine (see *19*) isolated from *Cynoglossum* species shows diuretic as well as hypotensive effects in rats, cats, and rabbits when injected s.c. (RAKSHAIN and MATS 1973).

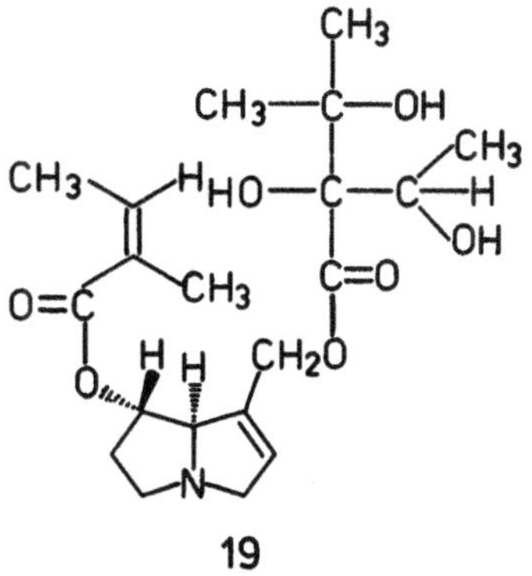

19

2.7.3 Semisynthetic Pyrrolizidines

Many pyrrolizidine alkaloids exert hepatic and pulmonary toxicity and carcinogenic effects in humans and animals. These toxic properties are related to certain structural features. An Indian group (see BAUMGARTH 1980, for references) synthesized about 120 pyrrolizidine derivatives, starting from natural alkaloids, and tested the resulted compounds pharmacologically. The most antihypertensive compounds are *N*-isopropyl-1-methylenpyrrolizidiniumbromide (see *20*) (in dogs 5–10 mg/kg, i.v., gives 50%–70% blood pressure reduction for 40–60 min) and retronamides, e.g., *N*-(*p*-hydroxybenzoyl)-retronamin (in dogs 0.5–5 mg/kg gives 37%–75% fall for 12–150 min).

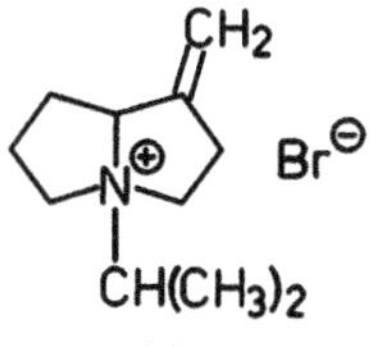

20

2.8 Tetramethylpyrazine

Tetramethylpyrazine (see *21*) has been isolated from the stem of *Jatropha podagria* (ODEBIYI 1980) and from the stem of *Ephedra sinica* (SUN 1983). OJEWOLE and ODEBIYI (1980, 1981) and SUN (1983) describe its hypotensive effect. The alkaloid inhibits the contractions of the rabbit, isolated, perfused, central ear artery induced by periarterial electrical stimulation or intraluminally administered noradrenaline. It reduces, like papaverine, the amplitude of the spontaneous myogenic contractions and noradrenaline-evoked contractions of the rat isolated portal vein. From these and other experiments it was concluded that tetramethylpyrazine probably causes hypotension in experimental animals by dilating blood vessels, and by acting as a nonspecific spasmolytic agent (like papaverine).

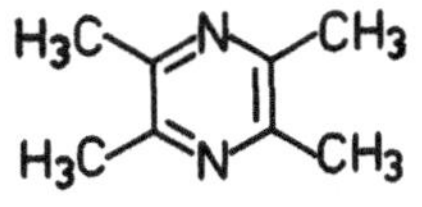

21

2.9 Steroid Alkaloids

Veratrum alkaloids (Sect. 2.2) are structurally steroid alkaloids. The hypotensive principle of *Conopharyngia pachysiphon* was elucidated as being 20-amino-3-β-hydroxy-5-pregnene-β-D-glucoside (DICKEL et al. 1959) and therefore also belongs to the steroid alkaloids.

3 Flavonoids

Flavonoids are derivatives of 2-phenylchromane. The main structural types differing in oxidation and substitution pattern of ring C are listed in Fig. 1.

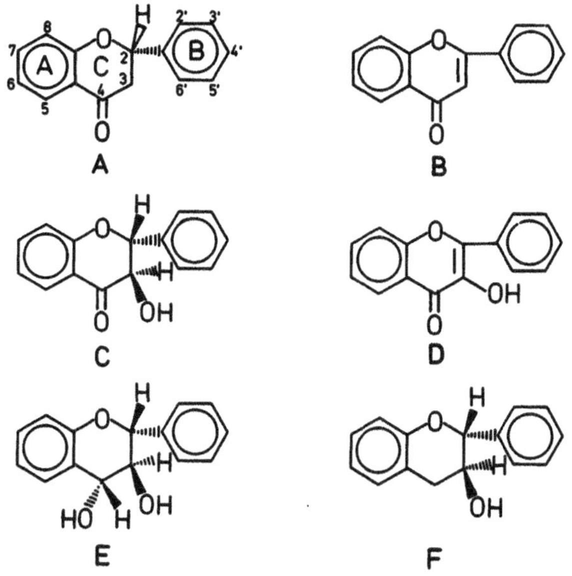

Fig. 1A–F. Structural variations of flavonoids due to different patterns of ring C. **A** flavanon; **B** flavon; **C** flavanonol; **D** flavonol; **E** flavan-3,4-diol; **F** catechin

More than 2000 naturally occurring flavonoids are derived from these basic types by various substituents, predominantly OH, OCH_3, O-sugar at the 5 and 7 positions in ring A or at 4′, 3′, 5′ positions in ring B. Further variations are C-glycosidation, C-alkylations, dimerization, and polymerization. Because of the structural varieties a typical pharmacological response of all flavonoids cannot be expected. Among the pharmacological properties reported for individual or groups of flavonoids are cardiovascular, antiviral, antiphlogistic, spasmolytic, and hepatoprotective activities (for review, see SPILKOVA and HUBIK 1988). In the following, only a few of the numerous reports concerning the antihypertensive activities will be mentioned briefly.

CHOU and LIAO (1982) isolated the flavonoids from *Melastoma candidum* f. *albiflorum* (Melastomaceae) and found hypotensive effects for kaempferol, afzelin, tilirosid, astragalin, kaempferol-3-0(2″,6″-*O*-di-*p*-cumaryl-)-β-D-glacto-pyranoside. The flavone icariin has been isolated from *Epimedium brevicornum* (Berberidaceae), which is used in Chinese folk medicine for treatment of arterial disorders and hypertension (YANG et al. 1980). Icariin has also been isolated from *Epimedium koreanum* (Berberidaceae) and proved effectively hypotensive in test rats (LIU et al. 1980). Luteolin was isolated as an hypotensive compound (WEI et al. 1980) from the seed coat of *Arachis hypogaea* (Fabaceae). Astragalin (see also CHOU and LIAO 1982) and isoquercitrin (FUNAYAMA and HIKINO 1979) are the hypotensive compounds from the leaves of *Diospyros kaki* (Ebenaceae). Vitexin from the flowers of *Ochrocarpus longifolius* (Hypericaceae) and *Arnebia hispissima* (Boraginaceae) is strongly hypotensive (administrated i.v.) in guinea pigs and rabbits. This effect is claimed to arise from the ability to block the vegetative ganglia (PRABHAKAR et al. 1981).

In a series of papers (NOMURA and FUKAI 1980; NOMURA et al. 1981, 1982, 1983) (FUKAI et al. 1985) the chemistry of the root barks of different *Morus* species was studied and the isolated compounds were listed for their hypotensive action. Among the compounds tested, kuwanon G (NOMURA and FUKAI 1980), a flavone, containing a condensed dihydrochalcone partial structure, produces significant hypotension in the rabbit (1 mg/kg, i.v.); sanggenon (NOMURA et al. 1981), with a similar structure, is equally effective; intravenous injection of mulberrofuran C (1 mg/kg) (NOMURA et al. 1982), a 2-arylbenzofuran derivative, produces significant hypotension (37 mmHg fall) in a rabbit (male, 3.3 kg) anestetized with pentobarbital sodium; kuwanon M (NOMURA et al. 1983) has a hypotensive effect in SHR (2 mg/kg, i.v.); a single intravenous injection of mulberrofuran F and G (both 1.1 mg/kg) causes a marked depressor effect in rabbits (26 and 16 mmHg, respectively) (FUKAI et al. 1985).

The peels of the fruits from various citrus and other *Rutaceous* species are rich sources for flavonoids. MATSUBARA et al. (1983, 1984, 1985) and KUMAMOTO et al. (1986) tested extracts and individual compounds of these peels and found many flavonoids that lower blood pressure when injected (~10 mg/kg, i.v.) into SHR. Other hypotensive compounds from *Citrus hassaku* and *Citrus sinensis* (orange) are phenylpropanoid glycosides (SAWABE et al. 1986).

Synthesis and antihypertensive activity of (3-phenyl-flavonoxy) propanolamines without β-adrenoceptor antagonism was described by WU et al. (1987).

The most active compound of the series (see *22*) lowers blood pressure at a dose of 8 mg/kg, p.o., in SHR. The effects are of long duration when tested at doses higher than the minimally active ones. No indication of cumulative effects is observed after its application orally for 18 consecutive days. Pharmacodynamic evaluation in rats fails to show any α-adrenergic blocking activity. The possibility exists that the antihypertensive activity of these flavonoid derivatives is related to modulation of sympathetic function by reducing noradrenergic neurotransmitter stores available for release during neuronal depolarization.

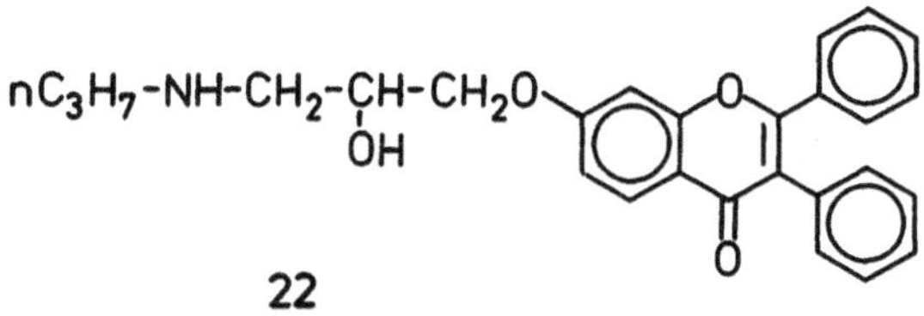

22

A semisynthetic derivative of rutoside (troxerutin, tri- and tetraethylrutoside) was clinically tested (3 g daily orally for 1 month) in 20 people with moderate hypertension (GUÉGUEN-DUCHESNE et al. 1987). After this period, a significant decrease in whole blood viscosity was observed, with a decrease in fibrinogen, and rouleaux formation visualized by scanning electron microscopy. The authors conclude that troxerutine therapy may be of value in the hyperviscosity situations which may accompany hypertension.

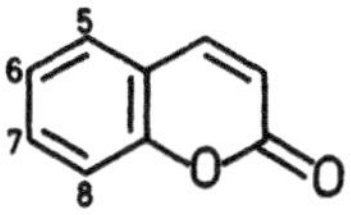

23

4 Coumarins

Coumarins (see *23*) are benzopyrane derivatives biogenetically derived by lactonization of *o*-hydroxy cinnamic acid. The aromatic ring may be substituted in different positions. The toxicity of coumarine varies from animal species to animal species; dogs tolerate at the most 10 mg over a short period; rats tolerate daily doses (50 to 100 mg/kg body weight, orally) throughout a lifetime without impairments. It requires further research to ascertain whether the use of small amounts of coumarin by humans is indeed harmful (LINDNER 1979).

4.1 Scoparone

Scoparone (6,7 dimethoxy-coumarin) has been isolated from different plant species, e.g., *Artemisia scoparia* and *Fagara macrophylla.* A strong hypotensive activity has been demonstrated in anesthetized normotonic animals (cats, dogs, rats) as well as with hypertonic dogs. The activity is dose dependent and can be observed immediately after application (i.v. or duodenal). Scoparone (10 mg/kg) causes a better and longer depression (58%, 160 min) than methyldopa (12%, 120 min). LD_{50} values (mg/kg) are as follows: rat 292 (p.o.), 190 (i.p.); mouse 280 (p.o.), 225 (i.p.). Scoparone causes a peripheral vasodilation, shows spasmolytic and relaxing activity for smooth muscle, and has weak sedative and anticonvulsant activity. Other coumarins tested were less potent (see BAUMGARTH 1980, and literature cited therein).

4.2 Scopoletin

OJEWOLE and ADESINA (1983) studied the mechanism of the hypotensive effect of scopoletin isolated from the fruit of *Tetrapleura tetraptera*. They mention that scopoletin probably produces hypotension in laboratory animals through (a) its smooth muscle relaxant activity, by which means it presumably dilates blood vessels, and (b) by acting as a nonspecific spasmolytic agent (like papaverine).

4.3 Osthole

When testing over 1500 plants including Japanese and Chinese herbal medicines for calcium-blocking activity, *Cnidii monnieri* was found to be the most effective in the initial screening test. Its active principle was osthole (7-methoxy-8-dimethylallyl-coumarin) (YAMAHARA et al. 1985).

4.4 Obtusoside

Coumarins isolated from *Haplophyllum* species all exhibit spasmolytic and hypotensive activities. Obtusoside was the most potent although its hypotensive effect did not last as long as that of other compounds (AMINOV and VAKHABOV 1985).

4.5 4-(2-Benzo(b)furanyl)coumarins

HAMMANTGAD et al. (1986) synthesized several 4-(2-benzo(b)furanyl)coumarins and tested them for biological activity. One (see *24*) had antiinflammatory, analgesic, and hypotensive activities.

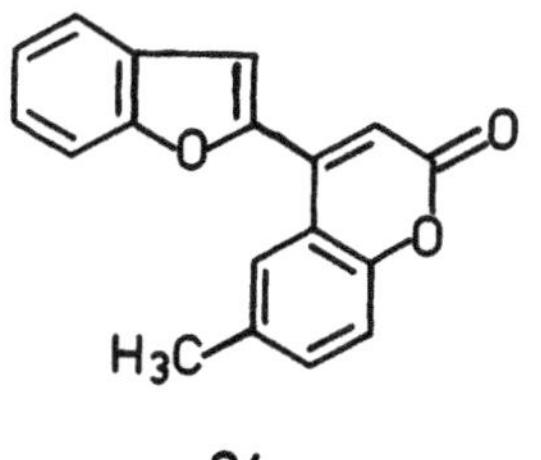

24

5 Lignans and Tannins

Lignans consist of two phenylpropane units linked by a C-C bond between the carbon atoms 2 and 2′ of the propanoid side chain. The best known lignans are those from *Podophyllum peltatum* which have antimitotic activity and are used in cancer treatment.

5.1 Pinoresinol Diglucoside

Tu-Chung (*Eucommia ulmoides*) extract has long been known as a tonic for old people. Oral administration of Tu-Chung bark tea or wine to hypertensive patients leads to improvement after 2–4 months in 93.6% of 62 cases. (SIH et al. 1976). Several investigators have confirmed the hypotensive action of aqueous and ethanol extracts of Tu-Chung in dogs, cats, rabbits, rats, guinea pigs (e.g., KIN and TING 1956). SIH et al. (1976) identified and synthesized pinoresinol di-β-D-glucoside (see *25*) as the major antihypertensive principle.

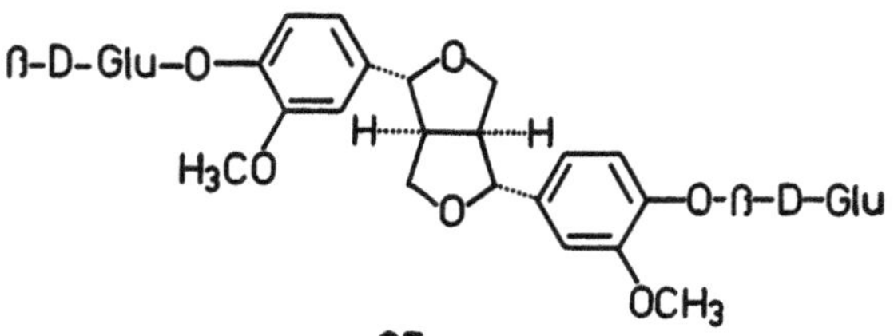

25

5.2 Lignans from Arctium lappa

Hot aqueous extracts of more than 150 Chinese herbal medicines were tested by ICHIKAWA et al. (1986) for their Ca^{2+} antagonist activity using the taenia coli of guinea pigs. Potent activity existed in the extracts of the fruits of *Arctium lappa* (Compositae; Japanese name: gobushi). By fractioning the extract it was found that this activity stemmed from those fractions containing lignans. The respective lignans were isolated, and their Ca^{2+} antagonist activity, and antihypertensive effects on SHR were reported alone with those of related compounds. The assay results demonstrate that of 33 lignans tested, 17 had significant inhibitory potency. Butanolides (see *26*) usually have stronger than *bis*-tetrahydrofuranes

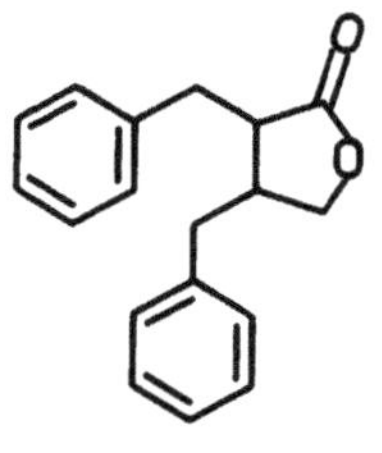

26

such as stegans (see *27*). The tetrahydrofurans (see *28*) and aryltetranaphthalenes (see *29*) had no significant activity. The most potent substance in the test system was trachelogenin (see *30*), a typical butanolid. A wide range of substituents on the aromatic rings (hydroxy, methoxy, or methylendioxy group) did not modify the measured inhibitory potencies, except for glucosides which cause large losses of activity in all types. Trachelogenin (*30*), having a high Ca^{2+} antagonist activity, is also highly potent in SHR. It has a relatively long-lasting antihypertensive effect.

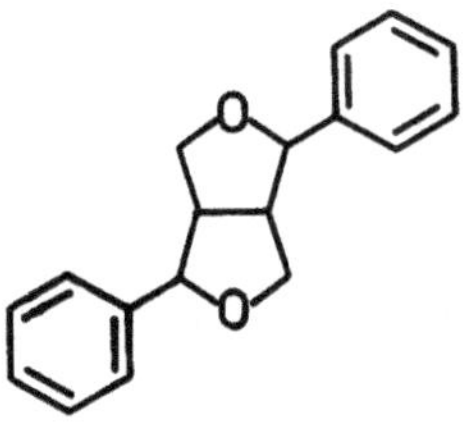

27

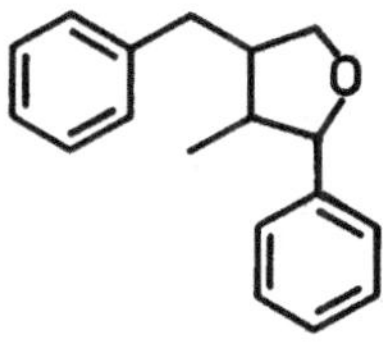

28

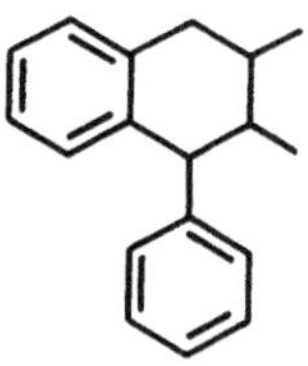

29

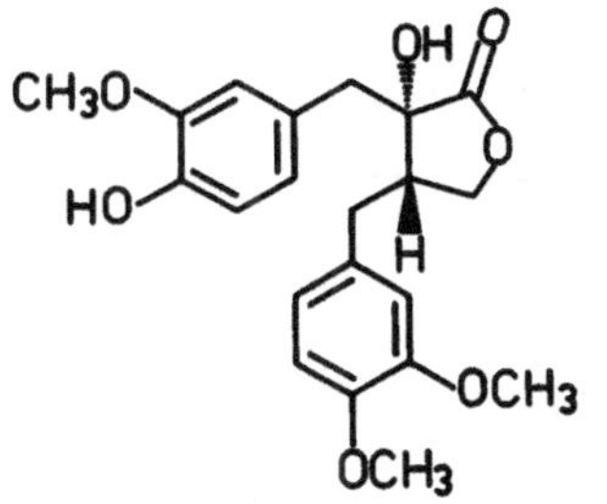

30

5.3 Bis-tetrahydrofurans (= 3,7-dioxabicyclo (3.3.0)-octane)

A Japanese patent (NISHIBE and NARITA 1986) describes hypotensive pharmaceuticals containing substituted *bis*-tetrahydrofurans (see *31*).

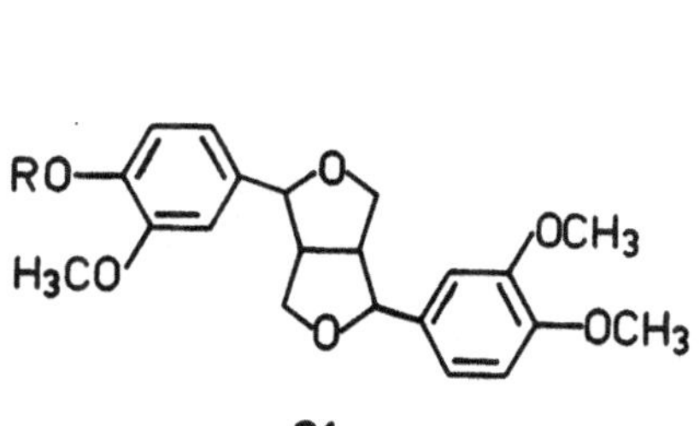

31

5.4 Tannins

An aqueous extract of *Acacia catechu*, a plant known to contain a high quantity of tannins, produces a dose-dependent decrease in blood pressure in both anesthetized dogs and rats. From pharmacological antagonist studies it was concluded that the action is probably bradykinin-related, resulting from vasodilatation (SHAM et al. 1984).

Hot water-methanol (50:50) extracts of different plants considered to have a hypotensive effect were tested for inhibitory effects on hog kidney ACE (INOKUCHI et al. 1984). Of 65 samples tested, 14 showed reproducible inhibition in the preliminary screening. The most potent fractions of *Arecae semen*, *Ephedrae herba*, *Epimedii herba*, *Polygoni avicularis herba*, *Potentillae herba*, and *Rhei rhizoma* show more than 90% inhibition at a concentration of 20 μg/ml. In two subsequent papers the authors tested isolated tannin samples (INOKUCHI et al. 1985) and a purified extract of *Areca catechu* that contains a tannin fraction (INOKUCHI et al. 1986). The tannin fraction (Areca II-5-C) showed the most potent ACE inhibitory activity in vitro. Oral administration of Areca II-5-C to SHR produces a lasting, dose-related, antihypertensive effect, and the responses obtained with doses of 100 and 200 mg/kg are comparable to those of captopril at doses of 30 and 100 mg/kg.

6 Terpenoids

6.1 Oleuropein from Olea europea

MAZET (1938) described treatment with olive extract of 38 patients suffering from hypertension. Eight did not respond to the treatment while the rest showed a lowering of both systolic and diastolic blood pressure. PETKOV and MANOLOV (1972) determined oleuropein (see *32*) as an active principle. Pure oleuropein

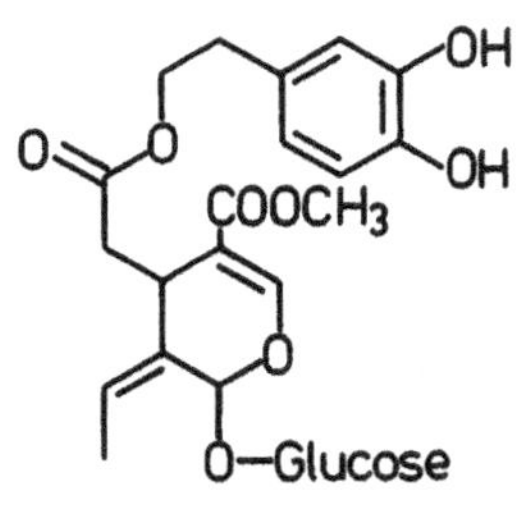

32

reduces blood pressure in dogs with induced hypertension (10–30 mg/kg, i.v.) and in anesthetized cats. They suggest that the effect is due to both central and peripheral actions. WEBER (1983), however, points out that the glycoside is unstable and that alcoholic and water extracts do not contain any intact glycoside. A reexamination of *Olea europea* for hypotensive activities should also take lignans (Sect. 5) into consideration (CHIBA et al. 1979).

6.2 Sesquiterpenes

Sesquiterpenes from *Arnica montana*, dihydrohelenalinacetat and helenalinacetat, were reported as hypotensive agents (LIST and FRIEBEL 1974). However, as these substances have severe toxic side effects, *Arnica* is not recommended for internal use.

The essential oil from *Nardostachys jatamansii* (Valerianaceae) and one of its main products, valeranone (= jatamansone), causes a pronounced hypotension in dogs (0.1–1.0 mg/kg of the oil, i.v.) for several hours (ARRORA et al. 1958) and in humans (2.5–10 mg/day valeranone) (ARRORA and ARRORA 1964).

6.3 Diterpenes from Ericaceous plants

Diterpenoids from *Ericaceous* plants have been described repeatedly as antihypertensive agents (e.g. TRUNZLER 1970; Von KÜRTEN et al. 1971; HUANYUAN et al. 1981). However, these compounds must be classified into the group of highly toxic agents because of their extremely high cardiotoxicity to mammals. The action may be due to a specific increase in membrane permeability to sodium ion. The acute toxicity correlates exactly with the cardiotonic toxicity (MAGER et al. 1981).

6.4 Forskolin

Forskolin (see *33*) is a diterpene derivative isolated from the Indian plant *Coleus forskohli*. Forskolin lowers blood pressure in dogs and cats and also in SHR and renal hypertensive rats (LINDNER et al. 1978).

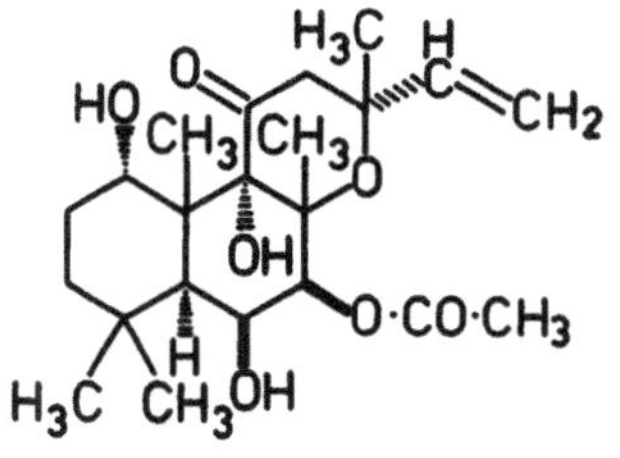

33

The cardiovascular effects of forskolin seem to be mediated by a direct stimulatory action on the catalytic unit of sarcolemmal adenylate cyclase.

It has been shown that forskolin is a potent and powerful activator of human myocardial adenylate cyclase and produced maximal effects that were 4.8-fold (normally functioning left ventricle) and 6.1-fold (failing left ventricle) greater than isoproterenol. Forskolin is a potent positive inotrope in failing human myocardium, producing a stimulation of contraction that is similar to isoproterenol (BRISTOW et al. 1984).

In view of the rapid development of tolerance toward β_1-receptor stimulation, forskolin, with its receptor-independent mechanism of action, may be advantageous for the treatment of severe heart failure. Application of forskolin in congestive heart failure appears to be safe and may represent a new therapeutic approach particularly for long-term treatment to prevent development of β-receptor down-regulation (BAUMANN et al. 1987).

7 Various Compounds from Lower Plants and Microorganisms

Microorganisms have been and still are largely looked to as a source of antibiotic and antitumor compounds. The richness and variability in their natural products have been used to a lesser extent for other biological activities.

7.1 Extracts and Compounds from Actinomycetales

Different ACE inhibitors have been isolated from Actinomycetales. An antihypertensive peptide of molecular weight 2200 is manufactured by fermentation of the *Streptomyces* strain 1647-P2 (Fujirebio inc. 1983). An amino acid with a molecular formula $C_{11}H_{23}N_5O_7$ was isolated from the culture filtrate of *Streptomyces* ATCC 36069. The compound produces a dose-related inhibition of the pressor response to angiotensin I in rats. It also inhibits ACE (HUANG 1984). SINGH et al. (1984) isolated a mixture of muramoyl derivatives from *Nocardia orientalis*. The mixture as well as three of the identified pure compounds are hypotensive and possess ACE inhibitory activity.

Foroxymithine, a piperazindion derivative (see *34*), was isolated from *Streptomyces zaomyceticus* MG 325-CF7 (UMEZAWA et al. 1985) and from *S. nitrosporeus* (NAGANAWA et al. 1985). It inhibits ACE with an IC_{50} value of 7 μg/ml. The inhibitory effect is completely abolished by $ZnCl_2$. It reduces blood pressure in hypertensive rats. Further ACE inhibitors were isolated from *Actinomyces* 937 ZE-1 (FUJIREBICO INC. 1983), from *Actinomadura* species (KIDO et al. 1984; KOGUCHI et al. 1986), and from *Micromonospora halophytica* (KASE et al. 1987). The two compounds from the last species were oligopeptides containing (*R*)-1-amino-2-(4-hydroxyphenyl)ethylphosphonic acid. A novel anti-hypertensive substance (see *35*) was manufactured by cultivation of *Streptomyces pactum* S 48727 (MATSUMOTO et al. 1986).

7.2 Lipopolysaccharide from Pasteurella multocida

Pasteurella multocida lipopolysaccharides (LPSs) reduce arterial blood pressure and heart rate in rats; this decrease begins 3–5 min after i.v. injection, reaches a peak within 30–50 min, and reverts to basal values within 2–3 h depending on the dose (0.3–1.2 mg/kg). LPS treatment changes neither phenylephrine nor angiotensin II pressor responses and reflex bradycardia.

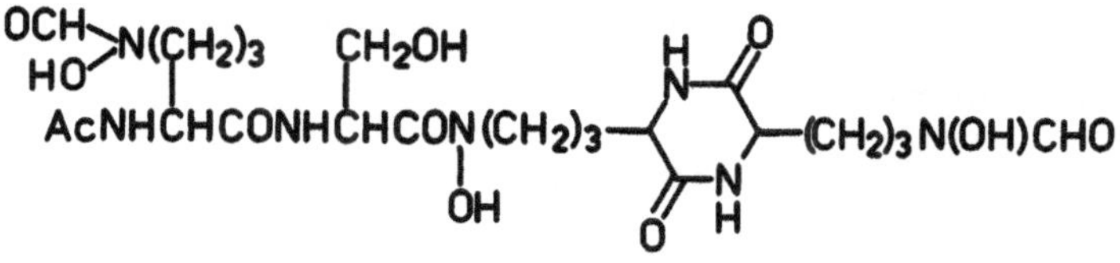

34

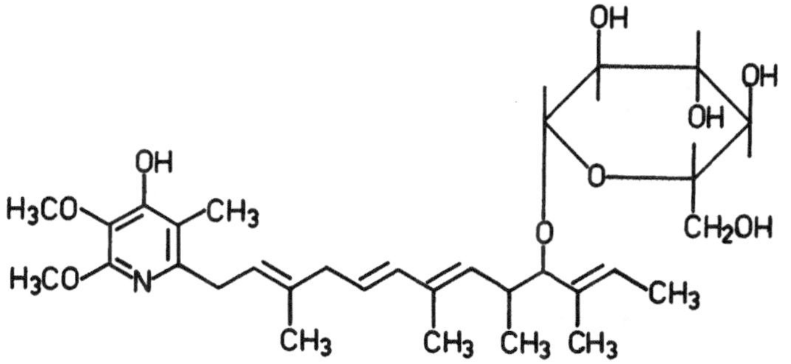

35

7.3 Extracts of Fungi

An aqueous extract of *Pleurotus sajor-caju* has a hypotensive effect in rats. Intravenous infusion of the extract into rats causes a decrease of the mean systemic blood pressure in a dose-dependent manner (TAM et al. 1986). The culture medium of *Fomes japonicus* (reishi fungus) was pulverized and treated with a mixture containing cellulase, protease, and glycosidase. The treated material was extracted with hot water. The extract contains a number of physiologically active compounds, including hypotensive compounds, and is used as a herb medicine and a health drink base (NAGAOKA 1985).

7.4 Extracts and Compounds from Algae

A glycoprotein has been isolated from *Chlorella* cell walls which on administration (5 mg/kg, i.p.) to hypertensive rats reduces blood pressure from 185 to 150 mmHg (DOI et al. 1983). Ethanol-treated *Euglena* cells are a highly digestable, protein- and amino acid-rich food material having hypotensive and anticholesterol activities (KITAOKA and KURAGANO 1985).

The extract of a commercial preparation of "nekombu" the basal parts of the blades of a laminariaceous algae has been fractionated and its hypotensive activity measured in urethane-anesthetized rats by i.v. administration. Two of the commercial preparations contain fairly large quantities of histamine (0.04% and 0.11%) (FUNAYAMA and HIKINO 1981b). GREGSON et al. (1979) isolated prostaglandin E_2 as the active principle from the red alga *Gracilaria lichenoides*.

8 Extracts and Compounds from Animals

8.1 Snake Venoms

In a project aimed at the discovery of new hypotensive peptides from snake venoms that are not related to ACE, 9 out of 66 filtered snake venoms showed an immediate hypotensive effect in normotensive rats. Five were venoms from viperids, 3 from elapids, and 1 from a crotalid (*Crotalus atrox*). A decapeptide of *C. atrox* shows hypotensive effects in SHR. The ACE-inhibiting effect of the decapeptide is secondary (POLITI et al. 1985). The major *N*-benzoyl-L-arginine Ethylesster hydrolase from the venom of *Heloderma horridum* (Mexican beaded lizard) was purified and characterized (ALAGON et al. 1986). Its activity vs. peptide amide substrates and human high-molecular-weight kininogen suggests a similarity to the family of kallikreins. Injection of the enzyme (2–16 μg/kg) into anesthetized rabbits leads to a rapid, dose-dependent, transient decrease of the arterial blood pressure.

8.2 Polypeptides from Sea Anemones

Extraction of *Anemonia sulcata* with water or an aqueous organic solvent and purification of the extract yield two peptides (molecular weight 3000–5000) that have marked antihypertensive activity with no neuro- or cardio-toxicity. Intravenous injection of 1 μg/kg of the peptides into cats or dogs decreases arterial blood pressure by 6% and 52%, respectively.

8.3 Lysophosphatidyl Choline from Cervus elaphus L. var. xanthophygus

The unossified horn of *Cervus elaphus* L. var. *xanthophygus*, called "Rokujo", has been used in Chinese medicine. By the use of SHR as a screening system, two hypotensive compounds were isolated from an alcohol extract (TSUJIBO et al. 1987). One was identified as lysophosphatidyl choline (LPC). Eleven LPCs with $C_{10:0}$ to $C_{20:0}$ fatty acids were studied for their antihypertensive effect. All except for those with $C_{10:0}$ and $C_{20:0}$ are active. In particular, $C_{14:0}$ and $C_{16:0}$ LPC show rather potent activity. On the other hand, of six LPCs with unsaturated fatty acids, only $C_{16:1}$ (3 mg/kg) shows any hypotensive effect.

9 Various Plants from Which an Active Principle Has Not Yet Been Unambiguously Identified

9.1 Crataegus species

Crataegus preparations are largely used in minor forms of coronary heart disease, minor forms of heart failure, and cardiac arrhythmia (AMMON and HÄNDEL 1981 a–c). The effect of various *Crataegus* preparations and constituents, especially flavonoids, oligomeric procyanidins, and saponins, on blood pressure in experimental animals was reviewed by AMMON and HÄNDEL (1981b). Intravenous administration of alcoholic extracts normally leads to a decrease of blood pressure in a range of 10–60 mmHg. The duration of this effect, when recorded in the original literature, is only a few minutes. If flavan polymers and oligomeric procyanidins (in a range of 1–5 mg/kg) and high doses of total saponins (50–100 mg) are administered, a decrease in blood pressure is observed for 1–4 h.

Extracts (made with glycerol-ethanol) of different plant parts of *C. oxyacantha* given orally at 125 or 25 mg dry matter/kg produce bradycardia in normal rats, lower arterial pressure in normal and in hypertensive rats, and protect rats against aconitine-, $BaCl_2$-, and chloroform-adrenalin-induced cardiac arrhythmias (OCCHIUTO et al. 1986).

In a clinical test over 6 weeks with a *Crataegus* preparation (Crataegutt) containing 30 mg of an extract of *Crataegus monogyna* and *Crataegus oxyacantha*, a slight reduction of systolic (-4.5 mmHg) and diastolic (-1.9 mmHg) blood pressure was observed (IWAMOTO et al. 1981).

9.2 European Mistletoe

Extracts of European mistletoe (*Viscum album*) are contained in about 20 medical preparations which are used in the Federal Republic of Germany as regulators of blood pressure. The indication can be attributed to observations by GAULTHIER and CHEVALIER (1907) who noted a blood pressure reduction when mistletoe extracts were injected intravenously. BIJLSMAN (1927) ascribed the blood pressure-reducing effect to the dilatation of the coronary and peripheral vessels. As mistletoe extracts show a high toxicity when parenterally administered, investigators have often tried to separate the toxic principle of the mistletoe from the hypotensive principle (for review, see LUTHER and BECKER 1987).

Acetylcholine, histamine, and α-aminobutyric acid have been claimed to be the active principles; however, their concentrations are too small to explain the observed lowering of the blood pressure. In the meantime, it is known that the toxic component, viscotoxin, leads to a marked blood pressure decrease when injected i.v. The present clinical research data (PORA et al. 1957) and pharmacological tests (LUTOMSKI 1985) mention hypotensive effectiveness even when given orally; however, more tests are necessary. So far, no substance group or single substance has been confirmed in the mistletoe which can account for a hypotensive effect with oral administration.

The commission of the German Federal Drug Administration stated in 1984: "The blood pressure lowering effects of mistletoe and the therapeutic effectiveness in mild forms of hypertension require an examination."

9.3 Garlic

Fresh garlic and various preparations and combinations with other plant extracts are used as folk remedies for various heart and arteriosclerotic diseases including hypertension. From experimental data there is good evidence that fresh garlic or oily extracts lower serum cholesterol and triglyceride values in test animals and also in humans (for review, see LUTOMSKI 1980; BECKER 1985). The antihypertensive activity is less well documented. PETKOV (1979) related hypotensive activity to vascular smooth muscle effects. No active ingredient causing these effects has as yet been isolated from garlic.

9.4 Further Plants Used in Folk Medicine to Treat Hypertension

Numerous other plants have been reported from the literature to have hypotensive effects. PETKOV (1979) in his review lists more than 50 different species. Fourteen other plants not mentioned in the present review are listed by VILLAR et al. (1986). In a phytochemical and biological screening of Saudi medicinal plants, 12 from 20 tested for hypotensive activity in normotensive rabbits were active (MOSSA et al. 1983). The high positive response (60%) may be partially due to the content of flavonoids, which are ubiquitous in green plants. RIBEIRO et al. (1986) tested 32 popular medicinal plants for their proposed diuretic and/or antihypertensive properties in conscious, restrained rats. Besides *Allium cepa* bulbs and *Olea europea* leaves described above, *Hedychium coronarium* leaf blades are also active. Extracts of *Sambucus ebulus* show a short hypotensive effect and are diuretic (PETKOV et al. 1979; PETKOV and MARKOVSKA 1981). The active principle has not been isolated. VIDRIO et al. (1982) found a blood pressure-lowering effect of relatively low doses of lyophilized ethanol extracts of *Cecropia obtusifolia* (Moraceae). It is interesting in view of its delayed onset and long duration. Extracts of *Sideritis mugronensis* (Lamiaceae) show hypotensive effects in rats (ALCAREZ et al. 1982). *Arachis hypogea* (peanut) pods are used in the form of a decoction as a popular remedy against hypertension. In pharmacological experiments, dose-dependent hypotensive activity has been demonstrated in rats while guinea pigs and rabbits provided inconsistent results (CAPASSO 1983). Hypotensive components from green tea are reviewed by IMURA (1985). Four plants, *Amelanchier ovalis*, *Prunus spinosa*, *Juniperus communis* and *Urtica dioica*, used to treat hypertension show a lowering of arterial blood pressure in rats (25 mg/kg, i.v.) of 30%, 27%, 22%, and 32%, respectively (LASHERAS et al. 1986).

In China, an aqueous extract of *Ilex pubescens* is available for parenteral administration and is used for the treatment of cardiovascular diseases. Among its several pharmacological actions, it is known to be hypotensive. YANG and PANG (1986) tested its direct vasorelaxing effect. In rats, the extract produces two consecutive hypotensive responses. The early response does not involve the adrenergic, cholinergic, histaminergic, prostaglandinergic, or bradykinergic systems. The second response is abolished by antihistamines or repeated injection of the extract (tachyphylaxis). In dogs, only the late response is seen, and it is blocked by antihistamines. It seems that when given intravenously, *Ilex pubescens* extract releases histamine.

A methanol extract of *Olax gambecola* produces a dose-dependent reduction in blood pressure in anesthetized normotensive rats and SHR (PARRY et al. 1986). There are marked similarities between the acetylcholine- and *Olax*-induced depressor responses.

Summary

This review shows that many plants have a presumed antihypertensive activity. Pharmacological data are still scarce and in many cases superficial. In most cases toxicological data are missing. Their use in folk medicine is by oral intake of water extracts (tea) or alcoholic extracts, whereas pharmacological data, if available, are mostly from parenteral application. When an active substance has been found in a natural organism, it should be applied in pure form or the respective extract should be standardized for this ingredient. Otherwise, there is a high risk that the patient will be given an ineffective or toxic drug. The analysis of natural sources for antihypertensive activities still remains an interesting task for research. It should be kept in mind that *Rauwolfia* alkaloids, for some time the most prominent antihypertensive agents, and forskolin, an interesting pharmacological tool, are natural substances. The relatively high recent rate of patents acquired on naturally occurring hypotensive substances suggests that they may become the future drugs for treating hypertensions.

References

Achenbach H, Raffelsberger B, Addae-Mensah I (1982) Alkaloide in Tabernaemontana-Arten. VIII. Tabernulosin und 12-Demethoxytabernulosin, zwei neue Alkaloide vom Picrinin-Typ aus Tabernaemontana glandulosa. Liebigs Ann Chem 830–841

Alagon A, Possani LD, Smart J, Schleuning WD (1986) Helodermatine, a kallikrein-like, hypotensive enzyme from the venom of Heloderma horridum horridum (Mexican beaded lizard). J Exp Med 164:1835–1845

Alcarez MJ, Esplugues J, Villar A (1982) Acivité pharmacodynamique de Sideritis mugronensis. II. Action sur la pression artérielle. Etude sur organe isolé. Plant Med Phytother 16:147–156

Altavilla D, Chisari M, Foca A, Mastroeni P, Caputi AP (1984) Hypotensive effect of Pasteurella multocida lipopolysaccharide in conscious rats. IRCS Med Sci 12:542–543

Aminov SD, Vakhabov AA (1985) Pharmacology of some coumarins isolated from the plant Haplophyllum (in Russian). Dokl Akad Nauk SSSR 44–45 [referred to in CA (1986) 105:122600g]

Ammon HPT, Händel M (1981a) Crataegus, Toxicologie und Pharmakologie. I. Toxicität. Planta Med 43:105–120

Ammon HPT, Händel M (1981b) Crataegus, Toxicologie und Pharmakologie. II. Pharmakodynamik. Planta Med 43:209–239

Ammon HPT, Händel M (1981c) Crataegus, Toxicologie und Pharmakologie. III. Pharmakodynamik und Pharmakokinetik. Planta Med 43:313–322

Arrora RB, Arrora CK (1964) Hypotensive and tranquilizing activity of jatamansone (valeranone), a sesquiterpene from Nardostachys jatamansi. 2nd International Pharmacological Meeting, Prague [referred to in CA (1965) 62:2151]

Arrora RB, Singh KP, Das PK, Mistry PN (1958) Prolonged hypotensive effect of the essential oil of Nardostachys jatamansi. Arch Int Pharmacodyn Ther 113:367–376

Banning JW, Salman KN, Patil PN (1982) A pharmacological study of two bisbenzylisoquinoline alkaloids, thalistyline and obamegine. J Nat Prod 45:168–177

Baumann G, Ningel K, Sattelberger U, Permanetter B, Busch U, Felix S (1987) Cardiovascular effects of forskolin (HL-32) in patients with idiopathic congestive cardiomyopathy—a comparative study with dobutamine and sodium nitroprusside. Eur J Physiol 400 (Suppl 1):R16

Baumgarth M (1980) Neue pharmakologisch interessante Naturstoffe. Planta Med 39:327–335

Becker H (1985) Knoblauch-nur Gewürz oder auch Phytopharmakon? Dtsch Apoth Z 125:1677–1688

Beress L, Doppelfeld JS, Etschenberg E, Graf E, Henschen-Edman A, Zwick J (1985) Polypeptides from sea anemones and their use as blood pressure lowering agents. Ger.Off.DE 3,324,689 (Cl. C07C103/52), 17 Jan [referred to in CA (1985) 102: 209417k]

Bijlsman UG (1927) L'action du Viscum album, gui blanc, sur les organes de la circulation sanguine. Arch Neer Sci Exactes Nat 6:142–145

Bristow MC, Ginsburg R, Strosberg A, Montgomery W, Minobe W (1984) Pharmacology and inotropic potential of forskolin in the human heart. J Clin Invest 74:212–223

Capasso F (1983) Hypotensive effect of extracts of *Arachis hypogaea* L. pods. Fitoterapia 54:273–274

Chang CC, Wang CK, Li CC, Shao JT, Pei YC, Chiang MY, Li T, Hsu TC (1964) Pharmacological studies on magnoflorine, a hypotensive principle from tu qing mu xiang. Yao Hsueh Pao 11:42–49 [referred to in CA (1964) 68:3590]

Chiba M, Okabe K, Hisada S, Shima K, Takemoto T, Nishibe S (1979) Elucidation of the structure of a new lignan glycoside from Olea europea by carbon13 nuclear magnetic resonance spectroscopy. Chem Pharm Bull (Tokyo) 27:2868–2873

Chou CJ, Liao C (1982) Phytochemical and pharmacological studies on the flower of Melastoma candidum D. Don forma albiflorum J.C. Ou kno Li Chung-kuo I Yao Yen Chiu So Yen Cin Pao Kao 69–129 [referred to in CA (1983) 98:77988j]

Dickel D, Lukas R, MacPhillamy HB (1959) A new hypotensive steroid alkaloid from Conopharyngia pachysiphon. J Am Chem Soc 81:3154–3155

Doi H, Shima M, Kawabata Y, Yorita M, Kanamori M (1983) Detection of antihypertensive glycoprotein from Chlorella (in Japanese). Kyoto-furitsu Daigaku Gakujutsu Hokuku, Nagaku 35:138–143 [referred to in CA (1984) 101:147417d]

Francesco C (1983) Hypotensive effective of extracts of Arachis hypogea L. Pods. Fitoterapia 54:273–274

Fujirebio Inc (1983) Angiotensin I containing inhibitor IS 83. Jpn Kokai Tokkyo Koho JP 58, 177, 920 (83, 177, 920) (Cl. A61K37/64) [referred to in CA (1984) 101:5549z]

Fukai T, Hano Y, Hirakura K, Nomura T, Uzawa J, Fukushima K (1985) Structures of two natural hypotensive Diels-Alder type adducts, mulberrofurans F and G, from the cultivated mulberry tree (Morus Chou KOIDZ.) Chem Pharm Bull (Tokyo) 38:3195–3204

Funayama S, Hikino H (1979) Hypotensive principles of Diospyros kaki leaves. Chem Pharm Bull (Tokyo) 27:2865–2868

Funayama S, Hikino H (1981a) Hypotensive principles from plants. Heterocycles 15:1239–1256

Funayama S, Hikino H (1981b) Hypotensive principle of Laminaria and allied sea-weeds. Planta Med 41:29–33

Funayama S, Yoshida K, Konno C, Hikino H (1980) Structure of kukoamine A, a hypotensive principle of Lycium chinense root barks. Tetrahedron Lett 21:1355–1356

Gaulthier R, Chevalier J (1907) Action physiologique du gui (Viscum album). C R Acad Sci Paris 145:941–942

Gregson RP, Marwood JP, Quinn RJ (1979) The occurrence of prostaglandins PGE_2 and PGF_2 in a plant–The red alga Gracilaria lichenoides. Tetrahedron Lett 46:4505–4506

Guéguen-Duchesne M, Durand F, LeGoff MC, Genetet B (1987) Troxerutine on the haemorheological parameters of subjects with moderate hypertension. 2 International Symposium on plant flavonoids in biology and medicine, Aug 31–Sept 3, Strasbourg

Hammantgad SS, Kulkarni MV, Patil VD, Diwan PV, Kulkarni DR (1986) Synthesis and pharmacological properties of some 4-(2-benzo(b)furanyl)coumarins. Indian J Chem [B] 25:779–781 [referred to in CA (1987) 106:196201r]

Hikino H, Shimoyama N, Kasahara Y, Takahashi M, Konno C (1982) Structures of mahuannin A and B, hypotensive principles of *Ephedra* roots. Heterocycles 19:1381–1384

Hikino H, Ogata M, Konno C (1983a) Structure of ferulylhistamine, a hypotensive principle of Ephedra roots. Planta Med 48:108–110
Hikino H, Ogata K, Konno C, Sato S (1983b) Hypotensive actions of ephedradines, macrocyclic spermine alkaloids of Ephedra roots. Planta Med 48:290–293
Huang L (1984) Antihypertensive compound 176 (Merck and Co., Inc., US). US 4,464,395 (Cl. 424-319; A61K31/195), Aug [referred to in CA (1984) 101:189720c]
Huanyuan M, Yuanshu T, Fuding N, Guofen L, Yibai F (1981) Rapid antihypertensive effect of rhomotoxin in 105 hypertension cases. Chin Med J [Engl] 94:733–736
Ichikawa K, Kinoshita T, Nishibe S, Sankawa U (1986) The Ca^{2+} antagonist activity of lignans. Chem Pharm Bull (Tokyo) 34:3514–3517
Imura K (1985) Hypotensive components in green tea. Seikatsu Eisei 29:163–172 [referred to in CA (1985) 103:128833m]
Inokuchi JI, Okabe H, Yamauchi T, Nagamatsu A (1984) Inhibitors of angiotensin-converting enzyme in crude drugs I. Chem Pharm Bull (Tokyo) 32:3615–3619
Inokuchi JI, Okabe H, Yamauchi T, Nagamatsu A, Nonaka GI, Nishioka I (1985) Inhibitors of angiotensin-converting enzyme in crude drugs II. Chem Pharm Bull (Tokyo) 33:264–269
Inokuchi JI, Okabe H, Yamauchi T, Nagamatsu A, Nonaka GI, Nishioka I (1986) Antihypertensive substance in seeds of Areca catechu L. Life Sci 38:1375–1382
Iwadare S, Shizuri Y, Sasaki K, Hirata Y (1976) Trichotomine from plants. Japan-Kokai 76 41,415 (Cl. A61K31/7011) [referred to in CA (1976) 85:25369]
Iwamoto M, Sato T, Ischizaki T (1981) Klinische Wirkung von Crataegutt[R] bei Herzerkrankungen ischämischer und/oder hypertensiver Genese. Planta Med 42:1–16
Kaczmarek F, Lutomski J, Wrocinski T (1962) Effect of vincamine, isovincamine, alkaloid, and nonalkaloid fractions of Vinca minor on blood pressure. Biul Inst Roslin Leczniczych 8:12–23 [referred to in CA (1963) 68:10634–10635]
Kase H, Kaneko M, Yamada K, Yasukawa T, Shirahata K, Sano H (1987) K-13, an inhibitor of angiotensin I-converting enzyme (ACE) from Micromonospora halophytica. J Antibiot (Tokyo) 40:450–454, 455–458
Kaken Pharmaceutical Co Ltd Jpn (1985) Pharmaceutical β-carboline derivative extraction from *Picrasma quassinoides*. Kokai Tokkyo Koho JP 60 58, 990 (85 58, 990) (Cl. C07D519/00) 05 Apr 1985 (referred to in CA (1985) 103:129042 q)
Kido Y, Hamakado T, Anno M, Miyagawa E, Motoki Y, Wakamiya T, Shibe T (1984) Isolation and characterization of 15 B 2 a new phosphorus containing inhibitor of angiotensin I-converting enzyme produced by Actinomadura sp. J Antibiot (Tokyo) 37:965–969
Kin KC, Ting KS (1956) Drugs for the treatment of hypertension. II. Toxicity and experimental therapy of Eucommia ulmoides. Acta Physiol Sinica 20:247–254 [referred to in CA (1957) 51:15788]
Kitaoka S, Kuragano T (1985) Protein-rich food materials from Euglena cells. Jpn Kokai Tokkyo Koho JP 60, 196, 157 (85, 196, 157) (Cl. A23L1/03) 4 Oct [referred to in CA (104:50127h)
Koguchi T, Yamada K, Yamato M, Okachi R, Nakayama K, Kase H (1986) K-4, a novel inhibitor of angiotensin I-converting enzyme produced by Actinomadura spiculosospora. J Antibiot (Tokyo) 39:364–371
Krayer O, Meilman E (1977) Veratrum alkaloids with antihypertensive activity. In: Gross F (ed) Antihypertensive agents. Springer, Berlin Heidelberg New York, pp 547–570 (Handbuch der experimentellen Pharmakologie, vol 3)
Kumamoto H, Matsubara Y, Iizuka Y, Okamoto K, Yokoi K (1986) Studies on physiologically active substances in citrus peel. IX. Structure and hypotensive effect of flavonoid glycosides in orange (Citrus sinensis Osbeck) peelings. Agric Biol Chem 50:781–783
Laguzza BC (1986) Ergoline derivatives (Lilly, Eli, and Co.). Eur. Pat. Appl. EP 185,491 (Cl. C07D457/02), 25 Jun [referred to in CA (1986) 105:134217w]
Lasheras B, Turillas P, Cenarruzabeita E (1986) Etude pharmacologique préliminaire de Prunus spinosa L. Amelanchier ovalis Medikus, Juniperus communis L. et Urtica dioica L. Plant Med Phytother 20:219–226
Lee JH, Park YH, Cho BH, Kim YJ, Kim JB, Kim CS, Cha YD, Kim YS (1986) The

effects of majarol on the blood pressure and heart rate in rats and isolated frog heart. Taehan Yakrihak Chapchi 22:34–44 [referred to in CA (1987) 106:95826t]
Lin BQ, Ma HS, Mou P (1980) Isolation and identification of icariin. Chung Ts'ao Yao 11:201 [referred to in CA (1981) 94:90117m]
Lindner E (1979) Toxikologie der Nahrungsmittel. Thieme, Stuttgart, p 75
Lindner E, Dohadwalla AN, Bhattacharya BK (1978) Positive inotropic and blood pressure lowering activity of a diterpene derivative isolated from Coleus forskohli: forskolin. Arzneimittelforschung 28:284–289
List PH, Friebel B (1974) Neue Inhaltsstoffe der Blüten von *Arnica montana*. Arzneimittelforsch 24:148–151
Liu BQ, Ma HS, Mou P (1980) Isolation and identification of icariin. Chung Ts'ao Yao 11–201 (referred to in CA (1981) 94:90 117 m)
Luckner M (1984) Secondary metabolism in microorganisms, plants, and animals. 2nd edn. Springer, Berlin Heidelberg New York, pp 398–403
Luther P, Becker H (1987) Die Mistel. Botanik, Lektine, medizinische Anwendung. Springer, Berlin Heidelberg New York, pp 124–126
Lutomski J (1980) Die Bedeutung von Knoblauch und Knoblauch-Präparaten in der Phytotherapie. Pharm Unserer Zeit 9:45–50
Lutomski J (1985) Die Bewertung einer hypertensiven Wirkung der Mistelpräparate des Kneipp-Heilmittelwerks. Institut für Heilpflanzenforschung, Poznan
Mager PP, Seese A, Takeya K (1981) Structure-toxicity relationships applied to grayanotoxins. Pharmazie 36:381–382
Matsubara Y, Kumamoto H, Iizuka Y, Murakami T, Okamoto K, Miyake H, Yokoi K (1983) The structure and physiological activity of flavonoid and flavonoid glycosides in four citrus fruit peels. Tannen Yuki Kago–butsu Toronkai Koen Yoshishu 26:142–149 [referred to in CA (1984) 101:12057r]
Matsubara Y, Kumamoto H, Yonemoto H, Iizuka Y, Murakami T, Okamoto K, Miyake H, Yokoi K (1984) Structure and hypotensive effect of flavonoid glycosides in citrus fruit peels (in Japanese). Kinki Diagaku Igaku Zasshi 9:61–71 [referred to in CA (1985) 103:200745d]
Matsubara Y, Kumamoto H, Iizuka Y, Murakami T, Okamoto K, Miyake H, Yokoi K (1985) Studies on physiological active substances in citrus peels. II. Structure and hypotensive effect of flavonoid glycosides in citrus unshiu peelings. Agric Biol Chem 49:909–914
Matsumoto M, Nagaoka K, Asaoka T, Mogi K, Isomae K, Nakajima T (1986) Manufacture of antibiotic Ss 48727B. Jpn Kokai Tokkyo Koho JP 61,210,093 (86, 210, 093) (Cl. C07H15/26) 18 Sept [referred to in CA (1987) 106:174677y]
Mazet M (1938) Contribution à l'étude pharmacodynamique de la feuille d'olivier. Gaz Med Fr 1:39–41
Mossa JS, Al-Yahya MA, Al-Meshal IA, Tariq M (1983) Phytochemical and biological screening of saudi medicinal plants. Part 5. Fitoterapia 54:147–152
Murano T, Tanaka F (1957) Possible roles of the central nervous system in the action of morphine on blood pressure. Jpn J Pharmacol 6:94–104 [referred to in CA (1958) 52:3158]
Naganawa H, Hamada M, Takeuchi T (1985) Foromyxithine, a new inhibitor of angiotensin-converting enzyme, produced by actinomycetes. J Antibiot (Tokyo) 38:1813–1815
Nagaoka H (1985) Production of reishi fungus extracts. Jpn Kokai Tokkyo Koho JP 60,149,528 (85, 149, 528) (Cl. A61K35-84) 7 Aug [referred to in CA (1986) 104:128205d]
Nishibe S, Narita T (1986) Pharmaceuticals containing hypotensive 3,7-dioxabicyclo (3.3.)-octane derivatives. Jpn Kokai Tokkyo Koho JP 61 12,624 (86 12,624) [referred to in CA (1986) 104:230475d]
Nishibe S, Tsukamoto H, Kinoshita H, Kitagawa S, Sakushima A (1986) Alkaloids from embryo of the seed of Nelumbo nucifera. J Nat Prod 49:547–548
Nomura T, Fukai T (1980) Kuwanon G, a new flavone derivative from the root barks of the cultivated mulberry tree (Morus alba L.). Chem Pharm Bull (Tokyo) 25:2548–2552

Nomura T, Fukai T, Hano Y, Uzawa J (1981) Structure of sanggenon C, a natural hypotensive Diels-Alder adduct from chinese crude drug "San-Bai-Pi" (Morus root barks). Heterocycles 16:2141–2148
Nomura T, Fukai T, Matsumoto J, Ohmori T (1982) Constituents of the cultivated mulberry tree. VIII. Components of root barks of Morus bombycis. Planta Med 46:28–32
Normura T, Fukai T, Hano Y, Ikuta H (1983) Kuwanon M, a new Diels-Alder adduct from the root barks of the cultivated mulberry tree (Morus Chou (Ser.) Koidz.). Heterocycles 20:585–591
Occhiuto F, Circosta C, Briguglio F, Tommasini A, de Pasquale A (1986) Comparative study on the cardiovascular activity of young shoots, leaves and flowers of Crataegus oxyacantha L. I. Electrical activity and arterial pressure in the rat. Plant Med Phytother 20:37–51
Odebiyi OO (1980) Antibacterial property of tetramethylpyrazine from the stem of Jatropha podagrica. Planta Med 38:144–146
Ojewole JAO, Adesina SK (1983) Mechanism of the hypotensive effect of scopoletin isolated from the fruit of Tetrapleura tetraptera. Planta Med 49:46–50
Ojewole JAO, Odebiyi OO (1980) Neuromuscular and cardiovascular actions of tetramethylpyrazine from the stem of Jatropha podagrica. Planta Med 38:332–338
Ojewole JAO, Odebiyi OO (1981) Mechanism of the hypotensive effect of tetramethylpyrazine, an amide alkaloid from the stem of Jatropha podagrica. Planta Med 41:281–287
Palm D, Hellenbrecht D, Quiring K (1987) Pharmakotherapie von Hypertonie, Hypotonie, obstruktiven Atemwegserkrankungen und vaskulären Kopfschmerzen. In: Forth W, Henschler D, Rummel W (eds) Allgemeine and spezielle Pharmakologie und Toxikologie, vol 1. B.I. Wissenschaftsverlag, Mannheim, pp 124–168
Parry O, Okwuasaba FK, Wkpenyoung KI, Ashra F CM (1986) Effects of Olax gambecola methanol extract on smooth muscle and rat blood pressure. J Ethnopharmacol 18:63–88
Perera P, Kanjanapothy D, Sandberg F, Verpoorte R (1985) Muscle relaxant and hypotensive activity of some Tabernaemontana alkaloids. J Ethnopharmacol 13:165–173
Petkov V (1979) Plants with hypotensive, antiatheromatous and coronarodilatating action. Am J Chin Med 7:197–236
Petkov V, Manolov P (1972) Pharmacological analysis of the iridoid oleuropin. Arzeimittelforschung 22:1476–1486
Petkov V, Manolov P. Paparlcora K (1979) Screening pharmacologique du Sambucus ebulus L. Plantes Med Phytother 13:134–138
Petkov V, Markovska V (1981) L'effet diurétique de Sambucus ebulus L. (Caprifoliacées). Plantes Med Phytother 15:172–182
Politi V, de Luca G, di Stazio G, Schinina E, Bossa F (1985) A new peptide from Crotalus atrox snake venom. Peptides [Suppl 3] 6:343–346
Pora A, Pop E, Rosca D, Rachu A (1957) Der Einfluβ der Wirtspflanze auf den Gehalt an hypotensiven und herzwirksamen Prinzipien der Mistel (Viscum album L.). Pharmazie 12:528–538
Prabhakar MC, Bano H, Kumar J, Shamsi MA, Khan MSY (1981) Pharmacological investigations on Vitexin. Planta Med 43:396–403
Quevauviller A, Foussard-Blanpin O, Sarrazin G, Bourrinat P, Nakaji Y (1969) Pharmacodynamics of the alkaloids from *Cinchona ledgeriana* leaves (in French) Ann Pharm Fr 27:397–402 [referred to in CA (1970) 72:65061b]
Rakshain KV, Mats MN (1973) Pharmacological properties of alkaloids of two species of Cynoglossum. Rast Rusur 9:418–420 [referred to in CA (1974) 80:22615h]
Ribeiro RDA, Margardia M, de Melo RF, de Barros F, Gomes C, Trolin G (1986) Acute antihypertensive effect in conscious rats, produced by some medicinal plants used in the state of Sao Paulo. J Ethnopharmacol 15:261–269
Sakai T, Iwata K, Utaka M, Takeda A (1987) A convenient synthesis of oudenone, a hypotensive compound from *Oudemansiella radicata.* Bull Chem Soc Jpn 60:1161–1162

Sawabe A, Matsubara Y, Kumamoto H, Iizuka Y, Okamoto K (1986) Structure and physiological activity of phenylpropanoid glycosides of hassaku (*Citrus hassaku* Hort.) and orange (*Citrus sinensis* Osbeck.) peels (in Japanese). Nippon Nogei Kagaku Kaishi 60:593–599 [referred to in CA (1986) 105:222728u]

Schlittler E (1977) The chemistry of antihypertensive agents. In: Gross F (ed) Antihypertensive Agents. Springer, Berlin Heidelberg New York, pp 13–86 (Handbuch der experimentellen Pharmakologie, vol 34)

Sham JSK, Chiu KW, Pang PKT (1984) Hypotensive action of *Acacia* catechu. Planta Med 172–180

Sih CJ, Ravikumar PR, Huang FC, Buckner C, Whitlock J Jr (1976) Isolation and synthesis of pinoresinol diglucoside, a major antihypertensive principle of Tu-Chung. J Am Chem Soc 98:5412–5413

Singh P, Bush K, Slusarchyk DS (1984) ACE inhibitors produced from Nocardia orientalis (Squibb E R and Sons, Inc. US). US 4,474,693 (Cl. 260-112.5R; C07C103/52), 2 Oct [referred to in CA (1984) 102:60775r]

Spilkova J, Hubik J (1988) Biologische Wirkung von Flavonoiden. Pharm Unserer Zeit 17:1–9

Sun J (1983) Novel active constituents of Ephedra sinica (in Chinese). Zhongcaoyao 14:345–346, 350 [referred to in CA (1983) 99:330]

Tam SC, Yip KP, Fung KP, Chang ST (1986) Hypotensive and renal effects of an extract of the edible mushroom Pleurotus sajor-caju. Life Sci 38:1155–1161

Tamada M, Endo K, Hikino H (1978) Maokonine, hypertensive principle of *Ephedra* roots. Planta Med 34:291–293

Tamada M, Endo K, Hikino H (1979) Structure of ephedradine B, a hypotensive principle of Ephedra roots. Heterocycles 12:783–786

Trunzler G (1970) Über eine blutdrucksenkende Substanz aus Rhododendron. Phys Med Rehabil 11:14–19

Tsujibo H, Miyake Y, Maruyama K, Inamori Y (1987) Hypotensive compounds isolated from alcohol extract of the unossified horn of Cervus elaphus L. var. xanthopygus Milne-Edwarg (Rokujo). I. Isolation of lysophosphatidyl choline as a hypotensive principle and structure activity study on related compounds. Chem Pharm Bull (Tokyo) 35:654–659

Tulyaganov TS, Ibragimov AA, Yunusov SY, Vakhabov AA, Aminov SD, Sultanov MB (1984) Nitraria komarovii alkaloids. VIII. Synthesis and pharmacological properties of nitramarine alkaloid (in Russian). Khim Farm Zh 18:1474–1476 [referred to in CA (1985) 102:128811g]

Umezawa H, Takeuchi T, Aoyagi T, Hamada M, Ogawa K, Iinuma H (1985) Physiologically active substance foroxymithine, a process and microorganisms for its use as medicament (Microbiochemical Research Foundation) Eur.Pat.Appl. EP 162,422 (Cl.C12P21/02), 27 Nov [referred to in CA (1986) 104:107913t]

Vidrio V, Garcia-Marquez F, Reyes J, Soto RM (1982) Hypotensive activity of Cecropia obtusifolia. J Pharm Sci 71:475–476

Villar A, Paya M, Terencio MC (1986) Plants with antihypertensive action. Fitoterapia 57:131–145

Von Kürten S, auf dem Keller S, Pachaly P, Zymalkowski F, Tauberger G, Moussawi M (1971) Über Inhaltsstoffe verschiedener Rhododendron-Arten und ihre Kreislaufwirkung. Arch Pharm (Weinheim) 304:753–762

Weber D (1983) Contribution à l'étude de l'action antihypertensive de la feuille d'olivier, l'oleuropeine principe actif antihypertenseur? Thesis, Faculty of Pharmacy, University of Montpellier

Wei CH, Yu SC, Kou CT, Ho HH, Mou CF (1980) Isolation and identification of the active principles of the shells of *Arachis hypogaea*. Yao Hsueh T'ung Pao 15:44 (referred to in CA (1981) 95:49 262 n)

Wu ESC, Cole TE, Davidson TA, Blosser JC, Borrelli AR, Kinsolving CR, Milgate TE, Parker RB (1987) Flavones. I. Synthesis and antihypertensive activity of (3-Phenylflavonoxy)propanol-amines without β-adrenoceptor antagonism. J Med Chem 30:788–792

Yamahara J, Miki S, Murakami H, Sawada T, Fujimura H (1985) Screening test for

calcium antagonists in natural products and the active principles of Cnidii monnieri (in Japanese). Yakugaku Zasshi 105:449–458 [referred to in CA (1985) 103:48042n]
Yang CH, Liu HK, Wu CL (1980) Chemical constituents of xinyeyinyanghuo (Epimedium brevicornum). Chung Ts'ao Yao 11:444 [referred to in CA (1981) 94: 127211r]
Yang ML, Pang PKT (1986) The vascular effects of Ilex pubescens. Planta Med 262–265
Zakirov UB, Kamilov IK (1967) Pharmacology of the alkaloid hemanthamine (in Russian). In: Kamilov IK (ed) Farmakologya alkaloidov glikozidov. Izd. Fan Uzb.SSR, Taschkent, pp 123–126 [referred to in CA (1969) 70:2215t]
Zuger O (1986) Pharmaceutical 9,10-dihydrogenated ergot alkaloid-containing compositions. Br UK Pat. Appl. GB 2,170,407 (Cl. A61K31/48) 5 Feb [referred to in CA (1987) 106:38482d]

CHAPTER 20

Stepwise Treatment of Hypertension

A. ZANCHETTI

CONTENTS

1 Philosophy of the Stepwise Approach to Antihypertensive Treatment

The dilemma whether to treat or not to treat a mild hypertensive patient is thought to be one of the most difficult issues in the management of hypertension. It is intimately connected with the equally important and difficult decisions about adding an antihypertensive drug to the nonpharmacological measures and which substance to use. Indeed, the decision to commence treatment is influenced by the knowledge of the properties and characteristics of the drugs and, on the other hand, by the multiplicity of antihypertensive agents available. These often have different mechanisms of action and pharmacological properties, and the doctor is in the embarrassing position of having to decide which drug should be prescribed first for each individual patient. Are there guidelines that we can offer about choosing the most suitable compound or about combining compounds when necessary?

There is no doubt that the most rational approach would be to match the pharmacological properties of the drug with the pathophysiological alterations of the patient. However, it must be conceded that in doing this two sets of difficulties are met, one relating to the patient, the other to the drug (ZANCHETTI 1980, 1985b).

The pathophysiological profile of the patient is complex and variable (ZANCHETTI, 1985b). Arterial pressure is regulated through a multiplicity of factors. Although technological progress has made many of these regulatory factors measurable (hemodynamic variables, cardiac performance, reflex neural control, number and sensitivity of various receptors, membrane transport, renal function, and hormonal responses), even the assessment of only a few of these factors in all or most hypertensive patients is hardly conceivable. Inferring the whole pathophysiological pattern from a single marker (e.g., renin, catecholamines, membrane markers) is arbitrary and misleading. Finally, that different pathophysiological patterns may underlie the slight rise in blood pressure in different subsets of mild hypertensive subjects is an assumption which, though attractive, is as yet unproven. If there are difficulties in profiling the pathophysiological pattern of the individual patient, there are also uncertainties in identifying all the mechanisms of action of antihypertensive drugs, the pharmacological properties of which are often multiple (ZANCHETTI, 1980, 1985b). Even the mechanism of action of long and widely used compounds such as the diuretics and β-blockers is still debated.

The practical impossibility of obtaining a satisfactory pathophysiological profile of the hypertensive patient in order to choose the most suitable drug has strengthened the trend toward formulating and using stepped-care programs. The philosophy behind the stepwise approach to the treatment of hypertension is based on the following concepts: What really matters in antihypertensive treatment is blood pressure reduction, not the means or mechanisms by which blood pressure is reduced; lowering of blood pressure should be slow and gradual, using agents likely to be efficacious with a minimum of untoward effects; therapy should be simple, starting generally with a single drug at low dose, later progressing to more complex therapeutic regimens (see WHO Expert Committee 1978).

There is some soundness in this philosophy. First, there is no proof that the benefit of antihypertensive therapy results from something other than lowering of elevated blood pressure. Second, it places due emphasis on the possible occurrence of side effects, which should be kept to a minimum. Third, implicit in the pragmatic philosophy of the stepped-care approach are the beliefs that the success of antihypertensive therapy has to be assessed by the response of the patient and that it is the balance of individual benefits and disadvantages that will influence the therapeutic regimen. In a condition such as mild to moderate hypertension, the best way of reducing blood pressure is by doing this slowly and progressively, and there is no better way to *predict* the outcome than by measuring the response (ZANCHETTI 1985b, 1987a).

Stepped-care programs, however, are often criticized as being too rigid, with guidelines that should apply to all patients while clinical practice is obviously based on an individualized approach. These two opposite aspects, i.e., the useful pragmatism versus the risk of rigidity and dogmatism, must be carefully considered when discussing traditional stepped-care programs and suggesting modifications for the current treatment of hypertension.

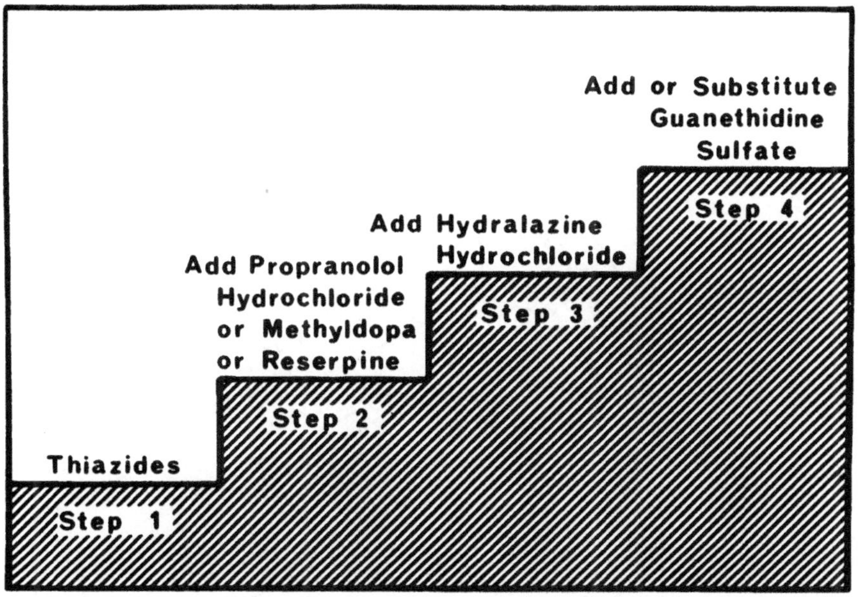

Fig. 1. Stepped-care antihypertensive program suggested by the US Joint National Committee on Detection, Evaluation, and Treatment of High Blood Pressure (1977) (by courtesy of *JAMA*)

2 Traditional Stepped-Care Programs

Figure 1 shows the first stepped-care program suggested by the US Joint National Committee on Detection, Evaluation, and Treatment of High Blood Pressure (1977). Although published in 1977 this program reflects the therapeutic habits of the 1960s and early 1970s, when undoubtedly thiazide diuretics were the best tolerated amongst the few antihypertensive compounds available. Therefore, it provides rather rigid guidelines, giving no choice for starting antihypertensive therapy other than using a thiazide and suggesting the administration of large doses of thiazides before resorting to an additional agent. The rigidity of these recommendations has probably complicated the outcome and the interpretation of most of the large trials of therapeutic intervention, which were all planned in the 1960s and 1970s.

Only 1 year after the American guidelines appeared, international experts convened by the WHO formulated more flexible recommendations (WHO Expert Committee 1978), suggesting a first choice between either a thiazide diuretic or a β-blocker. This stepped-care program is illustrated in Fig. 2, from which it can easily be appreciated that a larger number of choices and combinations were provided to the physician. These recommendations were endorsed in a memorandum from a WHO/ISH meeting in 1983 and were accepted, although as late a 1984, by the US Joint National Committee on Detection, Evaluation,

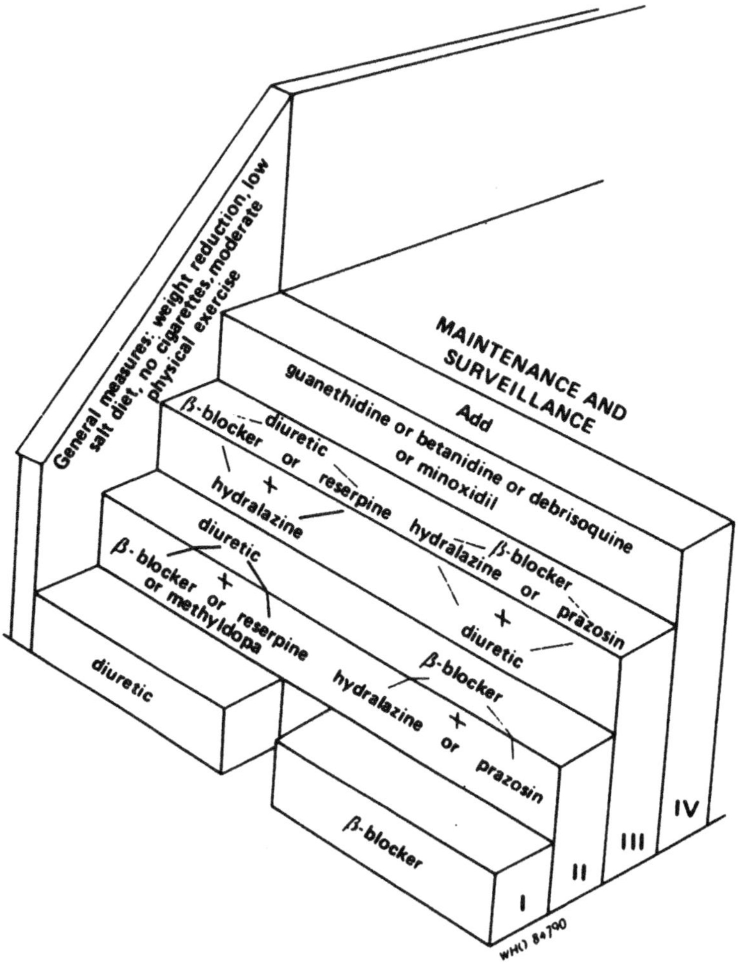

Fig. 2. Stepped-care antihypertensive program suggested by the WHO Expert Committee (1978) (by courtesy of WHO)

and Treatment of High Blood Pressure. Figures 2 and 3 show that the 1984 American guidelines are very similar to those suggested by the WHO in 1978.

The rationale for guidelines such as these is the following: (a) diuretics and β-blockers induce only a limited number of untoward effects, so that both classes of antihypertensive agents seemed to be suitable for widespread use; (b) many antihypertensive drugs (e.g., centrally active compounds, vasodilators) lead to sodium and water retention and therefore require to be combined with a diuretic; (c) traditional vasodilators, such as hydralazine, although in principle the most rational approach to a condition characterized by widespread vasoconstriction, have to be relegated to the second or, more often, third step, because

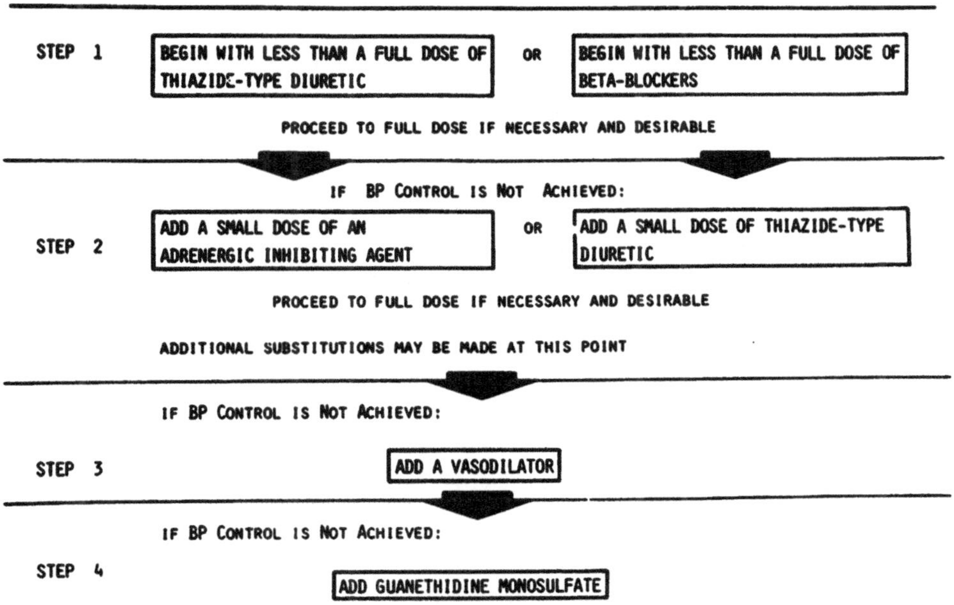

Fig. 3. Stepped-care antihypertensive program suggested by the US Joint National Committee on Detection, Evaluation, and Treatment of High Blood Pressure (1984) (by courtesy of Arch Int Med)

their sodium-retaining action and reflex sympathetic activation of the heart most often require their combination with a diuretic and a β-blocker (ZANCHETTI 1985a).

Since 1978 data have accumulated that have challenged some of these statements and weakened some of these opinions (ZANCHETTI 1985a). The opinion that diuretics and β-blockers induce only minor and infrequent untoward effects has been partly disputed by the recently published results of the Medical Research Council Working Party on Mild Hypertension (1981, 1985). As shown in Fig. 4, during the 5 years of this trial (which enrolled some 18 000 patients) about 23% of men and 13% of women had to be withdrawn from treatment with bendrofluazide, and 19% of men and 20% of women from treatment with propranolol because of untoward effects.

Awareness has been acquired not only of the success but also of the failures and limitations of current antihypertensive regimens (ZANCHETTI 1987b). In this context, concern has been expressed about the metabolic effects of diuretics and, to some extent, of β-blockers (HANSSON et al. 1984).

Finally, several new classes of antihypertensive drugs, notably the ACE inhibitors and calcium antagonists, have received extensive clinical testing in the past 10 years and cannot any longer be ignored when guidelines for antihypertensive treatment are formulated.

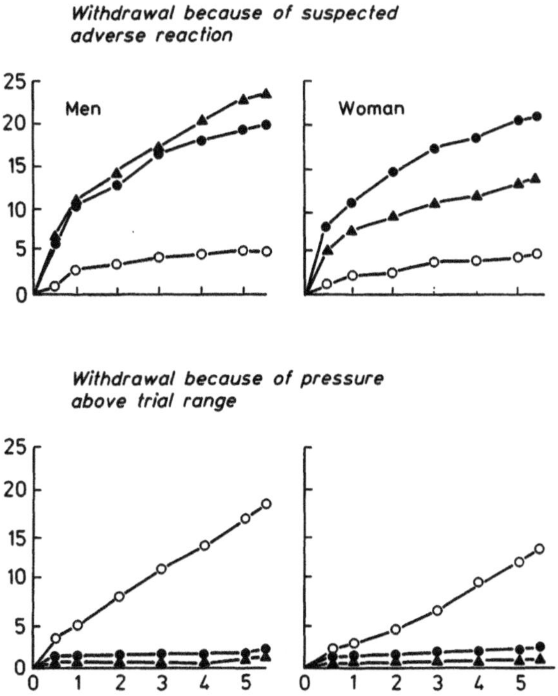

Fig. 4. Cumulative percentage withdrawals from randomized treatment over time in the study by the Medical Research Council Working Party (1985), caused by suspected adverse reactions to antihypertensive therapy (*above*) or by a rise in pressure above the mild hypertension range (*below*). *Solid circles*, propranolol; *solid triangles*, bendrofluazide; *open circles*, placebo (by courtesy of *Br Med J*)

3 Which Steps in 1988?

3.1 Has Stepwise Treatment of Hypertension Become Obsolete?

The availability of many drugs suitable for the treatment of hypertension makes it necessary to reconsider whether the guidelines first formulated in 1978 are still valid today and also poses the more radical question, whether any stepwise approach may be obsolete now and better replaced by an individualized approach. The problem should be discussed by first addressing the question whether drugs traditionally classified as first choice still qualify as such (a question essentially directed to diuretics) and then considering which of the new classes may qualify as additional choices for commencing antihypertensive treatment.

3.2 Diuretics

In the MRC trial diuretics were associated with a considerable proportion of adverse effects (Medical Research Council Working Party 1981, 1985), but it should also be recognized that the thiazide doses employed in this study were rather large. Awareness of the failures and limitations of diuretic-based antihypertensive therapy may be tempered by consideration of some findings of recent, controlled, therapeutic trials. In the patients in the MRC trial who received a rather large dose of diuretic for several years, average changes in serum cholesterol and blood glucose, through statistically significant, were on the whole small and were reversible up on the withdrawal of the medication (Medical Research Council Working Party 1981, 1986). Their impact on the patient's health is difficult to evaluate. Three major studies performed in the last decade to compare the effectiveness of diuretic-based or β-blocker-based therapy in preventing cardiovascular complications of hypertension have shown that diuretic-based treatment fares at least as well as β-blocker-based treatment (Medical Research Council Working Party, 1985; IPPPSH Collaborative Group 1985; Wilhelmsen et al. 1987). The recently completed study of the European Working Party on Hypertension in the Elderly has found that cardiovascular mortality and morbidity can be reduced by a diuretic-based treatment (Amery et al. 1985).

Finally, encouraging data for the use of diuretics were also found by further analysis of the study by the Medical Research Council Working Party (1988). As shown by Fig. 5, for similar systolic blood pressure values achieved by diuretic therapy and by placebo, stroke incidence is lower in the patients receiving a diuretic. This seems to suggest a protective effect of diuretics against stroke, additonal to the protection provided by mere lowering of blood pressure. However, Fig. 6 shows that quite different results were reported by the investigators of the Australian trial on mild hypertension (Management Committee 1982): a comparison of total terminating events occuring for the same level of diastolic blood pressure in patients receiving active treatment or placebo revealed a better outcome for the placebo patients.

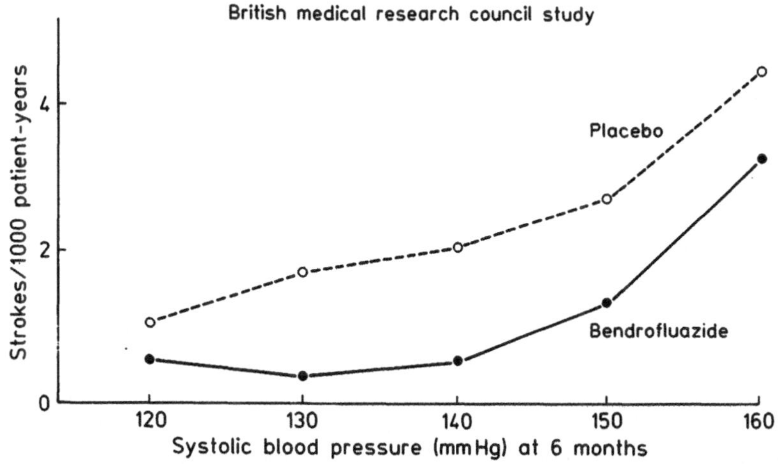

Fig. 5. Incidence of strokes in patients given placebo (*open circles*) or bendrofluazide, a diuretic (*solid circles*), according to systolic blood pressure level measured 6 months after treatment began. Redrawn from data from the study by the Medical Research Council Working Party (1988, by courtesy of *Br Med J*)

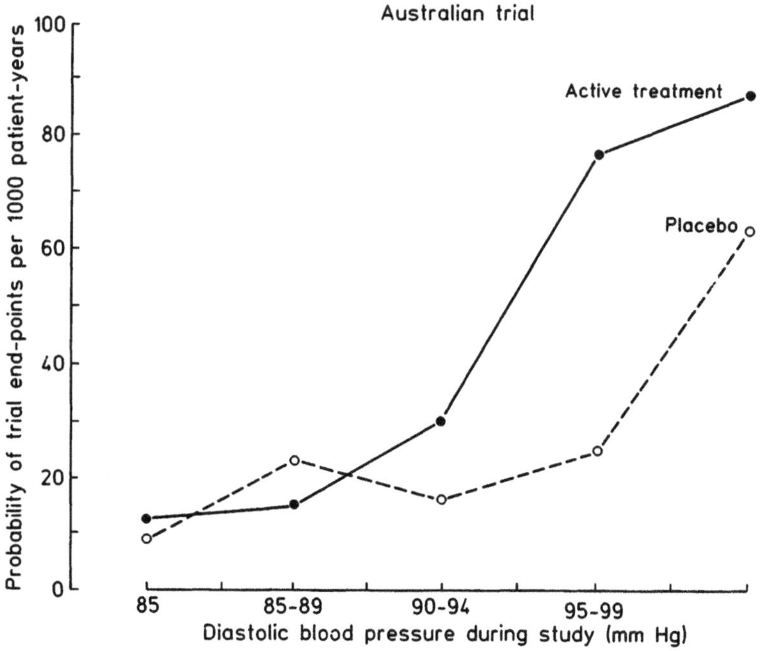

Fig. 6. Probability of the incidence of trial endpoints in patients given placebo (*open circles*) or active treatment (*solid circles*) in the Australian Therapeutic Trial in Mild Hypertension (Management Committee, 1982). Data plotted versus average diastolic blood pressure level measured during treatment. (From Doyle 1987, by courtesy of Williams & Wilkins)

In conclusion, although diuretics have certainly lost the exclusive or prominent role they used to enjoy in traditional stepped-care programs, they are among the few classes of antihypertensive agents for which the ability of reducing cardiovascular morbidity and mortality in hypertension has been demonstrated in controlled trials. Despite the recognized limitations of diuretics, especially when used in too large doses, it would be unwarranted at this stage to exclude these compounds from possible choices when antihypertensive therapy is started.

3.3 β-Adrenergic Blockers

As for diuretics, the MRC trial has shown β-blockers, or at least propranolol, to be less universally well-tolerated agents (especially by women) than previously thought. Their adverse effects, however, have not been substantially more numerous than those reported by patients receiving a thiazide diuretic (Medical Research Council Working Party 1981, 1985). The question can also be raised as to whether some of the adverse effects (e.g., lethargy and fatigue) reported by subjects receiving propranolol would have been equally prevalent with a non-lipophilic β-blocker that does not cross the blood-brain barrier.

As to the question of efficacy, both β-blocker- and non-β-blocker-based treatments are found equally effective on cardiovascular mortality and morbidity in the IPPPSH study (IPPPSH Collaborative Group 1985). In the MRC study, propranolol significantly reduces cardiovascular morbidity and mortality as compared with placebo (Medical Research Council Working Party 1985). In this study, however, the β-blocker was slightly less effective than the thiazide diuretic in the prevention of strokes. Nonetheless, in non-smokers (but not in smokers) stroke incidence was lower in the patients receiving propranolol than in patients receiving a placebo for the same levels of systolic blood pressure achieved by treatment, an observation that suggests that not only diuretics but also β-blockers may exert a protective effect against stroke in addition to the protection afforded by blood pressure lowering (Medical Research Council Working Party 1988).

As to the important question of a "cardioprotective" action of β-blockers in hypertension, available evidence is conflicting. This hypothesis has not been substantiated by either the MRC (Medical Research Council Working Party 1985, 1988) or the IPPPSH trial (IPPPSH Collaborative Group 1985), with the only exception of male nonsmokers, a subgroup in which both studies reported some reduction in coronary events under β-blocker treatment. On the other hand, the HAPPHY study (WILHELMSEN et al. 1987) was unable to show any cardioprotective effect of β-blockers over diuretics in both male smokers and nonsmokers, whereas the recent MAPHY study reported a significant reduction of coronary mortality in male hypertensive patients treated with a β-blocker as compared with patients treated with a diuretic, the cardioprotective effect being present in both smokers and nonsmokers, and even greater in smokers (WIKSTRAND et al. 1988).

Some indirect support for a cardioprotective action of β-blockers comes from a recent noncontrolled study by CRUICKSHANK et al. (1987): in their 939 hypertensive patients treated for 10 years with a β-blocker, mortality due to myocardial infarction was found to be very close to that of a reference normal population.

In conclusion, β-blockers together with diuretics are among the classes of antihypertensive drugs for which the ability to reduce cardiovascular morbidity and mortality has been demonstrated by controlled trials. Although they are not universally well-tolerated compounds, and their "cardioprotective" effect is still open to question, they certainty still qualify among the drugs of first choice for antihypertensive treatment.

3.4 Calcium Antagonists

Calcium antagonists (nifedipine and other dihydropyridines, verapamil, and diltiazem) have attracted great clinical interest because they are direct vasodilators (thereby appropriately correcting the hemodynamic abnormality in hypertension), which are suitable for monotherapy and do not require combination with a diuretic, β-blocker, or both (ZANCHETTI 1987c). In fact, calcium antagonists possess a distinct natriuretic and diuretic activity, well evident during the first few days of administration but not subsequently overcome by sodium-retaining mechanisms (Zanchetti and Leonetti 1985). Reflex tachycardia is absent with verapamil (Leonetti et al. 1980) and transient with nifedipine (Erne et al. 1983). Several million patients have been treated for many years with calcium antagonists, and the incidence of adverse effects with the most widely used compounds (nifedipine, verapamil, diltiazem) seems moderate and at least comparable to that seen with diuretics and β-blockers. A recent multicenter study compared the effects of the calcium antagonist nitrendipine and of the β-blocker propranolol on various parameters of quality of life and showed the calcium antagonist to have less effect on vigor and fatigue and partner's sexual satisfaction than the β-blocker (Zachariah 1987). Finally, calcium antagonists have been shown not to exert any untoward effect on glucose homeostasis and serum lipids (Trost and Weidmann 1987).

As to the problem of "cardioprotection", it has been remarked that calcium antagonists have many of those properties that led to the development of the concept for β-blockers (Bühler et al. 1985). It is true that, while secondary prevention by β-blockers in patients recovering from myocardial infarction is well documented (Yusuf et al. 1985), a similar action by calcium antagonists is controversial, although available clinical and experimental data suggest that the timing of intervention may be critical (Nayler et al. 1987). Furthermore, animal studies have shown that calcium is involved in experimental atherogenesis in a way that may be interfered with by calcium antagonists (Weinstein and Heider 1987; Chobanian 1987). Obviously, the antiatherogenetic properties of calcium antagonists await confirmation from studies on humans.

In summary, there appear to be several good reasons why calcium antagonists may also be considered as first-step choices in the treatment of hypertension.

3.5 Angiotensin-Converting Enzyme Inhibitors

ACE inhibitors are also vasodilating compounds that can be used in monotherapy. The two compounds captopril and enalapril have now been administered to several million patients for many years, showing effectiveness in blood pressure reduction and remarkable overall safety, provided the right doses are administered to patients with uncomplicated hypertension (Jenkins et al. 1985; McFate Smith et al. 1984). Care should be taken, however, in excluding patients with renovascular hypertension (Brunner et al. 1987). ACE inhibitors also appear to be relatively free of symptoms (such as fatigue, sleepiness, and dizziness) that are frequently reported with antihypertensive therapy. In a comparative trial with methyldopa and propranolol, captopril fared significantly better as far as various parameters of "quality of life" (including assessment of well-being and sexual activity) are concerned (Croog et al. 1986). Enalapril has been shown to preserve recent memory better than atenolol (Lichter et al. 1986). Furthermore, ACE inhibitors have never been shown to influence lipid metabolism adversely (see Amery et al. 1987).

As to the problem of "cardioprotection", although no evidence is available on the effect of ACE inhibitors on the incidence of coronary events in hypertension, evidence is accumulating on actions of these compounds that might be defined, at least indirectly, as cardioprotective: regression of left ventricular hypertrophy, improvement of coronary blood flow and coronary reserve, protection against ischemia- or reperfusion-induced cardiac arrhythmias, ventricular remodelling (SLEIGHT and ZANCHETTI 1988).

On the whole, there appear to be reasons for including ACE inhibitors among possible first-step drugs for the treatment of hypertension. Although no long-term, controlled trial of mortality and morbidity has been performed with them, as well as with calcium antagonists, it is fair to say that the presently available information on the clinical use of the two new classes of antihypertensive agents is at least comparable to that available on β-blockers in 1978, when they were suggested as an alternative first step to diuretics (WHO Expert Committee, 1978).

3.6 Other Classes of Antihypertensive Drugs

α-Adrenergic blockers, notably prazosin, have been used for many years with successful reduction of blood pressure and limited side effects. The greatest advantage of prazosin appears to be its property of favorably influencing the lipid profile (LEREN 1987); one disadvantage is the need for a cautious titration of the initial dose in order to avoid first dose postural hypotension. New compounds in this class, like doxazosin, might present easier titration and longer duration of action (BAEZ et al. 1986). Among the new α-blockers, urapidil possesses an interesting hybrid mechanism of action, combining peripheral α-receptor blockade with a central antihypertensive influence, possibly mediated through the stimulation of brainstem S_1-serotoninergic receptors (FOZZARD and MIR 1987). This S_2-serotonin antagonist, ketanserin, is also successfully used as antihypertensive agent and is being tested for the treatment or prevention of vascular disease, in line with the role serotonin is known to exert on platelet-vessel interaction (VANHOUTTE et al. 1988).

Obviously, with all new classes and new antihypertensive compounds firm recommendations of general use as a possible first choice in treatment have to await accumulation of considerable controlled clinical experience.

4 A Liberal Approach to Antihypertensive Therapy

4.1 Can Individualized Therapy Coexist with the Stepwise Approach?

When the first stepped-care programs were proposed, the number of effective and safe antihypertensive agents was limited, and this made these schemes easy to suggest and employ. Several classes of antihypertensive drugs now available lend themselves to commencing antihypertensive therapy, even in mild hypertensives. An indisputable advantage of having a wide array of antihypertensive agents is that it makes it possible to choose the agent most suitable to the individual patient. Obviously, the question immediately arises whether individualized therapy can coexist with the stepwise approach. How can we choose amongst the multiple possibilities? Should we perhaps return to the pathophy-

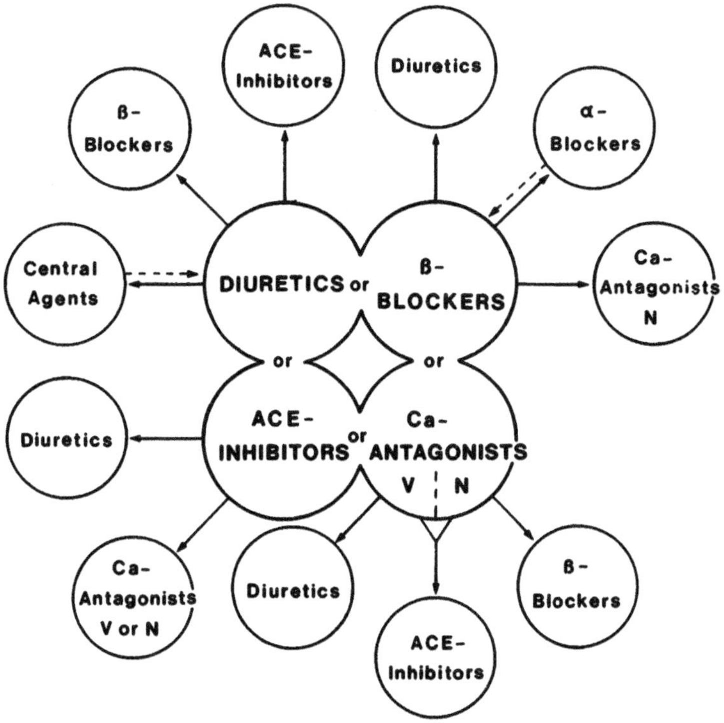

Fig. 7. Liberal stepped-care program. Treatment is usually started with one of the four classes of agents indicated in the *center* of the figure. The *dashed arrows* indicate the additional possibilities of other classes of agents that can be used for initial therapy. (From ZANCHETTI 1987a, by courtesy of Raven Press)

siological approach to selection of treatment, an approach whose difficulties were stressed at the beginning of this chapter?

Figure 7 illustrates a scheme that I first suggested in 1985 at the Königstein WHO/ISH meeting on mild hypertension (ZANCHETTI 1987a). The substance of this scheme has recently been adopted by the 1988 report by the US Joint National Committee on Detection, Evaluation, and Treatment of High Blood Pressure. The underlying philosophy of this scheme is that the individualized, liberal approach does not necessarily conflict with the stepwise approach. If in the scheme of Fig. 7 the step design seems graphically lost, preserved is the stepwise philosophy of proceeding from simple to more complicated means, from smaller to larger doses, from monotherapy to combinations of two or more drugs, but here associated with the concept of multiple simple choices available to the physician as well as to the patient.

The physician has the choice of starting treatment with a thiazide diuretic, a β-blocker, an ACE inhibitor, or a calcium antagonist, and sometimes also with small doses of other antihypertensive drugs. The choice among these various classes will first be made on simple clinical evaluation of existing contraindications or limited indications of the various compounds and of coexisting risk factors or pathological changes in the patient. As simple examples, β-blockers will not be chosen in subjects with chronic obstructive bronchial disease or peripheral obstructive arterial disease; thiazides will not be the first choice in a diabetic patient; coexisting dyslipidemia will favor ACE inhibitors, calcium antagonists, and α-blockers; coexisting ischemic heart disease will suggest the use of β-blockers or of calcium antagonists; cigarette smoking (if the patient does not follow the necessary advice to stop this habit) might suggest a limited usefulness of β-blockers (but we have seen above that the evidence is controversial). Other possible simple criteria of choice will be race (there is evidence that American blacks are more responsive to thiazides and possibly to calcium antagonists) or age (there are indications of a slightly reduced hypotensive effectiveness of β-blockers and of greater effectiveness of ketanserin in the elderly, while thiazides and calcium antagonists appear to be at least equally, if not more, effective in elderly as in younger hypertensives). As many patients have uncomplicated mild to moderate hypertension without concomitant risk factors, the first choice will often rely on the habits and confidence of the physician influenced by the following considerations: (a) If the physician pre-eminently trusts the results of controlled clinical trials, then his or her first choice will be centered on either diuretics or β-blockers, as these are the only two classes by which a reduction in cardiovascular morbidity and mortality has been proven. (b) If the physician's pre-eminent criterion is avoidance of adverse effects, then preference will probably go to an ACE inhibitor. (c) If concern about the possible consequences of metabolic effects is predominant, then the choice will be among ACE inhibitors, calcium antagonists, and α-blockers. (d) Whenever cost for the individual or for the society matters, then a thiazide will be the obvious first choice.

4.2 Up-Stepping, Side-Stepping, Down-Stepping

Independently of the criteria or considerations influencing these multiple choices, the liberal stepwise guidelines suggested now should be seen, as illustrated in Fig. 8, as an array of parallel staircases, in each of which the first step is represented by administration of a single drug, the second by a combination of two drugs, the third by a combination of three drugs. While in traditional stepped-care programs only upwards movements are suggested (see, for instance, Fig. 1), here *up-stepping* along the same staircase, *side-stepping* from one to another staircase or between multiple choices in the combination steps in a given staircase, and even *down-stepping* from a more complicated to a simpler and better tolerated therapy are all possible.

The general guidelines are the following. (a) Small doses of any agent should be used to start with, and the doses should not be increased subsequently beyond those suggested by the dose-response curves known for each agent or beyond the level at which adverse effects appear. (b) If efficacy is insufficient or symptoms arise, the physician has the choice of either switching to another first-step compound or reducing the dose of the original agent and combining it with

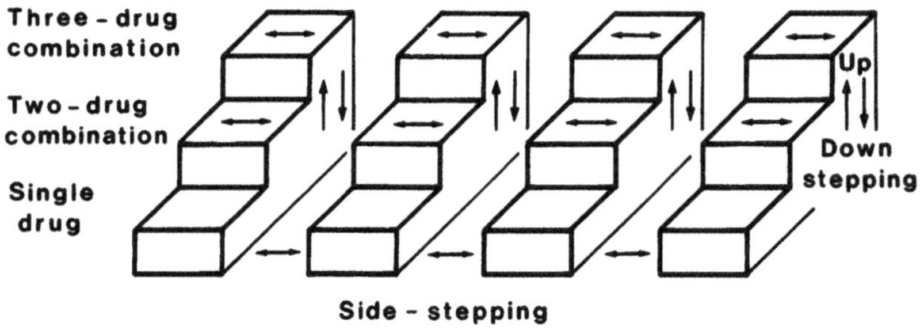

Fig. 8. Stepwise treatment of hypertension represented as an array of parallel staircases with possibilities for up-stepping, side-stepping, and down-stepping at each step

another agent. Both increased efficacy and a reduction of adverse reactions will often be achieved by the combination of two active agents at small doses. Some of the most reasonable and best tested combinations are indicated in the scheme of Fig. 7, which, however, is far from being complete and will be updated with the inclusion of new classes of compounds. (c) If efficacy is insufficient or symptoms arise from a drug combination, one of the drugs should be changed according to rational pharmacological and clinical criteria. (d) A three-drug combination should be used only when two drugs fail to achieve the goal of a satisfactory response. (e) Excessive blood pressure lowering or excessive disturbances should lead to down-stepping, i.e., passing from a more complicated to a simpler therapy, from higher to smaller doses, or from a more active to a less active compound. (f) In clinical antihypertensive practice, the choice of any drug amongst the several ones available is a tentative one, to be confirmed, corrected, or abandoned on the basis of the response of the patient. Most of the aspects of the patient's response are susceptible to clinical measurements, and they include not only blood pressure reduction but also the subjective and metabolic adverse effects, favorable or unfavorable physiological responses, and the arrest or reversal of secondary cardiovascular and renal changes.

5 Can Antihypertensive Therapy be Stopped?

If down-stepping of antihypertensive therapy is conceivable, the question arises as to whether, how often, and for how long, in patients whose blood pressure has been made normal by drugs down-stepping can be brought to full withdrawal from previous therapy. This is obviously a very important question both practically and theoretically: on one side, patients would like to know whether antihypertensive therapy is or is not a burden for life, once it is started; on the other hand, investigators are interested in understanding whether and how hypertensive mechanisms can prolongedly or permanently be reset by therapy.

Investigators have been intrigued by the possibility that blood pressure might prolongedly remain normal after withdrawal from long-term therapy since the early times of effective antihypertensive treatment. PAGE and DUSTAN (1962)

Table 1. Persistence of normal blood pressure after withdrawal of drug treatment

Study	Patients withdrawn[a] (*n*)	Pretreatment or hypertension severity	Criteria for normal blood pressure	Patients normalized at intermediate time		Patients normalized at end of observation time		
				%	Time	*n*	%	Time
Page and Dustan (1962)	27	severe				9	33	6 months–5 years
Thurm and Smith (1967)	69	mild-moderate	DBP≤ 90	36	5 months	16	23	10–42 months
Dustan et al. (1968)	65	mild-malignant	–	–	–	2	3	>8 years
Veterans Administration (1975)	60[b]	DBP 90–129	DBP≤ 95	16	6 months	9	15	72 weeks
						0	0	5 years[c]
Boyle et al. (1979)	20	moderate	DBP<100			2	10	31 weeks
Levinson et al. (1982)	24	DBP 90–109	DBP≤ 90	46	6 months	5	21	1 year
Maland et al. (1983)	31[b]	mild	DBP≤ 90			20	74	1 year
Finnerty (1984)	59	mild	DBP≤ 85			36	60	30 months
Langford et al. (1985)	159[b]	mild-severe	DBP≤ 95	53	26 weeks		40	56 weeks
Medical Research Council (1986)	192[b]	DBP 90–109	DBP< 90	45–56[d]	1 year		27–54[d]	2 years
Stamler et al. (1987)	44[b]	two-thirds mild	DBP≤ 90	50	1 year		5	4 years
Van Kruijsdijk et al. (1987, cited by Fletcher et al. 1988)	289	mild	DBP< 95	60	3 months		48	1 year

DBP, diastolic blood pressure.
[a] Only patients withdrawn from active treatment are indicated.
[b] Studies with additional control groups with treatment maintained or dietary treatment (not included in table).
[c] Follow-up cited by Freis (1987).
[d] Percentages cited are lowest and highest reported for groups separated by gender and drug withdrawal.

were the first to report a study of 27 patients in whom withdrawal from drugs was attempted, and then Perry et al. (1966) reported on 16 of their 316 treated hypertensive patients who has prolonged remissions of their hypertension when treatment was interrupted. Several other studies of treatment withdrawal have been published subsequently, the most recent ones being continuations of some of the large controlled therapeutic trials, such as the MRC trial on mild hypertension and the Hypertension Detection and Follow-up Program (HDFP) (see Fletcher et al. 1988).

If the results are analyzed, as in Table 1, for the percentage of patients with blood pressure still in the "normal" range after prolonged interruption of drug treatment, almost all studies have shown that a proportion of previously treated patients could maintain normal blood pressure values. The variable proportion of normalized patients seems to depend on the severity of hypertension before treatment was started and on the duration of the period of observation after the end of treatment.

Most of the earlier studies included rather severely affected (Page and Dustan 1962; Perry et al. 1966; Dustan et al. 1968) or a mixture of milder and more severe hypertensive patients (Veterans Administration Cooperative Study Group on Antihypertensive Agents 1975). This accounts for the very small proportion of prolongedly normalized patients (from 3% to 15%). The Veterans Administration study of 1975 found that the rise of diastolic blood pressure after withdrawal from treatment was proportional to the level of diastolic blood pressure before treatment (Fig. 9), and the recent study of HDFP patients by Langford et al. (1985) showed that, at about 1 year after drug withdrawal, 55% of mild hypertensive patients still had diastolic blood pressures ≤95 mmHg, whereas this criterion was met in only 25% of severe hypertensive patients.

The duration of the follow-up period without treatment is also a crucial factor. Those studies with a prolonged follow-up and providing data at different intermediate times indicate that the proportion of patients maintaining normal blood pressure progressively declines with the duration of follow-up: it was 36% at 5 months and 23% at 10–42 months in the study by Thurm and Smith (1967); 18% at 6 months, 15% at about 18 months, and 0% at 5 years in the study by the Veterans Administration Cooperative Study Group on Antihypertensive Agents (1975) (see also Freis 1987); 46% at 6 months and 21% at 1 year in the second Veterans Administration study (Levinson et al. 1982); 60% at 3 months and 48% at 1 year in the general practice study of Van Kruijsdijk et al. (1987, cited by Fletcher et al. 1988); 53% at 6 months and 40% at 1 year in the HDFP patients follow-up by Langford et al. (1985). The group 2 curve in Fig. 10, referring to the HDFP patients studied by Stamler et al. (1987), shows the progressive decline of the proportion of normalized patients from 50% at 1 year to only 5% at 4 years after withdrawal from drug therapy.

The data from the Medical Research Council Working Party (1986) add some further information in that the rate of rise of blood pressure after stopping treatment depends on pretreatment blood pressure only in men who received a thiazide. Finally, two trials on HDFP patients (Langford et al. 1985; Stamler et al. 1987) also included groups of patients in whom withdrawal from drug

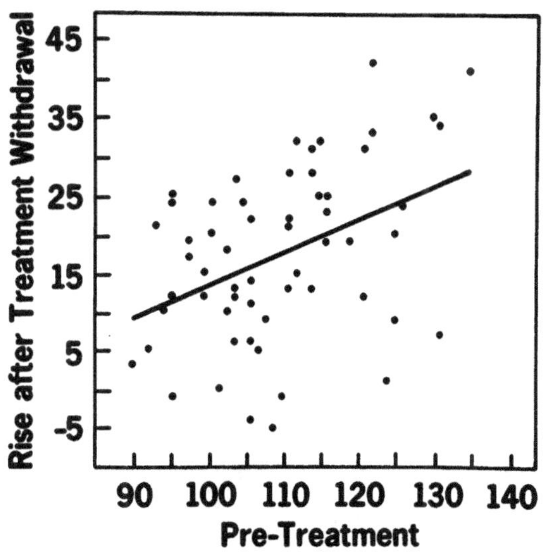

Fig. 9. Changes in diastolic blood pressure after discontinuation of treatment is shown on the *ordinate*. Level of diastolic blood pressure prior to beginning treatment is indicated on the *abscissa*. The degree of rise after discontinuing active treatment with drugs is correlated with the level of pretreatment diastolic blood pressure. Data from the study by the Veterans Administration Cooperation Study Group on Antihypertensive Agents (1975, by courtesy of Circulation)

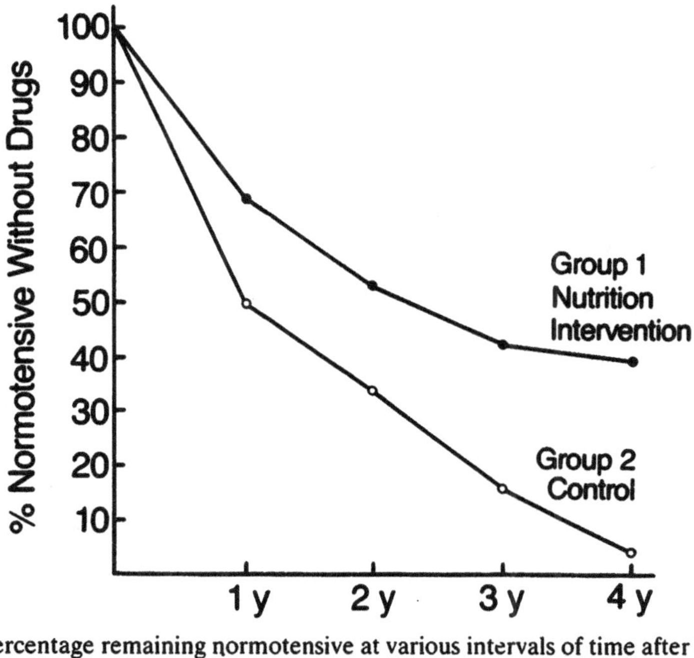

Fig. 10. Percentage remaining normotensive at various intervals of time after withdrawal from antihypertensive drug therapy: *Group 1* with added nutritional intervention, *Group 2* without nutritional intervention. (From STAMLER et al. 1987, by courtesy of JAMA)

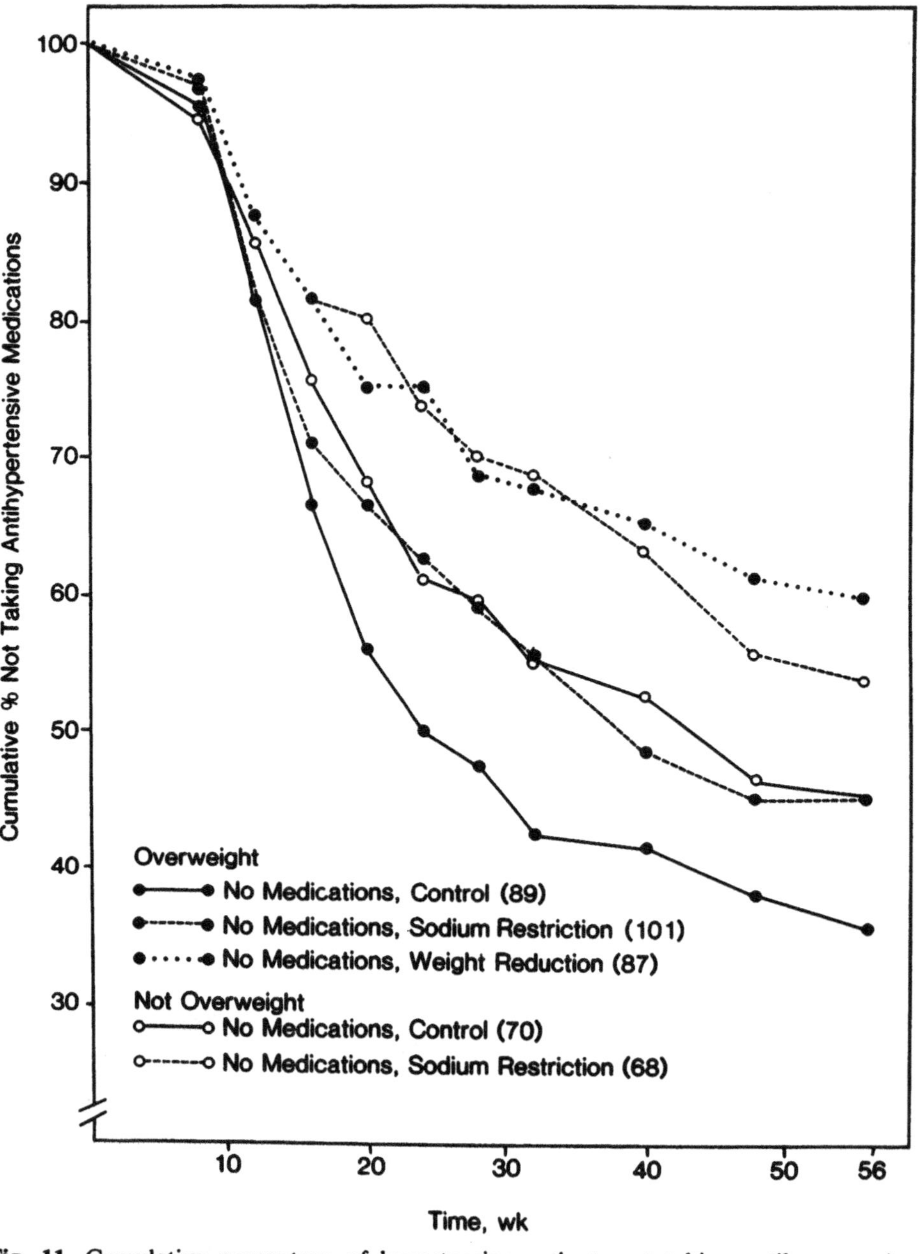

Fig. 11. Cumulative percentage of hypertensive patients not taking antihypertensive medications at various time intervals after withdrawal from drug therapy. (From Langford et al. 1985, by courtesy of JAMA)

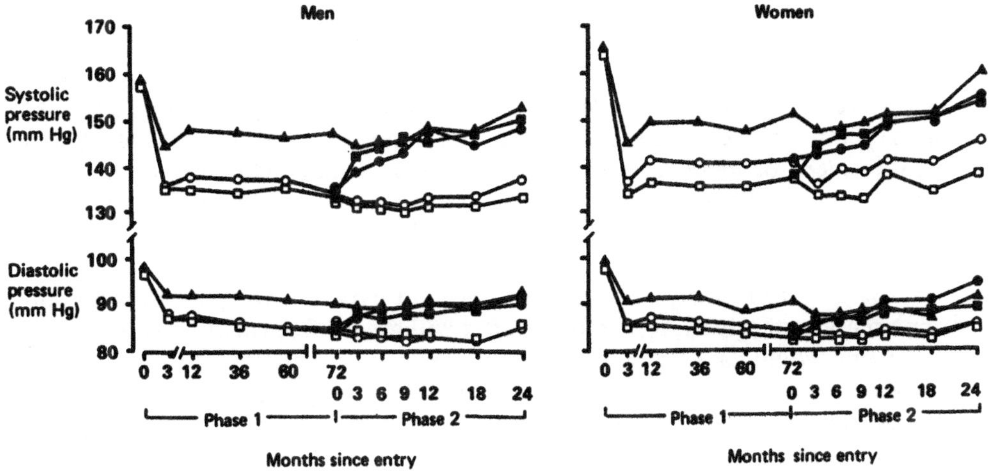

Fig. 12. Course of mean systolic (*above*) and diastolic (*below*) blood pressures in men (*left*) and women (*right*) during *phase 1* (treatment with either active drugs or placebo) and *phase 2* (previous treatment either withdrawn or continued). *Open squares*, bendrofluazide continued; *solid squares*, bendrofluazide withdrawn; *open circles*, propranolol continued; *solid circles*, propranolol withdrawn; solid triangles, placebo withdrawn (closely similar to placebo continued data, not shown). (From Medical Research Council Working Party 1986, by courtesy of Br Med J)

therapy was combined with various dietary measures. In both trials (Dietary Intervention Study in Hypertension, DISH, see LANGFORD et al. 1985; Hypertension Control Program, HCP, see STAMLER et al. 1987) dietary measures, particularly those leading to weight loss, were found to increase significantly the proportion of patients who could prolongedly stop antihypertensive medication (Figs. 10 and 11).

This appears to suggest that suitably prolonged antihypertensive therapy can exert a normalizing effect on blood pressure that extends itself for a considerable time, although probably not permanently, after withdrawal from therapy in a significant proportion of patients, especially with mild hypertension.

However, a different type of analysis leads to more cautious conclusions. Figure 12, from the study by the Medical Research Council Working Party (1986), shows the average systolic and diastolic blood pressure values of men and women withdrawn from prolonged treatment with either the diuretic bendrofluazide or the β-blocker propranolol and compares their blood pressure values with those of patients who were in the placebo arm of the study (and either continued placebo or were withdrawn from placebo). It is clear from Fig. 12 that within 3–9 months after drug withdrawal the average systolic and diastolic blood pressure values had reached the average values of placebo patients. If about 50% of patients withdrawn from active medication still had diastolic blood pressures lower than 90 mmHg, the same was the case for placebo patients. It is a well-known phenomenon, already described in the 1982 report by the Management Committee of the Australian Trial in Mild

Hypertension and in the principal results of the Medical Research Council Working Party (1985), that from 18% to 50% of patients initially entered as mild hypertensive and randomized to placebo treatment spontaneously lower their blood pressure to below the values used to define mild hypertension. This has been taken as a consequence of the alarm pressor reaction caused by the measurement of blood pressure by a doctor or a nurse (Mancia et al. 1983, 1987), which is frequent and large enough to move a consistent proportion of normotensive subjects transiently into the mild hypertensive range (Zanchetti 1988).

It is therefore likely that most of the mild hypertensive patients who still remain normotensive several months after withdrawal from active treatment are those who would have become normotensive under placebo or no treatment and therefore represent subjects incorrectly defined as hypertensive when treatment was commenced. The slow return toward pretreatment blood pressure values, however, cannot only be explained by an incorrect diagnosis of mild hypertension, as it has also been observed in patients with more severe hypertension and in studies, such as those by the Veterans Administration Study Group (1975) and Levinson et al. (1982), in which greater care had been taken to avoid including "false" mild hypertensive.

In summary, the available studies suggest the following conclusions. (a) A considerable proportion of those subjects, mostly originally defined as mild hypertensive, who remain normotensive 1 or 2 years after withdrawal from active treatment, consists of subjects inappropriately defined as mild hypertensive when treatment was commenced. (b) The slow return of blood pressure to pretreatment levels, which is observed not only in mild but also in more severe hypertensive patients and lasts much longer than the pharmacokinetic properties of any antihypertensive agent can account for, may depend on resetting of the blood pressure control mechanisms. These probably include more mechanisms than the arterial baroreflex whose resetting was implied in the original publication by Page and Dustan (1962). (c) Especially in more severe and complicated hypertensive patients and in those in whom pretreatment blood pressure reappears only after a long interval of time, it is likely that persistent normalization after withdrawal from medication is due to regression of structural components of hypertension, such as myocardial or vascular hypertrophy, induced by long-term, active, antihypertensive treatment. (d) When "false" or "transient" hypertensive patients are excluded, all studies with a sufficiently long follow-up indicate that at a distance of weeks, months, and more rarely years, withdrawal from medication is unavoidably followed by the reappearance of hypertension.

In medical practice the following guidelines can be suggested. In mild hypertension cautious down-stepping and eventually withdrawal from antihypertensive medication can be attempted when blood pressure has long been normalized: this might reveal subjects improperly diagnosed and treated or might allow a transient interruption of drug therapy for a number of subjects, especially if drug withdrawal is accompanied by appropriate dietary measures. Even in more severe hypertension, careful down-stepping and withdrawal from medication may be feasible after prolonged successful therapy, especially when regression of the cardiovascular consequences of hypertension has been documented. In all cases, withdrawal of medication can only be done under the careful supervision of a physician and if the patient's blood pressure is monitored at rather frequent intervals in order to reinstitute therapy as soon as it becomes necessary.

Summary

When the first stepped-care programs were proposed, the number of effective and safe antihypertensive agents was limited, and this made these schemes easy to suggest and employ. Several classes of antihypertensive drugs now available lend themselves to the start of therapy, even in mild hypertensives. This makes it possible to choose the agent most suitable to the individual patient. The obvious question is whether individualized therapy can coexist with the stepwise approach. The liberal stepwise guidelines suggested now should be seen as an array of parallel staircases, in each of which the first step is represented by the administration of a single drug, the second by a combination of two drugs, the third by a combination of three drugs. Up-stepping along the same staircase, side-stepping from one staircase to another, and down-stepping from a more complicated to a simpler and better tolerated therapy (and sometimes cautious interruption of therapy) are all possible.

References

Amery A, Birkenhäger WH, Brixho P, Bulpitt C, Clement D, de Ruyttere M, de Schaepdrijver A, et al. (1985) Mortality and morbidity results from the European Working Party on High Blood Pressure in the Elderly trial. Lancet 1:1349–1354

Amery A, Fagard R, Stassen J (1987) Recent data on changes in lipid metabolism induced by hypotensive drugs. Curr Opin Cardiol 2:769–774

Baez MA, Garg DC, Jallard NS, Weidler DJ (1986) Antihypertensive effect of doxazosin in hypertensive patients: comparison with atenolol. Br J Clin Pharmacol (Suppl 1) 21:63S–68S

Boyle RM, Price ML, Hamilton M (1979) Thiazide withdrawal in hypertension. J R Coll Physicians Lond 3:172–173

Brunner H, Waeber B, Nussberger J (1987) Renal effects of converting enzyme inhibition. J Cardiovasc Pharmacol [Suppl 3] 9:S6–S14

Bühler FR, Müller FB, Linder L, Bolli P (1985) Antihypertensive therapy and myocardial infarction: focus on calcium antagonists. J Hypertens [Suppl 2] 3:S95–S98

Chobanian A (1987) Effects of calcium channel antagonists and other antihypertensive drugs on atherogenesis. J Hypertens [Suppl 4] 5:S43–S48

Croog SH, Levine S, Testa MA, Brown B, Bulpitt CJ, Jenkin CD, Klerman GL, Williams GM (1986) The effect of antihypertensive therapy on quality of life. N Engl J Med 314:1657–1664

Cruickshank JM, Pennert K, Sörman AE, Thorp JM, Zacharias FM, Zacharias FJ (1987) Low mortality from all causes, including myocardial infarction, in well-controlled hypertensives treated with a beta-blocker plus other antihypertensives. J Hypertens 5:489–498

Doyle A (1987) When and how to treat hypertension. In: Hunyor SN (ed) Cardiovascular drug therapy. William and Wilkins, Baltimore, pp 136–141

Dustan HP, Page IH, Tarazi RC, Frohlich ED (1968) Arterial pressure responses to discontinuing antihypertensive drugs. Circulation 37:370–379

Erne P, Bolli P, Bertel O, Hultén L, Kiowski W, Müller FB, Bühler F (1983) Factors

influencing the hypotensive effects of calcium antagonists. Hypertension 5:96–102
Finnerty FA (1984) Step-down treatment of mild systemic hypertension. Am J Cardiol 53:1304–1307
Fletcher AE, Franks PJ, Bulpitt CJ (1988) The effect of withdrawing antihypertensive therapy: a review. J Hypertens 6:431–436
Fozzard JR, Mir AK (1987) Are 5HT receptors involved in the antihypertensive effects of urapidil (Abstr)? Br J Clin Pharmacol 90:24
Freis ED (1987) Can drug treatment be stopped? In: Strasser T, Ganten D (eds) Mild hypertension: from drug trials to practice. Raven, New York, pp 251–256
Hansson L, Lowenstein J, Zanchetti A (eds) (1984) Coronary heart disease: hvpertension and other risk factors. Am J Med [Suppl 2A] 76
IPPPSH Collaborative Group (1985) Cardiovascular risk and risk factors in a randomized trial of treatment based on the beta-blocker oxprenolol: the International Prospective Primary Prevention Study in Hypertension (IPPPSH). J Hypertens 3:379–392
Jenkins AC, Dreslinski GR, Tadros SS, Groel JT, Fand R, Herczeg SA (1985) Captopril in hypertension: seven years later. J Cardiovasc Pharmacol [Suppl 1] 7:S96–S101
Langford HG, Blaufox MD, Oberman A, Hawkins CM, Curb JD, Cutter GR, Wassertheil-Smoller S, et al. (1985) Dietary therapy slows the return of hypertension after stopping prolonged medication. JAMA 253:657–664
Leonetti G, Sala C, Bianchini C, Terzoli L, Zanchetti A (1980) Antihypertensive and renal effects of orally administered verapamil. Eur J Clin Pharmacol 18:375–382
Leren P (1987) Comparison of effects on lipid metabolism of antihypertensive drugs with alpha- and beta-adrenergic antagonist properties. Am J Med [Suppl 1A] 82:31–35
Levinson PD, Khatri IM, Freis ED (1982) Persistence of normal BP after withdrawal of drug treatment in mild hypertension. Arch Intern Med 142:2265–2268
Lichter I, Richardson PJ, Wyke MA (1986) Differential effects of atenolol and enalapril on memory during treatment for essential hypertension. Br J Clin Pharmacol 21: 641–646
Maland LJ, Lutz LJ, Castle CH (1983) Effects of withdrawing diuretic therapy on blood pressure in mild hypertension. Hypertension 5:539–544
Management Committee (1982) The Australian Therapeutic Trial in Mild Hypertension: untreated mild hypertension. Lancet 1:185–191
Mancia G, Bertinieri G, Grassi G, Parati G, Pomidossi G, Ferrari A, Gregorini L, Zanchetti A (1983) Effects of blood pressure measurement by the doctor on patient's blood pressure and heart rate. Lancet 2:695–698
Mancia G, Parati G, Pomidossi G, Grassi G, Casadei R, Zanchetti A (1987) Alerting reaction and rise in blood pressure during measurement by physician and nursse. Hypertension 9:209–215
McFate Smith W, Kulaga SF, Moncloa F, Pingeon R, Walker JF (1984) Overall tolerance and safety of enalapril. J Hypertens [Suppl 2] 2:113–117
Medical Research Council Working Party (1981) on Mild to Moderate Hypertension: Adverse reactions to bendrofluazide and propranolol for the treatment of mild hypertension. Lancet 2:539–543
Medical Research Council Working Party (1985) MRC trial of treatment of mild hypertension: principal results. Br Med J 291:97–104
Medical Research Council Working Party (1986) on Mild Hypertension: Course of blood pressure in mild hypertensives after withdrawal of long-term antihypertensive treatment. Br Med J 293:988–992
Medical Research Council Working Party (1988) Stroke and coronary heart disease in mild hypertension: risk factors and the value and treatment. Br Med J 296:1565–1570
Nayler WG, Panagiotopoulos S, Elz JS, Sturrock WJ (1987) Fundamental mechanisms of action of calcium antagonists in myocardial ischemia. Am J Cardiol 59:75B–83B
Page IH, Dustan HP (1962) Persistence of normal blood pressure after discontinuing treatment in hypertensive patients. Circulation 25:433–436
Perry HM, Schroeder HA, Catanzaro FJ, Moore-Jones D, Camel GH (1966) Studies on the control of hypertension. VI. Mortality, morbidity, and remissions during twelve years of intensive therapy. Circulation 33:958–972
Sleight P, Zanchetti A (eds) (1988) The renin-angiotensin system and the heart. Am J

Med [Suppl 3A] 84
Stamler R, Stamler J, Grimm R, Gosch FC, Elmer P, Dyer A, Berman R, et al. (1987) Nutritional therapy for high blood pressure. Final report of a four-year randomized controlled trial—the Hypertension Control Program. JAMA 257:1484–1491
Thurm RH, Smith WM (1967) On resetting of "barostats" in hypertenssive patients. JAMA 201:301–304
Trost BN, Weidmann P (1987) Effects of calcium antagonists on glucose homeostasis and serum lipid in non-diabetic and diabetic subjects: a review. J Hypertens [Suppl 4] 5:S81–S104
US Joint National Committee on Detection, Evaluation, and Treatment of High Blood Pressure (1977) A comparative study. JAMA 237:255–261
US Joint National Committee on Detection, Evaluation, and Treatment of High Blood Pressure (1984) The 1984 report. Arch Intern Med 144:1045–1057
US Joint National Committee on Detection, Evaluation, and Treatment of High Blood Pressure (1988) The 1988 report. Arch Intern Med 148:1023–1038
Vanhoutte P, Amery A, Birkenhäger W, Breckenridge A, Bühler F, Distler A, Dormandy J, et al. (1988) Serotoninergic mechanisms in hypertension. Focus on the effects of ketanserin. Hypertension 1:111–133
Veterans Administration Cooperative Group on Antihypertensive Agents (1975) Return of elevated blood pressure after withdrawal of antihypertensive drugs. Circulation 51:1107–1113
Weinstein DB, Heider JG (1987) Antiatherogenic properties of calcium antagonists. Am J Cardiol 59:163B–172B
WHO Expert Committee (1978) Arterial hypertension. WHO Tech Rep Ser 628
WHO/ISH (1983) Guidelines for the treatment of mild hypertension. Bull WHO 61: 53–56
Wikstrand J, Warnold I, Olsson G, Tuomilethto J, Elmfeldt D, Berglund G (1988) Primary Prevention with metoprolol in patients with hypertension. Mortality results from the MAPHY study. JAMA 259:1976–1982
Wilhelmsen L, Berglund G, Elmfeldt D, Fitzsimons T, Holzgreve H, Hosie J, Hörnkvist P-E, et al. (1987) Beta-blockers versus diuretics in hypertensive men: main results from the HAPPHY trial. J Hypertens 5:561–572
Yusuf S, Peto R, Lewis J, Collins R, Sleight P (1985) Beta-blockade during and after myocardial infarction: an overview of randomized trials. Prog Cardiovasc Dis 27:353–371
Zachariah PK (1987) Quality of life with antihypertensive medication. J Hypertens [Suppl 4] 5:S105–S110
Zanchetti A (1980) Rational approaches to clinical therapy. In: Turner P (ed) Clinical pharmacology and therapeutics. MacMillan, London, pp 270–274
Zanchetti A (1985a) A re-examination of stepped-care: a retrospective and prospective. J Cardiovasc Pharmacol [Suppl 1] 7:S126–S131
Zanchetti A (1985b) Which drug to which patient? J Hypertens [Suppl 2] 3:S57–S63
Zanchetti A (1987a) Step-wise treatment: Which step first? In: Strasser T, Ganten D (eds) Mild hypertension: from drug trials to practice. Raven, New York, pp 243–249
Zanchetti A (1987b) Current drug treatment of hypertension: problems and perspectives. Ann Life Ins Med 81:149–155
Zanchetti A (1987c) Role of calcium antagonists in systemic hypertension. Am J Cardiol 59:130B–136B
Zanchetti A (1988) What blood pressure level should be treated? In: Laragh JH, Brenner BM (eds) Hypertension: pathophysiology, diagnosis, and management. Raven, New York (in press)
Zanchetti A, Leonetti G (1985) Natriuretic effect of calcium antagonists. J Cardiovasc Pharmacol [Suppl 4] 7:S33–S37

CHAPTER 21

Prognosis of Treated and Untreated Hypertension

T. STRASSER

CONTENTS

1 Natural History of Hypertension

It is worth recalling, not only as a mere curiosity, that as recently as the student years of today's senior physicians, small doses of phenobarbitone were the best available treatment for hypertension. Phlebotomy and leeches were considered the last recourse in intractable cases, at least in some parts of Central Europe, when combinations of hypnotics, garlic extracts, and mistletoe failed to reduce blood pressure, and the patient, bleeding severely from the nose, was irreparably heading towards uremic death.

The meaning of such reminiscences is that information on the true natural history of hypertension must be sought in the prepharmacotherapeutic era. With the advent of anti-hypertensive drugs, modern treatment of severe hypertension became ethically mandatory in the 1950s, and that of moderate hypertension by the end of the 1960s, allowing no more observations on the natural course of these forms of the disease. The answer, if any, to the question whether the prognosis of mild hypertension is improved by drug treatment was left for the 1980s.

The grave prognosis of severe untreated hypertension can be assessed from a number of early major publications. FRANT and GROEN (1950) published, with considerable delay due to World War II, a 9-year follow-up study of 418 patients with arterial hypertension, examined in 1931 and 1932 and reassessed in 1940/1941. They found a nearly fourfold excess mortality in the highest pressure group and a more than sevenfold excess mortality in middle-aged men. Of all deaths 41% were due to heart disease (unspecified), 15% to renal failure, and 9% to stroke.

Similar findings were reported by BECHGAARD (1946) from a follow-up of 1038 patients for 4–11 years. Men below age 50 had an excess mortality of 875%; the average for all ages was 288%. Hypertensive heart disease was the most frequent cause of death; coronary thrombosis contributed 7.8%, stroke 13.6%, and renal failure 8.1% of all deaths — a pattern of mortality that has definitely changed since the advent of antihypertensive drugs.

The most often quoted source of information of early times is the SOCIETY OF ACTUARIES (1959) report, based on 4 900 000 insurance policies (most of them from the prepharmacotherapy era) with an average duration of 7.2 years and 102 000 cases of death. In this huge sample drawn from clinically healthy populations the ratio (percent) of actual to expected mortality is as shown in Table 1.

It is understandable that in view of the distressingly poor prognosis of hypertensive patients, especially of younger males in the upper pressure range, possibly thousands of Smithwick's operations (extensive dorsolumbar splanchnicectomy) were carried out in the 1940s (SMITHWICK 1955), without clear information whether the prognosis of those patients improved or not. At best, it could be stated:

"Thus it may well be that the overall reduction of blood pressure during any 24-hour period may be quite significant and the time taken away from the destructive and sclerosing effect of the elevated pressure contributed towards increasing longevity". (PAGE 1946)

It will never be known whether sympathectomy did improve the prognosis of hypertension, since this type of treatment was abandoned long before controlled trials were introduced. By the same token, the value of thiocyanate may never be elucidated, albeit for different reasons: although a very potent hypotensive agent shown since 1906, it seems to be an "orphan" drug, so cheap that industry

Table 1. Mortality of men according to blood pressure, expressed as ratio (percent) of actual to expected mortality (Society of Actuaries 1959); ratio 100 indicates average expected mortality

Systolic blood pressure	Ratio	Diastolic blood pressure	Ratio
88–97	78	48–67	83
98–127	88	68–82	97
128–137	118	83–87	129
138–147	155	88–92	150
148–157	194	93–97	188
158–167	244	98–102	234
168–177	242		
178–192	191		

may not be sufficiently interested in it — besides the fact that the use of this drug is technically difficult.

2 Prognosis of Hypertension, Derived from Prospective Epidemiological Studies

Epidemiological studies (e.g., KEYS 1980; Italian Research Group 1986) are an important source of information on the risk associated with various blood pressure levels and hence with hypertension. Unlike the retrospective study of the Actuarial Societies, these epidemiological investigations have the advantage of the methodologic rigor of prospective studies which follow a predesigned protocol. They may have the disadvantage that effective treatment of hypertension already existed at the time of these studies, and therefore some of the subjects observed may have been receiving antihypertensive treatment. However, it is unlikely that the results of these studies are biased in any significant way, since other epidemiological investigations have shown that despite the availability of antihypertensive drugs, only a small fraction of hypertensive subjects in the general population had been treated effectively — at least up to the 1970s (STRASSER 1980).

Statistical analyses of the rich data base of such studies allow for detailed probability estimates of the incidence of major morbid events associated with a number of risk factors, including blood pressure. The probabilities can be calculated independently for each risk factor, as well as for their combinations. The Framingham study (GORDON et al. 1971; KANNEL and GORDON 1973) is the most frequently quoted. For estimating the risk of coronary heart disease and of cerebrovascular disease in daily practice by the nonepidemiologist, handbooks have been developed (KANNEL and GORDON 1973; MEDALIE and GOLDBOURT 1973; KANNEL and DAWBER 1974; CAPOCACCIA et al. 1980); these provide probability tables for the incidence of myocardial infarction and stroke according to age, sex, blood pressure, serum cholesterol levels, smoking, etc. No such tables have been developed for other complications of hypertension, such as hypertensive heart or renal failure, but these have become rare since the introduction of the modern antihypertensive agents, leaving stroke and myocardial infarction as the main hazards for hypertensive patients.

Figure 1 presents a nomograph based on one such handbook (GORDON and KANNEL 1973) depicting the relative and absolute risks of developing clinically manifest coronary heart disease for men at various ages, initial levels of systolic pressure, serum cholesterol levels, and according to smoking status. The nomograph shows that — implicitly, in untreated persons — (a) the probability of myocardial infarction increases exponentially with blood pressure levels; (b) the slope of risk increment associated with blood pressure does not depend on age; (c) the risk increment for smoking and serum cholesterol decreases with age; and, perhaps the most important point, (d) the prognosis of hypertensive patients should be assessed in the light of a combination of their risk factors.

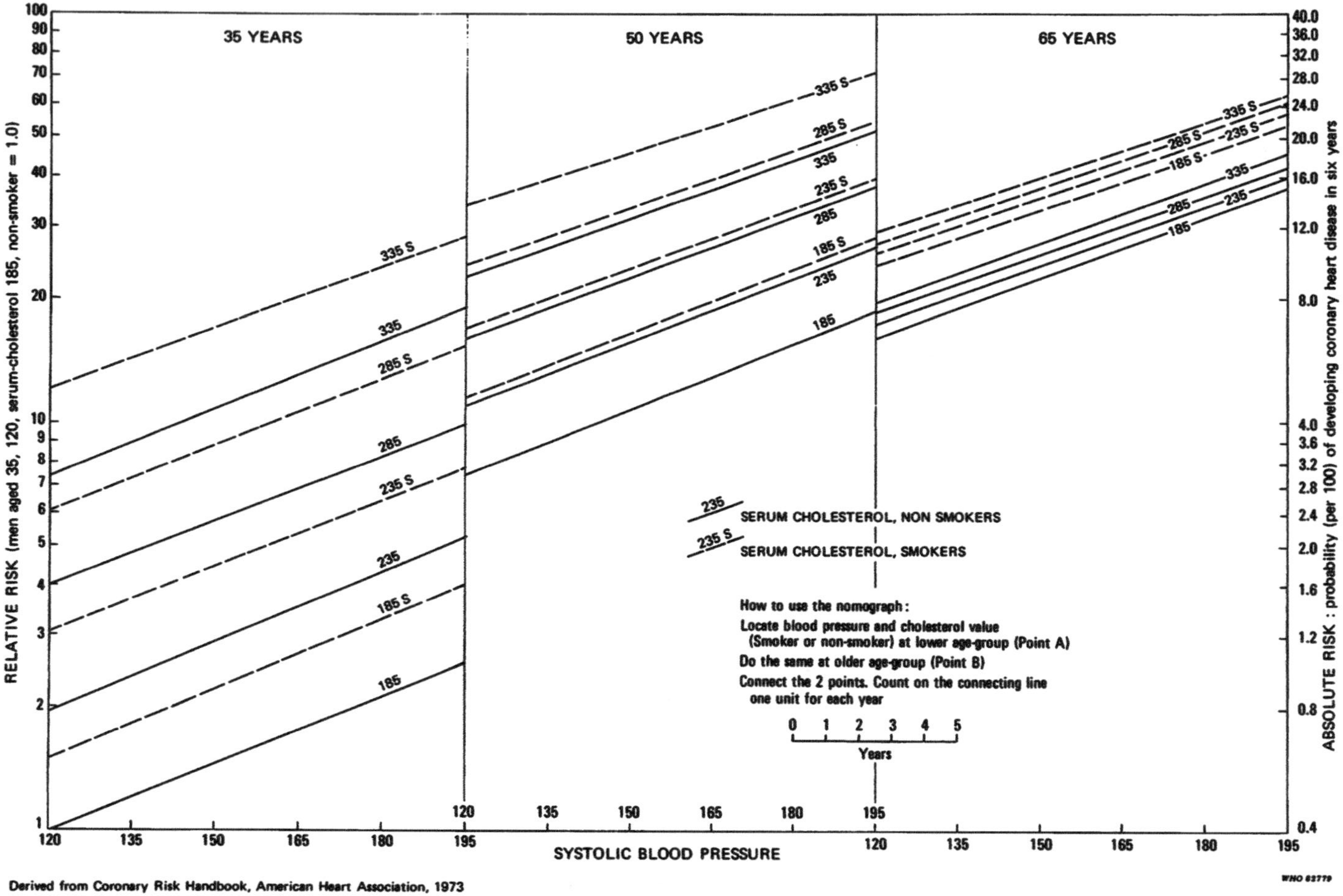

Derived from Coronary Risk Handbook, American Heart Association, 1973

Fig. 1. Nomograph for coronary risk estimates. Probabilities of developing clinical coronary heart disease in the next 6 years in 35–65-year-old males as a function of systolic blood pressure, serum cholesterol levels, and smoking. The probability increases exponentially with blood pressure; the risk increment attributable to blood pressure does not depend on age; however, the total risk, i.e., the prognosis of the patient, is a complex function, depending on a combination of several major risk factors. (From GORDON and KANNEL 1973)

3 Assessment of Prognosis in Clinical Trials

3.1 Rationale for Trials

Modern therapeutic research is hardly conceivable without controlled clinical trials. The less certain the benefit of treatment, the greater the importance of carrying out a controlled trial. In the early days of antihypertensive pharmacotherapy, when the diagnosis of malignant hypertension was equivalent to a death sentence, any effective antihypertensive agent was welcomed and accepted without the prior application of a controlled trials; treatment results were only compared with earlier experience such as described in Sect. 1 (e.g., BURNETT and EVANS 1955; MCMICHAEL and MURPHY 1955).

The prognosis of malignant hypertension has radically changed. A recent review of 100 patients with bilateral retinal hemorrhages and/or exudates, observed between 1974 and 1983 (BING et al. 1986), showed that survival rates for malignant hypertension nowadays differ little from those in the general population, provided that adequate treatment is started early enough to prevent renal damage.

In less clear-cut situations, however, controlled trials were needed. To decide whether treatment improves the prognosis of patients with uncomplicated, symptomless, benign primary hypertension, HAMILTON et al. (1964) observed 61 patients, half of them untreated controls, for an average time of 4 years. The average blood pressures were 226/134 mmHg and, as one would prognosticate today, the outcome in the control group was catastrophic: of the 31 controls, 7 patients had strokes, 6 developed cardiac complications, and (only) 3 suffered myocardial infarction. Among the treated patients there were 5 complications (3 strokes), but all except one occurred in patients with poor blood pressure control. If the latter are counted with the untreated group, the result is a rate of 57% complications (several of them fatal) among the untreated patients, compared with a 4% complication rate in the group in which the blood pressure had effectively been lowered. The prognosis in treated, moderately severe hypertension thus was some 15 times better than in similar patients left without treatment.

3.2 Mild Hypertension Trials

Obviously, the above figures apply only to patients with the blood pressure levels described, receiving treatment as specified in the particular publication. The effect of treatment on patients with less severe blood pressure elevations had yet to be explored.

During the quarter of a century that followed, a variety of trials were carried out at lower and lower pretreatment levels of blood pressure, on ever increasing numbers of subjects — and with more and more marginal results. A total of at least 19 therapeutic trials have been described in a great number of publications (WOLFE and LINDEMAN 1966; Veterans Administration Cooperative Study Group on Antihypertensive Agents 1967, 1970; PERRY 1977; MCFATE SMITH 1977; Co-operative Randomized Controlled Trial 1973; Hypertension Detection

Table 2. Summary of results of trials in the treatment of mild hypertension

No.	Study reference	n	BP	No of events		Rate/100 years		PER	TQ	Comments
				a	c	a	c	$c-a$	c/a	
1.	Hamilton et al. (1964)	61	229/131	1	20	0.96	14.28	13.32	14.87	Small numbers. Trial not blind
2.	Wolfe and Lindeman (1966)	87	178/109	2	21	2.52	25.25	22.73	10.02	BP remained high in two "treated patients
3.	Veterans Administration (1967)									
4.	Veterans Administration (1970)									
5.	Subgroup (a)	210	xx/105–114	8	35	2.46	9.79	7.33	3.98	Men only
6.	Subgroup (b)	170	xx/90–104	14	21	5.01	7.69	2.68	1.53	Men only
7.	Cooperative Randomized Controlled Trial (1973)	116	xx/109	3	14	2.58	12.06	9.48	4.67	Single-blind
8.	McFate Smith (1977)	389	148/99	56	90	4.14	6.56	2.42	1.58	Hospital-based
9.	HDFP (1979); Stratum I	7825	152/96	231	291	5.90	7.40	1.50	1.25	Mortality, all causes, community-based
10.	Management Committee (1980) Australian Trial	3427	157/100	91	127	1.05	1.26	0.21	1.20	Fatal plus nonfatal events
11.	Helgeland (1980)	785	156/97	25	34	1.23	1.79	0.56	1.45	Fatal plus nonfatal events
12.	Multiple Risk Factor Intervention Trial (1982)	1510	xx/100+	25	45	2.98	3.24	0.26	1.29	Multiple risk intervention; only hypertensive subjects analyzed; special versus

13. Multiple Risk Factor Intervention Trial (1982)	1676	xx/95–99	43	39	5.18	4.61	−0.57	0.89	usual care; mortality, all causes.
14. Multiple Risk Factor Intervention Trial (1982)	2338	xx/90–94	47	31	4.06	2.61	−1.45	0.64	
15. HDFP (1982)	10940	159/101	102	158	0.37	0.58	0.27	1.56	Strokes, fatal and nonfatal
16. HDFP (1984)	7141	152/96	307	355	1.73	1.99	0.26	1.15	Coronary heart disease, fatal and non-fatal
17. HDFP (1984)	1839	xx/108	84	103	1.79	2.29	0.50	1.28	Coronary heart disease, fatal and nonfatal
18. Medical Research Council Working Party (1985)	17354	158/98	286	352	0.60	0.74	0.14	1.23	All cardiovascular events
19. Medical Research Council Working Party (1985)	17354	158/98	60	109	0.13	0.23	0.10	1.77	All strokes
20. AMERY et al. (1985a,b, 1986)	840	182/101	135	149	6.90	7.60	0.70	1.10	Elderly patients, all causes of death
21. AMERY et al. (1985a,b, 1986)	840	182/101	21	31	1.10	1.60	0.50	1.45	Stroke only
22. COOPE and WARRENDER (1986)	884	196/99	84	121	4.55	5.88	1.33	1.29	Elderly patients, primary care

HDFP, Hypertension Detection and Follow-Up Program Cooperative Group; xx, average systolic blood pressure not indicated in available publication; *a*; actively treated group; *c*, control group.

PER stands for prevented events rate. This value presents the "net" effect of treatment. It is obtained by subtracting the event rate observed in the actively treated group from that in the placebo group. Note that the value is expressed in *rates*, not in percentage reduction; the latter expression, according to our opinion, often gives an exaggerated impression of treatment efficacy. TQ stands for therapeutic quotient. It is obtained by dividing the event rate in the placebo group by the rate observed in the actively treated group. This value is a relative measure of treatment efficacy, indicating how many times the treated group is better off than the placebo group. Being a relative measure, it is suitable for the comparison of various treatment regimens or of the effects of one such regimen measured by different end points. To make a circumspect judgement on treatment outcomes at various levels of blood pressure, both the absolute (PER) and relative (TQ) values should be taken into account.

and Follow-up Program Cooperative Group 1979, 1982 a, b, 1984, Management Committee 1980; HELGELAND 1980; MORGAN et al. 1980; SPRACKLING et al. 1981; Multiple Risk Factor Intervention Trial Research Group 1982; Medical Research Council Working Party 1985; AMERY et al. 1985 a, b, 1986; COOPE and WARRENDER 1986).

The results of those trials which can be compared with other studies on the basis of the published papers are presented in Table 2. It should be emphasized that comparisons between the trials are difficult. While some differences between trials are meaningful, such as different pretreatment blood pressure levels, other discrepancies, such as different ways of assessing average blood pressure levels are regrettable and detract from the comparability of such trials (STRASSER 1982). These and other difficulties, and the wish to clarify the message to be derived from all these trials, have stimulated a number of authors to publish comparisons, reviews, syntheses, or meta-analyses of the mild hypertension therapeutic trials (WHO/ISH Mild Hypertension Liaison Committee 1982; STAMLER and STAMLER 1983; MIALL et al. 1983; STRASSER 1986, 1987; STRASSER et al. 1983; CUTLER and FURBERG 1985; SACKS et al. 1985; WILCOX et al. 1986; LABARTHE 1986; MACMAHON et al. 1986a; BOISSEL and MOLEUR 1987; ROSE 1987; WEBER 1987; ROBERTSON 1987). Most of these papers conclude that drug treatment of mild hypertension prevents stroke but that it has only a slight effect on the incidence of coronary heart disease.

3.3 Measures of Prognosis

The differences between the treated and untreated patient groups are usually expressed in percentage reduction of end points or morbid events. This is not the best way of expressing the effects of treatment or, for that matter, the prognosis of treated patients compared with untreated ones. For example, stating that by treatment "incidence has been reduced by 20%" may mean the saving of 50 out of 1000 patients with a 25% morbidity, rate on may mean the saving of one single patient out of 1000 treated cases, when incidence is only 0.5%.

There are two legitimate ways of expressing such prognostic differences: (a) the *rate* at which expected events (deaths, complications) are prevented by treatment (prevented events rate, PER) and (b) the *quotient* (or ratio) of events in treated and untreated patients (therapeutic quotient, TQ). These concepts are used for assessing the outcomes of therapeutic trials in mild hypertension (STRASSER 1987).

PER is an absolute measure of the improvement of prognosis due to treatment, i.e., of the utility of the treatment. It gives the numbers of complications or deaths averted by treatment, calculated for 100 observation years. It provides information on the improvement of the prognosis of a given patient, in terms of statistical probabilities.

TQ is a relative measure that serves for comparing the prognosis of patients treated at various blood pressure levels, or that of patients undergoing various types of treatment at similar blood pressure levels.

These measures allow comparisons between trials. They also allow one to express the prognosis of a given patient in probabilistic terms.

3.4 Synthesis of Trial Results

It is not possible to pool the results of the numerous trials on the treatment of hypertension; as mentioned, there are too many differences in study design, inclusion and exclusion criteria, sample size definition of endpoints, degree of blood pressure lowering, and drug usage to allow for a joint analysis of a classic type. Nevertheless, when relating the above prognostic indicators to pretreatment blood pressures, a clear pattern emerges-despite the considerable "noise". Figure 2 shows an exponential correlation between blood pressure and the TQ

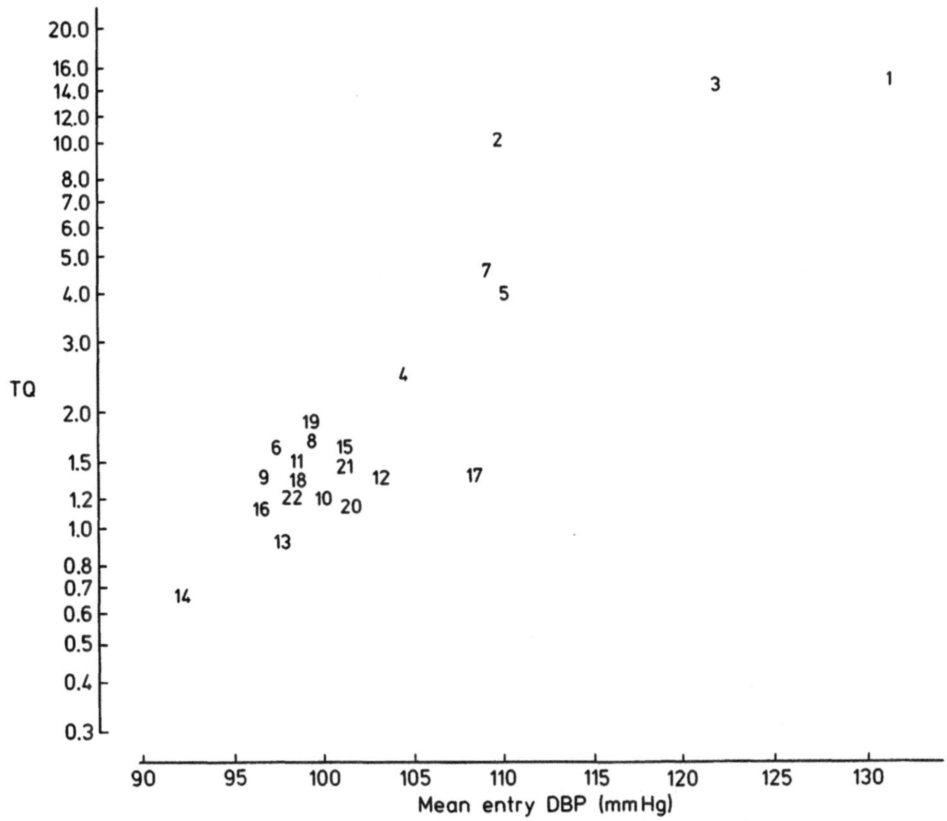

Fig. 2. Relationship between the therapeutic quotient (*TQ*) and mean entry diastolic blood pressure (*DBP*) in different therapeutic trials (1–22). TQ is calculated as the ratio of event rates in treated and untreated (controls) patients. The *number* refer to the trials as listed in Table 2. The higher the initial blood pressures, the better the effects of treatment (and the prognosis), as compared with the untreated patients. A TQ value of 1.0 means that there is no difference in this respect between treated and untreated groups. TQ values below 1.0 indicate that the treated groups are worse off than the control groups

values. Although in some instances the actual values are only approximations, the trend is clear.

This phenomenon is not unexpected. It is the natural consequence of the fact that the risk of hypertension itself is an exponential function, as shown by epidemiologic observations, an example of which is given in Fig. 1. Obviously, the higher the risk, the more the prognosis can be improved by treatment; conversely, if a risk is only slightly elevated, prognosis can be improved only marginally by eliminating the risk. By the same token, when studying the effects of treatment in mild hypertension, the numbers of subjects (the sample size) required to demonstrate these effects grow exponentially with decreasing pressures, as pointed out earlier (STRASSER 1980). The limits of demonstrability of treatment effects in mild hypertension are thus rapidly reached, leaving the perplexed with the issue whether there is no demonstrable treatment effect or no effect at all—clearly, a classic example of a semantic argument.

In conclusion, therapeutic trials in mild hypertension confirmed that the lower the pretreatment blood pressure, the less the patient's prognosis will improve under the influence of drug treatment. Mild hypertension (90–100 mmHg diastolic blood pressure) is a zone of marginal differences between the prognosis of treated and untreated patients.

3.5 Comments on the Meaning of Marginal Effects

It may be useful to translate the somewhat abstract and academic concept of PER into the colloquial language of medical practice. As an example, a PER value of 0.21 (Australian trial, 1980, item 10 in Table 2) means that 2.1 events (fatal and nonfatal strokes and infarctions) were prevented per 1000 patient-years of treatment. In other terms, the gain equals one prevented event per 500 patient-years, or, out of a group of 500 patients treated, each year only 1 would enjoy the benefit of having avoided an infarction or a stroke.

In still other terms, having in mind the long-term perspectives of hypertension treatment, in the course of say 20 years only 25 cases of infarction or stroke could be prevented in a group of 500 patients with mild hypertension. A practising physician having 40 patients with mild hypertension among his clientele would have the opportunity of "seeing" one prevented event among these patients every 12–13 years. Expressed as benefits, these probabilities are discouragingly low and do not seem to justify drug treatment in mild hypertension.

However, the same probabilities can be expressed inversely, as the risk of nontreatment, i.e., if therapy is withheld. Still taking the results of the Australian trial for basis of the estimates, a patient with mild hypertension would have the odds of 1:5000 of developing a fatal or nonfatal infarction or stroke within the next year, if left untreated. This does not seem to be a negligible risk. It is of the same order of magnitude as the risk of smoking 20 cigarettes per day. Although it is four times lower than that of a fatal accident for motorcyclists, it is approximately 30 times higher than the risk of a fatal accident for car drivers (STRASSER 1986).

An epidemiologist may have still another view of the same phenomenon. Assuming a prevalence rate of 5% in the general population (mild hypertension is a very common condition), the number of "events" potentially prevented by pharmacotherapy of mild hypertension amounts to 5000 per year for a population of 20 million, that of a medium-sized country. This is a radically different interpretation of the same underlying fact.

In conclusion, the marginal effects of drug treatment in mild hypertension may be interpreted in a number of different ways. Cautious considerations from multiple viewpoints are needed when making a clinical descision on the basis of available scientific information on the prognosis of treatment of untreated mild hypertension. Not all elements of such a decision are ponderable.

4 Special Issues

4.1 Hypertension Treatment in Stroke Survivors

Elevated blood pressure is a powerful risk factor for stroke (WELIN et al. 1987). Stroke definitely occurs less frequently in treated than in untreated hypertensive patients, as shown in Table 2. However, the question arises whether the prognosis of hypertensive patients who have already suffered a stroke will be improved with antihypertensive therapy. It may be assumed that such treatment will preserve the patient from a second, perhaps fatal stroke. On the other hand, it may also be assumed that lowering of (elevated) blood pressure in a patient with severely impaired cerebral circulation will further jeopardize the perfusion of brain tissue. Few studies have been carried out in this domain, and the problem seems to be unresolved.

CARTER (1970) studied 97 hypertensive patients surviving an ischemic-type stroke. Mortality rates at the end of 2–5 years of follow-up were 26% in the treated and 46% in the untreated group; the rates of nonfatal recurrences were 14% in the treated and 23% in the controls. However, the prognosis did not improve in elderly patients.

BEEVERS et al. (1973) reported that in a group of 162 hypertensive patients who had recovered from stroke, the recurrence rate of stroke was closely related to the adequacy of control of hypertension.

The Hypertension-Stroke Cooperative Study Group (1974) observed 452 stroke survivors with blood pressures 140–220 over 90–115 mmHg for a mean period of 3 years. Half the patients received antihypertensive drug treatment, and half received placebo. While, as expected, congestive heart failure occurred less frequently in the treated group, there was no difference in the rates of stroke recurrences in the two groups; this finding can also be interpreted as an incentive for giving antihypertensive treatment to stroke patients to improve their prognosis in general, regardless of the prognosis concerning recurrent stroke.

4.2 Does the Treatment of Mild Hypertension Prevent Myocardial Infarction?

It has been stated repeatedly (MacMahon et al. 1986b; Rose 1987; Weber 1987) and with disappointment that the treatment of mild hypertension reduces only slightly, if at all, the incidence of coronary heart disease. The overall reduction of myocardial infarction incidence rates in the mild hypertension trials seems to be around 9%. The question arises: is this unexpectedly little? Calculations show that this finding should not be surprising. In mild hypertension trials, by definition, blood pressure reductions are slight; the corresponding reduction of the risk of coronary heart disease cannot be great. For example, in the Framingham study (Gordon et al. 1971) the difference between the risk of myocardial infarction at 180 and at 160 mmHg systolic blood pressure is 15%; according to the Israel Civil Servants Study (Medalie and Goldbourt 1973) an approximately 20% difference in myocardial infarction incidence should be expected between systolic blood pressures of 175 and 160 mmHg. In the Italian study (Capocaccia et al. 1980) there is a 9% difference in the risk of myocardial infarction occurring at 180 compared with 160 mmHg. This latter figure is equal to the values observed, as mentioned, in the mild hypertension trials in general.

It should be added that patients on placebo treatment participating in trials run lower risks of morbid events than persons with similar characteristics who are not study participants. Lower than usual incidence rates of coronary heart disease were observed in, among others, the clofibrate primary prevention trial (Committee of Principal Investigators 1978). Due to such a nonspecific effect of care through trial, the observed differences between actively treated and control groups can become factitiously small.

In conclusion, the slight improvement of prognosis regarding myocardial infarction observed in *mild* hypertension trials is consistent with the modest magnitude of blood pressure reductions. Additionally our ability to demonstrate benefit may be mitigated by the positive effects of participation in a trial which affects placebo-treatment patients.

4.3 Can Treatment Worsen the Prognosis in Mild Hypertension?

In Fig. 2 one value of the therapeutic quotient is below 1.0, in other words, actively treated patients were worse off in this particular group than placebo-treated patients. While there are several explanations of this phenomenon, including the possibility of direct side-effects of the drugs used, the question arises whether lowering of blood pressure per se below a certain threshold may be harmful. Some researchers (Anderson 1978; Cruickshank et al. 1987a, b) are challenging the assertion, "the lower the pressure, the better."

Because, as shown, in the range of mild hypertension the risk attributable to blood pressure is relatively small, and because only few myocardial infarctions are prevented by treating mild hypertension, the certitude of the conclusions drawn in this pressure range is diminished, unless the number of observations is very great. This word of caution should be taken into account in the considerations that follow. By re-examining some of the unsmoothed data from the Framingham study, ANDERSON (1978) concluded that, unlike systolic pressures, diastolic pressures below about 90 mmHg fit poorly the "the lower, the better" model and have little or no prognostic significance. More recently, CRUICKSHANK et al. (1987a, b) found a J-shaped relationship between diastolic pressures achieved by treatment and death from myocardial infarction and stroke in the lower blood pressure tertile of 939 patients; the mean diastolic pressure in this group was slightly below 80 mmHg, with 11 fatal infarctions, while in the middle tertile mean diastolic blood pressure was 87 mmHg, with 9 fatal infarctions. Obviously, the numbers of events were rather small.

The assumption of a J-shaped relationship between the incidence of myocardial infarction (and of stroke) may or may not be correct; the information seems to be insufficient. However, it is judicious to assume that, as can be concluded also from Fig. 2, the prognosis of hypertensive patients may not be improved by lowering diastolic pressure below 90 mmHg Overtreatment does not improve prognosis.

5 Therapeutic Attitudes

Having reviewed the prognosis of treated and untreated hypertension at various levels of blood pressure, the practical implications of the findings should be discussed as well. There is no doubt that drug treatment with antihypertensive agents improves considerably the prognosis of patients with severe and moderate blood pressure elevations. Whether such treatment is appropriate in patients with mild hypertension remains to be clarified. "To treat or not to treat?" has been the topic of many general reviews and editorials, and a number of symposia have been dedicated to this subject. However, we do not think that it is appropriate to ask the question in such a categorical mode. Pharmacotherapy, though by far the most efficient in lowering high blood pressure, is not the only way of treatment. Even simple observation by the physician may have a therapeutic effect (although sometimes a negative one). Therefore, instead of the categorical alternative, the question to be asked is rather: How to treat?

A joint committee of the World Health Organization and the International Society of Hypertension has repeatedly formulated the guidelines for the definition of treatment of mild hypertension. These guidelines are based on the best available knowledge at the time and are being revised periodically, in the light of newly arising information and experience.

The 1986 Guidelines (WHO/ISH Mild Hypertension Liaison Committee 1986) are summed up in Fig. 3. They take into account two dimensions: average blood pressure levels obtained by repeated measurements (important because of short-term blood pressure fluctuations) *and* time trends, assessed through 3-month (6-month) observation periods. They do not take into account the time during which blood pressure has been elevated before treatment, a value rarely available but probably important for secondary organ damage and prognosis. Thus, in mild blood pressure elevations, no immediate decision is recom-

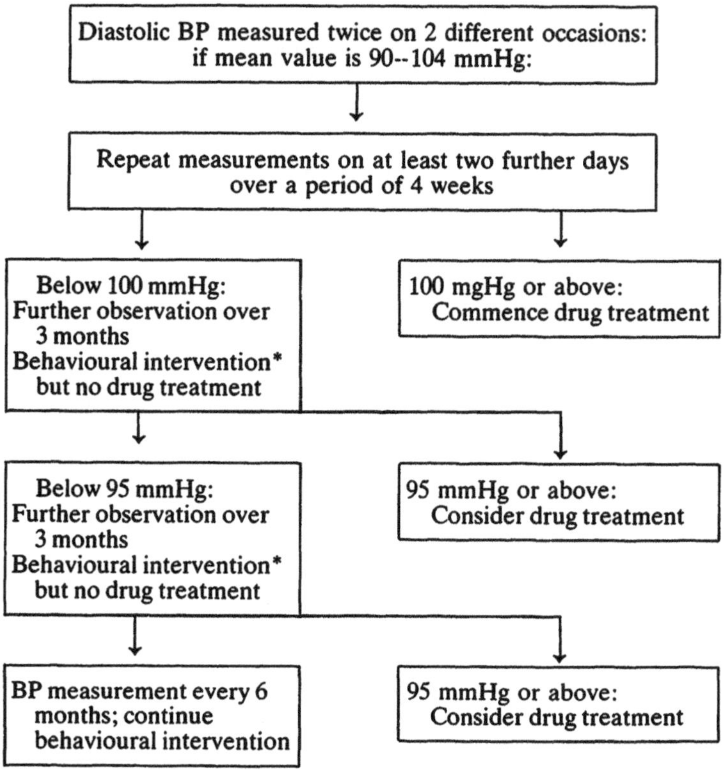

**Behavioural intervention*: Advice against smoking; dietary intervention, preferably in a structured programme, to lower the blood pressure, to lower serum cholesterol, and to control diabetes.

Fig. 3. Guidelines for the treatment of hypertension. (From WHO/ISH Mild Hypertension Liaison Committee 1986)

mended; the choice of treatment is a process that takes time. Behavioral intervention is recommended in all cases. It consists of advice against smoking and dietary intervention, preferably in a structured program, to lower blood pressure, to lower serum cholesterol, and to control diabetes. The (somewhat arbitrary) blood pressure value that should trigger off the adjunction of antihypertensive drug treatment is an average value of 95 mmHg after one or two 3-month observation periods.

For details, such as the influence of age, systolic pressure, or choice of drugs, the reader is referred to the full text of the guidelines (WHO/ISH Mild Hypertension Liaison Committee 1986). These seem to fit reasonably well the conclusions derived from the mild hypertension trials analyzed here, although the conclusions may vary according to the philosophy of the person who is interpreting the facts. It seems, however, that one more concept should be introduced, that of optimization. The question from the 1980s (How to treat?) should evolve in the 1990s into: How to treat best?

The optimal ways of treatment not only of mild but of any degree of hypertension, still have to be defined. At present, with the very wide gamut of antihypertensive drugs available, multiple choices and combinations are possible, and guindance is needed, especially for the practising physician, on how to make the best choice. But what does "best" mean? Is it treatment leading to the greatest lowering of blood pressure at the least cost in terms of side effects? Or at the cheapest expenditure for treatment? Or measured by the longest life expectancy? Or resulting in the best "quality of life"? Or should be patient be asked to choose a combination of all these criteria that would come closest to his or her own individual value system?

Introducing the concept to optimization into the treatment of hypertension thus brings up many new questions. It is unlikely that these could be answered by further clinical trials of the classic type. Imaginative innovations are needed.

6 Conclusions and Summary

Effective pharmacotherapy of hypertension has developed only during the past few decades. Clinical observations from the prepharmacotherapeutic era provide information on the natural history of hypertension and document well the poor prognosis of severe, untreated hypertension. Epidemiological studies have established the (exponential) relationship between blood pressure values and the probability of occurrence of complications; this relationship is somewhat less clear when getting closer to the "normal" blood pressure range.

The prognosis of severe hypertension is completely changed with treatment. Today the crux of the problem of hypertension therapeutics is whether the prognosis of patients with *mild* hypertension is improved by treatment. To answer this question, numerous controlled trials have been carried out during the past 2 decades. A summary to their results shows that, as may have been expected, the improvement of prognosis corresponds more or less to the risk attributable to hypertension. With decreasing risk, the prognostic benefit of drug treatment fades out; the treated individuals' probability of faring better than their untreated peers dwindles.

As there is no clear cutting point between "high" and "normal" blood pressure but rather a zone of transition, there can be no clear distinction between the prognosis of treated and untreated patients in this pressure range. A synthesis of the outcomes of various therapeutic trials indicates that this zone of transition is situated around 170–150 over 95–90 mmHg, values included in the range of mild hypertension.

While the patients' risk attributable to hypertension is being diminished by antihypertensive treatment, the individual's prognosis as regards cardiovascular diseases depends on a mosaic of risk factors. The less severe the initial blood pressure elevation, the greater the *relative* impact of the other cardiovascular risk factors such as lipid profile and smoking on the individual's prognosis. To improve the prognosis of a subject with mild hypertension beyond the limits of benefits achievable by antihypertensive drug therapy, all cardiovascular risk factors present in the particular individual should be dealt with.

References

Amery A, Birkenhager W, Brixko P, Bulpitt C, Clement D, Deruyttere M, de Schaepdryver A, et al. (1985a) Mortality and morbidity results from the European Working Party on High Blood Pressure in the Elderly Trial. Lancet 1:1349–1354

Amery A, Birkenhager W, Brixko P, Bulpitt C, Clement D, de Leeuw P, de Plaen JF, et al. (1985b) Influence of hypotensive drug treatment in the elderly hypertensives: study terminating events in the Trial of the European Working Party on High Blood Pressure in the Elderly. J Hypertens [Suppl 3] 3:S501–S508

Amery A, Birkenhager W, Brixko R, Bulpitt C, Clement D, Deruyttere M, de Schaepdryver A, et al. (1986) Efficacy of antihypertensive drug treatment according to age, sex, blood pressure, and previous cardiovascular disease in patients over the age of 60. Lancet 2:589–592

Anderson RW (1978) Re-examination of some of the Framingham blood-pressure data. Lancet 2:1139–1141

Bechgaard P (1946) Arterial hypertension. A follow-up study of one thousand hypertensives. Nyt Nordisk Copenhagen

Beevers DG, Fairman MJ, Hamilton M, Harpur JE (1973) Antihypertensive treatment and the course of established cerebral vascular disease. Lancet 1:1407–1409

Bing RF, Heagerty AM, Russell GI, Swales JD, Thurston H (1986) Prognosis in malignant hypertension. J Hypertens [Suppl 6] 4:S42–S44

Boissel JP, Moleur P (1987) Problems with intervention trials in hypertension. Am Heart J 114:1018–1024

Burnett CF, Evans JA (1955) Drug therapy in hypertension with haemorrhagic retinitis. N Engl J Med 253:395–398

Capocaccia R, Farchi G, Moriotti S, Menotti A, Verdecchia A (1980) Manuale del rischio coranorico. Associazione Nationale Centri per le Malattie Cardiovascolari, Udine

Carter AB (1970) Hypertension therapy in stroke survivors. Lancet 1:485–489

Committee of Principal Investigators (1978) A co-operative trial in the primary prevention of ischaemic heart disease using clofibrate. Br Heart J 40:1069–1118

Coope J, Warrender TS (1986) Randomised trial of treatment of hypertension in elderly patients in primary care. Br Med J 293:1145–1151

Co-operative Randomized Controlled Trial (1973) Control of moderately raised blood pressure. Br Med J 3:434–436

Cruickshank JM, Thorp JM, Zacharias FJ (1987a) Benefits and potential harm of lowering high blood pressure. Lancet 1:581–584

Cruickshank JM, Pennert K, Sorman AE, Thorp JM, Zacharias FM (1987b) Low mortality from all causes, including myocardial infarction in well controlled hypertensives treated with beta-blocker plus other antihypertensives. J Hypertens 5:489–498

Culter JA, Furberg CD (1965) Drug treatment trials in hypertension: A review. Prev Med 14:499–518

Frant R, Groen J (1950) Prognosis of vascular hypertension. A nine year follow-up study of four hundred and eighteeen cases. Arch Intern Med 85:727–750

Gordon T, Kannel WB (1973) Coronary risk handbook. Estimating risk of coronary heart disease in daily practice. American Heart Assoc, New York

Gordon T, Sorlie P, Kannel WB (1971) Coronary heart disease, atherothrombotic brain infarction, intermittent claudication—multivariate analysis of some factors related to their incidence, Framingham Study, 16-year follow-up, sect 27. US GPO, Washington

Hamilton M, Thompson EN, Wisnievski TKM (1964) The role of blood pressure control in preventing complications of hypertension. Lancet 1:235–238

Helgeland A (1980) Treatment of mild hypertension: A five year controlled drug trial. Am J Med 69:725–732
Hypertension Detection and Follow-Up Program Cooperative Group (1979) Five year finding of the Hypertension Detection and Follow-Up Program. I. Reduction in mortality of persons with high blood pressure, including mild hypertension. JAMA 242:2562–2571
Hypertension Detection and Follow-Up Program Cooperative Group (1982a) Five year findings of the Hypertension Detection and Follow-Up Program. III. Reduction in stroke incidence among persons with high blood pressure. JAMA 247:633–638
Hypertension Detection and Follow-Up Program Cooperative Group (1982b) The effect of treatment on mortality in "mild" hypertension. Results of the Hypertension Detection and Follow-Up Program. N Engl J Med 307:976–980
Hypertension Detection and Follow-Up Prgram Cooperative Group (1984) Effect of stepped care treatment on the incidence of myocardial information and angina pectoris. 5-year findings of the Hypertension Detection and Follow-Up Program. Hypertension [Suppl 1] 6:198–206
Hypertension Stroke Cooperative Study Group (1974) Effect of antihypertensive treatment on stroke recurrence. JAMA 229:409–418
Italian Research Group (1986) Seven Countries Study: Twenty-five year incidence and prediction of coronary heart disease in two Italian rural population studies. Acta Cardiol (Brux) 41:283–299
Kannel WB, Dowber TR (1974) Stroke risk handbook. Estimating risk of stroke in daily practice. American Heart Association, New York
Kannel WB, Gordon T (eds) (1973) The Framingham Study: An epidemiological investigation of cardiovascular disease. DHEW, Washington (Publication no (NIH) 74)
Keys A (1980) Seven countries. A multivariate analysis of death and coronary heart disease. Harvard University Press, Cambridge/MA
Labarthe D (1986) Mild hypertension: the question of treatment. Annu Rev Public Health 7:193–215
Macmahon SW, Cutler JA, Furberg CD, Payne GH (1986a) The effects of drug treatment for hypertension on morbidity and mortality from cardiovascular disease: A review of randomized controlled trials. Prog Cardiovasc Dis [Suppl 1] 39:99–118
MacMahon SW, Culter JA, Neaton JD, Furberg CD, Cohen JD, Kuller LH, Stamler J (1986b) Relationship of blood pressure to coronary and stroke morbidity and mortality in clinical trials and epidemiological studies. J Hypertens [Suppl 6] 4:S14–S17
Management Committee (1980) The Australian Therapeutic Trial in Mild Hypertension. Lancet 1:1261–1267
McFate Smith W (1977) Treatment of mild hypertension. Results of a ten-year intervention trial. US Public Health Service Co-operative Study Group. Circ Res [Suppl 1] 40:98–105
McMichael J, Murphy EA (1955) Methonium treatment of severe and malignant hypertension. J Chronic Dis 1:527–535
Medalie JH, Goldbourt M (1973) Estimated probabilities of men aged 40 and over developing a first myocardial infarction in five years. Israel Ischemic Heart Disease Study. National Heart Institute USA, Bethesda, Ministry of Health Israel, Hadassah Medical Organization, Jerusalem
Medical Research Council Working Party (1985) MRC trial of treatment of mild hypertension: principal results. Br Med J 291:97–104
Miall WE, Greenberg G, Brennan PJ (1983) Controlled clinical trials in mild hypertension. Acta Med Scand [Suppl] 686:67–74
Morgan TO, Adams WR, Hodgson M, Gibberd RW (1980) Failure of therapy to improve prognosis in elderly males with hypertension. Med J Aust 2:27–31
Multiple Risk Factor Intervention Trial Research Group (1982) Multiple Risk Factor Intervention Trial. Risk factor changes and mortality results. JAMA 248:1465–1477
Page IH (1946) Arterial hypertension. In: Stroud WD (ed) The diagnosis and treatment of cardiovascular disease. Davis, Philadelphia, pp 1413–1453
Perry HM (1977) Treatment of mild hypertension. Preliminary results of a two-year

feasibility study. Circ Res [Suppl 1] 40:180–187
Robertson JIS (1987) Hypertension and coronary risk: Possible adverse effects of antihypertensive drugs. Am Heart J 114:1051–1054
Rose G (1987) Review of primary prevention trials. Am Heart J 114:1014–1017
Sacks HD, Charlmers TC, Ancona Berk A, Reitman D (1985) Should mild hypertension be treated? An attempted meta-analysis of the clinical trials. M Sinai J Med (NU) 52:265–270
Smithwick RH (1955) Hypertensive vascular disease. Results and indications for splanchnicectomy. J Chronic Dis 1:477–496
Society of Actuaries (1959) Build and blood pressure study. Society of Actuaries, Chicago
Sprackling ME, Mitchell JRA, Short AH, Watt G (1981) Blood pressure reduction in the elderly: a randomized controlled trial of methyldopa. Br Med J 283:1151–1153
Stamler R, Stamler J (1983) "Mild" hypertension: risks and strategy for control. Prim Cardiol 9(10):150–166; 9(11):12–25
Strasser T (1980) Hypertension related to health care-research priorities. WHO Regional Office for Europe, Copenhagen (EURO reports and studies, vol 32)
Strasser T (1982) Research policies in mild hypertension and the role of the WHO/ISH Liaison Committee, Clin Sci 63:427s–430s
Strasser T (1986) Mild hypertension studies: A synthetic view. In: Hofmann H, Schrey A (ed) Bluthochdruck: Prävention kardiovaskulärer Risiken—Control of arterial hypertension in the prevention of cardiovascular disease. Schattauer, Stuttgant
Strasser T (1987) Inferences from drug trials: Risks, probabilities, ethics and decision taking. In: Strasser T, Ganten D (eds) Mild hypertension: From drug trials to practice. Raven, New York
Strasser T, Raymond L, Jeanneret O (1983) Prévention cardio-vasculaire: Limites de la pharmacothérapie de l'hypertension artérielle. Med Soc Prev 28:216–217
Veterans Administration Cooperative Study Group on Antihypertensive Agents (1967) Effects of treatment on morbidity of hypertension. Results in patients with diastolic blood pressures averaging 115 through 129 mmHg. JAMA 202:116–122
Veterans Administration Cooperative Study Group on Antihypertensive Agents (1970) Effects of treatment on morbidity in hypertension. II. Results in patients with diastolic blood pressure averaging 90 through 114 mmHg. JAMA 213:1143–1152
Weber MA (1987) Cardiovascular outcomes of treating high blood pressure. Am Heart J 114:964–968
Welin L, Swärdsudd K, Wilhelmsen L, Larsson B, Tibblin G (1987) Analysis of risk factors for stroke in a cohort of men born in 1913. N Engl J Med 317:521–526
WHO/ISH Mild Hypertension Liaison Committee (1982) Trials of the treatment of mild hypertension. An interim analysis. Lancet 1:149–156
WHO/ISH Mild Hypertension Liaison Committee (1988) 1986 guidelines for the treatment of mild hypertension. Memorandum from a WHO/ISH meeting. Bull WHO 64:31–35
Wilcox RG, Mitchell JRA, Hampton JR (1986) Treatment of high blood pressure: should clinical practice be based on results of clinical trials? Br Med J 293:433–437
Wolfe FW, Lindeman RD (1966) Effects of treatment in hypertension. Results of a controlled study. J Chronic Dis 19:227–240

CHAPTER 22

Toxicity Testing of Antihypertensive Drugs

D.A. EICHLER and D.P. CLOUGH

CONTENTS

1 Introduction

The routine methods employed in the toxicity testing of pharmaceuticals are described and discussed in many textbooks and other publications. Nevertheless, this contribution commences with a brief account of the current methods and principles in order to provide a background for the discussion of a number of findings attributed to an exaggeration of the pharmacological activity of antihypertensive agents during toxicity studies. These findings are either reported in the scientific literature or, in some instances, were made in our own laboratories. On rare occasions it has been necessary to refer to the Federal Drug Administration's (FDA) *Summary basis of approval*, reflecting the problem of the pharmaceutical industry's general diffidence towards the open publication of toxicological data.

Some changes are clearly attributable to the mode of action of antihypertensives and are recorded frequently during toxicity studies. They include tachycardia, to which dogs administered vasodilators are especially sensitive; bradycardia as induced by β-adrenergic antagonists; and polydipsia, polyuria and electrolyte imbalance when testing diuretics. Activities such as these are familiar to the cardiovascular pharmacologist examining relatively low dose levels over short periods. However, when high doses of some classes of antihypertensive agents are administered daily, often over extended periods, during toxicity testing, additional changes may be observed which are frequently less predictable. This chapter considers a number of such changes.

2 Toxicity Testing

The modern methods of toxicity testing for pharmaceuticals are well-established. They are accepted by all major regulatory authorities, and national guidelines differ mainly in such details as the duration of multidose general toxicity studies required for a given duration of dosing in humans (see Sect. 2.1) or the precise design of reproductive toxicity studies (see Sect. 2.4). Nevertheless, during product development for international registration, care must be taken to ensure that these variations are recognised and studies designed to prevent financially and ethically undesirable duplication. In addition to "regulatory" toxicology, mechanistic investigations are frequently undertaken, often requiring a multidisciplinary approach, to elucidate the underlying causes of adverse reactions. As discussed in Sects. 3 and 4 these are often unexpected, unusual and possibly linked to the pharmacological properties of the drug. This section describes the various toxicity studies which provide core information during the testing of antihypertensives and other pharmaceuticals developed for long-term therapy. In Sect. 2.6 the problems of predictivity are briefly discussed.

2.1 Multidose General Toxicity Studies

The repeated dose studies are designed to reveal target organ toxicity by administration from 2 or 4 weeks to 6, 12 or 18 months. They are undertaken sequentially, commencing with the shorter studies, and are closely phased with the clinical programme to ensure appropriate animal safety data are available before each major increment in human exposure. To obtain marketing authorisation in EEC countries, the intended duration of dosing to humans must be supported by multidose general toxicity studies, in rats and a non-rodent species, according to the following scheme:

Humans	*Animals* (two species)
Single/several dose(s) in 1 day	14 days
Repeated up to 7 days	4 weeks

Humans	*Animals* (two species)
Repeated up to 30 days	13 weeks
Repeated beyond 30 days	26 weeks

Japanese and American guidelines are more stringent and call for 12-month studies of drugs intended for long-term use. There is considerable debate among toxicologists about the usefulness of general toxicity studies beyond 26 weeks. LUMLEY and WALKER (1986), in a survey of data obtained directly from pharmaceutical companies, concluded that significant new findings are rarely made in studies of greater duration, but FREDERICK (1986) stated counter-arguments to support Canada's requirement for longer-term studies.

The laboratory rat is invariably chosen for multidose testing because of its well-documented responses to a wide variety of chemicals and its regulatory acceptability. For practical, scientific and historical reasons, the choice of a non-rodent is generally limited to the dog and several primate species. The route of administration is that proposed for humans, and any deviation from this must be supported by sound arguments. An example is the oral dosing of a drug proposed for topical application to humans which is known to be significantly absorbed through the skin.

Three dose levels are usually examined and chosen after considering such data as the reactions observed in previous studies, pharmacokinetic data and the intended clinical dose range. In the shorter term studies, the highest dose level is set, where practicable, to induce marked adverse effects in order to identify target organs at an early stage in the development process, and thus alert those conducting clinical trials. However, in longer term studies, the highest dose is set at a lower level to avoid marked toxicity, especially premature death, and to allow the expression of more insidious effects which may attend prolonged exposure. In multidose studies, the low dose level is usually set as a small multiple of the intended clinical dose, while the intermediate is the approximate geometric mean of the low and high dose levels. Safety margins can thus be defined by reference to the highest dose level showing no adverse effects, although differences in pharmacokinetic parameters between humans and the toxicity test species may make a comparison of other indices of systemic exposure more realistic.

The treatment groups, including vehicle controls, contain equal numbers of both sexes and are of an appropriate size to reveal toxic effects and allow assessment of their reversibility. Monitoring of the animals typically includes clinical condition, behaviour, body weight, food and water consumption, heart rate, electrocardiography, ophthalmoscopy, haematology, blood and urine biochemistry, urine microscopy and blood drug levels. Detailed autopsies are carried out on intercurrent deaths and at the end of the dosing and reversibility phases, and a comprehensive list of tissue samples is examined by light microscopy for pathological changes. Additional investigations, for example, the measurement of blood pressure or hormone levels or the use of the electron microscope may be appropriate in specific circumstances. This recognises the need to obtain as much relevant information as possible from these expensive and time-consuming experiments.

The principles and methods of multidose general toxicity testing are discussed at length by CHAN et al. (1984) and STEVENS and GALLO (1984).

2.2 Carcinogenicity Testing

An assessment of carcinogenic potential is usually required when a drug is intended for use for more than 6 months. However, even if the dosing regime is restricted, testing may be indicated if there are positive findings during mutagenicity studies (see Sect. 2.3), other members of the same therapeutic class are carcinogenic, the molecular structure suggests carcinogenic properties, or the drug or a metabolite is retained for a long period.

The experiments are designed to reveal carcinogenic potential during continuous administration by the route of proposed use over the life span of two species. For practical purposes, this restricts the choice to rodents with laboratory life spans of approximately 2 years, although circumstances may necessitate a supplementary study in a non-rodent species. Three dose levels are examined routinely, the highest being no greater than the maximum tolerated dose to ensure life-span exposure, the lowest a small multiple of the therapeutic dose, and the intermediate the approximate geometric mean.

Minimum group sizes of 50 animals per sex per dose level and 100 per sex as controls, with satellite groups for monitoring plasma drug levels and other laboratory investigations, are used. General health, body weight and food consumption are monitored regularly, but invasive investigations are confined to the satellite groups to avoid prejudicing the principal objective of investigating carcinogenic potential.

Careful autopsy and comprehensive histopathological investigations provide the essential data. All non-neoplastic, preneoplastic and neoplastic changes are recorded. Conclusions are drawn concerning the carcinogenic risk to humans not only from an increased incidence of tumours in treated animals but also taking into account such factors as the type of tumour, background incidences for the laboratory and strain, and the pharmacological properties of the candidate drug.

A more detailed account of the methods of carcinogenicity testing is given by ROBENS et al. (1984).

2.3 Mutagenicity Testing

Testing for mutagenicity is undertaken to reveal potential mutagenic hazards and to provide, relatively quickly and cost effectively, evidence of carcinogenic risk at an early stage in drug development. The close relationship between mutagens and carcinogens was recognised by AMES et al. (1973).

Genetic damage is known to occur at the level of individual genes or by inducing structural or numerical changes in the chromosomes. A variety of in vitro and in vivo tests are available which, if used in a correct combination, can reveal mutagenic potential. Four main categories of tests are conveniently recognised:

(a) Tests for gene mutations in prokaryotic systems (e.g. Ames test/*Salmonella typhimurium*);
(b) Tests for gene mutations in eukaryotic systems (e.g. yeasts);
(c) Tests for chromosomal aberrations in mammalian cell culture (e.g. human lymphocytes);
(d) Tests for genetic damage in vivo (e.g. micronucleus test in mice).

The EEC guidelines recommend that a test be performed from each of the four categories, and other major regulatory authorities from at least the first three categories. A considerable variety of mutagenicity tests of varying sensitivity and reliability is available. The interested reader is referred to BRUSICK (1984) for a comprehensive review of the principles, methods, data evaluation and approaches to risk assessment in this field.

2.4 Reproductive Toxicology

Examination of the effects of drugs on the wide variety of reproductive processes is an integral part of preclinical safety evaluation. Adverse changes are sought with respect to spermatogenesis and oogenesis, the ability to mate successfully, implantation, uterine nutrition, embryonic and fetal development, parturition, lactation, postnatal development and the reproductive capabilities of the offspring. These phases are tested in a short series of studies, the first of which examines all the above processes in rats, in variable detail, by dosing throughout gamete maturation, mating, pregnancy and lactation. The second study concentrates on teratogenicity: exposure to the drug during the period of embryonic development is examined in the rat and a non-rodent. The third study looks for adverse effects in the fetus and neonate during administration to rats in late pregnancy and during lactation.

The first in the above series, known as a fertility and general reproductive performance study, is of particular value in assessing fertility, mating activity and implantation. A proportion of the females are killed in late pregnancy to afford a gross assessment of effects on the uterine contents. The remaining females are allowed to deliver and suckle their offspring, and dosing of the mothers ceases at weaning (day 21 postpartum). The pups are observed for development, behavioural effects and their ability to reproduce.

The disadvantages of the fertility and general reproductive performance study include the inability to associate changes such as pre- and postnatal developmental effects with the exposure of a specific phase within the overall reproductive process. Moreover, treatment of the female before and during mating may enhance detoxification mechanisms, so reducing the capacity of a drug to damage the embryo or fetus. In view of such considerations, studies in pregnant rats and a non-rodent species, usually the rabbit, in which drug administration is conducted only during the most sensitive period of organogenesis, are considered essential to demonstrate teratogenic potential. Two species are routinely used, as responses may vary between species and strains. For example, thalidomide is markedly teratogenic in rabbits but not in rats or mice.

The effects of a drug on the fetus in late pregnancy and during lactation is tested in the rat in a peri- and postnatal study. Development and behavioural tests and the reproductive capabilities of the offspring may be studied.

The study designs described above are essentially those recommended in the United States of America and EEC countries. Japan differs principally in the dosing period of the first study (where this stops in early pregnancy), and an assessment of effects on the offspring is conducted as part of the rat teratology and peri- and postnatal studies. The total information obtained by Western and Japanese studies is broadly similar, and the data are mutually acceptable on scientific grounds.

As with multidose general toxicity studies, a minimum of three dose levels are compared with controls. However, the highest dose level should not cause marked maternal toxicity as this frequently induces secondary effects on the uterine contents or offspring which may erroneously lead to the conclusion that the drug was directly responsible for adverse findings.

The field of reproductive toxicology and the test methods employed are reviewed by DIXON and HALL (1984) and MANSON et al. (1984).

2.5 Miscellaneous Studies

Tests for acute (single dose) toxicity are undertaken in the early stages of drug development. For submissions in EEC countries it is only necessary to undertake these in two rodent species, but the requirement for additional data from a non-rodent species is expected by some regulatory authorities. Acute testing may indicate the probable effects of accidental or deliberate poisoning (and therefore its management), may assist in setting test dose levels for the first multidose study, and is important for hazard classification in relation to handling the drug substance. Skin irritancy and sensitisation studies in animals are also useful for classifying potential hazards, while parenteral formulations must be tested for local irritancy. Special tests for phototoxicity and photosensitisation may be of particular value for certain therapeutic classes, for example, non-steroidal, anti-inflammatory drugs.

Many drugs are believed to cause immunotoxic effects in humans and animals, and evidence of disturbances to the immune system can be observed during routine toxicity testing, for example, by alterations in lymphoid organ (spleen, thymus) weights and histology. However, adverse clinical effects in humans are ascribed to immunotoxicity frequently enough to stimulate the search for more precise screening systems. Developments in this field have been reviewed recently in detail by DESCOTES (1986).

2.6 Predictivity

It is a fact that many adverse effects encountered in humans cannot be predicted by conducting animal studies as currently practised. This is particularly so with respect to the subjective symptoms which may be reported, such as headache, chest pain or nausea, which animals cannot directly communicate to the experimenter. For such effects, data from clinical trials provide the only firm basis for determining the acceptability of a drug. Psychiatric effects present a similar and, frequently, closely related problem. Preclinical toxicity studies also fail to predict idiosyncratic responses. This may be either because research on a specific response has failed to demonstrate the effect in animals, or the response frequency is simply so low that statistical considerations preclude reliable detection.

There are, however, some examples of toxicity which were first observed in humans, were not of an idiosyncratic nature, and were reproduced subsequently in animals. The possibility of such a situation arising is minimised by careful study design and conduct and interpretation of the data. One important step that should be taken is to ensure adequate systemic exposure to the drug administered to a species with a metabolic pattern broadly comparable to humans. The necessary information should be available before choosing the non-rodent species for the chronic (≥ 6 months) studies which are pivotal to risk assessment.

Toxicity testing methods are under continuous review and subject to improvement wherever possible. Providing the studies are not regarded as "regulatory hurdles" to be overcome as quickly and as inexpensively as possible, preclinical toxicity studies will screen out potentially harmful compounds with a high degree of reliability, other than those giving rise to idiosyncratic reactions. When the data from all toxicity studies are assessed together with the safety pharmacology and clinical safety data for a drug which has reached the marketplace, considerable reassurance is afforded, which is further strengthened by appropriate postmarketing surveillance. However, before a solution to the problem of the non-predictivity of idiosyncratic reactions can be attained, further understanding is required of the reasons why only a very small proportion of the population is sensitive.

3 Expressions of Pharmacological Activity During General Toxicity Testing

This section describes examples of adverse effects ascribed to the pharmacological activity of agents under investigation in multidose general toxicity studies. The first part is concerned with a number of changes related to the kidneys induced by ACE inhibitors, and the second comprises a myocardial lesion commonly observed when testing vasodilators.

3.1 Renal Changes Associated with Angiotensin-Converting Enzyme Inhibitors

Functional and morphological renal changes have been reported during toxicity studies with ACE inhibitors in rodent and non-rodent species. Detailed information is available from a number of published studies for the marketed drugs, captopril and enalapril, and from our own experience with cilazapril (EICHLER, unpublished observations), which has completed its toxicological evaluation to satisfy international regulatory requirements for product registration. The breadth and depth of available information on the toxicology of other ACE inhibitors (e.g. SCH 31846, pentopril, quinapril, ramipril), however, are currently very variable. Nevertheless, sufficient data are accessible to support the argument that the renal findings discussed below commonly occur with this class of antihypertensive agents and result, in the main, from their pharmacological activity rather than by direct cytotoxicity.

3.1.1 Effects on Renal Tubule Integrity

Adverse morphological effects on the proximal tubules following repeated daily administration of ACE inhibitors in toxicity studies have been observed for captopril in rats (IMAI et al. 1981; HASHIMOTO et al. 1981), enalapril in dogs (BAGDON et al. 1985a; MACDONALD et al. 1987), pentopril in rats (GOODMAN et al. 1985), ramipril in rats (DONAUBAUER and MAYER 1988) and cilazapril in rats and marmosets. The effects range from minor changes, such as tubular dilatation and evidence of epithelial regeneration following earlier damage, to frank irreversible tubular necrosis. Such findings are commonly observed with a wide spectrum of dissimilar chemical agents (e.g. aminoglycoside and cephalosporin antibiotics, mercuric chloride, halogenated hydrocarbons) and are frequently due to direct cytotoxicity; this is unremarkable in view of the kidney's role as a major organ of concentration and elimination. However, it should be noted that the renal effects pertaining to ACE inhibitors occur at dose levels in animals far higher than those recommended for use in humans and therefore lack clinical significance.

The relationship between the mode of action of enalapril and renal tubule damage has been explored by MACDONALD et al. (1987). During routine toxicity testing it was observed that the dog is particularly sensitive, with an increasing severity of nephropathy occuring in multidose studies at 30 mg/kg per day and above. At a minimally nephropathic dose a pattern of proximal tubular necrosis is observed in which changes are recorded principally in the juxtamedullary region of the cortex. This contrasts to the pattern seen with many directly acting compounds in which damage occurs in the nephrons of the subcapsular region (MACDONALD et al. 1987). The investigators present data in which the daily administration of enalapril to dogs at 60 mg/kg for a week with or without physiological saline supplement demonstrates a marked reduction in the severity of tubular damage in the presence of saline. However, an increased incidence of animals with tubular basophilia (suggesting regeneration following an earlier injury) in the saline-supplemented group is observed. In single-dose experiments saline fails to exert a protective influence, while the incubation of enalapril with rabbit renal tubule tissue in an in vitro culture system indicates direct cytotoxicity. Based on the data from this series of studies, the investigators describe a two-component mechanism for the nephrotoxic action of enalapril in dogs. The first component comprises a direct cytotoxic effect by enalapril, and the second a response to the pharmacological action of the drug. During repeated application, the initial damage due to direct contact is exacerbated by the subsequent reductions in arterial pressure, possibly leading to ischaemic changes. If the fall in blood pressure is prevented by saline loading, the initial damage resolves spontaneously. Support for the second component is provided by BAGDON and BOKELMAN (1983) who showed that co-administration of hydrochlorothiazide to dogs results in a marked potentiation of the tubular damage. Also, BAGDON et al. (1985b) observed that rats, a species shown to be relatively insensitive to enalapril's renal action during routine toxicity studies, manifest adverse tubular changes when fed on a sodium-deficient diet. However, it is emphasised from the standpoint of enalapril's clinical safety that detectable renal impairment occurred neither in a 12-month toxicity study in the dog (BAGDON et al. 1985a) at a dose of 15 mg/kg per day (about 30-fold clinical dose) nor at any dose level in standard rat or primate toxicity studies (MACDONALD et al. 1987).

3.1.2 Effects on Blood Urea Levels

Uraemia was a consistent finding during our multidose toxicity studies with cilazapril in rodent and non-rodent species at dose levels greatly in excess of those ($\leq$0.1 mg/kg per day) administered to humans and is characteristic of other ACE inhibitors, as described below. Such a finding, particularly when accompanied by other indicators of renal impairment, often indicates directly induced nephropathy. Other indicators of nephropathy frequently include elevated plasma creatinine levels, decreased urine specific gravity and osmolality, and increased cellular content of the urine. However, as for the morphological changes of the proximal tubules discussed in Sect. 3.1.1, an alternative explanation must be sought for elevations of blood urea levels with ACE inhibitors when administered to animals, as they occur frequently in the absence of either direct (morphological) or indirect (body fluid indicators) evidence of renal perturbation in toxicity studies.

During the preclinical safety evaluation of cilazapril we observed that blood urea levels were elevated two- to fourfold over control values in the high dose groups (40–250 mg/kg per day) of all the multidose studies in rats and primates. Occasionally, they were also recorded in the mid-dose groups (4–125 mg/kg per day) of the rat studies. The absence of significant concurrent changes in renal function or morphology was a common feature. Onset of uraemia was characteristically early and maintained throughout the dosing period without a time-related increase in severity, and, where examined, the effect was rapidly reversible upon withdrawal of cilazapril administration. Recovery, however, did not occur in the 18-month rat toxicity study in which either marked, background, age-related nephropathy [common in chronic toxicity studies in laboratory rats (TURNBULL et al. 1985) or the duration of exposure to the drug, or both, may have been influencing factors.

Blood urea levels were measured during a 1-month study in rats in which cilazapril was administered at 100 mg/kg per day with or without the addition of sodium chloride to the drinking water. The presence of saline partially prevented uraemia after 2 weeks and wholly prevented it after 4 weeks.

Elevations in blood urea levels have been reported for captopril in rats (IMAI et al. 1981; HASHIMOTO et al. 1981), primates (SIBLEY et al. 1978) and dogs (KEIM 1980), for enalapril in rats and dogs (BAGDON et al. 1985a,b; MACDONALD et al. 1987) and for SCH 31846 in rats (LA ROCCA et al. 1986). They have also been reported for pentopril (GOODMAN et al. 1985), ramipril (DONAUBAUER and MAYER 1988) and quinapril (ANDERSON et al. 1984) in rats and dogs. Moreover, as with cilazapril, saline administration in rat studies with enalapril prevented uraemia induced in the absence of renal tissue damage. Conversely, when BAGDON et al. (1985b) administered enalapril at 90 mg/kg per day to rats on a sodium-deficient diet, an increase of approximately 10-fold over control values occurred, compared with 1.5-fold for the group receiving the same dosage but maintained on a standard diet. These observations indicate that uraemia, when seen in the absence of frank nephropathy during toxicity studies with ACE inhibitors, is related principally to the pharmacological activity of these agents.

When renal damage occurs, abnormal increases in blood urea levels are not generally observed until a total of 75% or more of the nephrons are unable to function normally (OSBORNE et al. 1975), indicating the considerable reserve capacity of the kidneys. However, the evidence suggests that uraemia in the absence of histological nephropathy, as observed with ACE inhibitors in animals, is probably related to haemodynamic changes in the kidney leading to a reduction in glomerular filtration pressure due to inhibition of ACE. If it is accepted that filtration pressure is dependent on blood pressure and the contractile state of the efferent glomerular arterioles, and as proposed by NISHIMURA and BAILEY (1982) the maintenance of muscle tone in these arterioles is a function of the renin-angiotensin system, then inhibition of the conversion of angiotensin I to angiotensin II by an ACE inhibitor should lower blood pressure and allow dilation of the efferent glomerular arterioles. Elevated blood urea levels could then be predicted in view of a resulting reduction in effective filtration due to a fall in filtration presure. An additional mechanism which would be expected to encourage a lowering of filtration pressure comprises the decrease in aldosterone secretion due to reduced angiotensin II production, which could act to lower blood pressure by allowing sodium loss and, therefore, blood volume reduction.

If the mechanisms described above do, indeed, operate, then removal of ACE inhibition should quickly restore normal, effective glomerular filtration. The return to normal blood urea levels following suspension of treatment with cilazapril during several of our toxicity studies suggests this to be the case.

3.1.3 Effects on the Juxtaglomerular Apparatus and Renal Vasculature

Morphological changes of the juxtaglomerular apparatus (JGA) of the kidney have been recorded during toxicity studies with cilazapril (baboon, cynomolgus monkey), captopril (rat, HASHIMOTO et al. 1981; rhesus monkey, ZAKI et al. 1982; mouse, KANETA et al. 1983; rabbit, OVERTURF et al. 1982, ramipril (rats, rhesus monkeys, and dogs, DONAUBAUER and MAYER 1988, SCH 31846 (rats and dogs, LA ROCCA et al. 1986), and spirapril (rats and dogs, SYBERTZ et al. 1987). These changes have been described variously as "proliferative" (= hyperplastic

= increase in cell numbers) or "hypertrophic" (= increase in cell size), or both, leading essentially to an increase in the size of the JGA. Characteristically, routine histological technique (light microscopy) shows a swelling of the glomerular afferent arteriole where it enters the glomerulus. HASHIMOTO et al. (1981), in a 12-month rat toxicity study with captopril at dosages up to 900 mg/kg per day, demonstrated that such changes are accompanied by significant increases in the number of renin granules in the JGA cells. This is expected following blockade of angiotensin II production. However, removal of a proportion of animals from treatment for 3 months at the end of the dosing period was attended by a marked size regression in the JGA and a reduction in renin content. A similar observation was made by ZAKI et al. (1982) when groups of rhesus monkeys were administered captopril at high dosages (150 and 450 mg/kg per day) for 12 months and a proportion removed from treatment for a further 6 months.

It is clear, therefore, that the JGA changes in the kidneys observed with the repeated dosing of captopril and other ACE inhibitors are an expression of their pharmacological action. Although the increase in size of the JGA may, in part be proliferative, it should not be regarded with unease because it is clearly reversible, and there is a mechanistic explanation.

A further renal effect, observed during toxicity studies with ACE inhibitors and usually associated with JGA hyperplasia and hypertrophy, comprises thickening of the glomerular afferent arterioles. In rats, this may extend upstream to the interlobular arteries, but experience with cilazapril indicates that it is less extensive in non-rodents. During the 12-month rat study previously referred to, HASHIMOTO et al. (1981) noted this effect on arterioles and arteries after 3 months' administration of captopril at 100, 300 and 900 mg/kg per day. After 12 months' administration, it was apparent also at the lowest dose level of 30 mg/kg per day but was confined to the arterioles in this group. At the end of the 3 month recovery phase it was observed that vascular thickening tended to decrease in incidence and severity, although it was still clearly apparent in males which received the two highest dose levels.

In a 12-month study in rats with enalapril at 10, 30 and 90 mg/kg per day, BAGDON et al. (1985b) observed neither JGA nor vascular changes in the kidney. However, in the discussion section of their paper they cited an unpublished report of a 1-month rat study which examined dose levels of 5,50,500 and 1500 mg/kg per day. At the two higher dosages in this study, increased numbers of renin granules were observed in the JGA cells, and the glomerular afferent arteriolar walls were thickened.

Our toxicity studies in rats and primates with cilazapril showed similar vascular changes to those described for captopril and enalapril and were generally proportional in degree of severity to study duration and dose level. They were most marked in the 18-month general toxicity and 24-month rat carcinogenicity studies in the mid and high dose groups receiving 4 or 40 mg/kg per day, respectively. In contrast, 4-week rat studies demonstrated that effects were only detectable at dose levels in excess of 100 mg/kg per day. No effect was evident in the low dose group of any study in any species.

HASHIMOTO et al. (1981) used electron microscopy to examine the renal vascular thickening and JGA changes seen in their 12-month captopril study in rats. They observed proliferation of the JGA with increased renin granularity and swelling and proliferation of smooth muscle cells with an increase in collagen fibrils. Glomerular afferent arterioles were noted to contain a high proportion of proliferating JGA cells in the region of the glomeruli, while more distally, the proliferation of smooth muscle cells comprised the principal change contributing to the thickening of the vessel wall. This description is at variance with that for cilazapril in which hypertrophy of the medial (smooth muscle) layer cells was described without any evidence of cell proliferation.

The mechanism responsible for the vascular thickening in the kidneys when ACE inhibitors are administered in overdosage is far from clear at this time, particularly if it occurs at some distance from the JGA. However, hypertrophy, with or without proliferation, of the JGA cells in the walls of the glomerular afferent arterioles, associated with decreased angiotensin II activity, are important factors in the thickening process in these vessels where they enter the glomeruli, both in rodents and non-rodents. Further upstream, well away from the JGA apparatus, HACKENTHAL et al. (1987) found renin-secreting cells scattered along the distal parts of the arterioles and the interlobular arteries. There is a far greater proportion of smooth muscle cells in the vessel wall than in the part of the arteriole proximal to the glomerulus, so that any change in the relatively few renin-secreting cells is unlikely to account for the total thickening process in rats.

Possible avenues of research into this vascular change might include further investigations of proliferative activity within the vessel wall, the effects of local renin concentrations on smooth muscle and any changes in haemodynamic characteristics peculiar to these vessels under conditions of gross ACE inhibitor overdosage. However, even at this stage, knowledge of the mode of action of ACE inhibitors, taken together with the highly specific changes described in the renal vascular system and the JGA, signifies that it is improbable that there is any direct action by these drugs on the wall of the blood vessels. If this were the case, then similar changes, which have not been observed, would be expected in other tissues and organs.

3.2 Myocardial Necrosis Associated with Vasodilating Antihypertensive Agents

Before considering the myocardial effect with vasodilators in detail, some more common indications of cardiac disturbances during toxicity studies with antihypertensive agents will be described briefly. In clinical terms, they range in severity from slight chronotropy without any serious implications for the health of the animals to marked arrhythmias leading to sudden death. Other cardiac parameters are not routinely monitored in the live animals because the invasive methods frequently required would conflict with the primary aim of toxicity studies. Such measurements are, therefore, left in the domain of the pharmacologist.

When changes in heart rate are moderate and the duration of dosing relatively short, routine toxicological methods only occasionally demonstrate morphological effects in the heart. However, in studies in which a significant period of tachycardia due to the pharmacological effects of a drug occurs after each daily dose, an increase in heart weight (myocardial hypertrophy) may be observed. This is frequently explained in the absence of pathological tissue changes as a response to an abnormal work load. An example of this was seen with nitrendipine in a 12-month toxicity study in the dog (HOFFMANN 1983). However, another calcium channel blocker, nicardipine, when examined in dogs for 6 months, was stated to have caused bradycardia, yet an increase in heart weight was recorded (BAKY 1985); no details are given with respect to the time of measurement in relation to dose administration, so a period of tachycardia shortly after each dose may have remained undetected.

The more common cardiac findings made during the toxicological evaluation of antihypertensive agents are either (a) readily anticipated because of the known pharmacological action of the compound under test (e.g. heart rate changes) or (b) not associated with tissue damage (eg. heart weight increase) within the limitations of standard toxicological procedures. It is proposed now to discuss in some detail the characteristic myocardial lesion consisting of frank, irreversible tissue damage which has been observed during the toxicological evaluation of a number of vasodilators. If considered superficially and without regard to the pharmacological properties of these compounds, this effect could suggest a direct cytotoxic action. However, as with the previously noted cardiac effects, there is strong evidence that the aetiology of this lesion is related to the mode of action of the agents.

3.2.1 Nature of the Lesion

The myocardial lesion, which may consist of many small, discrete or fewer, larger areas of necrosis, is characteristically located in the left ventricular papillary muscles or in the area of their junction with the left ventricular wall. The published literature includes the following examples of vasodilating antihypertensive agents associated with its induction:

Agent	Dog	Rat	Reference
Hydralazine	+	+	BALAZS and PAYNE 1971
Diazoxide	+	+	BALAZS et al. 1975
Minoxidil	+	+	HERMAN et al. 1979
Nitrendipine	+	−	HOFFMANN 1983
Nimodipine	+	−	SCHLUETER 1986
Nisoldipine	+	−	KAZDA et al. 1983
Amrinone	+	−	ALOUSI and DOBRECK 1983
Enoximone	+	−	DAGE et al. 1986
Milrinone	+	+	ALOUSI et al. 1985
Pinacidil	+	−	ARRIGONI-MARTELLI and FINUCANE 1985
S K & F 94120	+	NI	HARLEMAN et al. 1986

+, lesion present; −, lesion absent; NI, no information.

We give no information on the dose levels examined or the duration of the studies which, with the exceptions of hydralazine, diazoxide and minoxidil, are standard toxicity studies to current regulatory authority requirements. Although the dog is particularly sensitive in the production of this lesion, it is possible that the rat would be implicated more frequently if other drugs in the list were subjected to special studies such as those undertaken by BALAZS and his co-workers with hydralazine, diazoxide and minoxidil. Nevertheless, the rat toxicity studies employed significantly higher doses than those examined in the dog, so the relative sensitivity of the latter species is still signified by a dose-for-dose comparison.

Much of the early investigative work concerning the association between vasodilating antihypertensive agents and the induction of myocardial lesions in experimental animals was undertaken by BALAZS and his co-workers. In an early study with hydralazine in dogs, BALAZS and PAYNE (1971) demonstrated foci of fibrosis in the left ventricular papillary muscles of 2 out of 4 animals treated at 10 mg/kg per day orally for 5 days. During the dosing period, marked tachycardia and T-wave inversion were observed. When diazoxide was administered to dogs intravenously (BALAZS et al. 1975), 20 mg/kg per day on 2 or 3 days induced tachycardia, ST-segment depression and papillary muscle necrosis in the left ventricle: a single dose of 10 mg/kg or 20 mg/kg caused marked falls in blood pressure and increases in heart rate. The oral dosing of minoxidil to dogs by HERMAN et al. (1979) on two consecutive days at 0.5, 1 or 3 mg/kg per day was attended by hypotension and marked tachycardia lasting for up to 24 h following the second dose. Five of the eight animals which received 1 or 3 mg/kg per day demonstrated myocardial necrosis of the left ventricular papillary muscles with visible greyish lesions up to 10 mm in diameter. In a 4-week toxicity study in dogs with nisoldipine (KAZDA et al. 1983), myocardial scars were seen in the same area in the high-dose group (10 mg/kg per day) indicating an earlier necrotic event, and this finding was confirmed in a subsequent 3-month study in this species. In both studies tachycardia and sharp reductions in blood pressure were observed, with depression of the ST-segment of the electrocardiogram in several animals.

The presence of myocardial scars alone at the end of the dosing period in canine multidose toxicity studies suggests that damage occurs in the initial stages of the dosing period, and it is a feature of a number of vasodilators, including nisoldipine (KAZDA et al. 1983), milrinone (ALOUSI et al. 1985), nitrendipine (HOFFMANN 1983) and nimodipine (SCHLUETER 1986). However, this pattern is not consistent. In the case of amrinone (ALOUSI and DEBRECK 1983), histopathological examination of the heart after daily dosing for 1 year revealed left ventricular papillary muscle lesions, some of which were long-standing (with interstitial fibrosis) and others which were more recent, showing areas of necrosis surrounded by incipient fibrosis. It appears, therefore, that the development of resistance to myocardial necrosis during the repeated dose studies in dogs may vary in degree according to the antihypertensive agent under examination.

In studies with rats (BALAZS et al. 1981), a single intraperitoneal dose of hydralazine at 25 mg/kg gave a prolonged 60% decrease in blood pressure and a 40% increase in heart rate and produced lesions in the myocardium, essentially similar to those seen in dogs. Lower doses given on 2 consecutive days had similar effects, but the incidence and severity of the lesions were dosage-related. Histologically, they consist of areas of myocardial cell necrosis and degeneration accompanied by an inflammatory cell reaction. Occasionally, lesions were observed in the right ventricular myocardium, but only in those individuals showing very severe changes in the left ventricle. It was noted in these experiments that many lesions tended to be distributed around small coronary vessels. Similar myocardial changes were seen in rats administered diazoxide or minoxidil (BALAZS and WOLFF 1974).

A reduction in the severity of the lesion in rats was demonstrated by co-administration of propranolol or verapamil with hydralazine (BALAZS et al. 1981), although the degree of protection was greater with the β-adrenergic antagonist. Similarly, BALAZS et al. (1975) showed that propranolol reduces both tachycardia and the myocardial changes when administered with diazoxide to dogs, but the hypotensive action of the latter drug is not modified. A further example of the protective action of propranolol was demonstrated by ARRIGONI-MARTELLI and FINUCANE (1985) with pinacidil in dogs.

3.2.2 Mechanisms of Pathogenesis

The damage to the myocardium described above characteristically occurs at a specific site within the heart, that is, the left ventricle, and particularly in its papillary muscles. The agents responsible for the effect in animals, at dose levels generally well in excess of those recommended for clinical usage, are represented by a diversity of chemical structures, but with a common mode of pharmacological action. The diversity of chemical structure suggests it is improbable that cell necrosis in such specific circumstances and at such a specific site results from a direct effect. It is, therefore, more probable that the common pharmacological effect, vasodilation followed by hypotension, plays a critical role in the induction of this lesion.

The following account of the possible mechanisms involved draws substantially on those given in greater detail elsewhere, particularly by BALAZS (1981), BALAZS et al. (1981) and BALAZS and BLOOM (1982), who have made such significant contributions in this field.

The location of the damage corresponds with that known to be most sensitive to myocardial ischaemic injury. The left ventricular papillary muscles appear to be especially vulnerable because their oxygen requirements are high, due to the mechanically demanding function of supporting mitral valves in systole. However, they are poorly adapted to this role insomuch as their vascularisation is inferior when compared with other regions of the heart. It is probable, therefore, that hypoxia develops more readily and is more marked and of longer duration than in other parts of the myocardium when oxygen demand increases. When tachycardia occurs, an additional work load is placed on the heart, and this, together with reduced blood supply resulting from hypotension, is considered to be particularly disadvantageous for the left ventricular papillary muscles with their poorer levels of perfusion. Under such circumstances, cell death is anticipated, thus leading to the appearance of myocardial lesions at this site. The relatively marked reflex tachycardia in dogs, when compared with rats or primates, following the administration of vasodilating antihypertensive agents probably explains in part their greater susceptibility to myocardial necrosis.

The importance of a pharmacological basis to the pathogenesis of the myocardial lesion is further supported by the observation that propranolol exerts protection when administered with hydralazine to rats (BALAZS et al. 1981) and with diazoxide (BALAZS et al. 1975) or pinacidil to dogs (ARRIGONI-MARTELLI and FINUCANE 1985). This can be explained by the reduced tachycardia following blockade of the β-adrenoreceptors. Further support for the role of hypoxia in the pathogenesis of the lesion is provided by a study with the adrenergic bronchodilator isoproterenol in hamsters (KENNEDY et al. 1966). This agent induces left ventricular papillary muscle necrosis when administered to animals in overdosage, and the investigators found that protection occurs under conditions of hyperbaric oxygenation.

Intracellular calcium levels are considered to play a significant role in cell necrosis (FLECKENSTEIN 1971; BLOOM 1981). The importance of this in the aetiology of lesions induced by hydralazine in rats (BALAZS et al. 1981) is indicated in experiments which demonstrate exacerbation of the lesion when the rats are pretreated with dihydrotachysterol, an agent which increases plasma and myocardial calcium levels. Protection against this action is observed when verapamil is given, which would be expected to decrease calcium entry into the myocytes. Reduction in calcium entry by verapamil is also protective against hydralazine in this series of studies without modifying the latter's action in causing hypotension and tachycardia.

4 Expressions of Pharmacological Activity During Reproductive Toxicity Testing

Antihypertensive agents, in common with most other pharmaceuticals, are screened for immediate and delayed adverse effects on all stages of reproductive function, from the fertility of the parental generation (F_0) administered the test compound to the reproductive capacity of their offspring (F_1) and the development to weaning of the F_2 generation. The many facets examined during the course of these studies are routinely confined to the rat, with the notable exception of the test for teratogenic, embryolethal and fetotoxic potential which are also examined in a suitable non-rodent species, usually the rabbit. During the course of such studies with antihypertensive agents, various changes have been observed which are firmly or tentatively ascribed to exaggerated pharmacological effects. These range from reduced maternal competence in rats due to hypotension leading to an increased neonatal death rate as observed for cadralazine (DORIGOTTI and FERNI 1987) and the temporary distortion of the ribs of rats administered β-sympathomimetics due principally to fetal compression in utero (NISHIMURA et al. 1982; STERZ et al. 1985), to gross malformation of the offspring as observed for some diuretics.

This section is divided into two parts. The first discusses the fetotoxic potential of ACE inhibitors and the second part, malformations associated with carbonic anhydrase inhibiting and loop diuretics.

4.1 Fetotoxicity of Angiotensin-Converting Enzyme Inhibitors

Both captopril and enalapril are contraindicated in pregnancy. An important reason for this is the fact that teratology studies in the rabbit showed embryo- and/or fetotoxicity at dose levels close to those recommended for human use (data supplied under USA Freedom of Information Act: captopril NDA 18-343, enalapril NDA 18-998). The underlying mechanisms of fetotoxicity by ACE inhibitors have been investigated for captopril in rabbits by KEITH et al. (1982) and FERRIS and WEIR (1983), and in sheep by BROUGHTON PIPKIN et al. (1982). An ovine model was used subsequently to examine enalapril (BROUGHTON PIPKIN and WALLACE 1986).

KEITH et al. (1982) administered captopril orally at 2.5 or 5.0 mg/kg per day to groups of rabbits during the second half of the gestation period (days 15–30 inclusive). The combined fetal deaths comprised 86% from the captopril-treated groups (compared with 1% of control fetuses). This contrasts markedly with a cited teratology study (MYHRE 1978) in rats in which a dosage of 3000 mg/kg per day was not attended by fetal death. Such a comparison is not entirely valid, however, unless the rat study was of unusual design and administration of captopril was undertaken during the third trimester of pregnancy rather than the standard days 6–15 of gestation (term, 22 days). KEITH et al. (1982) recorded no structural abnormalities within the limitations of autopsy procedures on rabbit fetuses which died in utero at various stages of development. There was no evidence of severe maternal hypotension, while clinical and autopsy findings failed to reveal any changes which could suggest a fetal effect secondary to maternal toxicity. FERRIS and WEIR (1983) demonstrated that captopril caused fetal death (80%–93%, compared with 1% of controls) in rabbits when administered at 2.5 and 5.0 mg/kg per day from day 18 of gestation to parturition. This was associated with a marked reduction (approximately one-third) in uterine perfusion which was considered to result from a fall in uterine prostaglandin E synthesis attributed to blockade of angiotensin II.

In an experiment with sheep by BROUGHTON PIPKIN et al. (1982), captopril was administered intravenously as a single dose at 2.8–3.5 mg/kg in late pregnancy, between 119 and 133 days of gestation. Within 2 min, conversion of angiotensin I to angiontensin II was blocked in the mothers, and maternal and fetal basal systemic blood pressures subsequently declined. Maternal blood pressure returned to normal within 2 h, but the fetal blood pressure remained abnormally low for up to 2 days. At or toward the end of the gestation period (about 147 days), the five ewes gave birth to seven freshly dead lambs and one weak live birth. There was no evidence of abnormal growth in utero, and autopsy failed to reveal any gross abnormalities. The investigators discussed the possible mechanisms involved in the production of prolonged fetal hypotension. They argued that captopril might theoretically cross the placenta and the blood-brain barrier and exert a central effect. Captopril may also increase prostaglandin E_2 levels, lower peripheral resistance and block angiotensin II production, all of which could decrease placental, and therefore fetal, tissue perfusion. The possibility that captopril is cleared more slowly by the fetus, whose renal function is low compared with its mother, was considered by Broughton Pipkin et al. (1982) to be another possible factor.

A similar study in sheep with enalapril (Broughton Pipkin and Wallace 1986) resulted in fetal blood pressure reductions, but they were not prolonged as seen for captopril and were not followed by fetotoxicity. Direct measurement of enalapril in fetal blood shows that it never exceeds 9% of the maternal level, thus indicating very low placental transfer. The lipid solubility of enalapril is very low, so that significant transfer across placental and blood-brain barriers would not be anticipated. The investigators suggested that the fetal blood pressure effect may relate to changes in the utero-placental haemodynamics rather than, as suggested for captopril (Broughton Pipkin et al. 1982), by a direct pharmacological action of the drug. Nevertheless, if this is indeed the mode of action of enalapril in pregnant sheep, it still represents an example of a pharmacological effect, albeit secondary to the maternal response.

The above experiments in rabbits and sheep illuminate the problem of fetotoxicity in standard rabbit teratology studies with ACE inhibitors, and indicate that given the present state of knowledge, these agents should be the clinician's choice of last resort in pregnancy.

4.2 Teratogenesis of Diuretics

Skeletal malformations of the rat fetus following the administration of diuretics have been recorded for acetazolamide (Layton and Hallesy 1965; Holmes et al. 1988), dichlorphenamide (Hallesy and Layton 1967), ethoxzolamide (Wilson et al. 1968), indacrinone and furosemide (Robertson et al. 1981) and azosemide (Hayasaka et al. 1984). There is evidence that these malformations relate, at least in part, to the pharmacological activity of these agents, and this is now to be described.

4.2.1 Carbonic Anhydrase Inhibitors

An essentially identical fetal abnormality in rats is induced by the three structurally dissimilar diuretics, acetazolamide, dichlorphenamide and ethoxzolamide. These compounds, however, share a common mode of pharmacological action, that is, the inhibition of carbonic anhydrase. The defect as described for rats administered acetazolamide by Layton and Hallesy (1965) consists of missing skeletal elements in the right forelimb; a very low incidence of offspring show an effect in the left forelimb. When more severe deformity of the right also occurs. The abnormal pattern of skeletal elements in an affected limb ranges from a missing fifth digit to the absence of two or more digits, the corresponding metacarpals and the distal portion of the ulna, accompanied by a bowing of the radius resulting in an overall forearm shortening. The humerus is very rarely involved, and only where forearm defects are extreme. In view of its specificity and reproducibility, this defect has been the subject of a variety of investigations with acetazolamide.

HALLESY and LAYTON (1967) first suggested that the teratogenicity of acetazolamide in the rat is related to its only known pharmacological property, carbonic anhydrase inhibition. This hypothesis was supported by demonstrating that dichlorphenamide, a structurally dissimilar inhibitor, produces essentially similar malformations. Further credence to this line of reasoning was provided by WILSON et al. (1968), who showed ethoxzolamide to behave similarly: these investigators also defined a short period of maximum sensitivity on the 10th or 11th day of gestation. They concluded, however, that it was improbable that embryonic carbonic anhydrase inhibition was involved as this was not measurable before the 13th day, but their experiments did not exclude a possible role for this enzyme in maternal or extra-embryonic membranes. Maternal plasma analysis by WILSON et al. (1968) revealed metabolic acidosis and a sharp drop in potassium levels, but there were no other significant electrolyte disturbances. During the course of these studies in rats, supplementation with potassium failed to modify acetazolamide teratogenicity. Later experiments by HIRSCH et al. (1983) with embryos from two strains of mice showed that the most sensitive period (day 10) to acetazolamide coincided with higher levels of embryonic carbonic anhydrase than on day 12 when the embryos were insensitive.

ELLISON (1969) demonstrated that pregnant rats administered broadly similar doses of acetazolamide (0.6% in the diet, or 600 mg/kg subcutaneously on days 10 and 11 of gestation) compared to those examined by WILSON et al. (1968) lost 20–30% of their stored potassium. The plasma and muscle levels were most severely depleted, while hepatic levels increased. The possible role of potassium depletion was investigated by ELLISON and MAREN (1971) who, in contrast to WILSON et al. (1968), showed that the fetal defect in rats could be ameliorated or abolished if net maternal potassium loss is prevented by co-administration of postassium chloride or a potassium-sparing diuretic. However, hyperkalaemia was associated with exacerbation of the defect, indicating that maternal potassium depletion alone is not teratogenic per se. It was observed that hepatic potassium levels in the fetuses and mothers were increased by acetazolamide administration, and that they were greater in fetuses exhibiting the defect. The investigators concluded that a disturbance of potassium balance together with carbonic anhydrase inhibition is probably required to express teratogenicity.

The possibility that maternal acidosis, as measured by WILSON et al. (1968), plays a significant role in acetazolamide teratogenesis was dismissed by MAREN and ELLISON (1972). When they eliminated metabolic acidosis by sodium bicarbonate administration, the characteristic defect nevertheless occurred. However, WEAVER and SCOTT (1984) induced an identical right forearm defect in the pregnant mouse by exposure to carbon dioxide alone. They defined a threshold of 15% CO_2 for 8 h during a critical 16-h period of limb development

(12.00 h on day 9 to 16.00 h on day 10 of gestation) as being essential to produce the defect. The failure of previous investigators (Storch and Layton 1971; Ellison and Maren 1972) to induce teratogenicity is considered to be due to a combination of the examination of subthreshold conditions and species differences in carbon dioxide tolerance. Before undertaking the study with mice, Weaver and Scott (1984) subjected rats to 25% CO_2 for 16 h during the period of limb-bud development without success. Further evidence suggesting a common pathway in acetazolamide and carbon dioxide teratogenesis was obtained during these mouse studies, that is, a similar incidence of other abnormalities (kinked tail, rib anomalies, microphthalmia) was observed with both agents. The investigators argued that the increased maternal hypercapnia resulting from acidosis due to either carbonic anhydrase inhibition or exposure to carbon dioxide may lead to a reduction in intracellular pH which, in turn, can be correlated with decreased cell division in a variety of models. This could lead to defective development when such conditions are realised during limb-bud development.

Further support for an important role of carbonic anhydrase inhibition in the teratogenesis of acetazolamide is provided by the work of Ugen and Scott (1985, 1986), who demonstrated that the co-administration of vasoactive agents without known carbonic anhydrase inhibitory activity exacerbates the defect in rats. The vasoactive compounds serotonin, ergotamine and nicotine intensify the effect (Ugen and Scott 1985), while α-adrenergic antagonists (prazosin, phenoxybenzamine) eliminate the potentiating effect of the α-agonist phenylephrine (Ugen and Scott 1986). α-Adrenergic agents are known to modify uterine blood flow and vascular resistance (Greiss 1972). It was suggested that a hypoxic and/or hypercapnic embryonic environment could be produced, favouring a decreased intracellular pH, as discussed above (Weaver and Scott 1984), so potentiating the effects of acetazolamide in rats. Ugen and Scott (1986) suggested that high maternal plasma carbon dioxide concentrations induced by carbonic anhydrase inhibition may lead to the release of catecholamines from the maternal adrenal medulla. These could then act on the α-adrenergic receptors in the uterine vasculature, thus reducing blood flow.

The evidence summarised above favours the hypothesis that acetazolamide teratogenicity in rodents is related to its pharmacological activity: the inhibition of carbonic anhydrase leading to metabolic acidosis, possibly in concert with potassium loss, is probably an important factor in the production of the characteristic abnormality.

4.2.2 Loop Diuretics

Skeletal malformations were producted by high dosages of the loop diuretics furosemide (Robertson et al. 1981; Hayasaka et al. 1984), azosemide (Hayasaka et al. 1984) and indacrinone (Robertson et al. 1981) during teratology studies in rodents. Typically, the defect consists of "wavy" ribs with, at higher dose levels, distortion of the humerus and scapula. The affected forelimb is predominantly right-sided with indacrinone and furosemide (Robertson et al.

1981), as observed with carbonic anhydrase inhibitors (Sect. 4.2.1), but this was not indicated for azosemide by HAYASAKA et al. (1984). These latter investigators defined the sensitive periods for azosemide-induced skeletal abnormalities as days 15–17 and 12–15 of gestation for rats and mice, respectively.

Furosemide and azosemide are chemical analogues, but indacrinone has a distinctly different molecular structure. However, these compounds share the same mode of action on the loop of Henle which results in saluresis and potassium depletion.

ROBERTSON et al. (1981) co-administered the potassium-sparing diuretic amiloride with indacrinone to rats. This abolished the fetal scapular and forelimb abnormalities and reduced the incidence of "wavy" rib by 90% when compared with a concurrent group which received indacrinone alone. The investigators argued that it was probable that electrolyte imbalance, particularly potassium depletion, was an important common factor in the teratogenicity of both loop diuretics and carbonic anhydrase inhibitors. However, other studies (ELLISON and MAREN 1971) indicate that maternal potassium depletion is not primarily associated with azetazolamide teratogenicity (Sect. 4.2.1). In addition, studies by WEAVER and SCOTT (1984) and UGEN and SCOTT (1985, 1986) provide strong evidence of a critical role for carbonic anhydrase inhibition in the production of this defect (Sect. 4.2.1), an activity of no significance for loop diuretics. Moreover, although the defects caused by both types of diuretic are skeletal, they are morphologically distinct. The carbonic anhydrase inhibitors affect the forearm and the loop diuretics, the humerus, scapula and ribs. The difference between the lesions is further indicated by different periods of maximum sensitivity to drug-induced malformation, for example, in rats, this period is days 10–11 of gestation for acetazolamide (WILSON et al. 1968) and days 15–17 for azosemide (HAYASAKA et al. 1984). It seems probable, therefore, that there is a common pathway for the teratogenic action of carbonic anhydrase inhibitors, and this probably differs in some significant way from that of the loop diuretics. Nevertheless, there is strong evidence that the teratogenicity of both types of diuretics is, at least in part, related to their pharmacological activity.

5 Concluding Remarks

The prime purpose of this chapter, following a brief description of the principles and methods of toxicity testing, has been to illustrate the variety of anticipated and unexpected adverse changes encountered during such testing of antihypertensive drugs. We have considered a number of the more unusual effects in greater detail, and given evidence to signify relationships with pharmacological activity. It is probable that further research will indicate the aetiology of some or all of these findings to be complex interactions of many factors, including both pharmacological activity and direct damage of subcellular components by the drug administered in gross overdosage. This is already exemplified by the two-component mechanism proposed for renal damage by enalapril in the dog.

Summary

A brief description of the principles and methods of toxicity testing is presented. This is followed by consideration of a number of unexpected adverse changes encountered during the toxicity testing of antihypertensive drugs. It is concluded that while there is strong evidence signifying relationships between these changes and pharmacological activity, other factors, such as direct cellular damage by gross drug overdosage, may play important interactive roles.

Acknowledgement We wish to thank Mrs Susan Hicks for typing the manuscript.

References

Alousi AA and Dobreck HP (1983) Amrinone. In: Scriabine A (ed) Cardiovascular drugs, vol 1. Raven, New York, p 259 (New drugs annual)

Alousi AA, Fabian RJ, Baker JF, Stroshane RM (1985) Milrinone. In: Scriabine A (ed) New cardiovascular drugs, vol 3. Raven, New York, p 245

Ames BN, Durston WE, Yamasaki E, Lee FD (1973) Carcinogens are mutagens: a simple test system combining liver homogenates for activation and bacteria for detection. Proc Natl Acad Sci USA 70:2281

Anderson JA, Fitzgerald JE, Jayasekara U, Watkin JR, Aust AE, de la Iglesia FA (1984) Preclinical toxicological evaluation of an angiotensin II converting enzyme inhibitor of the tetrahydroquinoline series. Fed Proc 43:733

Arrigoni-Martelli E, Finucane J (1985) Pinacidil. In: Scriabine A (ed) New cardiovascular drugs, vol 3. Raven, New York, p 133

Bagdon WJ, Bokelman DL (1983) Toxicity of enalapril in dogs ameliorated by saline supplementation. Toxicology 3:130

Bagdon WJ, Bokelman DL, Stone CA (1985a) Toxicity study of MK 421 (enalapril maleate) (III) subacute, and one-year chronic studies in beagle dogs. Jpn Pharmacol Ther 13:467–518

Bagdon WJ, Bokelman DL, Stone CA (1985b) Toxicity study of MK 421 (enalapril maleate (II) subacute, chronic toxicity studies, saline supplementation, sodium-depletion studies in rats. Jpn Pharmacol Ther 13:425–466

Baky SH (1985) Nicardipine hydrochloride. In: Scriabine A (ed) New cardiovascular drugs, vol 3. Raven, New York, p 153

Balazs T (1981) Cardiotoxicity of adrenergic bronchodilator and vasodilating antihypertensive drugs. In: Balazs T (ed) Cardiac toxicology, vol 2. CRC Press, Boca Raton, p 61

Balazs T, Bloom S (1982) Cardiotoxicity of adrenergic bronchodilator and vasodilating antihypertensive drugs. In: van Stee EW (ed) Cardiovascular toxicology. Raven, New York, p 199

Balazs T, Payne BJ (1971) Myocardial papillary muscle necrosis induced by hypotensive agents in dogs. Toxicol Appl Pharmacol 20:442–445

Balazs T, Wolff F (1974) Cardiotoxic effects of vasodilating antihypertensive drugs and the use of beta-adrenoreceptor blocking agents. Br J Clin Pharmacol 1:182

Balazs T, Herman EH, Earl FL, Wolff FW (1975) Cardiotoxicity studies with diazoxide, reserpine, guanethidine, and combinations of diazoxide and propranolol in dogs. Toxicol Appl Pharmacol 33:498–504

Balazs T, Ferrans VJ, El-hage A, Ehrreich SJ, Johnson GL, Herman EH, Atkinson JC, West WL (1981) Study of the mechanism of hydralazine-induced myocardial necrosis in the rat. Toxicol Appl Pharmacol 59:524–534

Blooms S (1981) Reversible and irreversible injury: calcium as a major determinant. In: Balazs T (ed) Cardiac toxicology, vol 1. CRC Press, Boca Raton, p 179

Broughton Pipkin F, Wallace CP (1986) The effect of enalapril (MK 421), an angiotensin

converting enzyme inhibitor, on the conscious pregnant ewe and her foetus. Br J Pharmacol 87:533–542
Broughton Pipkin F, Symonds EM, Turner SR (1982) The effect of captopril (SQ14,225) upon mother and fetus in the chronically cannulated ewe and in the pregnant rabbit. J Physiol (Lond) 323:415–422
Brusick D (1984) Genetic toxicology. In: Hayes AW (ed) Principles and methods of toxicology. Raven, New York, p 223
Chan PK, O'Hara GP, Hayes AW (1984) Principles and methods of acute and subchronic toxicity. In: Hayes AW (ed) Principles and methods of toxicology. Raven, New York, p 1
Dage RC, Roebel LE, Gibson JP, Okerholm RA, Rolf CN (1986) Enoximone. In: Scriabine A (ed) New cardiovascular drugs, Vol 4. Raven, New york, p 63
Descotes J (1986) Immunotoxicology of drugs and chemicals. Elsevier, Amsterdam
Dixon RL, Hall JL (1984) Reproductive toxicology. In: Hayes AW (ed) Principles and methods of toxicology. Raven, New York, p 107
Donaubauer HH, Mayer D (1988) Acute, subchronic and chronic toxicity of the new angiotensin-converting enzyme inhibitor ramipril. Arzneimittel forsch 38:15–20
Dorigotti L, Ferni G (1987) Cadralazine. In: Scriabine A (ed) New cardiovascular drugs, vol 5. Raven, New York, p 155
Ellison AC (1969) Effects of acetazolamide on tissue cations. Proc Soc Exp Biol Med 130:893–897
Ellison AC Maren TH (1971) The effect of potassium metabolism on acetazolamide-induced teratogenesis. Johns Hopkins Med J 130:105–115
Ellison AC, Maren TH (1972) The effects of metabolic alterations on teratogenesis. Johns Hopkins Med J 130:87–94
Ferris TF, Weir EK (1983) Effect of captopril on uterine blood flow and prostaglandin E synthesis in the pregnant rabbit. J Clin Invest 71:809–815
Fleckenstein A (1971) Specific inhibitors and promoters of calcium action in the excitation-contraction coupling of heart muscle and their role in the prevention or production of myocardial lesions. In: Harris P, Oppie L (eds) Calcium and the heart. Academic, New York, p 135
Frederick GL (1986) The necessary minimal duration of final long-term toxicology tests of drugs. Fundam Appl Toxicol 6:385–394
Goodman FR, Weiss GB, Hurley ME (1985) Pentopril. In: Scriabine A (ed) New cardiovascular drugs, vol 3. Raven, New York, p 57
Greiss FC (1972) Differential reactivity of myoendometrial and placental vasculature: adrenergic responses. Am J Obstet Gynecol 112:20–27
Hackenthal E, Metz R, Buehrle CP, Taugner R (1987) Intrarenal and intracellular distribution of renin and angiotensin. Kidney Int [Suppl 20] 31:S4–S17
Hallesy DW, Layton WM (1967) Forelimb deformity of offspring of rats given dichlorphenamide during pregnancy. Proc Soc Exp Biol Med 126:6–8
Harleman JH, Joseph EC, Eden RJ, Walker TF, Major IR, Lamb MS (1986) Cardiotoxicity of a new inotrope/vasodilator drug (S K & F 94120) in the dog. Arch Toxicol 59:51–55
Hashimoto K, Imai K, Yoshimura S, Ohtaki T (1981) Toxicological studies of captopril, an inhibitor of angiotensin-converting enzyme 3. Twelve month studies on the chronic toxicity of captopril in rats. J Toxicol Sci [Suppl 2] 6:215–246
Hayasaka I, Uchiyama K, Murakami K, Kato Z, Tamaki F, Shibata T, Sugawara T, Hayashi M (1984) Teratogenicity of azosemide, a loop diuretic, in rats, mice and rabbits. Congenital Anomalies (Senten Ijo) 24:111–121
Herman E, Balazs T, Young R, Earl F, Krop S, Ferrans V (1979) Acute cardiomyopathy induced by the vasodilating antihypertensive agent minoxidil. Toxicol Appl Pharmacol 47:493–503
Hirsch KS, Wilson JG, Scott WJ, O'Flaherty EJ (1983) Acetazolamide teratology and its association with carbonic anhydrase inhibition in the mouse. Teratogenesis Carcinog Mutagen 3:2
Hoffmann K (1983) Toxicological studies with nitrendipine In: Scriabine A, Vanor S, Deck K (eds) Nitrendipine. Urban and Schwarzenberg, Baltimore, p 25

Holmes LB, Kawanishi H, Munoz A (1988) Acetazolamide: maternal toxicity, pattern of malformations, and litter effect. Toxicology 37:335–342

Imai K, Yoshimura S, Ohtaki T, Hashimoto K (1981) Toxicological studies of captopril, an inhibitor of angiotensin converting enzyme 2. One month studies on the subacute toxicity of captopril in rats. J Toxicol Sci [Suppl 2] 6:189–214

Kaneta M, Abe K, Ito T (1983) Juxtaglomerular cells in mice after long-term treatment with captopril: an electron microscopic study. Jpn Circ J 47:1071–1076

Kazda S, Garthoff BD, Ramsch KD, Schlueter G (1983) Nisoldipine. In: Scriabine A (ed) Cardiovascular drugs, vol 1. Raven, New York, p 243 (New drugs annual)

Keim GR (1980) Toxicology and drug metabolic studies of SQ 14,225 in animals. In: Case DB, Sonnenblick EH, Laragh JH (eds) Captopril and hypertension. Plenum, New York, p 137

Keith IM, Will JAI, Weir EK (1982) Captopril: association with fetal death and pulmonary vascular changes in the rabbit. Proc Soc Exp Biol Med 170:378–383

Kennedy JH, Alousi M, Homi J (1966) The protective effect of hyperbaric oxygenation upon isoproterenol-induced myocardial necrosis in syrian hamsters. Med Thorac 23:169–173

La Rocca PT, Squibb RE, Powell ML, Szot RJ, Black HE, Schwartz E (1986) Acute and subchronic toxicity of a nonsulfhydryl angiotensin-converting enzyme inhibitor. Toxicol Appl Pharmacol 82:104–111

Layton WM, Hallesy DW (1965) Deformity of forelimb in rats: association with high doses of acetazolamide. Science 149:306–308

Lumley CE, Walker SR (1986) A critical appraisal of the duration of chronic animal toxicity studies. Regul Toxicol Pharmacol 6:66–72

MacDonald JS, Bagdon WJ, Peter CP, Sina JF, Robertson RT, Ulm EH, Bokelman DL (1987) Renal effects of enalapril in dogs. Kidney Int [Suppl 20] 31:S148–S153

Manson JM, Zenick H, Costlow RD (1984) Teratology test methods for laboratory animals. In: Hayes AW (ed) Principles and methods of toxicology. Raven, New York, p 141

Maren TH, Ellison AC (1972) The effects of acetazolamide and amiloride on tissue electrolytes, with reference to the teratogenesis of carbonic anhydrase inhibition. J Pharmacol Exp Ther 181:212–218

Myhre JH (1978) Oral, stage II teratologic study in rats, study 7808. Squibb Memorandum, Nov 13, SQ 14225

Nishimura H, Bailey JR (1982) Intrarenal renin-angiotensin: system in primitive vertebrates. Kidney Int [Suppl 12] 22:S185–S192

Nishimura M, Iizuka M, Iwaki S, Kast A (1982) Repairability of drug-induced "wavy-ribs"in rat offspring. Arzneimittel forschung 32:1518–1522

Osborne CA, Finco DR, Locu DG (1975) Renal failure: diagnosis, treatment and prognosis. In: Ellinger SJ (ed) Textbook of veterinary internal medicine–diseases of dogs and cats. Saunders, Philadelphia, p 1465

Overturf ML, Sybers HD, Druilhet RE, Smith SA, Kirkendall WM (1982) Capoten-induced juxtaglomerular hyperplasia in rabbits. Res Commum Chem Pathol Pharmacol 36:169–172

Robens JF, Joiner JJ, Schueler RL (1984) Methods in testing for carcinogenicity. In: Hayes AW (ed) Principles and methods of toxicology. Raven, New York, p 79

Robertson RT, Minsker DH, Bokelman DL, Durand G, Conquet P (1981) Potassium loss as a causative factor for skeletal malformations in rats produced by indacrinone: a new investigational loop diuretic. Toxicol Appl Pharmacol 60:142–150

Schlueter G (1986) Toxicological investigations with nimodipine. Arzneimittel forschung 36:1733–1735

Sibley PL, Keim GR, Keysser CH, Kulesza JS, Miller MM, Zaidi IH (1978) SQ 14,225, an orally active inhibitor of angiotensin-converting enzyme: acute and subacute toxicity in animals. Toxicol Appl Pharmacol 45:315–316

Sterz H, Sponer G, Neubert P, Hebold G (1985) A postulated mechanism of beta-sympathomimetic induction of rib and limb anomalies in rat fetuses. Teratology 31:401–412

Stevens KR, Gallo MA (1984) Practical considerations in the conduct of chronic toxicity studies. In: Hayes AW (ed) Principles and methods of toxicology. Raven, New York, p 53

Storch TG, Layton WM (1971) The role of hypercapnia in acetazolamide teratogenesis. Experimentia 27:534–535

Sybertz EJ, Watkins RW, Ann HS, Baum T, La Rocca P, Patrick J, Leitz F (1987) Pharmacologic, metabolic, and toxicologic profile of spirapril (SCH 33844), a new angiotensin converting enzyme inhibitor. J Cardiovasc Pharmacol 10 (Suppl 7):S103–S108

Turnbull GJ, Lee PN, Roe FJC (1985) Relationship of body weight gain to longevity and to risk of development of nephropathy and neoplasia in sprague-dawley rats. Food Chem Toxicol 23:355–361

Ugen KE, Scott WJ (1985) Potentiation of acetazolamide induced ectrodactyly in wistar rats by vasoactive agents and physical clamping of the uterus. Teratology 31:273–278

Ugen KE, Scott WJ (1986) Acetazolamide teratogenesis in wistar rats: potentiation and antagonism by adrenergic agents. Teratology 34:195–200

Weaver TE, Scott WJ (1984) Acetazolamide teratogenesis: association of maternal respiratory acidosis and ectrodactyly in C57BL/6J mice. Teratology 30:187–193

Wilson JG, Maren TH, Takano K, Ellison A (1968) Teratogenic action of carbonic anhydrase inhibitors in the rat. Teratology 1:51–60

Zaki FG, Keim GR, Takii Y, Inagami T (1982) Hyperplasia of juxtaglomerular cells and renin localisation in kidneys of normotensive animals given captopril: electron microscopic and immunohistochemical studies. Ann Clin Lab Sci 12:200–215

CHAPTER 23

Traditions of Antihypertensive Therapy in Different Countries

CONTENTS

1 Continental Europe

R. LANG, H.M. STEFFEN, W. KAUFMANN

The therapy of hypertension has evolved over the past 50 years from the short-term care of a small number of hospitalized patients with severely elevated blood pressure and organ damage to a major community health problem involving a substantial proportion of the population with mild to moderate hypertension. In the beginning, severe side effects and toxicity of antihypertensive agents were accepted by patients and doctors as the price that had to be paid for this life-saving therapy. The results of recent therapeutic trials show the benefits of antihypertensive treatment for mild to moderate hypertension. This has changed the attitudes towards treatment. The aim of modern antihypertensive therapy is the reduction of the risk of cardiovascular disease. The management of hypertensive patients therefore has to include the minimization of other controllable risk factors such as diabetes, hypercholesterolemia, alcohol, and cigarette smoking. Blood pressure lowering can be achieved not only by pharmacological substances but also by non-drug methods, e.g., reduction of sodium intake, reduction of body weight, reduction of alcohol intake, increased physical activity, and meditation. These methods are part of an antihypertensive strategy with different priorities in the European countries.

The history of antihypertensive treatment is partly influenced by the availability of the different substances; however, the prescribing patterns vary from country to country for less obvious reasons.

1.1 Rauwolfia Drugs

Therapeutic applications of the whole root of *Rauwolfia serpentina* as a treatment for hypertension has been known in India for a long time. It was not until 1949 that the physicians in Western countries paid attention to this finding. *Rauwolfia* drugs have been used widely in the Federal Republic of Germany since the beginning of the 1950s, and they were the most prescribed drugs for hypertension even in the early 1970s in FRG, Italy, and Spain (Figs. 1, 5). Since then there has been a worldwide reduction in the use of *Rauwolfia* drugs. It is probable that the antihypertensive effects are related to both the central and peripheral actions of reserpine, while some of the side effects are clearly related to its action in the brain. Approximately 5% of the patients treated with *Rauwolfia* drugs must discontinue treatment because of intolerable side effects. Many patient will accept the sedation without complaint, but there may be psychotic depression. When the initially employed high dosage was decreased, the incidence of side effects diminished. Reserpine in combination with thiazide

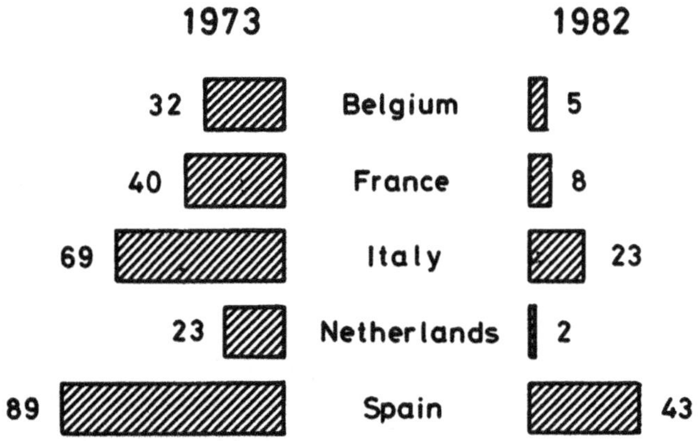

Fig. 1. Percentage of all prescriptions for antihypertensive agents that contained *Rauwolfia* (incl. combinations) in different European countries

diuretics is still widely used, especially in the German-speaking countries. Looking back, the introduction of reserpine into clinical use was the first step towards a modern pharmacological treatment of hypertension and correctly used, still is an inexpensive, effective treatment.

1.2 Diuretics

The mercurial diuretics were first used by parenteral administration to lower blood pressure in hypertensive patients. The discovery and development of thiazide compounds in the late 1950s constitute the next great contribution. The thiazide diuretics became the cornerstone of modern antihypertensive therapy, and a steady increase in clinical use can be observed for these drugs in most

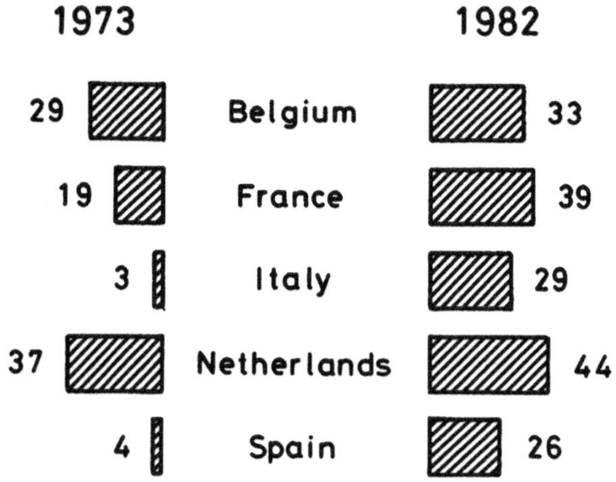

Fig. 2. Percentage of all prescriptions for diuretic antihypertensive agents in different European countries

European countries (Fig. 2). Recently, concern has emerged that thiazide diuretics may be atherogenic by worsening glucose tolerance and affecting lipoprotein metabolism. Furosemide was introduced in 1966, and its use has rapidly increased because of its potent diuretic action by inhibiting the ion transport at the ascending loop of Henle. As a parenterally applicable agent it has been used in cardiac emergencies since then. In patients with impaired renal function, furosemide is still the drug of choice in the treatment of hypertension.

With the introduction of spironolactone in Europe in 1960, triamterene in 1961, and amiloride in 1969, there have been important additions to the physician's antihypertensive armamentarium. The chief clinical use of these agents is in combination with the above-mentioned, more potent diuretics for the purpose of preventing hypokalemia, which thiazides or furosemide may produce. Spironolactone as an antagonist of aldosterone is the drug of choice in patients with primary hyperaldosteronism.

1.3 Ganglionic Blocking Drugs

Hexamethonium, pentolinium, and trimethaphan were widely used during the early 1950s. They are difficult to use in chronic antihypertensive therapy, causing usually severe side effects due to their parasympathetic blockade, e.g., constipation and paralytic ileus, but they provided effective treatment for most hypertensive emergencies in those days. A further improvement in drug development was the synthesis of agents capable of blocking selectively the sympathetic nervous system without the unwanted effect of parasympathetic blockade. The first of these drugs was guanethidine, an adrenergic blocking agent with a selective action at the peripheral sympathetic neuron, which was introduced in 1959. However, because of their marked side effects, mainly orthostatic hypotension, guanethidine as well as ganglionic blocking drugs were replaced in subsequent years by less troublesome antihypertensives.

1.4 Sympatholytica with a Central Action

Methyldopa was introduced in 1963 and is widely used throughout the world, whereas it never has reached great popularity in FRG. Methyldopa was regarded as an agent capable of filling the gap between the more potent ganglionic and adrenergic blockers and the diuretics or reserpine. Clonidine was discovered in 1962 and introduced into FRG in 1966, much earlier than in the English-speaking countries.

The main problem with the use of both drugs are their central side effects. In the late 1960s and early 1970s clonidine was recommended in Europe as one of the step 2 drugs, especially for the treatment of severe hypertension. However, as a consequence of its side effects, possible due to too high doses, their use declined in most European countries with the exception of Italy and Spain (Fig. 3). The pharmacological actions of clonidine and methyldopa on the medullary vasomotor control areas led to advances in the knowledge about the

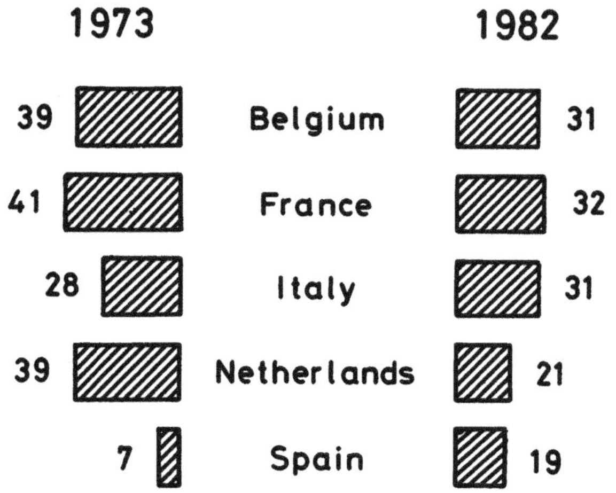

Fig. 3. Percentage of all prescriptions for antihypertensive agents that contained sympatholyticas with central/peripheral action and vasodilators in different European countries

mechanisms involved in the central control of blood pressure, and they became widely used research drugs.

1.5 Vasodilators

A further step in the treatment of hypertension, especially hypertensive emergencies, was the pharmacologically induced vasodilation by direct relaxation of the smooth muscle of peripheral arterioles. A number of vasodilator antihypertensive drugs (hydralazine, diazoxide, sodium nitroprusside, minoxidil) have this ability.

Hydralazine was introduced in 1951 as an arteriolar vasodilator. In the 1960s hydralazine lost popularity due to its unwanted side effects, but with the development of β-adrenoceptor blocking agents, interest was renewed. The risk of developing drug-induced lupus syndrome in approximately 5% of patients even at low dosages limits its use. Diazoxide, a potent arteriolar vasodilator, was introduced in 1973, showing its utmost efficacy in parenteral application in hypertensive crisis. Unacceptable toxicity, e.g., development of hyperglycemia, prevents its widespread clinical use.

Sodium nitroprusside was introduced for the treatment of hypertensive emergencies in 1974. Although the handling of the substance is difficult, as it can be given only parenterally, it is still today one of the drugs of choice for the treatment of pulmonary edema secondary to hypertensive heart disease. To avoid thiocyanate intoxication the thiocyanate levels are monitored during prolonged application in intensive care units.

Minoxidil, a potent, orally active arteriolar vasodilator, became generally available in the middle of the 1970s, making ambulatory therapy of patients with severe hypertension much more effective. One of its most undesirable side effects is hypertrichosis, which occurs in nearly all patients on prolonged therapy.

The percentage of prescriptions for sympatholytics and vasodilators has decreased in most countries (Fig. 3). However, in FRG this has been relative stable at approximately 3% for the prescription of vasodilators during the past 15 years. These drugs are still used in Europe as an effective alternative in the treatment of severe hypertension.

1.6 α-Adrenoceptor Antagonists

The classic α-adrenergic blocking agents phentalomine and phenoxybenzamine, which have been in use since the 1950s, are capable of blocking both the α_1- and α_2-adrenoceptors. They are of limited value in the management of hypertension and now are used only in the management of patients with pheochromocytomas. Besides troublesome adverse effects their blood pressure-lowering efficacy is only moderate. The selective α_1-adrenoceptor blocking agent prazosin was introduced in 1976 and is now widely used. Therapy with prazosin is considered to offer advantages especially in patients with accompanying congestive heart failure.

In recent years other selectively α_1-adrenoceptor blocking agents have been introduced (e.g., indoramin, urapidil) which, however, do not offer different therapeutic aspects. Although the principle of α-blockade has already been known for more than 30 years, the therapeutic role for the α-adrenoceptor blocking agents is still under discussion in Europe. On the one hand, they have marked side effects, e.g., orthostatic hypotension and fluid retention; on the other hand, they exhibit positive effects on glucose and lipoprotein metabolism which may be helpful in preventing atherosclerosis.

1.7 β-Adrenoceptor Antagonists

Propranolol was introduced as an effective antihypertensive drug in 1964. β-blocking agents have added an important therapeutic dimension to the treatment of hypertension. During the 1970s they became widely accepted in many European countries, representing the group of antihypertensive drugs with the greatest increase in prescriptions (Fig. 4). Finally, dozens of different β-blockers have become available in the 1980s, and the distinct preferences among β-blockers in different countries are mainly explained by marketing aspects.

The β-blocking agents have different pharmacological properties, e.g., cardioselectivity, intrinsic sympathomimetic activity, membrane stabilizing effect, solubility, and duration of action. Their blood pressure-lowering effect is equal regardless of the presence or absence of these associated pharmacological characteristics, and the overall hemodynamic and metabolic effects of the different β-blockers are similar. Specific pharmacological characteristics of these agents influence the selection of a particular drug in the clinical management of hypertensive patients with accompanying diseases.

More than 20 years of clinical experience with the use of β-blockers have made these agents the indispensable basic treatment in cases of uncomplicated

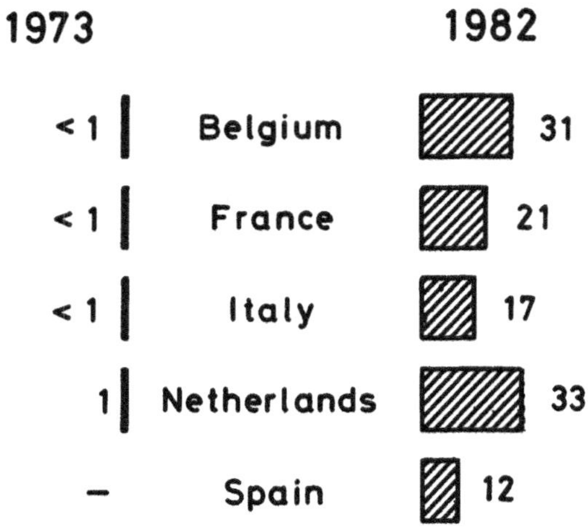

Fig. 4. Percentage of all prescriptions for antihypertensive agents that contained β-adrenoceptor antagonists in different European countries

hypertension. It has become clear that therapy employing these agents is much safer than initially expected.

Labetalol is a drug which differs from currently available adrenoceptor blocking agents because it blocks both α- and β-adrenoceptors. It has been suggested that labetalol may be an improvement in the therapy of severe hypertension and pheochromocytoma, an opinion which has not been generally accepted in Europe.

1.8 Calcium Antagonists

During the early 1960s the principle mechanisms of calcium antagonism were discovered, i.e., the inhibition of the cellular entry of calcium ions. Verapamil was introduced then primarily as an antiarrhythmic drug. Nifedipine was introduced in 1975 for the treatment of angina. Due to its pronounced arteriolar vasodilation it has been used increasingly as an antihypertensive drug. The effects of diltiazem, which was introduced during the late 1970s, seem to be intermediate to those of nifedipine and verapamil on pacemaker cells.

Oral application of nifedipine has become the treatment of choice in hypertensive crisis, leaving cerebral blood flow unchanged despite a marked fall in systemic blood pressure. It is considered an advantage that calcium antgonists do not interfere with the metabolism of glucose or lipoproteins and do not influence hepatic or renal function. Despite some disturbing side effects, e.g., dizziness, flushing, and headache, calcium antagonists are in comparison with other available antihypertensive agents well tolerated and are becoming the treatment of choice either in monotherapy or in combination. There is a steady increase in their use. In FRG the relative proportion of calcium antagonists in antihypertensive therapy rose from 1% in 1982 to 13% in 1987 (Fig. 5).

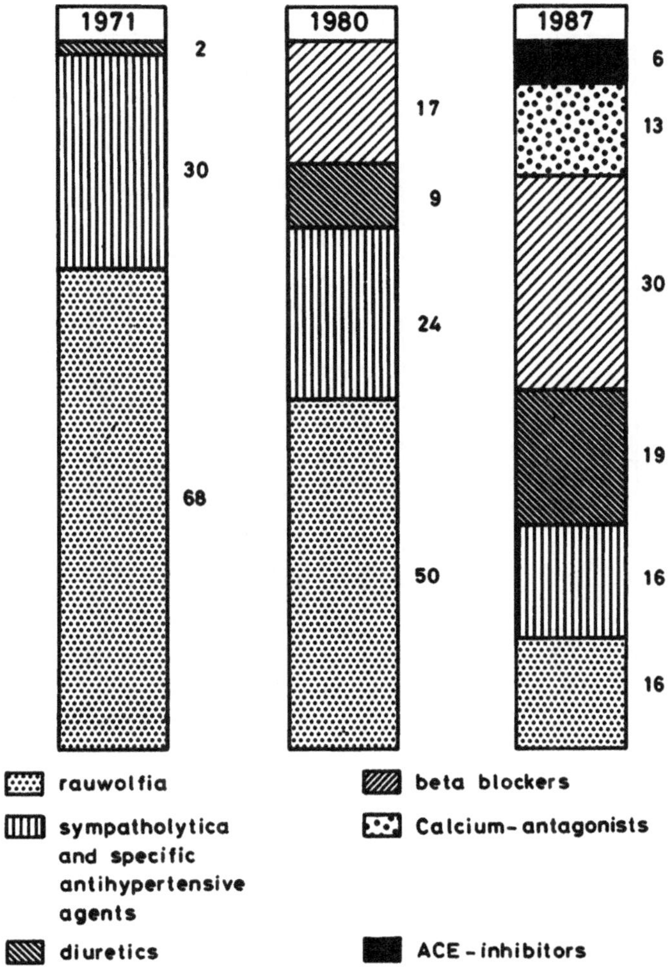

Fig. 5. Percentage of all prescriptions for antihypertensive agents in the Federal Republic of Germany

1.9 Converting Enzyme Inhibitors

The recognition of the importance of the renin-angiotensin system in hypertension has steadily increased since its discovery. In the diagnosis of angiotensin II-dependent hypertension the angiotensin receptor antagonist saralasin found temporarily clinical use. The orally applicable converting enzyme inhibitors captopril and enalapril were introduced in Europe in 1981 and 1984, respectively.

Converting enzyme inhibitors were initially used for severe forms of renovascular hypertension only at excessively high doses. Experience during the following years revealed that the blood pressure-lowering effect is independent of the pretreatment renin level. Thus, these drugs have been effective even in low renin hypertension and at low doses, which are well tolerated. A particular

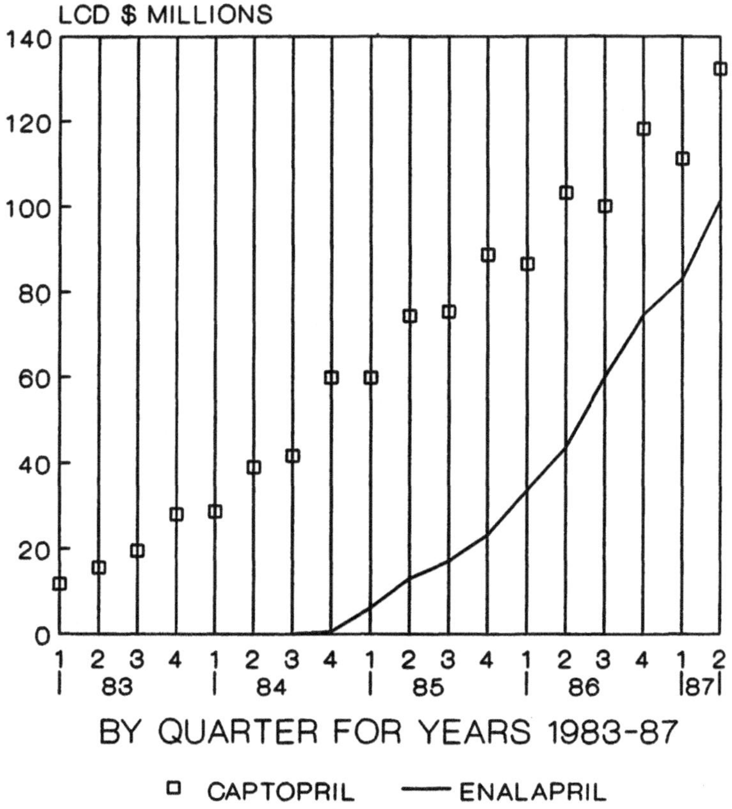

Fig. 6. Development of sales for angiotensin converting enzyme inhibitors in Europe

advantage of the converting enzyme inhibitor is that they do not cause reflex tachycardia while reducing the peripheral vascular resistance. Due to the venodilation concomitant with the arteriolar dilatation the use of converting enzyme inhibitors is especially beneficial in patients with hypertension and congestive heart failure. Within the past few years these drugs have become widely used, and the general acceptance of ACE inhibitors has led to their application even as monotherapy in mild hypertension in most but not all European countries. There is a rapid increase in the use of captopril and enalapril in most European countries (Fig. 6). Starting in 1981 with the sale of 1 million DM for captopril, the sales of converting enzyme inhibitors increased to 156 million DM in 1987, which was 16% of the total amount of the German antihypertensive drug market (978 million DM), whereas they represent only 6% of all antihypertensive prescriptions (Fig. 5).

References

Antonaccio MJ (ed) (1977) Cardiovascular pharmacology. Raven, New York
Birkenhäger WH, Reid JL (1984) Clinical pharmacology of antihypertensive drugs. In: Doyle AE (ed) Handbook of hypertension. Elsevier, Amsterdam
Bundesverband der Pharmazeutischen Industrie (1986) Basisdaten des Gesundheitwesens 1985/86. Bundesverband der Pharmazeutischen Industrie, Frankfurt
Davies DS, Reid JL (eds) (1975) Central action of drugs in blood pressure regulation. Pitman, London
Doyle AE, Bearn AG (eds) (1984) Hypertension and the angiotensin system. Raven, New York
Drayer JIM, Lowenthal DT, Weber MA (eds) (1987) Drug therapy in hypertension. Dekker, New York
Ganten D, Ritz E (eds) (1985) Lehrbuch der Hypertonie. Schattauer, Stuttgart
Genest J, Kuchel O, Hamet P, Cantin M (eds) (1983) Hypertension. McGraw-Hill, New York
Gessler U (ed) (1978) Differentialdiagnose und Therapie der Hypertonie. Aesopus, Lugano
Kaufmann W, Bönner G, Lang R, Meurer KA (eds) (1986) Primary hypertension. Springer, Berlin Heidelberg New york
Kobinger W, Ahlquist RP (eds) (1984) Alpha and beta adrenoceptors and the cardiovascular system. Excerpta Medica, Amsterdam
McMahon FG (ed) (1978) Management of essential hypertension. Futura, New York
Rosenthal J (ed) (1986) Arterielle Hypertonie. Springer, Berlin Heidelberg New York
Stumpe KO (ed) (1983) Therapie mit Antihypertensiva. Springer, Berlin Heidelberg New York

2 Scandinavia

L. Wilhelmsen

2.1 Introduction

Important prerequisites for the analysis of drug consumption over time and in different countries include defined criteria and a well-developed system for monitoring the sales of drugs. The Nordic Council on Medicines was established in 1974 with the aim to work for harmonization of legislation and administration in medicine in the Nordic countries, coordination of statistics, more effective interNordic reporting of adverse reactions, increased cooperation on drug information, and continued cooperation with the pharmacopeia. This agency has published Nordic Statistics on Medicines based upon sales statistics from 1975 to 1983 in three different volumes (published in 1979, 1982, and 1986). The different publications have covered 20%, 50%, and 80%, respectively, of medicines available in the Nordic countries. The work of the Council mirrors the interest in the Nordic countries in the epidemiology of drug usage, and it has encouraged studies into possible reasons for national differences.

2.2 Definitions

Of great importance for the work has been the classification of medicines according to the anatomical-therapeutic-chemical classification system (ATC system) and the technical characterization unit, the defined daily dose (DDD). These systems are also recommended by the WHO Drug Utilization Research Group (DURG).

In order to evaluate, discuss, or compare drug consumption in the individual countries, knowledge of the preparations classified in each ATC group is necessary. In addition, the DDDs used for the presentation of drug consumption must be available. In part 2 of Nordic Statistics on Medicine (Nordic Council on Medicines 1986) the DDDs for different drugs are stated. As examples it can be mentioned that the DDD for bendroflumethiazide is 2.5 mg, for hydrochlorothiazide 50 mg, and for the β-blocking agents, propranolol 160 mg, metoprolol 200 mg, and atenolol 100 mg.

It should, however, be emphasized that the ATC system and the DDD unit can only provide an approximate expression of how the drugs are used, as the drugs are often used for a variety of purposes and in different doses. β-Blocking drugs are for example used both as antianginal drugs and as hypotensive drugs, and diuretics are used both in the treatment of congestive heart failure and in hypertension, and the relative proportion used for these different indications may be difficult to calculate. However, in Sweden as in some other countries, a continued evaluation of all prescriptions in relation to diagnosis is carried out, so some information on the topic is available. The DDDs may differ from the prescribed daily doses (PDD) due to differences in traditions. However, at least for Norway and Sweden it has been shown that the DDDs agree reasonably well with currently PDDs (BAKSAAS 1984).

2.3 Results

Figure 1 shows a summary of the consumption of all hypotensive drugs from 1971 until 1980 according to BAKSAAS (1984), showing that Sweden had nearly twice as high a consumption as the other Nordic countries in 1971. The consumption increased for Denmark and Finland and was close to that of Sweden in 1980, whereas Norway and Iceland only had about two-thirds of that consumption in 1980. For comparison Northern Ireland and Czechoslovakia are shown, and these countries had a much lower consumption in 1971, and it did not rise as much as in the Nordic countries during the 10-year follow-up.

Prescription data according to a somewhat different classification system with hypotensives including antiadrenergic agents, agents acting on the arterial smooth muscles, agents acting on the renin-angiotensin system, and various

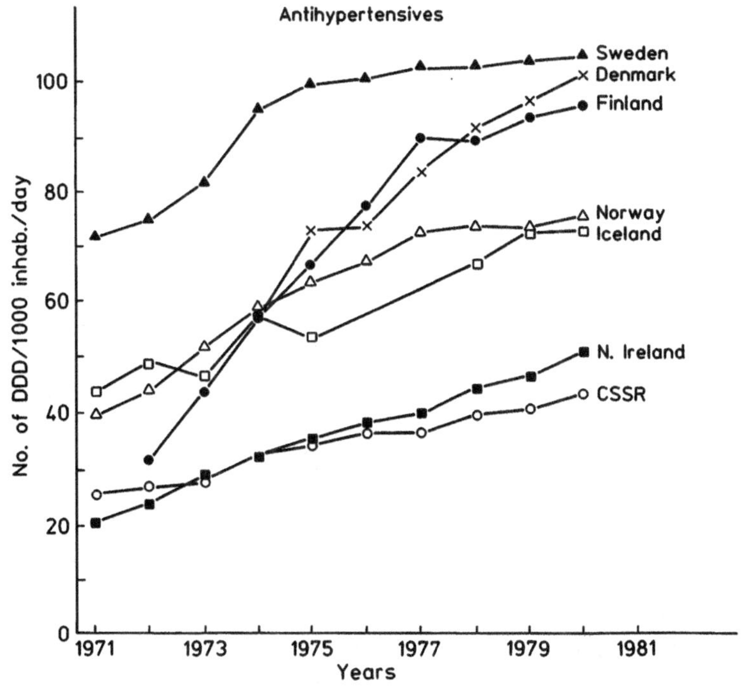

Fig. 1. Sales or prescription data (*N Ireland*) of drugs in seven European countries, 1971–1980, expressed as DDD per 1000 inhabitants per day (BAKSAAS 1984, used with permission)

combinations are given in Fig. 2. There have been increasing trends for Denmark, Norway, and Sweden, but somewhat decreasing trends for Finland, which on the other hand has a higher consumption than the other countries. Much of this difference is due to a higher prescription of agents acting on the renin-angiotensin system in Finland.

Figure 3 shows the prescription of β-blockers between 1971 and 1980 for the Nordic countries as well as Northern Ireland and Czechoslovakia. In Sweden about 14 times more β-blockers were prescribed in 1980 than in Czechoslovakia, more than twice as much as in Denmark and Northern Ireland, and about one and a half times the prescription rate in Finland, Iceland, and Norway.

Figure 4 gives the prescription for a more recent period for the previously mentioned hypotensive drugs, for diuretics, and for the β-blocking agents. In Sweden the prescription rate stabilized during the period 1979–1983, whereas it increased in the other Nordic countries, except for Denmark, to a level which in 1983 was close to that in Sweden. The selective β-blockers have gained ground and were prescribed to a much greater extent than the nonselective β-blockers, with the exception of Finland where nonselective β-blockers were still prescribed to about 40% in 1983. It can be seen that diuretics were used considerably more than β-blockers and other hypotensives, especially in Denmark.

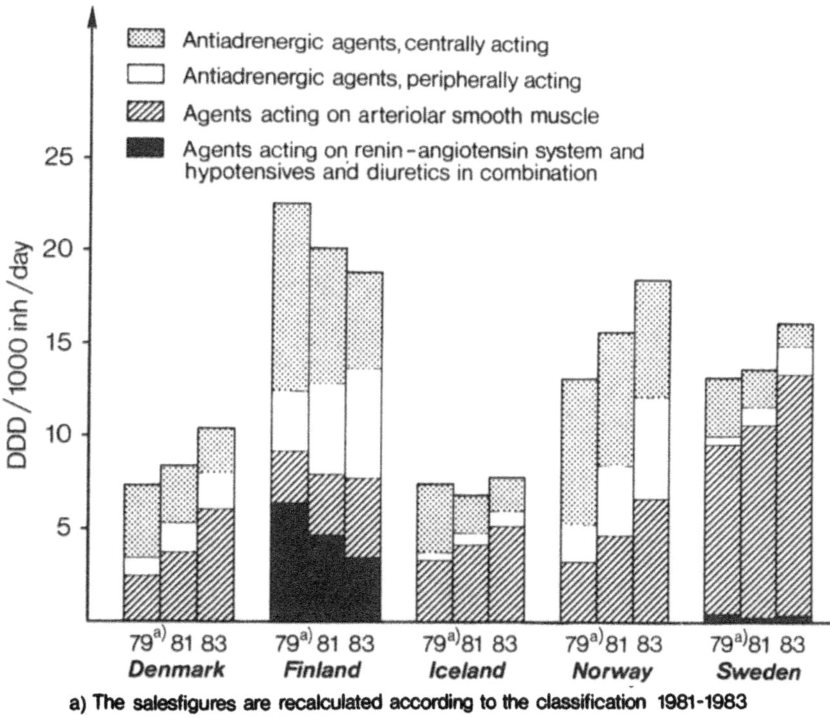

Fig. 2. Sales figures for antihypertensive drugs in Nordic countries 1979–1983 The fourth group (*solid bars*) includes both agents acting on the renin-angiotensin system and combinations of antihypertensives and diuretics (Nordic Council of Medicines 1986, used with permission).

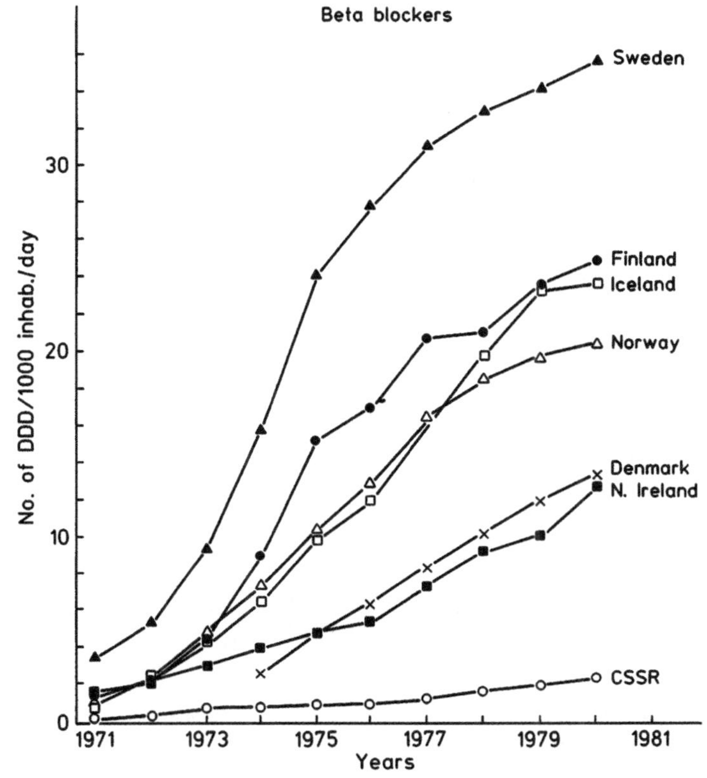

Fig. 3. Sales or prescription data (*N Ireland*) of β-blockers in seven European countries, 1971–1980 (BAKSAAS 1984, used with permission)

Prazosin, β-blockers, and calcium antagonists are gaining ground at the expense of methyldopa, while hydralazine was still used to a great extent in 1983. Clonidine was used in Finland, but very little in the other Nordic countries. The use of ACE inhibitors has increased rather rapidly recently in Sweden (Fig. 5).

β-Blockers, diuretics, calcium blockers, and ACE inhibitors are used for other indications than hypertension. Statistics in Sweden linking prescription to diagnosis indicate that about 75% of the β-blockers and 85% of the thiazides are used in the treatment of hypertension (Swedish Statistics on Medicines 1986). The drug profile in hypertension treatment based upon the same survey is given in Table 1 for the years 1979 and 1986. This table also shows the trend that more selective β-blockers, fewer diuretics, somewhat less hydralazine, and more ACE inhibitors and calcium channel-blocking drugs are being used.

2.4 Discussion

The majority of patients treated for hypertension have moderate hypertension, and the main aim of treatment is to try to prevent stroke, congestive heart

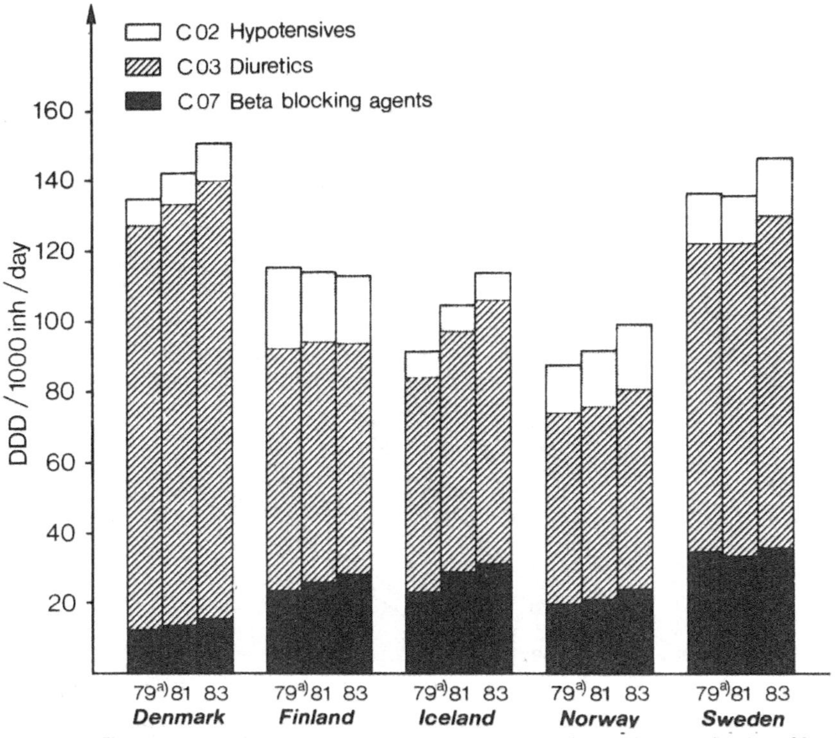

a) The salesfigures for hypotensives are recalculated according to the classification 1981-1983

Fig. 4. Sales figures for antihypertensives (according to definition in Fig. 2), diuretics, and β-blocking agents (Nordic Council of Medicines 1986, used with permission)

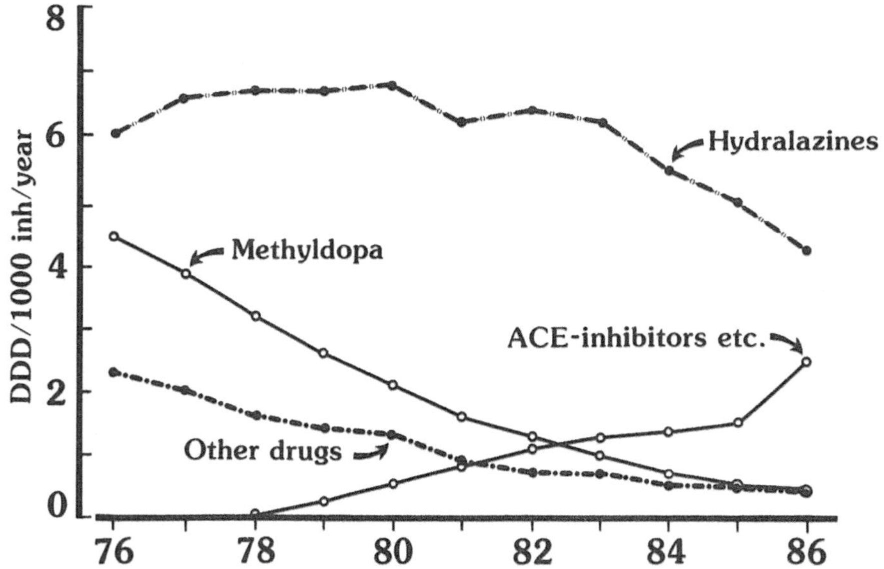

Fig. 5. Sales of some antihypertensive drugs in Sweden 1976–1986 (Swedish Statistics on Medicines 1986)

Table 1. Drug profile in hypertension management, Sweden

Drug	Percentage of drug-treated patients	
	1979	1986
β-Blockers	44	49
Nonselective	16	14
Selective	28	35
Diuretics	65	59
Bendroflumethiazide	24	21
Hydrochlorothiazide	11	9
Spironolactone	3	10
Combinations	13	15
Other diuretics	14	4
Hydralazine	13	9
ACE inhibitors	0	3
Calcium blockers	1	6
Potassium supplement	7	4
Other drugs	3	3

Percentage of patients not prescribed any drug was 3%. Number of preparations per drug-treated patient = 1.4.

failure, renal complications, and the most common sequel, coronary heart disease. For most of these diseases several factors contribute to the risk, and antihypertensive treatment is only one measure to prevent disease. The utilization of hypotensive drugs should preferably be related to the prevalence of hypertension in the specific community, but morbidity data that can be compared between countries are difficult to achieve. Therapeutic traditions may differ between prescribing physicians in various countries and may explain part of the reported differences in the use of drugs. In a recent study it was not possible to confirm that the different therapeutic attitudes in Northern Ireland, Norway, and Sweden are a major reason for the intercountry differences (GRIFFITHS et al. 1986). On the contrary, the threshold for treatment is lowest in Northeran Ireland, which also has the lowest total usage of these drugs. Thus, real differences in the prevalence rate of hypertension seem to be a more likely explanation for the difference, but even though that type of information seems rather easy to achieve, reliable data are not available.

The death rate from cardiovascular diseases, especially coronary heart disease, is considerably higher in Finland than in the other Nordic countries, and it is also rather high in Northern Ireland. This fact does not seem to explain the different prescription habits either.

There were marked differences in the type of different hypotensive drugs used, with a strong tendency to employ β-blocking drugs in Sweden and diuretics in Denmark. It may be that the positive results on morbidity and mortality in postinfarction trials with β-blockers (YUSUF et al. 1985) have been considered to be valid also in primary prevention and to a greater extent in Sweden than in the other countries. Other reasons, like suggestions that thiazides and β-blockers might interfere adversely with lipid metabolism, could have had greater impact on prescribing habits in some countries than in others. The importance of various opinion leaders among physicians might also be significant in this context.

Besides the possible medical implications of the use of different hypotensive drugs, there are clearly economic consequences. In 1980 Swedish expenses for hypotensive drugs were about 53% higher per capita than those in Norway and 58% higher than those in Denmark. The reason is to a large extent the different prescription rates for diuretics and β-blockers. The economic results of using cheaper drug profiles have been discussed by WAALER and HJORT (1982). In conclusion, the cost for treatment of hypertension is dependent upon the prevalence of the condition in the community, the treatment traditions regarding level of blood pressure at which treatment is started, and the choice of type of antihypertensive drugs because of the marked differences in costs between them.

References

Baksaas I (1984) Patterns in drug utilization—national and international aspects: Antihypertensive drugs. Acta Med Scand [Suppl] 683:59–66

Griffiths K, McDevitt DG, Andrew M, Baksaas I, Helgeland A, Jervell J, Lunde PKM, et al. (1986) Therapeutic traditions in Northern Ireland, Norway and Sweden. II. Hypertension. Eur J Clin Pharmacol 30:521–525

Nordic Council on Medicines (1979) Nordic statistics on medicines 1975–1977. Nordic Council on Medicines, Helsinki

Nordic Council on Medicines (1982) Nordic statistics on medicines 1978–1980. Nordic Council on Medicines, Uppsala

Nordic Council on Medicines (1986) Nordic statistics on medicines 1981–1983. Nordic Council on Medicines, Uppsala

Swedish Statistics on Medicines (1986) Diagnosis and therapy survey. Apoteksbolaget, Stockholm

Waaler HT, Hjort PF (1982) The consumption of blood pressure lowering drugs in the Nordic countries. In: Nordic Council on Medicines (ed) Nordic statistics on medicines 1978–1980. Nordic Council on Medicines, Uppsala, pp 195–215 (NLN publication no 8)

Yusuf S, Peto R, Lewis J, Collins R, Sleight P (1985) Beta-blockade during and after myocardial infarction: An overview of the randomized trials. Prog Cardiovasc Dis 5:335–371

3 United Kingdom

J.I.S. Robertson

Serious investigation into hypertension in the United Kingdom can be regarded as beginning with the experiment of Stephen Hales of Teddington. Hales (1733, cited by Smirk 1957, p. 4) cannulated the carotid artery of a conscious restrained horse and so made the first direct observation of intra-arterial blood pressure.

Richard Bright of Guy's Hospital in London showed the connection between cardiac and arterial hypertrophy and nephrosclerosis with albuminuria, observations which formed a basis for understanding the inter-relationships between raised arterial pressure and pathological changes in various organs (Bright 1827, 1836).

The very strong and influential modern British tradition in the cardiovascular field in general and of hypertension in particular stems notably from the laboratory of Thomas Lewis of University College Hospital, London, in the 1920s and 1930s. The work of this school established a sound investigational basis for understanding the physiology and pathophysiology of the cardiovascular system. Probably the most distinguished of Lewis' pupils was Pickering. The authority and prestige of Pickering especially ensured in the years that followed a sustained critical and essentially scientific creative interest. The pervasive influence of Lewis, Pickering and their successors spread well beyond the shores of the UK and is still evident in the third, fourth and fifth generations of research workers.

Two others who subsequently achieved considerable fame in the field of hypertension were McMichael and Smirk. Both McMichael and Smirk worked at University College Hospital in Lewis' time, although in other departments and not then on hypertension. They appear to have remained apart from Lewis and his group, although it is possible that provocative stimuli may have been exchanged, perhaps engendering some of the refreshing arguments that later took place between Pickering, McMichael, Smirk and their various schools.

With this background it is scarcely surprising that the discipline of clinical pharmacology took root in Britain and from the outset was deeply involved with cardiovascular medicine (Dollery 1987).

Such basic interest also guaranteed continual attention to the pathogenesis and both the surgical and, where appropriate, medical treatment of secondary forms of hypertension, notably phaeochromocytoma, aldosterone-secreting adenoma, aortic coarctation and renovascular hypertension, as well as of essential hypertension.

Central to present concepts of preventive antihypertensive therapy lies a celebrated and almost exclusively British controversy concerning the nature of essential hypertension, involving Pickering and Platt. The course of this dispute and its eventual resolution have been recounted by SWALES (1985). SWALES emphasizes the contrasting traditions inherited by Pickering and Platt, traditions which represent distinct philosophies stretching back to the nineteenth century. Pickering's early career was firmly based in experimental laboratory studies. Platt spent what he regarded as an educationally illuminating and formative 10 years in private practice. Pickering and Platt agreed that raised arterial pressure as such is predominantly responsible for the complications of hypertension. However, Pickering considered that, probably because of polygenic inheritance, blood pressure values within populations were distributed continuously, with no evident demarkation between "normal" blood pressure and "hypertension". By contrast Platt believed that a single gene with incomplete dominance was responsible for essential hypertension. According to this latter view blood pressures within the population were distributed bimodally, with the existence of a distinct hypertensive subset. After a stormy and entertaining debate, accompanied by vigorous polemic, vehement invective but little apparent rancour, the view of Pickering prevailed. The implications of this for the treatment of hypertension are evident. As blood pressure is continuously distributed in the population so, and proportionately, is the consequent risk of cardiovascular complications. The indications for and benefits to be derived from antihypertensive therapy follow the curve describing blood pressure and thus risk.

The Pickering/Platt controversy illustrated, not surprisingly, some contemporary British naivety of the understanding of certain genetic, statistical and pathophysiological issues, and its resolution required the rapid development of expertise in the defective areas. Such awakening of interest was wholly beneficial, and the derived benefits are being exploited even today. Proper epidemiological surveys of blood pressure were undertaken, with due attention being paid to standardization of the circumstances of measurement and the avoidance of bias in recording the readings. Continuous blood pressure measurements over 24 h were made, and techniques for undertaking these have subequently evolved steadily. The results have emphasized not only the continuous distribution of blood pressure within populations, but also its continual diurnal change in individuals (PICKERING 1968). Thus it is more appropriate to discuss the "tessitura" rather than the "level" of blood pressure in a person. Not surprisingly, risk has been shown to be more closely related to blood pressures as recorded continuously than to single readings made at intervals (WEBER 1987). From this work has evolved improved expertise in the design, conduct and interpretation of controlled intervention trials. Not least, interest has focused on the heritable factor or factors in arterial blood pressure, and their interplay with the environment in determining the tessitura of pressure in an individual.

It is against this background that the treatment of essential hypertension evolved in Britain. With contributions from such diverse, colourful and opinionated characters, it appears more appropriate to talk of "trends" or even "controversies" rather than "tradition" in this country. The acceptance or denial of a particular treatment has frequently been forceful, although the rational basis for this approach is not always evident. Such variations within one country perhaps help to explain in part the even bigger divergencies of therapeutic fashion between countries.

The earliest approaches were surgical: bilateral adrenalactomy and bilateral dorsolumbar sympathectomy. These were formidable procedures, with frequent complications and unpleasant side effects. Nevertheless, they showed the benefits to be derived in severely hypertensive patients from blood pressure reduction.

Moreover, sympathectomy paved the way for the autonomic ganglion blockers, of which hexamethonium, azamethonium and later pentolinium were employed therapeutically (BARLOW and ING 1948; PATON and ZAIMIS 1948). These effectively began the modern era of antihypertensive drug therapy. Despite their prominent side effects, the ganglion blocking agents and their successors, the adrenergic neuron antagonists, were enthusiastically and not always very critically espoused, notably by MCMICHAEL (1952), PLATT (1954), ROSENHEIM (1954), SMIRK (1957) and LEISHMAN (1959). Strangely, PICKERING (1968), although a champion of sympathectomy, seemed sometimes to evince less zeal in pursuing treatment with these early drugs.

The ambivalent combination of enthusiasm and critical denial has marked the British approach to antihypertensive drugs from those early days to the present. Reserpine, extensively employed in FRG, USA, Switzerland and elsewhere, fell foul of PLATT and SEARS (1956) and of SMIRK (1957), who reported severe depression and suicide in patients given the drug. Despite its efficacy, reserpine was described by PLATT and SEARS (1956) as a "dangerous drug", and it rapidly declined in favour in the UK as a consequence. Despite the subsequent demonstration that in lower doses the drug was both effective and well-tolerated, it never regained its position.

Reserpine is by no means alone in the UK in suffering from the vigour and eminence of detractors. Hydralazine similarly was early and possibly correctly tainted by the observation that it induces a lupus-like syndrome (PERRY and SCHROEDER 1954). Although hydralazine has since been shown to be, at least in the short term, effective and well-tolerated when given in association with a diuretic and a β-adrenoceptor blocker (MCAREAVEY et al. 1984), the lupus features remain too frequent for comfort (CAMERON and RAMSAY 1984).

Orally active diuretics were, quite soon in their era in antihypertensive therapy, subjected in the UK to a small but careful dose-response study (CRANSTON et al. 1963). The lessons of this were not absorbed perhaps as well as might have been, because the subsequent Medical Research Council (MRC) trial of antihypertensive treatment (Medical Research Council Working Party 1985) employed what many regard as an excessively high dose, 10 mg daily, of bendrofluazide. Herein is illustrated conspicuously the ambivalence of the British attitude. The MRC trial clearly demonstrated the wide range of metabolic, electrophysiological and symptomatic problems accompanying the use of thiazides (Medical Research Council Working Party 1981, 1983) but has also been interpreted as freeing these agents from suspicion of carrying serious adverse effects (RAMSAY 1985). Despite the assurances, I retain some concern that thiazides may be in part harmful as well as beneficial (ROBERTSON 1987).

The history of the introduction of β-blocking drugs in the treatment of hypertension in the UK is particularly intriguing. Their early development has been described in piquant detail by BLACK (1988). The antihypertensive effect of β-blockade was discovered as a result of an astute observation made by PRICHARD (1964). For several years PRICHARD's conviction that this could be a major contribution to the therapeutic repertoire was regarded by colleagues, critics and drug manufacturers variously with scepticism, derision and hostility (CRUICKSHANK and PRICHARD 1988). Nevertheless, PRICHARD was eventually vindicated. β-Blocking drugs do indeed have an antihypertensive action and are now established in the UK, as elsewhere, as agents of first choice in the treatment of essential hypertension. In 1988 BLACK was awarded the Nobel Prize, largely for his work in creating these drugs.

Regulatory attitudes to more recent classes of antihypertensive drugs have become increasingly severe in the UK in the past few years. The powerful vasodilator minoxidil is, rightly, reserved for cases of severe, resistant hypertension. ACE inhibitors are not officially recognized as initial therapy. No serotonin antagonist is registered in the UK.

This cautious British attitude to the therapy of essential hypertension is not restricted to drugs. The ready acceptance of moderate dietary salt restriction so widespread elsewhere has not been seen in the UK (SWALES 1988), although other dietary approaches, such as weight reduction, limitation of alcohol intake and potassium supplementation have been explored with interest. Indeed the roles of dietary factors both in pathogenesis and treatment have been critically reviewed by Beilin, an Englishman in origin although now working in Australia. BEILIN (1988) was so impressed by these influences in the pathogenesis of primary hypertension that he considers the term "essential" in this connection to be now obsolete.

At present in the UK, there is more accord on the broad strategies to be employed in treating hypertension. This is firmly based on drug therapy, with non-pharmacological means being supportive only. Rigid adherence to stepped-care programmes is out of favour (ROBERTSON and BALL 1989). Instead, the requirements and the response of the individual patient are paramount, with accent on administering the minimum effective number and doses of drugs. Nowadays, if one agent is ineffective, it is usually withdrawn and another substituted, rather than layering one type of drug on top of another in steps. However, the use of different agents conjointly can be of value in obtaining an adequate response while minimizing unwanted side effects.

The indications for the treatment of mild hypertension have recently been reviewed by a committee of the British Hypertension Society in a document which has achieved remarkable accord in view of the composition of the group (SWALES et al. 1989). Pharmacological therapy is recommended in adult men and women under 80 years of age whose 5th phase diastolic pressure remains at 100 mmHg or more over a period of observation of 3–4 months. Subjects with a diastolic blood pressure of 95–99 mmHg over this period should not usually be treated but carefully followed at intervals of 3–6 months. Those whose diastolic pressure is initially raised but falls to values below 95 mmHg should have their pressure measured annually. All patients must be warned against smoking and heavy alcohol intake. When indicated, dietary weight reduction is advised. Initial therapy with a thiazide diuretic or β-blocker is acceptable; other drugs may be added as necessary where these are ineffective, poorly tolerated or contra-indicated. The objective is a diastolic pressure of 85–90 mmHg in the absence of unacceptable side effects. These are current guidelines only; the advice is necessarily interim and will require regular revision.

The tradition of antihypertensive therapy in the UK has been predominantly one of controversy rather than accord. It will be surprising if these recommendations are accepted nationwide or remain extant for long.

Acknowledgement. I am particularly grateful to Lady Carola Pickering for her recollections of University College Hospital, London, in the 1930s.

References

Barlow RB, Ing HR (1948) Curare-like action of polymethylene bisquarternary ammonium salts. Nature 161:718
Beilin LJ (1988) Epitaph to essential hypertension: a preventable disorder of known aetiology? J Hypertens 6:85–94
Black J (1988) Beta-blockers in clinical practice. Livingstone, Edinburgh, pp v–vii
Bright R (1827) Reports of medical cases, selected with a view of illustrating the symptoms and cure of diseases by a reference to morbid anatomy. Longman, London
Bright R (1836) Tabular view of the morbid appearances in 100 cases connected with albuminous urine. With observations. Guy's Hosp Rep 1:380–392
Cameron HA, Ramsay LE (1984) The lupus syndrome induced by hydralazine: a common complication with low-dose treatment. Br Med J 289:410–412
Cranston WI, Juel-Jensen BE, Semmence AM, Handfield-Jones RPC, Forbes JA, Mutch LMM (1963) Effects of oral diuretics on raised arterial pressure. Lancet 2:966–970
Cruickshank JM, Prichard BNC (1988) Beta-blockers in clinical practice. Livingstone, Edinburgh, pp 3–8
Dollery C (1987) Jubilee editorial: hypertension. Br Heart J 58:179–184
Leishman AWD (1959) Hypertension treated and untreated: a study of 400 cases. Br Med J 1:1361–1368
McAreavey D, Ramsay LE, Latham L, McLaren AD, Lorimer AR, Reid JL, Robertson JIS, et al. (1984) "Third Drug" trial: comparative study of antihypertensive agents added to treatment when blood pressure remains uncontrolled by a beta-blocker plus thiazide diuretic. Br Med J 288:106–111
McMichael J (1952) The management of hypertension. Br Med J 1:933–938
Medical Research Council Working Party (1981) Adverse reactions to bendrofluazide and propranolol following treatment of mild hypertension. Lancet 2:539–543
Medical Research Council Working Party (1983) Ventricular extrasystoles during thiazide treatment: substudy of the MRC Mild Hypertension Trial. Br Med J 287:1249–1253
Medical Research Council Working Party (1985) MRC Trial of Treatment of Mild Hypertension: principal results. Br Med J 291:97–104
Paton WD, Zaimis E (1948) Curare-like action of polymethylene bis-quarternary salts. Nature 161:718
Perry HM, Schroeder HA (1954) A syndrome simulating collagen disease caused by 1-hydrazino-phthaline (apresoline). JAMA 154:670–673.
Pickering GW (1968) High blood pressure, 2nd edn. J & A Churchill, London
Platt R (1954) Hypertensive retinopathy and its medical treatment. Q J Med 23:441–449
Platt R, Sears HTN (1956) Reserpine in severe hypertension. Lancet 1:401–403
Prichard BN (1964) Hypotensive action of pronethalol. Br Med J 1:1227–1228

Ramsay LE (1985) Mild hypertension: treat patients, not populations. J Hypertens 3:449–455
Robertson JIS (1987) The large studies in hypertension: what have they shown? Br J Clin Pharmacol 24:3–14 S
Robertson JIS, Ball SG (1989) Hypertension. In: Julian DG, Poole-Wilson PW, Fox K, Camm AJ, Hall R (eds) Diseases of the heart. Baillière Tindall, London 1227–1292
Rosenheim ML (1954) The treatment of severe hypertension. Br Med J 2:1181–1193
Smirk FH (1957) High arterial pressure. Blackwell, Oxford, pp 532–535
Swales JD (1985) Platt versus Pickering: an episode in recent medical history. Keynes/ British Medical Association, London
Swales JD (1988) Non-pharmacological antihypertensive therapy. Eur Heart J [Suppl G] 9:45–52
Swales JD, Ramsay LE, Coope J, Pocock S, Robertson JIS, Shafer J, Sever P (1989) Treatment of mild hypertension: Recommendations of the British Hypertension Society. Br Med J 298:694–698
Weber MA (1987) Automatic blood pressure recorders and 24 hour monitoring. Curr Opin Cardiol 2:748–757

4 United States of America

N.M. KAPLAN

4.1 Introduction

In the United States of America, the treatment of hypertension has been characterized as early and aggressive. Although I would greatly prefer that "aggressive" be changed to a less threatening descriptive term such as "vigorous," the characterization is clearly correct: American physicians treat people with lower levels of hypertension more rapidly than do physicians in Europe (WHO Drug Utilization Research Group 1986). After surveying American practice, HART (1983) commented: "The question 'to treat or not to treat' need no longer be asked. A free-fire zone has been created above diastolic 90, in which we simply shoot everything that moves."

There are multiple likely explanations for the more widespread therapy of mild hypertension in the USA, than elsewhere (GUTTMACHER et al. 1981). These include:

- A more pioneering spirit that leads to a more liberal, activist attitude: in the face of a perceived problem, Americans want to do something quickly to correct it.
- A greater awareness of the dangers of hypertension and other cardiovascular riks. Witness the vigorous campaigns in the USA to stop cigarette smoking and reduce cholesterol levels. A well-funded and supported National High Blood Pressure Education Program, headquartered in Bethesda, Maryland, has been functioning for over 15 years to inform both the general public and the health professions about the widespread presence of uncontrolled hypertension and the dangers therefrom.
- A health care system (fee-for-service, unstructured, entrepreneurial) that encourages more contacts with professionals who are more than willing to provide therapies that patients want to receive.
- A greater affluence that allows more people to pay for their therapy.
- More doctors per unit of population than in any other country except Israel; the more doctors, the more medical care provided.
- Greater patient expectations for therapy which have encouraged physicians to practice "defensive" medicine both to satisfy their patients' desires and to avoid malpractice suits.
- Greater faith in modern technology and the new therapies that are available with less concern about possible long-term disadvantages.
- Extensive promotion by pharmaceutical companies that goes so far as to

provide gifts in payment for a physician's use of their product (GRAVES 1987). Such promotion may go too far, but advertising is certainly a well-accepted practice in this capitalistic society.

4.2 Quantitative Aspects

For whatever the reasons, the treatment of hypertension has spread rapidly in the last 15 years, so that it is now the leading indication for visits to physicians and for the use of prescription drugs (KOCH 1987). The rise in the number of visits to physicians for hypertension has far exceeded the rise in office visits for other reasons (IMS America 1986) (Fig. 1).

The absolute number and the relative proportion of the population who have been identified as being hypertensive and who have been given antihypertensive therapy has expanded considerably over the past 20 years (Table 1) (ROBERTS and MAURER 1977; ROWLAND and ROBERTS 1982).

4.3 Qualitative Aspects

American physicians, despite their unbridled enthusiasm to treat, have tended to be rather conservative in their choice of drugs, usually sticking to habits established in the 1960s and 1970s, particularly because these habits were blessed and codified by the recommendations of a group of experts selected by the director of the National Heart, Lung, and Blood Institute under the title of the Joint National Committee on Detection, Evaluation, and Treatment of High Blood Pressure (JNC). The recommendations of the successive JNC committees starting in 1977 are shown in Table 2 (Joint National Committee on Detection, Evaluation, and Treatment of High Blood Pressure 1977, 1980, 1984, 1988).

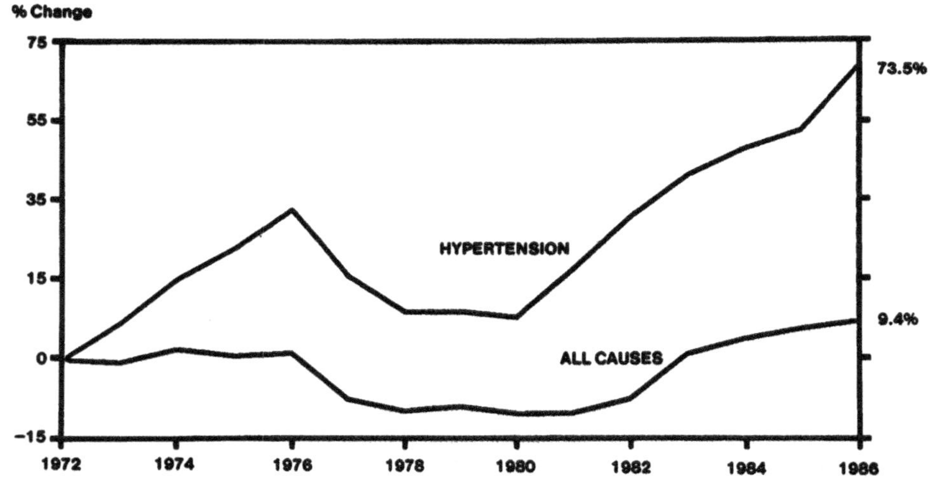

Fig. 1. Percent change in physician visits for hypertension and all other causes in the United States of America, 1972–1986. (From IMS AMERICA 1986)

Table 1. Findings of three hypertension surveys using data only from people 25–74 years of age (from KAPLAN 1986b)

	National Health Survery (1960–1962)	National Health and Nutrition Examination Survey I (1971–1975)	National Health and Nutrition Examination Survey II (1976–1980)
No. of people examined	6672	17 796	16 204
Percentage with BP ⩾ 160/95	20.3	22.1	22.0
Percentage of hypertensive patients aware of diagnosis	49	64	73
Percentage of hypertensive patients being treated	31	34	56
Percentage of hypertensive patients under control	16	20	34
References	ROBERTS and MAURER (1977)	ROBERTS and MAURER (1977)	ROWLAND and ROBERTS 1982)

Table 2. Drugs recommended in the first three Joint National Committee reports (From Kaplan 1986a)

	JNC I (1977)	JNC II (1980)	JNC III (1984)
Step 1	Thiazide	Thiazide	Thiazide or β-blocker
Step 2	Propranolol Methyldopa Reserpine	β-Blocker Clonidine Methyldopa Prazosin Rauwolfia	Adrenergic inhibitor or diuretic
Step 3	Hydralazine	Hydralazine	Hydralazine Minoxidil

The JNC overall plan has been labeled as step-care, involving the initiation of therapy with one drug and the stepwise addition of other drugs as needed to bring the blood pressure down to the goal, usually a diastolic blood pressure below 90 mmHg. Two reasons have been given for this approach: first, to ensure that drugs would be given in a systematic fashion, taking advantage of pharmacologic interactions; second, to minimize the potential for dose-related side effects, with the belief that smaller does of multiple drugs would be less bothersome than larger doses of single agents.

The first choice in the treatment protocol in the 1977 and 1980 JNC reports was a thiazide diuretic. In the 1984 report, β-blockers were given almost equal footing. In the 1988 report, calcium entry blockers and angiotensin-converting enzyme inhibitors were added to the choices for initial monotherapy.

Nonetheless, surveys of American physicians have clearly documented the supremacy of thiazide diuretics as the initial choice of therapy (Table 3) (Cloher and Whelton 1986). This survey was performed about 5 years ago. Since then sales of diuretics have slowed somewhat as sales of other agents have continued to rise, but hydrochlorothiazide is far and away the single most widely prescribed antihypertensive agent (Koch 1987).

As ACE inhibitors and calcium entry blockers became available and the advantages of α-blockers are more widely perceived, their use has begun to rise, but they are still far behind diuretics and β-blockers. The widespread advocacy of diuretics and β-blockers as noted in recent surveys of internal medicine academicians in university teaching hospitals (Kosecoff et al. 1985; Davidson and Meuleman 1986) suggets that physicians entering medical practice will continue to follow the traditions established over the past 10–15 years.

However, a steadily enlarging group of hypertension experts initially led by Laragh (1973) has called for a break from past traditions to a broader use of virtually all available agents, following two general principles: first, different types of patients may show better responses to one or another class of drugs (Kaplan 1986a); second, if the first choice does not work well or causes bothersome side effects, that choice should be stopped and drugs from another class chosen (Krakoff et al. 1987). The first principle will lead to the use of more

Table 3. Drugs recommended for first-step therapy of patients with mild hypertension (From CLOHER and WHELTON 1986)

	Family/ general practice (%)	Internal medicine practice (%)	Speciality medicine practice (%)	Weighted statewide estimate (%)[a]
Diuretics	92	89	87	90
β-Blockers	5	9	10	8
Others[b]	5	2	1	2

[a] Grand means based on the responses for the three practice settings that have been appropriately weighted according to the number of physicians in each practice setting within the state of Maryland.
[b] Reserpine, methyldopa, hydralazine, and guanethdidine.

drugs, breaking away from the "diuretic or β-blocker first" approach so widely used up until now. The second principle will lead to a "substitution" approach, rather than step-care.

Evidence that the "diuretic first then step-care" approach that has become so firmly entrenched in the treatment of hypertension in the United States of America has been reconsidered and that changes are beginning to occur can be recognized in summaries of reviews on drugs for hypertension published in the widely read and highly respected *Medical Letter* from 1974 to 1987 (ANONYMOUS 1974, 1977, 1984, 1987):

- 1974: Drug treatment should start with a thiazide-type diuretic; if this does not produce an adequate response, a second drug may be needed.
- 1977: Most *Medical Letter* consultants start treatment with a thiazide diuretic, and add another antihypertensive agent only if the diuretic does not produce an adequate response.
- 1984: Initial therapy with a diuretic or a beta-blocker is recommended for most hypertensive patients; other drugs can be added if the response is not adequate.
- 1987: A thiazide-type diuretic or a beta-blocker has generally been the first drug used for treatment of hypertension. An angiotensin-converting enzyme inhibitor or a calcium-entry blocker could also be used alone. If a second drug is necessary, and a diuretic was not used initially, most *Medical Letter* consultants would add a diuretic.

Obviously, a major change is occurring in the choices of drug used for the treatment of hypertension in the United States (ZUSMAN 1986; DUSTAN 1987; DZAU 1987). In addition, a number of experts have called for a more conservative overall attitude toward the institution of therapy, advocating that not all with a diastolic pressure above 90 mmHg need be actively treated (ALDERMAN 1980; KAPLAN 1981; FREIS 1982).

Here again, changes seem to be getting under way with increasing acceptance of these principles: (a) the need for a longer period of repeated blood pressure measurements before patients are labeled as hypertensive and started on drugs;

(b) the more vigorous use of various nondrug therapies; and (c) the institution of drugs only after a 3–6-month interval and only to those with a diastolic blood pressure above 95 mmHg (Kaplan 1987).

I feel certain that we in the USA are breaking away from established traditions with an increasing acceptance of these changes, toward a more conservative attitude about the institution of drug therapy but yet a more open attitude toward the choices of drugs that can be used once treatment is decided upon. Nonetheless, traditions die slowly, so that it will be some time before the "diuretic first then step-care" therapy of almost all with a diastolic blood pressure above 90 mmHg — early and aggressive therapy — will give way to a "multiple choice, substitution" approach.

References

Alderman MH (1980) Mild hypertension: new light on an old clinical controversy. Am J Med 69:653–655

Anonymous (1974) Drugs for hypertension. Med Lett 16:65–68

Anonymous (1977) Drugs for hypertension. Med Lett 19:21–24

Anonymous (1984) Drugs for hypertension. Med Lett 26:107–112

Anonymous (1987) Drugs for hypertension. Med Lett 29:1–6

Cloher TP, Whelton PK (1986) Physician approach to the recognition and initial management of hypertension: results of a statewide survey of Maryland physicians. Arch Intern Med 146:529–533

Davidson RA, Meuleman JR (1986) Initial treatment of hypertension: a questionnaire survey. J Clin Hypertens 4:339–345

Dustan HP (1987) Rational therapies for hypertension: is step 1 of stepped care archaic? Circulation 75:96–100

Dzau VJ (1987) Evolution of the clinical management of hypertension: emerging role of "specific" vasodilators as initial therapy. Am J Med [Suppl 1A] 82:36–43

Freis ED (1982) Should mild hypertension be treated? N Engl J Med 307:306–309

Graves J (1987) Frequent-flyer programs for drug prescribing. N Engl J Med 317:252

Guttmacher S, Teitelman M, Chapin G, Garbowski G, Schnall P (1981) Ethics and preventive medicine: the case of borderline hypertension. Hastings Center Rep 11: 12–20

Hart JT (1983) The practitioner's view. In: Gross F, Strasser T (eds) Mild hypertension: recent advances. Raven, New York, pp 365–374

IMS America (1986) National disease and therapeutic index. Ambler, Pennsylvania

Joint National Committee on Detection, Evaluation, and Treatment of High Blood Pressure (1977) Report of the Joint National Committee on Detection, Evaluation, and Treatment of High Blood Pressure: a cooperative study. JAMA 237:255–261

Joint National Committee on Detection, Evaluation, and Treatment of High Blood Pressure (1980) The 1980 report of the Joint National Committee on Detection, Evaluation, and Treatment of High Blood Pressure. Arch Intern Med 140:1280–1285

Joint National Committee on Detection, Evaluation, and Treatment of High Blood Pressure (1984) The 1984 report of the Joint National Committee on Detection, Evaluation, and Treatment of High Blood Pressure. Arch Intern Med 144:1045–1057

Joint National Committee on Detection, Evaluation, and Treatment of High Blood Pressure (1988) The 1988 report of the Joint National Committee on Detection, Evaluation and Treatment of High Blood Pressure. Arch Intern Med 148:1023–1038

Kaplan NM (1981) Whom to treat: the dilemma of mild hypertension. Am Heart J 101:867–870

Kaplan NM (1986a) Treatment of hypertension: drug therapy. In: Kaplan NM (ed) Clinical hypertension, 4th edn. Williams and Wilkin, Baltimore, pp 180–272

Kaplan NM (1986b) Hypertension in the population at large. In: Kaplan NM (ed) Clinical hypertension, 4th edn. Williams and Wilkins, Baltimore, pp 1–28

Kaplan NM (1987) Misdiagnosis of systemic hypertension and recommendations for improvement. Am J Cardiol 80:1383–1386

Koch H (1987) Highlights of drug utilization. In: National Center for Health Statistics (ed) Office Practice National Ambulatory Medical Care Survey, 1985. Public Health Service, Hyattville (Vital and Health Statistic no 134; DHHS publ no (PHS) 87-1250)

Kosecoff J, Fink A, Brook RH, et al. (1985) General medical care and the education of internists in university hospitals: an evaluation of the Teaching Hospital General Medicine Group Practice Program. Ann Intern Med 102:250–257

Krakoff LR, Phillips RA, Eison HB (1987) New directions for hypertenion therapy. Compr Ther 13:61–68

Laragh JH (1973) Vasoconstriction-volume analysis for understanding and treating hypertension: the use of renin and aldosterone profiles. Am J Med 55:261–274

Roberts J, Maurer K (1977) Blood pressure level of persons 6–74 years. Public Health Service, Hyattsville (Vital and Health Statistics no 203; DHEW publ no (HRA) 78-1648, ser 11)

Rowland M, Roberts J (1982) Advance data from Vital and Health Statistics no 84. Public Health Services, Washington

WHO Drug Utilization Research Group (DURG) (1986) Therapeutic traditions in Northern Ireland, Norway and Sweden. II. Hypertension. Eur J Clin Pharmacol 30:521–525

Zusman RM (1986) Alternatives to traditional antihypertensive therapy. Hypertension 8:837–842

5 Brazil

E.M. KRIEGER, L.O.T. NASCIMENTO, and O.L. RAMOS

5.1 Prevalence of Hypertension

Two surveys on the prevalence of hypertension in the Brazilian population were conducted. One study (DEBERT-RIBEIRO et al. 1981, 1982) analyzed the prevalence of hypertension in the labor force of the metropolitan area of Sao Paulo city (population of approximately 12 million people) while the second survey (ACHUTTI and MEDEIROS 1985; ACHUTTI et al. 1987) studied the prevalence of hypertension in the population of the state of Rio Grande do Sul (8.5 million people). The data from both studies are similar and show that the prevalence of hypertension in the adult population (20 years of age or older) is 12%. In blacks, the prevalence of hypertension is higher and the disease more severe than in whites. In general the information is not different from that published in North America and Europe. However, mortality from cardiovascular disease in Brazil has progressively increased over the past 50 years. In 1930, cardiovascular disease accounted for only 11.8% of total mortality, while in 1980 it represented 30.8%. When only the population older than 50 years of age is considered, cardiovascular disease accounts for 54.5% of the total mortality. Thus, hypertension in Brazil is currently considered to be a primary public health problem owing to its high prevalence and because cardiovascular disease is becoming a leading cause of death (RIBEIRO et al. 1988).

5.2 Treatment of Hypertension

Assuming a prevalence of 12% in the adult population of Brazil, one can calculate the total number of individuals with high blood pressure in 1987 to be 8.4 million (population of 140 million in which approximately 50% are aged 20 years or older). The knowledge of the degree of awareness, treatment, and control status is incomplete and fragmented. As an indirect evaluation, the total number of antihypertensive drugs used in Brazil in 1987 is presented in Table 1, derived from data obtained from two different sources: 70% of the drugs used were sold in pharmacies (International Marketing Service 1981–1987), while 30% were given free by the National Health System to treat hypertension (only diuretics, methyldopa, and β-blockers). Applying a correction factor to exclude the use of diuretics and β-blockers for diseases other than hypertension, and assuming that each individual with high blood pressure was treated by a single drug given in a dosage sufficient to control hypertension, and alo assuming that medication was maintained with full compliance, it can be estimated that 35% of all hypertensive

Table 1. Number of tablets of antihypertensive drugs delivered (sold or given) to the Brazilian population during 1987

Diuretics	697 237 500
β-Blockers	398 220 000
Methyldopa	263 916 500
Calcium antagonists	229 131 500
Tranquilizers	179 420 000
Reserpine	61 300 000
Clonidine	46 100 000
Prazosin	34 250 000
Converting enzyme inhibitors	27 020 000
Hydralazine	9 473 000
Minoxidil	2 460 000

See text for criteria of estimation.

patients in Brazil in 1987 could have been treated (3 million compared with 8.4 million). This figure is probably an overestimate considering that in a survey conducted in 1978 only 5.5% were found to be taking medication (DEBERT-RIBEIRO et al. 1981, 1982). Indeed, Fig. 1 shows that the calculated number of individuals that could have been treated (using the data on delivered antihypertensive agents) has increased consistently from 1981 to 1987. In 1981–1983 this estimation was 15%; in 1986 and 1987 the percentage had doubled to 30%.

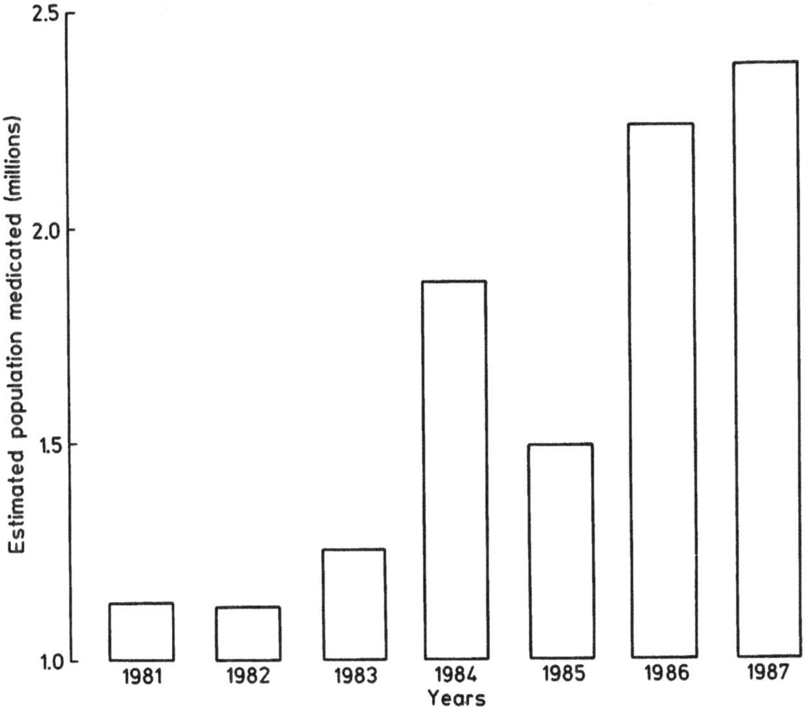

Fig. 1. Estimates of hypertensive patients that could have been treated considering the volume of antihypertensive drugs sold in pharmacies from 1981 to 1987 in Brazil (drugs given by the National Health System are not included)

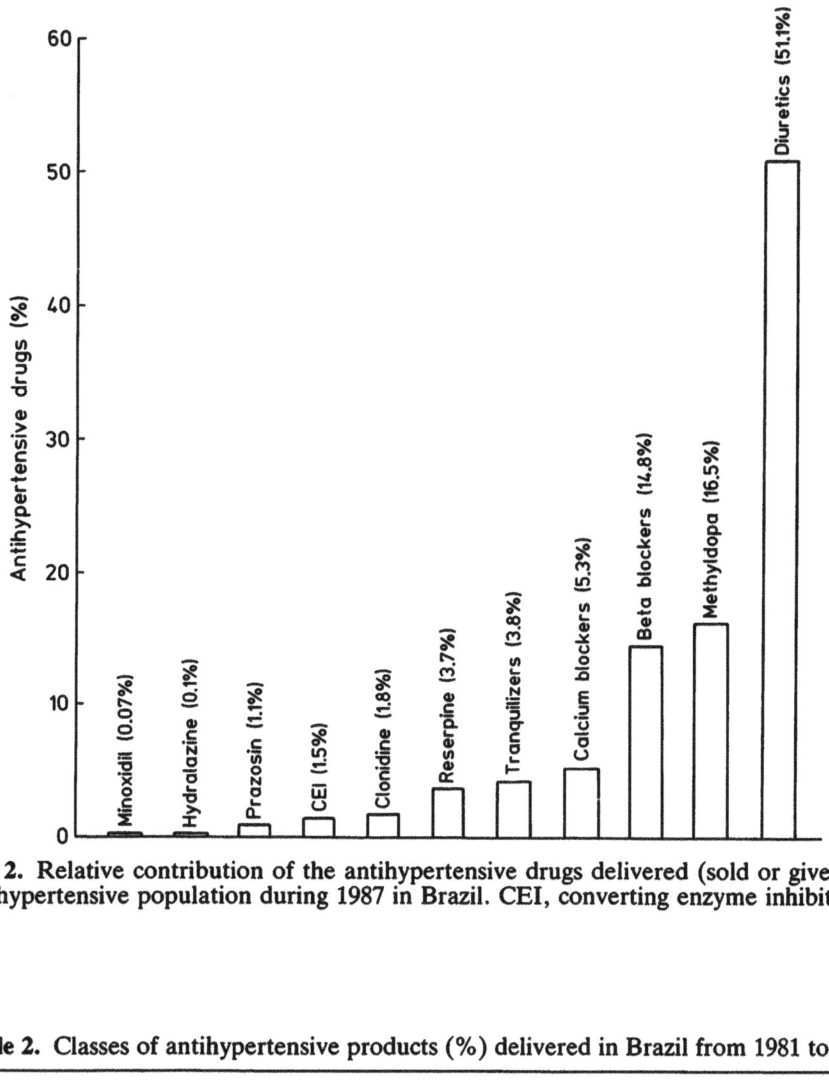

Fig. 2. Relative contribution of the antihypertensive drugs delivered (sold or given) to the hypertensive population during 1987 in Brazil. CEI, converting enzyme inhibitors

Table 2. Classes of antihypertensive products (%) delivered in Brazil from 1981 to 1987

	1981	1982	1983	1984	1985	1986	1987
Diuretics	42.6	43.9	43.5	34.9	52.1	51.5	51.1
Methyldopa	19.7	16.8	16.4	20.2	13.0	18.9	16.5
β-Blockers	7.3	10.7	11.5	20.2	13.7	10.3	14.8
Calcium antagonists	–	0.05	0.6	0.8	3.5	4.1	5.3
Tranquilizers	6.6	7.1	8.8	9.5	7.6	5.01	3.8
Reserpine	19.3	15.9	14.3	12.2	5.7	5.8	3.7
Clonidine	2.4	2.2	1.9	0.5	2.0	1.8	1.8
Converting enzyme inhibitors	0.2	0.3	0.4	0.3	0.7	1.2	1.5
Prazosin	1.5	1.7	1.9	1.3	1.8	1.3	1.1
Hydralazine	–	–	0.02	0.02	0.2	0.02	0.1
Minoxidil	–	0.02	–	0.02	0.2	0.2	0.07

See text for criteria of estimation.

5.3 Classes of Antihypertensive Drugs Used

To calculate the relative contribution of each class of antihypertensive drug, the number of tablets was corrected for the common dosage prescribed. Figure 2 shows that in 1987 more than 50% of the antihypertensive agents prescribed were diuretics, followed by methyldopa (16.5%) and β-blockers (14.8%). Minoxidil and hydralazine represented less than 0.1%, while prazosin, converting enzyme inhibitors, clonidine, reserpine, tranquilizers, and calcium blockers were between 1% and 5%. From 1981 to 1987 diuretics and methyldopa remained stable, while the contribution of β-blocker, calcium antagonists, and converting enzyme inhibitors progressively increased (Table 2). The percentages of clonidine, prazosin, minoxidil, and hydralazine were small and relatively constant from 1981 to 1987 while the use of reserpine and tranquilizers declined.

Summary

Hypertension is gaining attention as a public health problem in Brazil. Exact information is not available to evaluate the effectivenes of treatment or the number of individuals on adequate antihypertensive medication. Based on the number of tablets of antihypertensive agents delivered to the Brazilian population in 1987, it can be estimated that approximately 30% of the total number of hypertensives could have been treated. Diuretics account for more than 50% of the agents used, followed by methyldopa and β-blockers. The relative participation of calcium antagonists and converting enzyme inhibitors is still small but increasing, while the use of tranquilizers and reserpine is declining.

References

Achutti A, Medeiros AMB (1985) Hipertensão arterial no Rio Grande do Sul. Bol Saude 12:2–72

Achutti A, Costa E, Fischman A, Bassanesi S, Klein C (1987) Epidemiological survey on arterial pressure supporting preventing health program (Abstr). Rev Med Chile 109:435

Debert-Ribeiro MB, Ribeiro AB, Stabile Neto C, Chavess CC, Kater CE, Iunes M, Saragoça MAS, et al. (1981) Hypertension and economic activities in São Paulo, Brazil. Hypertension [Suppl 2] 3:II-233–II-237

Debert-Ribeiro MB, Ribeiro AB, Stabile Neto C, Anção MS, Saragoça MAS, Ramos OL, Iunes M, et al. (1982) Prevalencia da hipertensão na força de trabalho da Grande São Paulo: Influencia de idade, sexo e grupo etnico. Rev Assoc Med Bras 28:209–215

International Marketing Service (1981–1987) The pharmaceutical market of Brasil. International Marketing Service, ZUG

Ribeiro AB, Kohlmann O Jr, Marson O, Zanella MT, Ramos OL (1988) Hypertension: A major public health problem in Brazil. Drugs, (in press)

6 Union of Soviet Socialist Republics

I.K. Shkhvatsabaya†

Prevalence of arterial hypertension in Moscow among men aged 40–49 years is 14% and among men aged 55–59 years, 26%; among men aged 40–59 years it is 22%–28% in other Soviet cities. The proportion of hypertensive individuals aware of their condition is low (up to 57%); only 17% of the patients are treated, and only 10% have satisfactorily controlled hypertension.

In order to change this situation an All-Union Comprehensive Collaborative Research Program of Arterial Hypertension Control was launched in 1976. This program involves 27 research centers and covers 23 cities in the country. It provides for the use of nondrug therapy (in mild hypertension) and drug therapy using a four-step scheme similar to those in other countries.

In most of the Soviet collaborating centers the proportion of hypertensive patients aware of their disease has reached 75%–77%, the proportion receiving antihypertensive treatment has increased to 35%–40%, and the efficacy of this treatment has more than tripled (Britov 1984; Study Group of the All-Union Cooperative Program on Arterial Hypertension Prevention 1986).

Our experience indicates that nondrug measures alone such as restricted dietary salt intake, diminished total dietary intake for obese subjects, limitation or discontinuation of alcohol consumption, and increased physical activity can achieve a normalization or persistent reduction of blood pressure in mild hypertension.

A popular form of nondrug therapy has become the so-called psychorelaxation therapy (PRT): biofeedback-based behavioral therapy, suggestive procedures such as hypnosis and autogenic training, and progressive muscular relaxation (Aivazyan et al. 1987). The All-Union Cardiology Research Centre reported that a significant and sustained reduction in BP (by 10.3 and 8.0 mmHg for systolic and diastolic pressure, respectively) is achieved in patients at an early stage of hypertension through the use of PRT alone, without any pharmacotherapy. The 5-year follow-up has indicated that patients treated by PRT are much less likely to show progression of the disease and to develop complications. Regression of left ventricular hypertrophy may also occur. In patients with labile hypertension in whom PRT treatment was combined with the use of hypotensive drugs, the drugs were discontinued in 70%, and doses could be reduced in 46% with stable arterial hypertension.

---

† Professor Shkhvatsabaya died October 11th, 1988.

Three main groups of drugs are most frequently used:

1. Antiadrenergic drugs acting at different levels of the adrenergic system
2. Diuretics, of which the most widely used are thiazides
3. Vasodilators (hydralazine, α_1-postsynaptic adrenoreceptor blocking drug — prazosin, calcium entry blockers, and converting enzyme inhibitors) have become popular in recent years

In practice the decision to use a particular antihypertensive drug is based on the measurement of individual responsiveness to the drug in acute tests. Optimal conditions for these tests have been defined. The drug is first administered in a low dose and, if ineffective, a medium dose of the drug is given sublingually to improve its absorption.

In 60%–70% of patients the antihypertensive effect of a drug in an acute test has been shown to be similar to the effect in long-term treatment. The main differences between acute testing and long-term treatment are the development of major adverse reactions during long-term treatment.

Acute tests to determine a patient's sensitivity are performed for all vasodilators, diuretics, ACE inhibitors (captopril) and for other agents.

We use the acute furosemide test proposed by Nekrasova et al. (1986) to determine which patients should be treated with diuretics. This test involves administering furosemide for 2–3 days in a daily dose of 60–120 mg. On the 1st day two 40 mg doses are usually given. If the daily diuresis exceeds the initial level by more than 200%, the daily dose is decreased to 60 mg. If the diuresis does not exceed 200%, the dose is increased to 120 mg.

A decrease of mean blood pressure by 10–20 mmHg on days 2 or 3 of the furosemide test indicates that the patient's sensitivity is moderate, whilst a decrease by more than 20 mmHg indicates a high sensitivity.

The rather elaborate furosemide test permits not only the detection of patients sensitive to diuretics but also those who are prone to develop hypokalemia and who should be treated with a potassium-sparing diuretic, such as triamterene, amiloride, or spironolactone from the very beginning. Directly after the furosemide test, patients sensitive to diuretics are placed on thiazide therapy using hydrochlorothiazide, chlorthalidone, or clopamide.

The furosemide test has enabled us to identify two groups of patients. The first group shows good hypotensive responses to the acute test and is characterized by an initially subnormal PRA level and low blood aldosterone level, which rise slightly at the end of the test. The subsequent prolonged thiazide treatment results in a pronounced and persistent blood pressure reduction period. In the second group of patients a 3-day furosemide test has only a mild, if any, antihypertensive effect. These patients are characterized by an elevated PRA level, elevated plasma aldosterone concentration, and an increase in the pulse rate at the end of the test. These findings predict an inadequate antihypertensive effect of long-term diuretic therapy.

Our extensive experience with the furosemide test for screening of patients for diuretic therapy in the USSR serves as a warning against indiscriminate use of diuretics in arterial hypertension — a practice adopted in many countries such as the USA and Western Europe. This applies not only to diuretic monotherapy but also to combined therapies using a three-step scheme in which the basic drug is a diuretic.

About 15%–20% patients develop refractoriness to drugs which are taken for a long time, even when the treatment is carefully monitored and the drugs or their combinations have been selected on an individual basis. In such cases one usually tries to increase the dose of the antihypertensive drug, but this produces only a short-term effect and frequently promotes adverse reactions. We gradually discontinue antihypertensive drugs and revise the whole scheme of hypotensive therapy; the main drug is then selected using the acute tests.

To overcome refractoriness to drug therapy a number of methods are used such as intravenous infusions of the vasodilator prostaglandin E (PGE) and extracorporeal techniques of blood clearance (hemosorption, plasmapheresis, and less commonly isolated ultrafiltration of blood plasma). A basis for the use of PGE infusions has been provided by experimental studies which show that intravenous PGE causes a substantial blood pressure reduction by decreasing vessel tone, augmenting intra-organ bloodflow, and intensifying diuresis and natriuresis (NEKRASOVA et al. 1982, 1984; BESSEGHIR 1985; MCGIFF 1981; AKUNO et al. 1980; NAKANO et al. 1973; FABRE and VALLOTON 1983).

PGE increases the patients' sensitivity to thiazide diuretics, propanolol, clonidine, and to a lesser degree nifedipine (NEKRASOVA et al. 1984; LONIGRO et al. 1973). The indication for PGE infusions is the inefficiency of antihypertensive therapy including four or five drugs such as β-adrenergic blockers, calcium antagonists, antiadrenergic, and diuretic agents.

The Soviet-made PGE drug prostenon is given in three infusions at 24-h intervals. The infusion rate varies from 50 to 250 ng/kg per min and depends upon the patient's response. In two-thirds of patients with essential hypertension or secondary hypertension due to chronic glomerulonephritis or pyelonephritis, the hypotensive effect of infusions persists for 60 to 240 days.

Contraindications for use of the test include ischemic heart disease of functional classes III and IV, severe heart failure, pregnancy, metrorrhagia, uterine tumors, and acute inflammatory conditions of any etiology.

Extracorporeal techniques are used in patients with arterial hypertension due to parenchymatous renal disease without marked renal insufficiency or with malignant hypertension of any origin, in whom conventional antihypertensive therapy fails.

For plasmapheresis two sessions with a 3-day interval are carried out; the mean plasma volume removed per session is about 1600 ± 84 ml. After the first session the systolic and diastolic blood pressure falls in all patients, so that the dose of any antihypertensive drug can be lowered subsequently. The procedure is usually well-tolerated and is repeated after 3 days, since the hypotensive effect is of short duration. In patients with malignant arterial hypertension the level of proteinuria decreases by 60%, and diuresis and the effective renal blood flow increase slightly for an average of 2 weeks after the plasmapheresis. The beneficial effects should be considered to include enhanced sodium excretion and augmented diuresis, since sodium and fluid retention are difficult to control with diuretics in patients with refractory arterial hypertension (GIFFORD and TARAZI 1978; KUTSENKO and LEGKONOGOV 1987).

No less beneficial in the multimodality treatment of secondary malignant arterial hypertension is hemosorption. For this two or three sessions are performed with blood being perfused via a veno-venous circuit at a rate of 90–100 ml/min. The procedure results in improved appearance of the eyegrounds, a persistent fall in blood pressure, and diminished hypotensive drug dosages. Kidney function may improve in patients with early signs of renal failure.

References

Aivazyan TA, Zaitsev VP, Yurenev AP (1987) Results of relaxation therapy application in essential hypertension. Kardiologiia 8:34–36

Akuno T, Kondo K, Suzuki H, Saruta T (1980) Effects of prostaglandins E_2, I_2 and F_2, arachidonic acid and undomethacin on pressor responses to norepinephrine in conscious rats. Prostaglandins 19:855–864

Besseghir K (1985) Renal tubular action of prostaglandin E_2 on water and electrolyte excretion in the nonanesthetized chicken. J Pharmacol Exp Ther 233:823–829

Britov AN (1984) Control of arterial hypertension at the population level (in Russian). Klin Med (Mosk) 9:43–49

Fabre L, Valloton MB (1983) Prostaglandines et pression arterielle. Schweiz Med Wochenschr 113:1042–1049

Gifford RW, Tarazi RC (1978) Resistant hypertension: diagnosis and treatment. Ann Intern Med 88:661–665

Kutsenko AL, Legkonogov AV (1987) Hypotensive effect of plasmapheresis in patients with severe symptomatic arterial hypertension due to renal disease (in Russian). Bull VKNC AMN USSR 1:87–90

Lonigro AJ, Terragno NA, Maliket KU, et al. (1973) Differential inhibition by prostaglandins of the renal action of pressor stimuli. Prostaglandins 3:595–606

McGiff JC (1981) Prostaglandins, prostacyclin and thromboxanes. Annu Rev Pharmacol Toxicol 21:479–509

Nakano J, Chang A, Fisher R (1973) Effect of prostaglandins E_1, E_2, A_1, A_2 and F_2 on canine arterial blood flow, cerebrospinal fluid pressure and intraocular pressure. J Neurosurg 38:32–39

Nekrasova AA, Dzhusipov AK, Shkhvatsabaya IK (1982) Use of prostaglandine E_2 for the treatment of essential hypertension with high blood pressure levels (in Russian). Kardiologiia 9:37–41

Nekrasova AA, Dzhusipov AK, Chernova NA, Uchitel IA, Akhmetov MA (1984) Change of endocrine renal function in patients with essential hypertension combined with stable hypertension under the effect of PGE infusions (in Russian). Ter Arkh 7:89–93

Nekrasova AA, Suvorov YI, Chernova NA, et al. (1986) Water-salt metabolism in patients with stable essential hypertension and principles of diuretic treatment (in Russian). Kardiologiia 1:27–34

Study Group of the All-Union Cooperative Program on Arterial Hypertension Prevention (AUCPAHP) (1986) Results of secondary prevention of arterial hypertension (in Russian). Bull VKNC AMN USSR 1:56–62

7 China

L.S. Gong, W.Z. Zhang, and H. Wang

7.1 Introduction

Hypertension is the most common cardiovascular disease in China. Its prevalence is 7.7% according to the nationwide survey conducted in 1979–1980, using the WHO criteria and involving more than 4 million people above age 15 years (Lu et al. 1980). Thus, it can be estimated that about 30 million people in this country are afflicted with established hypertension, most of them (80%) having the mild form. Accelerated or malignant hypertension seems to be rare (3.9% of patients hospitalized during the period 1975–1984) (Wang and Zhang 1986). Elevated blood pressure, mainly systolic, is frequent in the elderly over age 60 (44%) (Zhu et al. 1987).

In China, cardiovascular disease associated with hypertension constitutes one of the major causes of death. Some 70% of patients suffering from stroke are hypertensive. In contrast to what is seen in most Western countries, the incidence of stroke is relatively high, 5 times that of myocardial infarction (Wu 1979). The mortality from stroke, in different regions, has been found to be 130–160 per 100 000 per year, and in one study, the relative risk for stroke in hypertensive patients was 32 times higher than in normotensives (Di et al. 1987).

Because of the large number of patients throughout the country and the clinical particularities of the disease, the health care system is faced with the difficult problem of the detection and treatment of hypertension. Although annual health examinations, including blood pressure measurement, are carried out in many places, especially in governmental institutions, universities, and large factories, which lead to the earlier detection and treatment of hypertension, the majority of patients are being treated and followed on an outpatient basis in clinics and hospital of different levels.

Apart from the popular Tai-Chi, a form of slow-movement exercise, and Qi-Gong, a form of relaxation, which are frequently practised by patients as well as by healthy people, the treatment of hypertension consists mainly of drug therapy. Most of the currently used antihypertensive drugs are available in China. Research on traditional Chinese medicine and screening for an effective antihypertensive herbal medicine has continued ever since the early 1950s.

7.2 Traditional Chinese Medicine

Using the traditional dialectical method of diagnosis, most of the patients with hypertension fall into two categories, namely those with deficiency of yin leading to hyperactivity of yang and those with deficiency of both yin and yang. Accordingly, and with the purpose of correcting the deficiency and to regain the equilibrium between yin and yang that is necessary for normal physiological functions, traditional herbal medicines known to possess these effects are being used in combination in the form of decoctions. The following medicines have been found to have some hypotensive action: Fangji (Radix *Stephaniae tetrandrae*), Gouteng (Ramulus *Uncariae cumuncis*), Balima (Fructus *Rhododendri mollis*), Chouwutong (Folium *Clerodendri trichotomi*), Luobuma (Folium *Apocyni veneti*), Qingmuxiang (Radix *Aristolochiae*), Yejuhua (Flos *Chrysanthemi indici*), Duzhong (Cortex *Eucommiae*), Gegen (Radix *Puerariae*). Active principles have been isolated from some of the plants and studied for their hypotensive action.

7.2.1 Tetrandrine

Tetrandrine is an alkaloid isolated from the root of *Stephaniae tetrandrae*. Pharmacological studies have shown that its hypotensive action may be related to its peripheral vasodilation mediated by inhibition of potential-dependent channels and prevention of the influx of calcium ions. Clinically, tetrandrine injected intravenously in a dose of 120–180 mg has a rapid blood pressure lowering effect in patients with severe hypertension or with hypertensive crisis. Given orally in doses of 100 mg three times a day, both standing and supine blood pressure can be decreased. Side effects are infrequent and usually mild, including nausea, anorexia, and epigastric discomfort (GAO et al. 1965).

7.2.2 Rhynchophylla

Rhynchophylla is an alkaloid isolated from *Uncariae cumuncis*. Pharmacological studies have shown that it inhibits the sympathetic nervous system and has antihypertensive effects in Goldblatt hypertensive rats (CHANG et al. 1987a). Clinical observations indicate that rhynchophylla given orally 15–30 mg three times a day can decrease blood pressure in patients with hypertension. No adverse effects were noted (CHANG et al. 1978b).

7.2.3 Rhomotoxin

Rhomotoxin was isolated from the fruit of *Rhododendron molle* G. Don. Pharmacological studies have shown that it stimulates the parasympathetic nervous system, thus slowing the heart rate and lowering blood pressure (MAO et al. 1982). Given by intravenous infusion in a dose of 1–3 mg, rhomotoxin was shown to be useful in hypertensive emergencies. Systolic and diastolic pressures decrease by 36% and 30%, respectively, and the effect lasts for 1–4 h. Side effects, which are short-lived, include a burning sensation of the skin and dry mouth.

7.3 Use of Antihypertensive Agents

7.3.1 Drug Combination

In the 1960s, the drugs available for the treatment of hypertension were essentially reserpine, hydrochlorothiazide, hydralazine, and guanethidine. Because of the quite frequent side effects of these agents, a combination of antihypertensives in small doses was thought to be more acceptable to patients. Different combinations of these antihypertensive compounds have been used, the most widely prescribed being the one containing mainly reserpine (0.032 mg), hydrochlorothiazide (3.2 mg), and hydralazine (3.2 mg). Another compound called CPF antihypertensive tablet is composed of clonidine (15 µg), hydralazine (8 mg), and hydrochlorothiazide (5 mg) (SHEN et al. 1986). Clinical observations suggest that these compounds may be effective in 60%–70% of patients with mild-to-moderate hypertension (efficacy was designed as a decrease in systolic blood pressure > 20 mmHg and/or a decrease in diastolic blood pressure > 10 mmHg). Side effects were few and mild, usually not necessitating interruption of treatment. SHEN et al. (1987) followed 142 patients treated with these compounds for 2 years. Echocardiographic studies showed improvement in cardiac function, decrease in total peripheral resistance and in the left ventricular mass, along with a significant decrease in blood pressure. There were no changes in serum cholesterol or triglyceride.

The rationale for the use of such combinations has been criticized, and beginning in the 1980s, monotherapy with β-adrenergic receptor blockers or calcium antagonists and the stepped-care regimen are used more and more frequently, especially in large medical centers.

7.3.2 Diuretics

Hydrochlorothiazide and chlorthalidone are the diuretics most commonly used in the treatment of hypertension but only rarely as first-line drug or as monotherapy. This may be due to the fact that unwanted side effects such as fatique and dizziness are frequently seen. The rate of efficacy was only 39% with hydrochlorothiazide (SHEN and WANG 1983). Recently, indapamide, an indoline derivative of chlorosulphonamide with minimal diuretic activity has been introduced into China. Preliminary clinical observations confirmed its efficacy in the treatment of mild hypertension (ZHAO et al. 1987).

7.3.3 β-Adrenergic Receptor Blockers

Among the β-blockers used for the treatment of hypertension, propranolol was practically the only drug prescribed after practolol was withdrawn from the market in the late 1970s. In recent years, however, there is a tendency to replace it by atenolol and metoprolol, while nadolol is used less often.

In an open study of 55 mild-to-moderate hypertensive patients treated with atenolol, 64% responded with a significant reduction in blood pressure, and in 42% of these, diastolic blood pressure was reduced to normal (SHEN et al. 1981). There was a further fall in blood pressure in those patients who had continued the treatment for more than 1 year. In another group of patients, atenolol was given together with hydrochlorothiazide. This combination yielded an efficacy rate of 86% (SHEN and WANG 1983).

In patients receiving atenolol, bradycardia and chest oppression were observed in as many as one-third. Echocardiographic studies showed a reduction of left ventricular systolic function in those patients who complained of chest oppression.

7.3.4 Calcium Antagonists

Although the three currently available calcium antagonists (nifedipine, verapamil, and diltiazem) seem comparable in their antihypertensive potency, nifedipine is the most widely prescribed, especially in patients with moderate to severe hypertension and in the elderly. The efficacy rate was reported to be as high as 90%, with a reduction of diastolic blood pressure to normal in 44% of patients.

Flushing, headache, and increase in heart rate were troublesome in around 30% of the patients. Tachycardia resulting from nifedipine could be alleviated by the concomitant use of β-blockers. The addition of verapamil to nifedipine produced a similar decrease in blood pressure and allowed a reduction in the dose of the latter (GONG et al. 1987a). However, the long-term safety of such a combination has not been assessed.

Recently, nitrendipine, nicardipine, and nimodipine have become available. Preliminary clinical observations have suggested that nitrendipine is as effective as nifedipine but with a more convenient once-a-day dosage (ZHANG et al. 1987).

7.3.5 Converting Enzyme Inhibitors

Captopril is the only converting enzyme inhibitor used in China. It was not found to be very effective as a monotherapy drug, with an efficacy rate of only 41% in the treatment of mild-to-moderate hypertension. The doses used were 25–100 mg three times a day. With such large doses, side effects including rash, leukopenia, nausea, vomiting, and impaired renal function occurred in about 25% of cases (WANG and ZHANG 1984). At present, the drug is given in smaller doses, i.e., 12.5–25 mg two to three times a day and often in combination with nifedipine or diuretics.

7.3.6 Other Antihypertensive Drugs

Clonidine and prazosin are used quite frequently for the treatment of hypertension, while α-methyldopa and minoxidil have not been found to be satisfactory, the latter because of hypertrichosis, tachycardia, and fluid retention, despite a favorable response of the blood pressure of patients with severe hypertension. Reserpine and hydralazine are mainly used as components of the antihypertensive compounds. Labetalol, both orally and intravenously, has proved to be effective in the treatment of established hypertension and hypertensive emergencies, respectively (WANG et al. 1986).

7.4 Present Status and Future Trends

From the above general picture of the antihypertensive agents used and studied in China, it appears that nifedipine is the preferred one to be given as the first choice drug. In younger patients, however, many physicians begin therapy with a β-blocker. Diuretics and captopril are usually considered as second or third line drugs. The majority of patients with mild-to-moderate hypertension are still given antihypertensive compounds. As a whole, the choice of antihypertensive agents is largely empirical. There are a few studies attempting to correlate treatment efficacy with certain clinical characteristics, such as cardiac structural and functional parameters (degree of left ventricular hypertrophy, compliance, total peripheral resistance) and plasma renin activity, that might be helpful in choosing the appropriate drugs (Zhang and Shen 1982).

A recent survey by questionnaire among 392 patients and physicians from 22 clinics showed that only 36% of the patients were taking the drugs as prescribed, and only 16% had their diastolic blood pressure reduced to below 90 mmHg (Gong et al. 1987b). Furthermore, during the period 1975–1984, the annual mortality from stroke has not decreased in Baoshan County, in the suburbs of Shanghai (Di et al. 1987). These results indicate a rather poor control of blood pressure. Indeed, the problem of patient's compliance to therapy has not been examined.

In order to improve the treatment of hypertension, several points are important and need to be solved: better patient education, along with better medical care at all levels, especially the primary health care levels; the assessment of the beneficial effect of the treatment of mild hypertension which accounts for the vast majority of patients, and of hypertension in the elderly; better use of currently available antihypertensive drugs in the concrete demographic and socioeconomic settings of China.

References

Chang TS et al. (1978a) Hypotensive action of rhynchophylla alkaloids and rhynchophylline (in Chinese). Nat Med J China 58:408–501

Chang TS et al. (1978b) Evaluation of the therapeutics effect of rhnchophylla alkaloid on hypertension by both Chinese traditional and western medical methods (in Chinese). Nat Med J China 58:750–753.

Di SD et al. (1987) Study on risk factors for stroke in patients with hypertension (in Chinese). Acta Univ Med Secondae Shanghai 7:339–342

Gao Y et al. (1965) Tetrandrine in hypertension, clinical observation and analysis of efficacy of treatment in 270 cases (in Chinese). Chin J Intern Med 13:504–507

Gong LS et al. (1987a) Changes of calcium ion in blood and platelet, and treatment of nifedipine and verapamil in combination in hypertension (in Chinese). Chin J Clin Pharmacol [Suppl]:38

Gong LS et al. (1987b) Survey on present status of antihypertensive therapy in 22 clinics in Shanghai (in Chinese). Shanghai Med J 10:97–98

Lu CQ et al. (1980) Preliminary report on general survey of hypertension of whole China in 1979 (in Chinese). Chin J Cardiol 8:165–169

Mao HY et al. (1982) Rhomotoxin pharmacologic action in lowering blood pressure and slowing heart rate. Chin Med J 95:311–318

Shen JQ, Wang LD (1983) Combined effect of hydrochlorothiazide and atenolol in antihypertensive therapy in 42 patients (in Chinese). Acta Pharmacol Sin 4:254–258

Shen JQ et al. (1981) Atenolol, a new beta-adrenergic blocking agent in treatment of hypertension, therapeutic effect and hemodynamic changes (in Chinese). Chin J Cardiol 9:94–98

Shen JQ et al. (1986) Therapeutic effects and echocardiographic changes in a long term treatment of essential hypertension with western versus Chinese plus western drugs (in Chinese). Shanghai Med J 9:501–505

Shen JQ et al. (1987) Observation of hemodynamic and echocardiographic changes in the treatment of essential hypertension with clonidine compound (in Chinese). N Drugs Clin Remedies 6:74–77

Wang HM et al. (1986) Clinical observation on severe hypertension treated by intravenous labetalol (in Chinese). Chin J Cardiol 14:28–30

Wang XM, Zhang WZ (1984) Collaborating action of captopril combined with diuretics in the treatment of mild and moderate hypertension (in Chinese). N Drugs Clin Remedies 3:150–152

Wang XM, Zhang WZ (1986) Clinical analysis of 48 cases of malignant hypertension (in Chinese). Acta Univ Med Secondae Shanghai 6:362–363

Wu YK (1979) Epidemiology and community control of hypertension, stroke and coronary heart disease in China. Chin Med J 92:665–670

Zhang WZ, Shen JQ (1982) Comparison of hemodynamic changes between atenolol and nifedipine in short term treatment of hypertension (in Chinese). N Drugs Clin Remedies 1:97–100

Zhang WZ et al. (1987) Immediate hemodynamic effects in the treatment of hypertension with nitrendipine (in Chinese). N Drugs Clin Remedies 6:78–79

Zhao LY et al. (1987) An observation of the clinical effects of indapamide on hypertension (in Chinese). Chin J Cardiol 15:333–337

Zhu YJ et al. (1987) Systolic hypertension in the elderly (in Chinese). Chin J Geriatr 6:246–247

8 Japan

Y. KAWANO and T. OMAE

8.1 Characteristics of Hypertensive Diseases in Japan

It has long been known that people in Japan have a high incidence of hypertension and consume large amounts of salt. Epidemiological studies in the 1950s revealed that the prevalence of hypertension was 39% and the average amount of daily salt intake was 26 g in 5301 adults in Akita, northeastern Japan, while they were 21% and 14 g, respectively, in 456 adults in Hiroshima, southwestern Japan (DAHL 1960). The prevalence of hypertension was said to be one of the highest in the world.

However, the levels of blood pressure and salt consumption in Japan have changed. According to the national survey by the Ministry of Health and Welfare (1983a), average blood pressure and the prevalence of hypertension in the adult population in 1980 were lower than those in 1961 and 1971. The average daily salt intake was 12.5 g in 1981, ranging from 10.5 g in the mid-western area to 14.8 g in the northeasthern area (Ministry of Health and Welfare 1983b). These trends are possibly caused by changes in dietary habits (decreased salt intake and increased protein and fat intake), improvement of the health care system, and increasing awareness of hypertension.

Stroke is the major complication of hypertension in Japan, and until the early 1980s it was the most frequent cause of death. The mortality rate from cerebral hemorrhage was particularly high and was higher than that from cerebral infarction. However, fatal stroke, especially cerebral hemorrhage, has markedly decreased in recent years, although it is still more common compared with its occurrence in Western countries. The Hisayama study, a long-term follow-up with autopsy verification in most of deceased (OMAE et al. 1981; OMAE 1985; UEDA et al. 1988) demonstrated a marked change in mortality figures in recent years (Fig. 1).

On the other hand, the mortality rate from ischemic heart disease in Japan has been much lower than in Western countries. It was about one-fifth of that in the United States of America and several European countries in the 1960s and 1970s (OWADA 1985). This may be attributed to lower serum cholesterol levels, although the average cholesterol level has increased during the past 20 years and reached nearly 200 mg/dl recently (ISOMURA 1987). However, the age-adjusted rate of mortality from ischemic heart disease showed some reduction during the period 1958–1978 (OWADA 1985).

The characteristics of hypertensive cardiovascular diseases in Japan are not due solely to racial differences but appear to be largely influenced by environ-

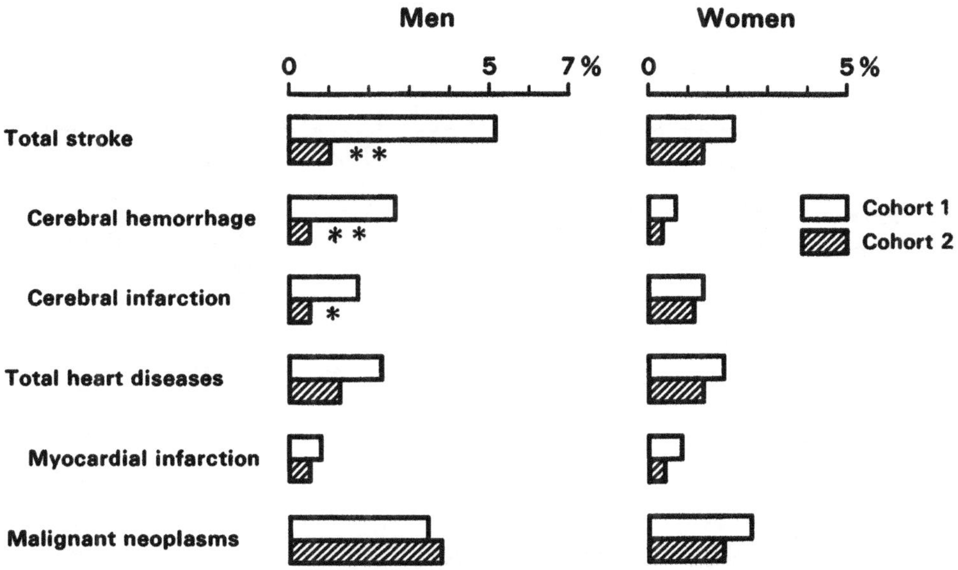

Fig. 1. Mortality rates from major diseases during 7 years after the beginning of follow-up in Hisayama. *Cohort 1*, 1621 persons aged 40 years or older at entry in 1961; *Cohort 2*, 2053 persons aged 40 years or older at entry in 1974; *, $P < 0.05$; **, $P < 0.01$

mental factors. The Ni-hon-san study compared the mortality figures among Japanese men in Hiroshima, Honolulu, and San Francisco and demonstrated the higher risk of cerebrovascular disease and the lower risk of ischemic heart disease in Hiroshima (KAGAN et al. 1974). Japanese men in Hiroshima had lower serum cholesterol levels than those in Hawaii and Los Angeles, and the prevalence of hypercholesterolemia (greater than 250 mg/dl) was 5.9% in Hiroshima, 26.8% in Hawaii, and 21.2% in Los Angeles (OWADA 1985).

8.2 Trends of Antihypertensive Therapy

As in Western countries, effective antihypertensive drugs were not available in Japan until the introduction of ganglionic blockade in 1951. Reserpine, hydralazine, and thiazide diuretics greatly contributed to the rapid expansion of drug therapy for hypertensive patients during the 1950s and 1960s. At the beginning of the 1970s, thiazides, sympatholytics such as reserpine and alpha methyldopa, and hydralazine were the major antihypertensive drugs.

Figure 2 shows the frequency of various types of antihypertensive drug prescribed and average blood pressure in hypertensive patients at the Hypertension Clinic of Kyushu University Hospital in Fukuoka during the period from 1971 to 1986 (OMAE et al. 1987). Diuretics were prescribed in more than 50% of hypertensive patients throughout the period. β-Blockers and α-blockers have become major pharmacological agents since the mid-1970s; their share was the largest among all types of antihypertensive agents in 1986. On the other hand, other sympatholytics and direct vasodilators such as hydralazine have been less

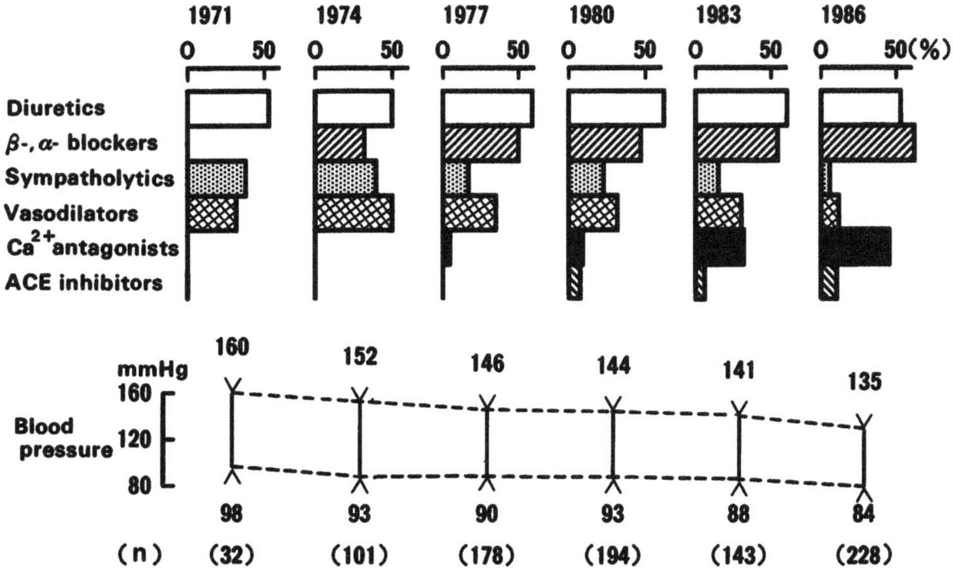

Fig. 2. Trends of antihypertensive medication (*above*) and levels of patients' blood pressure (*below*) at the Hypertension Clinic of Kyushu University Hospital. Some patients received more than one medication

frequently used in recent years. Calcium antagonists were introduced in the late 1970s, and their use became progressively more frequent. ACE inhibitors established their position in antihypertensive drug treatment in the 1980s. With an increasing number of drugs available, blood pressure levels in treated hypertensive patients decreased from 160/98 mmHg in 1971 to 135/84 mmHg in 1986. The same trends of antihypertensive drug therapy are seen in several other university hospitals in Japan (OMAE et al. 1987).

As a nonpharmacological therapy, restriction of dietary salt intake has been stressed. This may have contributed to the trend of decreasing salt consumption in the general population in Japan.

8.3 Current Antihypertensive Therapy

With the growing public attention directed to hypertension, a majority of Japanese people now have opportunities to have their blood pressure measured in mass screening programs, which have been operating in communities, companies, and schools. There are increasing numbers of treated hypertensive patients and decreasing numbers of unaware hypertensive sufferers.

Currently, various agents are approved for treatment of hypertension in Japan: 22 diuretics. 14 β-blockers including 2 α- and β-blockers, 4 α_1-blockers, 15 other sympatholytics including 4 centrally acting α_2-stimulants, 3 direct vasodilators, 4 calcium antagonists, and 4 ACE inhibitors. Table 1 shows the antihypertensive agents which were given to 1193 patients at the Hypertension-Nephrology Clinic of the National Cardiovascular Center in February 1987.

Table 1. Antihypertensive agents given to 1193 patients at the Hypertension-Nephrology Clinic of the National Cardiovascular Center in February 1987

Antihypertensive drug	Number of total prescriptions	Number of prescriptions as monotherapy
Diuretics	666 (30.3%)	99 (25.2%)
β-Blockers[a]	663 (30.1%)	141 (35.9%)
Calcium antagonists	613 (27.9%)	129 (32.8%)
ACE inhibitors	170 (7.7%)	21 (5.3%)
α_1-Blockers	37 (1.7%)	1 (0.3%)
α_2-Stimulants	31 (1.4%)	2 (0.5%)
Direct vasodilators[b]	20 (0.9%)	0 (0%)
Others[c]	1 (0%)	0 (0%)
Total	2211	393

[a] Including α-, β-blockers (32 total prescription, 14 for monotherapy).
[b] Hydralazine and related agents.
[c] Reserpine.

Diuretics, β-blockers, and calcium antagonists were used frequently, and ACE inhibitors shared the 4th position. Among the drugs prescribed as monotherapy, β-blockers and calcium antagonists outnumbered diuretics. Prescription of α_1-blockers, α_2-stimulants, and direct vasodilators was less frequent. This pattern of antihypertensive drug therapy is similar to that at several university hospitals, as cited perviously (OMAE et al. 1987), and may represent current antihypertensive therapy trends in Japan.

There is an increasing number of patients who measure their blood pressure at home since various electronic sphygmomanometers with high accuracy are commercially available at reasonable prices. Although the advantage of blood pressure measurement at home has not yet been established, information about both office and home blood pressure levels may provide a better antihypertensive treatment for the patients.

References

Dahl LK (1960) Possible role of salt intake in the development of essential hypertension. In: Bock KD, Cottier PT (eds) Essential hypertension. Springer, Berlin Gōttingen Heidelberg p 53

Isomura K (1987) An epidemiological study of the relationship between recent changes in the dietary habits of the young and old and cardiovascular disease (in Japanese). In: National Cardiovascular Center (ed) Annual Report of the Research on Cardiovascular Diseases 1986. National Cardiovascular Center, Suita p 550

Kagan A, Harris BB, Winkelstein W Jr, Johnson KG, Kato H, Syme SL, Rhoads GG, et al. (1974) Epidemiological studies of coronaty heart disease and stroke in Japanese men living in Japan, Hawaii and California: Demographic, physical, dietary and biochemical characteristics. J Chronic Dis 27:345–364

Ministry of Health and Welfare (1983a) Summary of national survey on circulatory disorders 1980. Report of national survey on circulatory disorders 1980. Japan Heart Foundation, Tokyo, p 17

Ministry of Health and Welfare (1983b) Summary of national survey on nutrition 1981 (in Japanese). Rinsho Eiyo 62:38–42
Omae T (1985) Pathophysiology and outcome of hypertensive subjects (in Japanese). J Jpn Soc Intern Med 74:401–405
Omae T, Ueda K, Kikumura T, Shikata T, Fujii I, Yanai T, Hasuo Y (1981) Cardiovascular deaths among hypertensive subjects of middle to old age: a long-term follow-up study in a Japanese community. In: Onesti G, Kim WE (eds) Hypertension in the young and the old. Grune and Stratton, New York, p 285
Omae T. Fukiyama K, Ishii M, Miura Y (1987) Current choice of antihypertensive drugs (in Japanese). Jpn J Hypertens 9:81–97
Owada K (1985) International comparison of mortality, morbidity and risk factors of cardiovascular diseases (in Japanese). In: National Cardiovascular Center (ed) annual Report of the Research on Cardiovascular Diseases 1984. National Cardiovascular Center, Suita p 1
Ueda K, Hasuo Y, Kiyohara Y, Wada J, Kawano H, Kato I, Fujii I, et al. (1988) Intracerebral hemorrhage in a Japanese community, Hisayama: incidence, changing pattern during long-term follow-up, and related factors. Stroke 19:48–52

CHAPTER 24

Listing of Antihypertensive Medications

V.F. MAURO

The following represents an attempt to compile a worldwide listing of commonly used antihypertensive medications. It should be emphasized that by no means is this listing complete. While care has been taken to ensure the accuracy of the information presented, the reader is advised that the authors, editors, reviewers, contributors, and publishers cannot be responsible for the continued currency of the information or for any errors or omissions in this chapter or for any consequences arising therefrom.

In Table 1 the antihypertensive medications are arranged by general pharmacological classification. Additionally, for each medication cited, the available dosage forms and strengths and general dosing guidelines are given. Available dosage forms and strengths and specific dosing guidelines may differ from country to country.

Table 2 lists commonly used brand names for antihypertensive agents cited in Table 1. Due to the tremendous number of medications and manufacturers, this table is by no means complete.

Table 3 is a listing of combination antihypertensive products and brand names available in the USA, some of which are available in other countries. This listing does not contain combination products available only outside the USA.

Table 4 is an alphabetized listing of brand and generic names. This table is helpful in determining the ingredients of an antihypertensive medication when only the brand name is known and in determining the general pharmacological classification of a medication when only the generic name is known.

The information contained in these tables is from manufacturer product literature whenever possible. Additional references utilized include: *Index Nominum, Inpharma, Martindale: The Extra Pharmacopoeia*, 28th edition, *Physician's Desk Reference, Rote Liste, USAN and the USP Dictionary of Drug Names*, and The 1988 Report of the Joint National Committee on Detection, Evaluation, and Treatment of High Blood Pressure. Arch Intern Med (1988) 148:1023–1038.

Acknowledgement. The assistance of Dr. Channing Hinman, Karen Kier, MS, and Patricia Gore in the preparation of this manuscript is appreciated.

Table 1. Listing of antihypertensives by pharmacological class

Drug	Dosage forms	Dosing guidelines
Angiotensin-Converting Enzyme Inhibitors		
Captopril	12.5, 25, 37.5, 50, & 100 mg tablets	Initial, 25 mg 2–3 times a day; increase as needed every 1–2 weeks; maximum dose 300–450 mg daily
Enalapril	5, 10, & 20 mg tablets	Initial 5 mg once daily; average maintenance dose 10–40 mg per day in 1 or 2 doses
	2.5 mg/2 ml vial	1.25 mg every 6 h IV
Lisinopril	5, 10 & 20 mg tablets	Initial 10 mg once daily; average maintenance dose 20–40 mg daily
Ramipril	1.25, 2.5, 5, & 10 mg capsules	Initial, 1.25–2.5 mg daily; increase to 10 mg daily as needed
β-Antagonists		
Acebutolol	200 & 400 mg capsules	Initially, 400 mg per day in 1 or 2 doses; maintenance, 400–800 mg per day in 1 or 2 doses
Alprenolol	50 mg tablet 200 mg sustained-release tablet	50 mg 4 times a day 200 mg once a day
Arotinolol*	5 & 10 mg tablets	10 mg twice a day; maximum dose 30 mg per day
Atenolol	25, 50, & 100 mg tablets	Initial, 50 mg once a day; if needed, increase to 100 mg QD after 1–2 weeks
Betaxolol	20 mg tablet	10–20 mg once a day
Bevantolol	75, 100, 200, & 400 mg tablets	Initial, 200 mg daily; maintenance, 200–400 mg daily
Bisoprolol	5 & 10 mg tablets	Initial 5 mg daily; increase to 20 mg daily as needed
Bopindolol	1 mg tablet	Initial, 1 mg daily; maintenance, 0.5–2 mg daily
Bunitrolol	10 mg tablet	10 mg three times a day
Bupranolol	50 & 100 mg tablets	Initial, 50–100 mg daily; increase daily dose by 50 mg each week as needed; maximum dose 400 mg daily
	200 mg sustained-release tablet	100–200 mg daily; increase to 400 mg daily, if needed
Carazolol	5 mg tablet	Initial, 5 mg once daily; average maintenance dose 5 mg three times daily
Carteolol	5 mg tablet	Initial, 10–15 mg daily in 2–3 doses; may increase to 30 mg daily in 2–3 doses as needed
Celiprolol	200 mg tablet	Initial, 200 mg daily; increase to 400 mg daily as needed

Table 1. (continued)

Drug	Dosage forms	Dosing guidelines
Cloranolol	5 mg tablet	2.5 mg 2–3 times daily; average daily dose 10–20 mg daily; maximum dose 45 mg daily
Labetalol*	100, 200, & 300 mg tablets	Initial 100 mg twice daily; maintenance, 200–400 mg twice daily
	5 mg/ml solution for injection in 20 and 40 ml vials	20 mg slowly IVP; may repeat as needed with 40–80 mg every 10 min; continuous infusion 2 mg/min
Levomoprolol	75 mg tablet	Initial, 75 mg daily; after 1 week, may increase to 150 or more daily as needed
Mepindolol	2.5 & 5.0 mg tablets	Initial, 5 mg daily; increase to 10 mg daily as needed
Metipranolol	10 & 20 mg tablets	20 mg 2 or 3 times a day
Metoprolol	50 & 100 mg tablets	Initial 100 mg per day in 1 or 2 doses; maintenance, 100–450 mg per day in 1 or 2 doses
	200 mg sustained-release tablet	100–200 mg daily
Nadolol	20, 40, 80, 120, & 160 mg tablets	Initial 40 mg once daily; usual maintenance, 40–80 mg once a day; maximum dose, 160–240 mg once a day
Oxprenolol	40 & 80 mg tablets	Initial, 40–80 mg twice a day; increase daily dose by 80–160 mg every 1–2 weeks as needed
	160 mg sustained-release tablet	Initial, 160 mg daily; increase to 320 mg daily, if needed
Penbutolol	40 mg tablet	Initial 40 mg daily; increase to 80 mg daily as needed
Pindolol	2.5, 5, 10, & 15 mg tablets	Initial 5 mg twice a day; maximum maintenance dose, 30 mg twice a day
	20 mg sustained-release tablet	20 mg daily
Propranolol	10, 20, 40, 60, 80, & 90 mg tablets; 20 mg/5 cc & 80 mg/cc oral solutions	Initial 40 mg twice a day; maintenance, 120–240 mg daily in 2–3 doses; maximum daily dose—640 mg
	60, 80, 120, & 160 mg sustained release capsules	80–240 mg daily
Sotalol	80, 160, 240, 320 & 480 mg tablets	Initial, 160 mg daily; increase by 80–160 mg every 2 weeks as needed; maximum dose, 640 mg daily
Talinolol	50 & 100 mg tablets	Initial, 50 mg 2–3 times daily; increase as needed to 300 mg daily in 2–3 doses

Table 1. (continued)

Drug	Dosage forms	Dosing guidelines
Tertatolol	5 mg tablet	5 mg daily
Timolol	5, 10, & 20 mg tablets	Initial, 10 mg twice a day; maintenance, 20–60 mg per day in 2 doses
Calcium Antagonists		
Diltiazem	30, 60, 90, & 120 mg tablets	Initial 30 mg 4 times a day; increase as needed to 180–360 mg per day in 3 or 4 doses
	90 mg sustained-release tablet; 60, 90 & 120 mg sustained-release capsules	Initial, 60–120 mg twice a day; may increase to 180–270 mg twice a day
	10 mg/2 ml & 25 mg/5 ml ampules	0.3 mg/kg slow IVP; 0.2–1.0 mg/min IV infusion
Felodipine	5 & 10 mg extended-release tablets	Initial, 5–10 mg daily; increase to 20 mg daily as needed
Gallopamil	25 & 50 mg tablets	50 mg 2–4 times a day
Nicardipine	20 & 30 mg capsules	Initial, 20 mg 3 times a day; maintenance, 60–90 mg per day in 2 or 3 doses
Nifedipine	10 & 20 mg capsules; 20 mg/ml oral solution	Initial, 10 mg 3 times a day; maintenance, 10–40 mg three times a day
	20 mg sustained-release capsule	20–40 mg twice a day
	30, 60, & 90 mg sustained-release tablets	Initial, 30–60 mg daily; maximum dose, 120 mg daily
Nitrendipine	10 & 20 mg tablets	Initial, 10–20 mg in 1 or 2 doses; maintenance, 20–60 mg per day
Verapamil	80 & 120 mg tablets	40–80 mg 3 times a day; increase to 120 mg 3 times a day if needed
	240 mg sustained-release tablet	120–480 mg daily in 1–2 doses
Central α-2 Agonists		
Clonidine	0.075, 0.1, 0.2, 0.3, & 0.5 mg tablets	Initial, 0.1 mg twice a day; gradually increase by 0.1–0.2 mg per day as needed; maximum dose, 2.4 mg per day
	0.25 sustained-release capsule	0.25–0.50 mg once daily
	0.1 mg, 0.2 mg, & 0.3 mg/24-h patches	Initial, 0.1 mg patch each week; maximum dose, two 0.3-mg patches each week
	0.1 mg/ml & 0.15 mg/ml ampules	0.15–0.3 mg IM or slow IVP; may repeat in 3–4 h if necessary

Table 1. (continued)

Drug	Dosage forms	Dosing guidelines
Guanabenz	4, 8, & 16 mg tablets	Initial, 4 mg twice a day; maximum dose, 32 mg twice a day
Guanfacine	1 mg tablet	Initial, 1 mg at bedtime; gradually increase to 2–3 mg per day if necessary
Lofexidine	0.15 & 0.2 mg tablets	Initial, 0.4–0.45 mg daily in 2 doses; gradually increase as needed to 1.2–1.35 mg per day in 2 or 3 doses
Methyldopa	125, 250, & 500 mg tablets; 250 mg/5 ml oral suspension	Initial, 250 mg 2 or 3 times a day; maintenance, 0.5–3 g per day in 2–4 doses
	250 mg/5 cc solution for injection	0.25–1 g every 6 h IV
Tiamenidine	0.5 & 1.0 mg tablets	Initial, 0.5 mg twice daily; increase as needed to 3 mg daily in 2–3 doses
Diuretics		
Amiloride	5 mg tablet	Initial, 5 mg daily; increase to 20 mg daily as needed
Azosemide	80 mg tablet	40–80 mg per day
Bendroflumethiazide (Bendrofluazide)	2.5, 5, & 10 mg tablets	Initial, 5–20 mg daily; maintenance, 2.5–15 mg daily
Benzthiazide	50 mg tablet	Initial, 50–100 mg daily in 2 doses; maximum maintenance dose, 200 mg per day
Benzylhydrochlorothiazide	4 mg tablet	Initial, 4–8 mg daily in two doses; increase to 20 mg daily in 2 doses as needed
Bumetanide	0.5, 1, 2, & 5 mg tablets	Initially, 0.5–2.0 mg as a single dose; May increase to 5–10 mg daily in 1–2 doses as needed
	0.25 mg/ml solution for injection	Initial, 0.5–1.0 mg IV or IM; may repeat every 2–3 h up to a maximum daily dose of 10 mg
Buthiazide (Butizide)	5 mg tablet	5–10 mg daily
Cancrenoate	200 mg/10 ml ampule	200 mg 2–3 times a day IV; maximum single dose 400 mg; maximum daily dose 800 mg
Chlorothiazide	250 & 500 mg tablets; 250 mg/5 ml oral suspension	125–500 mg daily
	500 mg powder for injection	0.5–2 g once or twice a day IV
Chlorthalidone	25, 50, & 100 mg tablets	12.5–50 mg daily
Clopamide	20 mg tablet	5–20 mg daily

Table 1. (continued)

Drug	Dosage forms	Dosing guidelines
Clorexolone	10 mg tablet	10–25 mg daily
Cyclopenthiazide	0.5 mg tablets	0.25–0.5 mg daily; maximum dose; 1.5 mg daily
Cyclothiazide	2 mg tablet	2 mg daily
Ethacrynic Acid	25 & 50 mg tablets	25–100 mg daily in 1–2 doses
	50 mg powder for injection	0.5–1.0 mg/kg slow IVP
Etozolin	200 & 400 tablets	200–400 mg daily
Fenquizone	10 mg capsule	10–20 mg every day
Furosemide (Frusemide)	20, 40, & 80 mg tablets; 40 mg/5 ml & 10 mg/ml oral solutions	20–40 mg daily; may need to increase in patients with chronic renal failure
	10 mg/ml solution for injection	20–80 mg IM or slow IVP
Hydrochlorothiazide	25, 50, & 100 mg tablets; 10 mg/ml & 100 mg/ml oral solutions	12.5–50 mg daily
Hydroflumethiazide	50 mg tablet	Initial, 50 mg twice a day; maintenance,50–100 mg daily
Indapamide	2.5 mg tablet	Initial, 2.5 mg daily; increase to 5 mg daily if necessary
Mefruside	25 mg tablet	Initial, 25–50 mg daily; increase to 100 mg daily as needed
Methyclothiazide	2.5 & 5 mg tablets	2.5–5 mg daily
Meticrane	150 mg tablet	150 mg once or twice daily
Metolazone	2.5, 5, & 10 mg tablets	2.5–5 mg daily
Piretanide	3 & 6 mg tablets	3–12 mg daily in 1–2 doses
	6 mg sustained-release capsule	6 mg once or twice a day
	6 mg/2 ml, 12 mg/5 ml, & 60 mg/20 ml ampules	Initial, 6–12 mg IVP once or twice a day; increase as needed
Polythiazide	1, 2, & 4 mg tablets	2–4 mg daily
Quinethazone	50 mg tablet	50–100 mg daily
Spironolactone	25, 50, & 100 mg tablets	50–100 mg daily
Triamterene	50 & 100 mg capsules	Initial, 100 mg twice a day; maintenance, 100–150 mg twice a day
Trichlormethiazide	2 & 4 mg tablets	2–4 mg daily
Tripamide	15 mg tablet	15 mg once or twice daily
Xipamide	10 & 40 mg tablets	10–40 mg daily

Table 1. (continued)

Drug	Dosage forms	Dosing guidelines
Ganglionic Blockers		
Azamethonium	5% solution for injection in 1 or 2 cc ampules	Maximum single dose, 150 mg; maximum daily dose, 450 mg
Mecamylamine	2.5 & 10 mg tablets	Initial, 2.5 mg twice a day; average maintenance dose, 25 mg per day divided in 3 doses
Pempidine	1 & 5 mg tablets	Initial, 2.5 mg 3 or 4 times a day; usual maintenance dose 10–80 mg per day in 4 doses
Pentolinium	10 & 40 mg tablets	10–20 mg every 12 h; gradually increase as needed; usual maintenance, 100–900 mg daily
	50 mg/10 ml ampule	1–2.5 mg SC every 12 h; gradually increase dose as needed; usual maintenance, 20–100 mg daily
Trimethaphan	500 mg/10 ml	Initial, 3–4 mg/min IV infusion; adjust rate as needed
Monoamine Oxidase Inhibitor		
Pargyline	10 & 25 mg tablets	25 mg once daily; usual maintenance, 25–50 mg daily; maximum daily dose, 200 mg
Peripheral Adrenergic Inhibitors		
Bethanidine	10 & 50 mg tablets	Initial, 10 mg 3 times daily; increase gradually by 5 mg three times daily as needed; average maintenance, 20–200 mg daily
Debrisoquine	10 & 20 mg tablets	Initial, 10 mg once or twice daily; increase daily dose by 10–20 mg every 3–4 days as needed; average maintenance, 40–120 mg daily
Guanadrel	10 & 25 mg tablets	Initial, 5 mg twice a day; average maintenance, 20–75 mg per day in 2 doses
Guanethidine	10 & 25 mg tablets	Initial, 10–20 mg daily; increase by 10 mg each week as needed; average maintenance, 30–100 mg daily
	10 mg/ml ampule	10–20 mg IM
Guanoclor	10 & 40 mg tablets	Initial, 5–10 mg twice daily; increase gradually, average maintenance dose is 10–120 mg daily
Guanoxan	10 & 40 mg tablets	Initial, 10 mg per day in 1 or 2 doses; increase weekly by 5–10 mg daily as needed

Table 1. (continued)

Drug	Dosage forms	Dosing guidelines
Postsynaptic α-Antagonists		
Bunazosin	0.5, 1, & 3 mg tablets	Initial, 1.5 mg per day in 2 or 3 doses; maximum daily dose, 12 mg per day in 2 or 3 doses
Doxazosin	1, 2, & 4 mg tablets	Initial, 1 mg daily; gradually increase as needed to maximum daily dose of 16 mg daily
Indoramin	25 & 50 mg tablets	Initial, 25 mg twice a day; maximum dose, 200 mg in 2 or 3 doses
Prazosin	1, 2, & 5 mg capsules	Initial, 1 mg 2 or 3 times daily; usual maintenance, 6–15 mg daily
	1, 2, 4, & 6 mg sustained-release capsules	1 mg daily; may increase up to 6 mg daily as needed
Terazosin	1, 2, & 5 mg tablets	Initial, 1 mg at bedtime; usual maintenance, 1–5 mg daily; maximum dose, 20 mg
Urapidil	30, 60, & 90 mg sustained-release capsules	30–60 mg daily; increase to 60 mg twice daily as needed
	25 mg/5 ml & 50 mg/10 ml ampules	25 mg slow IVP; may increase to 50–75 mg if needed; 15–30 mg/h IV infusion
Pre- and Postsynaptic α-Antagonists		
Phenoxybenzamine	1, 5, & 10 mg capsules	Initial, 10 mg twice a day; usual dose, 20–40 mg 2 or 3 times a day
Phentolamine	5 mg/ml, 10 mg/ml, & 50 mg/5 ml ampules	5 mg IV or IM
***Rauwolfia* Extracts and Derivatives**		
Alseroxylon	2 mg tablet	Usual dose, 1–8 mg daily
Deserpidine	0.25 mg tablet	Usual dose, 0.25 mg daily
Methoserpidine	5 & 10 mg tablets	Usual dose, 15–50 mg daily
Rescinnamine	0.25 & 0.5 mg tablets	Usual dose, 0.25–0.5 mg daily
Reserpine	0.1, 0.25 & 1.0 mg tablets	Usual dose, 0.1–0.25 mg daily
Whole root *Rauwolfia*	50 & 100 mg tablets	Usual dose, 50–100 mg daily
Syrosingopine	1 mg tablet	Usual dose, 0.5–3 mg daily

Table 1. (continued)

Drug	Dosage forms	Dosing guidelines
Serotonin Antagonist		
Ketanserin	20 & 40 mg tablets	Initial, 20 mg twice daily; after 1 month, may increase to 40 mg twice daily, if needed
	5 mg/ml solution for injection in 2 ml & 5 ml ampules	3 mg/min IVP until response of a maximum dose of 30 mg; continuous infusion 2–6 mg/h
		Also, 10 mg IM, may repeat after 30–45 min
Vasodilators		
Cadralazine	10, 15, & 20 mg tablets	Initial, 10 mg daily; increase to 30 mg daily as needed
Diazoxide	50 mg tablets; 25 & 100 mg capsules	0.4–1 g daily in 2 or 3 doses
	300 mg/20 ml injection	Initial, 1–3 mg/kg IV (maximum dose, 150 mg), repeat every 5-15 min as needed; maintenance, repeat initial dose every 4–24 h as needed
Dihydralazine	25 & 50 mg tablets	25–50 mg 3 times a day
	25 mg ampule	12.5–25 mg IM or 6.25–12.5 mg IV (maximum dose IV, 25 mg); repeat once or twice every 15–20 min as needed; IV infusion, 4–12.5 mg/h
Endralazine	5 & 10 mg capsules	5–10 mg twice a day
Hydralazine	10, 25, 50, & 100 mg tablets	Initial 10 mg 4 times a day; gradually increase to maximum dose 200–300 mg per day in 2 doses
	20 mg/ml ampule	20–40 mg IM or IVP
Minoxidil	2.5 & 10 mg tablets	Initial, 5 mg once a day; average maintenance, 10–40 mg per day; maximum dose, 100 mg per day
Nitroprusside	50 mg powder for injection	Initial, 0.25–0.5 μg/kg per min; increase by 0.25–0.5 μg/kg per min every 10 min until response or maximum dose of 10 μg/kg per min

* combined α- and β-antagonist

Table 2. Brand names of antihypertensive agents

Generic name	Brand names
Acebutolol	Acetanol Monitan Neptall Prent Rhodiasectral Sectral
Alprenolol	Alpresol Apllobal Aptine Aptol Gubernal Regletin Sinalol Vasoton Yobir
Alseroxylon	Angioserpina Iposalfa Rauwan Rauwiloid Ra-Valeas
Amiloride	Arumil Kaluril Midamor Modamide Nirulid Pandiuren
Arotinolol	Almarl
Atenolol	Antipressan Betablok Ibinolol Myocord Normiten Oraday Tenolone Tenormin Vericordin
Azamethonium	Ganlion Pentamini
Azosemide	Diart Diurapid Luret
Bendroflumethiazide	Aprinox Berkozide Centyl Esberizid Naturetin Neo-Naclex Notens Pluryl Polidiuril

Table 2. (continued)

Generic name	Brand names
	Salural Salures Sinesalin Sodiuretic Tesical Urinagen Urizide
Benzthiazide	Aquatag Exna Fovane Hydrex Marazide Proaqua
Benzylhydrochlorothiazide	Behyd 3 BT
Betaxolol	Kerlone
Bethanidine	Batel Bendogen Benzoxine Betaling Esbaloid Esbatal Eusmanid Hypersin Regulin
Bevantolol	Ranestol Sentiloc
Bisoprolol	Bisobloc Concor Detensiel Encor Isoten Monocor Soprol
Bopindolol	Sandonorm
Bumetanide	Aquazone Bonures Bumex Burinex Butinat Cambiex Diurama Fontego Fordiuran Lixil Lunetoron Segurex
Bunazosin	Detantol

Table 2. (continued)

Generic name	Brand names
Bunitrolol	Betrilol Stresson
Bupranolol	Betadran Betadrenol Looser Monobeltin Oxycardin Panimit
Buthiazide	Eunephran Saltucin
Cadralazine	Cadralin Cadraten
Cancrenoate	Aldactone Osiren Osirenol Osyrol Phanurane Sincomen Soldactone Spiroctan Venactone
Captopril	Acepril Acetan Capoten Capotena Captolane Cortensobon Dilabor Isopresol Lopirin Lopril Tensobon
Carazolol	Conducton
Carteolol	Endak Meptin Mikelan
Celiprolol	Cardem Selectol
Chlorothiazide	Azide Chlotride Diachlor Diubram Diurazide Diuret Diurigen Diuril Diurilix Diurone

Table 2. (continued)

Generic name	Brand names
	Saluretil Saluric
Chlorthalidone	Higrotona Hygroton Hylidone Igrolina Igroton Novothalidone Odemase Renon Thalitone Urid Uridon Urolin Zambesil
Clonidine	Catapresan Catapress Clonidin Clonilou Clonistada Drylon Hyposyn Ipotensium Paracefan Renalia Tensinova
Clopamide	Adurix Brinaldix
Cloranolol	Tobanum
Clorexolone	Nefrolan
Cyclopenthiazide	Navidrex
Cyclothiazide	Anhydron Doburil
Debrisoquine	Declinax Equitonil Tendor
Deserpidine	Harmonyl
Diazoxide	Eudemine Hyperstat Hypertonalum Proglicem Proglycem
Dihydralazine	Dihyzin Nepresol Nepressol
Diltiazem	Aralix Britiazim Cardizem

Table 2. (continued)

Generic name	Brand names
	Dilatem Diltikor Dilzem Hart Herbesser Masdil Tidiem Tilazem
Doxazosin	Carduran
Enalapril	Analept Conversin Convertin Enalten Enapren Hiopartel Innovace Levinezal Lotrial Megapres Naprilene Olivin Pres Rablas Reminal Renitec Supotron Vasotec Xanef
Endralazine	Miretilan
Ethacrynic Acid	Crinuryl Edecril Edecrin Edecrina Edecrine Hydromedin Reomax Taladren Uregyt
Etozolin	Elkapin
Felodipine	Agon Hydac Plendil
Fenquizone	Idrolone
Furosemide	Aluzine Aquamide Aquasin Arasemide Diural

Table 2. (continued)

Generic name	Brand names
	Diurolasa Dryptal Errolon Franyl Frucee Frusetic Frusid Furix Fur-O-Ims Hypo-Rapid Impugan Lasiletten Lasilix Lasix Laxur Moilarorin Neo-Renal Nicorol Novosemide Parksemide Promedes Seguril Sigasalur Uremide Urex Uritol Virifenemide
Gallopamil	Procorum
Guanabenz	Rexiten Wytens Wytensin
Guanadrel	Hylorel
Guanethidine	Antipress Dopom Ipotidina Ismelin Ismeline Solo-Ethidine Visutensil
Guanfacine	Entulic Estulic Hipertensal Tenex
Guanoclor	Vatensol
Guanoxan	Envacar Guanutil
Hydralazine	Alphapress Appresolin

Table 2. (continued)

Generic name	Brand names
	Aprelazine Apresolina Apresoline Dralzine Hyperazin Hyperex Ipolina
Hydrochlorothiazide	Atenadon Catiazida Chlorzide Chlothia Delco-Retic Diaqua Dichlotride Didral Diidrotiazide Direma Diruex Diucen-H Diuchlor Diursana-H Dixidrasi Esidrex Esidrix Hidrenox Hidrosaluretil Hydro-Aquil Hydro-Chlor Hydrodiuril Hydroma Hydrosaluric Hydro-Tl Hydro-Z Hydrozide Idrodiuvis Idrofluin Idrolisin Jen-Diril Lexor Loqua Maschitt Mictrin Natrimax Neo-Codema Neoflumen Neo Minzil Newtolide Novohydrazide Oretic Pantemon Ro-Hydrazide Tandiur Thiuretic

Table 2. (continued)

Generic name	Brand names
	Urirex Urozide
Hydroflumethiazide	Di-Ademil Diucardin Enjit Hydrenox Leodrine Rivosil Robezon Rontyl Saluron Salurona
Indapamide	Bajaten Extur Fludex Lozol Narix Natrilix Noranat
Indoramin	Baratol Vidora Wydora Wypres
Ketanserin	Serepress Sufrexal
Labetalol	Albetol Ipolab Labelol Labrocol Mitalolo Normadate Normodyne Opercol Presolol Pressalold Salmagne Trandate
Levomoprolol	Levotensin Omeral
Lisinopril	Carace Prinivil Zestril
Lofexidine	Lofetensin
Mecamylamine	Inversine Mevasine
Mefruside	Baycaron Mefrusal
Mepindolol	Caridian

Table 2. (continued)

Generic name	Brand names
	Corindolan Mepicor
Methoserpidine	Decaserpyl
Methyclothiazide	Aquatensen Duretic Enduron Endurona Thiazidil
Methyldopa	Aldomet Aldometil Alphamex Baypresol Dopamet Dopegyt Grospisk Hydopa Hyperpax Hy-Po-Tone Medimet Medomet Medopa Medopal Medopren Methopa Methoplain Metoras Mulfasin Novomedopa Presinol Sembrina
Meticrane	Arresten
Metipranolol	Betamann Disorat
Metolazone	Diulo Metenix Zaroxolyn
Metoprolol	Beloc Betaloc Cardiosel Denex Lopresor Lopressor Metoblock Prelis Selokeen Seloken Selopral
Minoxidil	Loniten Lonolox Prexidil

Table 2. (continued)

Generic name	Brand names
Nadolol	Corgard Nadic Solgol
Nicardipine	Cardene Cardepine Convertal Dacarel Loxen Nerdipina Nicarpin Nicodel Nimicor Perdipine Ridene Vasonase
Nifedipine	Adalat Adalate Aprical Calcibloc Carotrend Cordicant Corotrend Duranifin Nifcor Nifecard Nifedicor Nifedipat Nifelat Nife-Puren Pidilat Procardia Tibricol
Nitrendipine	Bayotensin Bayopress Tracil
Nitroprusside	Hypoten Nipride Nipruss
Oxprenolol	Oxanol Trasacor Trasicor
Pargyline	Eudatine Eutonyl
Pempidine	Pempidil Pempiten Synapleg Tenormal Viotil
Penbutolol	Betapressin Betapressine

Table 2. (continued)

Generic name	Brand names
	Betapressor
Pentolinium	Ansolysen Pentio
Phenoxybenzamine	Dibenzyline Dibenzyran
Phentolamine	Regitina Regitine Rogitine
Pindolol	Blocklin Carvisken Durapindol Pectobloc Pinadol Pinbetol Pyltelol Pynastin Viskeen Visken Visloc
Piretanide	Arelix Perbilen
Polythiazide	Drenusil Nephril Renese
Prazosin	Duramipress Eurex Hexapress Hypovase Minipress Peripress
Propranolol	Angilol Apsolol Arablock Avlocardyl Beprane Berkolol Beta-Neg Betaryl Beta-Tablinen Blocardyl Cardinol Caridolol Creanol Curanol Deralin Dociton Efektolol Elbrol Frekven Herzul

Table 2. (continued)

Generic name	Brand names
	Inderal Indobloc Kemi Noloten Oposim Pranix Pranolol Prano-Puren Prolol Pronovan Propabloc Propalong Propayerst Pylapron Sloprolol Sumial Tesnol Tonum
Quinethazone	Aquamox Hydromox
Ramipril	Tritace
Rescinnamine	Anaprel Cartric Cinnasil Moderil Rescimin
Reserpine	Lemiserp Mephaserpin Neo-Serp Rausan Rau-Sed Rauwifa Resedril Reselar Resercen Reserfia Reserpanca Reserpoid Sandril Sedaraupin Serpalen Serpasil Serpasol Serpate Serpresan Vio-serpine
Sotalol	Beta-Cardone Cormedigin Sotacor Sotalex
Spironolactone	Acelat

Table 2. (continued)

Generic name	Brand names
	Alatone Aldace Aldactone Aldopur Aquareduct Duraspiron Laractone Osiren Osyrol Sagisal Sincomen Spirix Spirocta Spiroctian Spiron Spirotone Supra-Puren
Syrosingopine	Aurugopin Londomin Neoreserpan Novoserpina Raunova Seniramin Siringina Siroshuten Syrogopin
Talinolol	Cordanum
Terazosin	Heitrin Hytrin Hytrinex
Tertatolol	Artex
Tiamenidine	Sundralen
Timolol	Betim Blocadren Blocanol Proflax Temserin Timacor
Triamterene	Diesse Diucelpin Dyrenium Dytac Jatropur Natrium Teriam Triamteril Urocaudal
Trichlormethiazide	Achletin Anatran Anistadin Aponorin

Table 2. (continued)

Generic name	Brand names
	Carvacron Chlopolidine Cretonin Diu-Fortan Diurese Esmarin Fluitran Flutra Intromene Kubacron Metahydrin Naqua Niazide Sanamiron Schebitran Tachionin Tolcasone
Trimethaphan	Arfonad
Tripamide	Normonal
Urapidil	Ebrantil Uraprene
Verapamil	Anpec Berkatens Calan Civicor Durasoptin Isoptin Rapam Securon Univer Vasolan Veramex Verelan Verpal
Whole Root *Rauwolfia*	Bagoserfia Hypercal Raudixin Rauval Rauwolfinetas Rawlini Rivadescin Serenol Serpetin Tensowolfia
Xipamide	Aquafor Aquaforil Aquaphor Aquaphoril Diurexan Imovance Zipex

Table 3. Antihypertensive combinations available in USA

I. Diuretic with:		
A. Rauwolfia derivatives		
Diupres 500	500 mg chlorothiazide	0.125 mg reserpine
Diupres 250	250 mg chlorothiazide	0.125 mg reserpine
Regroton	50 mg chlorthalidone	0.25 mg reserpine
Demi-Regroton	25 mg chlorthalidone	0.125 mg reserpine
Hydropres 50	50 mg hydrochlorothiazide	0.125 mg reserpine
Hydropres 25	25 mg hydrochlorothiazide	0.125 mg reserpine
Serpasil-Esidrix #2	50 mg hydrochlorothiazide	0.1 mg reserpine
Serpasil-Esidrix #1	25 mg hydrochlorothiazide	0.1 mg reserpine
Salutensin	50 mg hydroflumethiazide	0.125 mg reserpine
Salutensin-Demi	25 mg hydroflumethiazide	0.125 mg reserpine
Diutensen-R	2.5 mg methyclothiazide	0.1 mg reserpine
Renese-R	2 mg polythiazide	0.25 mg reserpine
Hydromox R	50 mg quinethazone	0.125 mg reserpine
Diurese-R	4 mg trichlormethiazide	0.1 mg reserpine
Metatensin #4	4 mg trichlormethiazide	0.1 mg reserpine
Naquival	4 mg trichlormethiazide	0.1 mg reserpine
Metatensin #2	2 mg trichlormethiazide	0.1 mg reserpine
Oreticyl Forte	25 mg hydrochlorothiazide	0.25 mg deserpidine
Oreticyl 50	50 mg hydrochlorothiazide	0.125 mg deserpidine
Oreticyl 25	25 mg hydrochlorothiazide	0.125 mg deserpidine
Enduronyl Forte	5 mg methyclothiazide	0.5 mg deserpidine
Enduronyl	5 mg methyclothiazide	0.25 mg deserpidine
Rauzide	4 mg bendroflumethiazide	50 mg *Rauwolifia serpentina*
Rautrax-N 400 mg KC1	4 mg bendroflumethiazide	50 mg *Rauwolifia serpentina*
Rautrax 400 mg KC1	400 mg flumethiazide	50 mg *Rauwolifia serpentina*
B. Vasodilators		
Apresazide 100/50	50 mg hydrochlorothiazide	100 mg hydralazine
Apresazide 50/50	50 mg hydrochlorothiazide	50 mg hydralazine
Apresazide 25/25	25 mg hydrochlorothiazide	25 mg hydralazine
Apresoline-Esidrex	15 mg hydrochlorothiazide	25 mg hydralazine
C. β-Blockers		
Tenoretic 100	25 mg chlorthalidone	100 mg atenolol
Tenoretic 50	25 mg chlorthalidone	50 mg atenolol
Corzide 80/5	5 mg bendroflumethiazide	80 mg nadolol
Corzide 40/5	5 mg bendroflumethiazide	40 mg nadolol
Timolide	25 mg hydrochlorothiazide	10 mg timolol
Inderide LA* 160/50	50 mg hydrochlorothiazide	160 mg propranolol
Inderide LA 120/50	50 mg hydrochlorothiazide	120 mg propranolol
Inderide LA 80/50	50 mg hydrochlorothiazide	80 mg propranolol
Inderide 80/25	25 mg hydrochlorothiazide	80 mg propranolol
Inderide 40/25	25 mg hydrochlorothiazide	40 mg propranolol
Lopressor HCT 100/50	50 mg hydrochlorothiazide	100 mg metoprolol
Lopressor HCT 100/25	25 mg hydrochlorothiazide	100 mg metoprolol
Lopressor HCT 50/25	25 mg hydrochlorothiazide	50 mg metoprolol

Table 3. (continued)

Normozide	25 mg hydrochlorothiazide	100 mg labetalol	
	25 mg hydrochlorothiazide	200 mg labetalol	
	25 mg hydrochlorothiazide	300 mg labetalol	
Trandate HCT	25 mg hydrochlorothiazide	100 mg labetalol	
	25 mg hydrochlorothiazide	200 mg labetalol	
	25 mg hydrochlorothiazide	300 mg labetalol	
D. Central α-2 agonists			
Aldoril D50	50 mg hydrochlorothiazide	500 mg methyldopa	
Aldoril D30	30 mg hydrochlorothiazide	500 mg methyldopa	
Aldoril-25	25 mg hydrochlorothiazide	250 mg methyldopa	
Aldoril-15	15 mg hydrochlorothiazide	250 mg methyldopa	
Aldoclor-250	250 mg chlorothiazide	250 mg methyldopa	
Aldoclor-150	150 mg chlorothiazide	250 mg methyldopa	
Combipres 0.3	15 mg chlorthalidone	0.3 mg clonidine	
Combipres 0.2	15 mg chlorthalidone	0.2 mg clonidine	
Combipres 0.1	15 mg chlorthalidone	0.1 mg clonidine	
E. ACE inhibitors			
Capozide 50/25	25 mg hydrochlorothiazide	50 mg captopril	
Capozide 25/25	25 mg hydrochlorothiazide	25 mg captopril	
Capozide 50/15	15 mg hydrochlorothiazide	50 mg captopril	
Capozide 25/15	15 mg hydrochlorothiazide	25 mg captopril	
Vaseretic	25 mg hydrochlorothiazide	10 mg enalapril	
F. Postsynaptic α-antagonists			
Minizide 5	0.5 mg polythiazide	5 mg prazosin	
Minizide 2	0.5 mg polythiazide	2 mg prazosin	
Minizide 1	0.5 mg polythiazide	1 mg prazosin	
G. Peripheral adrenergic inhibitor			
Esimil	25 mg hydrochlorothiazide	10 mg guanethidine	
H. MAO inhibitor			
Eutron	5 mg methyclothiazide	25 mg pargyline	
I. Veratrum alkaloid			
Diutensen	2.5 mg methyclothiazide	2 mg cryptenamine	
J. Reserpine and hydralazine			
Ser-Ap-Es	15 mg hydrochlorothiazide	0.1 mg reserpine	25 mg hydralazine
H. Other diuretics			
Moduretic	50 mg hydrochlorothiazide	5 mg amiloride	
Aldactazide	25 mg hydrochlorothiazide	25 mg spironolactone	
	50 mg hydrochlorothiazide	50 mg spironolactone	
Dyazide	25 mg hydrochlorothiazide	50 mg triamterene	
Maxzide-25MG	25 mg hydrochlorothiazide	37.5 mg triamterene	
Maxzide	50 mg hydrochlorothiazide	75 mg triamterene	
II. Reserpine with hydralazine			
Serpasil-Apresoline #2	50 mg hydralazine	0.2 mg reserpine	
Serpasil-Apresoline #1	25 mg hydralazine	0.1 mg reserpine	

* Long-acting

Table 4. Index to antihypertensive agents' generic and brand names (Generic names indicated by **bold** print; brand names indicated by normal print.)

Acebutolol β-Antagonist
Acelat see Spironolactone
Acepril see Captopril
Acetan see Captopril
Acetanol see Acebutolol
Achletin see Trichlormethiazide
Adalat see Nifedipine
Adalate see Nifedipine
Adurix see Clopamide
Agon see Felodipine
Alatone see Spironolactone
Albetol see Labetalol
Aldace see Spironolactone
Aldactazide contains hydrochlorothiazide and spironolactone
Aldactone see Cancrenoate and/or Spironolactone
Aldoclor contains chlorothiazide and methyldopa
Aldomet see Methyldopa
Aldometil see Methylopa
Aldopur see Spironolactone
Aldoril contains hydrochlorothiazide and methyldopa
Almarl see Arotinolol
Alphamex see Methyldopa
Alphapress see Hydralazine
Alprenolol β-Antagonist
Alpresol see Alprenolol
Alseroxylon *Rauwolfia* extract and derivative
Aluzine see Furosemide
Amiloride Diuretic
Analept see Enalapril
Anaprel see Rescinnamine
Anatran see Trichlormethiazide
Angilol see Propranolol
Angioserpina see Alseroxylon
Anhydron see Cyclothiazide
Anistadin see Trichlormethiazide
Anpec see Verapamil
Ansolysen see Pentolinium
Antipress see Guanethidine
Antipressan see Atenolol
Apllobal see Alprenolol
Aponorin see Trichlormethiazide
Appresolin see Hydralazine
Aprelazine see Hydralazine
Apresazide contains hydrochlorothiazide and hydralazine
Apresolina see Hydralazine
Apresoline see Hydralazine
Apresoline-Esidrex contains hydrochlorothiazide and hydralazine
Aprical see Nifedipine
Aprinox see Bendroflumethiazide
Apsolol see Propranolol
Aptine see Alprenolol
Aptol see Alprenolol
Aquafor see Xipamide
Aquaforil see Xipamide

Table 4. (continued)

Aquamide see Furosemide
Aquamox see Quinethazone
Aquaphor see Xipamide
Aquaphoril see Xipamide
Aquareduct see Spironolactone
Aquasin see Furosemide
Aquatag see Benzthiazide
Aquatensen see Methyclothiazide
Aquazone see Bumetanide
Arablock see Propranolol
Aralix see Diltiazem
Arasemide see Furosemide
Arelix see Piretanide
Arfonad see Trimethaphan
Arotinolol β-Antagonist
Arresten see Meticrane
Artex see Tertatolol
Arumil see Amiloride
Atenadon see Hydrochlorothiazide
Atenolol β-Antagonist
Aurugopin see Syrosingopine
Avlocardyl see Propranolol
Azamethonium Ganglionic blocker
Azide see Chlorothiazide
Azosemide Diuretic
Bagoserfia see Whole root *Rauwolfia*
Bajaten see Indapamide
Baratol see Indoramin
Batel see Bethanidine
Baycaron see Mefruside
Bayopress see Nitrendipine
Bayotensin see Nitrendipine
Baypresol see Methyldopa
Behyd see Benzylhydrochlorothiazide
Beloc see Metoprolol
Bendogen see Bethanidine
Bendroflumethiazide Diuretic
Benzoxine see Bethanidine
Benzthiazide Diuretic
Benzylhydrochlorothiazide Diuretic
Beprane see Propranolol
Berkatens see Verapamil
Berkolol see Propranolol
Berkozide see Bendroflumethiazide
Beta-Cardone see Sotalol
Beta-Neg see Propranolol
Beta-Tablinen see Propranolol
Betablok see Atenolol
Betadran see Bupranolol
Betadrenol see Bupranolol
Betaling see Bethanidine
Betaloc see Metoprolol
Betamann see Metipranolol
Betapressin see Penbutolol
Betapressine see Penbutolol

Table 4. (continued)

Betapressor see Penbutolol
Betaryl see Propranolol
Betaxolol β-Antagonist
Bethanidine Peripheral adrenergic inhibitor
Betim see Timolol
Betrilol see Bunitrolol
Bevantolol β-Antagonist
Bisobloc see Bisoprolol
Bisoprolol β-Antagonist
Blocadren see Timolol
Blocanol see Timolol
Blocardyl see Propranolol
Blocklin see Pindolol
Bonures see Bumetanide
Bopindolol β-Antagonist
Brinaldix see Clopamide
Britiazim see Diltiazem
3 BT see Benzylhydrochlorothiazide
Bumetanide Diuretic
Bumex see Bumetanide
Bunazosin Postsynaptic α-antagonist
Bunitrolol β-Antagonist
Bupranolol β-Antagonist
Burinex see Bumetanide
Buthiazide Diuretic
Butinat see Bumetanide
Cadralazine Vasodilator
Cadralin see Cadralazine
Cadraten see Cadralazine
Calan see Verapamil
Calcibloc see Nifedipine
Cambiex see Bumetanide
Cancrenoate Diuretic
Capoten see Captopril
Capotena see Captopril
Capozide contains hydrochlorothiazide and captopril
Captolane see Captopril
Captopril Angiotensin converting enzyme inhibitor
Carace see Lisinopril
Carazolol β-Antagonist
Cardem see Celiprolol
Cardene see Nicardipine
Cardepine see Nicardipine
Cardinol see Propranolol
Cardiosel see Metoprolol
Cardizem see Diltiazem
Carduran see Doxazosin
Caridian see Mepindolol
Caridolol see Propranolol
Carotrend see Nifedipine
Carteolol β-Antagonist
Cartric see Rescinnamine
Carvacron see Trichlormethiazide
Carvisken see Pindolol
Catapresan see Clonidine

Table 4. (continued)

Catapress see Clonidine
Catiazida see Hydrochlorothiazide
Celiprolol β-Antagonist
Centyl see Bendroflumethiazide
Chlopolidine see Trichlormethiazide
Chlorothiazide Diuretic
Chlorthalidone Diuretic
Chlorzide see Hydrochlorothiazide
Chlothia see Hydrochlorothiazide
Chlotride see Chlorothiazide
Cinnasil see Rescinnamine
Civicor see Verapamil
Clonidin see Clonidine
Clonidine Central α-2 agonist
Clonilou see Clonidine
Clonistada see Clonidine
Clopamide Diuretic
Cloranolol β-Antagonist
Clorexolone Diuretic
Combipres contains chlorothalidone and clonidine
Concor see Bisoprolol
Conducton see Carazolol
Conversin see Enalapril
Convertal see Nicardipine
Convertin see Enalapril
Cordanum see Talinolol
Cordicant see Nifedipine
Corgard see Nadolol
Corindolan see Mepindolol
Cormedigin see Sotalol
Corotrend see Nifedipine
Cortensobon see Captopril
Corzide contains bendroflumethiazide and nadolol
Creanol see Propranolol
Cretonin see Trichlormethiazide
Crinuryl see Ethacrynic Acid
Curanol see Propranolol
Cyclopenthiazide Diuretic
Cyclothiazide Diuretic
Dacarel see Nicardipine
Debrisoquine Peripheral adrenergic inhibitor
Decaserpyl see Methoserpidine
Declinax see Debrisoquine
Delco-Retic see Hydrochlorothiazide
Demi-Regroton contains chlorthalidone and reserpine
Denex see Metoprolol
Deralin see Propranolol
Deserpidine *Rauwolfia* extract and derivative
Detantol see Bunazosin
Detensiel see Bisoprolol
Di-Ademil see Hydroflumethiazide
Diachlor see Chlorothiazide
Diaqua see Hydrochlorothiazide
Diart see Azosemide
Diazoxide Vasodilator

Table 4. (continued)

Dibenzyline see Phenoxybenzamine
Dibenzyran see Phenoxybenzamine
Dichlotride see Hydrochlorothiazide
Didral see Hydrochlorothiazide
Diesse see Triamterene
Dihydralazine Vasodilator
Dihyzin see Dihydralazine
Diidrotiazide see Hydrochlorothiazide
Dilabor see Captopril
Dilatem see Diltiazem
Diltiazem Calcium antagonist
Diltikor see Diltiazem
Dilzem see Diltiazem
Direma see Hydrochlorothiazide
Diruex see Hydrochlorothiazide
Disorat see Metipranolol
Diu-Fortan see Trichlormethiazide
Diubram see Chlorothiazide
Diucardin see Hydroflumethiazide
Diucelpin see Triamterene
Diucen-H see Hydrochlorothiazide
Diuchlor see Hydrochlorothiazide
Diulo see Metolazone
Diupres contains chlorothiazide and reserpine
Diural see Furosemide
Diurama see Bumetanide
Diurapid see Azosemide
Diurazide see Chlorothiazide
Diurese see Trichlormethiazide
Diurese-R contains trichlormethiazide and reserpine
Diuret see Chlorothiazide
Diurexan see Xipamide
Diurigen see Chlorothiazide
Diuril see Chlorothiazide
Diurilix see Chlorothiazide
Diurolasa see Furosemide
Diurone see Chlorothiazide
Diursana-H see Hydrochlorothiazide
Diutensen contains methyclothiazide and cryptenamine
Diutensen-R contains methyclothiazide and reserpine
Dixidrasi see Hydrochlorothiazide
Doburil see Cyclothiazide
Dociton see Propranolol
Dopamet see Methyldopa
Dopegyt see Methyldopa
Dopom see Guanethidine
Doxazosin Postsynaptic α-antagonist
Dralzine see Hydralazine
Drenusil see Polythiazide
Drylon see Clonidine
Dryptal see Furosemide
Duramipres see Prazosin
Duranifin see Nifedipine
Durapindol see Pindolol
Durasoptin see Verapamil
Duraspiron see Spironolactone

Table 4. (continued)

Duretic see Methyclothiazide
Dyazide contains hydrochlorothiazide and triameterene
Dyrenium see Triamterene
Dytac see Triamterene
Ebrantil see Urapidil
Edecril see Ethacrynic Acid
Edecrin see Ethacrynic Acid
Edecrina see Ethacrynic Acid
Edecrine see Ethacrynic Acid
Efektolol see Propranolol
Elbrol see Propranolol
Elkapin see Etozolin
Enalapril Angiotensin converting enzyme inhibitor
Enalten see Enalapril
Enapren see Enalapril
Encor see Bisoprolol
Endak see Carteolol
Endralazine Vasodilator
Enduron see Methyclothiazide
Endurona see Methyclothiazide
Enduronyl contains methyclothiazide and deserpidine
Enduronyl Forte contains methyclothiazide and deserpidine
Enjit see Hydroflumethiazide
Entulic see Guanfacine
Envacar see Guanoxan
Equitonil see Debrisoquine
Errolon see Furosemide
Esbaloid see Bethanidine
Esbatal see Bethanidine
Esberizid see Bendroflumethiazide
Esidrex see Hydrochlorothiazide
Esidrix see Hydrochlorothiazide
Esimil contains hydrochlorothiazide and guanethidine
Esmarin see Trichlormethiazide
Estulic see Guanfacine
Ethacrynic acid Diuretic
Etozolin Diuretic
Eudatine see Pargyline
Eudemine see Diazoxide
Eunephran see Buthiazide
Eurex see Prazosin
Eusmanid see Bethanidine
Eutonyl see Pargyline
Eutron contains methyclothiazide and pargyline
Exna see Benzthiazide
Extur see Indapamide
Felodipine Calcium antagonist
Fenquizone Diuretic
Fludex see Indapamide
Fluitran see Trichlormethiazide
Flutra see Trichlormethiazide
Fontego see Bumetanide
Fordiuran see Bumetanide
Fovane see Benzthiazide
Franyl see Furosemide
Frekven see Propranolol

Table 4. (continued)

Frucee see Furosemide
Frusetic see Furosemide
Frusid see Furosemide
Fur-O-Ims see Furosemide
Furix see Furosemide
Furosemide Diuretic
Gallopamil Calcium antagonist
Ganlion see Azamethonium
Grospisk see Methyldopa
Guanabenz Central α-2 agonist
Guanadrel Peripheral adrenergic inhibitor
Guanethidine Peripheral adrenergic inhibitor
Guanfacine Central α-2 agonist
Guanoclor Peripheral adrenergic inhibitor
Guanoxan Peripheral adrenergic inhibitor
Guanutil see Guanoxan
Gubernal see Alprenolol
Harmonyl see Deserpidine
Hart see Diltiazem
Heitrin see Terazosin
Herbesser see Diltiazem
Herzul see Propranolol
Hexapress see Prazosin
Hidrenox see Hydrochlorothiazide
Hidrosaluretil see Hydrochlorothiazide
Higrotona see Chlorthalidone
Hiopartel see Enalapril
Hipertensal see Guanfacine
Hy-Po-Tone see Methyldopa
Hydac see Felodipine
Hydopa see Methyldopa
Hydralazine Vasodilator
Hydrenox see Hydroflumethiazide
Hydrex see Benzthiazide
Hydro-Aquil see Hydrochlorothiazide
Hydro-Chlor see Hydrochlorothiazide
Hydro-Tl see Hydrochlorothiazide
Hydro-Z Hydrochlorothiazide
Hydrochlorothiazide Diuretic
Hydrodiuril see Hydrochlorothiazide
Hydroflumethiazide Diuretic
Hydroma see Hydrochlorothiazide
Hydromedin see Ethacrynic Acid
Hydromox R contains quinethazone and reserpine
Hydromox see Quinethazone
Hydropres contains hydrochlorothiazide and reserpine
Hydrosaluric see Hydrochlorothiazide
Hydrozide see Hydrochlorothiazide
Hygroton see Chlorthalidone
Hylidone see Chlorthalidone
Hylorel see Guanadrel
Hyperazin see Hydralazine
Hypercal see Whole Root *Rauwolfia*
Hyperex see Hydralazine
Hyperpax see Methyldopa

Table 4. (continued)

Hypersin see Bethanidine
Hyperstat see Diazoxide
Hypertonalum see Diazoxide
Hypo-Rapid see Furosemide
Hyposyn see Clonidine
Hypoten see Nitroprusside
Hypovase see Prazosin
Hytrin see Terazosin
Hytrinex see Terazosin
Ibinolol see Atenolol
Idrodiuvis see Hydrochlorothiazide
Idrofluin see Hydrochlorothiazide
Idrolisin see Hydrochlorothiazide
Idrolone see Fenquizone
Igrolina see Chlorthalidone
Igroton see Chlorthalidone
Imovance see Xipamide
Impugan see Furosemide
Indapamide Diuretic
Inderal see Propranolol
Inderide contains hydrochlorothiazide and propranolol
Indobloc see Propranolol
Indoramin Postsynaptic α antagonist
Innovace see Enalapril
Intromene see Trichlormethiazide
Inversine see Mecamylamine
Ipolab see Labetalol
Ipolina see Hydralazine
Iposalfa see Alseroxylon
Ipotensium see Clonidine
Ipotidina see Guanethidine
Ismelin see Guanethidine
Ismeline see Guanethidine
Isopresol see Captopril
Isoptin see Verapamil
Isoten see Bisoprolol
Jatropur see Triamterene
Jen-Diril see Hydrochlorothiazide
Kaluril see Amiloride
Kemi see Propranolol
Kerlone see Betaxolol
Ketanserin Serotonin antagonist
Kubacron see Trichlormethiazide
Labelol see Labetalol
Labetalol β-Antagonist
Labrocol see Labetalol
Laractone see Spironolactone
Lasiletten see Furosemide
Lasilix see Furosemide
Lasix see Furosemide
Laxur see Furosemide
Lemiserp see Reserpine
Leodrine see Hydroflumethiazide
Levinezal see Enalapril
Levomoprolol β-Antagonist
Levotensin see Levomoprolol

Table 4. (continued)

Lexor see Hydrochlorothiazide
Lisinopril Angiotensin converting enzyme inhibitor
Lixil see Bumetanide
Lofetensin see Lofexidine
Lofexidine Central α-2 agonist
Londomin see Syrosingopine
Loniten see Minoxidil
Lonolox see Minoxidil
Looser see Bupranolol
Lopirin see Captopril
Lopresor see Metoprolol
Lopressor see Metoprolol
Lopressor HCT contains hydrochlorothiazide and propranolol
Lopril see Captopril
Loqua see Hydrochlorothiazide
Lotrial see Enalapril
Loxen see Nicardipine
Lozol see Indapamide
Lunetoron see Bumetanide
Luret see Azosemide
Marazide see Benzthiazide
Maschitt see Hydrochlorothiazide
Masdil see Diltiazem
Mazide contains hydrochlorothiazide and triameterene
Mecamylamine Ganglionic blocker
Medimet see Methyldopa
Medomet see Methyldopa
Medopa see Methyldopa
Medopal see Methyldopa
Medopren see Methyldopa
Mefrusal see Mefruside
Mefruside Diuretic
Megapres see Enalapril
Mephaserpin see Reserpine
Mepicor see Mepindolol
Mepindolol β-Antagonist
Meptin see Carteolol
Metahydrin see Trichlormethiazide
Metatensin contains trichlormethiazide and reserpine
Metenix see Metolazone
Methopa see Methyldopa
Methoplain see Methyldopa
Methoserpidine *Rauwolfia* extract and derivative
Methyclothiazide Diuretic
Methyldopa Central α-2 agonist
Meticrane Diuretic
Metipranolol β-Antagonist
Metoblock see Metoprolol
Metolazone Diuretic
Metoprolol β-Antagonist
Metoras see Metoprolol
Mevasine see Mecamylamine
Mictrin see Hydrochlorothiazide
Midamor see Amiloride
Mikelan see Carteolol
Minipress see Prazosin

Table 4. (continued)

Minizide contains polythiazide and prazosin
Minoxidil Vasodilator
Miretilan see Endralazine
Mitalolo see Labetalol
Modamide see Amiloride
Moderil see Rescinnamine
Moduretic contains hydrochlorothiazide and amiloride
Moilarorin see Furosemide
Monitan see Acebutolol
Monobeltin see Bupranolol
Monocor see Bisoprolol
Mulfasin see Methyldopa
Myocord see Atenolol
Nadic see Nadolol
Nadolol β-Antagonist
Naprilene see Enalapril
Naqua see Trichlormethiazide
Naquival contains trichlormethiazide and reserpine
Narix see Indapamide
Natrilix see Indapamide
Natrimax see Hydrochlorothiazide
Natrium see Triamterene
Naturetin see Bendroflumethiazide
Navidrex see Cyclopenthiazide
Nefrolan see Clorexolone
Neo Minzil see Hydrochlorothiazide
Neo-Codema see Hydrochlorothiazide
Neo-Naclex see Bendroflumethiazide
Neo-Renal see Furosemide
Neo-Serp see Reserpine
Neoflumen see Hydrochlorothiazide
Neoreserpan see Syrosingopine
Nephril see Polythiazide
Nepresol see Dihydralazine
Nepressol see Dihydralazine
Neptall see Acebutolol
Nerdipina see Nicardipine
Newtolide see Hydrochlorothiazide
Niazide see Trichlormethiazide
Nicardipine Calcium antagonist
Nicarpin see Nicardipine
Nicodel see Nicardipine
Nicorol see Furosemide
Nifcor see Nifedipine
Nife-Puren see Nifedipine
Nifecard see Nifedipine
Nifedicor see Nifedipine
Nifedipat see Nifedipine
Nifedipine Calcium antagonist
Nifelat see Nifedipine
Nimicor see Nicardipine
Nipride see Nitroprusside
Nipruss see Nitroprusside
Nirulid see Amiloride
Nitrendipine Calcium antagonist
Nitroprusside Vasodilator

Table 4. (continued)

Noloten see Propranolol
Noranat see Indapamide
Normadate see Labetalol
Normiten see Atenolol
Normodyne see Labetalol
Normonal see Tripamide
Normozide contains hydrochlorothiazide and labetalol
Notens see Bendroflumethiazide
Novohydrazide see Hydrochlorothiazide
Novomedopa see Methyldopa
Novosemide see Furosemide
Novoserpina see Syrosingopine
Novothalidone see Chlorthalidone
Odemase see Chlorthalidone
Olivin see Enalapril
Omeral see Levomoprolol
Opercol see Labetalol
Oposim see Propranolol
Oraday see Atenolol
Oretic see Hydrochlorothiazide
Osiren see Cancrenoate and/or Spironolactone
Osirenol see Cancrenoate
Oreticyl contains hydrochlorothiazide and deseripidine
Oreticyl Forte contains hydrochlorothiazide and deseripidine
Osyrol see Cancrenoate and/or Spironolactone
Oxanol see Oxprenolol
Oxprenolol β-Antagonist
Oxycardin see Bupranolol
Pandiuren see Amiloride
Panimit see Bupranolol
Pantemon see Hydrochlorothiazide
Paracefan see Clonidine
Pargyline Monoamine oxidase inhibitor
Parksemide see Furosemide
Pectobloc see Pindolol
Pempidil see Pempidine
Pempidine Ganglionic blocker
Pempiten see Pempidine
Penbutolol β-Antagonist
Pentamini see Azamethonium
Pentio see Pentolinium
Pentolinium Ganglionic blocker
Perbilen see Piretanide
Perdipine see Nicardipine
Peripress see Prazosin
Phanurane see Cancrenoate
Phenoxybenzamine Pre- and postsynaptic α-antagonist
Pentolamine Pre- and postsynaptic α-antagonist
Pidilat see Nifedipine
Pinadol see Pindolol
Pinbetol see Pindolol
Pindolol β-Antagonist
Piretanide Diuretic
Plendil see Felodipine
Pluryl see Bendroflumethiazide
Polidiuril see Bendroflumethiazide

Table 4. (continued)

Polythiazide Diuretic
Pranix see Propranolol
Prano-Puren see Propranolol
Pranolol see Propranolol
Prazosin Postsynaptic α-antagonist
Prelis see Metoprolol
Prent see Acebutolol
Pres see Enalapril
Presinol see Methyldopa
Presolol see Labetalol
Pressalold see Labetalol
Prexidil see Minoxidil
Prinivil see Lisinopril
Proaqua see Benzthiazide
Procardia see Nifedipine
Procorum see Gallopamil
Proflax see Timolol
Proglicem see Diazoxide
Proglycem see Diazoxide
Prolol see Propranolol
Promedes see Furosemide
Pronovan see Propranolol
Propabloc see Propranolol
Propalong see Propranolol
Propayerst see Propranolol
Propranolol β-Antagonist
Pylapron see Propranolol
Pyltelol see Pindolol
Pynastin see Pindolol
Quinethazone Diuretic
Ra-Valeas see Alseroxylon
Rablas see Enalapril
Ramipril Angiotensin converting enzyme inhibitor
Ranestol see Bevantolol
Rapam see Verapamil
Rau-Sed see Reserpine
Raudixin see Whole root *Rauwolfia*
Raunova see Syrosingopine
Rausan see Reserpine
Rautrax contains flumethiazide, *Rauwolifia serpentina*, and KCl
Rautrax-N contains bedroflumethiazide, *Rauwolifia serpentina*, and KCl
Rauval see Whole root *Rauwolfia*
Rauwan see Alseroxylon
Rauwifa see Reserpine
Rauwiloid see Alseroxylon
Rauwolfinetas see Whole root *Rauwolfia*
Rauzide contains bendroflumethiazide and *Rauwolifia serpentina*
Rawlini see Whole root *Rauwolfia*
Regitina see Phentolamine
Regitine see Phentolamine
Regletin see Alprenolol
Regroton contains chlorthalidone and reserpine
Regulin see Bethanidine
Reminal see Enalapril
Renalia see Clonidine
Renese see Polythiazide

Table 4. (continued)

Renese-R contains polythiazide and reserpine
Renitec see Enalapril
Renon see Chlorthalidone
Reomax see Ethacrynic Acid
Rescimin see Rescinnamine
Rescinnamine *Rauwolfia* extract and derivative
Resedril see Reserpine
Reselar see Reserpine
Resercen see Reserpine
Reserfia see Reserpine
Reserpanca see Reserpine
Reserpine *Rauwolfia* extract and derivative
Reserpoid see Reserpine
Rexiten see Guanabenz
Rhodiasectral see Acebutolol
Ridene see Nicardipine
Rivadescin see Whole root *Rauwolfia*
Rivosil see Hydroflumethiazide
Ro-Hydrazide see Hydrochlorothiazide
Robezon see Hydroflumethiazide
Rogitine see Phentolamine
Rontyl see Hydroflumethiazide
Sagisal see Spironolactone
Salmagne see Labetalol
Saltucin see Buthiazide
Salural see Bendroflumethiazide
Salures see Bendroflumethiazide
Saluretil see Chlorothiazide
Saluric see Chlorothiazide
Saluron see Hydroflumethiazide
Salurona see Hydroflumethiazide
Salutensin contains hydroflumethiazide and reserpine
Salutensin-Demi contains hydroflumenthazide and reserpine
Sanamiron see Trichlormethiazide
Sandonorm see Bopindolol
Sandril see Reserpine
Schebitran see Trichlomethiazide
Sectral see Acebutolol
Securon see Verapamil
Sedaraupin see Reserpine
Segurex see Bumetanide
Seguril see Furosemide
Selectol see Celiprolol
Selokeen see Metoprolol
Seloken see Metoprolol
Selopral see Metoprolol
Sembrina see Methyldopa
Seniramin see Syrosingopine
Sentiloc see Bevantolol
Ser-Ap-Es contains hydrochlorothiazide, reserpine, and hydralazine
Serenol see Whole root *Rauwolfia*
Serepress see Ketanserin
Serpalen see Reserpine
Serpasil see Reserpine
Serpasil-Apresoline contains hydralazine and reserpine
Serpasil-Esidrix contains hydrochlorothiazide and reserpine

Table 4. (continued)

Serpasol see Reserpine
Serpate see Reserpine
Serpetin see Whole root *Rauwolfia*
Serpresan see Reserpine
Sigasalur see Furosemide
Sinalol see Alprenolol
Sincomen see Cancrenoate
Sinesalin see Bendroflumethiazide
Sinocomen see Spironolactone
Siringina see Syrosingopine
Siroshuten see Syrosingopine
Sloprolol see Propranolol
Sodiuretic see Bendroflumethiazide
Soldactone see Cancrenoate
Solgol see Nadolol
Solo-Ethidine see Guanethidine
Soprol see Bisoprolol
Sotacor see Sotalol
Sotalex see Sotalol
Sotalol β-Antagonist
Spirix see Spironolactone
Spirocta see Spironolactone
Spiroctan see Cancrenoate
Spiroctian see Spironolactone
Spiron see Spironolactone
Spironolactone Diuretic
Spirotone see Spironolactone
Stresson see Bunitrolol
Sufrexal see Ketanserin
Sumial see Propranolol
Sundralen see Tiamenidine
Supotron see Enalapril
Supra-Puren see Spironolactone
Synapleg see Pempidine
Syrogopin see Syrosingopine
Syrosingopine *Rauwolfia* extract and derivative
Tachionin see Trichlormethiazide
Taladren see Ethacrynic Acid
Talinolol β-Antagonist
Tandiur see Hydrochlorothiazide
Temserin see Timolol
Tendor see Debrisoquine
Tenex see Guanfacine
Tenolone see Atenolol
Tenoretic contains chlorthalidone and atenolol
Tenormal see Pempidine
Tenormin see Atenolol
Tensinova see Clonidine
Tensobon see Captopril
Tensowolfia see Whole root *Rauwolfia*
Terazosin Postsynaptic α-antagonist
Teriam see Triamterene
Tertatolol β-Antagonist
Tesical see Bendroflumethiazide
Tesnol see Propranolol
Thalitone see Chlorthalidone

Table 4. (continued)

Thiazidil see Methyclothiazide
Thiuretic see Hydrochlorothiazide
Tiamenidine Centrai α-2 agonist
Tibricol see Nifedipine
Tidiem see Diltiazem
Tilazem see Diltiazem
Timacor see Timolol
Timolide contains hydrochlorothiazide and timolol
Timolol β-Antagonist
Tobanum see Cloranolol
Tolcasone see Trichlormethiazide
Tonum see Propranolol
Tracil see Nitrendipine
Trandate see Labetalol
Trandate HCT contains hydrochlorothiazide and labetalol
Trasacor see Oxprenolol
Trasicor see Oxprenolol
Triamterene Diuretic
Triamteril see Triamterene
Trichlormethiazide Diuretic
Trimethaphan Ganglionic blocker
Tripamide Diuretic
Tritace see Ramipril
Univer see Verapamil
Urapidil Postsynaptic α-antagonist
Uraprene see Urapidil
Uregyt see Ethacrynic Acid
Uremide see Furosemide
Urex see Furosemide
Urid see Chlorthalidone
Uridon see Chlorthalidone
Urinagen see Bendroflumethiazide
Urirex see Hydrochlorothiazide
Uritol see Furosemide
Urizide see Bendroflumethiazide
Urocaudal see Triamterene
Urolin see Chlorthalidone
Urozide see Hydrochlorothiazide
Vaseretic contains hydrochlorothiazide and enalapril
Vasolan see Verapamil
Vasonase see Nicardipine
Vasotec see Enalapril
Vasoton see Alprenolol
Vatensol see Guanoclor
Venactone see Cancrenoate
Veramex see Verapamil
Verapamil Calcium antagonist
Verelan see Verapamil
Vericordin see Atenolol
Verpal see Verapamil
Vidora see Indoramin
Vio-serpine see Reserpine
Viotil see Pempidine
Virifenemide see Furosemide
Viskeen see Pindolol
Visken see Pindolol

Table 4. (continued)

Visloc see Pindolol
Visutensil see Guanethidine
Whole root *Rauwolfia* *Rauwolfia* extract and derivative
Wydora see Indoramin
Wypres see Indoramin
Wytens see Guanabenz
Wytensin see Guanabenz
Xanef see Enalapril
Xipamide Diuretic
Yobir see Alprenolol
Zambesil see Chlorthalidone
Zaroxolyn see Metolazone
Zestril see Lisinopril
Zipex see Xipamide

Subject Index

GPSR Compliance

The European Union's (EU) General Product Safety Regulation (GPSR) is a set of rules that requires consumer products to be safe and our obligations to ensure this.

If you have any concerns about our products, you can contact us on ProductSafety@springernature.com

In case Publisher is established outside the EU, the EU authorized representative is:

Springer Nature Customer Service Center GmbH
Europaplatz 3
69115 Heidelberg, Germany

Batch number: 10761693

Printed by Printforce, the Netherlands